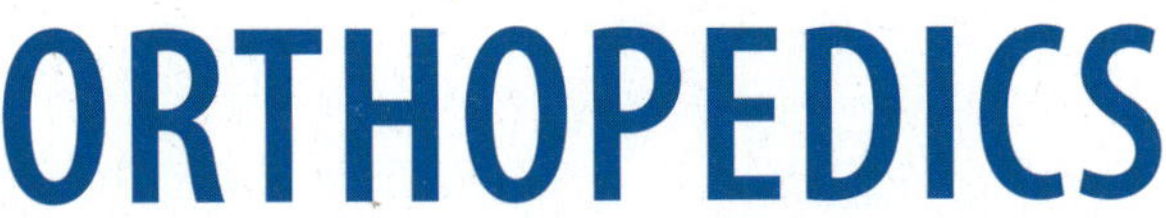
ORTHOPEDICS
(A Postgraduate Companion)

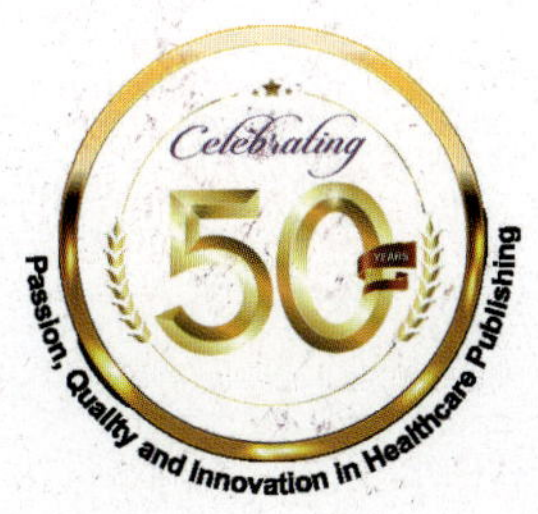
Celebrating
50 YEARS
Passion, Quality and Innovation in Healthcare Publishing

ORTHOPEDICS

(A Postgraduate Companion)

Second Edition

VOLUME 1

(Col) Samar Kumar Biswas
MBBS MS (Gen Surgery) MS (Ortho) FAISF (Swiss)
Professor Emeritus
Department of Orthopedics
Padmashree Dr DY Patil Medical College
Hospital and Research Center
Pune, Maharashtra, India

Foreword
KH Sancheti

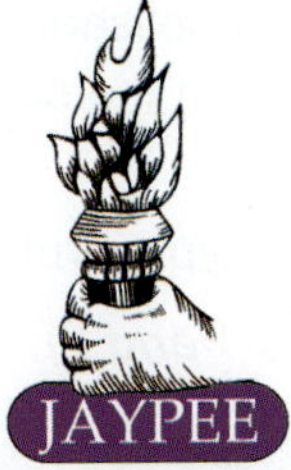

JAYPEE BROTHERS MEDICAL PUBLISHERS
The Health Sciences Publisher
New Delhi | London

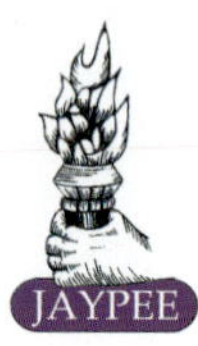

Jaypee Brothers Medical Publishers (P) Ltd

Headquarters
Jaypee Brothers Medical Publishers (P) Ltd
4838/24, Ansari Road, Daryaganj
New Delhi 110 002, India
Phone: +91-11-43574357
Fax: +91-11-43574314
Email: jaypee@jaypeebrothers.com

Overseas Office
J.P. Medical Ltd
83 Victoria Street, London
SW1H 0HW (UK)
Phone: +44 20 3170 8910
Fax: +44 (0)20 3008 6180
Email: info@jpmedpub.com

Website: www.jaypeebrothers.com
Website: www.jaypeedigital.com

Inquiries for bulk sales may be solicited at: jaypee@jaypeebrothers.com

Orthopedics (A Postgraduate Companion) (Volumes 1 and 2)

First Edition: 2013
Second Edition: **2020**

ISBN 978-93-89188-27-1

Printed at: Samrat Offset Pvt. Ltd.

Dedicated to

My parents

My teachers

My family, and

My beloved PG students

Contributors

Anurag Garg
MS (Gen Surgery) MCh CVTS Fellow in Vascular Surgery (UK)
Senior Professor and Head
Department of Cardiovascular and Thoracic Surgery
Padmashree DY Patil Medical College
Pune, Maharashtra, India

Ashish Devgan
MS (Ortho) Fellow in Arthroscopy Shoulder Knee and Wrist
Senior Professor and Unit Chief
Department of Orthopedics
PGIMS and Pt BDS University of Health Sciences
Rohtak, Haryana, India

BB Dogra
MS (Gen Surgery) MCh Plastic and Reconstructive Surgery
Senior Professor and Head
Department of Plastic Surgery
Padmashree DY Patil Medical College
Pune, Maharashtra, India

Ganesh Reddy
MS (Orth) Fellow in Arthroplasty & Arthroscopy
Associate Professor
Department of Orthopedics
Narayana Medical College
Nellore, Andhra Pradesh, India

Mahendra Bendre MS (Gen Surgery)
Senior Professor and Head of Unit
Department of General Surgery
Padmashree DY Patil Medical College
Pune, Maharashtra, India

Mahendra Reddy
MS (Ortho) Fellow in Arthroplasty and Arthroscopy
Joint Replacement Specialist
Assistant Professor
Department of Orthopedics
Santhiram Medical College and General Hospital
Nandyal, Andhra Pradesh, India

Mukesh Phalak
MS (Ortho) Fellow in Spine Surgery (Mumbai) and
Trauma center (Mumbai)
Professor
Department of Orthopedics
Padmashree DY Patil Medical College
Pune, Maharashtra, India

Rahul Mehta
MS (Ortho) Fellow in Minimally Invasive
Spine Surgery (Mumbai, Korea and Japan)
Assistant Professor
Department of Orthopedics
SSV Medical College
Ujjain, Madhya Pradesh, India

Sarang Begalvi Sethi
Fellow in Arthroplasty and Arthroscopy (UK)
Associate Professor
Department of Orthopedics
Belgaum Medical College
Belgaum, Karnataka, India

Best Wishes

It gives me immense pleasure to pen a few lines of greetings and good wishes to Dr (Col) Samar Kumar Biswas for this book.

I know Dr Biswas over the last fifteen years, when he joined as a Professor and Head, Department of Orthopedics in Padmashree Dr DY Patil Medical College, Hospital and Research Center, Pune, Maharashtra, India. In a short span of time, he became a popular Professor among undergraduate as well as postgraduate students for his excellent teaching practices. The classes and clinics of Dr Biswas were well attended and appreciated by the students. Even students from other institutions, in and around Pune, were also interested in attending his lectures. He has been honored with 'Best Teacher Award'.

Dr Biswas has a dynamic personality. He has good relations with his colleagues, who revere him for his vast knowledge and pleasant personality.

As Albert Einstein aptly said, 'The only source of knowledge is experience.' Dr Biswas has put his vast teaching experience in this book to share his knowledge for the betterment of the postgraduate students. I am sure that his book will also become as popular among the students as were his teachings.

I congratulate Dr Biswas for this book and wish him all the success in future endeavor.

Dr PD Patil
Honorable President
Padmashree Dr DY Patil Vidyapeeth
Pune, Maharashtra, India

Foreword

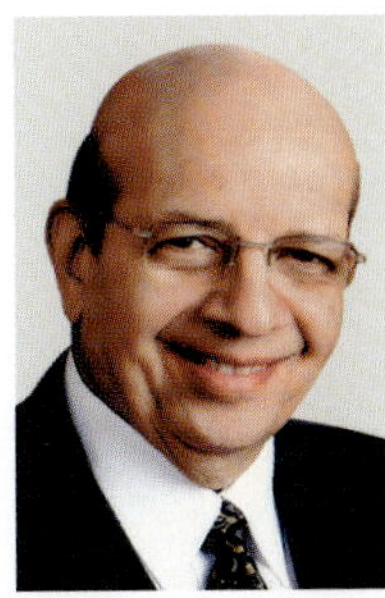

As a student, whenever I found information on any topic to be scattered and incomplete, I often had to refer to many books to get a complete picture. Nowadays, information available on any subject is enormous. A book that is comprehensive and covers every topic from A to Z was deeply needed to make the life of the postgraduate students easier. I think Dr (Col) Samar Kumar Biswas has been successful in accomplishing this feat.

I have gone through his book and I found that each region is adequately covered, from anatomy to the latest advances in surgical management. There is a lot of emphasis on basic principles and clinical examination, both of which are very close to my heart. This book eliminates the need to refer to a separate book on clinical skills. He has addressed controversies without bias and the sections on 'Recent Advances' is updated with current literature. The sections on 'Congenital Anomalies and Trauma' are a pleasure to go through. All recent classifications have been included and topics, like 'Scaphocapitate Fracture Syndrome,' have been explained in a lucid and clear manner.

A section on 'General Surgery' is given which would rival any general surgery textbook, means a student has to deal with one less book. The information is with special reference to the orthopedic students, so that this extra nonetheless essential knowledge is easy to grasp.

The real surprise, however, is the chapter on the Spine. Dr Biswas has truly done justice to this complicated and difficult topic.

I would encourage every postgraduate student to take advantage of this wonderful book. I have already decided to keep copies of this book in our institute's library.

I congratulate Dr Biswas for his vision and his tireless efforts to convert it into a reality.

Padma Vibhushan Dr KH Sancheti
MS PhD (Ortho) FRCS (Edinburgh) FICS FACS (USA)
Sancheti Institute for Orthopedics and Rehabilitation
Pune, Maharashtra, India

Preface to the Second Edition

After seeing the popularity of the book among the postgraduate students and junior surgeons as well as some healthy suggestions from seniors verbally communicated, I got prompted to write a second edition with the addition of certain new chapters and revision of certain old chapters and include certain important topics of general surgery related to trauma.

Addition of some new techniques like arthroscopy as well as arthroplasty written by experts in those fields.

This has definitely increased the value of the book and I am sure it will be appreciated and accepted at all levels.

(Col) Samar Kumar Biswas

Preface to the First Edition

I got inspired to write a book, mainly for the postgraduate students, while teaching them and examining the postgraduate candidates during examinations of various universities, as a postgraduate teacher and examiner over the last fifteen years. I felt the necessity of a book describing regions, like hip, knee, elbow, etc. right from the anatomy and development of the regions to trauma, tumors, infections and even reconstruction or replacement of the part in one chapter. There is lack of such a book, as a guide for postgraduate students in market today. Orthopedics today is not just a crude way of treating with plasters, screws and plates, it is advancing day-by-day with new techniques and concepts of management from noninvasive to minimally invasive. This has been possible also from early diagnosis for proper institution of appropriate treatment, to join the patients back to their jobs early. Keeping the above, I have prepared the seminar topics accordingly, for my postgraduate students and guided them in making the seminars. I have also included the recent advances and concepts on the subjects, even by consulting the Internet. I have given special emphasis on the clinical methods of examination in detail, as during most of the examinations, postgraduate students are asked to demonstrate the clinical tests and signs.

Hence, by taking the name of Lord Ganesha, I made a fair attempt to prepare this book, describing the topics region-wise, encompassing from the very basics to most recent advances in that particular subject.

I will consider my attempt to be successful only when this book will be welcomed by the postgraduate students, as a constant companion while preparing their tough subject and will help them in becoming a successful orthopedic clinician.

(Col) Samar Kumar Biswas

Acknowledgments

At the outset, I want to acknowledge my family members, my wife Mrs Smriti Biswas, my daughter Snigdha Dutta and my son Somnath Biswas, for their constant inspiration and selfless encouragement and cooperation, without these, I would not have been able to complete this impossible work, of writing this book.

I want to acknowledge the continuous help from my beloved postgraduate students, especially Drs Tanveer Singh Bhutani, Mahendra Kumar Reddy, Praful Kilaru, Ganesh Kumar Reddy, Dhyan Patel and Shalin Maheswari, in preparing and editing the manuscript of this book. I also want to acknowledge Drs Himanshu Bhugra, Tushar Chaudhari, K Charith Nagarjuna, Abhishek and Manoj for continuous support and help in preparing and editing the manuscript of the 2nd edition of the book.

My special thanks to my students, my colleagues, Assistant Professor, Dr Rahul Salunkhe; Dr Samir Deshmukh and Dr Abhijit Shroff. My thanks also goes for some of my favorite students, my colleagues, Professor, Dr Suahs Kamble; Associate Professor, Dr Amit Swamy; Professor, Dr Anil Salgia; Dr Subhash Puri for their continuous inspiration in writing this book for postgraduate students.

I want to acknowledge and thank from the bottom of my heart all contributors as authors Drs Mukesh Phalak, BB Dogra, Anurag Garg, Mahendra Bendre, Professor Ashish Devgan, SK Jain, Rahul Mehta and Sarang Begalvi Sethi for their valuable contribution to improve the quality and value of the book.

I also want to express my thanks to Ms Usha and Ms Vaishnavi, the clerks of our Orthopedics department, for helping in preparing the data.

I will be failing in my duty, if I do not remember our Honorable President Dr PD Patil, without his blessings and best wishes I could not have completed this work.

My special acknowledgments go for Dr (Brig) Amarjit Singh, Vice Chancellor and Dr BS Mane, Registrar of our prestigious university Padmashree Dr DY Patil, Medical College and Vidyapeeth, Pune, Maharashtra, India.

My special gratitude goes for our artist Mr Pomaji, who has taken pain-taking task of making beautiful illustrations for this book.

While writing the manuscript of certain topics of seminars and recent advances, I have gone through various articles and studies done by authors in Pubmed and taken certain portions of the text in the manuscript like, Systemic approach to limping child, Surgical site infection, 3-D Bioprinting, Mechanobiology. I have tried to contact the authors and got verbal permission from some authors who could be contacted. But many could not be contacted personally.

Hence, I am taking this opportunity to express my heartfelt gratitude and sincerely acknowledge their help in preparing this book.

I take this opportunity to thank Shri Jitendar P Vij (Group Chairman), Mr Ankit Vij (Managing Director), Ms Chetna Malhotra Vohra (Associate Director–Content Strategy), Ms Kritika Dua (Senior Development Editor) and all the staff of M/s Jaypee Brothers Medical Publishers (P) Ltd, New Delhi, India.

Contents

VOLUME 1

SECTION 1: GENERAL ORTHOPEDICS

SECTION 2: GENERAL SURGERY RELATED TO ORTHOPEDICS

SECTION 3: REGIONAL ORTHOPEDICS

VOLUME 2

SECTION 4: RECENT ADVANCES (SEMINAR) IN ORTHOPEDICS

SECTION 5: SEMINARS IN ORTHOPEDICS

SECTION

1

General Orthopedics

- History of Orthopedics
- Bone
- Anomalies Related to Development of Bones
- Genetic Disorders
- Metabolic Disorders
- Endocrine Disorders
- Blood Disorders
- Gouty Arthritis
- Degenerative and Inflammatory Disorders
- Infections in Orthopedics
- Bone Tumors
- Gait Analysis

CHAPTER 1

History of Orthopedics

OBJECTIVES

- Important Figures in Orthopedics
- Total Joint Replacement

INTRODUCTION

Orthopedics, like many specialties, has developed through a necessity. A necessity to correct deformity, restore function, and alleviate pain. Orthopedic surgeons have developed an ability to prevent major losses of bodily functions and indeed they can prevent an otherwise inevitable death. They seek perfection of their art, by ensuring that the patient reaches optimal condition in the shortest period of time by the safest possible method.

HISTORY

Ancient Egypt

- Splints have been found on mummies and they were made of bamboo, reeds, wood, or bark, and padded with linen
- There is also evidence of the use of crutches, with the earliest known record of the use of a crutch coming from a carving made in 2830 BC on the entrance of a portal on Hirkouf's tomb
- In the Papyrus (a book), the examination of peripheral limbs was described
- In this Papyrus, injuries were classified according to their prognosis into three categories:
  1. An ailment, which they would treat
  2. An ailment that they would contend
  3. An ailment, which they would not treat
- The Papyrus also mentioned many cases and the treatment involved.

Ancient Greece

- Many principles behind conditions and their treatment have been attributed to the ancient Greece
- They could be regarded as the first to use a scientific approach
- They were also the first to document in detail their history and developments
- Hegetor of Alexandria (100 BC), described in detail the anatomical relations of the hip joint and was the first to record a description of the ligamentum teres
- In Corpus Hippocrates (it is named after Hippocrates, who is known as the Father of Medicine), dislocation of the shoulder was described together with the various methods used in reduction and correction of club foot
- Hippocrates had a thorough understanding of fractures. He knew the principles of traction and counter traction. He developed special splints for fractures of the tibia, similar to external fixation.

Roman Era

- Another respected roman figure of Greek origin by the name of Galen (129–199 BC) "Father of Sports Medicine"
- He gave a good account of the skeleton and the muscles that move it
- He first recorded a case of cervical ribs
- He described bone destruction, sequestration, and regeneration in osteomyelitis, and sometimes performed resection in such cases
- During this Greco-Roman period, there were also attempts to provide artificial prosthesis
- It is said that both linen and catgut sutures were used for the procedures, during this period
- Various drills, saws, and chisels were also developed during this period.

Arab Era

- Although, the Arab practices were regarded as an extension of those of the Greeks, the use of Plaster of Paris (POP) in the 10th century was significant
- With the addition of water to a powder of anhydrous calcium sulfate, a hard crystalline material was produced
- It was not until the 12th century that Europe began to awake gradually from its dark ages
- Until the 16th century, all developments remained within the shadow casted by Hippocrates.

IMPORTANT FIGURES IN ORTHOPEDICS

Ambroise Paré (1510–1590) (Fig. 1)

- Most famous surgical figure of the 16th century and the Father of French Surgery
- Used ligature, for large vessels in amputations
- Used a tourniquet in his amputations
- Paré designed scoliosis corset and clubfoot boot.

Nicolas Andry (1658–1742) (Fig. 2)

- Father of Orthopedics
- He coined the term, "Orthopedics" (Greek word Orthos, means straight and Paed, means child) in 1741

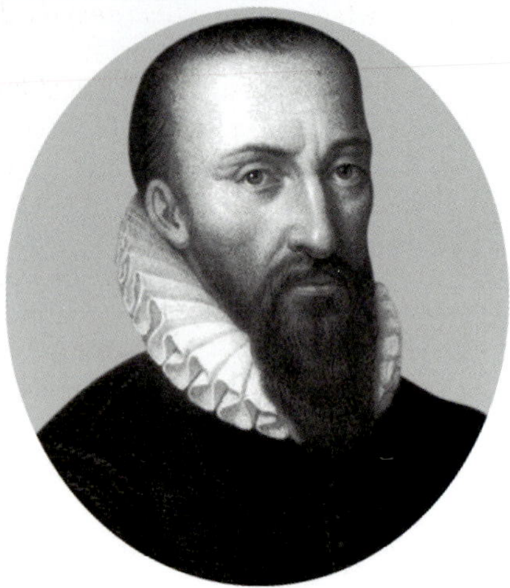

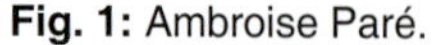

Fig. 1: Ambroise Paré.

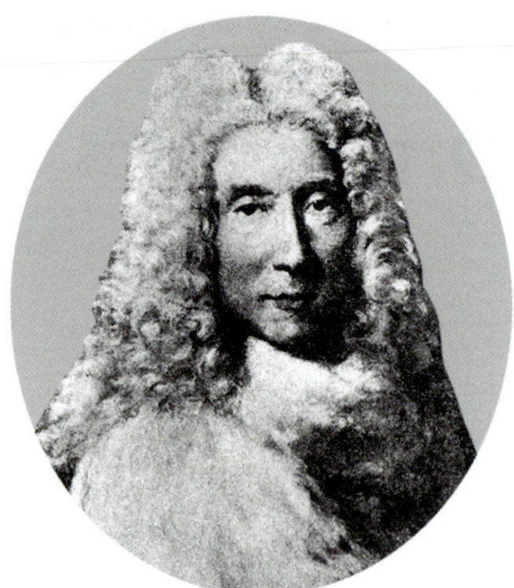

Fig. 2: Nicolas Andry.

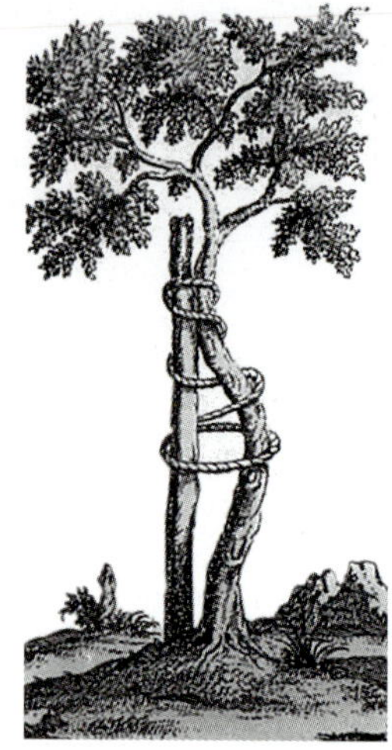

Fig. 3: Andry Tree—a symbol for orthopedics.

- He published, a famous book called "Orthopedia" or the "Art of Correcting and Preventing Deformities in Children"
- He gave the symbol "Andry Tree" (Fig. 3), which has been adopted worldwide, as the symbol for orthopedics.

Percival Pott (1714–1788)

- Percival Pott (Fig. 4) was born in the Threadneedle Street of Cockney
- He obtained grand diploma of Barber Surgeon's Company in 1736 from St Bartholomew's Hospital and was soon appointed to the staff of the same hospital 8 years later
- He is best known for the fracture that bears his name, Pott's fracture, as he was the first to give a good description of this ankle fracture
- In 1756, Pott sustained a broken leg after fall from his horse. It is often assumed that his injury was the same one that later came to be known as Pott's fracture, but in reality Pott's broken leg was much more serious compound fracture of femur
- As he laid in the mud, he sent a servant to buy a door from nearby and had himself placed on the door. Surgeons cleaned the wound and discussed amputation, but Pott insisted to splint the leg and recovered completely
- In 1775, Pott found an association between exposure to soot and high incidence of scrotal cancer. This was the first occupational link to cancer
- Pott was the first person, to demonstrate that malignancy could be caused by environmental carcinogen
- Pott's most famous work is on the paraplegia of spinal tuberculosis, where he stressed that the condition was not related to spinal cord compression, but associated with strumous disorders in the lungs. This is known as Pott's paraplegia. His account of tuberculosis paraplegia was first published in 1779.

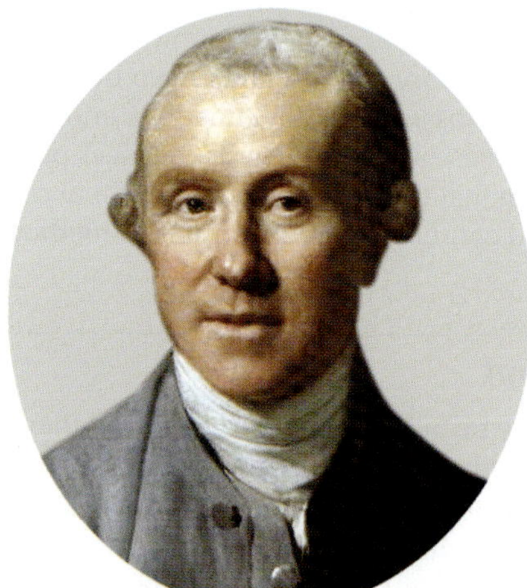

Fig. 4: Percival Pott.

John Hunter (1728–1793)

- John Hunter's (Fig. 5) saying "do not think, try the experiment", has inspired generations of modern surgeons
- He described how to assess power in a weak muscle
- He believed that healing depends on the body innate power and that the surgeon's task was to aid this

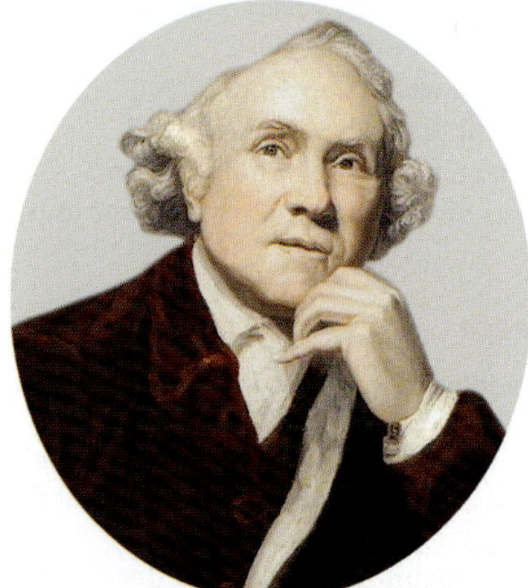

Fig. 5: John Hunter.

- He studied loose bodies in joints, pseudoarthroses, and fracture healing.

William Hey (1736–1819)

- Subacute osteomyelitis of the tibia was described by him and he advocated deroofing of the lesion

- In 1773, Hey (Fig. 6) banged his knee getting out of the bath and many attributed his subsequent interest in the knee to this
- He coined the phrase "Internal Derangement of the Knee", and described meniscal injuries
- Hey described loose bodies and introduced tarsometatarsal amputation.

Abraham Colles (1773–1843)

- Abraham Colles (Fig. 7) was responsible for much of the early scientific development of surgery in Ireland and was the leading Irish surgeon of his time
- On January 4, 1802, when only 29 years of age, he was elected as President of the Royal College of Surgeons in Ireland
- He was the first to tie the first stage of the right subclavian artery for a large axillary aneurysm in 1811
- Best known for his description of Colles' fracture in 1814.

Colles' Fracture

In his classical paper, "On Fracture of the Carpal Extremity of the Radius" in 1814, when no X-rays were available, he had described accurately the classical deformity following the fracture of lower end of radius, which is known as "Colles' fracture" after him.

Colles' Fascia

In the perineum, the middle fascia of the urogenital triangle, the attachments of which served to confine within strict limits extravasation of urine from a ruptured urethra is known as "Colles' fascia".

Colles' Ligament

It is the name sometimes given to the small triangular fascia that springs from the pubic crest and iliopectineal line and passes upwards and inwards toward the linea alba, under cover of the internal pillar of the external abdominal ring.

Colles' Law

- In 1837, Colles published a book entitled "Practical Observations", on the venereal disease and on the use of mercury. In a chapter, dealing with syphilis in infants, he made an observation that later became known as Colles' law, which can be stated as, "a child born of a mother, who is without any obvious venereal symptoms and which, without being exposed to any infection subsequent to its birth, shows this disease. When it is a few weeks old, this child will infect the most healthy nurse, whether she suckles it or merely handles and dresses it and yet this child is never known to infect its mother, even though she suckles it, while it has venereal ulcers on the lips and tongue"
- He clearly observed the apparent immunity of the mother, but could not have guessed that she already had the disease in a mild form. It was nearly 70 years later that the *Fritz Schaudinn* discovered *Spirochaeta pallida* and the serological test devised by Wassermann
- This work on venereal disease was his last important contribution.

Antonius Mathijsen (1805–1878)

Antonius Mathijsen (Fig. 8), was a Dutch military surgeon, who in 1851 invented the POP bandage, which has become so important in orthopedic practice.

Hugh Owen Thomas (1834–1891)

- Hugh Owen Thomas (Fig. 9) is known as Father of British Orthopedics
- He was the eldest of five sons born to a well-known bonesetter at that time
- He could not even work with his father and never held a hospital appointment
- He treated all his patients at home
- His practice was so busy that he started his rounds at 5 o'clock or 6 o'clock in the morning and never left his home for other than professional purposes. Thomas would designate Sunday, as his free day and hundreds of patients from the country would surround his house in order to be treated
- The people of Liverpool knew Thomas as a short and quick man. A man who always wore a black coat buttoned up to the neck and a sailor's cap pulled over a damaged eye. A cigarette was also seen constantly in his mouth
- Thomas contributions include:
  - Thomas splint
  - Thomas wrench

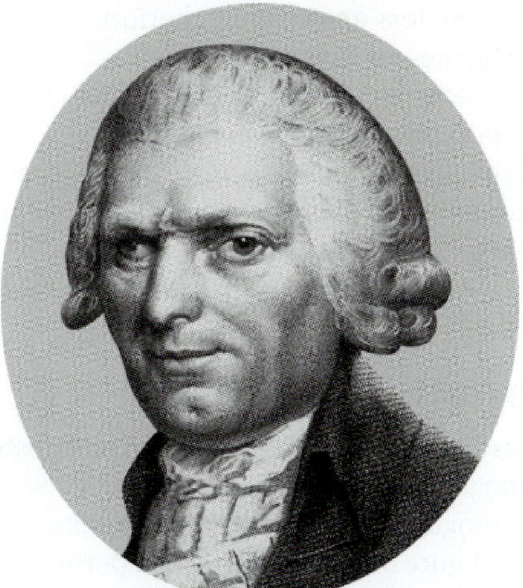

Fig. 6: William Hey.

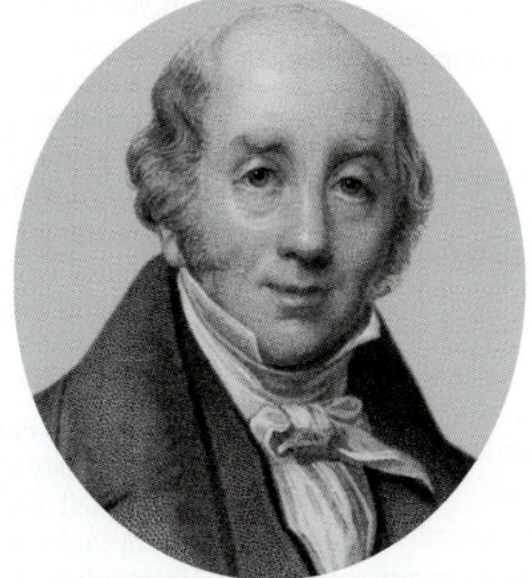

Fig. 7: Abraham Colles.

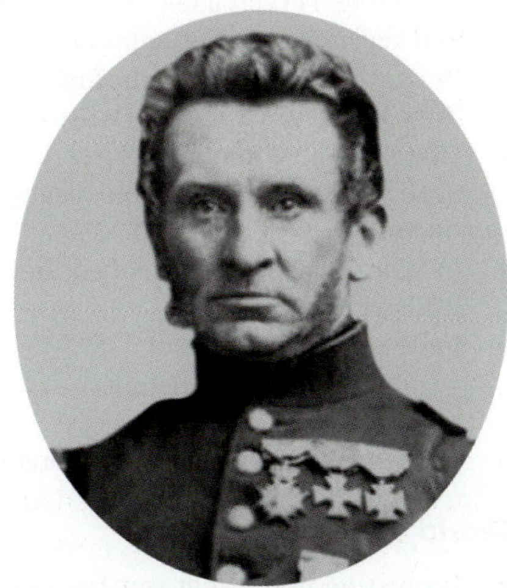

Fig. 8: Antonius Mathijsen.

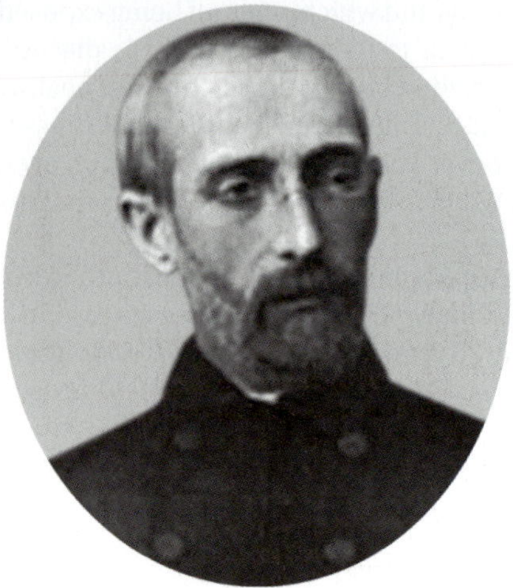

Fig. 9: Hugh Owen Thomas.

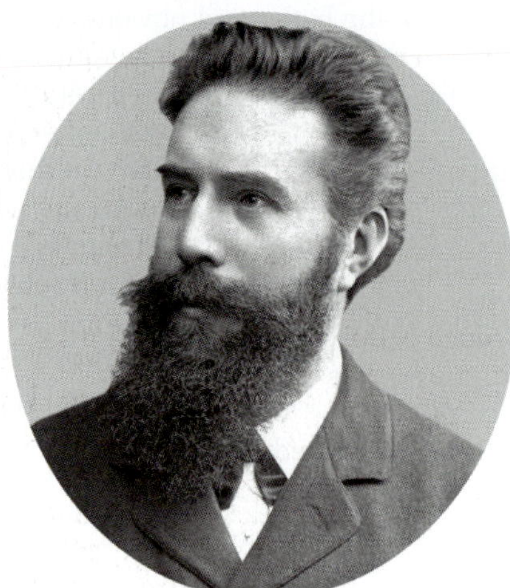

Fig. 10: Wilhelm Conrad Roentgen.

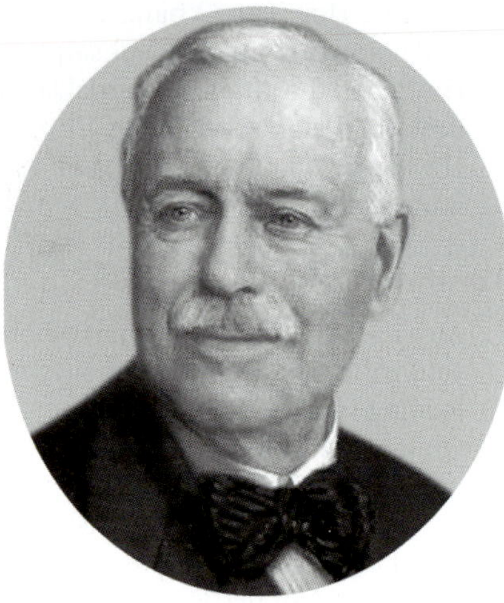

Fig. 11: Sir Robert Jones.

  - Cervical collar
  - Metatarsal bar
  - Heel wedge
  - Knee splint
- Many of these are still in use, such as the Thomas splint
- He was the first to demonstrate concealed flexion of the hip joint and a way of unmasking this, by performing the "Thomas test".

The Modern Era (20th Century Orthopedics)

The discovery of the X-ray almost marked 1900 and orthopedics was only now being seen, as a true specialty of its own.

Wilhelm Conrad Roentgen (1845–1923)

- Roentgen (Fig. 10) was a professor of physics at Wurzburg, his discovery of X-rays (Roentgen rays) and their use has been a huge contribution to orthopedics
- The first radiography that Roentgen took was of his wife's hand on December 22nd 1895. This was allegedly her Christmas present
- Roentgen received the Nobel Prize for his discovery in 1901.

Sir Robert Jones (1857–1933)

- Jones (Fig. 11) was a nephew of the great Hugh Owen Thomas and became one of his apprentices in Liverpool
- In 1896, Jones published the first report of the clinical use of an X-ray to locate a bullet in a wrist
- His textbook "Orthopedic Surgery" is said to be the first to have dealt systematically with the diagnosis and treatment of fresh fractures
- In World War I, Jones headed the orthopedic section of the British forces
- Jones was an advocate of:
  - Tendon transplantation
  - Bone grafting
  - Other conservative and restorative procedures.

World War I

- It must be noted that war has played an important part in orthopedic history
- Many of our greatest contributors were military surgeons
- It is interesting to note that many of the achievements during and after World War I were not related directly to traumatic injuries received at war
- Orthopedics was definitely seen as a separate specialty, after World War I and that this was the first major war, where aseptic techniques were saving many more lives than in the past wars.

Thomas Porter McMurray (1888–1949)

- In the chain of great surgeons that followed Hugh Owen Thomas, came Thomas Porter McMurray (Fig. 12), who worked for Robert Jones
- His operative dexterity was renowned, for he could remove an entire meniscus in 5 min and disarticulate a hip in 10 min
- He introduced his sign for a torn meniscus, McMurray's sign.

McMurray's Osteotomy

An operation was also named after him, as McMurray was the first to perform a displacement osteotomy, for ununited fractures of the femoral neck and arthrosis of the hip.

World War II

- The knowledge learnt in fighting World War I, helped in treating the casualties of World War II
- In World War II, there were less amputations performed, less gangrene, and better measures for fixation of fractures
- We must not forget the importance of penicillin (whose effects were discovered by Sir Alexander Fleming, in 1928)
- The Germans needed quick measures, to restore their fighters, to optimal fighting potential and developed a number of nailing procedures, during this period
- Together with this, the Americans were now making more contributions than ever before.

Willis Campbell (1880–1941)

- Campbell (Fig. 13) was the main advocate of interpositional arthroplasty at that time
- Campbell used a free autogenous transplant of fascia lata
- Campbell was also a key figure in bone grafting and performed inlay full thickness grafts, for nonunion bones fixed with screws of beef bone

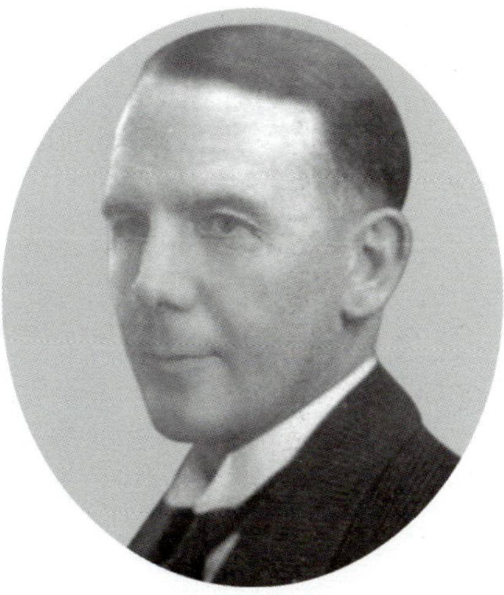

Fig. 12: Thomas Porter McMurray.

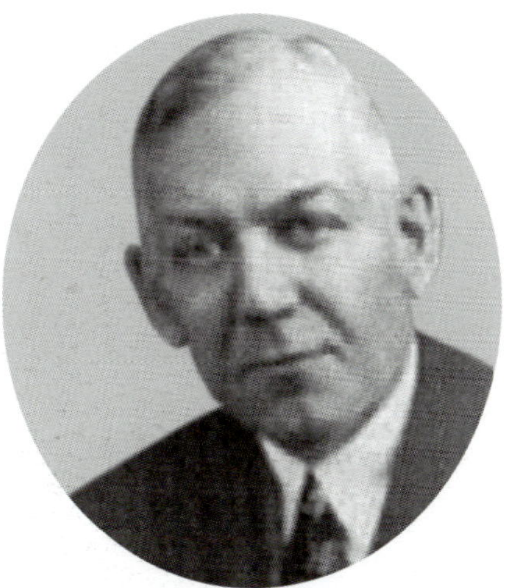

Fig. 13: Willis Campbell.

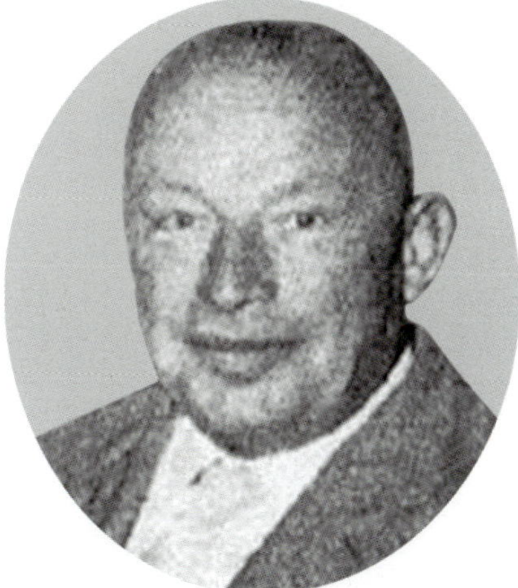

Fig. 14: Gerhard Kuntscher.

- He published three volumes:
  1. A monograph, "Orthopedics of Childhood", 1927
  2. A textbook, "Orthopedic Surgery", 1930
  3. His last publication was "Operative Orthopedics", in 1939.

Gerhard Kuntscher (1900–1972)

- Gerhard Kuntscher (Fig. 14) served in the German army during the World War II and published his revolutionary procedure in the opening months of the war
- His work was concerned with the intramedullary nailing of fractures of the shafts of long bones and his name is associated with the nail.

Martin Kirschner (1879–1942) (Fig. 15)

- Known for his methods of fixation, in particular for the Kirschner or K-wire
- He also performed the first successful pulmonary embolectomy.

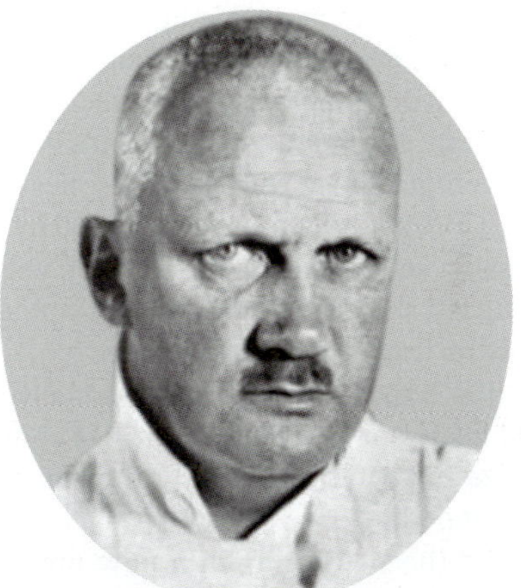

Fig. 15: Martin Kirschner.

Sir Reginald Watson-Jones (1902–1972)

- Watson Jones (Fig. 16) was born in Brighton, England on March 1902
- He acquired an interest in the field of medicine after about with typhoid fever
- He was graduated from the University of Liverpool in 1922
- He decided to pursue orthopedics, following an operation to remove hemangioma from his leg
- During World War II, he was among the leading teachers in fracture therapy
- He was responsible for and was the first editor of the British volume of the Journal of Bone and Joint Surgery (JBJS) and retained the post through four decades
- He was the orthopedic surgeon for England's King and Queen
- Watson-Jones published "Fractures and Joint Injuries" in 1940, which remained a standard reference for several decades and was considered as a bible of the fracture and joint injuries. It was translated into many languages.

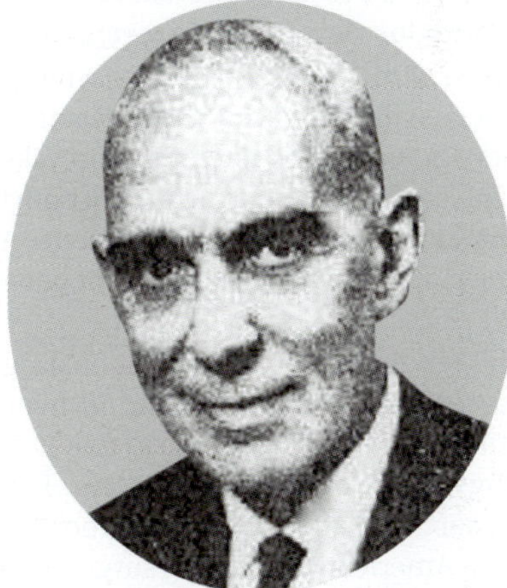

Fig. 16: Sir Reginald Watson–Jones.

Austin T Moore (1899–1963)

- Moore (Fig. 17) performed the first metallic hip replacement. He had replaced for the first time, the entire upper portion of the femur with a vitallium prosthesis
- Over the years, the design of the prosthesis and the procedure improved. Consequently, there is one type of prosthesis called the Austin-Moore, which is still used today.

Gavriil A Ilizarov (1921–1992)

- G Ilizarov (Fig. 18) was born in the Caucasian Mountains and did not attend school until he was 12 years old, because his family had no money for shoes

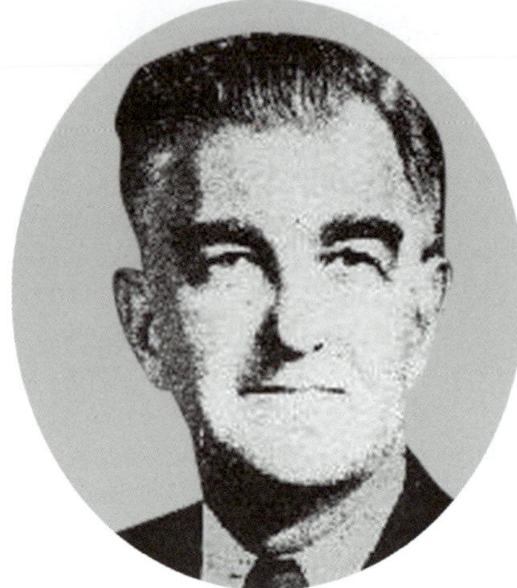

Fig. 17: Austin T Moore.

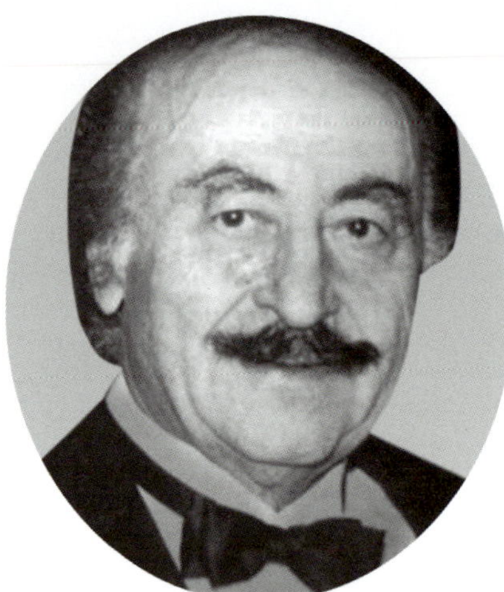

Fig. 18: Gavriil A Ilizarov.

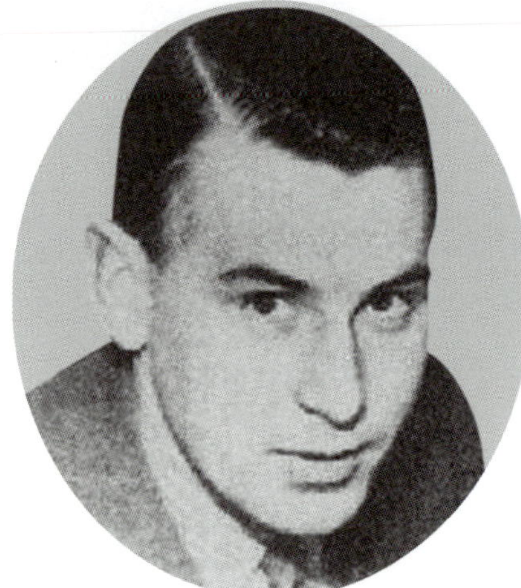

Fig. 19: H Lowry Rush.

- He graduated from Simferopol Medical School, which had been moved during the war to the Soviet near east
- During World War II, he was evacuated to Dolgovka, near Kurgan and ran a hospital single handed, where working conditions were primitive with no antibiotics and inadequate equipment. The operating room was heated by a wood fire
- Injured Russian soldiers came through the village and this is when he started developing his famous apparatus, circular frame for distraction osteogenesis
- His theory that bone would grow, if gradually distracted and his external fixator of circular steel haloes connected by rods and bone-fixating wires, produced dramatic results not seen before in orthopedics
- His work was the beginning of a new medical paradigm, the conservation and exploitation of the unlimited natural plasticity of bone
- Although Dr Ilizarov's results were astonishing, his theory was contrary to orthodox views on bone regeneration
- His reputation remained confined to Siberia, until 1967, when he successfully treated the Russian Olympic high jumper, Valery Brumel, who after a motorcycle accident, had chronically infected nonunited fractures of both legs, even after 14 operations, by the best surgeons in Moscow. After treatment by Ilizarov, he completely healed and went onto jump again in competition
- From then, his reputation soared into national and international prominence and by 1984, he presided over a new 1,000 bed, Scientific Center for Reconstructive Orthopedics and Traumatology, with over 350 surgeons, 1,500 nurses, 60 doctorate researchers, and 24 operating rooms
- By 1986, North American orthopedic surgeons had learned the Ilizarov techniques from Europeans, who had worked directly with him and were performing Ilizarov limb-saving operations
- The use of his methods is widespread. The North American Association for the Study and Application of the Methods of Ilizarov (ASAMI) now includes over 200 surgeons.

After the Wars

- In the years following the war, orthopedic surgeons sought to perfect their treatment of fractures, in particular with the use of metallic pins and wires for fixation
- With the introduction of alloys that could be used effectively, there was also a new wave of prosthesis, which are developing for treatment of arthritis as well as problematic fractures
- Antibiotics have greatly improved and so have our diagnostic devices and material, to replace arthritic hip surfaces. The acrylic provided a smooth surface, but unfortunately tended to become loose.
- In 1950s, Charnley devised effective methods of replacing both the femoral head and acetabulum of the hip. He first used teflon implant for acetabular component, but when it failed, he tried polyethylene, which worked wonderfully well. In order to obtain fixation of this polyethylene socket as well as the femoral implant to the bone, Charnley borrowed polymethyl methacrylate from the dentists. This substance, known as bone cement, was mixed during the operation then used as a strong grouting agent to firmly secure the artificial joint to the bone. Truly this was the birth of "total hip replacement"
- In the last 10 years, there had been considerable effort.

H Lowry Rush (1879–1965) (Fig. 19)

Used pins made of especially hardened stainless steel, for treating long bone fractures.

Sir John Charnley (1911–1982)

- Sir John Charnley (Fig. 20) wrote a classic book on the nonoperative approach to fractures, "Closed Treatment of Common Fractures"
- Sir Charnley is, however, renowned, as the effective innovator of the total hip replacement and development of a self-curing acrylic bone cement
- Many of the total hip replacements that he performed in the 1960s are still sound and serving their patients effectively.

Amulya Kumar Saha (1913–1994)

Professor Amulya Kumar Saha was born in 1913 in Pabna in undivided India (now in Bangladesh). After graduating both in science and medicine from Calcutta University, he underwent surgical training under Professor LM Banerji, the then legendary surgeon of India in his time, he joined British Indian Army during World War II, was serving in Burma and in Middle East, as surgical specialist and quickly promoted to rank of major.

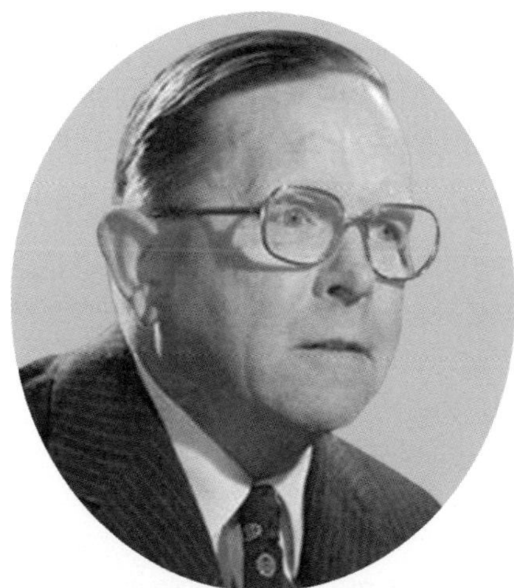

Fig. 20: Sir John Charnley.

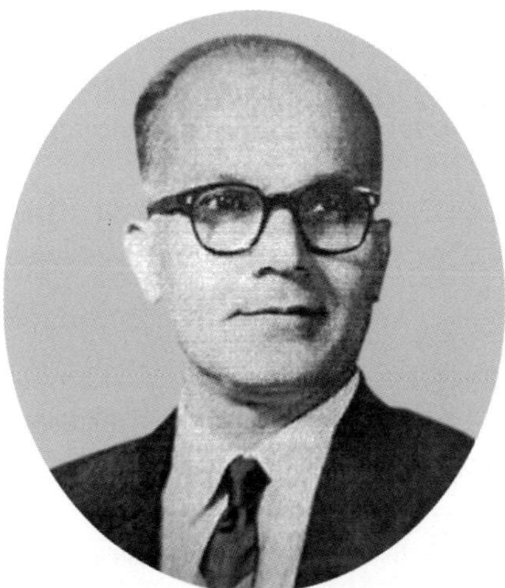

Fig. 21: Prof Amulya Kumar Saha.

After demobilization, he went to United Kingdom for additional study and training in surgery and got qualified with titles of Fellowship of The Royal College of Surgeons (FRCS) (Eng), FRCS (Edin), and Mch. Ortho (L`Pool) in 1948. He became interested in shoulder mechanism while assisting Professor SK Basu at the Indian Museum in 1940. He delivered his first dissertation to the Liverpool orthopedics group in 1948. Thereafter, the shoulder was one of his abiding interest (Fig. 21).

After return to India, he joined as Reader in Surgery at Gwalior Medical College. Subsequently, he joined Nilratan Sircar Medical College and University of Calcutta as Associate Professor of surgery, served from 1949 to 1955 and then promoted to post of Professor Director in the department of surgery and served till 1963, subsequently he became honorary consultant orthopedic surgeon from 1964 to 1972. In 1972, he became Professor emeritus of orthopedics. During his time, only orthopedic surgery was just becoming recognized as a specialty in India. In fact, he was largely instrumental in popularizing orthopedics in Calcutta and training a number of younger surgeons in this field. Professor Saha's major contribution to orthopedic research and clinical orthopedic practice is in relation to the shoulder joint. While at Nilratan Sircar Medical College, he conducted extensive studies on the functional anatomy of the shoulder joint from anatomic, anthropologic, morphologic, radiologic, and electromyographic, as well as mathematic, points of views. As a result of these studies, he published his work on the zero position of the glenohumeral joint in 1950. In 1957, he was invited by the Royal College of Surgeons of England to deliver a Hunterian Lecture, "Zero-position of the Glenohumeral Joint: its Recognition and Clinical Importance." At about this time (1954), he became interested in the study of recurrent dislocation of the shoulder joint and in rehabilitating patients with paralysis of the shoulder following poliomyelitis. He was convinced that dynamic stability was essential during various stages of elevation of the shoulder joint with versatile ranges of movements. He postulated that there are three main factors that maintain the dynamic stability of the fully developed shoulder joint—(1) normal retrotilt of glenoid articular surface in relation to the axis of the scapula; (2) the optimum retrotorsion of the humeral head in relation to the shaft; and (3) balanced power of the horizontal steerers. Based on these principles, he evolved his operations for treatment of recurrent dislocation of the shoulder joint, which he considered to be primarily due to lack of dynamic stability during abduction. In some cases of recurrent anterior dislocation of the shoulder joint, there was no history of injury, and in many cases, no Bankart lesion was demonstrable. He was of the opinion that the Bankart lesion possibly was not the cause of recurrent anterior dislocation and occurred from lack of the stabilizing factors and superimposed trauma. In other words, some shoulder joints are more prone than others to undergo spontaneous dislocation, with or without minimal stress. Based on these considerations, he evolved his operations—(1) glenoid neck osteotomy to increase the retrotilt of the glenoid (modified Meyer Burgdorff), when it was demonstrated radiologically that the glenoid retrotilt was diminished or there was actual antetilt; (2) decreasing the retrotorsion of the humeral head by rotation osteotomy of the upper shaft of the humerus, when there was excessive retrotorsion demonstrable by special radiograms; and (3) augmenting the power of the horizontal steerers by transferring the tendon of the latissimus dorsi to the posterior aspect of the humeral neck. He published several monographs, one of which was translated into German in 1978. For the postpoliomyelitis paralyzed and flail shoulder, Professor Saha developed his techniques of multiple muscle transfers based on his concept of dynamic stability of the shoulder; this work was described in a supplement to Acta Orthopaedica Scandinavica in 1967. This concept and its application have been included in many books on the shoulder, including Campbell's Operative Orthopedics. In addition to his great interest in surgery of the paralyzed shoulder, he also devoted his efforts to the rehabilitation of the paralyzed hip following poliomyelitis, using various original muscle transfer techniques to increase muscle power around the hip. He published a number of articles on this subject in Indian journals. Professor Saha was also interested in partial and total shoulder arthroplasty and was working in this field at the time of his retirement. He designed a removable metal prosthesis based on his concept of dynamic stability of the shoulder, which uses available muscles to provide motor power to the shoulder. Lately, this prosthesis has been modified by one of his colleagues to include a high-density polyethylene cover. In addition to the subjects already mentioned, Professor Saha was interested in various other aspects of orthopedics and was first and foremost an excellent clinician and versatile surgeon. He is held in high esteem by his colleagues and students. He is a past president of the Indian Orthopedic Association, an honor that he very much cherished. He was also the recipient of DSc 295 Who's Who in Orthopedics (Anatomy) and Coats Gold Medal of the Calcutta University for original research. Professor Saha was an active member of the Société Internationale de Chirurgie Orthopédique et de Traumatologie (SICOT) and attended many of its meetings, presenting papers on the shoulder. He was invited by several universities in the United States, the United Kingdom, and Japan to deliver lectures about his work on the shoulder joint.

ZERO POSITION OF THE GLENOHUMERAL JOINT: ITS RECOGNITION AND CLINICAL IMPORTANCE

Hunterian Lecture delivered at the Royal College of Surgeons of England

On

10th July 1957

by

AK Saha BSc M Ch Orth (Liverpool) FRCS FRCS (E)

Professor of Surgery, Nil Ratan Sircar Medical College, Calcutta University

INTRODUCTION

The time has come to take stock of the accumulated knowledge on shoulder movements.

The glenohumeral joint is a ball and socket joint, the head of the humerus having a bigger articular surface with a smaller radius and the glenoid a smaller articular surface with a bigger radius. Participation of the accessory joints in shoulder movements have long been recognized (Morris, 1879; Cathcart, 1884, and Lockhart, 1930). Till recently *(vide infra)* the movements at these and the glenohumeral joints were believed to be phasic and compartmental.

The occurrence of reverse rotations during flexion and abduction (Martin, 1933; Codman, 1934; and McGregor, 1937) led to the concept of locking with rotation as a mechanism to get past the natural barriers. The plane of the scapula, though a changing plane in a strict sense, replaced the coronal plane as the plane of reference (Johnston, 1937). Later still Milch (1938 and 1949) described the cone arrangement of muscles when the arm is lifted overhead. In this position, the muscles lose all rotatory power and this suggested the technique of reduction of the shoulder dislocation in the overhead vertical position of the arm. Inman *et al.* (1944) established the pattern of movements of the accessory joints. They are continuous though they occur at varying rates at different phases of elevation. The function of depressors on the head of the humerus was established. They keep the head in contact with the glenoid during elevation.

ANATOMICAL CONSIDERATIONS

The glenohumeral joint surfaces are not perfectly spherical. Rotundity is near perfection at the central part of the two articular areas. There are individual variations and variations with age, though their exact relation has not been established (Fig. 22). Spherometry has also established three types of joints: Type A—the glenoid has a bigger radius than that of the humerus; Type B—both have more or less the same radii; and Type C—the glenoid has a smaller radius than that of the humerus (Fig. 23). In Type A, the contact of the adjoining articular surfaces is by a small area, in Type B, by a much bigger surface and in Type C, the contact is mainly by the margin of the glenoid labrum and the adjoining articular surface. Impression studies of the contact surfaces with the help of lamp.

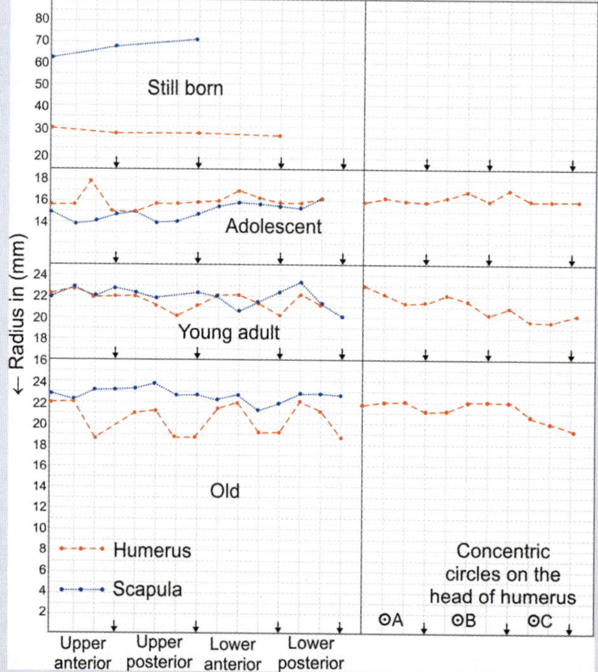

Fig. 22: Graph shows the radii of curvatures of the humeral head and glenoid cavity. Fresh specimens from dead bodies were used. Dotted and continuous lines represent radii of humerus and glenoid, respectively. *Left hand* series gives the radii in stillborn mature babies, adolescents, young adults, and old, and these were taken in four quadrants. They are seen to be too irregular to be called spherical surfaces. The disparity between the articular surfaces can be seen. Graphs on the *right hand* side represent radii on two concentric bands and a central circle on the heads of the humerii used in the previous determination. The radii are more uniform toward the central part of the articular surface in all than toward the periphery.

Black in different positions of elevation has shown three types corresponding with the three types of joints. The contact surfaces do not take uniform impression nor are these identical in different positions of elevation in the same joints. These confirm the irregular nature of the articular surfaces.

The contact area migrates in a characteristic way on the humeral articular surface and less so on the glenoid cavity particularly in the Type C joint in the different phases of elevation (Fig. 24). The anatomical axis of the head and neck bears two angles with the axis of the shaft, 16° in the coronal (retrotorsion angle) and about 130° in the sagittal plane (neck-shaft angle). With abduction, the contact area is exhausted in the plane of elevation before 90° is reached. How then is the rest of the movement at the glenohumeral joint carried out? This is possible by rolling or gliding, analogous to dislocation action within physiological range. This movement would be difficult if the head of the humerus was set on the top of the shaft in a "drum stick" fashion as in quadrupeds. In man with the development of erect posture, the upper limb has come to stay vertical and parallel to the body. So, he has developed the neck-shaft and the retrotorsion angulations just mentioned. These structural changes have helped him in another way. The rotation of the shaft gives gliding effect at the articular end till the constantly changing mechanical axis approximates to the anatomical axis in the "zero position" of the glenohumeral joint (*vide infra*).

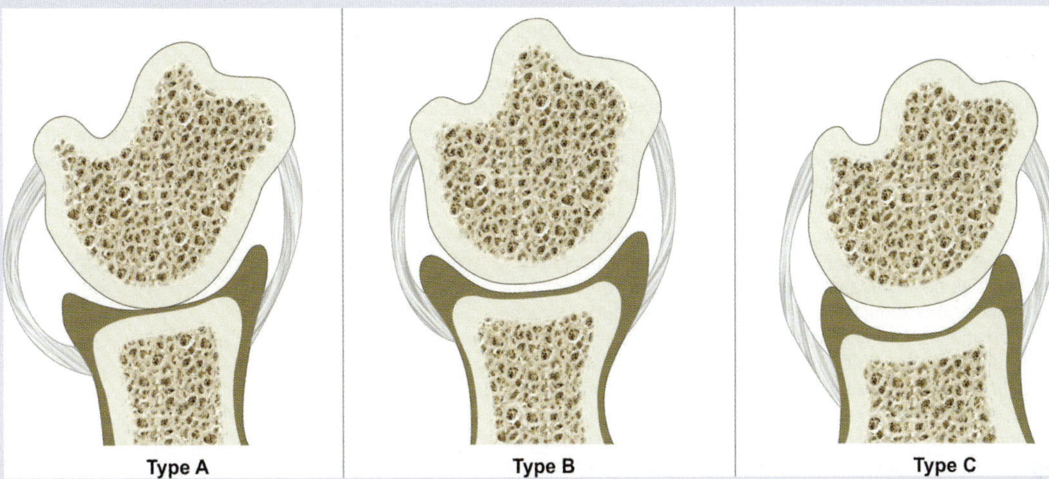

Fig. 23: The three types of joints and their contact surfaces.

Acromion locking during elevation does not take place in any phase of abduction in a healthy joint. The external rotation of the shoulder is necessary even after acromionectomy during abduction.

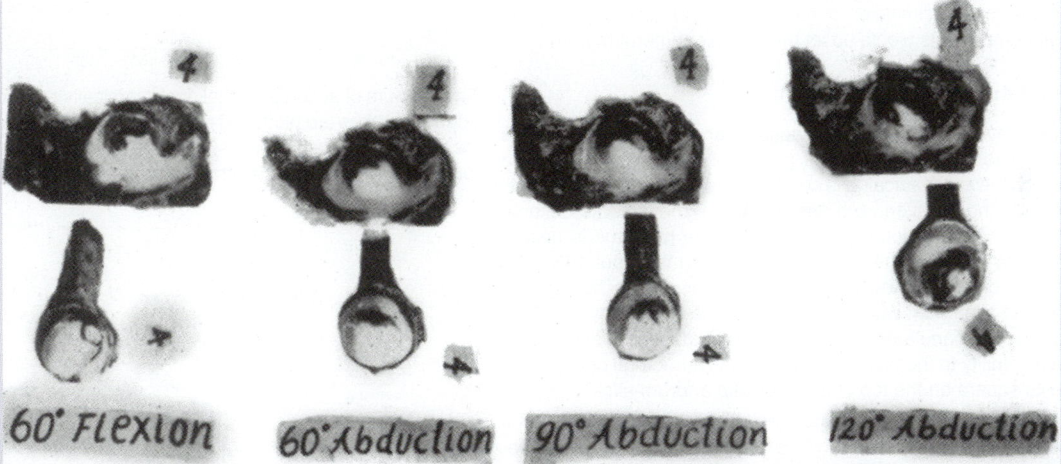

Fig. 24: Lamp black contact impression photographs of the glenoid and humerus at 60° of flexion and abduction, 90° of abduction and 120° of abduction in a typical Type C joint. These irregular circular contact bands hardly migrate in the glenoid with different elevations though they do so on the head of the humerus.

Shoulder Movements

Movements at the glenohumeral joint may be analyzed as follows:

- Movement on a fixed contact point, area, or band (hinging). There is no change of mechanical axis.
- Movements that bring about change of contact point, area of band—this has been referred to as gliding, rolling, or physiological dislocation action. There is change of mechanical axis with this type of movement.
- Movement of rotation—even if it takes place on a circular band contact, pressure would be distributed equally on all points of the contact surface. Here there is no change in mechanical axis.

One or all of these may be necessary to bring about elevation in any direction.

The nature of the "breast-stroke" movement at the glenohumeral joint has never been dealt with analytically. "Breast-stroke" movement is a combination of gliding (rolling) and some amount of hinging movements. Its range diminishes with the elevation of the arm.

Rotation of the arm and rotation at the glenohumeral joints are not identical till the mechanical axis corresponds with the anatomical axis of the shaft of the humerus. It has been seen that rotation of the arm, which is equivalent to gliding at the glenohumeral joint steadily diminishes with the raising of the limb. Rotation at the glenohumeral joint is equivalent to circumduction with vertical position of the extremity. Its range also shows steady diminution with lifting of the limb.

Why the above three movements diminish as the arm is raised is understandable when it is seen that the contact area changeover brings about alteration in the mechanical axis. This, when the movements are "Zero", corresponds most closely to the anatomical axis of the shaft. In this position, most of the rotatory power of the muscles is lost.

Muscle Power

Action potentials and frequency discharges recorded during abduction and flexion by eight-channel electromyography have shown that besides the prime movers acting in a particular direction, other muscles also show activity to varying degrees. This accessory power is essential—(1) to fix the glenohumeral joint, (2) help gliding and thus bring about change of contact surface, and (3) move the accessory joints. For deeper muscles, coaxial needle electrodes were used. Unsuspected muscles like the latissimus dorsi and the subclavius are seen to come into play during elevation.

During abduction, the supraspinatus and the deltoid are known to be prime movers. The remaining six muscles, infraspinatus, teres minor, teres major, subscapularis, pectoralis major (sternal), and latissimus dorsi also show variable amount of contraction starting at about 30° (Fig. 25). The power of the internal rotators balances the power of the external rotators so that the algebraic sum of their power does not alter the rotation state of the humeral head up to about 60° elevation. The power till then is utilized only for fixation of the head against the glenoid. Above 60° the external rotators gain more power, which is utilized for gliding purposes. The main internal rotator, the subscapularis, has toward the end of elevation only gliding and fixation action. Above 120°, the power of the internal rotators again exceeds that of the external rotators.

In flexion, adjustment of the shoulder girdle takes place at a slightly earlier phase to make elevation at the glenohumeral joint easy (Fig. 26). From the very onset, the internal rotators are more powerful than the external rotators and at the peak (120°) are twice as powerful as the external rotators. The events are explained on the same lines as in abduction. The glenohumeral articular surfaces change by rotation of the shaft in the initial and end stages of flexion movement.

In movements at the accessory joints, we notice that the subclavius plays a major role in both abduction and flexion. The subclavius rotates the clavicle-crankshaft in an anticlockwise direction (looked at from its outer end) and indirectly adjusts the scapula to bring about the desired elevation. Electromyographic studies show that the movement just mentioned takes place at an earlier phase in flexion (Fig. 27). The rotation of the clavicle crankshaft is maximal between 150° and 180° during abduction. During flexion, rotation of the clavicle starts at 30° of elevation and is maximal at an earlier phase.

Scapulohumeral rhythm is an essential component of the sequence of events taking place during elevation of the shoulder. So accurate is the balance and adjustment that even slightest disturbance by way of spasm of any particular muscle, pain from any cause, limitation of movement, and disturbance in the mechanism of joint components would upset the scapulohumeral rhythm.

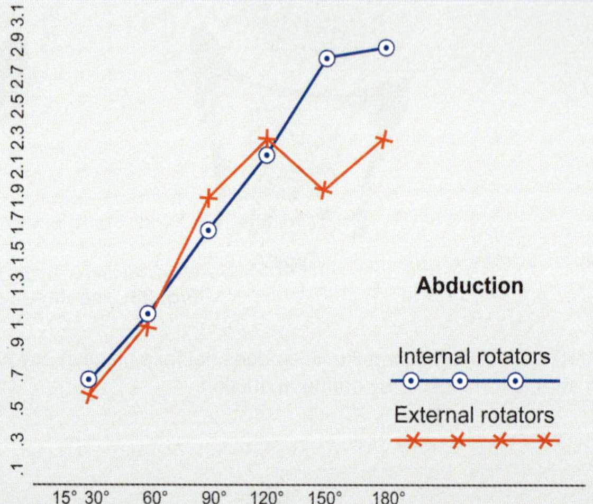

Fig. 25: Sum of action potential of anatomically recognized internal and external rotators are plotted at different phases of abduction. Continuous line with crosses represents summated action potential of external, and continuous line with circles that of internal rotators.

"Zero-position" of the Glenohumeral Joint

The position during elevation in coronal or sagittal plane, in fact in any plane where there is no further rotation, no active gliding of the joint surfaces and circumduction; where the mechanical axis corresponds to the anatomical axis of the shaft; where gliding, rotation, and "breast stroke" movements become identical is known as "zero-position." In this position, the humerus is neither internally nor externally rotated. The humerus is elevated to about 165° with individual variations and is in the newly acquired scapular plane. The humeral shaft axis roughly is in alignment with the scapular spine in this position. This is the relative position of scapula and humerus, which is seen in fast-moving quadrupeds to give stability to the joint. This has brought structural change, the articular surface sits square on the top of the shaft like a "drum-stick".

In the unimpacted fracture of the surgical neck, it has been shown that, if released from the influences of the lower by elevation in any plane, the upper fragment assumes the "zero-position."

Bearing of the anatomical observations on the etiology of the recurrent dislocation of the shoulder. Alternative method of treatment on the basis of the concept.

In the Type C joint, the humeral articular surface is not in contact with the depth of that of the glenoid cavity. The circular-band-contact, in this joint, is affected mostly by the glenoid labrum with much less excursion and change of contact band in glenoid cavity than in the other two types. So, the physiological dislocation action, bringing about change of contact band on humeral articular surface, will, in these cases, throw maximum pressure on some portion of the glenoid labrum depending on the direction of the motion. If the power of the subscapularis, which brings about this in the terminal phases of abduction is insufficient due to various causes including incoordination from sudden contraction of the prime movers and other muscles, it may throw extra burden on the anterior and/or inferior part of the labrum thus causing it to be detached from its bony attachment. It is distinct from other types of dislocation where the tear is in the capsule and is capable of healing, but in this type of subluxation, the detached rim cannot heal by itself by reattachment.

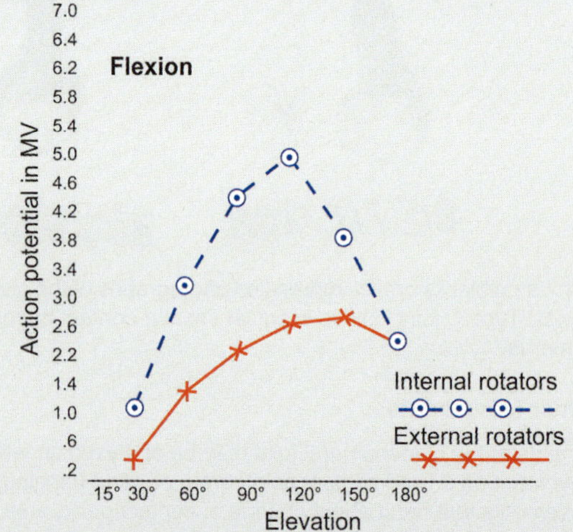

Fig. 26: Sum of action potential of anatomically recognized internal and external rotators are plotted at different phases of flexion. Continuous line with crosses represents summated action potential of external, and dotted line with circles that of internal rotators.

To my mind recent views on the pathology of the recurrent dislocation cannot effectively explain (1) the groove on the humeral head and (2) in some cases, splitting and attenuation of the glenoid labrum at the site of detachment analogous to the finding of a medial meniscus tear.

With this untreated and detached glenoid labrum, further unguarded elevation with external rotation may result in forward migration of the head of the humerus when actually there should be a backward rolling.

Repeated many times, the subscapularis further elongates and its active rolling action progressively deteriorates, resulting in more frequent recurrences. The feeling of something giving way and locking in that position is due to muscle spasm from riding of the head on the edge of the bony glenoid (subluxation). The characteristic groove on the head, if present, makes slipping easier.

The main principles on which treatment of this condition would be based are thus:

- Actual repair of the lesion, i.e. reattachment of the detached labrum to the bony glenoid;
- Shortening and "double breasting" of the subscapularis to increase its power;
- Block or check operations, either by bone, tendon, or fascia; and
- Development of extra power to aid the physiological dislocation action of the subscapularis by muscle transplantation.

On the basis of this last principle, a new operative procedure was developed for the cure of the recurrent dislocation of the shoulder. The method consists of transplantation of the insertion of the latissimus dorsi on the posterior aspect of the greater tuberosity so that during abduction, the muscle will assist the subscapularis to draw the humeral head backwards and prevent its forward slipping. This muscle was chosen in view of its synergistic action, checked electromyographically during the later stages of abduction of the arm overhead.

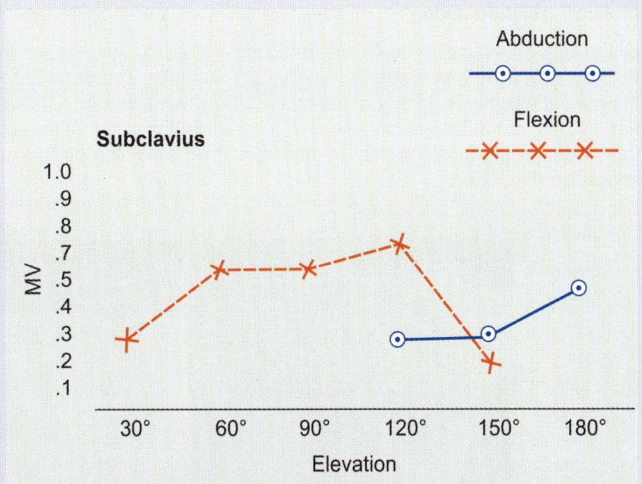

Fig. 27: The diagram represents the action potential in millivolts (MV) of subclavius at different phases of abduction and flexion. Dotted line with crosses represents action potential during flexion and continuous line, action potential during abduction.

The operation was performed by us on a cured epileptic with a bilateral recurrent dislocation where the right side had been treated by the Bankart procedure by one of our colleagues 1 year before.

The patient last seen about 1 year from the date of operation has full use of the limb and there has been no recurrence. The operation has been tried only in a single case, so it is too early to pass any definite opinion but the result suggests that it is worth trying in other cases of recurrent dislocation of the shoulder.

Clinical Application of "Zero-position" in the Treatment of Dislocation of the Shoulder

It is suggested that in treating dislocation of the head of the humerus, the detrimental effect of the rotators, chiefly of the subscapularis, can be effectively eliminated when the limb is brought into the "zero-position". A single force exerted along the axis of the humerus when the limb is in "zero-position" can thus be made to oppose the combined action of all the musculature in spasm.

Method

The patient lies on the table supine, and the surgeon takes his position at the head end and on the side of the dislocation. Usually, an anesthetic is not necessary except in cases of an old dislocation or a neurotic individual. The surgeon gently abducts the arm to bring it in the "zero-position", i.e. 165° overhead and 45° in front of the coronal plane with the medial epicondyle pointing forwards and medially. Slight traction in this direction suffices to reduce the dislocation in recent cases. In older cases, an assistant fixes the patient by putting both his hands round the waist. As the surgeon exerts sustained traction, the head goes back to its original position, pushed by the thumb if necessary. An associated fracture of the greater tuberosity, if present, falls into place during this maneuver.

After the dislocation is reduced, early motion is encouraged in all directions except in abduction in an uncomplicated case. To check abduction, the patient is provided with a figure of eight bandage round the affected arm and the trunk, which acts as a "check" ligament. Every third or fourth day greater degree of abduction is permitted by increasing the length of this "check" ligament. After 21 days from the date of reduction, the sling is taken off and all movements are allowed.

To give full range of mobility, exercises such as swinging the arm at the shoulder or wall climbing exercises are prescribed and within 15 days, the patient gets back the full use of the injured limb.

Unimpacted Fracture of the Surgical Neck of the Humerus: Displacement of the Proximal Fragment

Difference of opinion exists regarding the displacement of the upper fragment. The fragment is abducted, slightly flexed, and rotated. The rotational displacement is generally believed to be fully external but according to a few, it is moderately externally rotated and others internally rotated. With the hanging position of the upper extremity, the fragment is fully internally rotated if it is free from the influence of the distal fragment. The fully internally rotated position of the proximal fragment is proved by comparing it with the identical anteroposterior radiograph of a 45° abducted and internally rotated normal shoulder. In both, the greater tuberosity hides most of the head of the humerus. Secondly, in a true lateral view of the glenohumeral joint, the radiograph of the upper fragment is a replica of its anteroposterior view with the greater tuberosity pointing toward the sternum. The curve of the head is directed toward the vertebral column and the greater tuberosity toward the sternum. This is true for epiphyseal separation and upper third fracture.

The displacements of the proximal fragment are dependent on the position of the limb. As the distal segment of the limb is raised, the abduction displacement steadily increases till it assumes the "zero-position". This new displacement may appropriately be termed absolute abduction.

It is further seen that while changing to the absolute position, the proximal fragment, which in its initial position was fully internally rotated, gradually derotates, i.e. rotates laterally and in the final position, it is neither internally nor externally rotated (Figs. 28A to D).

In the treatment of unimpacted fracture of the neck of the humerus, closed reduction is always preferred to the various open methods. Frankau's (1933) method has not proved satisfactory. Perfect anatomical alignment with elimination of rotation deformity is only possible with the help of the "zero-position".

Method of Reduction

Under light general anesthesia, the arm is lifted so as to allow the proximal fragment to assume the absolute position, i.e. "zero-position". In this position, the fragment is neither rotated internally nor externally. The distal humeral segment is now adjusted to perfect alignment by comparing the direction of the medial epicondyle to that of the sound side when the latter is lifted to the same position. Alignment thus being achieved, apposition is obtained by firm traction of the limb till the ends hitch against each other. In the majority of instances, especially elderly persons in whom the fracture is common, this end-to-end apposition may be maintained by impaction by firm compressive force. The arm is then brought down and tested for the stability of impaction (Fig. 28E).

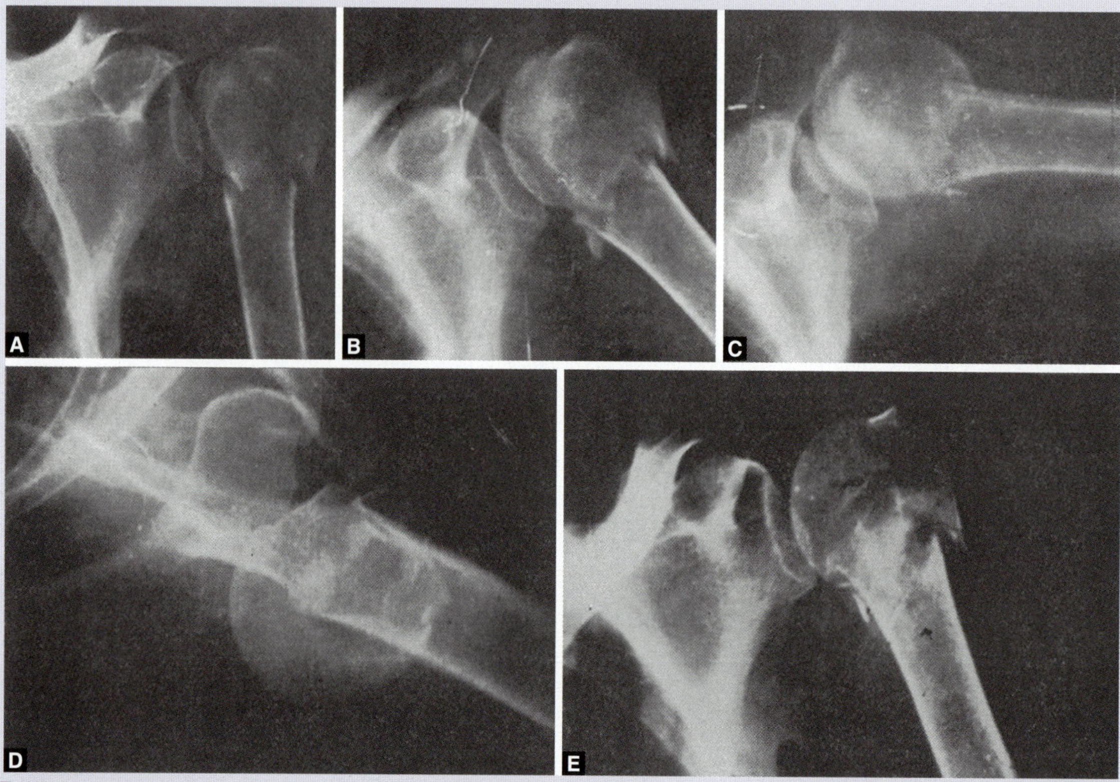

Figs. 28A to E: (A) Anteroposterior skiagram of the shoulder shows unimpacted fracture of the surgical neck. The upper fragment is internally rotated. (B) Derotation of the proximal fragment with 45° of abduction is seen. Outline of the head is visible as an area medial to the tuberosity. (C) Further elevation has brought in relief the greater part of the head. (D) Elevation to the zero-position has brought the whole of the head outline as would be seen in an ordinary anteroposterior skiagram of the shoulder. (E) Skiagram shows impaction after reduction in the "zero-position". There is some comminution of the fragments during the impaction.

In all our cases, possible future disimpaction was prevented by a three-inch overlapping adhesive strapping between the flexed elbow and the top of the shoulder. Cases where there is some comminution are not stable; reduction and fixation is obtained by fixed skin traction over specially constructed iron sidebars with a cross loop incorporated in a plaster jacket. A preliminary plaster jacket is applied with a cross bar over the affected shoulder. Specially constructed sidebars with a cross loop at the distal ends are incorporated in the plaster. Fixed skin traction is applied with the shoulder in the "zero-position" (Fig. 29). Some of our cases were given mobile skin traction with the help of a Balkan frame and/or Thomas' arm splint. This is especially necessary for very well-built individuals. After 6–8 weeks of fixation, the movements are allowed till full function is obtained.

Upper Humeral Epiphyseal Separation and Fracture of the Upper Fourth of the Shaft of the Humerus

In the upper humeral epiphyseal separation, the internal rotation deformity of the upper fragment is not so well demonstrated owing to the poor development of the tuberosity region. The normal upper humeral epiphysis sits like a beret on the proximal diaphyseal end in the anteroposterior view. The presence of rotation deformity masks this appearance. When the rotation deformity is eliminated in the "zero-position", this picture reappears. With alignment of the fragments in this position, slight or moderate traction brings about perfect apposition (Figs. 30A to C).

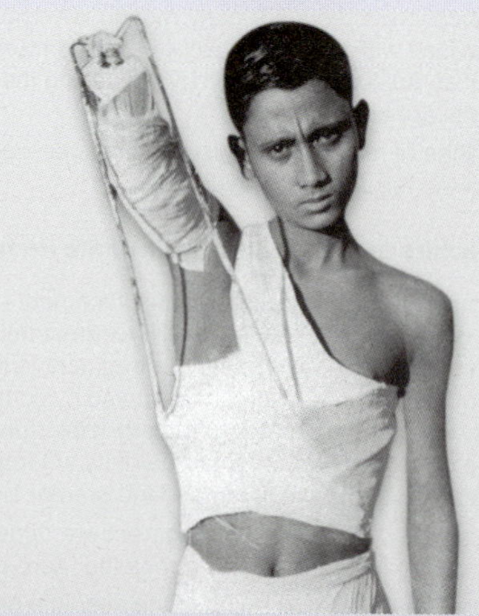

Fig. 29: It shows the method of fixed traction on side bars incorporated in a plastic jacket in the zero-position.

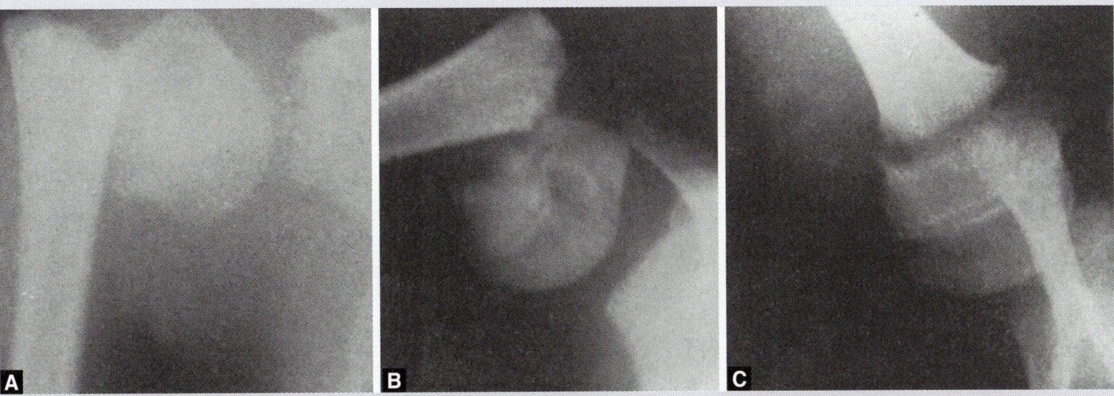

Figs. 30A to C: (A) Epiphyseal separation in an anteroposterior view. (B) Elevation of the distal segment derotates the proximal fragment. (C) The typical cap-appearance of the proximal segment appears in the "zero-position". The fracture is completely reduced with traction.

Maintenance of reduction has not been possible in our series of cases by impaction. The limb has to be kept under traction for a period of 3 weeks by one of the methods outlined above till clinical union is obtained. The subsequent management is on the same lines as unimpacted fracture of the surgical neck.

Upper Fourth Fracture of the Humeral Shaft

In the upper fourth shaft fracture, the displacements are similar. Reduction and fixation are on the same lines. The period of fixation till clinical union is a little longer and varies from 4 to 6 weeks (Figs. 31A to C).

CONCLUSION

The present day concept of the mechanism of the shoulder joint has been outlined. Anatomical peculiarities have been shown to explain the etiology of recurrent dislocations and a new line of treatment has been advocated.

The "zero-position" has been defined and its clinical use in the treatment of dislocations, unimpacted abduction fractures of the surgical neck, epiphyseal separations, and upper fourth shaft fractures has been described.

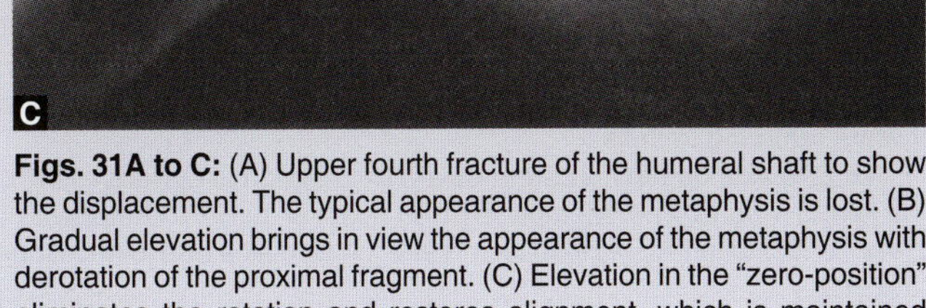

Figs. 31A to C: (A) Upper fourth fracture of the humeral shaft to show the displacement. The typical appearance of the metaphysis is lost. (B) Gradual elevation brings in view the appearance of the metaphysis with derotation of the proximal fragment. (C) Elevation in the "zero-position" eliminates the rotation and restores alignment, which is maintained by traction.

DONATIONS

The following generous donations have been received during the last month:

£10,000—the Simon Marks Charitable Trust (first of seven equal annual instalments).

General Fund:

£1,000—the Prudential Assurance Co. Ltd. (who have expressed the hope that it may be repeated in subsequent years).

Seven-year Covenant for £428 l ls. 6d. p.a. Johnson and Johnson (Gt. Britain) Ltd.

£105—British Glues and Chemicals Ltd. (per Mr LJ Williams).

£100—the Littlewood Charitable Trust (further gift).

Down House:

£100 Josiah Wedgwood & Sons Ltd.

Donations for Chairs in the Great Hall:

DH Sandell, FRCS; JT Chesterman, FRCS. (2).

APPOINTMENT OF FELLOWS AND MEMBERS TO CONSULTANT POSTS

WS Foulds, MB, Ch B, DO, FRCS, Consultant Ophthalmologist, United Cambridge Hospitals and the East Anglian Regional Hospital Board.

Barry O'Donnell, FRCS, M Ch, FRCSI, Consultant Surgeon, Our Lady's Hospital for Sick Children, Crumlin, Dublin.

Richard Rowlandson, FRCS, Consultant Thoracic Surgeon, Brook Hospital, Shooters Hill and Preston Hall, Maidstone, Kent.

REFERENCES

1. Cathcart CW. Movements of the shoulder girdle involved in those of the arm on the trunk. J Anat Physiol. 1884;18:211-8.
2. Codman EA. The shoulder: Rupture of the Supraspinatus Tendon and Other Lesions in or about the Subacromial Bursa. Boston: Thomas Todd Co; 1934.
3. Evans FG, Krahl VE. Amer J Anat. 1945;76:330.
4. Frankau C. Lancet. 1933;2:750.
5. Inman VT, deC M Saunders JB, Abbot, LC. Observations on the function of the shoulder joint. J Bone Joint Surg. 1944;26:1-30.
6. Johnston TB. The movements of the shoulder joints: a plea for the use of the "plane of the scapula" as the plane of reference for movements occurring at the humeroscapular joint. Br J Surg. 1937;25:252.
7. Lockhart RD. Movements of the normal shoulder joint and of a case with trapezius paralysis studied by radiogram and experiment in the living. J Anat. 1930;64:288.
8. Martin CP. The cause of torsion of the humerus and of the notch on the anterior edge of the glenoid cavity of the scapula. J. Anat. 1933;67:573-82.
9. Martin CP. The movement of the shoulder-joint with special reference to rupture of the supraspinatus tendon. Am J Anat. 1940;66:213-34.

10. McGregor L. Rotation at the shoulder: a critical inquiry. Br J Surg. 1937;24:425-38.
11. Milch H. Treatment of dislocation of the shoulder. Surgery. 1938;3:732-40.
12. Milch H. The treatment of recent dislocations and fracture-dislocations of the shoulder. J Bone Joint Surg. 1949;31A: 173-80.
13. Morris H. The anatomy of the joints of men. London, J. A. Churchill: Creative Media Partners, LLC; 1879
14. Perkins G. Fractures. Oxford: Oxford University Press. 1940.
    --- and Watson Jones R. *Proc Roy Soc Med.* 1936;29:1055.
15. Saha AK. Mechanism of shoulder movements and a plea for the recognition of "zero position" of glenohumeral joint. Indian J Surg. 1950;12:153-65.
16. Saha AK, Das NN, Chakravarty BG. Studies on electromyographic changes of muscles acting on the shoulder joint complex. Calcutta Med J. 1956;53:409-13.
17. Saha AK, Saha MR, Chakravarty BG. Anatomical and mechanical observation on the glenohumeral joint. Calcutta MED J. 1957;54;48-53.

Pioneers in Rheumatology

Dr KT Dholakia: Pioneer of Joint Replacement Surgery in India

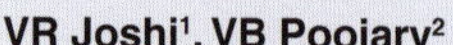

VR Joshi[1], VB Poojary[2]

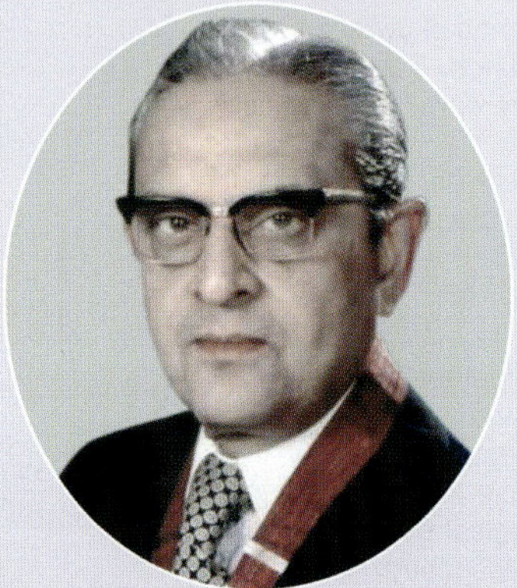

Dr Kandarp Tuljashankar Dholakia was born on 12th August 1920 in Rajkot, Gujarat. His father was a teacher and mother, Sukhwa Ben, was the homemaker. He lost his father at the age of 2 years and was brought up by his maternal uncle who was a doctor in the state medical service. This may be one reason for his taking up medicine.

After completing his schooling at various towns, because of transfers of his maternal uncle in the erstwhile Bombay Residency, Dr Dholakia moved to Mumbai for higher education. He studied at St. Xavier's college, Mumbai (Bombay), passed inter science in 1938, and joined Seth GS Medical College Mumbai to pursue medicine. He secured MBBS in 1943 and MS (General Surgery) in 1945; following this, he went to England for higher education on a Government of India Foreign Scholarship. He was one of the three candidates selected for the fellowship. The final selection involved interview with Viscount Wavell, the then Viceroy of India. Dr Dholakia obtained MCh orthopedics from the University of Liverpool and FRCS from the Edinburg, both in the year 1948. He then visited orthopedic centers in the continent and attended the First International Conference on Poliomyelitis held in New York, before returning to India.

Dr Dholakia began his career as a polio surgeon at Children's orthopedic hospital of "Society for Rehabilitation of Crippled Children". Subsequently, he joined King Edward Memorial (KEM) hospital as Hon. Orthopedic Surgeon. He was appointed as Professor and Chief of Orthopedic Surgery in the year 1952. He left KEM Hospital in 1972. Dr Dholakia had joined Bombay Hospital in the year 1956. He remained associated with Bombay Hospital till the end.

Dr Dholakia was a hard-working individual, a tough task master, a perfectionist (he would often read the operation before coming to surgery), and a strict disciplinarian. He pioneered joint replacement surgery and scoliosis surgery in India. With a single mindedness of purpose, he established and raised orthopedic surgery to great heights. Many of todays leading lights of the specialty were trained by him. He was a good mentor and supported his juniors in their work. One of his students says—"he learnt more from him than from the degrees". Dr Dholakia was an astute clinician and caring to his patients. His mere presence and touch would make patients and the relations confident that the problem would be resolved. He was truly a gifted individual.

For his invaluable contributions to the growth and progress in Orthopedics, Dr Dholakia was decorated with many honors and recognitions. These include Dhanwantari Award (1982), Purkyne Medal of Czech (1988), International Master Surgeons Award of the International College of Surgeons (1994), and Orthopaedic Surgeon of the Millennium Award [Orthopaedic Association of South Asian Association for Regional Cooperation (SAARC) countries]. He delivered prestigious lectures—MacMurray lecture Liverpool; Keynote address World Orthopaedic Concern (WOC) Nigeria; Guest oration Beijing; Guest oration Moscow; Dr Kini, Dr Borges, Dr Katrak, Dr Ginde, and Dr Mukhopadhya Orations. He was President of many associations including Indian Orthopaedic Association (1968), SICOT (1978), and Association of Surgeons of India (1982). He was awarded Padma Shri by President VV Giri in 1973.

Dr. Dholakia had a towering personality (literally and figuratively). He had a commanding voice and was an effective speaker. His interests included music, cricket, travel, and photography.

Dr Dholakia died on 17th June, 2004 after a prolonged illness. He is survived by his 91-year-old wife Saroj, a gynecologist.

Acknowledgments

Authors thank Dr Mrs Saroj Dholakia, Dr LN Vora, Dr HR Jhunjhunwala, and Dr Sanjay Agarwala for their invaluable help.

[1]Director, [2]Former, Research Administrator, Research Department, PD Hinduja National Hospital and MRC, Mahim, Mumbai, Maharashtra

Indian Journal of Plastic Surgery

Home Current issue Instructions Submit article

Kaushik S. Dr. B.B. Joshi—A visionary Hand Surgeon. Indian J Plast Surg. 2011;44(2):176-7.

Dr Brij Bhushan Joshi was one of the pioneers of hand surgery not only in India but also was renowned for his knowledge, ingenuity, and innovativeness the world over.

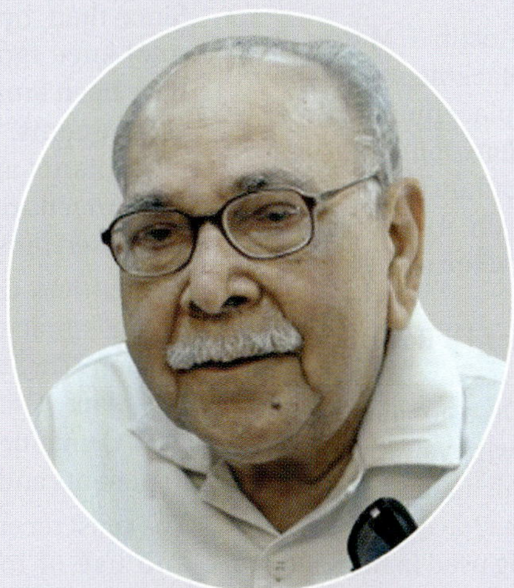

Dr BB Joshi

Dr Joshi started his medical education at the prestigious KEM Medical College in Lahore, then in undivided India, and later completed the degree course at the Grant Medical College and Sir JJ Group of Hospitals, Bombay. He was the first MS in Orthopedic surgery not only from Bombay University but also in India. He then moved to Delhi and was the youngest Chief of Surgery, at the age of 27 years, at the Lady Irwin Hospital, Delhi.

In 1962, his love for the city where he did his medical education brought him back to Bombay. He joined the Mahatma Gandhi Memorial (MGM) Hospital in Parel, Bombay, where he worked tirelessly till he retired in 1986. Working at the MGM Hospital meant dealing with a deluge of hand injuries, as it was an ESIS Hospital. Workers, injured in factories and at their work places came with a wide spectrum of challenging problems. Many patients came with severely crushed and mutilated hands. Dr Joshi had no formal training in hand surgery, as none existed in the country then. This led him to realize early in life that he had to find his own solutions to these peculiar and varied problems.

This was a blessing in disguise, for he was forced to invent his own techniques. When Dr Joshi was presented with a blind patient who had fingertip injury of all his fingers, he felt that this made the patient doubly blind as he could now neither see nor feel! This made him design his own sensory flaps for fingertips to give patients a chance to work with their hands again. Mr Guy Pulvertraft recognized the genius of Dr Joshi and encouraged him to take his work to a wider audience. Dr Joshi was a reluctant speaker but he had brilliant original material which was obvious when he mesmerized the audience in the first meeting of the Indian Society of Surgery of the Hand (ISSH) and later in England before an august international audience in 1973. He offered eight new sensory flaps that he had devised and earned instant and enduring respect of top hand surgeons of the world.

Dr Joshi believed that in hand Surgery even the best surgical work would not produce desired results, unless it was complemented by appropriate postoperative splintage and physiotherapy. His work on simple and economic splints for the hand (using scrap materials like rubber tubing, chicken wire, aluminum strips, and rubber bands) bears the hallmark of his genius. He concentrated on total rehabilitation of the patient, both physical and mental. He trained patients, who were skilled laborers, in a small workshop in the hospital, to fashion splints out of cheap and readily available material. One of his handicapped patients now has a small-scale industry making these splints at an affordable cost!

Always a visionary and always ahead of his time, retirement from MGM Hospital gave him the opportunity to explode to his fullest potential. Realizing the importance of minimally invasive surgery and external fixators, he could not imagine to deny his patients these twin benefits just because the cost of the available gadgets were exorbitant. Once the mini blocks, from inside an electric plug, were put in his hands, there was no looking back. The effort he has made to devise a whole system of external stabilization, around the humble yet versatile and economical link joint, was been phenomenal. What started as a simple fracture holding frame developed into a whole system that encompassed not only the treatment of trauma but also the correction of various congenital and acquired deformities, bums contractures and reconstruction of the thumb.

The versatility of this creation, spilled over to the feet when a patient's parent demanded correction of the clubfoot along with the ongoing treatment for radial club hand. The genius' mind set to work and the congenital talipes equinovarus (CTEV) frame was created. The results were very encouraging and it is now accepted worldwide as a modality to treat clubfeet not amenable to nonoperative methods. Over 300 workshops, to teach the orthopedic and plastic surgeons the scope and versatility of the external fixation device, were conducted by him and his prodigies all over the world and today the JESS techniques are an established and popular technique amongst all hand surgeons.

Dr Brij Bhushan Joshi was a one-man institution and his students are doing brilliantly today to address the unfortunate victims of hand trauma all over India. His generosity is exemplified by the fact that he chose not to patent the JESS fixator, so that it could be made available to a larger section of the medical fraternity and it can be kept affordable for the masses. His wish for "Vidyadaan" is being fulfilled by his associates in the form of a series of books showcasing his monumental work, with the hope that many surgeons, who read these books, will find the light of knowledge to guide them in their clinical decision making.

The entire collection of Dr Joshi's books and original files and photographs of his patient records were donated to the library of Ganga Hospital, Coimbatore. Anyone interested in them can do so in the hospital library.

Articles from Indian Journal of Plastic Surgery: Official Publication of the Association of Plastic Surgeons of India is provided here courtesy of *Wolters Kluwer—Medknow Publications*

TOTAL JOINT REPLACEMENT

Hip

- In 1925, a surgeon in Boston, Massachusetts, MN Smith Petersen MD, molded a piece of glass into the shape of a hollow hemisphere, which could fit over the ball of the hip joint and provide a new smooth surface for movement. While proving biocompatible, the glass could not withstand the stress of walking and quickly failed
- Frederick R Thompson of New York and Austin T Moore of South Carolina, separately developed replacements for the entire ball of the hip. This type of hip replacement, called hemiarthroplasty, only addressed the problem of the arthritic femoral head (the ball). The diseased acetabulum (hip socket) was not replaced. While very popular in the 1950s results remained unpredictable and arthritic destruction of the socket persisted
- As early as 1938, Dr Jean Judet and his brother, Dr Robert Judet of Paris, attempted to use an acrylic and research done, in trying to improve the methods of fixation. Occasionally, it has been found that cement fixation breaks down over time. Due to this, implants with textured surfaces, which allow bone to grow into them have been developed. These have been used experimentally in animals and are now being used in humans. The results of these cementless joints look very promising, when utilized in the correct circumstances.

Knee

- The first attempt at total knee arthroplasty was a prosthesis, which was really a hinge fixed to the bones with stems into the medullary canals (the hollow marrow cavity). These hinges provided good short-term pain relief, but function was not always great due to the limitations of motion and were abandoned
- McKeever (1957) and Macintosh (1958 and 1964) tried to treat arthritis of the knee with a metal spacer, which was placed between the bones of the knee to eliminate the rubbing of irregular surfaces on each other. These implants achieved some success, but were not predictable and many patients continued with significant symptoms
- Surgeons at Massachusetts General Hospital made a prosthesis in the shape of the femoral half of the knee joint. This mould type arthroplasty helped in relieving symptoms, but was neither predictable nor were the results always lasting
- During the late 1960s, a Canadian orthopedist, Frank Gunston from Sir John Charnley's Hip Center, developed a metal or plastic knee replacement, which secured to the bone with cement. This was really the first metal and plastic knee and the first with cement fixation (1968). Hence, the era of total knee arthroplasty had begun
- In 1972, another Englishman living in New York City, John Insall, MD, designed what has become the prototype for current total knee replacements. This was prosthesis, made of three components, which would resurface all three surfaces of the knee, i.e. the femur, tibia, and patella (kneecap). They were all fixed with bone cement and the results were outstanding. This was the first total knee complete with specific instrumentation, to help with accurate bone cutting and implantation
- Since then, by reviewing the cases of patients, who have had total knee replacements, further significant improvements have been introduced. Today with metal backing of the plastic components, an increased inventory of appropriate sizes of implants and markedly better instruments, to perform the procedure, knee replacement results have equaled or surpassed those of hip replacement
- Cementless fixation, using prosthesis with a textured and porous surface, into which bone can grow, may provide biologic fixation. That is, the bone grows into the prosthesis and holds it in place. This may be more durable than cement used in the past. Cementless total knee arthroplasty is currently being used in patients and the results look very promising
- The most recent significant change has been the development and use of total knee implants that are gender specific developed by Dr Bertin.

Minimal Invasive Surgery

- Endoscopy was first described by Hippocrates in Greece (460–375 BC). He made reference to a rectal speculum
- Pioneering work in the field of arthroscopy began, as early as the 1920s, with the work of Eugen Bircher
- Japanese surgeon Masaki Watanabe, receives primary credit for using arthroscopy, for interventional surgery
- History is very important to any surgeon, particularly an orthopedic surgeon. An orthopedic surgeon has once again been presented with advancing technology. This technology must be applied to the surgeon's practice, but it is best applied only when the surgeon has an underlying knowledge of the history of his art. He must be aware of the way surgeons in the past have contributed to orthopedics and more importantly, of the mistakes that they have made in the process. A surgeon, who makes same mistake that was made by someone before him, is surely seen as poorly educated. So is he, who states that he has developed a technique that no one has thought of before, as chances are, that it has been thought of in the past
- For orthopedics to advance in an optimal manner, it is clear that attention must be paid to its history. Past is our foundation for future developments, we must build upon it, so that we too can act as a stable foundation for future generations.

CHAPTER

2 Bone

OBJECTIVES

- Bone Structure
- Fracture
- Bone Grafting

BONE STRUCTURE

Introduction

Mammalian bones (including humans) are constructed of two types of grossly recognizable bones termed "cortical" and "cancellous" respectively.

Cortical Bone

Cortical bone (Fig. 1) is dense and solid, and grossly resembles ivory. In the arch typical long bone, the cortical type bone forms the cortex, which is a solid tubular structure that comprises the outer shell of the bone.

Cancellous Bone

Cancellous bone (Fig. 2) describes the bone structure that is found within the center of the long bones.

Cortical bone has tremendous strength approximating that of tempered steel. Its main function is to provide a rigid structure, which can provide a platform for the attachment of skeletal muscles. Due to its rigidity, cortical bone allows vertical posture. Cortical bone has a low surface to volume ratio, a fact that is important regarding its role in skeletal remodeling and calcium ion homeostasis.

Cancellous bone demonstrates a tremendously high surface to volume ratio, and grossly it resembles the porous structure of a sponge. This accounts for the alternative designation of cancellous bone as "spongy bone". Cancellous bone is found within the marrow cavities of long and flat bones. It is principally concerned with transmitting the forces, directed across synovial joints from the articulating surface to the adjacent metaphyseal and diaphyseal cortical bone. Since the surface to volume ratio of cancellous bone is large, so it has an important role to play in calcium ion homeostasis. The importance of cancellous bone in calcium homeostasis is exemplified by the fact that 99% of the total body calcium is stored within the skeleton.

The terms cortical and cancellous, describe the gross arrangement of bone tissue. Microscopically, bone is composed of cells and extracellular matrix. Bone is unique among all human tissues, due to its calcified matrix. This is formed by the crystallization of calcium hydroxyapatite crystals [$Ca_{10}(PO_4)_6(OH)_2$] within the extracellular matrix that surrounds the bone cells.

Functionally, there are four types of bone matrix cells, as shown in Figure 3.

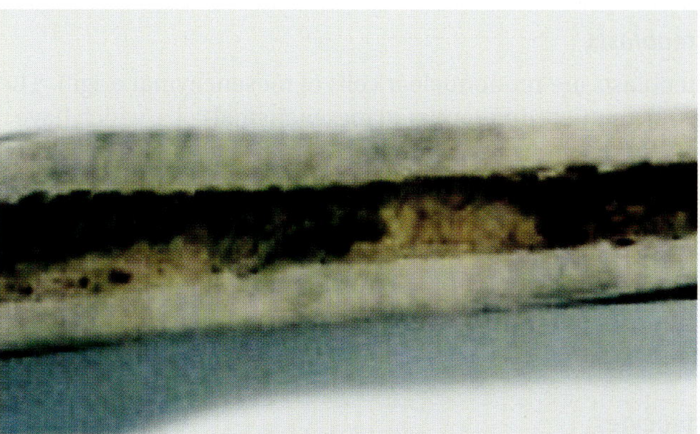

Fig. 1: Normal cortex.

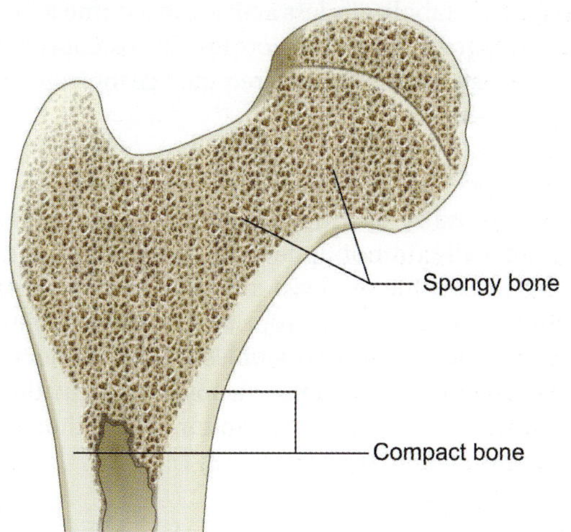

Fig. 2: Cancellous bone in the femoral head.

Osteoclasts

Osteoclasts are syncytial multinucleated cells of monocyte origin. These cells reabsorb calcified bone matrix. They perform this function while attached to mineralized bone within a concave depression called a Howship's lacuna. Osteoclasts are able to reabsorb bone, by selectively producing an extremely low pH within the immediate microenvironment of their action (the Howship's lacuna). The acidification of the extracellular space results from the intracellular production of H^+ ions, by carbonic anhydrase II.

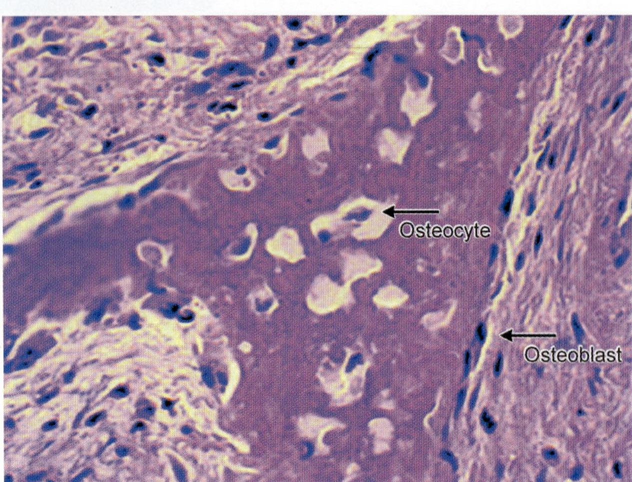

Fig. 3: Normal cells of bone.

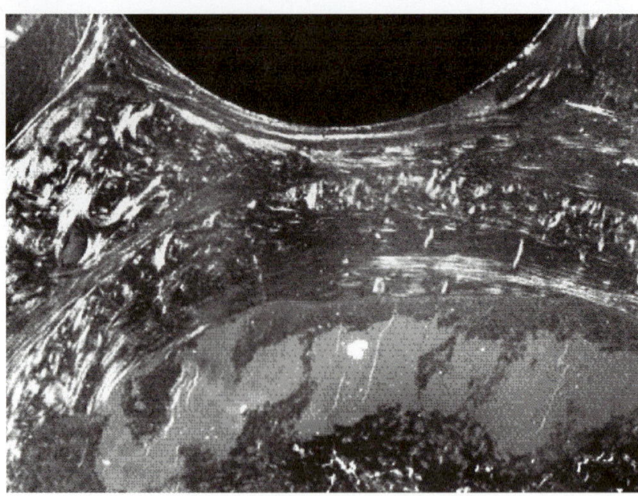

Fig. 4: Woven and lamellar bone.

Osteoblasts

Osteoblasts are mononuclear cells of mesenchymal origin. These are the uniquely differentiated mesenchymal cells, which have the capacity to synthesize and mineralize bone matrix. Osteoblasts typically operate in groups and functionally are often arranged on the external surface of a segment of cortical or cancellous bone, on which they are active. The periosteum, which is the fibrous membrane that surrounds the external nonarticulating aspect of bones, contains cells that may differentiate into functional osteoblasts.

Osteocytes

As bone matrix formation proceeds, some of the osteoblasts get surrounded by the matrix that they have formed. When this occurs, the cells become metabolically less active and assume an inactive appearance. They are termed as osteocytes. The osteocytes are the same cells as the osteoblasts; they merely change their appearance and function.

Osteoprogenitor Cells

These are functionally undifferentiated mesenchymal cells that morphologically do not appear to be differentiated (they microscopically resemble the least differentiated mesenchymal cell, the fibroblast). Under the appropriate stimulation, these cells may differentiate into functional osteoblasts. Many of the cells that reside within the periosteum of adults (a nonactive structure under normal circumstances) are osteoprogenitor cells, although these cells are found throughout the bones.

Bone Matrix*

It is composed of an inorganic phase (calcium hydroxyapatite) and an organic phase. The organic phase consists predominantly of type I collagen, however, there are numerous additional protein and proteoglycan structural components of bone matrix. These include:

- Osteonectin
- Osteocalcin
- Protein growth factors
- Various glycosaminoglycans.

The structural strength (and therefore its mechanical function) of any bone is determined by the following parameters:

- The volume of bone matrix
- The type of bone matrix (woven or lamellar, as shown in Figure 4)
- The degree of mineralization of the matrix
- The structural arrangement of the matrix.

Alterations in any of these parameters will result in a potentially mechanically dysfunctional skeleton.

Types of Bone Matrix

- *Woven bone:* The collagen fibrils, which have been manufactured by osteoblasts, are distributed within the matrix in a haphazard arrangement in bone. This type of bone matrix is rapidly formed, however, it is mechanically weak. Woven bone is the first bone matrix formed in enchondral and intramembranous bone formation, during skeletal growth and development. Woven bone is always abnormal in the context of the mature skeleton, suggesting an abnormal pattern of bone formation. The finding of woven bone in the mature skeleton, while abnormal, is completely nonspecific.
- *Lamellar bone:* It is a bone, in which the collagen fibrils that are manufactured and secreted into the extracellular space, by the osteoblasts, having an orderly arrangement in "curving linear arrays." This is mechanically, more sound matrix. It is the type of bone found in the mature skeleton. Within the cortex, the lamellar bone is functionally arranged as virtually solid tubes, centered upon a capillary in the cortex. These tubular structures are termed haversian systems or osteons. Within the marrow cavity, the lamellar bone forms linear anastomosing trabeculae (cancellous or trabecular bone).

Bone Remodeling

- The change in size, composition, and arrangement of the components of the skeleton that occur in embryological development and growth is called "bone modeling." During this time, it is obvious that the skeleton is active, by virtue of the striking changes in size and shape of its components. When skeletal maturity is reached (i.e. when growth ceases), there is an apparent cessation of its activity. This apparent inactivity is

*Bone matrix (for the purposes of this section the word bone refers to microscopic tissue, i.e. cells and extracellular matrix)

erroneous. The skeleton remains one of the most active organs of the body (do not be fooled, simply because the skeleton fails to alter its shape or manufacture some noxious liquid, gas, or solid, like many of the other viscera). In fact, the activity of osteoclasts and osteoblasts persist throughout life. This activity, within the mature skeleton is termed "bone remodeling".

- The functional unit of bone remodeling is formed by the sequential coordinated activities of osteoclasts, osteoprogenitor cells, osteoblasts, and finally osteocytes.
- A group of osteoclasts commences bone resorption, by attaching to a mineralized bone surface. Each individual cell acidifies the local extracellular space and secretes active lysozomal enzymes, which enzymatically breaking down the bone matrix. These enzymes include serine proteases, collagenases, and tartrate resistant acid phosphatase (the latter can be measured within serum and its level crudely reflects osteoclastic activity). The enzymatic destruction of the bone matrix releases various proteins, including growth factors, previously stored during bone formation. These, in addition to cytokines, manufactured the osteoclasts themselves and other cells, recruit adjacent osteoprogenitor cells to become osteoblasts. In general, osteoclasts function as groups that resorb cones of bone termed cutting cones (Fig. 5).
- The osteoblasts, which typically function in groups, enter the resorption defect created by the osteoclasts and manufacture new bone matrix of either woven or lamellar type. As the cells become entrapped within the bone matrix, they are transformed to osteocytes.
- This sequential activity of osteoclast resorption, followed by osteoblastic bone formation is constantly occurring within the skeleton at all times. Since the surface to volume ratio of cancellous bone is so much greater than that of cortical bone, this presents a greater area for bone remodeling. In fact, studies have estimated that up to 25% of the cancellous bone of humans may be remodeled each year, under normal circumstances. In comparison, 3% of cortical bone is remodeled annually. Under normal circumstances, the net effect of these sequences of bone resorption and formation resulted in as such no overall change in skeletal mass. This process, whereby the degree of new bone formation is linked to the preceding bone resorption, is termed "coupling".

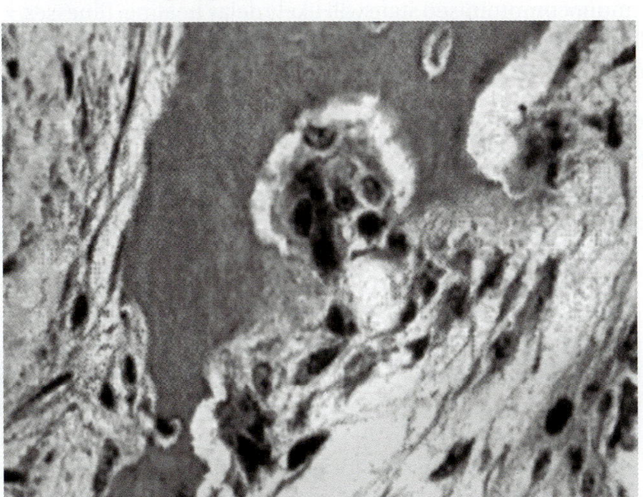

Fig. 5: Cutting cone.

Factors Affecting Bone Remodeling

There are three broad categories of conditions that result in altered bone remodeling. These can be classified as:

1. *Metabolic activity of the relevant cells:* In practice, inborn metabolic dysfunction of cells, involved in bone remodeling is extremely rare and in addition to affecting "remodeling", these disorders typically have profound effects on growth and development (skeletal modeling). In contrast, acquired metabolic abnormalities of these cells are relatively common and account for the most common of all metabolic bone diseases, such as osteoporosis.
2. *Calcium homeostasis and nutritional status:* Calcium ions are required for numerous intracellular enzymatic reactions. Extracellular calcium levels are stringently maintained within a narrow range. Since the skeleton is the repository of 99% of the body's calcium, it is clear that circumstances affecting calcium homeostasis can have major effects on remodeling activities too. In this regard, the level of hormones, "parathyroid hormone" and "vitamin D", may have major effects on the skeleton. In general terms, parathyroid hormone stimulates osteoclastic activity and recruitment of osteoclast precursors (monocytes) to become osteoclasts, producing a net increase of osteoclastic function.
3. *Physical stress: Bone* is not unique in its ability to react to altered physical stress (the myocardium reacts by hypertrophy of cells, when it faces altered systolic pressures), however the extent and precision of the skeletal reaction, to physical stress is unique among all viscera. "Wolff's law", states that bone (an individual bone or group of bones) remodels itself, based upon the physical stresses placed upon it. The denser bones that are present within the dominant arms of professional tennis players, best exemplify this. Conversely, bones that lose their physical stressors for any reason typically become more lucent reflecting a net resorptive state.

Regardless of which of the above factors pertain in any circumstance, the osteoclasts, osteoprogenitor cells, osteoblasts, and osteocytes, always mediate remodeling activities within the skeleton. It has become increasingly clear that cytokines, manufactured by these cells, acting in a paracrine and autocrine fashion, actually mediate the activities of all these cells. The interleukin family of cytokines appears particularly important in this regard, especially regarding the function of osteoclasts.

FRACTURE

Introduction

A fracture may be defined as any break in continuity of a bone's structure. Fractures are virtually always associated with soft tissue injury and the healing process, which occurs with fracture repair, inevitably will have major effects on these structures. However, for the purposes of this discussion, comments will be confined to the sequence of events, which occur at the time of bone injury and subsequently with bone healing.

The following is a brief glossary of terms pertaining to fractures:

- *Closed fracture*: In this, the skin overlying the fracture bone is intact.
- *Complete fracture*: In this, a full thickness break of the affected bone.
- *Comminuted fracture*: It is a fracture that results in multiple separated bone fragments.

- *Compound fracture*: It is a fracture in which the skin overlying the fracture is broken.
- *Avulsion fracture*: It is a fracture due to pulling of a tendon or ligament at its insertion site.
- *Greenstick fracture*: It is an incomplete fracture of the shaft of a long bone in the immature skeleton.
- *Pathologic fracture*: It is a fracture occurring in abnormal bone (for any reason). In clinical practice, this is often used to describe fractures through bone tumors.
- *Stress fracture*: It is an undisplaced fracture, usually involving a part of the cortex of bone that occurs due to excess loading. Stress fractures are sometimes referred to as "fatigue fractures".

Fracture Healing

A fracture occurs, when the continuity of a bone is broken and local blood supply is interrupted. If the overlying soft tissues are also injured, fracture healing may be delayed or disrupted, particularly in anatomic regions with decreased vascular networks, such as the tibial diaphysis. Bone is unique in its ability to regenerate itself. Healing occurs, via reactivation of embryologic processes, resulting in the formation of bone, not scar. Fracture healing can be described in three conceptual stages. An understanding of the timing and mechanisms associated with each stage is important in planning fracture treatment. The stages are:

Inflammation

This begins immediately after bone injury, with the formation of a local hematoma or fibrin clot. There is local cell death, where vessel disruption has resulted in ischemia, usually at the very ends of the fractured bone. Over the course of the next few days, this area becomes infiltrated by inflammatory cells and is characterized by local swelling and warmth. The inflammatory cells release lysozomal enzymes and other mediators that attract pluripotent cells to the area. They also act to remove necrotic tissue. Fibroblasts, mesenchymal cells, and osteoprogenitor cells appear and may transform nearby tissues. The fracture is tender and may be grossly mobile to physical examination at this stage. Inflammation is at its peak, after 48 hours following a fracture.

Repair

The reparative phase begins a few days after the injury, with the arrival of mesenchymal cells, which are able to differentiate into fibroblasts, chondroblasts, and osteoblasts. The repair phase persists for several months. It can be divided into two distinct phases, i.e. soft and hard callus formation.

Soft callus formation

It lasts for approximately 6 weeks from the time of injury. During this preliminary stage of repair, pain and swelling subside and bony fragments become united by fibrous and cartilaginous tissue and woven bone is formed. While this creates some stability, the fracture may still angulate at this stage if not held with stable external support, such as a cast or external fixator or internal support provided by plates, screws, or intramedullary devices.

Hard callus formation

During this second stage of repair, woven bone is transformed into lamellar bone and this takes approximately 3 months.

Remodeling

Remodeling is the process, by which bone is removed in tiny increments and then replaced by new bone. After a fracture, remodeling may continue for months or even years. The adult human skeleton continuously replaces itself at rate of 10–18% per year. The rate of remodeling is accelerated in children and during fracture repair. In addition to being an essential part of fracture healing, remodeling plays an important role in calcium homeostasis. During the remodeling phase, the woven bone is converted to lamellar bone and the medullary canal is reconstituted. During this phase, bone responds to loading characteristics, according to Wolff's law. Some angular deformities may correct during this stage, in children with sufficient growth remaining (up to 5° per year of growth remaining).

The efficiency of bone healing is determined by the following parameters:

- The general health of the patient, in particular the patient's nutritional status
- The presence or absence of preexisting skeletal conditions, either localized or generalized
- The number of fragments in the fracture
- The alignment of the fracture fragments
- The presence and extent of adjacent soft tissue injury
- The presence of intervening soft tissue between the bone fragments
- The presence or absence of infection at the fracture site.

Systemic Factors Affecting Bone Healing

Various local and systemic factors affect the duration and effectiveness of the healing process. Abnormalities in any of these areas may lead to abnormally slow healing (delayed union) or failure to heal (nonunion). These factors include:

Age

Young patients heal rapidly and have a remarkable ability to remodel and correct angulation deformities. These abilities decrease, once skeletal maturity is reached.

Nutrition

A substantial amount of energy is needed for fracture healing to occur. An adequate metabolic stage with sufficient carbohydrates and protein is necessary.

Systemic Diseases

Diseases like osteoporosis, diabetes, and those causing an immunocompromised state will likely delay healing. Illnesses, like Marfan's syndrome and Ehlers-Danlos syndrome, cause abnormal musculoskeletal healing.

Hormones

Thyroid hormone, growth hormone, calcitonin, parathyroid hormone (PTH), and others play significant roles in bone healing. Corticosteroids impede healing through many mechanisms:

- *Thyroid hormones:* They affect bone growth and maturation. Maturation of skeleton is mainly dependent on thyroid hormone. The growth action of growth hormone is potentiated by T4. Thyroid hormone promotes the release of calcium from bone. Hyperthyroidism causes bone resorption, leading to osteopenia, hypercalcemia, and hyperphosphaturia, etc. The rates of calcium deposition and resorption in bone is increased by several folds and returned to normal with treatment of hyperthyroidism. However, resorption always exceeds formation. In hypothyroidism, a state of secondary hyperparathyroidism develops and renal tubular resorption of phosphate is decreased. There is increased urinary excretion of hydroxyproline due to collagen breakdown, as a result of bone destruction.

- *Calcitonin:* It is released from C cells of thyroid. Its function is to inhibit bone resorption and to reduce tubular resorption of calcium. It is therapeutically used in conditions of excessive bone resorption, like osteoporosis, Paget's disease, and renal osteodystrophy.
- *Parathyroid hormone (PTH):* The hormone carries out following functions:
  - Maintains blood calcium levels, by resorption of bone, promoting tubular resorption of calcium and acting with vitamin D, to promote intestinal absorption of calcium
  - Encourages glomerular filtration of calcium and phosphate ions
  - Stimulates osteoclasis
  - Lowers serum phosphorus levels, by inhibiting tubular reabsorption of phosphate from glomerular filtrate
  - Directly affects dissolution of bone
  - Increases solubility of calcium and phosphate
  - Inhibits mineralizing effect of vitamin D.
- *Growth hormone*: Proliferation and hypertrophy of chondrocytes, in the epiphyseal growth plate are controlled by growth hormone. An abnormal increase in growth hormone, leads to proliferation of cartilage cells in the epiphyseal plate. It may continue even beyond the usual time of skeletal maturation and epiphyseal closure. Also, subperiosteal ossification is increased, resulting in increased cortical thickness.
- *Estrogen*: Estrogen is thought to stimulate calcium absorption and to protect bone from unrestrained action of PTH. Estrogen withdrawal leads to bone depletion and osteoporosis.
- *Androgen*: It affects anabolic proteins, which is exerted on muscles, skeleton, sex organs, and other structures. When testosterone is administered to a child, it results in early growth spurt, but skeletal maturation is accelerated, leading to premature epiphyseal fusion, resulting in shortened stature.
- *Adrenal corticosteroids*: In excess, they can cause pernicious type of osteoporosis due to combination of increased bone resorption, diminished bone formation, decreased intestinal calcium absorption from intestine, and increased calcium excretion. Collagen synthesis may also be defective.

Drugs

Nonsteroidal anti-inflammatory drugs (e.g. ibuprofen) and antibiotics (ciprofloxacin), depress healing.

Smoking

Found to decrease the process of bone healing.

Local Factors Affecting Fracture Healing

Type of Bone

Cancellous (spongy) bone fractures are usually more stable, involve greater surface areas, and have a better blood supply than the cortical (compact) bone fractures. Cancellous bone heals faster than the cortical bone.

Degree of Trauma

The more extensive the injury to bone and surrounding soft tissues, the poorer the outcome. Mild contusions with local bone trauma will heal easily, whereas severely comminuted injuries with extensive soft tissue, damage heal poorly.

Vascular Injury

Inadequate blood supply impairs healing. Especially, vulnerable areas are the femoral head, talus, and scaphoid bones.

Degree of Immobilization

The fracture site must be immobilized for vascular ingrowth and bone healing to occur. Repeated disruptions of repair tissue, especially to areas with marginal blood supply or heavy soft tissue damage will impair healing.

Intra-articular Fractures

These fractures communicate with synovial fluid, which contains collagenases that retard bone healing. Joint movement will cause the fracture fragments to move further impairing union. When intra-articular fractures are comminuted, the fragments tend to float apart, owing to loss of soft tissue support.

Separation of Bone Ends

Normal apposition of fracture fragments is needed for union to occur. Inadequate reduction, excessive traction, or interposition of soft tissue, will prevent healing.

Infection

Infections cause necrosis and edema, take away energy from the healing process, and may increase mobility of the fracture site.

Local Pathology

Any disease process that weakens the musculoskeletal tissues, like osteoporosis or osteomalacia, may impair union.

Primary Bone Healing

- In this kind of healing, callus is not formed at all and requires rigid stabilization, with or without compression of the bone ends.
- Rigid stabilization suppresses the formation of callus, in either cancellous or cortical bone.
- Primary bone healing can be divided into gap healing and contact healing. Union occurs in both the types.

Gap Healing

Gap healing occurs in two stages. These are:

- Firstly, the width of the gap is filled by direct bone formation. An initial scaffold of a woven bone is laid down, followed by formation of a lamellar bone as support. The orientation of the new bone formed in this first stage is transverse, to that of the original lamellar bone orientation.
- In the second stage, which happens after several weeks, longitudinal Haversian remodeling, reconstructs the necrotic fracture ends and leads the newly formed bone, to replace the woven bone with osteons of the original orientation. In the end, the normal bone structure results.

Contact Healing

- Contact healing occurs, where fragments are in direct apposition and osteons can grow across the fracture site, parallel to the longitudinal axis of the bone.

- When fracture fragments are in contact, osteoclasts on one side of the fracture, undergo a tunneling resorptive response, forming cutting cones that cross the fracture line.
- This tunneling, allows the penetration of capillaries and eventually the formation of new Haversian systems. These blood vessels are then accompanied by endothelial cells and osteoprogenitor cells for osteoblasts, leading to the production of osteons across the fracture line, eventually leading to regeneration of the normal bone architecture.

Secondary Bone Healing

It occurs when there is no rigid fixation of the fractured bone ends, which leads to the development of a fracture callus. It includes an inflammatory phase, a reparative phase, and a remodeling phase.

Complications during Fracture Healing

Early Complications

Local

- *Vascular injury:* This can cause external or internal hemorrhage.
- *Visceral injury:* This can cause damage to vital organs, like kidneys, intestine, or bladder.
- Neural damage.
- Injury to surrounding tissue.
- *Hemarthrosis:* There is blood in the joint.
- *Compartment syndrome:* Due to bleeding, the blood gets accumulated in the closed compartment, formed by fascia and bone. When this accumulation is too much, with increase in intracompartmental pressure in closed compartment, which does not expand, pressure is produced, on the surrounding tissues, leading to ischemia or lack of oxygen, following a poor blood supply.
- Wound contamination that could lead to infection.

Systemic

- Fat embolism
- Shock
- Thromboembolism
- Acute respiratory distress.

Late Complications

Local

- *Delayed union:* The bone takes more time to heal than the normal limit. Union occurs, eventually with or without augmentation procedure.
- *Nonunion:* There occurs a complete cessation of fracture healing process, clinically and radiologically, beyond the stipulated optimum time for healing, for that particular bone, site of fracture, type of fracture and age. In this case, fracture would not heal without any intervention (surgical), like open reduction and internal fixation augmentation procedure, like bone grafting.

Nonunion as defined by FDA panel (1986): A fracture is said to be nonunited, when at least 9 months have passed since injury and when the last 3 months have elapsed, without progress in healing, clinically and radiologically. Exception, e.g. fracture neck femur, 3 months, since injury (and not 9 months). Local causes of nonunion are illustrated in Table 1 and types on nonunion are explained in Table 2.

TABLE 1: Different causes of nonunion.

Essential local causes of nonunion (DISCO)
Distraction
Especially, by gravity or excessive traction. For nonunion of tibia, additional reasons can be delayed weight bearing and distal third fracture
Infection
Inadequate fixation, ill-advised operation and insufficient Immobilization
Segmental fractures
Soft tissue interposition, severe soft tissue damage
Comminuted fractures
Open fractures

TABLE 2: Different types of nonunion.

Types of nonunion
Hypertrophic type *Due to mechanical failure:* Vascularity not compromised. They are rich in callus. They result from insecure fixation, inadequate immobilization and premature weight-bearing *Elephant foot nonunion:* Hypertrophic and rich in callus Horse hoof nonunion: Mildly hypertrophic and poor in callus. They result from unstable fixation with plates and screws
Oligotrophic nonunion • Callus is absent. They occur after major displacement of fracture or distraction of fragment
Atrophic type • *Due to biological failure:* Vascularity is compromised • *Torsion wedge nonunion:* It is characterized by presence of an intermediate fragment, in which the blood supply is decreased or absent. The intermediate fragment has united to one main fragment and not to other • *Comminuted nonunion:* It is characterized by presence of one or more intermediate fragments • *Defect nonunion:* It is characterized by loss of a fragment of the diaphysis of a bone. Ends of the fragments are viable, but union across the defect is impossible and end in becoming atrophic

- *Malunion:* The fracture unites with fragments in unacceptable position, leading to deformity and other potential problems of malalignment.
- Joint stiffness.
- *Contractures of soft tissue:* This may include tendon, ligaments, joint capsule, and skin.
- *Myositis ossificans:* This is a term used for abnormal ossification of soft tissues. If present around joint, it may limit the range of motion.
- Avascular necrosis.
- *Algodystrophy or Sudeck's atrophy (refer to chapter on CRPS in wrist and hand):* It is neurovascular disturbance following abnormal behavior of sympathetic nervous system.
- *Osteomyelitis (refer to chapter on osteomyelitis):* It is infection of bone and medulla.
- Growth disturbance or deformity, leading to limb length discrepancy.
- Pressure ulcers, following cast.
- Pin tract infection.
- Volkmann's ischemia and ischemic contracture (refer to chapter on VIC in elbow).

Systemic

- *Gangrene:* It may occur due to vascular injury, failed vascular repair, or as a complication of a plaster cast.
- *Tetanus:* This may occur as a result of contamination by tetanus spores, at the time of injury.
- Septicemia.

BONE GRAFTING

Introduction

A bone graft is a transfer of living bone tissue.

Mechanism

Three biological mechanisms are involved in bone grafting, these are discussed here.

Osteogenesis

It is the production of a new bone, by proliferation, osteoid production, and mineralization.

Osteoconduction

It is the production of new bone and migration of local osteocompetent cells, along a conduit, e.g. fibrin, blood vessel, or even certain alloplast material, like hydroxyapatite. New bone originates from the endostium or residual periostium of the host bone.

Osteoinduction

It is the formation of bone, by stem cells transforming into osteocompetent cells by bone morphogenetic protein (BMP). It inducts the recipient tissue cells, to form periostium and endostium.

Indications

- Delayed unions, nonunions, osteotomies, and arthrodeses
- Replacement of lost cortical segments
- Cavities or defects, secondary to cysts or neoplasia.

Types of Grafts

Autograft

- Taken from same individual
- Allows for osteogenesis, osteoinduction, and osteoconduction
- Free (10%) or vascularized (90%).

Isograft

Taken from same family.

Allograft

From same species.

Xenograft

From different species.

Sources of Grafts

Cancellous Bone

- Taken from metaphyseal regions
- Has increased surface area
- Has 80% porosity.

Cortical Bone

- Increased mechanical strength
- Has 10% porosity
- Frequently corticocancellous grafts are used.

Osteochondral

Cartilage attached to parent bone.

Composite Bone Graft

A composite bone graft is made up of hydroxyapatite (HA) crystals, tricalcium phosphate (TCP), and bone marrow.

Vascularized Grafts (Corticocancellous)

- Increased cell survival
- Increased patient morbidity
- Generally for large bony defects.

Sites for Graft Collection

- Cancellous bone metaphyses, e.g. olecranon, distal tibia, etc.
- Cortical bone graft, e.g. ribs, fibula, iliac crest, tibia, etc.

Techniques for Graft Collection

- Aseptic collection
- Avoid oscillating equipment
- Place directly onto the host bone, as air kills the cells
- Place into blood soaked sponge, as saline kills cells
- Be generous
- Implant in stable and sterile environment
- Can regraft in eight weeks.

Process of Graft Healing

- Inflammation
- *Revascularization:* Takes more time for cortical grafts because of less porosity
- *Osteoinduction*: Decreased with cortical grafts
- *Osteoconduction:* Decreased with cortical grafts
- Remodeling.

Healing of Allografts

- "Creeping substitution"
- Basic bone remodeling, at graft host interface
- Bone resorption is followed by bone production
- May take years.

Harvesting Grafts from Different Bones

Ribs

- Indicated for costochondral graft, to restore pseudoarticulation of the temporomandibular joint (TMJ) or to replace a missing part of the anterior mandible, to reconstruct a functional articulation.
- The rib is usually, fifth or sixth, the typical one.
- The sixth rib has the distal origin of the pectoralis major muscle and dissection transects the muscle minimally.
- Right rib is always preferred because:
  - It could be contoured to fit either side of the mandible or facial bones
  - Postoperative pain is less likely to be confused with cardiogenic pain.

Surgical access

- Incision is placed in the inframammary crease, to hide the scar.
- Sharp dissection is carried through full thickness of skin, subcutaneous tissues, and the muscle, to expose the rib periostium and chest wall cortex.
- The periosteum is incised from 1 cm onto the rib cartilage, to the full desired length, the anterior border of the latissimus dorsi muscle, about 12 cm.
- Reflected carefully from the chest wall cortex, around the inferior and superior rib edges to the pleural cortex periostium, using a maxillofacial surgery periosteal elevator, rather than Doyen rib stripper.
- This is to avoid creating pleural tear because of the irregularities and bony projections, to which periostium and lung pleura are firmly attached, leading to pneumothorax.
- A releasing incision made at right angle to the rib incision, carried to the rib edges, help in reflecting the perichondrium and gaining access to the cartilage.
- The cartilage is separated first, by scalpel blade and the proximal part is cut with a saw or rib cutter, after lifting the rib and carefully separating any adherent periosteal membrane from the pleural cortex.
- The closure is layered as periostium, subcutaneous tissue, dermis, and lastly skin.
- Drain is not necessary.
- The length of the cartilage is related to the growth of the graft, not to the prevention of bony ankylosis.

Disadvantages

- Longer length, creates a longer lever arm, promoting separation (2–3 mm).
- Associated with overgrowth.
- Incorporation of the perichondrium or periostium sleeve, in the graft does not enhance survival or stability of the graft.
- In children, the cartilage is easily separated from bone sleeve, thereby reducing the chance of separation.
- In adult, the cartilage is firmly incorporated to the bone.
- Increases the probability of pneumothorax.
- It is recommended that a 2–3 mm of cartilage length, without adherent periostium or perichondrium for both costochondral growth grafts in children and articulation graft in adult.

Iliac Crest

- The lateral approach to the anterior ilium gives most effect on the gait.
- The medial anterior approach involves the large iliacus muscle, which is not necessary for normal gait, but large medial hematoma might produce gait disturbances.

Surgical access

- Incision should be placed 1 cm posterior to the anterosuperior iliac spine and extend to the iliac tubercle.
- It should be placed lateral to the bony prominence, to prevent irritation by tight cloths or belt.
- Proceed down to bone medial to the muscles, tensor fascia lata and gluteus medius and lateral to the iliacus and the external abdominal muscles.
- Cancellous bone is available in the anterior ilium within the upper 2–3 cm, between the tubercle and the anterosuperior iliac spine.
- "Trap door" is one of the most common osteotomy used for anterior ilium harvest.
- During closure, strict attention should be followed in order to reorient and reposition the muscles in their original positions.
- A drain is required because of the dead space and should be placed within the bony cavity.

Tibia

- The extensive subcutaneous surface of the tibia makes it an accessible donor site for bone grafts.
- The tibial plateau is an excellent reservoir for cancellous bone.
- It can provide up to 40 cc of bone, without affecting the structural support of the tibia.

Bone Harvesting

Indications

Small bony defects include:

- Nonunion
- Osteotomy defects
- Dentoalveolar defects
- Sinus lift procedure.

Surgical Access

- Could be done under local anesthesia.
- Incision over the lateral tubercle, best accomplished by flexing the leg at the knee joint.
- It is 6–10 mm, from the skin and dissection is made through the thin subcutaneous tissue.
- Sharp dissection is done to reflect the tensor fascia lata band and make 1 cm opening into the cortex. The cancellous bone could be harvested, lateral and inferior to the midline, to avoid damage to the knee.

Bone Graft Substitutes

- Demineralized bone matrix
- Porous calcium phosphorus ceramics
- Collografts
- Orthografts
- Hydroxyapatite cement
- Platelet gel
- Bone marrow cells
- Bone morphogenic protein
- Composite bone graft.

Properties of Bone Graft Substitutes

- Should be osteoconductive
- Should have load bearing capacity
- Should allow attachment, spreading, division, and differentiation of cells, to produce lamellar bone on its mineral surface.

Demineralized Bone Matrix

It is produced by acid extraction of bone and has a variable amount of bone morphogenic protein. It is available as paste, powder, and gel, with no intrinsic strength (allomatrix).

Porous Calcium Phosphate Ceramics

- Hydroxyapatite ($Ca_{10} (PO_4)_6 (OH)_2$)
- Tricalcium phosphate ($Ca_3 (PO_4)_2$).

Collografts

- These are granular composites of hydroxyapatite and tricalcium phosphate, with added dermal collagen.
- Used with autogenous bone marrow, aspirate to have both osteoconductive and osteoinductive agents.

Orthografts

- They are made of pure tricalcium phosphate.
- It is resorbed by dissolution.

Hydroxyapatite Cement

- It is a mixture of inorganic calcium phosphate and water. Setting time is 10–20 minutes.
- It can be contoured to fill any bony defect before setting.
- It bears minimal load.
- It is replaced by host bone at the rate of 3–4 mm in 6–8 months, by cell mediated response.
- It gives no adverse effects on bone remodeling.

Autologus Platelet Concentrate (Platelet Gel)

This product is harvested from blood. It has multiple growth factors (osteoinductive) and may be combined with matrix, to enhance bone formation.

Ceramics

- These are derived from marine corals that are porous and brittle, have variable resorption, and are often used for augmentation of fractures.
- It is highly crystalline hydroxyapatite porous material, which mimics human cancellous bone in appearance and architecture.
- Bone regenerates into the pores.
- Preparation is done by hydrothermal conversion reaction, where organic material is washed out.
- *Advantages:* Biocompatible, with no inflammatory reaction.
- *Disadvantages:* Weak, brittle, unable to bear cyclical loading and fixation required with grafting.

Bone Morphogenic Protein

- It was discovered by Dr Marshall Urist.
- It is osteoconductive in nature.
- Bone morphogenic protein (BMP) can be produced, concentrated and placed in the body, where bone formation is needed.
- They stimulate regular cells, into bone forming cells.
- It can be used for:
  - Intractable nonunion
  - Large bone defects
  - Massive trauma
  - Old infection
  - Excision of tumors
  - Congenital malformations.

Composite Bone Graft

- Composite bone graft is made up of hydroxyapatite (HA) crystals, tricalcium phosphate (TCP), and bone marrow.
- Composite bone grafting consists of combination of osteoconductive matrix and bioactive agents that provide osteoinductive and osteogenic properties.
- Thus, the osteoconductive substrates become a delivery system for bioactive agents, requiring less chemotaxis and less migration of osteoblasts progenitor cells to graft site.
- The composite bone graft is nonantigenic, noncarcinomatous, and noninfective.
- Advantages include:
  - It is useful, when large quantities of bone are required to bridge a bone defect.
  - Useful in pediatric and geriatric age groups.
  - Have good osteoinductive and osteoconductive properties.
  - No donor site morbidity, in contrast to autograft.
  - Healing time of fracture and consolidation of bone was almost same as autograft.
  - Easy availability of composite bone grafts in all sizes and shapes, facilitate better and more compact packing of bone defect.

CHAPTER

3 Anomalies Related to Development of Bones

OBJECTIVES

- Classification of Developmental Disorders
- Limb Anomalies
- Osteogenesis Imperfecta
- Achondroplasia
- Hypochondroplasia
- Metaphyseal Chondrodysplasia (Dysostosis)
- Osteopetrosis (Marble Bones, Albers-Schonberg Disease)

CLASSIFICATION OF DEVELOPMENTAL DISORDERS

The grouping used here is a convenient way of dividing the various clinical syndromes.

Disorders of Cartilage and Bone Growth

- *Dysplasias with predominantly physeal and metaphyseal changes:*
  - Hereditary multiple exostosis
  - Achondroplasia
  - Hypochondroplasia
  - Metaphyseal chondrodysplasia
  - Dyschondroplasia (enchondromatosis, Ollier's disease)
- *Dysplasias with predominantly epiphyseal changes:*
  - Multiple epiphyseal dysplasia
  - Spondyloepiphyseal dysplasia
  - Dysplasia epiphysealis hemimelia
  - Chondrodysplasia punctata (stippled epiphysis)
- *Dysplasias with predominantly metaphyseal and diaphyseal changes:*
  - Metaphyseal dysplasia (Pyle's disease)
  - Craniometaphyseal dysplasia
  - Diaphyseal dysplasia
  - Craniodiaphyseal dysplasia
  - Osteopetrosis
  - Pyknodysostosis
  - Candle bones, spotted bones, and striped bones
- *Combined and mixed dysplasias:*
  - Spondylometaphyseal dysplasia
  - Pseudoachondroplasia
  - Diastrophic dysplasia
  - Cleidocranial dysplasia
  - Nail-patella syndrome
  - Craniofacial dysplasia.

Connective Tissue Disorders

- *Generalized joint laxity*
- *Ehlers-Danlos syndrome*
- *Osteogenesis imperfecta (brittle bones)*
  - Mild
  - Lethal
  - Severe
  - Moderate
  - Fibrodysplasia ossificans progressiva.

Storage Disorder and Metabolic Defects

- Mucopolysaccharidoses
- Hurler's syndrome
- Hunter's syndrome
- Morquio-Bralisford syndrome
- Gaucher's disease
- Homocystinuria
- Alkaptonuria
- Congenital hyperuricemia.

Chromosome Disorders

- Down's syndrome
- Thoracospinal anomalies
- Elevation of the scapula
- Limb anomalies.

LIMB ANOMALIES

Introduction

Localized malformations of limbs include extra bones, absent bones, hypoplastic bones, and fusions. Complete absence of bones is called "amelia", almost complete absence (a mere stub remaining) "phocomelia" and partial absence "ectromelia". Defects may be transverse or axial. In the hands and feet brachydactyly, syndactyly, polydactyly, and symphalangism are among the many possibilities.

The embryonal limb buds appear at about 26th day of gestation. By the 30th day, upper limb starts differentiating into its three segments (upper arm, forearm, and hand) and in the lower limb, the same process occurs shortly afterwards. By the end of the 6th week, the embryo acquires a recognizable human form. The upper limb is fully formed by 12 weeks and the lower limb by 14 weeks. During this period, the muscles and nerves also develop and by the 20th week joint movement becomes possible.

Most of the malformations, involving limb reductions are due to embryonal insult, between the fourth and sixth week of gestation. Some are genetically determined and these usually have an autosomal dominant pattern of inheritance.

Classification

Various classifications of limb deficiencies have been proposed, but none is completely satisfactory. Some veer towards the purely descriptive, others go into almost obsessive detail, based on topographical and morphological features. Their usefulness lies in the elaboration of an agreed terminology, which will aid communication and permit sensible auditing of the results of various forms of treatment.

Some of the important disorders are referred to below and further details appear in the section on Regional Orthopedics.

Clinical Features

Radial Deficiency

Absence or hypoplasia of the radius may occur alone or in association with visceral anomalies or (more rarely) certain blood dyscrasias. Sometimes, the thumb is missing too and the elbow is often abnormal. In about half the cases, the condition is bilateral.

The forearm is short and bowed and the hand is underdeveloped and markedly deviated towards the radial side (radial club hand). In some cases, the thumb is absent.

The clinical deformity may look bizarre, but children often acquire excellent function. If these seem unlikely, operative reconstruction may be advisable.

Ulnar Deficiency

Hypoplasia of the distal end of the ulna is usually seen as a part of generalized dysplasia, but occasionally it occurs alone. The radius is bowed (as if growth is tethered on ulnar side) and the radial head may dislocate and along with wrist, deviated medially. If the function is severely disturbed, only then the wrist stabilization should be advised.

Congenital absence of the ulna is extremely rare. The forearm deformity is not as marked as in radial deficiency, but overall function is severely restricted. Operative reconstruction may provide some improvement.

Transverse Deficiency of the Arm

Transverse deficiency of the distal part of the arm will leave a stump below a normal elbow. This can be managed by fitting prosthesis, with a mechanical facility for grasp.

Femoral Deficiency (Congenital Short Femur)

In its most benign form, femoral dysplasia consists merely of shortening of the bone, with a normal hip and knee. This can be dealt with, by limb lengthening procedures, if shortening is very marked, then by adding a distal orthosis.

Dysplasia of the Distal Third

Although uncommon, sometimes this occurs with synostosis of the knee. Since the hip permits normal weight-bearing, so this condition can be managed by limb lengthening operations.

In most cases, it is the proximal third, which is under developed or absent. This results in a two-fold problem of shortening of the limb and defective weight-bearing, at the hip.

Various grades of proximal femoral dysplasia are encountered. There may be coxa vara with moderate shortening of the shaft. This can be dealt with, by corrective osteotomy and limb lengthening. Severe degrees of coxa vara, sometimes associated with pseudarthrosis of the neck, may result in marked shortening of the femur. In the worst set of cases, most of the femoral shaft is missing, the knee is situated at thigh level and the foot hangs, where the knee is normally expected to be. If the deformity is bilateral and symmetrical, walking is possible and some individuals acquire remarkable agility. However, they may still seek treatment, to overcome the severe cosmetic problem. Unilateral deformities are not only unsightly, but also very disabling. Effective limb lengthening is out of the question and fitting prosthesis to a short limb, with flexion deformities of hip and knee with a foot jutting forwards, where the knee hinge of the prosthesis will lie is a daunting prospect. In the past, there was some enthusiasm for the Van Nes operation, i.e. fusion of the knee and 180° rotational osteotomy of the leg bones, to get the foot facing back to front and the ankle substituting for the knee, followed by fitting an "above knee" prosthesis. However, the trick is easier and looks better in drawings than in real life and the procedure is seldom done nowadays. One alternative is to fuse the knee in a functional position, amputate the foot, and fit a suitable prosthesis. The earlier this is done, the better the outcome.

Tibial Deficiency

Congenital absence of the tibia is extremely rare. When it occurs, it is usually associated with other anomalies of the limbs. The ankle is nonexistent and the foot is in varus. It is quite possible to construct a functioning one bone leg, by transposing the fibula and fusing it to the center of the femoral articular surface. Once the fusion is achieved, a Syme's amputation can be performed. This should be done as soon as the fibula has developed sufficiently, to permit fusion at the knee. If the procedure fails or if the associated abnormalities turn out to be more severe than expected, proximal amputation can be undertaken at a later stage.

Fibular Deficiency

Mild fibular dysplasia causes little shortening or deformity. However, complete absence of the fibula, leads to considerable shortening of the leg, bowing of the tibia and valgus deformity of the unsupported ankle. There may also be absence of the fourth and fifth rays of the foot and underdevelopment of the entire limb. Sometimes, if only the distal fibula is absent, there is a fibrous band in its place. Excision of this remnant may permit correction of the valgus deformity. If the overall limb length is markedly affected and the foot deformity intractable, distal amputation of the leg may be needed.

Congenital Pseudarthrosis of the Tibia

This rare condition is usually diagnosed in early infancy. The child may be born with a fractured tibia or the bone may be attenuated and then get fractured some months later. In either cases, the fracture fails to unite or heals very poorly, only to get fractured again, shortly afterwards. By the age of 2 years, the leg is noticeably short and bowed anteriorly. By then, it has become obvious that this is an intractable condition, which will not yield to ordinary forms of fracture treatment. X-ray shows a gap or marked thinning of the tibial shaft. Sometimes, the fibula also is affected.

Biopsy of the abnormal segment may show histological features of neurofibromatosis and other stigmata of this condition are present in about half of those affected.

Treatment is likely to be prolonged. Simple immobilization will certainly fail and internal fixation, with bone grafting succeeds occasionally. Better results have been achieved, by correcting the deformity, bone grafting the fracture and immobilizing the tibial fragments in a circular external fixator (the Ilizarov technique). Success has been claimed for extension of the abnormal segment and replacement by a vascularized fibular graft (Weiland et al. 1990).

Congenital Tibial Bowing

Congenital tibial bowing compromises a spectrum of disorders, with significant differences in both etiology and prognosis for the different types (Crawford and Schorry, 1999).

Posteromedial tibial bowing is a relatively benign condition, which resolves spontaneously as the child grows. However, the leg may end up shorter than normal, requiring epiphysiodesis on the opposite side, to counteract the limb length inequality.

Anteromedial bowing is almost always associated with fibular deficiency and congenital defects of the foot or some type of femoral dysplasia. Treatment depends on the presence or absence (and severity) of the associated disorders and varies from reconstructive procedures of the ankle to (in the worst cases) amputation.

Anterolateral tibial bowing, with failure of normal tubularization may be the forerunner of localized osteolysis and eventual fracture, with persistent nonunion and pseudarthrosis of the tibia. Corrective osteotomy should be avoided because of the high risk of nonunion. When the bone is intact, treatment consists of bracing, until the bone matures. If a fracture occurs, treatment is same, as for congenital pseudarthrosis.

Pseudarthrosis of the Clavicle

A child sometimes presents with a painless lump over the clavicle and X-rays confirm the presence of a nonunited fracture or pseudarthrosis. The condition is not really comparable to pseudarthrosis of the tibia and is thought to be due to pressure by the subclavian artery, on the developing bone. In every reported universal case, the right side has been affected, except in the presence of dextrocardia. Treatment, if required is by excision and grafting.

Synostosis

The various types of interosseous fusion (radioulnar, tibiofibular, carpal, or tarsal) are discussed in the relevant chapters. They rarely cause significant disability, except tarsal synostosis (which may be associated with spastic flat foot) or radioulnar fusion, which limits forearm supination (a considerable disability, if both forearms are affected). In spastic flat foot, division or removal of the bony bridge, may improve symptoms. Radioulnar fusion resists any form of operative mobilization because of the associated soft tissue involvement. However, the bones can be osteotomized and rotated to leave the hand in a more functional position.

Digital Anomalies

There are numerous digital anomalies, e.g. missing digits, extra digits, or split deformities of the hand or foot, which may occur in isolation, in combination with each other or as part of a generalized dysplasia. Short digits seldom require any form of treatment. Extra digits, if simply hanging by a neck of skin, can be amputated at any time. The more complex anomalies, which involve not only bone, but also the associated muscles and neurovascular structures, may be treated by operative reconstruction, when the child is 3–4 years old, but only after painstaking assessment and by someone experienced in this branch of surgery.

MUCOPOLYSACCHARIDOSES

Introduction

The polysaccharide glycosaminoglycans (GAGs) form the side chains of macromolecular proteoglycans, a major component of the matrix in bone, cartilage, intervertebral disks, synovium, and other connective tissues. Defunct proteoglycans are degraded by lysosomal enzymes. Deficiency of any of these enzymes causes a hold up on the degradative pathways. Partially degraded GAGs, accumulate in the lysosomes in the liver, spleen, bones, and other tissues and spill over in the blood and urine, where they can be detected by suitable biochemical tests. Confirmation of the enzyme lack can be obtained by tests on cultured fibroblasts or leukocytes.

Clinical Features

Depending on the specific enzyme deficiency and the type of GAG storage, a number of different clinical syndromes have been defined. All except, Hunter's syndrome (an X-linked recessive disorder), are transmitted as autosomal recessive. As a group they have certain recognizable features, such as excessively short stature with vertebral deformity, coarse facies, hepatosplenomegaly and (in some cases) mental retardation. X-rays show bone dysplasia, affecting the vertebral bodies, epiphyses, and metaphyses. Typically, the bones have a spatulate appearance.

There is superficial similarity to spondyloepiphyseal dysplasia (SED) and spondylometaphyseal dysplasia. However, careful observation reveals several points of difference and the diagnosis can be confirmed, by testing for abnormal GAG excretion or demonstrating the enzyme deficiency in blood cells or cultured fibroblasts.

At least ten different disorders are recognized, here only the three important conditions will be described.

Hurler's Syndrome (MPS 1)

Infants look normal at birth, but over the next 2–3 years they gradually develop a typical appearance. They are undersized, with increasing kyphosis, hepatosplenomegaly, coarse facies, protruding tongue, defective hearing, and mental retardation. Speech is very poor, joints are stiff, and walking is delayed. There may be corneal opacities, respiratory difficulty, and cardiac anomalies. X-rays usually show unmistakable features, such as hypoplastic epiphyses and vertebral bodies, poorly modeled metaphyses, short but wide metacarpals, underdeveloped mandible, spatulate ribs and clavicles, flared iliac blades, shallow acetabuli, and coxa valga. Cardiac or respiratory complications usually cause death in later childhood.

Hunter's Syndrome (MPS II)

This is also a recessive disorder, but X-linked, so all patients are male. Clinical features are similar to those of Hurler's syndrome, but are less severe. Suspicious features usually appear at about 3 years, cardiorespiratory complications gradually become more severe and death usually occurs in middle or late teens.

Morquio-Brailsford Syndrome (MPS IV)

Development seems normal for the first year or two, although walking may be delayed. Thereafter, the child begins to look dwarf, with a moderate kyphosis, short neck, and protuberant sternum. There is marked joint laxity and progressive genu valgum. Suitable tests will reveal a conductive hearing loss. However, the face is unaffected and intelligence is normal. X-rays of the spine, show the typical ovoid, hypoplastic vertebral bodies, which end up abnormally flat (platyspondyly) and peculiarly pointed, anteriorly. Odontoid hypoplasia is usual. A marked manubriosternal angle (almost 90°) is pathognomonic. By the age of 5 years, the femoral head epiphyses are underdeveloped and flat, along with abnormally shallow acetabula. The long bones are of normal width, but the metacarpals may be short and broad, having pointed proximal ends.

Management

- There is yet no specific treatment for the mucopolysaccharide disorder. However, enzyme replacement and gene manipulation are possible in the future.
- Hurler's syndrome has very poor prognosis, but the complications (e.g. respiratory infection) may need treatment.
- Morquio's syndrome presents several orthopedic problems. Genu valgum may need correction, by femoral osteotomy, though this should be delayed till growth has ceased. Coxa valga and subluxation of the hips, if symmetrical, may need femoral or acetabular osteotomy. Atlantoaxial instability may threaten the cord and require occipitocervical fusion. All the spondylodysplasias carry a risk of atlantoaxial subluxation, during anesthesia. Intubation and special precautions are needed during operation.

OSTEOGENESIS IMPERFECTA

Introduction

Also termed as, fragilitas ossium, idiopathic osteopsathyrosis or periosteal dysplasia. It is a hereditary condition and is characterized by:

- Fragility of bones, with tendency to fractures and bowing
- Deafness
- Blueness of sclerae
- Laxity of joints
- Tendency to improve with age.

Etiology

- The pattern of inheritance is autosomal dominant in postnatal cases and autosomal recessive in prenatal cases.
- Each and every child of an affected parent has a 50% chance of inheriting the faulty gene and of having osteogenesis imperfecta.
- However, this can also be a result of spontaneous genetic mutation.

Pathogenesis and Pathology

- Primary defect is the failure of osteoblasts formation.
- Very few osteoblasts appear and osteoid formation is minimal.
- Some of calcified cartilage may undergo direct metaplasia to bone.

Features of Bones

Features of bones are shown in Figure 1. These are described as follows:

- Periosteum is thick, but cambium layer is thin.
- Bone is short and thin.
- Epiphysis is bulbous.
- Cortex is thin and medullary contents are fatty and fibrous.
- Deformity results from fractures and bending.
- Callus formation is abundant, except in severe cases.

Classification

The types of osteogenesis imperfecta are given in Table 1.

Sillence and Danks Classification

Sillence and Danks classification is depicted in Table 2.

Shapiro's Classification

Shapiro's classification is depicted in Table 3.

Falvo's Classification of Osteogenesis Imperfecta

Type 1: Osteogenesis Imperfecta Tarda

- Presence of bowing of long bones (Fig. 1).

Type 2: Osteogenesis Imperfecta Tarda

- No bowing of long bones
- Fractures may be present in both types, but less in type 2.

TABLE 1: Types of osteogenesis imperfecta.

Fetal/prenatal/ congenital form (Osteogenesis imperfecta gravis)	• Multiple fractures present at birth • In severe forms, infant may be stillborn or die in first few weeks • Skull feels like membranous bag of bones
Infantile form	• Less severe • Skull is thin and globular-like hydrocephalic • Multiple fractures + • If child survives first few years, prognosis is good • Child is normal at birth
Adolescent form (Osteogenesis imperfecta tarda)	• Fractures due to trivial trauma in childhood • Later, tendency to fracture is lost • Prognosis is good

TABLE 2: Sillence and Danks classification of osteogenesis imperfecta.

Type	*Inference*	*Description*
1 A	Autosomal dominant	Without dentinogenesis imperfecta; blue sclerae
1 B	Autosomal dominant	With dentinogenesis imperfecta; blue sclerae
2 (Osteogenesis imperfecta gravis)	Autosomal recessive	Lethal type; blue sclerae and blue line on gums severe crumpled bones; marked absence of ossification; perinatal death
3	Autosomal recessive	Severe bone fragility; multiple fractures; severe growth retardation, sclerae change from blue to white with age
4 A	Autosomal dominant	Without dentinogenesis imperfecta; variable severity to fractures and deformity more severe than type 1
4 B	Autosomal dominant	With dentinogenesis imperfecta; variable severity of fractures and deformity more severe than type 1

TABLE 3: Shapiro's classification.

Type	Description	Deaths
Osteogenesis imperfecta congenita A	*In utero*/birth fractures, short, broad, crumpled femora and ribs	94%
Osteogenesis imperfecta congenita B	*In utero*/birth fractures, normal long bone contours, no chest deformity	8%
Osteogenesis imperfecta tarda A	Fractures after birth, but before walking	0%
Osteogenesis imperfecta tarda B	Fractures after walking	0%

TABLE 4: Normal value of inorganic pyrophosphate.

0–14 weeks	6 μg/dL
15–24 weeks	18 μg/dL
25 weeks to term	13 μg/dL

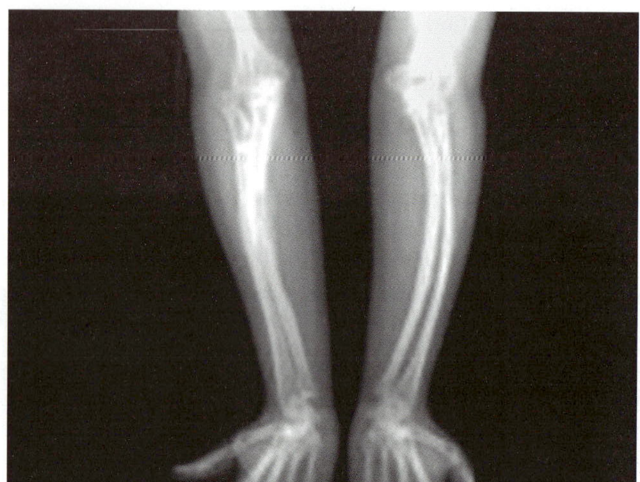

Fig. 1: X-ray, showing features of bones.

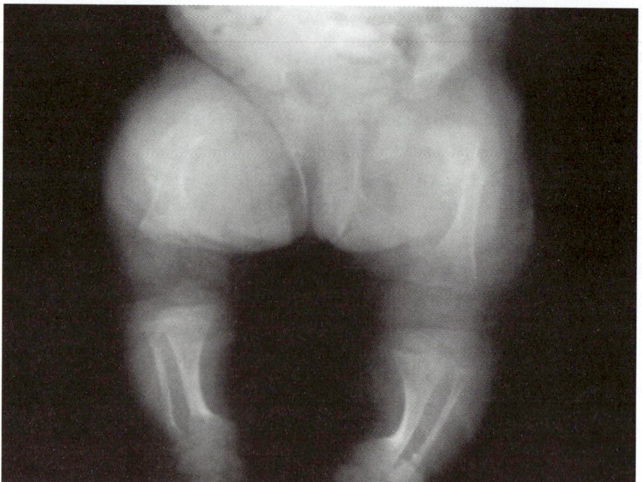

Fig. 2: X-ray, showing generalized osteoporosis in osteogenesis imperfecta.

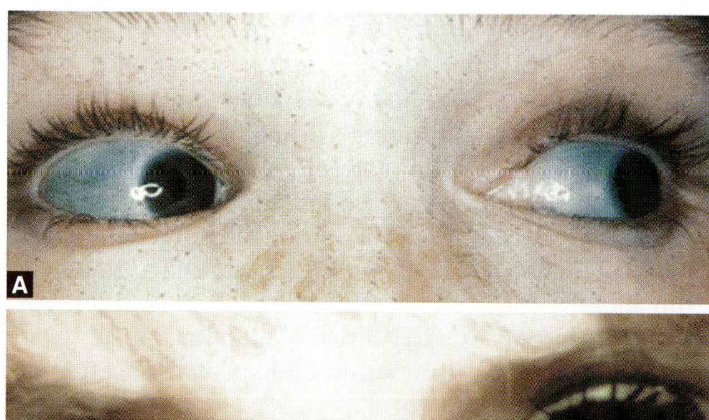

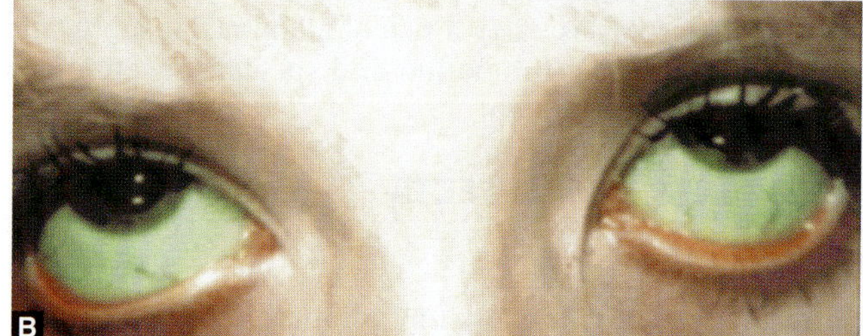

Figs. 3A and B: Deep indigo color of sclerae or blue sclerae, is one of the clinical features, associated with osteogenesis imperfecta.

Clinical Features

- Condition may vary from mild to severe.
- Onset occurs from any time before birth, to late adolescence and rarely in adults.
- Patients present, with blue sclera and blue line on gums, dentinogenesis imperfecta, and generalized osteoporosis (Fig. 2).
- Osteoporosis gives rise to bowing of bones and multiple spontaneous fractures seen in severe cases.
  Characteristic features include:
  - Healing occurs readily, with deformity.
  - Abundant callus formation is seen.
  - Tendency to fractures, lessens with age.
- *Deafness:* Hearing decreased in 80% patients by third decade of life. Can be caused by otosclerosis
- *Laxity of joints:* Increased tendency to strains and dislocations.
- Blue sclerae (Figs. 3A and B) is present in 92% cases. A fairly deep indigo color is seen.
- Dentinogenesis imperfecta, with characteristic blue line along the gums, more pronounced on the lower gums (Fig. 4).
- Feeble musculature.
- *Dwarfing:* Due to deformities of lower limbs and spine.

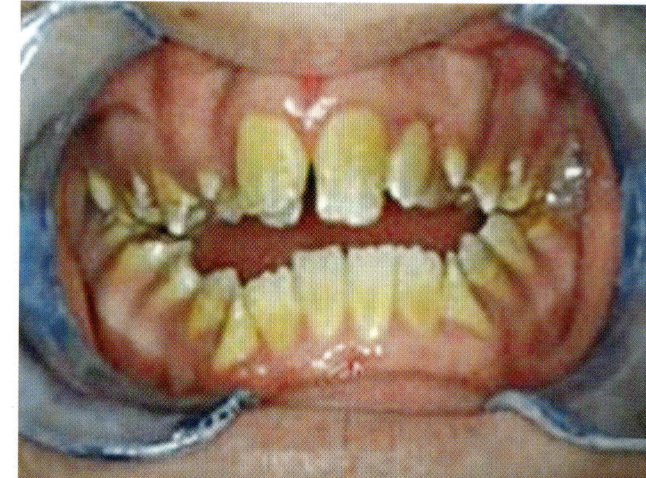

Fig. 4: Dentinogenesis imperfecta with blue line on gums.

- *Broad skull:* Parietal and occipital bones are prominent and is called "Crâne-à-rebord."
- *Poorly calcified deciduous teeth:* Permanent teeth are normal.

- Normal blood chemistry.
- X-ray findings
  - Skeleton is osteoporotic
  - Long bones appear thin and elongated, with thinned cortices and bulbous epiphyses (Fig. 5).
  - Thinning of the outer cortex of the skull as seen in the X-ray skull lateral view (Fig. 6), a characteristic picture seen in osteogenesis imperfecta.
- The normal values of inorganic pyrophosphate are given in Table 4.

Treatment

- Protection of child, until tendency for fractures decreases.
- Adequate vitamin intake for deposition.
- Guard against overdosage of vitamin D, which leads to decalcification.
- Administration of estrogen and androgens, may be helpful.
- Severe deformities of long bones may be corrected, by multiple osteotomies through the metaphyses as well as through shaft of the bone and threading the fragments on an intramedullary rod.
- *Bailey and Buboy's method (Fig. 7):* Telescoping medullary rod is used, which elongates as growth occurs.
- *William's method:* Retrograde nailing is done, by fixing an extension to distal end of rod and driving the nail through the heel.

ACHONDROPLASIA

Introduction

This is the most common form of abnormally short stature. Adult height is usually around 122 cm (48 inches). Severe, disproportionate shortening of the limb bones is diagnosed by X-ray before birth.

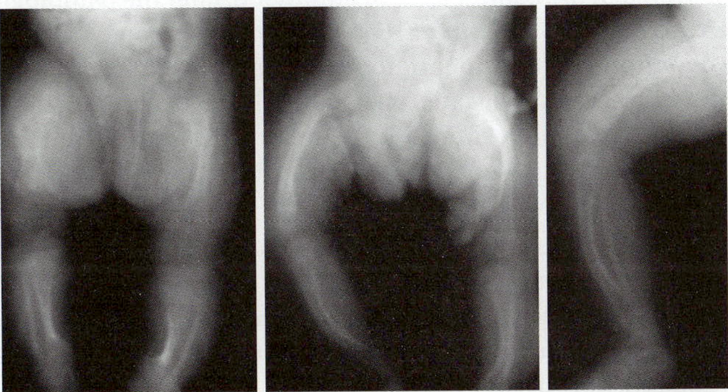

Fig. 5: X-ray findings, in patients with osteogenesis imperfecta.

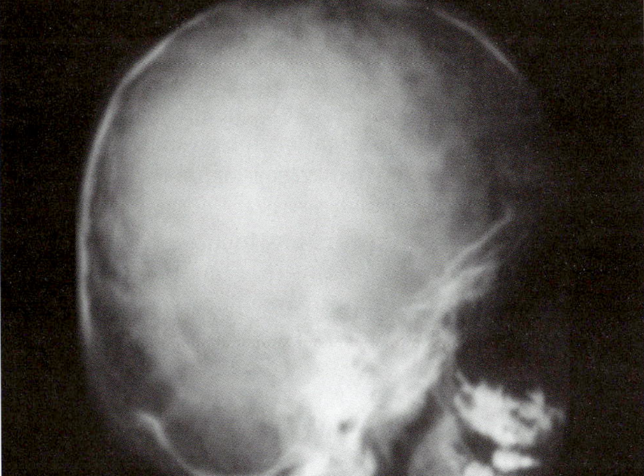

Fig. 6: X-ray, showing thin skull.

Pathology

This is an abnormality of endochondral longitudinal growth. The physes show diminished and less regular cell proliferation, which accounts for the bone formation, is unaffected hence the normal growth of the skull vault and the periosteal contribution to bone width.

Clinical Features

The abnormality is obvious in the childhood, as growth is severely stunted, the limbs (particularly the proximal segments) are disproportionately short and the skull is quite large, with prominent forehead and saddle shaped nose. The finger appears stubby and somewhat splayed (trident hands). Joint laxity is common. Many infants have a thoracolumbar kyphosis, but this almost always disappears in a year or two. Mental development is normal.

By early childhood, the trunk is obviously disproportionately long in comparison to the limbs. The standing posture is typical, i.e. the back is excessively lordotic, the buttocks are prominent, the hip flexed, the legs bowed and elbows are bent.

During adulthood, shortening of the vertebral pedicles may lead to lumbar spinal stenosis and disk prolapse, which is quite common and has exceptionally severe effects. Cervical spine stenosis, may cause typical features of cord compression.

X-ray

The tubular bones are short, the metaphyses wide, and the physeal lines somewhat irregular; however, the epiphyses are usually normal. Although the proximal limb bones are disproportionately affected (rhizomelia), changes are also seen in wrists and hands, where the metaphyses are broad and cup-shaped. The pelvic cavity is small (too small for a normal delivery) and the iliac wings are flared, producing an almost horizontal acetabular roof. The skull vault is large, but the base is rather short and the forearms magnum smaller than usual. The pelvic cavity is small (too small for normal delivery) and the iliac wings are flared, producing an almost horizontal acetabular roof. The skull vault is large, but the spinal cord is reduced in size. These features are clearly defined on computed tomography (CT) or magnetic resonance imaging (MRI).

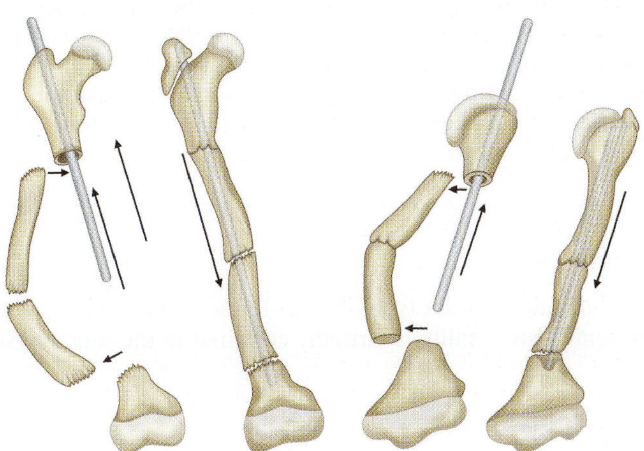

Fig. 7: Bailey and Buboy's method.

Diagnosis

Achondroplasia should not be confused with any other types of short limbed dwarfism. In some (e.g. Morquio's disease) the shortening affects distal segments more than proximal and there may be widespread associated abnormalities. Others (e.g. pseudoachondroplasia and the epiphyseal dysplasias) are distinguished by the fact that the head and face are quite normal, whereas the epiphyses show characteristic changes on X-ray examination.

Genetics

Achondroplasia occurs, in about one in 25,000 births. There is autosomal dominant inheritance, however because few achondroplastic people have children, over 80% cases are sporadic. The fault has been shown to be point mutation in the gene coding for fibroblasts growth factor receptor three, which apparently plays a role in endochondral cartilage growth.

During childhood, operative treatment may be needed for lower limb deformities (usually genu varum). Occasionally, the thoracolumbar kyphosis fails to correct itself. If there is significant deformity (angulation of more than 40°), by the age of 5 years, there is a risk of cord compression and operative correction, may be needed.

During adulthood, spinal stenosis may require decompression. Intervertebral disk prolapse, superimposed on a narrow spinal canal, should be treated as an emergency.

Advances in the method of external fixation have made leg lengthening a feasible option. This is best achieved by chondrodiatasis of the physis or callotis of the shaft. However, there are drawbacks, like complications, including nonunion, infection and nerve palsy, which may be disastrous and the cosmetic effect of long legs and short arms, may be less pleasing than anticipated. It is essential that the details of the operation, its aims, limitations, and the patient (and where appropriate with the parents) should be carefully discussed and prioritized, as anesthesia carries a greater than usual risk and requires expert supervision.

HYPOCHONDROPLASIA

This has been described as a very mild form of achondroplasia. However, apart from shortness of stature (with the emphasis on proximal limb segments) and noticeable lumbar lordosis, there is little to suggest any abnormality, the head and face are not affected and many of those with hypochondroplasia pass for normal stocky individuals. X-rays may show slight pelvic flattening and thickening of long bones. The condition is transmitted as autosomal dominant. Those affected, sometimes ask for limb lengthening and after careful discussion, this may be done, with a considerable chance of success.

METAPHYSEAL CHONDRODYSPLASIA (DYSOSTOSIS)

Introduction

This term describes a type of short-limbed dwarfism, in which the bony abnormality is virtually confined to the metaphyses. The epiphyses are unaffected, but the metaphyseal segments adjacent to the growth plates are broadened and mildly scalloped, somewhat resembling rickets. There may be bilateral coxa vara and bowed legs, as patients tend to walk with a waddling gait. Apart from the lordotic posture, the spine is normal. The main deformities are around the hips and knees.

There are several forms of metaphyseal chondrodysplasia. The best known Schmid type has the classic features described above, with autosomal dominant inheritance. Another group (McKusick type) is associated with sparse hair growth and is sometimes complicated by Hirschsprung's disease. Inheritance shows an autosomal recessive pattern. It is thought that these cases may represent an entirely distinct entity. The rarest (and most severe) of all, Jansen type is usually sporadic and may be associated with deafness.

Operative correction (osteotomy) may be needed for coxa vara or tibia vara.

OSTEOPETROSIS (MARBLE BONES, ALBERS-SCHONBERG DISEASE)

Osteopetrosis is one of several conditions, which are characterized by thickening and increased radiographic density of the bone, differences in the pattern of inheritance, the age of presentation and the distribution of the clinical and X-ray changes, shows that they are genetically distinct conditions.

Osteopetrosis Tarda

The common form of osteopetrosis is a fairly benign, autosomal dominant disorder that seldom causes symptoms and may only be discovered in the adolescence or adulthood, after the pathological fracture or when an X-ray is taken for other reasons, hence the designation tarda. Appearance and function are unimpaired, unless there are complications, like pathological fracture or cranial nerve compression, due to bone encroachment or foramina. Sufferers are also prone to bone infections, particularly of the mandible, after tooth extraction.

X-rays show increased density of all the bones, such as cortices are widened, leaving narrow medullary canals, sclerotic vertebral end plates produce a striped appearance (Rugger Jersey spine), the skull is thickened, and the base density is sclerotic. Treatment is required, only if complications occur.

Osteopetrosis Congenita

This rare, autosomal recessive form of osteopetrosis, present at birth and causes severe disability. Bone encroachment on marrow results in pancytopenia, hemolysis, anemia, and hepatosplenomegaly. Foraminal occlusion may cause optic or facial nerve palsy. Repeated hemorrhage or infection, usually leads to the death in early childhood.

Treatment, in recent years has focused on the methods of enhancing bone resorption. This has been achieved by transplanting marrow from normal donors, suggesting that the condition is due to lack of marrow cells that control osteoclastic activity.

CHAPTER

Genetic Disorders 4

OBJECTIVES

- Introduction to Genetics
- Patterns of Inheritance
- Gene Mapping and Genetic Markers
- Prenatal Diagnosis
- Childhood Diagnosis
- Management of Genetic Disorders
- Down's Syndrome (Trisomy-21)
- Marfan's Syndrome
- Turner's Syndrome
- Ehlers–Danlos Syndrome

INTRODUCTION TO GENETICS

History of Genetics

People have known about inheritance for a long time, as evident from the following facts:

- Children resemble their parents
- Domestication of animals and plants, selective breeding for good characteristics
- Sumerian horse breeding records
- Bible and hemophilia.

Old Ideas

Despite knowing about inheritance in general, a number of incorrect ideas had to be generated and overcome before modern genetics could arise. All lives come from other lives. Living organisms are not spontaneously generated from nonliving material. Big exception though is origin of life itself.

Species concept: Offspring arises only when two members of the same species mate. Monstrous hybrids do not exist. Organisms develop by expressing information carried in their hereditary material. As opposed to "preformation", the idea that in each sperm (or egg) is a tiny, fully-formed human that merely grows in size. Male and female parents contribute equally to the offspring. Ancient Greek idea, male plants a "seed" in the female "garden".

Mid-1800s Discoveries

Three major events in the mid 1800s directly led to the development of modern genetics. Some of the major related discoveries are:

1859: Charles Darwin publishes *The Origin of Species, which* describes the theory of evolution by natural selection. This theory requires heredity to work.

1866: Gregor Mendel publishes his experiments in plant hybridization, which lays out the basic theory of genetics. It is widely ignored until 1900.

1871: Friedrich Miescher isolates "nucleic acid" from pus cells.

1900: Rediscovery of Mendel's work by Robert Correns, Hugo de Vries, and Erich von Tschermak.

Major Events in the 20th Century

1902: A Garrod discovers that alkaptonuria, a human disease, has a genetic basis.

1904: G Bateson discovers linkage between genes. He also coins the word "genetics".

1910: Thomas Hunt Morgan proves that genes are located on the chromosomes (using Drosophila).

1944: Oswald Avery, Colin MacLeod, and Maclyn McCarty, show that DNA can transform bacteria, demonstrating that DNA is the hereditary material.

1953: James Watson and Francis Crick determine the structure of the DNA molecule, which leads directly to knowledge of how it replicates.

1966: Marshall Nirenberg solves the genetic code, showing that three DNA bases code for one amino acid.

2001: Sequence of the entire human genome is announced.

"Blending" Theory of Inheritance

Before Mendel's work, the most popular theory of inheritance stated that the qualities of the parents blended to form the qualities of the child. Under this theory, one tall parent and one short parent would produce a child of medium height. Most ordinary observations seemed to support this hypothesis, which rejected the notion of discrete units of inheritance (i.e. genes). However, this theory was poorly equipped to deal with such phenomena, as two brown-eyed parents giving birth to a blue-eyed baby.

Early Genetics

The study of genetics began with observations made by Gregor Mendel. After noticing that the flowers of his pea plants were either violet or white, Mendel began to study the segregation of heritable traits.

Because the principles established by Mendel form the basis for genetics, the science is often referred to as Mendelian genetics. It is also called classical genetics to distinguish it from another branch of biology known as molecular genetics.

Mendel devised two fundamental principles of inheritance:

1. *Mendel's principle of segregation:* The factors of inheritance (genes) normally are paired, but are separated or segregated in the formation of gametes (eggs and sperm).
2. *Mendel's principle of independent assortment:* Each factor's distribution in the gametes is not related to the distribution of any other factor. This principle is not strictly true due to the organization of genes on chromosomes.

Mendel's Observations

- Mendel made numerous important observations in his exhaustive study of pea plants characteristics. He elaborated an important distinction between dominant and recessive traits through his work with pea plants.
- By studying the characteristics of pea plants, such as their height, seed shape, seed color, flower position, and other traits.
- This discussion will use height as a primary example. Mendel first crossbred one tall, true-breeding plant with one short, true-breeding plant. Contrary to the blending theory, all the offspring were tall. In terms of genotype, the original tall plant was "TT" (two dominant alleles; homozygous), the short plant was "tt" (two recessive alleles; homozygous) and the second generation plants were " Tt" (one dominant and one recessive allele; heterozygous).
- When Mendel next time allowed these plants to self-fertilize, he found that the short trait reappeared in the third generation. The ratio of tall to short plants was almost exactly 3:1. Their genotypes were in ratio of 1:2:1 [one short (tt), two tall (Tt) and one tall (TT)].

Limitations of the Mendelian System

The simple system of Mendelian genetics is very powerful and serves to explain the inheritance patterns of numerous traits. However, many traits are controlled by many genes acting in tandem, and thus do not obey strict Mendelian patterns (although their constituent genes may). Furthermore, many human traits are strongly influenced by the environment as well, therefore their phenotypes cannot be said to be Mendelian (though the genetic components may be). In sum, Mendelian patterns are important, but cannot be applied universally. Individual traits must be researched to find out, if they obey typical Mendelian patterns.

What is Gene?

A gene is an information entity. It is a sequence of DNA that codes for a single genetic instruction. Usually, this instruction is the sequence of a protein, but a gene may also serve to activate or deactivate other genes, in a cell or in neighboring cells. Every aspect of our species is constructed based on information encoded in genes. The genes themselves do very little, they are information storage molecules. It is the cytological machinery of our cells, passed from one generation to the next, that translate these instructions into a living organism. The effects of every gene depend both upon other genes and on the environment.

What is an Allele?

An allele is one variant of a gene. Many genes have two, several, or many different variants of the same basic genetic information. Some alleles are minor differences that do not significantly affect the organism, while others cause profound changes.

Example: Nucleotide substitutions in the third codon position often produces no change at all, because they code for the same transfer RNA and thus the same protein is produced:

- In humans CCU, CCA does not cause a change, both triplets code for proline. Other substitutions may produce profound effects.
- Sickle cell anemia is caused by a single nucleotide substitution, GAG to GUG changes normal hemoglobin to hemoglobin, that "sickles" under.
- In humans, a cell's nucleus contains 46 individual chromosomes or 23 pairs of chromosomes. Half of the chromosomes come from one parent and half come from the other parent.
- Chromosomal DNA contains other things besides genes:
  - Centromere (where the mitotic spindle attaches)
  - Telomeres (special structures on the ends of chromosomes)
  - Origins of replication (where copying of DNA starts)
  - Pseudogenes (nonfunctional, mutated copies of genes)
  - Transposable elements AKA transposons (intranuclear parasites)
  - Genes that make small RNAs and not proteins.
- The set of all genes that specify an organism's traits is known as the organism's genome. The genome for a human cell consists of about 100,000 genes. The gene composition of a living organism is its genotype. For a person's earlobe shape, the genotype may consist of two genes for attached earlobes or two genes for free earlobes or one gene for attached and one gene for free earlobes. The physical expression of the genes is referred to as the phenotype of a living thing. If a person has attached earlobes, the phenotype is "attached earlobes." If the person has free earlobes, the phenotype is "free earlobes." Even though three genotypes for earlobe shape are possible only two phenotypes (attached earlobes and free earlobes) are possible.
- As you remember, diploid organisms have two sets of redundant genetic information and two copies of every gene.
  - An individual is homozygous at a locus, if they have two alleles for a gene and heterozygous at that locus, if they have different copies.
- Dominant alleles mask the effect of a recessive allele at that locus they are expressed in the homozygous or the heterozygous state.
- Recessive alleles are only expressed in the homozygous state.
- *Example:* Alleles for albino coloration in many animals result from recessive alleles. Thus, for albino coat color in mice, individuals with either one or two copies A (dominant) allele have brown fur. Therefore, "AA" and "Aa" have brown fur. Note that "Aa" individuals can pass on the allele, even though they do not express it themselves, they are carriers. Individuals with two copies of the albino allele, "aa" have white fur.
- Some alleles of medical interest, when rare, recessive alleles are usually in the heterozygous state and not subject to natural selection, human populations harbor quite a few harmful, recessive alleles at low frequencies.
- For instance, a rare, autosomal recessive allele on chromosome 7 disrupts the normal migration of neurons, leading to an abnormally thick and smooth cerebral cortex and reduced cerebellum, and hippocampus and brainstem causing a condition called lissencephaly. It is typical of these conditions for an affected individual to be born to normal parents.
- Dominant alleles, by contrast are generally manifested in the parents. For instance, ectrodactyly, a condition where the

affected individual has severely deformed digits, is caused by a dominant allele. It runs in families, conspicuously.

- Codominance (sometimes called incomplete dominance) is the allelic interaction, where in the heterozygous state, both alleles are expressed (for attributes) or the heterozygote is in between the phenotypes of the homozygous individuals for those alleles (in the case of measurable characters). Thus, the heterozygote has a unique phenotype. For example, in chickens, black feather color is codominant with white feather color. Heterozygous chickens have black and white feathers in a checkered pattern.
- *Mitosis:* Mitosis, the duplication of the genetic material within a eukaryote cell, is worth mentioning here because of what it *is* and what it *is not*. A cell gives rise to two smaller but genetically identical copies of itself. It is a duplication of the genetic complement of a eukaryote cell. Since it is usually followed by cell division, it can lead to growth, in a multicellular organism, or asexual reproduction, in a single-celled organism. It is not a means of producing gametes. In sexual organisms, mitosis is peripheral to sexual reproduction, it serves to give rise to cell types which ultimately "kill themselves off" by splitting and splitting again into four, very different cells.
- *Meiosis:* Meiosis is that process, by which a single diploid cell gives rise to four genetically different, haploid cells. It works like this (forget the phases):
  - The diploid progenitor duplicates its genetic material, thus every chromosome is composed of two identical chromatids joined at the centromere (this happens before meiosis starts).
  - Each chromosome finds its match, to form "matching pairs" of homologous chromosomes. This process which occurs during the first of the two meiotic divisions is unique to meiosis, it does not occur during mitosis.
  - Four strands (two homologous chromosomes, composed of two identical strands each) cluster in structures sometimes called tetrads, along a plane in the center of the dividing cell. A process called "crossing over" may occur at this time.
  - First division, homologous chromosomes separate.
  - Spindle fibers drag them to opposite poles of the cell. The cell then divides. Where chromosome ends up is completely random and is not influenced by the fate of the other chromosomes around it. The cell then divides.
  - Second division, chromatids separate.
  - Spindle fibers drag them to opposite poles of the cell. The cell then divides. This gives you four, genetically different, daughter cells from a single parent.
- *Errors in meiosis:* Errors in meiosis have the potential to produce unusual phenotypes in the offspring.
- The most common meiotic error is nondisjunction, where an entire homologous pair of chromosomes migrates to the pole of a cell, without splitting.
- If this happens to a single pair, it causes either a trisomy or a monosomy in the resulting offspring.
- If it happens to the entire genome, it can produce triploid or even tetraploid offspring.
- The human condition of Down's syndrome results from a trisomy at chromosome 23, a trisomy at chromosome 18, 13, or the sex chromosomes, is also survivable. In humans, trisomies for other chromosomes are not usually viable.
- In other organisms, triploids and tetraploids may be viable.

PATTERNS OF INHERITANCE

What is Inheritance?

Inheritance is the transfer of characteristics from parents to their offspring, e.g. hair, eye, and skin color.

What is Inheritance Patterns?

Inheritance patterns trace the transmission of genetically encoded traits, conditions, or diseases to offspring.

Modes of Inheritance

- Single gene or Mendelian
- Multifactorial
- Mitochondrial.

Single Gene or Mendelian Inheritance

- Genetic conditions caused by a mutation in a single gene follow predictable patterns of inheritance within families.
- Single gene inheritance is also referred to as Mendelian inheritance, as they follow transmission patterns that he observed in his research on peas.
- There are four types of Mendelian inheritance pattern:
  - Autosomal dominant
  - Autosomal recessive
  - X-linked dominant
  - X-linked recessive
- *Autosomal:* The gene responsible for the phenotype is located on one of the 22 pairs of autosomes (nonsex determining chromosomes).
- *X-linked:* The gene that encodes for the trait is located on the X chromosome.
- *Dominant:* Conditions that are manifest in heterozygotes (individuals with just one copy of the mutant allele).
- *Recessive:* Conditions are only manifest in individuals who have two copies of the mutant allele (are homozygous).

Autosomal Dominant

- Dominant conditions are expressed in individuals, who have just one copy of the mutant allele.
- Affected males and females have an equal probability of passing on the trait to offspring.
- Affected individuals have one normal copy of the gene and one mutant copy of the gene, thus each offspring has a 50% chance on inheriting the mutant allele.
- As shown in this pedigree (Fig. 1), approximately half of the children of affected parents inherit the condition and half do not.
- *Autosomal dominant diseases:* The most common diseases are:
  - Achondroplasia
  - Marfan's syndrome
  - Brachydactyly
  - Ehlers-Danlos syndrome
  - Osteogenesis imperfecta
  - Neurofibromatosis.

Autosomal Recessive

- Recessive conditions are clinically manifest only when an individual has two copies of the mutant allele.
- When just one copy of the mutant allele is present, an individual is a carrier of the mutation, but does not develop the condition.

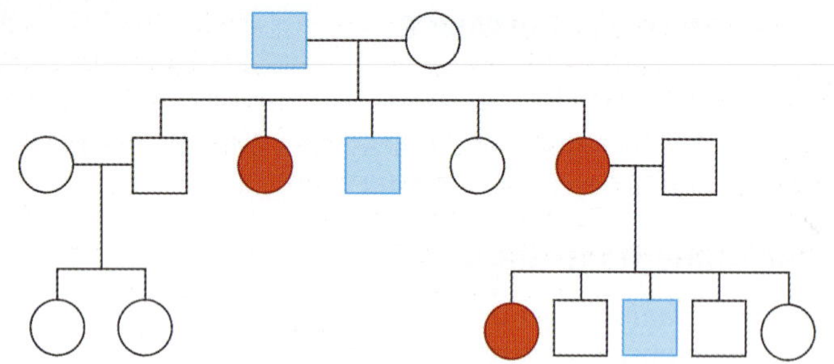

Fig. 1: Pedigree chart showing the transfer of the mutant genes to offsprings.

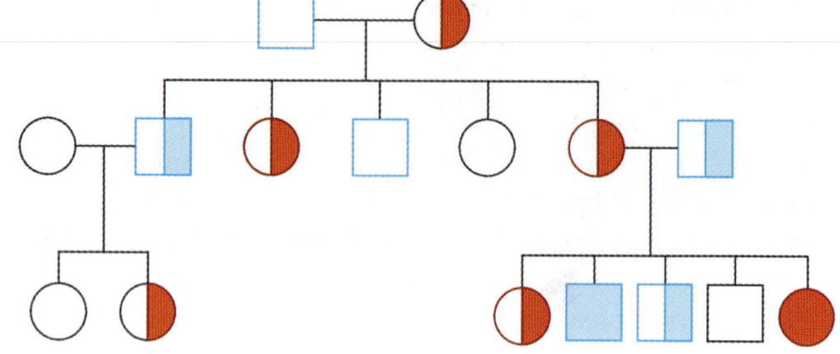

Fig. 2: Pedigree chart showing each child has a 25% chance of being homozygous wild-type (unaffected); a 25% chance of being homozygous mutant (affected); a 50% chance of being heterozygous (unaffected carrier).

- Females and males are affected equally by traits transmitted by autosomal recessive inheritance.
- When two carriers mate, each child has a 25% chance of being homozygous wild-type (unaffected), a 25% chance of being homozygous mutant (affected) or a 50% chance of being heterozygous (unaffected carrier) (Fig. 2).
- *Autosomal recessive diseases:* Most common diseases are:
  - Chondrodystrophia calcificans
  - Hurler's syndrome
  - Tay-Sachs disease
  - Phenylketonuria
  - Cystic fibrosis.

X-linked Recessive

- X-linked recessive traits are not clinically manifest, when there is a normal copy of the gene.
- All X-linked recessive traits are fully evident in males because they only have one copy of the X chromosome, thus do not have a normal copy of the gene to compensate for the mutant copy.
- For that same reason, women are rarely affected by X-linked recessive diseases, however they are affected, when they have two copies of the mutant allele.
- As the gene is on the X chromosome, there is no father to son transmission, but there is father to daughter and mother to daughter and son transmission. If a man is affected with an X-linked recessive condition, all his daughters will inherit one copy of the mutant allele from him.
- *X-linked recessive diseases (Fig. 3):* Some of these diseases are:
  - Duchenne dystrophy
  - Fragile X syndrome
  - Hemophilia A.

X-linked Dominant

- As the gene is located on the X chromosome, there is no transmission from father to son, but there can be transmission from father to daughter.
- All daughters of an affected male will be affected, since the father has only one X chromosome to transmit.
- Children of an affected woman have a 50% chance of inheriting the X chromosome with the mutant allele.
- X-linked dominant disorders are clinically manifest when only one copy of the mutant allele is present.
- *X-linked dominant diseases (Fig. 4):* Most common diseases are:
  - Chondrodysplasia punctata
  - Hypophosphatemic rickets
  - Vitamin D resistant rickets
  - Morquio's osteochondrodystrophy.

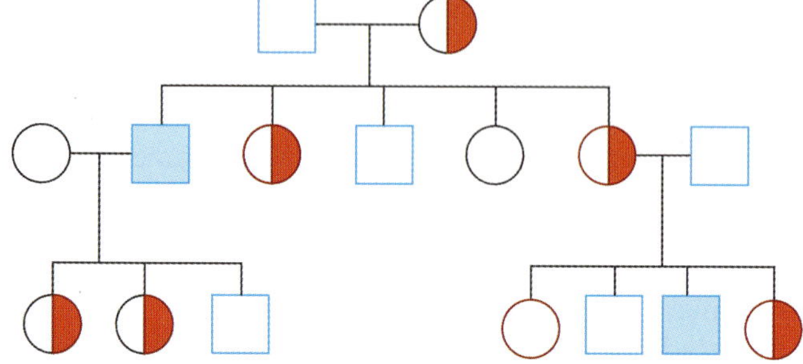

Fig. 3: Pedigree chart for X-linked recessive gene transmission.

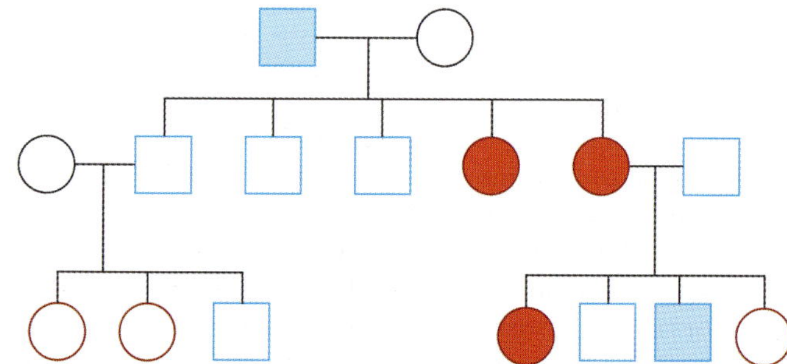

Fig. 4: Pedigree chart for X-linked dominant transmission of genes.

Multifactorial Inheritance

- Most diseases have multifactorial inheritance patterns. As the name implies, multifactorial conditions are not caused by a single gene, but rather are a result of interplay between genetic factors and environmental factors.
- Diseases with multifactorial inheritance are not genetically determined, but rather a genetic mutation may predispose an individual to a disease.
- Other genetic and environmental factors contribute to whether or not the disease develops.
- Numerous genetic alterations may predispose individuals to the same disease (genetic heterogeneity). For instance, coronary heart disease risk factors include high blood pressure, diabetes, and hyperlipidemia. All of those risk factors have their own genetic and environmental components.
- Thus, multifactorial inheritance is far more complex than Mendelian inheritance and is more difficult to trace through pedigrees.
- *Multifactorial inheritance diseases:* Most common examples are:
  - Cleft lip or palate
  - Club foot
  - Congenital dislocation of hip
  - Congenital heart disease

- Coronary artery disease
- Hypertension
- Diabetes mellitus
- Schizophrenia.

Mitochondrial Inheritance

- Mitochondria are organelles found in the cytoplasm of cells.
- Mitochondria are unique in that they have multiple copies of a circular chromosome.
- Mitochondria are only inherited from the ovum, thus only females can transmit the trait to offspring, however, they pass it onto all of their offspring.
- The primary function of mitochondria is conversion of molecule into usable energy.
- Thus, many diseases transmitted by mitochondrial inheritance affect organs with high-energy use, such as the heart, skeletal muscle, liver, and kidneys.
- *Mitochondrial inheritance disease:* Maternally inherited diabetes and deafness (MIDD) is a disorder with this type of inheritance pattern.

GENE MAPPING AND GENETIC MARKERS

Gene Mapping

Gene mapping is an intensively developing area of modern genetics that is highly relevant to studies of the organization of the human genomes. Its narrow scope is building of genetic maps, providing a basis for medical and human genetics. Its broader scope is to open up new possibilities to a better understanding of the anatomy of the genome and its organization principles.

Comparative gene mapping has offered new prospects for the research of the patterns, produced by evolving linkage groups, chromosomes, and single gene associations that brought closer to examination of a fundamental biological problem that "Do genes combine randomly or not into linkage groups?" and for the research of, may be the role of natural selection in their combination.

Genetic mapping, also called linkage mapping, can offer firm evidence that a disease transmitted from parent to child is linked to one or more genes. It also provides clues about which chromosome contains the gene and precisely where it lies on that chromosome. Genetic maps have been used successfully to find the single gene responsible for relatively rare inherited disorders, like cystic fibrosis and muscular dystrophy. Maps have also become useful in guiding scientists to the many genes that are believed to interact to bring about more common disorders, such as asthma, heart disease, diabetes, cancer, and psychiatric conditions.

Genetic distance, which is expressed in centimorgans, is a measure of the likelihood of crossover between two loci. Two loci are 1 cm apart, if there is a 1% probability of crossover during meiosis in males and perhaps twice as many during meiosis in females. Feasibility of human linkage analysis was revolutionized by demonstration of genetic variation in the size of fragments generated, by digestion of normal human DNA with restriction endonuclease. Restriction fragment length polymorphisms (RFLPs) are the consequences of DNA sequence polymorphisms and inherited according to Mendelian principles.

Restriction enzyme digestion and southern blotting, makes it possible to utilize these polymorphisms as genetic markers for sites within genomes. If one of the base pairs in the recognition sequence for restriction enzyme differs between individual copies of the genome or if there is a length variation in DNA, then there will be variation in the size of DNA fragments generated by restriction enzyme digestion. Genetic linkage can be assesed between any group of markers, one of which genes may represent a mutation that causes a diseases of phenotype.

For autosomal gene, each individual inherits one copy of each chromosome from each parent. Based on the following methods:

- Chromosomal and regional assignments of genes were made.
- Genes were ordered on physical and genetic maps (Fig. 5).

Restriction Fragment Length

Polymorphisms Process

- Blood sample extracted.
- It is digested by restriction enzyme and separated by gel electrophoresis.
- Double stranded DNA is denatured and is converted to single stranded.
- Then blotted on solid membrane (southern transfer) and hybridized with radio probe.
- On X-ray exposure specific DNA fragment can be seen (Fig. 6).

Variable number of tandem repeat (VNTR) polymorphisms (Fig. 7).

- Restriction enzymes cleave DNA on two different chromosomes, on either sides of the tandem repeat sequence.
- Radioactive probes hybridized to the DNA.
- They undergo complementary base pairing.
- Autoradiography reveals fragments of different length.
- DNA is applied to gel.
- Electrophoresis is done.
- DNA is blotted with the help of salt solution by capillary action.
- DNA is transferred to filter.
- It is then hybridized with unique nucleic acid probe.
- Then unbound probe is removed.
- Exposure to X-ray produces the desired auto-radiogram.

See Western blot method for proteins (Fig. 8).
See Northern blot method for RNA (Fig. 9).
See Southern blot method for DNA (Fig. 10).

Approaches Used to Build Genetic Maps

- Interspecific cell hybridization
- Radiation hybridization
- In situ hybridization

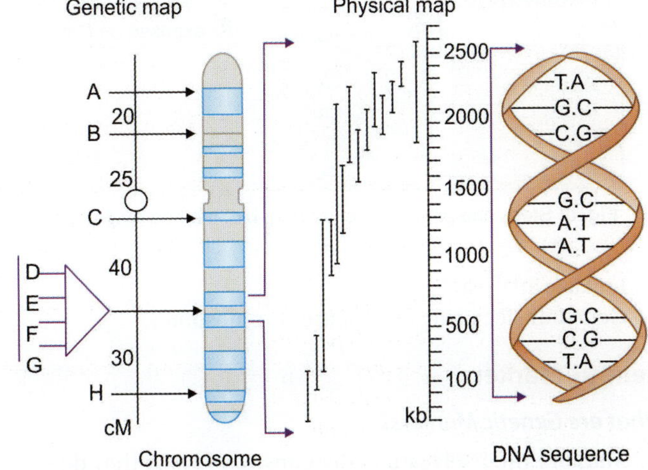

Fig. 5: Genes order, as shown on genetic and physical maps.

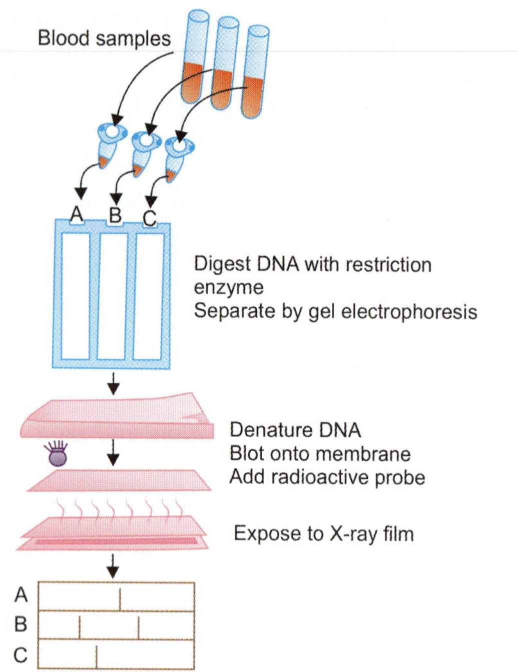

Fig. 6: Steps of RFLP process.

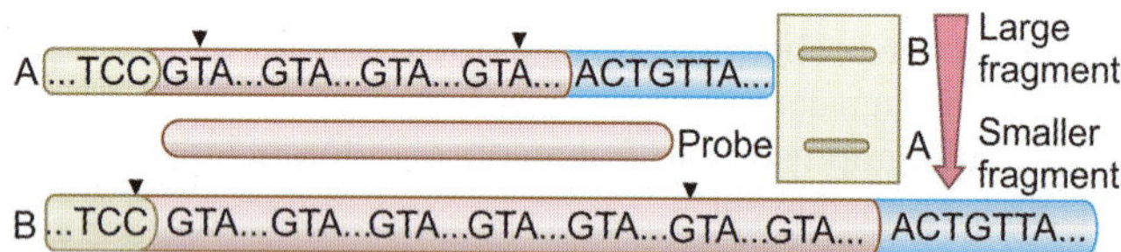

Fig. 7: VNTR polymorphisms: Restriction enzyme cleave DNA on two different chromosomes—(A) Smaller chromosomal segment; (B) Larger segment.

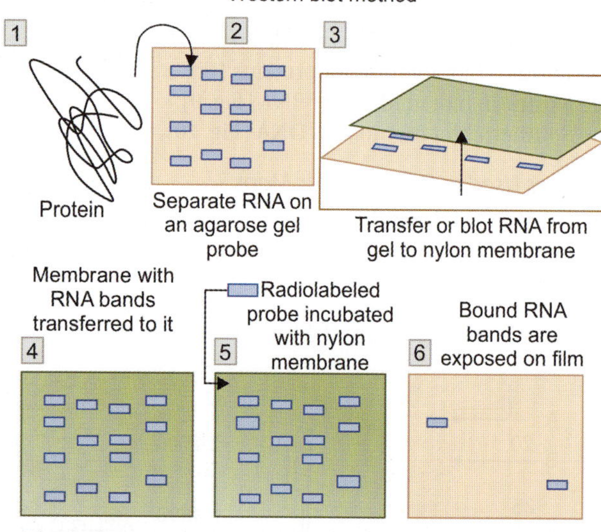

Fig. 8: Steps and procedure of western blot method for proteins.

- Linkage analysis
- Gene transfer, using metaphase chromosomes.

Genetic Markers

What are Genetic Markers?

- Markers themselves usually consist of DNA that does not contain a gene.

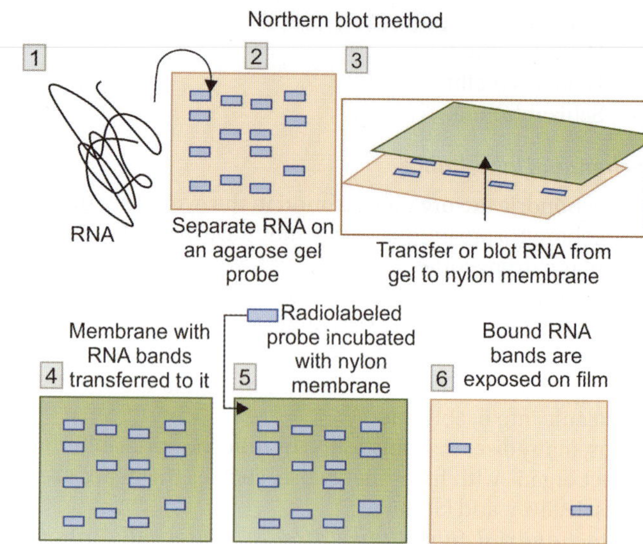

Fig. 9: Steps and procedure of northern blot method for RNA.

- They can tell a researcher the identity of the person a DNA sample came from. This makes markers extremely valuable for tracking inheritance of traits through generations of a family and markers have also proven useful in criminal investigations and other forensic applications.
- Although, there are several different types of genetic markers, the type most used on genetic maps today is known as a "microsatellite map".
- However, maps of even higher resolution are being constructed using single-nucleotide polymorphisms or SNPs (pronounced "snips").
- Both types of markers are easy to use with automated laboratory equipment; so researchers can rapidly map a disease or trait in a large number of family members.
- Development of high-resolution, easy-to-use genetic maps, with the Human Genome Project (HGP) successful sequencing and mapping human genome has revolutionized genetic research.
- The improved quality of genetic data has reduced the time required to identify a gene from a period of years to, in many cases, a matter of months or even weeks.

How Do Researchers Create a Genetic Map?

- Researchers collect blood or tissue samples from family members, where a certain disease or trait is prevalent.
- Using various laboratory techniques, the scientists isolate DNA from these samples.
- Then it is examined for unique patterns of bases, seen only in family members who have the disease or trait.
- These characteristic molecular patterns are referred to as polymorphisms or markers.
- Before researchers identify gene responsible for disease or trait, DNA markers can tell them roughly where the gene is on chromosome.
- This is possible because of a genetic process known as recombination.
- As eggs or sperm develop within a person's body, the 23 pairs of chromosomes within those cells exchange or recombine genetic material.

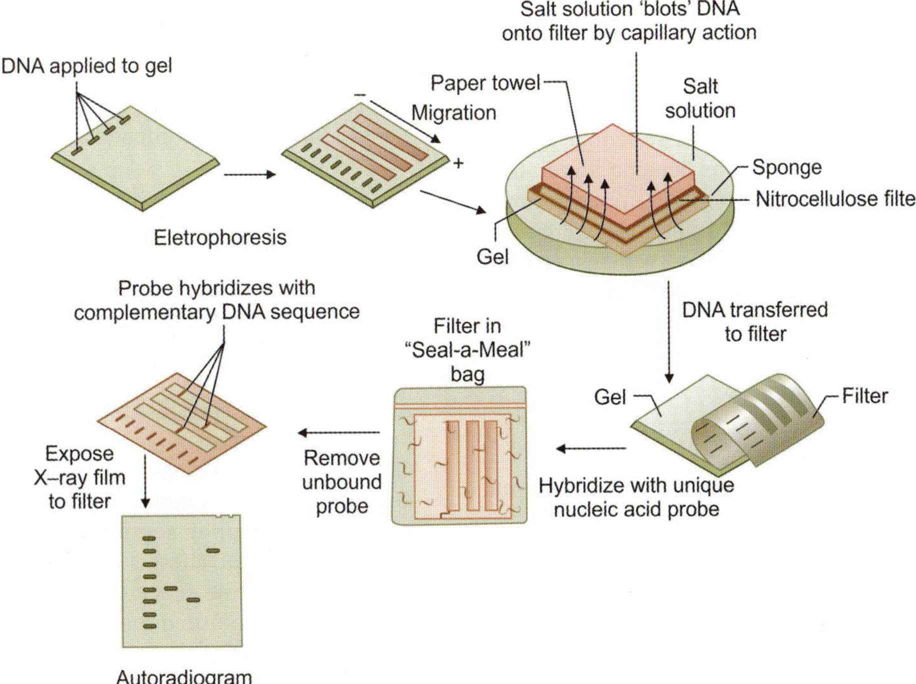

Fig. 10: Steps and procedure of southern blot method for DNA.

- If a particular gene is close to DNA marker, the gene and marker will likely to stay together during the recombination process and passed on together from parent to child.
- If each family member with a particular disease or trait also inherits a particular DNA marker, chances are high that gene responsible for the disease lies near that marker.
- The more DNA markers on a genetic map, the more likely that one will be closely linked to a disease gene and the easier it will be for researchers to zero-in on that gene.
- One of the first major achievements was to develop dense maps of markers spaced evenly across the entire collection of human DNA.

Clinical Relevance (Table 1)

TABLE 1: Genetic diseases, type of chromosomal aberration and the genes or chromosomes involved.

Diseases	*Aberration*	*Chromosome*
Ewing's sarcoma	Translocation	11q24 and 22q12
Germ cell tumor	Isochromosome	12p
Sarcoma, synovial	Translocation	Xp11 and 18q11

PRENATAL DIAGNOSIS

Introduction

Many genetic disorders can be diagnosed before birth, thus improving the chances of treatment or at worst, giving the parents the choice of selective abortion. Ultrasound imaging is harmless and is being done almost routinely. On the other hand, test that involve amniocentesis or chronic villous sampling, carry a risk of injury to fetus and are therefore used only when there is reason to suspect some abnormality. Indications are:

- Maternal age over 35 years or an unduly high paternal age.
- A previous history of chromosome abnormalities or genetic abnormalities amenable to biochemical diagnosis.
- To confirm noninvasive test, suggesting an abnormality.

Maternal Screening

Fetal neural tube defect is associated with increased level of alpha fetoproteins in amniotic fluid and to lesser extent in maternal blood. Women with positive blood test may be given the option of further investigation by amniocentesis. It has also been noted that abnormally low level of alpha-fetoprotein (AFP) are associated with Down's syndrome.

Amniocentesis

Under local anesthesia a small amount (200 mL) of fluid is drawn from amniotic sac with a needle and syringe. The procedure is usually carried out between 14th and 18th weeks of pregnancy. The fluid can be directly examined for AFP and desquamated fetal cells can be collected and cultured for chromosomal studies and biochemical tests for enzymes disorders.

Chorionic Villus Sampling

Under ultrasound screening, a fine needle catheter is passed through cervix and a small sample of chorionic is sucked out. This is usually done between 8th and 10th weeks of pregnancy. Mesenchymal fibroblast can be cultured and can be used for chromosomal studies, biochemical test, and DNA analysis. Rapid advances in DNA technologies have made it possible to diagnose sickle cell anemia and hemophilia during early pregnancy.

Fetal Imaging

By the 18th week of pregnancy, high resolution ultrasonography may show anatomical abnormalities, such as open neural tube defect and short limb. In late pregnancy, X-ray examination will reveal any marked change in bone density and multiple fractures.

CHILDHOOD DIAGNOSIS

Introduction

It is a difficult task for a physician to determine whether the disease with which the patient is afflicted, is genetic in origin. Towards the end, accurate diagnostic steps become imperative. Retarded growth, disproportionate length of the upper or lower trunk, childhood deformity, and any malformations are the most commonly encountered conditions in childhood, which need to be corrected in the pediatric age group itself, to avoid any disability in the adulthood.

Predisposing Factors

- An abnormal fetus detected in intrauterine life by ultrasonography (USG).
- A child with mental retardation or delayed physical and mental milestones.
- An infant with single or multiple malformations.
- When it is suspected that the disease is either an inherited metabolic disorder, a single-gene disorder, or a chromosomal disorder.
- Consanguinity marriage.
- History of multiple miscarriages.
- Exposure to teratogens.

History

- A thorough detailed history and physical examination are essential.
- A detailed history about the individual's prenatal period, labor, delivery, and documentation of family relationships, i.e. charting the pedigree are useful.
- In pedigree charting, gender of each individual and the relationship between individuals should be indicated using standard pedigree symbols.
- In patients with X-linked recessive disorders, the history of the male relatives on the mother's side of the family is important; the age should be recorded along with the history of the presence or absence of any disease.

Examination

- In the clinical examination, attention should be paid to physical variations or minor abnormalities, which can provide clues to diagnosis.
- Following physical examination, relevant routine laboratory tests, such as blood examination, ECG, imaging studies, special molecular cytogenic studies, molecular biochemical tests, etc. are carried out.
- Routine tests usually enable recording of physical features, such as cardiac anomalies or musculoskeletal deformities.
- Chromosomal analysis helps to establish diagnosis in cases, such as failure to thrive, developmental delay, multiple malformations, sexual dysmorphism, mental retardation, etc.
- Specific recombinant DNA tests enable the detection of mutation and establish diagnosis.

Prenatal Diagnosis

- Prenatal diagnosis includes both screening and diagnostic tests.
- A popular screening test used for prenatal diagnosis is an assay of maternal serum alpha-fetoprotein, at 15 weeks of gestation.
- The diagnostic tests can be used for two purposes:
  - Analysis of fetal tissues, e.g. aminocentesis, chorionic villus sampling (CVS), cordocentesis and in *in vitro* fertilization (IVF) diagnosis.
  - Visualization of the fetus, e.g. USG.

Clinical Features

- Retarded growth and shortness of stature.
- Disproportionate length of trunk and limbs.
- Localized malformations (dysmorphism).
- Soft-tissue contracture.
- All the skeletal dysplasias affect growth, although this may not be obvious at birth.
- Children should be measured at regular intervals and a record kept of height and length of lower segment (pubic symphysis to heel) and upper segment (pubis to cranium), head circumference, and chest circumference.
- Failure to reach the expected height for the local population group should be noted and marked shortness of stature is highly suspicious.
- The normal upper segment ratio changes gradually from about 1.5:1, at the end of the first year to about 1:1 at puberty.
- Shortness of the stature with normal proportions is not necessarily abnormal, but it is also seen in endocrine disorders, which affect the different parts of the skeleton more or less equally.
- By contrast, small stature with disappropriate shortness of the limbs is characteristic of skeletal dysplasia, the long bones being more markedly affected than the axial skeleton.
- The different segments of the limbs also may be disproportionately affected.
- The subtleties of:
  - Rhizomelia proximal segments (humeri and femora).
  - *Mesomelia:* Short middle segments (forearms and legs).
  - *Acromelia:* Stubby hands and feet.
- Dysmorphism (a misshapen part of the body) is the most obvious in the face and hands.
- There is a remarkable consistency about these changes, which makes for a disturbing similarity of appearance in members of a particular group.
- Local deformities, such as kyphosis, valgus or varus knees, bowed forearms, and ulnar deviated wrists result from disturbed bone growth.

Radiological Findings

- Presence of any above features calls for a limited radiograph survey. Anteroposterior views of the skull and thoracolumbar spine.
- Fractures, deformity in bones, tumors, etc.
- Epiphyseal dysplasia and spinal deformities may be obvious, especially in the older child.
- Sometimes a complete survey is needed and it is important to know, which portion of the long bone (epiphysis, metaphysis, or diaphysis) is affected.
- With severe and varied changes in the metaphyses, periosteal new bone formation or epiphyseal separation always consider the possibility of non-accidental fractures. The battered baby syndrome.

Special Investigations

- In most cases, the diagnosis can be made without laboratory tests.
- Routine blood and urine is helpful in excluding metabolic and endocrine disorders, such as rickets and pituitary, or thyroid dysfunction.
- Special tests are also available to identify specific excretory metabolites in the storage disorders, and specific enzyme activity can be measured in the serum, blood cells or cultured fibroblasts.

MANAGEMENT OF GENETIC DISORDERS

Genetic Consultation

Definition or Purpose

- To relay information on diagnoses, prognoses, risk, implication, options, test, therapy, services, and mode of inheritance for genetic disorder
- To maintain confidentiality
- For accurate diagnosis
- To relieve anxiety
- To provide management.

Reasons for Reference

- Advanced maternal age (AMA)
- Previous family history
- Single gene defect
- Chromosomal anomalies
- Multifactorial disorders
- Cancer history
- Repeated miscarriages
- Infertility
- Abnormal prenatal diagnosis
- Teratogen exposure.

Ideal Consultation Schedule

Session 1

- Obtain family and medical history
- Available options and test
- Cost of test
- Collection of samples
- Schedule next session.

Session 2

- Discuss test results
- Explain mode of inheritance
- Explain risk to future children and other family members; anhydrase activity in erythrocytes, counseling for autosomal dominant and recessive inheritance
- Similarly, the other genetic disorders are counseled based on their inheritance pattern.

Counseling

- *Achondrogenesis*: The recurrence risk for siblings for type 1B is one in four, whereas for type 2 it is much lower.
- *Achondroplasia*: Counseling is for autosomal dominant inheritance. When both parents have this disease, there is one chance in four that each of their children will be affected homozygotes—almost all such infants die before or after birth.
- *Hereditary multiple exostosis:* Counseling is on the basis of autosomal dominant inheritance with variable expression.
- *Osteogenesis imperfecta:* Counseling is for autosomal dominant inheritance for type 2.
- *Osteopetrosis:* Measuring the level of carbonic.

Treatment and Therapy

- Fetal surgery:
  - Open fetal surgery
  - Laser treatment
- Prenatal stem cell and gene therapy.

Fetal Surgery

Fetal surgery is a unique field in maternal-fetal medicine, detecting birth defects prenatally has allowed physicians to provide better perinatal care, but many of these babies were already too sick to treat them successfully after they were born. This dilemma led to the development of fetal surgery.

Open Fetal Surgery

- Repairing birth defects in the womb.
- Open fetal surgery involves cutting into the mother's abdomen and uterus in order to operate on the fetus, to remove abnormal masses or patch an opening.
- Fetal surgery places special demands on caregivers, to ensure safety for two patients, the mother and the fetus.
- Adzick, in his first article, described fetal surgeries for two life-threatening defects:
  - Lung masses, which may compress the developing heart, leading to heart failure
  - Sacrococcygeal teratomas, which can lead to heart failure or a fatal hemorrhage before birth.
- Adzick, in his second article, described fetal surgery for myelomeningocele. To repair a myelomeningocele, fetal surgeons shield the developing spinal cord by closing the defect with the fetus's own tissue.

Laser Treatment

- Another application of fetal surgery is for twin-twin transfusion syndrome, occurring in 10–15% of identical twins.
- In this condition, one fetus grows at the expense of its twin because of abnormal blood vessel connections in their shared placenta.

Procedure: Selective Laser Photocoagulation

In this procedure, using a viewing instrument called a fetoscope, the fetal surgeon employs a laser to seal off the blood vessels that carry hazardous blood flow between the two fetuses, thus shutting off dangerous twin-to-twin connection.

Prenatal Stem Cell and Gene Therapy

- The greatest future impact of fetal treatments probably lies in nonsurgical approaches—prenatal stem cell therapy and gene therapy.
- In contrast to the relatively rare anatomical defects addressed in fetal surgery, cell and gene therapy offer the possibility of treating many genetic diseases before birth, including sickle cell anemia, immune deficiency disorders, and some types of muscular dystrophy.

In Utero Hematopoietic Stem Cell Transplantation

- It focuses on stem cells that develop into all the types of cells found in the blood.
- The keystone of this approach is the fetal immune system's unique tolerance of transplanted cells.
- Flake's strategy involves, using prenatal stem cell transplants to achieve tolerance of foreign cells, which are incorporated into the fetal circulation.
- This sets the stage for postnatal transplant of therapeutic blood cells from the same donor that will not be rejected by the infant's immune system.
- The specific characteristics of severe combined immunodeficiency (SCID) make this disease uniquely amenable to a prenatal stem cell approach.
- At present, research in animal models is progressing toward using in utero hematopoietic stem cell transplantation (IUHCT) to treat other immune deficiency diseases, the hemoglobin disorders sickle cell anemia and thalassemia, and lysosomal storage diseases (genetic disorders in which the lack of an enzyme causes metabolic chemicals to accumulate to toxic levels in cells).
- Some diseases that progress to irreversible organ damage may offer targets for prenatal gene therapy, in which physicians deliver therapeutic DNA to correct a genetic defect.
- Proof-of-principle studies in animals have produced preclinical successes for prenatal gene therapy in cystic fibrosis, Duchenne's muscular dystrophy, Pompe disease, and the lysosomal storage disease, Sly syndrome.
- There have also been promising animal studies in types of hemophilia.
- As with postnatal gene therapy, important safety issues remain to be solved before prenatal gene therapy can be offered in the clinic.
- Fetal gene therapy is still in the early experimental stage, said Flake, while noting great progress in this field.

Ex Utero Intrapartum Therapy

- The *ex utero intrapartum therapy* (EXIT) procedure is a partial delivery, in which the fetus is partially removed from the uterus, but remains attached to the circulation carried by the umbilical cord and placenta, so that surgeons can correct airway blockages before performing a full delivery.
- It is a partial delivery, which buys time for fetal surgery eventually.
- Clinicians at Children's Hospital of Philadelphia, USA have the world's most extensive experience in performing the EXIT procedure.

Set-Up

In order to carry out these procedures, there should be a multidisciplinary team and sophisticated imaging technologies, used to assess patients referred to the center and the facilities should include a "special delivery unit" for mothers carrying babies, with known birth defects.

DOWN'S SYNDROME (TRISOMY-21)

Introduction

- It is a chromosomal disorder caused by the presence of all or part of an extra 21st chromosome.
- It is named after John Langdon Down, the British physician who described the syndrome in 1866.
- The disorder was identified as a chromosome 21 trisomy, by Jerome Lejeune in 1959.
- The condition is characterized by a combination of major and minor differences in structure.

Incidence

- The incidence of Down syndrome is estimated as 1 per 800 to 1,000 births.
- Although, it is statistically much more common with elderly females.

Genetics

- Trisomy-21 (47 and + 21), frequency of occurrence is about 94%. The frequency of trisomy increases with increasing maternal age (Figs. 11 and 12)
- Robertsonian translocation, involving chromosome 21, approximately 3–4%, not related to maternal age (Figs. 13A and B)
- Trisomy-21 mosaicism: 2–3% cases.

Clinical Features (Fig. 14)

- Brachycephaly
- Up-slanting palpebral fissures

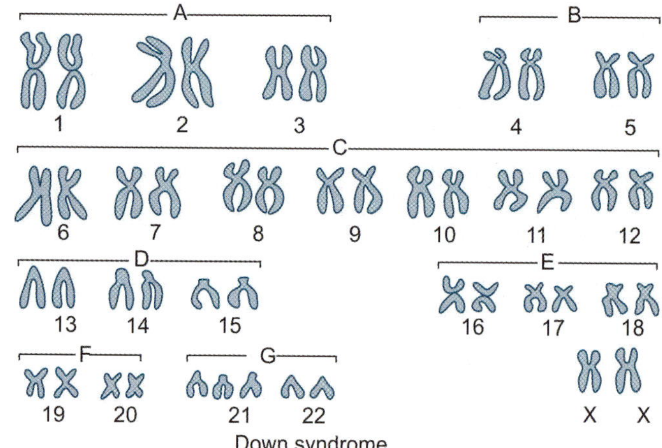

Fig. 11: Presentation of different chromosomal pattern in Down's syndrome (21st chromosome showing trisomy).

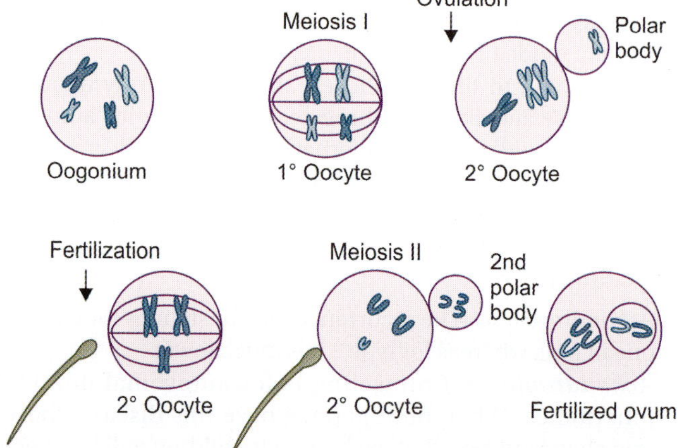

Fig. 12: Chromosomal nondisjunction in meiosis I, resulted in trisomy.

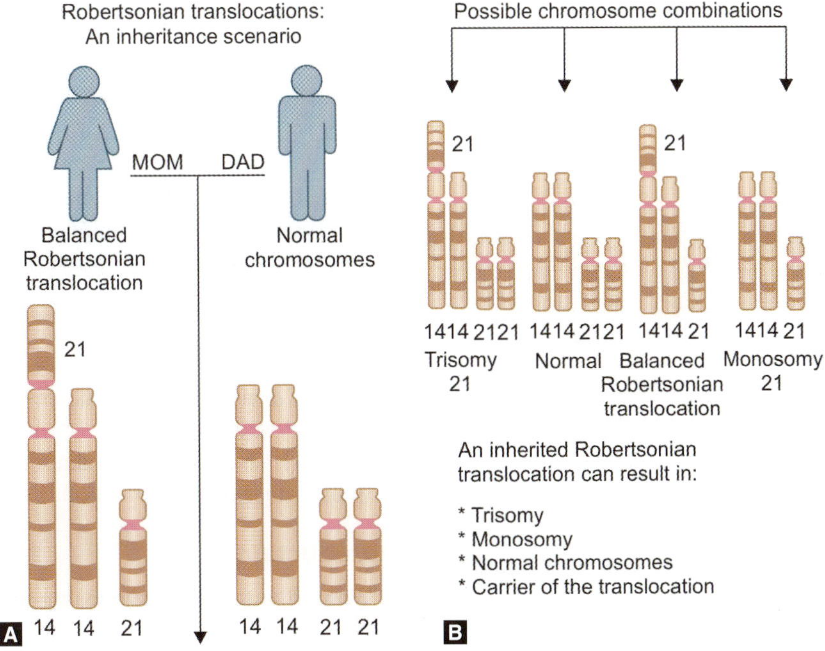

Figs. 13A and B: Robertsonian translocation—(A) Showing an inheritance scenario; (B) Possible chromosomal combinations.

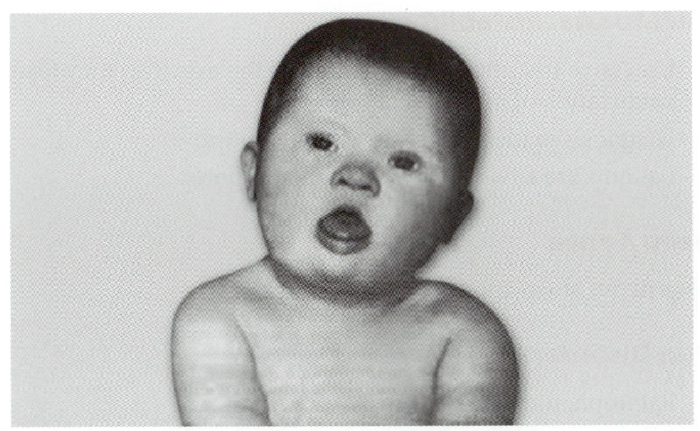

Fig. 14: A child suffering from Down's syndrome, with protruding tongue, open mouth and other presentable clinical features of Down's syndrome.

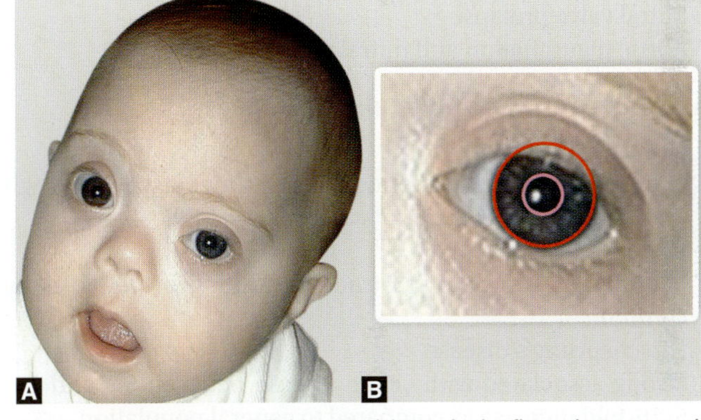

Figs. 15A and B: Brushfield spots (shown in the figure between red circles around iris).

- Epicanthal folds
- Brushfield spots (Figs. 15A and B)
- Flat nasal bridge
- Folded or dysplastic ears
  - Open mouth
  - Protruding tongue
  - Short neck
  - Excessive skin at the nape of neck
  - Extremities
  - Short broad hands
  - Short fifth finger
  - Incurved fifth finger
  - Transverse palmar crease
  - Space between first and second toe
  - Hyperflexibility of joints.

Neonatal Features

- Flat facial profile
- Poor Moro reflex
- Excessive skin at the nape of neck
- Slanted palpebral fissures
- Hypotonia
- Hyperflexibility of joints
- Dysplasia of pelvis
- Anomalous ears
- Dysplasia of midphalanx of fifth finger
- Transverse palmar crease (Figs. 16A and B).

Mental Retardation

- Almost all Down syndrome babies are mentally retarded.
- Mildly to moderately retarded.
- Starts in the first year of life.
- Average age of sitting (11 months) and walking (26 months), which is twice the typical normal age.
- Child starts speaking first word at 18 months.
- IQ declines through the first 10 years of age, reaching a plateau in adolescence that continues into adulthood.

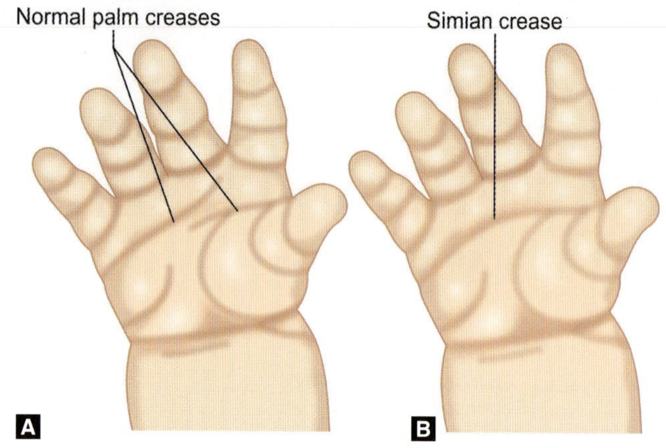

Figs. 16A and B: Transverse palmar crease, a typical neonatal feature of Down's syndrome.

Heart Diseases

Fifty percent of Down syndrome patients have heart disease, most common defects include:
- Atrioventricular septal defect
- Ventricular septal defect
- Secundum atrial septal defect
- Patent ductus arteriosus
- Tetrology of Fallot
- Mitral valve prolapse
- Aortic regurgitation and mitral regurgitation.

Gastrointestinal Abnormalities

- Only in 5% of cases
- Duodenal atresia or stenosis, sometimes associated with annular pancreas in 2.5% of cases
- Imperforate anus
- Esophageal atresia, with tracheoesophageal fistula is less common
- Hirschsprung's disease
- Strong associated with celiac disease between 5% and 16%, 5–16-fold increase as compared to general population.

Growth

- Body weight, length, and head circumference are less in Down syndrome.
- Reduced growth rate.
- Prevalence of obesity is greater in Down syndrome.
- Weight is less than expected for length in infants with Down syndrome and then increases disproportionally, so that they are obese by the age of 3–4 years.

Eye Problems

Most common disorders are:
- Refractory error (35–76%)
- Strabismus (25–57%)
- Nystagmus (18–22%)
- Cataract occur in 5% of newborns
- Frequency increases with age.

Hearing Loss

- Unilateral or bilateral
- Conductive, sensorineural, or mixed
- Otitis media is a frequent problem.

Hematologic Disorders

- The risk of leukemia is 1–1.5%.
- 65% of newborn have polycythemia, resulting in hypoglycemia.
- Risk of acute myeloid leukemia and acute lymphocytic leukemia is also much higher than the general population.
- Transient leukemia, exclusively affects newborn. It is asymptomatic with spontaneous resolution in 2–3 months.
- Vesiculopustular skin eruptions are common and resolve with disorder.

Endocrine Disorder

- *Thyroid disease:* Hypothyroidism occurs more frequently than hyperthyroidism.
- *Diabetes:* The risk of type 1 diabetes is three times greater than that of the general population.

Reproduction

- Women with Down syndrome are fertile and may become pregnant.
- Nearly all males with Down syndrome are infertile. The mechanism is impairment of spermatogenesis.

Atlantoaxial Instability

- Excessive mobility of atlas (C1) and the axis (C2) may lead to subluxation of the cervical spine.
- Diagnosis made by lateral neck radiograph.
- Patients are advised, to avoid contact sports.

Sleep Apnea

Obstructive sleep apnea is more common.

Skin Disorder

- Palmoplantar hyperkeratosis
- Seborrheic dermatitis
- Fissured tongue
- Cutis marmorata
- Geographical tongue
- Xerosis.

Mortality

- Median age of death for Down syndrome patients was 25 years in 1983 and with the advancement of medicine field the survival age has been increasing at the rate of 1.7 years per year.
- Improved survival is because of increased placements of infants in homes and changes in treatment for common causes of death.
- Most likely cause of death is congenital heart disease, dementia, hypothyroidism, and leukemia.
- Survival is better for males and blacks.

Counseling

- It may begin, when a prenatal diagnosis is made.
- Discuss the wide range of variability in manifestation and prognosis.

- Medical and educational treatments and interventions should be discussed.
- Initial referrals for early intervention, informative publications, parent groups, and advocacy group.

Diagnosis

- Prenatal screening
- Genetic testing, such as amniocentesis, chorionic villus sampling (CVS) or percutaneous umbilical cord blood sampling (PUBS)
- *If no screening:* It is recognized from the characteristic phenotypic features, confirmed by karyotype.

Examination at Birth

- Particular attention to physical signs.
- Evaluation of the red reflex can help identify congenital cataracts. Movement of the eyes should be observed to identify strabismus.
- Constipation should raise concerns for Hirschsprung's disease and feeding problems should prompt intense education, to ensure adequate input and nutrition.
- Ultrasound of the heart (echocardiogram) should be done immediately.
- Complete blood count should be done in order to identify preexisting leukemia immediately, in order to identify congenital heart disease.

Investigation

- *Growth based:* Measurements should be plotted on the appropriate growth chart for children with Down syndrome. This will help in prevention of obesity and early diagnosis of celiac disease and hypothyroidism.
- *Cardiac disease:* All newborns should be evaluated by cardiac echo for congenital heart disease in consultation with pediatric cardiologist.
- *Hearing:* Brainstem auditory evoked responses (BAERs) testing is to be done in the newborn periodically in every 6 months until 3 years of age and then annually.
- *Eye disorders:* An eye exam should be performed in the newborn period or at least before 6 months of age, to detect strabismus, nystagmus and cataracts.
- *Thyroid function:* Normal values in newborn versus values in Down syndrome should be done in newborn period and should be repeated at 6 and 12 months and then annually.
- *Celiac disease:* Screening should begin at 2 years. Repeat screening, if signs/symptoms develop.
- *Hematology:* Complete blood count with differential at birth, to evaluate for polycythemia as well as WBC.
- *Atlantoaxial instability:* X-ray for evidence of atlantoaxial instability or subluxation at 3–5 years of age.
- *Alzheimer's disease:* Adult with a Down syndrome has earlier onset of symptoms. When diagnosis is considered, thyroid disease, and possible depression should be excluded.

Management

- Treatment of individuals with Down syndrome depends on the particular manifestations of the disorder.
- For instance, individuals with congenital heart disease may need to undergo major corrective surgery soon after birth.
- Other individuals may have relatively minor health problems requiring no therapy.

Plastic Surgery

- It has sometimes been advocated and performed on children with Down syndrome, based on the assumption that surgery can reduce the facial features associated with Down syndrome, therefore decreasing social stigma and leading to a better quality of life.

Example: Facial reconstruction and glossectomy (tongue reduction).

Cognitive Development

- Individuals with Down syndrome differ considerably in their language and communication skills.
- Low gain hearing aids other amplification devices can be useful for language and learning.
- Individualized speech therapy can target specific speech errors, increase speech intelligibility, and in some cases encourage advanced language and literacy.
- Augmentative and alternative communication (AAC) methods, such as pointing, body language, objects, or graphics are often used to aid communication.

Follow-up

- As children with Down syndrome grow, their progress should be plotted on a growth chart, in order to detect deviations from expected growth. Special growth charts are available so that children with Down syndrome can be compared with other children with Down syndrome.
- Thyroid function testing should be performed at 6 months and 12 months of age as well as yearly, thereafter.
- Evaluation of the ears for infection as well as objective hearing tests should be performed at every visit.
- Formal evaluation for refractive errors requiring glasses should be performed at least every 2 years with subjective vision assessments with each visit.
- After the age of three, an X-ray of the neck should be obtained to screen for atlantoaxial instability.
- As the child ages, yearly symptom screening for obstructive sleep apnea should be performed.

MARFAN'S SYNDROME

Introduction

- Marfan's syndrome is an inherited connective-tissue disorder, transmitted as an autosomal dominant trait (Figs. 17A and B).
- It is noteworthy for its worldwide distribution, relatively high prevalence, clinical variability, and pleiotropic manifestations, some of which are life-threatening.
- Cardinal features of the disorder include tall stature, ectopia lentis, mitral valve prolapse, aortic root dilatation, and aortic dissection.
- About three quarters of patients have an affected parent and new mutations account for the remainder.

Pathophysiology

- Marfan's syndrome results from mutations in the *Fibrillin-1 (FBN1) gene* on chromosome 15, which encodes for the glycoprotein fibrillin.

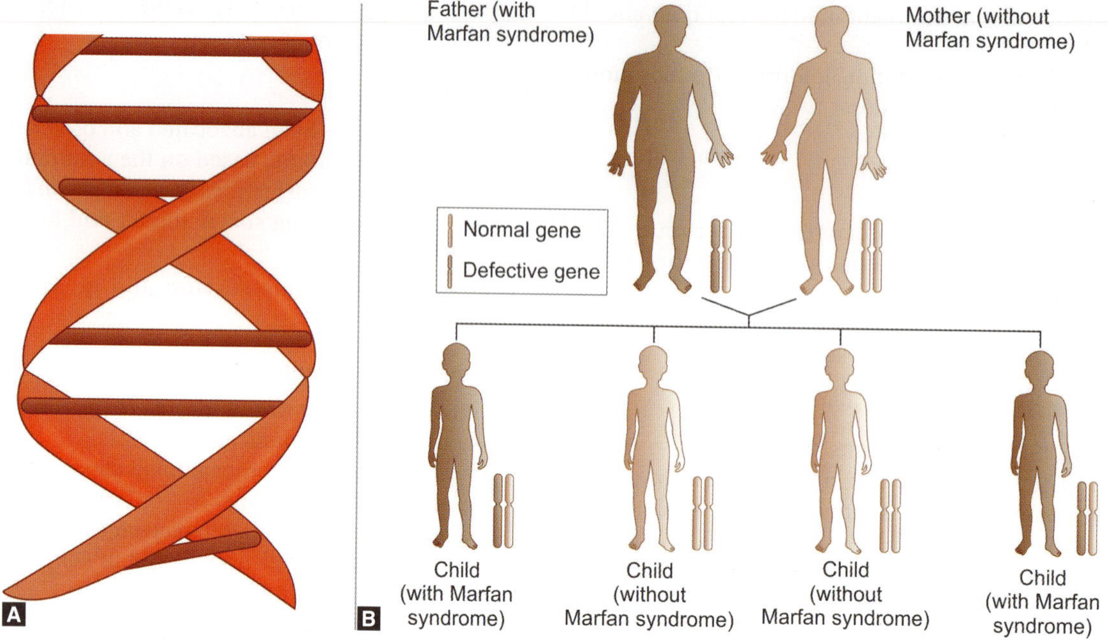

Figs. 17A and B: Inheritance of Marfan's syndrome or transfer as autosomal dominant trait.

- Fibrillin is a major building block of microfibrils, which constitute the structural components of the suspensory ligament of the lens and serve as substrates for elastin in the aorta and other connective tissues.
- Abnormalities involving microfibrils weaken the aortic wall. Progressive aortic dilatation and eventual aortic dissection occurs.
- Likewise, deficient fibrillin deposition leads to reduced structural integrity of the lens zonules, ligaments, lung airways, and spinal dura.
- Recent studies have suggested that abnormalities in the transforming growth factor-beta (TGF)-signaling pathway may also involve in the development of the Marfan's phenotype. The gene defect ultimately leads to decreased and disordered incorporation of fibrillin into the connective tissue matrix.
- *Frequency:* Marfan's syndrome is one of the most common single-gene malformation syndromes with incidence of about 1 in 10,000 individuals.
- No geographic predilection is known.
- *Race:* Marfan's syndrome is panethnic.
- *Sex:* No sex predilection is known.
- *Age:* Marfan's syndrome may be diagnosed prenatally, at birth or well into adulthood. Neonatal presentation is associated with a more severe course than that associated with other presentations.
- Most clinical features are specific to age and some features may not manifest, until relatively late in life. This feature may make diagnosis in a child difficult.
- *Mortality and morbidity:* Cardiovascular disease (aortic dilatation and dissection) is the major cause of morbidity and mortality. Progression from mitral valve prolapse to mitral regurgitation, often in conjunction with tricuspid prolapse and regurgitation is the most common cause of infant morbidity. If untreated, Marfan's syndrome is highly lethal. The average age at death is 30–40 years.
- Death after infancy usually involves ascending aortic dissection and chronic aortic regurgitation. Dissection generally occurs at the aortic root and is uncommon in childhood and adolescence.

Clinical History

- Marfan's syndrome is currently diagnosed using criteria based on an evaluation of the family history, molecular data, and six organ systems.
- The diagnosis cannot be based on molecular analysis alone because molecular diagnosis is not generally available, mutation detection is imperfect and not all FBN1 mutations are associated with Marfan's syndrome.
- Due to this, Berlin criteria is used for diagnosis of Marfan.
- In 1995, a group of the world's leading clinicians and investigators in Marfan's syndrome proposed revised diagnostic criteria, which is known as the Ghent criteria, which identify major and minor diagnostic findings.
- The major criteria include the following:
  - A first-degree relative (parent, child, or sibling), who independently meets the diagnostic criteria.
  - Presence of an FBN1 mutation known to cause Marfan's syndrome.
  - In family members, major involvement in one organ system and involvement in a second organ system.
  - If the family and genetic histories are not contributory, major criteria in two different organ systems and involvement of a third organ system are required, to make the diagnosis (organ system criteria described in physical).

Skeletal Findings

Affected patients are usually taller and thinner than their family members. Their limbs are disproportionately long compared with the trunk (dolichostenomelia), as shown in Figures 18, 19 and 21.

Major Criteria

- Pectus excavatum that requires surgery or pectus carinatum (Fig. 20).

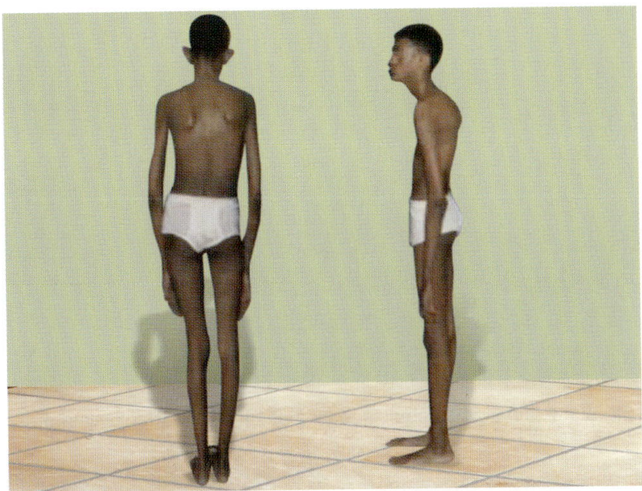

Fig. 18: Skeletal findings in Marfan's syndrome, Note tall and thin build, disproportionately long arms and legs and kyphoscoliosis.

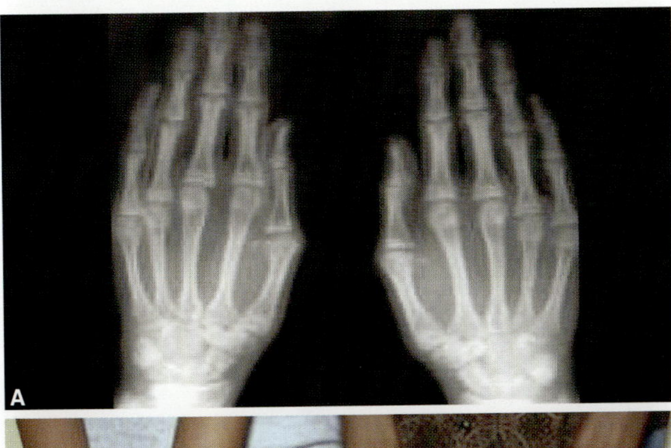

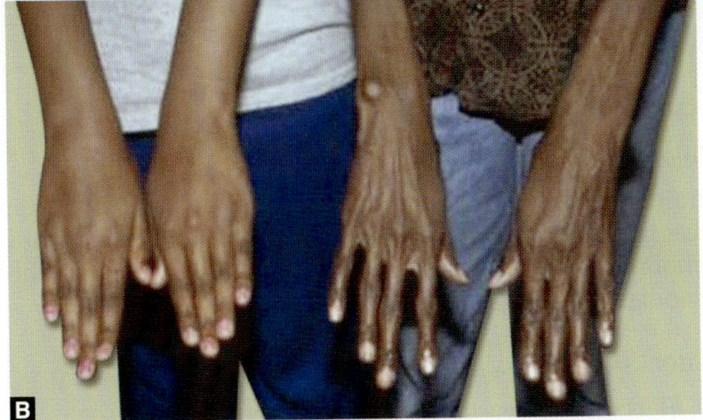

Figs. 19A and B: Arachnodactyly in Marfan's syndrome—(A) X-ray findings; (B) Comparison of normal hands with the Marfan's syndrome patient.

- *Pectus excavatum of moderate severity:* Reduced upper-to-lower body segment ratio (0.85 vs. 0.93) or arm span-to-height ratio greater than 1.05. Arms and legs may be unusually long in proportion to the torso.
- *Positive wrist (walker) and thumb (Steinberg) signs (Figs. 22 to 24): Two* simple maneuvers may help demonstrate arachnodactyly. First, the thumb sign is positive if the thumb, when completely opposed within the clenched hand, projects beyond the ulnar border. Second, the wrist sign is positive if the distal phalanges of the first and fifth digits of one hand overlap when wrapped around the opposite wrist.

Scoliosis greater than 20°: More than 60% of patients have scoliosis. Progression is most likely with curvature of more than 20° in growing patients.

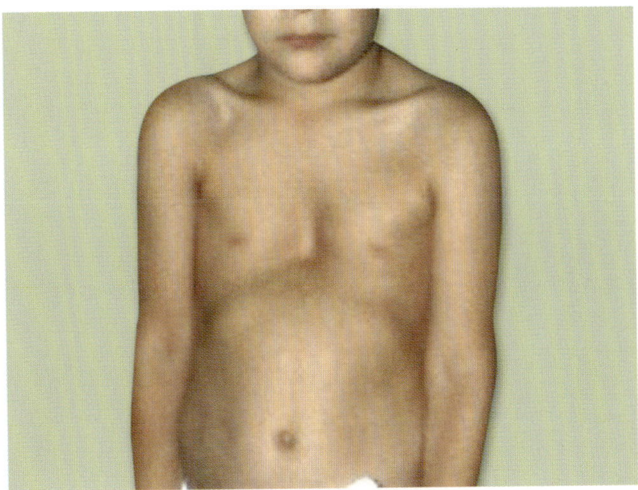

Fig. 20: Pectus excavatum.

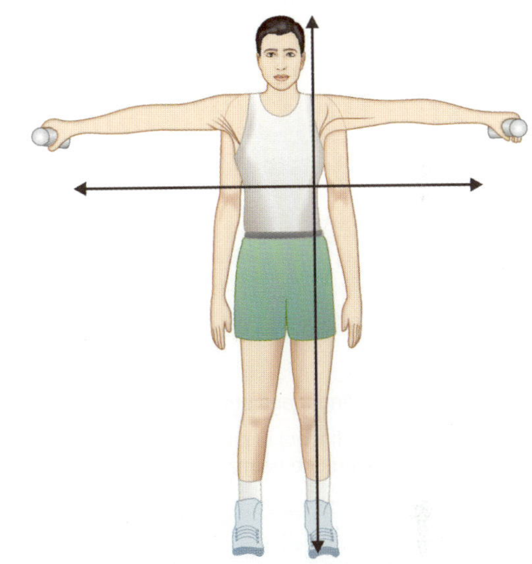

Fig. 21: This person in the figure with Marfan's syndrome is tall and thin and has an arm span that exceeds his height.

- Reduced extension of the elbows (less than 170°).
- Medial displacement of the medial malleolus, resulting in pes planus. Pes planus is best diagnosed by examining the foot from behind. A valgus deviation of the hind foot indicates pes planus.
- *Protrusio acetabuli of any degree:* This is a deformity of the hip joint, in which the medial wall of the acetabulum invades the pelvic cavity with associated medial displacement of the femoral head and is ascertained using radiography. Protrusio acetabuli affects 31–100% of patients to varying degrees (Fig. 25).
- Clinical manifestations include hip joint stiffness and progressive limitation in activity related to joint pain, a waddling gait, limited range of motion, flexion contracture, a pelvic tilt, with a resulting hyperlordosis of the lumbar spine, and eventual osteoarthritic changes. Local progressive protrusion can lead to early hip pain and osteoarthritis.

Minor Criteria

- Pectus excavatum of moderate severity
- Scoliosis less than 20°
- Thoracic lordosis

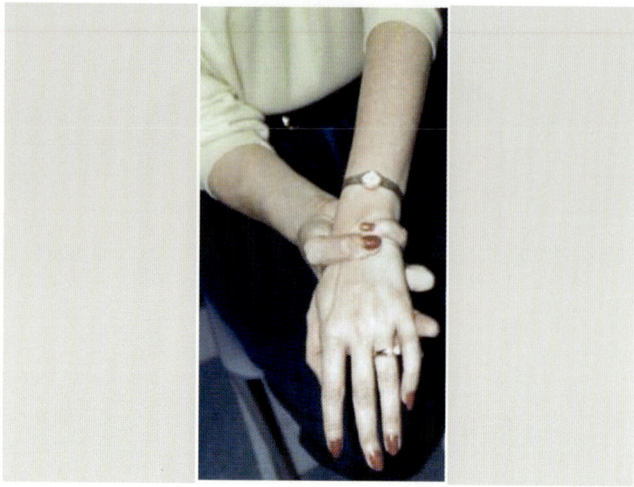

Fig. 22: Positive wrist (walker) sign, demonstrates arachnodactyly.

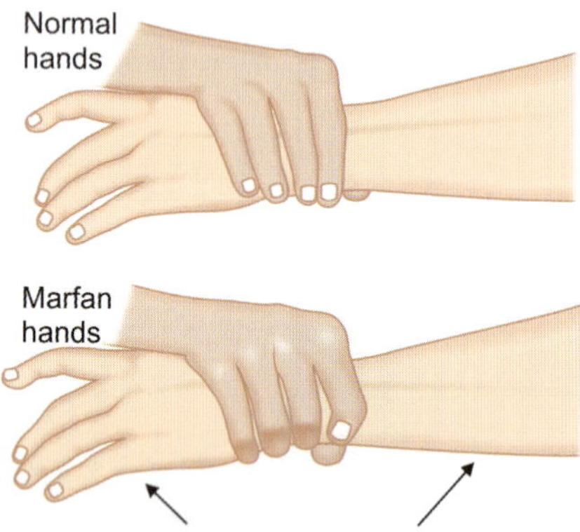

Fig. 23: Elongated arm and fingers in patient with Marfan's syndrome, compared to normal hands.

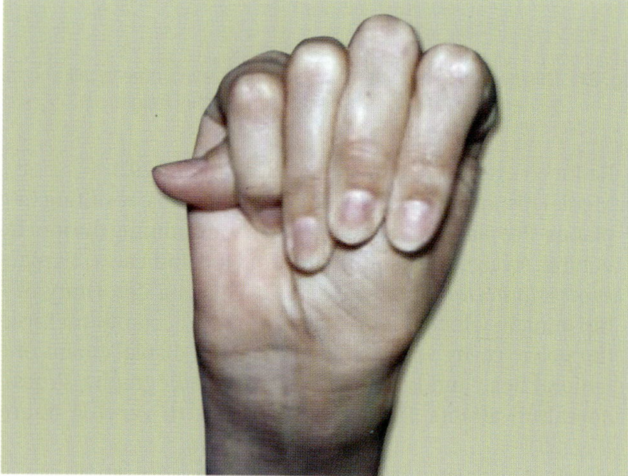

Fig. 24: Steinberg sign or positive thumb sign.

- Joint hypermobility (Fig. 26)
- Highly arched palate
- Dental crowding
- Typical facies (malar hypoplasia, enophthalmos, retrognathia, down-slanting palpebral fissures)
- For the skeletal system to be involved
- At least two major criteria or one major criterion plus two minor criteria must be present.

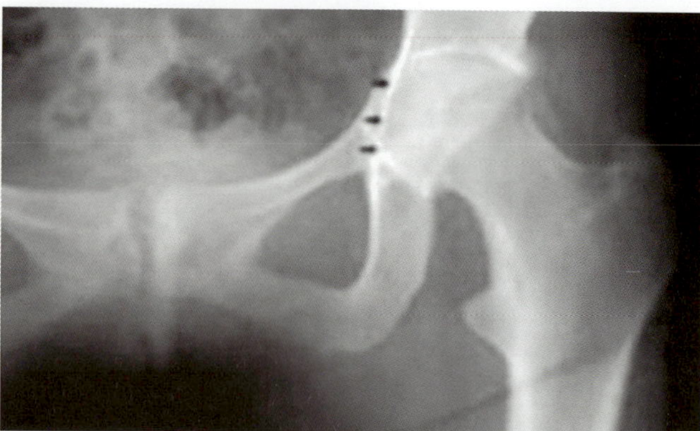

Fig. 25: Protrusio acetabuli, seen in patient with Marfan's syndrome.

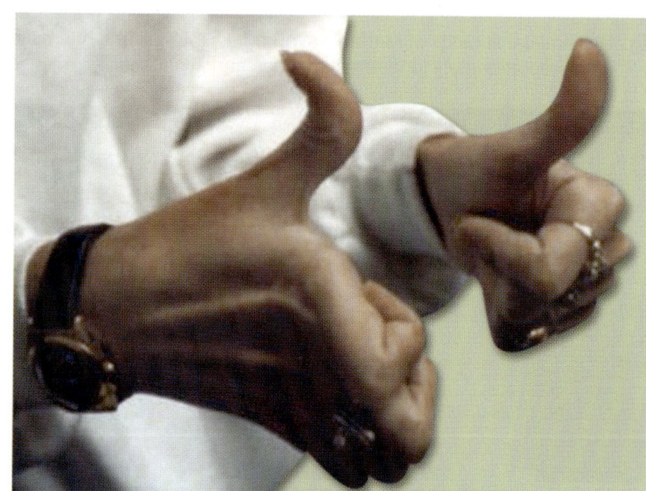

Fig. 26: Hypermobility of finger joints.

Ocular Findings

Major Criteria

The major criterion is ectopia lentis. About 50% of patients have lens dislocation. The dislocation is usually superior and temporal. This may present at birth or develop during childhood or adolescence (Figs. 27A and B).

Minor Criteria

- Flat cornea (measured by keratometry).
- Increased axial length of the globe (measured by ultrasound).
- Cataract in patients younger than 50 years.
- Hypoplastic iris or hypoplastic ciliary muscle that causes decreased miosis.
- Nearsightedness regardless of whether the lens is in place the most common refraction error is myopia due to elongated globe.
- Glaucoma (patients less than 50 years).
- Retinal detachment.
- At least two minor criteria should be present.

Cardiovascular Findings

Cardiovascular involvement is the most serious problem associated with Marfan's syndrome.

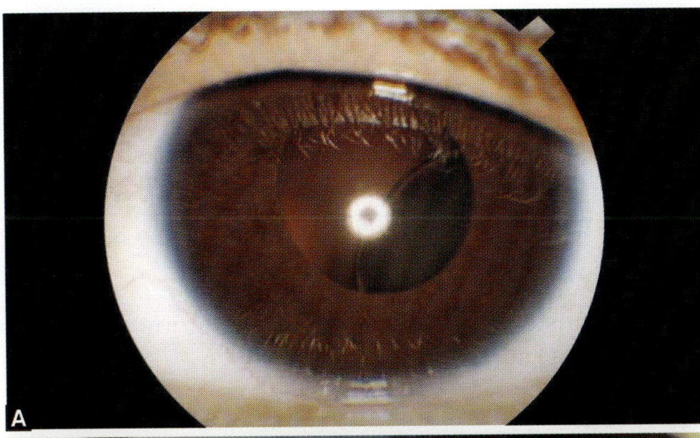

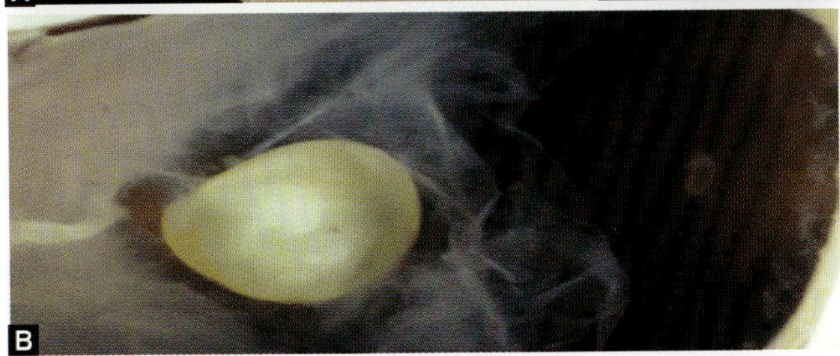

Figs. 27A and B: Ectopia lentis—dislocated eye lens.

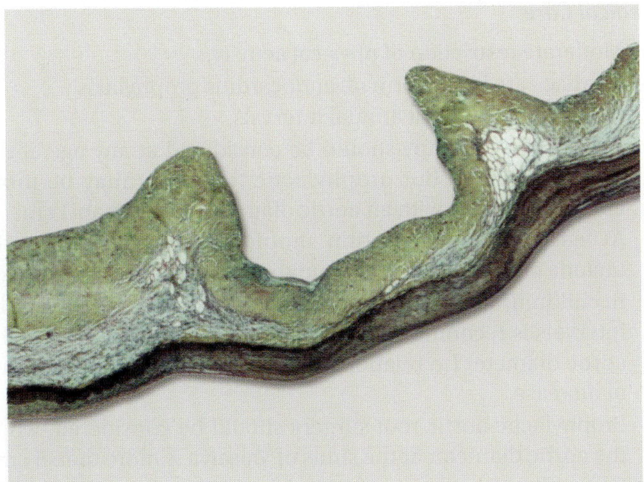

Fig. 28: Manifestation of Marfan syndrome—myxomatous degeneration of the aortic valve.

Major Criteria

- Aortic root dilatation involving the sinuses of Valsalva. Its prevalence in Marfan's syndrome is 70–80%.
- Aortic dissections involving the ascending aorta.

Minor Criteria

- *Mitral valve prolapse (55–69%):* Midsystolic clicks.
- Dilatation of proximal main pulmonary artery in the absence of peripheral pulmonic stenosis or other cause.
- Calcification of mitral annulus (patients less than 40 years).
- Dilatation of abdominal or descending thoracic aorta (patients less than 50 years).
- For the cardiovascular system to be involved, a major, and a minor criterion must be present.
- Micrograph demonstrating myxomatous degeneration of the aortic valve, is common (Fig. 28).

Lungs

- Marfan's syndrome is a risk factor for spontaneous pneumothorax.
- The lung becomes partially compressed or collapsed. This can cause pain, shortness of breath, cyanosis, and, if not treated, death.
- Marfan's syndrome has also been associated with sleep apnea and idiopathic obstructive lung disease.

Central Nervous System

- Another condition that can reduce the quality of life for an individual, though not life-threatening is dural ectasia, the weakening of the connective tissue of the dural sac, the membrane that encases the spinal cord.
- Symptoms that can occur are lower back pain, leg pain, abdominal pain, and other neurological symptoms in the lower extremities or headaches. Such symptoms usually diminish when the individual lies flat on his or her back.
- Other spinal issues associated with Marfan include degenerative disk disease, and spinal cysts.
- *Dural findings:* For the dura, only one major criterion is defined, "dural ectasia" must be present and confirmed using CT or MRI.
- Dural ectasia is a common feature of Marfan's syndrome. The prevalence of dural ectasia among patients with Marfan's syndrome is 65–92%.
- Dural ectasia is defined as a ballooning or widening of the dural sac, often associated with herniation of the nerve root sleeves out of the associated foramina. Dural ectasia most frequently occurs in the lumbosacral spine (Fig. 29).

Skin and Integumentary Findings

- For skin and integument, only minor criteria are noted.
- Minor criteria include the following:
  - Striae atrophicae in the absence of marked weight changes, pregnancy, or repetitive stress. Stretch marks are usually found on the shoulder, mid back and thighs.
  - Excessive skin elasticity (Fig. 30).
  - Stretch marks (striae atrophicae) in the lower back.
  - Recurrent or incisional hernia.

Differential Diagnoses

- Ehlers-Danlos syndrome
- Fragile X syndrome
- Gigantism and acromegaly
- Hyperpituitarism
- Hyperthyroidism
- Klinefelter syndrome.

Laboratory Studies

- As no common mutations have been identified, genetic testing includes screening the entire *FBN1* gene.
- DNA testing cannot exclude a diagnosis of Marfan's syndrome.
- By 1998, *137 FBN1* mutations had been characterized in patients with Marfan's syndrome. Mutations are distributed throughout the *FBN1* gene.

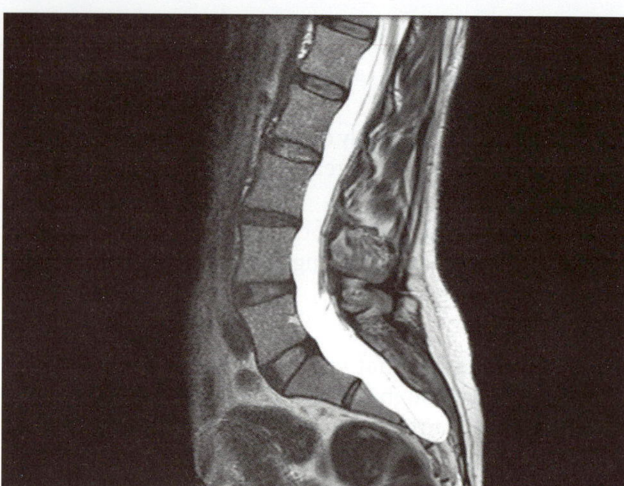

Fig. 29: Dural ectasia in the lumbosacral region.

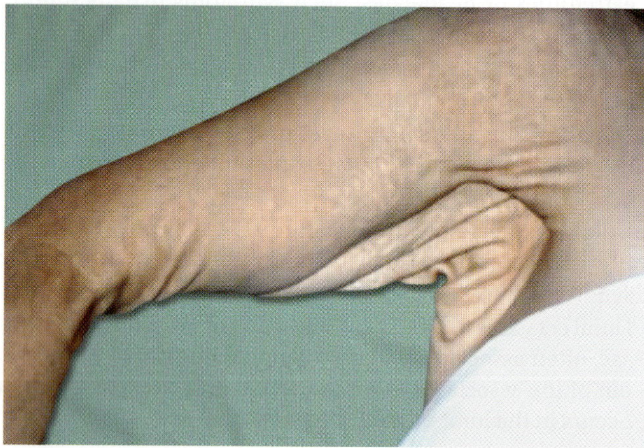

Fig. 30: Excessive skin elasticity, seen in Marfan's syndrome.

Imaging Studies

Radiography

- Chest radiography should be focused on apical blebs. Chest radiographs may also be of value in detecting a thoracic aortic dissection, by demonstrating enlargement of the aortic and cardiac silhouette.
- Pelvic radiography is required only if a positive finding of protrusio acetabula is needed for the diagnosis.

Echocardiography

- Cross-sectional echocardiography is a common tool in the diagnosis and management of aortic root dilatation.
- Standard echocardiography is valuable in assessing mitral valve prolapse, left ventricular size, and function, function of the tricuspid valve, and left atrial size.

Computed Tomography and Magnetic Resonance Imaging

- Magnetic resonance imaging (MRI) is the best choice for assessing chronic dissection of any region of the aorta. It should be performed in any patient at any age who has an aortic root dimension of more than 150% of the mean for their body surface area.
- CT or MRI of the lumbosacral spine may be needed to detect dural ectasia.
- Presence of dural ectasia requires one major criterion or both minor criteria.
- *Major criterion:* Sagittal width of the dural sac at S1 or below, which is greater than the sagittal width of the dural sac above L4.
- *Minor criteria:* Nerve root sleeve at L5 of more than 6.5 mm in diameter or at S1 of more than 3.5 mm.

Aortography

Many still consider this procedure, the criterion standard for diagnosing acute aortic dissection.

Other Tests

Histologic Findings

- Immunohistologic evaluation of the skin for abnormal fibrillin has been reported, but is not widely available.
- This is partly due to the high incidence of false-positive results in patients with other connective-tissue disorders.
- Electron microscopy of fibrillin from cultured fibroblasts has shown a substantial increase in fraying of microfibrils in patients with Marfan's syndrome.

Treatment

Medical Care

- Moderate restriction of physical activity.
- Cardiac care in the form of, endocarditis prophylaxis.
- Echocardiography at annual intervals.
- Beta-blocker therapy should be considered at any age, if the aorta is dilated, but prophylactic treatment may be more effective in those with an aortic diameter of less than 4 cm.
- At least annual evaluation should be offered and should include clinical history, examination, and echocardiography.
- In children, serial echocardiography at 6 months to 12 months intervals is recommended and the frequency depends on the aortic diameter (in relation to body surface area) and the rate of increase.
- Prophylactic aortic root surgery should be considered, when the aortic diameter at the sinus of Valsalva is more than 5 cm.
- Counseling for pregnancy 50% risk of transmitting the disease to offsprings.

Other Therapy

- Anticoagulant medications, such as warfarin are needed after artificial heart-valve placement.
- Progesterone and estrogen therapy have been used to induce puberty and reduce the patient's ultimate height, if hormonal treatment is begun before puberty, but no conclusive data are yet available to show whether this therapy reduces scoliosis.
- Conservative treatment of protrusio acetabuli mostly involves physiotherapy, by forcible stretching (stress fractures of the femoral neck due to stretching are documented), weight extension on an abduction frame, local heating, and re-education concerning daily activities.
- Myopia is treatable with refraction.
- Patients with flat feet may wear shoes with adequate arch support.
- Psychological counseling is helpful for families coping with feelings of denial, anger, blame, depression, or guilt.

Future Therapeutic Strategy

Transforming growth factor (TGF) antagonism is a general strategy against aneurysm progression in patients with Marfan's syndrome and other disorders of the TGF signaling network.

Scoliosis Surgery

- Severe scoliosis requires surgery. Bracing has a limited role in treating the most severe form of infantile scoliosis.
- Surgery should not be performed on a child younger than 4 years because many patients with large curves before this age spontaneously die of cardiac complications. Results of spinal fusion are better in children older than 5 years.
- Indications for surgery in adults include pain, neurologic signs, and thoracic curves greater than 45°, which can cause restrictive lung disease.

Protrusio Acetabuli Surgery

This is directed at arresting progression, relieving pain, and restoring the function of the hip through hip replacement with bone grafting of the medial acetabular cavity, in older patients and closure of the triradiate cartilage in a child or adolescent.

Pectus Repair

The shape of the front of the thorax becomes stable and established by mid adolescence. Therefore, repair of pectus excavatum to improve respiratory mechanics should be delayed, until then to lessen the risk of recurrence. Pectus carinatum repair is mainly performed.

Pneumothorax Therapy

Chest tube is an appropriate initial therapy. After one recurrence, a more aggressive approach involving bleb resection and pleurodesis is recommended.

Diet

No special diet is needed.

Activity

- In general, patients can remain fully active unless their symptoms limit them. Patients should be discouraged from participating in demanding sports because several Marfan's syndrome patients have suddenly died from ruptured aortic aneurysm.
- To protect against pneumothorax, patients should avoid the rapid decompression associated with quick ascents in elevators, scuba diving, and flying in unpressurized aircraft.
- Patients should avoid activities involving isometric work, such as weightlifting, climbing steep inclines, participating in gymnastics, and performing pull-ups.
- No strenuous activities and sports.

Complications

- Complications that affect the aorta are the primary cause of death.
- Aortic dissection.
- Mitral valve prolapse may be the most common cause of death with Marfan's syndrome.
- Bacterial endocarditis.
- Severe pectus excavatum can compromise cardiac and pulmonary function.
- Rarely the retina may detach.

Prognosis

- The patient's prognosis depends on the severity of cardiovascular complications and is mainly determined by progressive dilation of the aorta, which potentially leads to aortic dissection and death at a young age.
- Improved detection, timely, and improved surgical techniques and the prophylactic use of beta-blockers, all are helping to prolong survival. The average lifespan is now about 70 years.

TURNER'S SYNDROME

Turner's syndrome or congenital female hypogonadism is a rare abnormality caused by a defect in one of the X chromosomes. Those affected are phenotypically females, with a normal vagina and uterus, but the ovaries are markedly hypoplastic or absent.

Clinical Features

- Short stature
- Webbing of the neck
- Barrel chest
- Increased carrying angle of the elbows
- Cardiovascular and renal abnormalities are common, they have primary amenorrhea and hypogonadism leads to early onset osteoporosis.

Treatment

Estrogen replacement from puberty onward.

EHLERS–DANLOS SYNDROME

Introduction

The syndrome is named after two doctors, Edverd Ehlers of Denmark and Henri Alexander Danlos of France. Ehlers–Danlos syndrome (EDS) is characterized by hyperelasticity of the skin and hypermobility of joints.

Epidemiology

Incidence: 1 in 5,000 births

Race: Higher incidence in blacks

Sex: Affects both males and females of all racial and ethnic backgrounds

Types: The most commonly occurring type is the hypermobility type, followed by classical type. The other types of EDS are very rare (Table 2).

Etiology

- Ehlers–Danlos syndromes are a group of inheritable connective tissue disorders. There are problems of collagen formation and affect the musculoskeletal system, either by bone weakness (osteogenesis imperfecta) or soft tissue weakness (Marfan's, homocystinuria, EDS, etc.)
- In EDS, there appear to be disorganization of the cross linkages due to reduction of the enzymes lysyl hydroxylase.

TABLE 2: Different types of EDS, their clinical features and associated defects.

Type	*Typical features*	*Inheritance*	*Gene defect*	*Protein defect*
Classic (EDS1-Severe and EDS2-MILD)	Skin hyperextensibility and fragility, joint hypermobility tissue fragility manifested by widened atrophic scarring	AD AR	COL5A1 COL5A2 COL1A1 COL1A2	Collagen 5
Hypermobile (EDS3)	Joint hypermobility moderate skin involvement, absence of tissue fragility	AD	TNX	Tenascin
Vascular (EDS4)	Marked reduced life span due to spontaneous rupture of internal organs such as arteries and intestines	AD	COL3A1	Collagen 3
X-linked (EDS5)	Similar to classic type 2	XR	Unknown	Unknown
Ocular-scoliotic (EDS6)	Severe muscular hypotonia after birth, progressive kyphoscoliosis, rupture of eye globe and arteries	AR	PLOD1	Def. of procollagen lysine 5 dioxygenase activity
Arthrochalasia (EDS7)	Cong. b/l dislocation of hip, hypermobile joints, osteopenia	AD	COL1A1 COL1A2	Mutation that prevents cleavage of N pro- peptides
Periodontotic (EDS8)	Premature loss of permanent teeth	AD	Unknown	Unknown

(AD: autosomal dominant; AR: autosomal recessive; XR: X-linked recessive)

Clinical Features

- *Skin:* Skin changes vary from thin and velvety to skin, that is either dramatically hyperextensible, e.g. "rubber man syndrome" (Fig. 31) or easily torn or scared. Patients with classical EDS develop characteristic "cigarette paper scars" (Fig. 32).
- *Ligaments and joint changes:* Laxity and hypermobility of joints vary from mild to unreducible dislocations of hip and other large joints. In mild forms, patients learn to reduce dislocations by limiting physical activity (Figs. 33A to C).

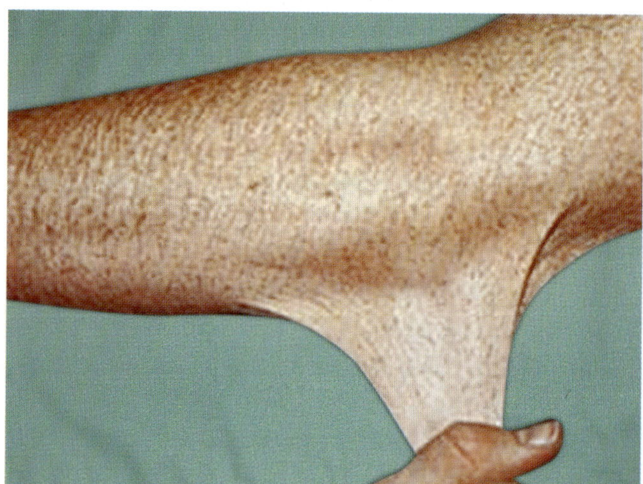

Fig. 31: Rubber man syndrome, with dramatically hyperextensible skin.

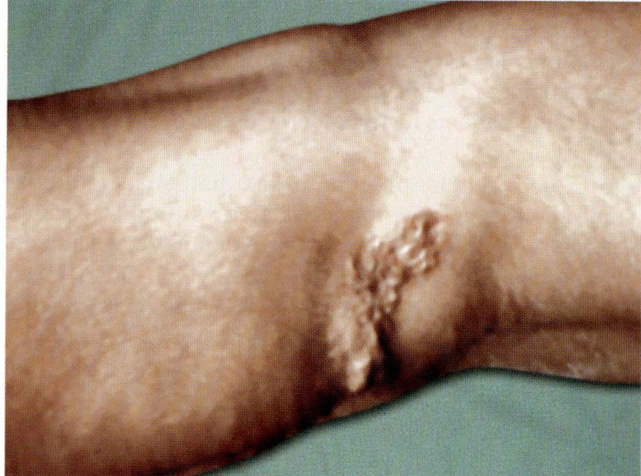

Fig. 32: Cigarette paper scars, as seen in patients with EDS.

Other Features

- Flat feet
- High and narrow palate, resulting in dental crowding
- Fragile blood vessels, resulting from cystic medial necrosis with tendency towards aneurysm
- Abnormal wound healing and scar formation
- Early onset of osteoarthritis
- Low muscle tones and muscle weakness
- Cardiac effects, like dysautonomia accompanied by valvular heart diseases, such as mitral valve prolapse
- Myalgia and arthralgia
- Osteopenia
- Congenital talipes equinovarus (CTEV), especially in the vascular type
- Deformities of the spine, such as scoliosis, kyphosis, occipitoatlantoaxial hypermobility, etc.
- Nerve compression disorders, e.g. carpal tunnel syndrome (CTS), acroparesthesia, neuropathy, etc.
- Raynaud's phenomenon
- Otosclerosis
- Functional bowel disorders
- Delayed development of motor skills, such as sitting, walking, and standing.

Diagnosis

- Based on clinical criteria, both DNA and biochemical studies can be used to help identify affected individual. In some cases, a skin biopsy has been found to be useful in confirming a diagnosis. Unfortunately, these tests are not sensitive enough to identify all individuals with EDS.
- If there are multiple affected individuals in a family, it may be possible to perform prenatal diagnosis using a DNA information technique known as linkage study.

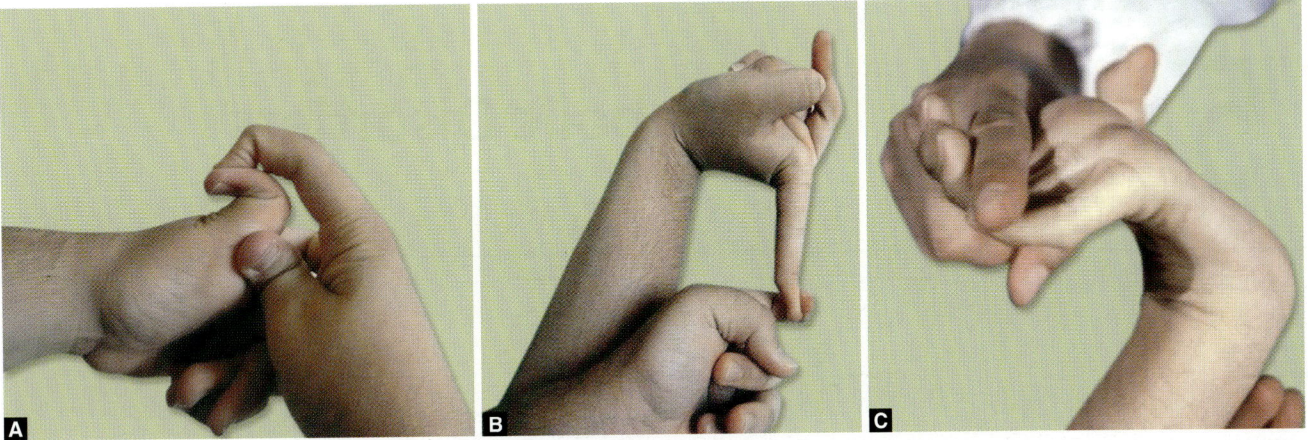

Figs. 33A to C: Excessive laxity and hypermobility of joints, seen in patients with EDS.

Differential Diagnosis

There are several disorders that have some of the characteristics of EDS:

- In cutis laxa the skin is loose, hanging, and wrinkled. In EDS, the skin can be pulled away from body, but is elastic and returns to normal when let go.
- In Marfan's syndrome, the joints are very mobile but skin elasticity not seen. In the past, Menkes disease a copper metabolism disorder was thought to be a form of EDS.

Treatment

- Surgical repair and tightening of joint ligaments require careful evaluations of individual patients, as the ligaments frequently do not hold sutures.
- Patients with easily prone to bruises, should be evaluated for bleeding disorders.
- Patients with type 4 EDS and members of families should be evaluated at regular intervals for detection of aneurysm.

Prognosis

- The outlook of individuals with EDS depends on the type of EDS, with which they have been diagnosed. Symptoms vary in severity, even within one subtype and the frequency of complications changes on individual basis.
- Some individuals have negligible symptoms, while others are severely restricted in their daily life. Those with blood vessels involvement have an increased risk of fatal complications.

CHAPTER

5 Metabolic Disorders

OBJECTIVES

- Osteoporosis
- Scurvy
- Rickets
- Renal Rickets
- Osteomalacia
- Ochronosis (Alkaptonuric Arthritis)
- Fluorosis
- Mucopolysaccharidoses
- Gaucher's Disease

OSTEOPOROSIS

Introduction

Osteoporosis is a bone disease, in which bone tissue is normally mineralized, but the amount of bone is decreased. The structural integrity of trabecular bone is impaired and cortical bone becomes more porous and thinner.

WHO Definition

It is a reduction in bone mass density (BMD), beyond a standard deviations value of "2" from the mean, for a given age, sex, and given site of the bone. It indicates weak bones, prone for getting fractured.

Risk Factors

Nonmodifiable

- Female sex
- Advanced age
- History of fractures
- Dementia.

Modifiable

- Smoking
- Alcoholism
- Low body weight
- Low calcium
- Estrogen deficiency
- Decreased physical activity.

Classification of Nordin (1964)

Generalized

- Primary
- Secondary.

Classification of Riggs and Melton (1988)

Primary Osteoporosis

Type 1:

- Postmenopausal 51–70 years
- Sex ratio of female:male = 5:2
- Mainly trabecular bone
- Vertebral fractures are more common
- Parathyroid hormone (PTH) decreased
- Calcium absorption decreased
- Cause is related to menopause.

Type 2:

- Senile
- *Age:* Greater than 70 years
- *Sex ratio:* Female to male ratio is 2:1
- Both cortical and trabecular bone
- Mainly fracture of neck of femur and intertrochanteric fractures
- PTH increased
- Calcium absorption decreased
- Cause related to aging.

Secondary Osteoporosis

Hormonal:

- Hypogonadism
- Hyperadrenocorticism
- Thyrotoxicosis
- Hyperprolactinemia
- Diabetes mellitus.

Nutritional:

- Calcium deficiency
- Malabsorption
- Malnutrition
- Alcoholism
- Scurvy
- Liver disease
- Vitamin D deficiency.

Drugs:

- Glucocorticoids
- Thyroxine excess
- Anticonvulsants
- Heparin
- Cytotoxic drugs
- Alcohol
- Lithium.

Metabolic diseases:
- Osteogenesis imperfecta
- Ehlers-Danlos syndrome
- Homocystinuria
- Marfan's syndrome.

Other causes:
- Multiple myeloma
- Rheumatoid arthritis
- Mastocytosis
- Thalassemia
- Pregnancy.

Localized Osteoporosis

- Disuse osteoporosis
- Sudecks osteodystrophy
- Transient osteoporosis
- Regional migratory osteoporosis
- Idiopathic chondrolysis of hip.

Clinical Features

- Low backache, usually mild
- Loss of height
- Thoracic kyphosis
- Fractures.

Chronic pain in osteoporosis is due to:
- Vertebral fracture
- Kyphosis and scoliosis, with stretching of ligaments
- Iliocoastal friction syndrome.

Physical Examination

- Careful measurement of height
- Detection of kyphosis
- Blue sclera, thin skin
- Hepatosplenomegaly (systemic disease)
- Skin pigmentation (Cushing's syndrome).

Differential Diagnosis

Differential diagnosis is shown in Table 1
- Hyperparathyroidism
- Paget's disease
- Osteomalacia
- Osteogenesis imperfecta
- Multiple myeloma
- Secondary tumors.

TABLE 1: Differential diagnosis of secondary osteoporosis.

	Ca	*PO_4*	*ALP*
Osteoporosis	N	N/decreased	N
Hyperparathyroidism	Increased	Decreased	Increased
Paget's	N/increased	N/decreased	Increased
Osteomalacia	N/decreased	Decreased	Increased
Osteogenesis imperfecta	N	N	N/increased
Multiple myeloma	N/increased	N/decreased	N

(N: normal; ALP: alkaline phosphatase; Ca: calcium; PO_4: phosphate)

Laboratory Investigations

- Blood routine examination
- Serum calcium
- Serum phosphorus
- 24 hours urine calcium
- Alkaline phosphatase (ALP)
- Increased serum calcium
  - Hyperparathyroidism
  - Malignancy
- Decreased serum calcium
  - Malnutrition
  - Osteomalacia
- If calcium level is increased, test PTH levels
- If increased, it indicates hyperparathyroidism
- If decreased, it indicates malignancy
- Increased levels of parathyroid hormone related protein (PTHP), leads to malignancy
- *Urine calcium:* If low, i.e. less than 50 mg/24 hours, causes osteomalacia, malnutrition and malabsorption
- *High urine calcium:* Greater than 300 mg/24 hours
- Causes
- Increased renal calcium leak
  - Males with osteoporosis
- Absorptive hypercalciuria
  - Idiopathic
  - Granulomatous disease
- Malignancy and diseases, with increased bone turnover
- Thyroid stimulating hormone (TSH): To rule out hyperthyroidism
- Urinary free cortisol, e.g. Cushing's disease
- Urine, Bence Jones proteins (myeloma).

Biochemical Markers

Bone Formation Markers

- Serum bone specific ALP
- Serum osteocalcin
- Serum probe peptide of type I procollagen.

Bone Resorption Markers

- Urine hydroxyprolene
- Serum tranexamic acid phosphatase
- Serum bone sialoprotein
- Urine and serum cross-linked biochemical markers
- Immunoassay of pyridinoline.

Uses of Biochemical Markers

- Monitoring response to treatment
- Resorption marker is used
- Measure 4–6 months prior and after starting the treatment.

X-ray

- Postmenopausal osteoporosis
- Trabecular resorption and cortical resorption
- Senile osteoporosis
- Endosteal resorption
- Hyperparathyroidism
- Subperiosteal resorption
- Osteoporosis produces, increased radiolucency of vertebral bone

- Approximately 30–80% of bone tissue must be lost, before a recognizable abnormality can be detected on spinal radiographs
- Lesions less than 2 cm, may escape detection.

Vertebral Osteoporosis (Fig. 1)

- Cod fish vertebra
- Kyphosis
- Fractures
- Kleer Koper score:
  - Grade 0: Normal
  - Grade I: Biconcave deformity
  - Grade II: Wedge deformity
  - Grade III: Compression deformity
- Assessed from lateral view of spine T4 to L5.

Bone Mass Density

Indications

- Estrogen deficient women are at risk of osteoporosis
- Vertebral abnormalities on X-ray
- Steroid treatment, greater than 3 mg and greater than 7.5 mg of prednisone
- Primary hyperparathyroidism
- Monitoring response to treatment.

Histological Method

It is given by Beck and Nordin.

- Sample is taken from iliac crest biopsy
- Scoring is based on amount of bone present per unit area of biopsy sample. This is illustrated in Table 2.

Management

Prophylaxis

- Calcium: 1–1.5 g/day
- Vitamin D: 400–800 IU/day
- Weight-bearing and gravity resistant exercises
- Avoid alcohol, cigarette
- Moderate phosphate intake
- Prophylactic agents
  - Alendronate (5 mg)
  - Raloxifene (60 mg).

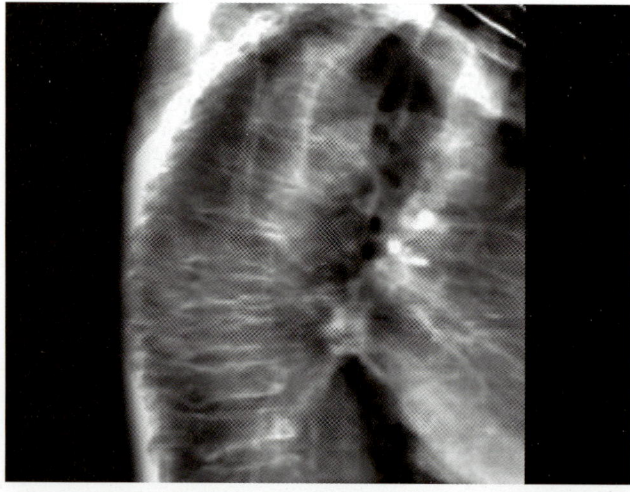

Fig. 1: X-ray, showing vertebral osteoporosis.

Antiresorptive Agents

- *Hormone replacement therapy (HRT):* Estrogen and progesterone.
- Bisphosphonates, e.g. etidronate, alendronate, pamidronate, zoledronate, etc.
- Calcitonin.
- Tibolone.

Hormone Replacement Therapy

- *Dose:* 0.625 mg/day
- *Duration:* At least 5 years, to reduce risk of fractures
- *Timing:* Start HRT at perimenopause, for at least 5 years and start at late 60s.

Bisphosphonate

Mechanism of Action

They bind to the surface of hydroxyapatite crystals and inhibit its resorption and digestion of bone by osteoclast.

Example: Alendronate

- *Dose:* 10 mg/day
- *Side effects*
  - Gastrointestinal intolerance
  - Esophagitis
  - Bone pain.

Selective Estrogen Receptor Modulators

Raloxifene

- *Dose:* 60 mg/day.
- Reduces the occurrence of vertebral fracture by 30–50%.
- Not associated with increasing risk of uterine cancer or benign uterine disease.

Tamoxifene

Calcitonin

- *Dose:* Nasal spray, containing 200 IU/day
- Not for prevention of osteoporosis
- Analgesic affects on bone pain
- *Mechanism of action:* Inhibit osteoclast activity by direct action on osteoclast calcitonin receptor
- Action on cortical bone is doubtful.

TABLE 2: Histological scoring (Beck and Nordin), based on the amount of bone present per unit area of bone biopsy sample.

Score assigned	*Bone percentage per unit area of biopsy sample*
Score 1	6%
Score 2	9%
Score 3	12%
Score 4	14%
Score 5	16%
Score 6	18%
Score 7	21%
Score 8	24%
Score 9	27%

(Normally score >5)

Orthopedic Management

Prophylactic Measures

- Avoid lifting heavy weight
- Avoid lifting weight in forward bending position
- Pectoral stretching, deep breathing and back extension exercises
- Avoid kyphotic posturing
- Low healed soft shoes and walking aids.

Rehabilitation in Established Osteoporosis

- Improve posture
- Relieve pain
- Activity and ambulation
- Low self-esteem and depression have to be treated.

Treatment

- Improve posturing
- Superficial heat, like infrared therapy
- If pain persists, penetrating heat, like ultrasound or shortwave diathermy
- If pain still persists, rule out malignancy
- Back strengthening extension exercises.

Types of Osteoporosis

Steroid Induced Osteoporosis

- Most common cause, therapeutic dose
- Depends on dose and duration of treatment
- Bone loss is more, during early months of treatment
- Trabecular bone severely involved.

Mechanism of Action

- Inhibit osteoblast
- Increase resorption
- Decrease calcium absorption from gastrointestinal tract (GIT)
- Increase urinary calcium dose.

Prevention

- Use low dose
- Prefer topical and inhaled route
- Risk factor reduction.

Treatment

Bisphosphonates.

Idiopathic Osteoporosis

- Idiopathic juvenile osteoporosis, between 8 years and 14 years, abrupt appearance of bone pain, fracture after minimal trauma.
- *Causes*
  - Malabsorption of calcium
  - High urinary calcium loss.
- Vertebrae on X-ray
  - Regular biconcavity, with large disk space
- Usually self limited
- No response to vitamin D or calcium therapy.

Transient (Regional) Osteoporosis

- Rare
- Affects large joint
- Femoral head, most common site
- Young to middle age
- Male more than female
- In female
  - Left hip, most common site
  - In third trimester of pregnancy
- Resolve spontaneously in 4–6 months.

Regional Migratory Osteoporosis

- Mainly knee, ankle, foot are involved
- Males, affected more than females
- Between 30 and 50 years
- Involvement of each joint lasts 9 months
- Recurrence in other joints occurs successively or be separated by 2 years or more.

Indices of Osteoporosis

Bone Mineral Density

- Bone mineral density (BMD), a measure of bone density, reflecting the strength of bones, as represented by calcium content.
- Bone mineral density (BMD) is scored by two measures:
  - T-score
  - Z-score.

T-score

The T-score is a comparison of a patient's BMD, to that of a healthy 30-year-old, of the same sex and ethnicity. This value is used in postmenopausal women and men over aged 50 because it better predicts, risk of future fracture. The criteria of the WHO are:

- *Normal:* A T-score of 1.0 or higher
- *Osteopenic:* Less than 1.0 and greater than 2.5
- *Osteoporotic:* 2.5 or lower, meaning a bone density that is two and a half standard deviations below the mean of a 30-year-old woman.

Z-score

The Z-score is the number of standard deviations; a patient's BMD differs from the average BMD of their age, sex, and ethnicity. This value is used in premenopausal women, men under the age of 50 and in children.

Spinal Deformity Index

- The spinal deformity index (SDI), described by Minne, et al. and Genant, et al. is an assessment tool that integrates both number and severity of fractures, by summing the vertebral fracture grades along the spine from T4 to L4.
- Lateral radiographs of the spine should be taken.
- Assessment of each vertebra from T4 to L4 should be performed.
- Grading scale is as follows:
  - Grade 0: Normal
  - Grade I: Mild (a decrease in a height of a vertebra of 20–25%)
  - Grade II: Moderate (a decrease of 25–40%)
  - Grade III: Severe (a decrease of 40% or more) fracture.
- A spinal deformity index (SDI) is calculated, by adding the grade of each vertebra from T4 to L4.
- The SDI value can vary between zero (no fracture) to 39 (all the assessed vertebrae are grade 3).
- SDI is a good predictor of incident vertebral fractures.
- Patients with highest SDI should receive highest priority to treatment.

Strength Index

- Reflection of both bone mass and structural architecture.
- Calculated as section modulus × bone mineral, apparent density.
- Section modulus is an estimate of the ability of distal radius to withstand bending forces.
- Bone mineral (BM) apparent density is tissue mineral content or cortical area.
- Low calculated strength index (STI) and section modulus is a more accurate predictor of fracture risk than BMD.
- SI, which reflects both bone density and bone size, appears to predict the risk of future fragility-related fractures (at distal radius).
- Femur strength index (FSTI), predicts hip fracture, independent of bone density, and hip axis length.
- Femur strength index (FSTI), calculated as the ratio of estimated compressive yield strength of the femoral neck to the expected compressive stress of a fall, on the greater trochanter.

Hip Axis Length (Fig. 2)

- Hip axis length (HAL) has been reported to be an independent predictor of hip fracture.
- HAL provides the length of hip axis and the variance from the expected values, based on that patient's height. Every standard deviation (SD) above the average length or expected length represents a 1.8 fold higher risk for hip fracture.

Stiffness Index

- Ultrasonographic stiffness index of calcaneum, is a noninvasive indicator of osteoporosis
- Different stiffness index (SI) values and risk of accompanied osteoporosis are illustrated in Table 3.

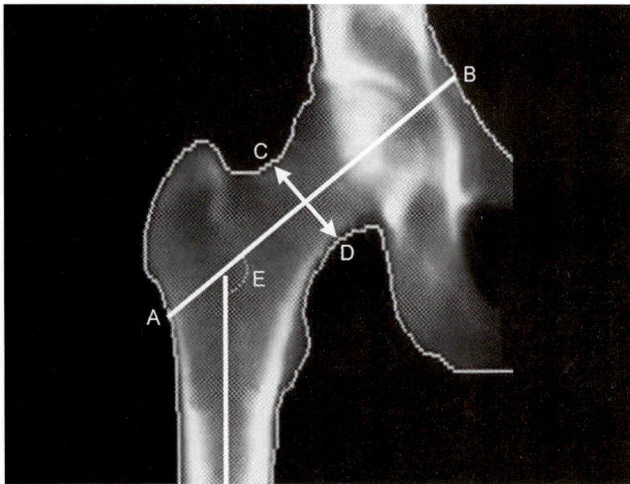

Fig. 2: Line AB, represents the HAL (see the chapter), line CD represents femoral neck diameter, and E is the neck-shaft angle.

TABLE 3: Stiffness index values and its interpretations.

Value of SI	*Interpretation*
<57%	High risk of having osteoporosis
57–77%	Moderate risk of having osteoporosis
>78%	Low risk of having osteoporosis

- *Stiffness index is calculated using the following formula:* Stiffness index = broadband ultrasound attenuation (BUA) + speed of sound (SOS).

Singh Index

- The Singh index, which describes trabecular patterns in the proximal femur, has been used as a predictor for hip fractures and as an indicator of osteopenia.
- *Grading*

  Grade VI: All normal trabecular groups are visible. Upper end of femur seems to be completely occupied by cancellous bone.

  Grade V: Principal tensile and principal compressive trabeculae are accentuated. Ward's triangle appears prominent.

  Grade IV: Principal tensile trabeculae are markedly reduced, but can still be traced from lateral cortex to upper part of the femoral neck.

  Grade III: There is a break in the continuity of the principal tensile trabeculae, opposite the greater trochanter. This grade indicates definite osteoporosis.

  Grade II: Only principal compressive trabeculae stand out prominently, remaining trabeculae have been essentially absorbed.

  Grade I: Principal compressive trabeculae are markedly reduced in number and are no longer prominent.

SCURVY

Definition

It is a nutritional disorder, caused by deficiency of vitamin C (ascorbic acid) and is characterized clinically, by a generalized hemorrhagic tendency.

Daily recommended intake:

- 0 to 1 year: 35 mg
- 1 year to adults: 40 mg.

Etiology

- Most frequent between 5 and 10 months, in artificially fed children.
- Vitamin C deficient diet (especially in old age, with restricted diet).
- When seen with rickets, it is called Barton's disease.

Pathology

- Inability to form normal intercellular collagen and organic bone matrix.
- Hemorrhagic tendency due to fragility of capillary walls due to poor intercellular cement substance.
- *Sites include:*
  - Extra skeletal sites are gums, intestine, conjunctiva, skin, bladder, and kidney.
  - Skeletal sites are subperiosteal and marrow bleeding, particularly in metaphysis and especially, adjacent to actively growing epiphysis.
  - Within bone, subperiosteal hemorrhage is characteristic, with ballooning of periostium resembling tumor.
- *Later it can get:*
  - Completely resorbed
  - Replaced by fibrous tissue
  - Ossified, forming fine periosteal trabeculations.

- Hemorrhage, within metaphysis near metaphysioepiphyseal junction, can interfere with in-growth of osteoblasts into calcified cartilage, resulting in failure of conversion of calcified cartilage into ossified bone.
- So, excess of calcified cartilage accumulates and appears as a characteristic dense line on X-ray known as "White Line of Fraenkel".
- Metaphysis in response to hemorrhage, undergoes hyperemia causing increased resorption of bone, forming dark zone of radiolucency (*Scurvy line*), adjacent to Fraenkel's line.
- In epiphysis, a zone of calcified cartilage is formed, encircling the bony centrum, which is known as "Wimberger's line".
- Weakening of epiphysiometaphyseal junction can occur, which can lead to fractures and complete/incomplete epiphyseal separation.
- Hemorrhage in medullary cavity, undergoes fibrous organization and replacement of hematopoietic tissue. This causes secondary anemia.
- Fractures can easily occur, through metaphysis in children and diaphysis in adults.
- Osteoporosis of alveolar bone can cause loosening of teeth.

Clinical Features

Infants

- Irritable, restless, night cries, pale, and febrile.
- Extremities are held immobile, due to muscular spasm (pseudoparalysis). Any attempt to move the limbs, causes the child to cry.
- Subperiosteal hemorrhages are caused, forming palpable and soft, extremely tender swelling, fixed to bone.
- Gums are bluish, swollen, tender, and bleeds on touch.
- Petechial or ecchymosis hemorrhage in skin and mucous membrane.
- Hematemesis or hemoptysis may develop.
- Epiphyseal separation in lower end of femur, upper end of tibia, and upper humerus.
- *Scorbutic rosary:* Due to costochondral separation.
- Severe cases, show anorexia, weight loss, anemia, hyperpyrexia, pneumonia, and even death.

Adults

- Petechiae in skin and conjunctiva
- Bleeding gums, with bluish discoloration
- Alveolar loose teeth
- Anorexia and weight loss
- Pain and tenderness, over bony structures
- A fracture, with minimal trauma is suggestive.

Diagnosis

Laboratory

Serum ascorbic acid level, less than 0.5 mg/dL (Normal 0.7–1.2 mg/dL).

Radiologically

- White line of Fraenkel
- Scurvy line (also called Trummerfeld's zone of rarefaction)
- *Pelkan spur:* A small bony spur, protruding from lateral or medial border of epiphysiometaphysis junction
- Ground glass translucency of bones, due to generalized osteoporosis
- *Pencilling of cortex:* Cortex is thinned out, leaving out a mere pencil streak
- *Wimberger's line:* Epiphysis is outlined, as a rim standing out against a rarefied body, with pencilling
- Epiphyseal separation or fracture
- Ribs, show subluxation at costochondral junction (scorbutic rosary)
- Large subperiosteal hematomas produce regional increase in soft tissue density. Calcification of hematoma occurs later, appearing as a shell enveloping the shaft
- Fissuring and fracture above calcified cartilage, in the metaphysis is common. Diaphyseal fractures are less common.

Differential Diagnosis

- Rickets
- Osteomalacia
- Acute osteomyelitis
- Osteogenesis imperfecta
- Septic arthritis
- Pseudoparalysis, may resemble poliomyelitis
- Other bleeding disorders.

Treatment

- Ascorbic acid tablets 500–1,000 mg, daily for 1 week.
- Vitamin C rich foods (citrus fruits, e.g. orange, lemon, etc.).
- Immobilization of fracture and painful joints with plaster splints.

RICKETS

Introduction

It is a metabolic disease of childhood, in which the osteoid, the organic matrix of bone fails to mineralize, due to interference with calcification mechanism. It commonly occurs between 6 months and 2 years.

Causes

Four main causes are:

- Vitamin D deficiency
- Reduced dietary intake
- Reduced amount of sunlight
- Pigmented skin

Other Causes

Malabsorption

It occurs due to:

- Celiac disease
- Hepatic osteodystrophy.

Renal disease

- Glomerular failure
- Renal osteodystrophy.

Antiepileptic drugs

They favor the formation of hepatic enzyme, which prevents conversion of calciferol.

Types of Rickets

Fetal Rickets

Children born to osteomalacic mother.

Infantile Rickets (Nutritional Rickets)

Most common form seen between 6 months and 3 years. Rarely seen before 6 months of age.

Late Rickets or Rachitic Tarda

Late onset rickets, familial, vitamin D resistant rickets.

Clinical Features

Symptoms

- Complains of bone pain during rest.
- Excessive perspiration in upper half of the body
- Weakness of proximal muscle of the lower limb produces waddling gait
- Irritability of central nervous system produces convulsion, laryngismus, spasmophilia, Chovsteck's sign, opisthotonos, etc.

Signs

Different body parts show following signs:

Skull
- Broadened forehead
- Skull square (caput quadratum)
- Frontal and parietal bossing
- Craniotabes is ping pong sensation on compressing the membranous bone of the skull.

Chest
- Pigeon chest due to prominent sternum
- Narrow chest
- Rickety rosary (enlargement of costocondral junction)
- Harrison's sulcus due to diaphragmatic pull on the soft ribs.

Abdomen
Protrubent abdomen (pot belly), develops due to weakness and hypotonia of muscles.

Spine
When the child starts sitting, he may develop kyphosis in thorax and lumbar spine scoliosis. Lordotic deformity, may develop when child starts walking.

Pelvis
Pelvic deformity with retardation of growth. Pelvic inlet is narrowed, by forward projection of promontory. Pelvic outlet is narrowed, by forward projection of caudal part of sacrum and coccyx. Changes become permanent in females, leading to obstetric problems.

Muscles: Lacking tone.

Extremities
- Epiphyseal enlargement of wrist and ankle
- Enlarged epiphysis can be seen or palpated, but cannot be seen on X-ray, as it consists of cartilage and uncalcified osteoid tissue
- Softened bones are vulnerable to bend and cause deformity like knock-knee or bow leg
- Decreased stature, giving rise to rachitic dwarfism.

Other features
Delayed dentition, deficient dental enamel, and secondary anemia, etc.

Laboratory Findings

- Calcium level is normal or deceased (due to compensatory hyperparathyroidism)
- Serum phosphorous is low
- Alkaline phosphates is normal
- Urinary calcium is low
- Serum 25-hydroxycholecalciferol is decreased.

Differential Diagnosis

- Acute poliomyelitis
- Congenital syphilis
- Septic arthritis
- Infantile scurvy.

Treatment

Prevention

- Adequate exposure of sunlight and consumption of milk and cheese.
- Daily requirement of vitamin D is 10 μg (400 IU).

Active Treatment

- Oral or parental administration of vitamin D is preferred, as follows:
  - *In active stage:* 15,000 μg (600,000 IU)
  - *In milder cases:* 50–150 μg (20,00–6,000 IU)
- Adequate intake of calcium is ensured
- It takes 2–4 weeks for X-ray healing.

RENAL RICKETS

Renal Osteodystrophy

This is the term given to the bone changes, which accompany chronic renal failure. The changes are due to a combination of hyperparathyroidism and osteitis fibrosa, osteomalacia, osteosclerosis, periosteal new bone formation, osteoporosis, and growth disturbances in children.

Clinical Features

- Children are always stunted in growth, often to a degree not equaled, by any other form of infantilism
- Less body weight
- May show infantilism and dwarfism
- Bone pain
- Muscle weakness
- Softening of bone causes skeletal deformity, like thoracic kyphosis and lumbar scoliosis
- Pruritus in skin, due to extraskeletal calcification
- Interstitial keratitis and conjunctivitis in eye.

Pathophysiology

Normal vitamin D metabolism is shown in Flowchart 1.

Abnormal Vitamin D Metabolism

- The major active metabolites of vitamin D is 1,25(OH) 2D3 (calcitriol) which is produced by 1- hydroxylation within the kidney.

Flowchart 1: Vitamin D metabolism.

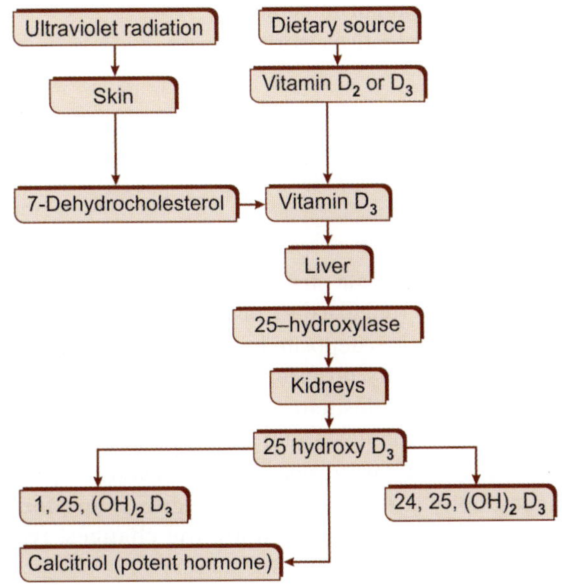

- Serum level of calcitriol is decreased when the glomerular filtration rate drops below 40 mL/min and is very low in end-stage renal failure.
- Lack of calcitriol leads to diminished intestinal calcium absorption, retardation of skeletal growth, and defective mineralization.
- A further vitamin D metabolite, 1-alpha, 25(OH)2D3 and 24R, $25(OH)_2D_3$ is also produced by the kidney. Low levels of this compound in renal failure may contribute to abnormalities of bone homeostasis.

Abnormal Calcium and Phosphate Metabolism

- In chronic renal failure (CRF), due to loss of renal tissue, the ability of body to excrete phosphate is diminished.
- Increased phosphate lowers the ionized serum calcium and tends to cause extraskeletal calcification, by raising the calcium and phosphate product.

Abnormal Parathyroid Hormone (PTH) Metabolism

- Pure hyperparathyroidism or fibro-osteoclasis is still the most common form of renal bone disease.
- Excretion of PTH degradation products is reduced in renal impairment.

Aluminum Toxicity

- Patients on dialysis accumulate a number of trace elements from the dialysis fluid
- Aluminum has been shown to be important in the pathogenesis of osteomalacia.

Pathological Changes in Kidneys

Kidney Lesions

- Kidney lesions occur, due to total renal insufficiency, as found in chronic glomerulonephritis, focal nephritis and congenital cystic disease, where there is reduced glomerular function, with failure to excrete phosphorus, as well as general uremia, and acidosis.
- The main skeletal change is an osteitis fibrosa, with little osteoid formation, either as rickets or as osteomalacia.

Tubular Insufficiency

- The resorption of phosphorus, amino acids, glucose, electrolytes, and water is impaired, particularly from the proximal convoluted tubules.
- If there is disease of the distal tubules, there is disturbance of potassium and creatinine secretion in the urine.
- There is marked disturbance in the general acid-base regulation of the body, by alteration in bicarbonate, ammonium, and hydrogen ions concentrations.

Syndromes Related to Renal Rickets

Snapper and Nathan (1957) reviewed the renal lesions and gave rise to the following syndromes:

Lignac–Fanconi Syndrome

- In this syndrome, there is proximal tubular deficiency, with polydipsia, polyuria, anorexia, and vomiting.
- The children exhibits rickets and dwarfism and usually die before puberty.
- Hyperphosphaturia, with a low serum phosphate level, but normal calcium level.
- Massive dosage of vitamin D, may improve skeletal disorder.

Renal or Hyperchloremic Acidosis

- Primary defect is in the distal tubules, which fails to resorb water and to secrete ammonium.
- Excrete large amount of sodium, potassium, and calcium.
- Marked disturbances in acid-base mechanism.
- Skeletal changes of either osteitis fibrosa or rickets are caused by excessive mobilization of calcium, from bone.
- Condition can be improved, by administering excessive alkalizing salts, ammonium, or calcium chlorides, and vitamin D.

Characteristics of Different Types of Rickets

Various characteristics of different types of rickets are illustrated in Table 4.

Treatment

- Ingested phosphate load is reduced by administration of oral phosphate binding compounds.
- *Active treatment:* Oral or parental administration of vitamin D is preferred.
  - *In active stage:* 15,000 µg (600,000 IU)
  - *In milder cases:* 50–150 µg (2,000–6,000 IU)
- Adequate intake of calcium is ensured.
- Parathyroidectomy.
- Renal transplantation.

OSTEOMALACIA

Definition

It is an adult counterpart of rickets characterized by failure of mineralization and an excess of osteoid due to interference of calcium metabolism.

Etiology

- Decreased vitamin D absorption from intestine
- Derangement of vitamin D and phosphorous metabolism.

TABLE 4: Characteristic features of different types of rickets.

Vitamin-D	*Renal deficiency*	*Renal tubular*	*Renal glomerula*
Family history	–	+	–
Myopathy	+	–	+
Growth defect	±	++	++
Serum			
Ca		N	
P			
Alkaline phosphate			
Urine			
Ca			
P			
Osteitis fibrosa	±	+	++
Other	Dietary deficiency or malabsorption	Aminoaciduria	Renal failure anemia

Clinical Features

- Generalized skeletal pain and muscle weakness
- Acute pain due to fracture
- Other symptoms may be related to causative factor like GIT, renal, dietary
- Deformities like scoliosis, khyphosis, coxa vara, protrusion of acetabula, trefoil pelvis, knock knee, etc. are encountered.

Radiological Features

- Reveals generalized demineralization of bone
- Loss of transverse trabeculae
- No subperiosteal resorption of bone
- Presence of losers line are characteristic of osteomalacia.

Looser's line: Also called as pseudofracture, Milkman's line. Fracture heals by defective callus. Sometimes only an evidence of osteomalacia is left in treated cases.

- Common sites are axillary border of scapula, ramus of pubis or ischium, neck of femur, ribs
- *Spine:* The bodies of spine are biconcave codfish spine
- Hip shows protrusio acetabuli and triradiate pelvis.

Laboratory Findings

- Serum calcium is normal or increased
- Serum phosphatase is normal or increased
- ALP is increased
- Serum PTH is increased.

Treatment

- Calcium is given at 0.5–3 g/day
- Vitamin D 10,000 IU/day
- High protein diet.

OCHRONOSIS (ALKAPTONURIC ARTHRITIS)

- Homogentisic acid is an aromatic acid, formed from incomplete breakdown of the amino acids tyrosine and phenylalanine in the body.
- It has affinity for certain tissues, particularly cartilages, which becomes brittle and disintegrates.
- Secondary degenerative arthritis ensues.

Etiology

- Congenital and inherited, as a Mendelian recessive tract
- Occurs in the offsprings of consanguineous parents.

Pathology

- Homogentisic acid is a strong reducing agent, which when oxidized is converted to a dark pigment.
- Tissues in which it is deposited are sclera, ligaments, tendons and cartilages of ears, nose, joints, and intervertebral disk.
- Cartilage loses its elasticity, becomes brittle, and has poor resistance to mechanical strain.
- Cracks easily and is worn away by friction and compression.
- Exposed bony surfaces, undergo sclerosis, and formation of marginal exostoses, which are the changes, typical of degenerative arthritis.
- Intervertebral disks, particularly in lumbar area, degenerate and calcify.
- Disk space decreases and opposing surface of vertebral bodies become irregular sclerotic.

Clinical Features

First Phase: Simple Alkaptonuria

Child passes urine, which on exposure to air turns black.

Second Phase: Ochronosis

Deposit of ochre. Colored deposits in bone, cartilage, tendon sheath, pinna of ear. Sclera slate colored patches.

Third Phase

Alkaptonuric arthritis patient develops, generalized pain, and stiffening of spine, peripheral joints, like hip and knee. Perspirations stain the clothing.

X-ray Findings

- Disks appear eliptical, thin and, calcified wafer like
- Opposing vertebral bodies are sclerotic and spurred
- Evidence of degenerative arthritis is seen in large joints.

Laboratory Findings

- Homogentisic acid is a strong reducing agent that is oxidized on exposure to air and turns the urine black.
- Heating or addition of alkali, fasten the reaction.
- Cooper solution (Benedict's or Fehling's) is reduced.
- Fermentation tests are negative.
- Diagnostic test is the bluish-green coloration, produced by the addition of a drop of dilute ferric chloride solution to urine.

Treatment

Reduction of intake of food, containing tyrosine and phenylalanine plus administration of high dosage of vitamin C will reduce excretion of homogentisic acid, but have no effect on progression of the disease.

FLUOROSIS

Fluorine in very low concentration, 1 part per million (ppm) or less, has been used to reduce the incidence of dental caries. At slightly higher levels (2–4 ppm) it may produce mottling of the teeth. It is a condition, which is fairly common in those parts of the world, where fluorine appears in the soil and drinking water. In some areas, notably parts of India and Africa, where fluorine concentrations in the drinking water may be above 10 ppm, chronic fluorine intoxication (fluorosis) is endemic and widespread skeletal abnormalities are occasionally encountered in the affected population. Mild bone changes are also sometimes seen in patients, treated with sodium fluoride for osteoporosis.

Fluorine directly stimulates osteoblastic activity, fluoroapatite crystals are laid down in bone and these are unusually resistant to osteoclastic resorption. Other effects are thought to be due to calcium retention, impaired mineralization, and secondary hyperparathyroidism. The characteristic pathological features in severe cases are subperiosteal new bone accretion and osteosclerosis, most marked in the vertebrae, ribs, pelvis, and the forearm and leg bones, together with hyperostosis at the bony attachments of ligaments, tendons, and fascia in these areas. Despite the apparent thickening and density of the skeleton, tensile strength is reduced and the bone fractures occur more easily, under bending and twisting loads.

Patients complain of backache, bone pain, and joint stiffness. Examination may show thickening of the tubular bones. Sometimes, the first clinical manifestation is a stress fracture. In the worst cases, there may be deformities of the spine and lower limbs, hyperostosis can lead to vertebral canal encroachment, and resultant neurological defects.

The typical X-ray features are osteosclerosis, osteophytosis, and ossification of ligamentous and facial attachments. Changes are most marked in the spine and pelvis, where the bones become densely opaque.

In full blown cases, the diagnosis should be obvious, but the rarity of the condition leads to it being overlooked. X-ray features at individual sites can be mistaken for those of Paget's disease, idiopathic skeletal hyperostosis, renal osteodystrophy, or osteopetrosis.

There is no specific treatment for this condition. After exposure ceases, it still takes years for bone fluoride to be excreted. If there is evidence of osteomalacia and secondary hyperparathyroidism, this can be treated with calcium and vitamin D.

MUCOPOLYSACCHARIDOSES

Introduction

- Mucopolysaccharidoses are a group of metabolic disorders, caused by an absence or malfunctioning of lysosomal enzymes, needed to breakdown molecules called glycosaminoglycans, long chains of sugar carbohydrates, in each of our cells that help to build bone, cartilage, tendons, corneas, skin, and connective tissues. Glycosaminoglycans (formerly called mucopolysaccharides) are also found in the fluid that lubricates our joints.
- People with a mucopolysaccharidosis (MPS) disease either do not produce enough of one of the eleven enzymes, required to break down these sugar chains into simpler molecules or they produce enzymes that do not work properly.
- Over time, these glycosaminoglycans collect in the cells, blood, and connective tissues. The result is permanent, progressive cellular damage, which affects appearance, physical abilities, organ, and system functioning and in most cases, mental development.
- The mucopolysaccharidoses are part of the lysosomal storage disease family.
- Affects 1 in 25,000 babies.
- It is an autosomal recessive disorder, except MPS II, which shows X- linked recessive inheritance.

Clinical Features

- The clinical features may not be apparent at birth, but may appear later, as storage of glycosaminoglycans affects bone, skeletal structure, connective tissues, and organs.
- Neurological complications may include damage to neurons, as well as pain and impaired motor function, resulting from compression of nerves or nerve roots in the spinal cord or in the peripheral nervous system.
- Depending on the MPS subtype, affected individuals may have normal intellect or profoundly retarded, may experience developmental delay or may have severe behavioral problems.
- Many individuals have hearing loss, either conductive, neurosensitive, or both.
- Communicating hydrocephalus is common in some of the mucopolysaccharidoses.
- The cornea often becomes cloudy from intracellular storage and glaucoma, along with degeneration of the retina, which also may affect the patient's vision.
- Physical symptoms generally include:
  - Coarse or rough facial features (including a flat nasal bridge, thick lips, and enlarged mouth and tongue).
  - Short stature with disproportionately short trunk (dwarfism), dysplasia (abnormal bone size and/or shape) and other skeletal irregularities.
  - Thickened skin.
  - Enlarged organs, such as liver (hepatomegaly) or spleen (splenomegaly).
  - Hernias.
  - Excessive body hair growth.
  - Short and often claw-like hands.
  - Progressive joint stiffness.
  - Carpal tunnel syndrome.
- Recurring respiratory infections are common.
- Many affected individuals also have heart disease.
- Another lysosomal storage disease, often confused with the mucopolysaccharidoses is mucolipidosis. In this disorder, excessive amounts of fatty materials (lipids) are stored, in addition to sugars. Persons with mucolipidosis may share some of the clinical features, associated with the mucopolysaccharidoses (certain facial features, bony structure abnormalities, and damage to the brain) and increased amounts of the enzymes, needed to break down the lipids are found in the blood.

Types

- There are seven distinct clinical types and numerous subtypes of the mucopolysaccharidoses that have been identified and are shown in Table 5.

TABLE 5: Types of mucopolysaccharides and associated symptoms.

Type	*Main disease*	*Deficient enzyme*	*Accumulated products*	*Symptoms*
MPS I	Hurler syndrome	-L-iduronidase	Heparan sulfate Dermatan sulfate	Mental retardation Micrognathia Coarse facies Macroglossia Retinal degeneration Corneal clouding Cardiomyopathy
MPS II	Hunter syndrome	Iduronate sulfatase	Heparan sulfate Dermatan sulfate	Mental retardation (similar, but milder, symptoms to Hurler syndrome is also X-linked recessive, as opposed to autosomal recessive)
MPS III	Sanfilippo syndrome A Sanfilippo syndrome B Sanfilippo syndrome C	Heparan sulfamidase N-acetylglucosaminidase Acetyl-CoA:alpha-glucosaminide acetyltransferase	Heparan sulfate	Developmental delay Severe hyperactivity Spasticity
	Sanfilippo syndrome D	N-acetylglucosamine 6-sulfatase		Motor dysfunction Death by the second decade
MPS IV	Morquio syndrome A	Galactose-6-sulfate sulfatase	Keratan sulfate Chondroitin 6-sulfate	Severe skeletal dysplasia
	Morquio syndrome B	-galactosidase	Keratan sulfate	Short stature, motor dysfunction
MPS VI	Maroteaux- Lamy syndrome	N-acetylgalactosamine-4-sulfatase	Dermatan sulfate	Severe skeletal dysplasia, Short stature, Motor dysfunction, Kyphosis, Heart defects
MPS VII	Sly syndrome	-glucuronidase	-glucuronidase	Hepatomegaly Skeletal dysplasia Short stature Corneal clouding Developmental delay
MPS IX	Natowicz syndrome	Hyaluronidase	Hyaluronic acid	Nodular soft-tissue masses around joints Episodes of painful swelling of the masses Short-term pain Mild facial changes Short stature Normal joint movement Normal intelligence

- Although each MPS differs clinically (Table 5), most patients generally experience a period of normal development, followed by a decline in physical and/or mental function.

MPS I

- MPS I is divided into three subtypes, based on severity of symptoms:
  - MPS I H
  - MPS I S
  - MPS I H-S
- All three types result from an absence of or insufficient levels of the enzyme, -L-iduronidase.
- Children born to an MPS I parent, carry the defective genes.

MPS I H

- Also called Hurler's syndrome or -L-iduronidase deficiency.
- It is the most severe of the MPS I subtypes.
- Developmental delay is evident by the end of the first year and patients usually stop developing between age of 2–4 years.
- This is followed by progressive mental decline and loss of physical skills.
- Language may be limited, due to hearing loss and an enlarged tongue.
- In time, the cornea became clouded and retina may begin to degenerate.
- Carpal tunnel syndrome and restricted joint movement are common.
- Affected children may be quite large at birth and appear normal, but may have inguinal or umbilical hernias.
- Many children develop a short body trunk and a maximum stature of less than 4 feet.
- Distinct facial features (including flat face, depressed nasal bridge and bulging forehead) become more evident in the second year.
- By age of 2 years, the ribs have widened and are oar-shaped.
- The liver, spleen, and heart are often enlarged.
- Children may experience noisy breathing and recurring upper respiratory tract and ear infections.
- Feeding may be difficult for some children and many experience periodic bowel problems.
- Children with Hurler's syndrome, often die before 10 years of age from obstructive airway disease, respiratory infections, and cardiac complications.

MPS I S (Scheie Syndrome)

- It is the mildest form of MPS I.
- Symptoms generally begin to appear after 5 years, with diagnosis most commonly made after age of 10 years.
- Children with Scheie syndrome have normal intelligence or may have mild learning disabilities, some may have psychiatric problems.

- Glaucoma, retinal degeneration, and clouded corneas may significantly lead to impaired vision.
- Other problems include Carpal tunnel syndrome or other nerve compression, stiff joints, claw hands and deformed feet, a short neck, and aortic valve disease.
- Some affected individuals also have obstructive airway disease and sleep apnea. Persons with Scheie syndrome can live into adulthood.

MPS I H-S (Hurler-Scheie Syndrome)

- It is less severe than Hurler's syndrome alone.
- Symptoms generally begin between 3 and 8 years.
- Children may have moderate mental retardation and learning difficulties.
- Skeletal and systemic irregularities include short stature, marked smallness in the jaws, progressive joint stiffness, compressed spinal cord, clouded corneas, hearing loss, heart disease, coarse facial features, and umbilical hernia.
- Respiratory problems, sleep apnea, and heart disease may develop in adolescence.
- Some persons with MPS I H-S need continuous positive airway pressure during sleep, to ease breathing.
- Life expectancy is generally into the late teens or early twenties.

MPS II

- MPS II, Hunter's Syndrome or iduronate sulfatase deficiency is caused by lack of the enzyme iduronate sulfatase.
- Hunter's syndrome has two clinical subtypes and (since, it shows X-linked recessive inheritance) is the only one of the mucopolysaccharidoses, in which the mother alone can pass the defective gene to a son.
- The incidence of Hunter's syndrome is estimated to be 1 in 100,000–150,000 male births.

MPS II A

- It is more severe form of Hunter's syndrome.
- Children share many of the same clinical features associated with Hurler syndrome (MPS I H), but with milder symptoms.
- Onset of the disease is usually between 2 and 4 years of age.
- Developmental decline is usually noticed in the ages of 18–36 months, followed by progressive loss of skills.
- Other clinical features include coarse facial features, skeletal irregularities, obstructive airway and respiratory complications, short stature, joint stiffness, retinal degeneration (but no corneal clouding), communicating hydrocephalus, chronic diarrhea, enlarged liver and spleen, and progressive hearing loss.
- Whitish skin lesions may be found on the upper arms, back, and upper legs.
- Death from upper airway disease or cardiovascular failure usually occurs by age of 15 years.

MPS II B

- Physical characteristics of MPS II B are less obvious and progress at a much slower rate.
- Diagnosis is often made in the second decade of life.
- Intellect and social development are not affected.
- Skeletal problems may be less severe, but Carpal tunnel syndrome and joint stiffness can restrict movement and height is somewhat less than normal.
- Other clinical symptoms include hearing loss, poor peripheral vision, diarrhea and sleep apnea, although respiratory and cardiac complications, can contribute to premature death. Persons with MPS II B may live into their 50s or beyond.

MPS III

- MPS III, Sanfilippo syndrome, is marked by severe neurological symptoms.
- These include progressive dementia, aggressive behavior, hyperactivity, seizures, some deafness and loss of vision, with an inability to sleep for more than a few hours at a time.
- This disorder tends to have three main stages:
  1. During the first stage, early mental and motor skill development may be somewhat delayed. Affected children show a marked decline in learning between 2 and 6 years, followed by eventual loss of language skills, and loss of some or all hearing. Some children may never learn to speak.
  2. In the second stage, aggressive behavior, hyperactivity, profound dementia, and irregular sleep, may make children difficult to manage, particularly those who retain normal physical strength.
  3. In the last stage, children become increasingly unsteady on their feet and most are unable to walk by age of 10 years.
- Thickened skin and mild changes in facial features, bone, and skeletal structures become noticeable with age.
- Growth in height usually stops by age of 10 years.
- Other problems may include, narrowing of the airway passage in the throat and enlargement of the tonsils and adenoids, making it difficult to eat or swallow. Recurring respiratory infections are common.
- There are four distinct types of Sanfilippo syndrome, each caused by alteration of a different enzyme, needed to completely breakdown the heparan sulfate sugar chain.
- Different types of MPS III syndromes are:
  1. *Sanfilippo A:* It is the most severe of the MPS III disorders and is caused by the missing or altered enzyme heparan N-sulfatase. Children with Sanfilippo A, have the shortest survival rate among those, with the MPS III disorders.
  2. *Sanfilippo B:* Caused by the missing or deficient enzyme, alpha-N-acetylglucosaminidase.
  3. *Sanfilippo C:* Results from the missing or altered enzyme acetyl-Ca alpha-glucosaminide acetyl- transferase.
  4. *Sanfilippo D:* This is caused by the missing or deficient enzyme, N-acetylglucosamine 6-sulfatase.
- Little clinical difference exists between these four types, but symptoms appear most severe and seem to progress more quickly in children with type A. The average duration of Sanfilippo syndrome is 8–10 years, following onset of symptoms. Most persons with MPS III live into their teenage years and some live even longer.
- The incidence of Sanfilippo syndrome (for all four types combined) is about one in 70,000 births.

MPS IV

- MPS IV, Morquio syndrome, is estimated to occur in 1 in 700,000 births.
- Its two subtypes result from the missing or deficient enzymes, N-acetylgalactosamine 6-sulfatase (Type A) or beta-

galactosidase (Type B) needed to break down the keratan sulfate sugar chain.
- Clinical features are similar in both types, but appear milder in Morquio type B.
- Onset is between age of 1 and 3 years.
- Neurological complications include spinal nerve and nerve root compression, resulting from extreme, progressive skeletal changes, particularly in the ribs and chest, conductive and/or neurosensitive loss of hearing and clouded corneas.
- Intelligence is normal, unless hydrocephalus develops and is not treated.
- Physical growth slows and often stops between 4 and 8 years.
- Skeletal abnormalities include a bell-shaped chest, a flattening or curvature of the spine, shortened long bones, along with dysplasia of the hips, knees, ankles, and wrists.
- The bones that stabilize the connection between the head and neck can be malformed (odontoid hypoplasia), in these cases, a surgical procedure called spinal cervical bone fusion, can be life-saving.
- Restricted breathing, joint stiffness, and heart diseases are also common.
- Children with more severe form of Morquio syndrome may not live beyond their twenties or thirties.

MPS VI

- Children with MPS VI, Maroteaux-Lamy syndrome, usually have normal intellectual development, but share many of the physical symptoms found in Hurler's syndrome.
- It is caused by the deficient enzyme N-acetylgalactosa-mine 4-sulfatase and Maroteaux-Lamy syndrome, has a variable spectrum of severe symptoms.
- Neurological complications include clouded corneas, deafness, thickening of the dura, and pain caused by compressed or traumatized nerves and nerve roots.
- Growth is normal at first, but stops suddenly around 8 years.
- By age of 10 years, children have developed a shortened trunk, crouched stance, and restricted joint movement.
- In more severe cases, children also develop a protruding abdomen and forward curving spine.
- Skeletal changes (particularly in the pelvic region) are progressive and limit movement.
- Many children also have umbilical or inguinal hernias.
- Nearly, all children have some form of heart disease, usually involving valve dysfunction.
- An enzyme replacement therapy was tested on patients with MPS VI and was successful in that it improved growth and joint movement.

MPS VII

- MPS VII, Sly syndrome, one of the least common forms of the mucopolysaccharidoses, is estimated to occur in less than 1 in 250,000 births.
- The disorder is caused by deficiency of the enzyme beta-glucuronidase.
- In its rarest form, Sly syndrome causes children to be born with hydrops fetalis, in which extreme amounts of fluid are retained in the body.
- Survival is usually a few months or less.
- Most children, with Sly syndrome are less severely affected.
- Neurological symptoms may include mild to moderate mental retardation by 3 years of age, communicating hydrocephalus, nerve entrapment, corneal clouding, and some loss of peripheral and night vision.
- Other symptoms include short stature, some skeletal irregularities, joint stiffness, and restricted movement, with umbilical and/or inguinal hernias.
- Some patients may have repeated bouts of pneumonia during their first years of life.
- Most children with Sly syndrome live into the teenage or young adult years.

MPS IX

- As of 2001, only one case of MPS IX, Natowicz syndrome or online Mendelian inheritance in man (OMIM), had been reported.
- The disorder results from hyaluronidase deficiency.
- Symptoms include nodular soft tissue masses located around joints, with episodes of painful swelling of the masses and pain that ended spontaneously within 3 days.
- Pelvic radiography, showed multiple soft tissue masses and some bone erosion. Other traits included mild facial changes, acquired short stature, as seen in other MPS disorders, and normal joint movement and intelligence.

Diagnosis

- By clinical examination
- Urine tests (excess mucopolysaccharides are excreted in the urine)
- Enzyme assays
- Prenatal diagnosis, using amniocentesis and chorionic villus sampling, can verify if a fetus either carries a copy of the defective gene, or is affected with the disorder
- Genetic counseling can help parents, who have a family history of the mucopolysaccharidoses, determine if they are carrying the mutated gene that causes the disorders.

Treatment

- Currently, there is no cure for these disorders.
- Medical care is directed at treating systemic conditions and improving the person's life quality.
- Physical therapy and daily exercise may delay joint problems and improve the ability to move.
- Changes to the diet will not prevent disease progression, but limiting milk, sugar, and dairy products, has helped some individuals experiencing excessive mucus.
- Surgery to remove tonsils and adenoids may improve breathing among affected individuals, with obstructive airway disorders and sleep apnea. Some patients may require surgical insertion of an endotracheal tube to aid breathing.
- Surgery can also correct hernias, help to drain excessive cerebrospinal fluid from the brain and free nerves and nerve roots compressed by skeletal and other abnormalities.
- Corneal transplants may improve vision among patients, with significant corneal clouding.
- Enzyme replacement therapy (ERT) is currently being tested. Enzyme replacement therapy has proven useful, in reducing non-neurological symptoms and pain.

- Bone marrow transplantation (BMT) and umbilical cord blood transplantation (UCBT) have had limited success in treating the mucopolysaccharidoses. Abnormal physical characteristics, except for those affecting the skeleton and eyes, may be improved, but neurological outcomes have varied. BMT and UCBT are high-risk procedures and are usually performed only after family members receive extensive evaluation and counseling.

GAUCHER'S DISEASE

The genetic disorder, first described by Gaucher over 100 years ago is now known to be caused by lack of a specific enzyme, which is responsible for the breakdown and the excretion of the cell membrane products from defunct cells. This is a classical example of a lipid storage disease, for which the pathogenesis has been painstakingly worked out, leading to the development of an effective treatment.

Each time one of the cells in the body dies, a glucocerebroside is released from the cell membrane. Before it can be excreted, the glucoside bond holding the glucose molecule, has to be split by a specific enzyme, glucosylceramide beta-glucosidase. If this enzyme is lacking, the glucocerebroside cannot be excreted and instead is stored in the lysosomal bodies of macrophage of reticuloendothelial system, notably in the marrow, spleen, and liver. Accumulation of these abnormal macrophage leads to enlargement of the spleen and liver, along with secondary changes in the marrow and bone.

Most patients suffer from a chronic form of disorder, with changes predominantly in the marrow, bone, and spleen and varying degree of pancytopenia (Type I). A rare form of the disease affecting central nervous system (Type II) appears in infancy and usually causes death within a year. Type III is a subacute disorder, characterized by the appearance of hepatosplenomegaly in childhood and skeletal and neurological abnormalities during adolescence.

Like other storage disorders, Gaucher's disease is transmitted as an autosomal recessive trait. Males and females are affected equally with relative high incidence in Jewish people of Ashkenazi descent. The phenotype is associated with a large number of different gene defects, five of which appear in the majority of cases.

Clinical Features

In the most common form of disease (Type 1), patients present in the childhood or adult life with anemia, thrombocytopenia, and hepatosplenomegaly or bone pain, about two-thirds of affected people develop skeletal abnormalities. Older patients may develop back pain due to vertebral osteopenia and compression fractures. Femur neck fractures also are not uncommon, however diaphyseal fractures are rare. The hematocrit and platelet counts are usually diminished. A suggestive finding (when positive) is elevation of serum acid phosphatase level. The diagnosis can be confirmed by demonstrating low glucocerebrosidase activity in blood or by identifying abnormal gene mutations in DNA tests.

A common complication is osteonecrosis, usually of femoral head, but sometimes in the femoral condyles, the proximal head of humerus or the bones around the ankle. The patients (usually a child or adolescent) may present with an acute bone crisis, with unrelenting pain, local tenderness, and restriction of movement, accompanied by pyrexia, leukocytosis, and elevated erythrocyte sedimentation rate (ESR). The clinical features resemble, those of osteomyelitis or septic arthritis, indeed Gaucher's disease predisposes to bone infection and this may be a source of confusion.

Imaging

X-rays show a variable pattern of radiolucency or patchy density, more marked in cancellous bone. The distal end of femur may be expanded, producing Erlenmeyer flask appearance. A skeletal survey, may lead to reversal of osteonecrosis of femoral head, femoral condyles, talus, or humeral head.

A radioisotope bone scan may help to distinguish a crisis episode from infection, the former is usually "Cold" and the latter is "Hot". MRI is the most reliable way of defining marrow involvement.

Treatment

Bone pain may need symptomatic treatment. For the acute crisis analgesic medication and bed rest are followed by nonweight-bearing walking with crutches. Specific therapy, is now available (albeit costly) in the form of replacement enzyme, alglucerase. This has been shown to reverse the blood changes and reduce the size of the liver and the spleen. The bone complications also are diminished.

Osteonecrosis of the femoral head, usually result in progressive deformity of the hip. However, most patients manage quite well with symptomatic treatment and surgery should be deferred for as long as possible.

CHAPTER

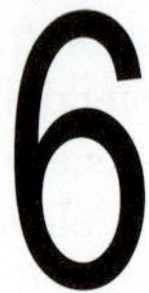

Endocrine Disorders

OBJECTIVES

- Hypothyroidism
- Hyperparathyroidism
- Hypopituitarism
- Hyperpituitarism
- Hypervitaminosis

HYPOTHYROIDISM

Hypothyroidism takes various forms depending on the age of onset. These are explained here, with associated clinical features.

Congenital Hypothyroidism (Cretinism)

- It may be caused by developmental abnormalities of thyroid, but it also occurs in endemic form in areas of iodine deficiency.
- Unless the condition is treated immediately (diagnosis at birth is not easy), the child becomes severely dwarfed and mentally retarded.
- X-ray may show irregular epiphyseal ossification.
- Treatment with thyroid hormone is essential.

Juvenile Hypothyroidism

- It is usually less severe than congenital type.
- Growth and sexual development are retarded and the child may be mentally subnormal.
- X-rays show the typical epiphyseal "fragmentation" appearance.
- Treatment with thyroid hormone may reverse these changes.

Adult Hypothyroidism (Myxedema)

- It may result from some primary disorder of thyroid function (including Hashimoto's disease) or from iatrogenic suppression, following treatment for hyperthyroidism.
- The onset is slow and there may be long period of nonspecific symptoms, such as weight increase, a general lack of energy, and depression.
- Later complications, include deafness, thinning of hair, muscle weakness, nerve entrapment syndromes, and joint pain, sometimes associated with calcium pyrophosphate dehydrate crystal deposition.
- Treatment with thyroxine is effective and will have to be continued for life.

HYPERPARATHYROIDISM

Introduction

Excessive secretion of parathyroid hormone (PTH) may be primary (usually due to an adenoma or hyperplasia), secondary (due to persistent hypocalcemia) or tertiary (when secondary hyperplasia leads to autonomous over activity).

Pathology

Overproduction of PTH enhances calcium conservation, by stimulating tubular absorption, intestinal absorption, and bone resorption. The resulting hypercalcemia, leads to an increase in glomerular filtration of calcium, so there is hypercalciuria, despite the augmented tubular resorption. Urinary phosphate also is increased due to suppressed tubular resorption. The main effects of these changes are seen in the kidney, as calcinosis, stone formation, recurrent infection, and impaired function. There may also be calcification of soft tissues.

There is a general loss of bone substance. In more severe cases, osteoclastic hyperactivity produces subperiosteal erosions, endosteal cavitation, and replacement of the marrow spaces, by vascular granulations and fibrous tissue (osteitis fibrosa cystica). Hemorrhage and giant cell reaction within the fibrous stroma, may give rise to brownish, tumor-like masses, whose liquefaction leads to fluid-filled cysts.

Primary Hyperparathyroidism

Primary hyperparathyroidism is quite common, the usual cause is a solitary adenoma in one of the small glands.

Patients are middle-aged (40–65 years) and women are affected, twice as often as men. Many remain asymptomatic and are diagnosed only because routine biochemistry tests unexpectedly reveal a raised serum calcium level.

Clinical Features

They are mainly due to hypercalcemia, anorexia, nausea, abdominal pain, depression, fatigue, and muscle weakness. They may develop polyuria, kidney stones, or nephrocalcinosis due to chronic hypercalciuria. Some complaint of joint symptoms, due to chondrocalcinosis. Only a minority (probably less than 10%) present, with bone disease and this is usually generalized osteoporosis rather than the classic features of osteitis fibrosa, bone cysts, and pathological fractures.

X-rays show signs of osteoporosis (sometimes including vertebral collapse) and areas of cortical erosion. Hyperparathyroid "brown tumors", should be considered in the differential diagnosis of atypical cyst-like lesions of long bones. However, the classic and almost pathognomonic feature, which should always be sought, is subperiosteal cortical resorption of the middle phalanges. Nonspecific features of hypercalcemia are renal calculi, nephrocalcinosis, and chondrocalcinosis.

Biochemical tests show hypercalcemia, hypophosphatemia and a raised serum PTH concentration. Serum alkaline phosphatase is raised with osteitis fibrosa. Diagnosis involves the exclusion of other causes of hypercalcemia (multiple myeloma, metastatic disease, sarcoidosis), in which PTH levels are usually depressed. Hyperparathyroidism also comes into the differential diagnosis of all types of osteoporosis and osteomalacia.

Treatment is usually conservative and includes adequate hydration and decreased calcium intake. The indications for parathyroidectomy are marked and unremitting hypercalcemia, recurrent renal calculi, progressive nephrocalcinosis, and severe osteoporosis. Postoperatively, there is a danger of severe hypocalcemia due to brisk formation of new bone (the Hungry bone syndrome). This must be treated promptly, with one of the fast acting vitamin D metabolites.

Secondary Hyperparathyroidism

Parathyroid over secretion is a predictable response to chronic hypocalcemia. Secondary hyperparathyroidism is seen, therefore, in various types of rickets and osteomalacia and accounts for some of the radiological features in these disorders. Treatment is directed at the primary condition.

HYPOPITUITARISM

Pituitary Dysfunction

The posterior lobe of the pituitary gland has no influence on the musculoskeletal system. The anterior lobe is responsible for the secretion of pituitary growth hormone, as well as the thyrotropic, gonadotropic, and adrenocorticotropic hormones. Abnormalities may affect the production of some of these hormones and not others, thus there is no single picture of pituitary deficiency or pituitary excess. Moreover, the clinical effects are determined in part, by the stage in skeletal maturation, at which the abnormality occurs.

Hypopituitarism Etiology

Anterior pituitary hyposecretion, may be caused by intrinsic disorders, such as infarction or hemorrhage in the pituitary, infection, and intrapituitary tumors or by extrinsic lesions (such as a craniopharyngioma), which press on the anterior lobe of the pituitary. In some cases, there may also be features, due to posterior lobe dysfunction (e.g. diabetes insipidus) and space occupying lesions, are likely to have other intracranial pressure effects, such as headache or visual field defects. In childhood and adolescence, two distinct clinical disorders are encountered.

Childhood

In the Lorain syndrome, the predominant effect is on growth. The body proportions are normal, but the child fails to grow (proportionate dwarfism). Sexual development may be unaffected. The condition must be distinguished from other causes of short stature, i.e. hereditary or constitutional shortness, which is not as marked as childhood illness or malnutrition rickets and the various bone dysplasias, which generally result in disproportionate dwarfism.

In Fröhlich's adiposogenital syndrome, the effects include those of gonadal hormone deficiency. There is delayed skeletal maturation, associated with adiposity and immaturity of the secondary sexual characteristics. Weakness of the physes combined with disproportionate adiposity, may result in epiphyseal displacement (epiphysiolysis or slipped epiphysis) at the hip or knee.

Adults

Panhypopituitarism causes a variety of symptoms and signs, including those of cortisol and sex hormone deficiency. The only important skeletal effect is premature osteoporosis.

Investigations

These should include direct assays and tests for hormone function.

X-rays

X-rays of the skull may show expansion of the pituitary fossa and erosion of the adjacent bone. CT and MRI may reveal the tumor.

Treatment

Treatment will depend on the cause and the degree of dwarfism. If a tumor is identified, it can be removed or ablated. A word of warning, the sudden reactivation of pituitary function, after removal of a tumor may result in slipping of the proximal femoral epiphysis. Awareness of this risk will make for early diagnosis and if necessary, surgical treatment of the epiphysiolysis. Growth hormone deficiency has been successfully treated, by the administration of biosynthetic growth hormone (somatotropin). The response should be checked, by serial plots on the growth chart.

HYPERPITUITARISM

Over secretion of pituitary growth hormone, is usually due to an acidophillic adenoma. However, there are rare cases of growth hormone secretion, by pancreatic (and other) tumors. The effects vary according to the age of onset.

Gigantism

Over secretion of growth hormone in childhood and adolescence, causes excessive growth of entire skeleton. The condition may be suspected quite early and it is important to track the child's development, by regular clinical and X-ray examinations. In addition to being excessively tall, patients may develop deformity of the hip, due to epiphyseal displacement (epiphysiolysis). There may be mental retardation and sexual immaturity. Treatment is directed at early removal of the pituitary tumor.

Acromegaly

Over secretion of pituitary growth hormone in adulthood causes enlargement of the bones and soft tissues, but without the very marked elongation, which is seen in gigantism. The bones are thickened, rather than lengthened. Due to appositional growth, there is also hypertrophy of articular cartilage, which leads to enlargement of the joints. Bones, such as the mandible, clavicle, ribs, sternum, and scapulae, which develop secondary growth centers in late adolescence or early adulthood, may go on growing longer than usual. Thickening of the skull, prominence of the orbital margins, overgrowth of the jaw, and enlargement of the nose, lips and the tongue produce the characteristic facies of acromegaly. The chest is broad and barrel-shaped and the hands and feet are large. Thickening of the bone ends may causes secondary osteoarthritis. About 10% of acromegalics develop diabetes and cardiovascular disease more commonly than usual.

Treatment

The indications for operation are the presence of a tumor in childhood and cranial nerve pressure symptoms at any age. Trans-sphenoidal surgery has a high rate of success, provided the diagnosis is made reasonably early and the tumor is not too large.

Mild cases of acromegaly can be treated by administering growth hormone suppressants (a somatostatin analog or bromocriptine, a dopamine agonist).

HYPERVITAMINOSIS

Hypervitaminosis A

- Occurs in children, following excessive dosage.
- In adults, it seldom occurs except in explorers, who eat Polar bear's liver.
- There may be bone pain and headache and vomiting, due to raised intracranial pressure.
- X-ray shows increased density in the metaphyseal region and subperiosteal calcification.

Hypervitaminosis D

- Occurs, if too much vitamin D is given.
- It exerts a PTH like effect and so as in the underlying rickets, calcium is withdrawn from bones, but metastatic calcification occurs.
- In treatment, the dose of vitamin D must be properly regulated and the infant should be given a low calcium diet, but plentiful fluids.

CHAPTER

7 Blood Disorders

OBJECTIVES

- Hemophilia in Orthopedics

INTRODUCTION

The most common presentation of blood disorder in orthopedics is hemophilia and conditions simulating hemophilia.

HEMOPHILIA IN ORTHOPEDICS

Definition

It is characterized by a bleeding diathesis due to the defect in the clotting mechanism of the blood.

Coagulation Factors of Blood

• Factor I:	Fibrinogen
• Factor II:	Prothrombin
• Factor III:	Tissue thromboplastin (tissue factor)
• Factor IV:	Ionized calcium (Ca^{2+})
• Factor V:	Labile factor or proaccelerin
• Factor VI:	Unassigned
• Factor VII:	Stable factor or proconvertin
• Factor VIII:	Antihemophilic factor
• Factor IX:	Plasma thromboplastin component, Christmas factor
• Factor X:	Stuart–Prower factor
• Factor XI:	Plasma thromboplastin antecedent
• Factor XII:	Hageman factor
• Factor XIII:	Fibrin-stabilizing factor

Types of Hemophilia

• *Hemophilia A:*	Due to the deficiency of factor VIII (Antihemophilia factor)
• *Hemophilia B:*	Due to deficiency of factor IX (Christmas factor)
• *Hemophilia C:*	Due to deficiency of factor XI (Plasma thromboplastin antecedent)
• *von Willebrand's disease:*	When both Factor VIII and platelet are deficient

Conditions Simulating Hemophilia

Von Willebrand's Disease

It is named after a Finnish Physician Erik von Willebrand, it is an autosomal dominant genetic disorder caused by lack of or defective von Willebrand factor (vWF, a clotting protein). Von Willebrand factor binds factor VIII, a key clotting protein, which is required for platelet adhesion. Hence, both factor VIII and platelet are deficient or defective. It is treated by desmopressin and more recently recombinant vWF.

Bernard-Soulier Disease (Hemorrhagiparous Thrombocytic Dystrophy)

It is a rare autosomal recessive disease caused by deficiency of glycoprotein 1b (GP 1b), which is the receptor of vWF. It is characterized by abnormally large platelets (giant platelet disorder).

Idiopathic Thrombocytopenic Purpura

It is defined as primary thrombocytopenia (<50,000/mm^3) with normal bone marrow and absence of other pathologies that can lead to a low platelet count, clinically manifested by formation of spontaneous bruises (purpura), petechiae, bleeding from mucosal membranes (e.g. nose, gums) and hematomas. In more than half cases of idiopathic thrombocytopenic purpura (ITP), autoantibody against the platelets is found in the blood.

Treatment consists of corticosteroids, platelet infusion, thrombopoietin receptor agonists (e.g. romiplostim), and splenectomy.

Vitamin K Deficiency

Vitamin K is a fat-soluble vitamin that changes into active form in liver. Activated vitamin K is then used to carboxylate, thus activate factors II, VII, IX, X, protein C and S. The inability to activate the clotting cascade may lead to hemorrhagic disorders. Vitamin K deficiency may occur by disturbed intestinal uptake or by intake of vitamin K antagonist such as warfarin.

The above conditions described simulate hemophilia clinically by presenting hemorrhages in muscles and different tissue planes and joints. The causes and presentation of the condition with specific investigation and treatment have already been described in brief.

Clinical Features

The common orthopedic manifestations are:

- Hemorrhage into the following structure
  - Joints

- Muscles
- Peripheral nerves
- Hemophilic cyst (Fig. 1).

Hemorrhages into Joint

There is a sudden attack of hemarthrosis in joint, following minimal trauma. The bleeding occurs not only inside the synovial cavity of joint, but also intraosseous hemorrhages from subchondral bone. In later stage, destruction of cartilage takes place with fibrous ankylosis and deformity. Knee, elbow, ankle, and hip are commonly involved.

Hemorrhages into Muscle

Bleeding into iliacus, results in lump in iliac fossa and flexion deformity of hip, due to spasm of muscles. In calf, it gives rise to equinus deformity. In forearm, it produces Volkmann ischemic contracture (VIC) occasionally.

Hemorrhages into Nerves

Nerve lesion occurs due to intraneural hemorrhages.

Hemophilic Cyst

The bleeding forms cysts in various planes of muscles, fasciae or in bones (pseudotumor). The clinical picture in Figure 2 is showing, swollen, warm and painful joint, causing contractures and deformities. Knee is commonly involved.

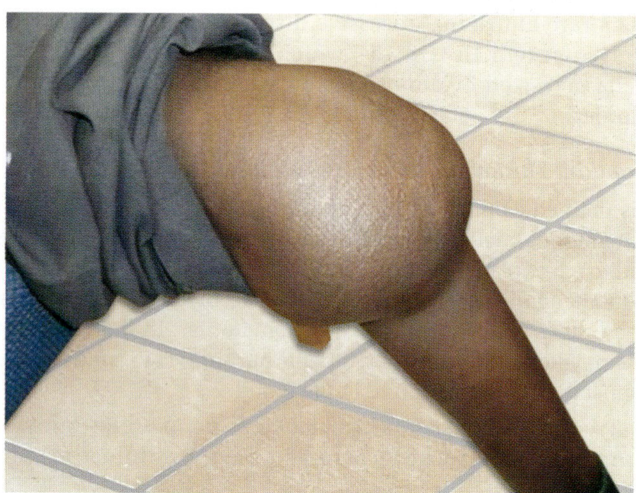

Fig. 1: Hemorrhage into the joint (knee).

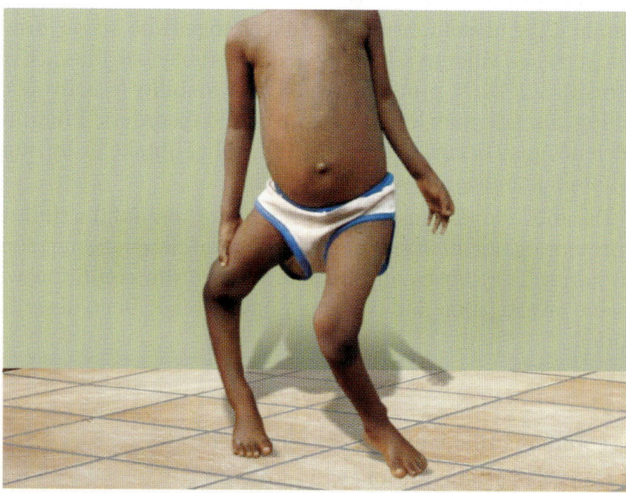

Fig. 2: "Wind swept deformity" of knee joint.

Stages of Joint Involvement

Stage I

Trauma to joint, hemarthrosis, with mild to severe effusion.

Stage II

- Articular damage is present, with, widening of intercondylar notch
- Due to subchondral cysts, joint space is reduced and squaring of patella is present
- Patient may have subluxation of tibia and lateral rotation.

Stage III

- Patient is bed-ridden, with joint severely deformed and ankylosed
- Late arthritic changes, with subluxation of tibia.

Laboratory Findings

- Bleeding time and prothrombin time are normal
- Deficiency of factor VIII and IX
- Plasma thromboplastin time is elevated
- Blood HIV should be tested in hemophilia, as transfusion related AIDS is a well-recognized complication of hemophilia.

Radiological Findings

Early Stage

Distended synovium, no para-articular skeletal deformity.

Intermediate Stage

Persistent boggy swelling and osteoporosis, with subchondral cyst are present. Squaring of patella is present and intercondylar notch of femur, along with trochlear notch is widened.

End Stage

- Joint is disorganized. Subchondral cysts are large and fibrous ankylosis is present.
- Pseudotumor is seen as cystic, expansile, and lucent, soft tissue swellings, eroding the cortex (Fig. 3).

Management

This varies according to stage.

Acute Stage

- Factor VIII is replaced
- Joint aspiration is done
- Immobilized with splint.

Late Cases

- Prolonged immobilization, with caliper or splint is recommended.
- Trial aspiration.

Surgical Methods

- Fresh frozen plasma and blood transfusion
- Synovectomy
- Osteotomy, for severe flexion contracture

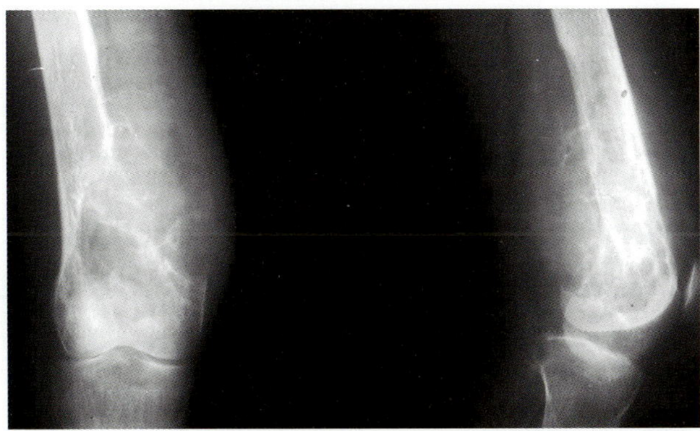

Fig. 3: X-ray showing, pseudotumor in a joint, as cystic, expansile and lucent, soft tissue swellings, eroding the cortex.

- Arthrodesis
- Lengthening or release, for contractures
- Joint replacement.

Surgical Approach

Principle of Surgery in Hemophilia

- HIV and inhibitors of factor VIII (antibodies) must be assayed in serum preoperatively.
- Factors VIII replacement, must be started 45 minutes to 1 hour before surgery and continue till suture removal.
- Factor VIII levels in serum must be maintained at 100% for the first week, following surgery and at 50–75% during the second weeks.
- Tourniquets should be used, wherever possible.
- Sharp dissection is preferred, blunt dissection should be avoided.
- Drains should not be used.
- Bulky dressing should be used.
- Physiotherapy should be continued, under the coverage of factor VIII.

CHAPTER

8 Gouty Arthritis

OBJECTIVES

- Pseudogout (Chondrocalcinosis)
- Hydroxyapatite Crystals Deposition Disease

INTRODUCTION

Gout is a hereditary condition of disturbed uric acid metabolism, in which sodium urate salts are deposited in articular, periarticular, and subcutaneous tissues. It is characterized by recurring attacks of acute arthritis, with intervals of freedom from pain.

ETIOLOGY

Actual cause is unknown. Predisposing causes are:

- *Hereditary (Heredity):* Occurs in families.
- *Sex:* Males predominantly affected and in females, usually occur at menopause.
- *Age:* Second to fourth decade. It is common in the age of 40 years..
- *Adrenal cortex activity:* An adequate amount of cortical steroids counteracts gouty attack.
- *Vascular changes:* Extremity involved by acute gouty arthritis, displays increased blood flow and amplitude, suggesting vascular disturbance, as the cause of extreme pain.
- *Disturbed electrolyte equilibrium:* Marked diuresis that precedes acute attacks of gout.
- *Decreased urinary 17-ketosteroids:* Formed from metabolism of adrenocortical and testicular androgens. Reduction below 3 mg/24 hours is a constant finding in gout.

PATHOLOGY

- Sodium urate crystals are deposited on the surface of and replacing articular cartilage.
- Articular cartilage is eroded; the subchondral bone is replaced in well-circumscribed punched-out areas, by crystalline deposits.
- Pannus of granulation tissue, grows over the articular surface, invades and replaces the cartilage and may bridge the joint to opposite articular surface, producing fibrous ankylosis.
- Irregularity of joint surfaces leads to secondary degenerative arthritis.
- Urate crystals are deposited in the synovial membrane, periarticular soft tissues, and subcutaneous tissues.
- Microscopically, deposits are surrounded by an inflammatory reaction, fibrous tissues, and giant cells.
- Urate salts are found in articular cartilage, bone marrow, synovial membrane, joint capsules, ligaments, periosteum, tendons, bursae, subcutaneous, and intramuscular tissues.
- Metatarsophalangeal joint of big toe is predisposed.
- Next affected parts are intertarsal joints, ankles, fingers, and the wrist.
- Cause of death is usually cerebral or coronary disease, or nephrosclerosis with uremia.

CLINICAL FEATURES

- Serum urate level exceeds 6 mg/dL.
- Initial attack is acute and may be precipitated by trauma, dietary indiscretions (high fat diet), drugs (liver extract), surgical operations, exposure to cold, and withdrawal of adrenocorticotropic hormone (ACTH).
- *Attack:* Sudden onset, frequently at night.
- *Joint:* Swollen, red, and tender. May mimic cellulitis. Pain is excruciating.
- Inflammation may involve a nonarticular urate deposit, such as a subcuatenous tophus or in a bursa.
- *Constitutional symptoms*: Fever, tachycardia, and headache.
- Attacks last from a few days to several weeks before it subsides, with complete restoration of function of the joint.
- Desquamation is involved up to final stage.
- Intervals between attacks, may vary in length, they tend to become progressively shorter and the intensity of succeeding attacks, become progressively severe.
- Small deposits of urate salts, in subcutaneous tissues are seen as a pearly white appearance. Characteristic location for these deposits is about ears.
- Tophi may increase in size and assume large globular shapes, distending the overlying skin and rupturing it, to form a chronically discharging sinus, exuding milky white material.
- Main complication is due to deposits of urate crystals in the kidneys. Impairment of renal function, due to chronic glomerulonephritis and interstitial nephritis, leads to uremia and death.

DIAGNOSIS

Main diagnostic factors include:

- Family history of gouty arthritis
- Repeated attacks, with intervals of freedom from pain
- Renal disturbance
- Hyperuricemia
- Satisfactory response to adequate dose of colchicines.

LABORATORY FINDINGS

- *Blood:* Leukocytosis, increased erythrocyte sedimentation rate (ESR).
- Increased concentration of sodium urate. Normal level is less than 5 mg/dL.
- Microscopic examination of joint fluid include:
  - Sodium biurate crystals, found in joint aspirates
  - Needle shaped crystals, show strong negative birefringence, when viewed under polarizing microscope digested by uricase
  - It helps in differentiating from pseudogout, in which rhombic calcium phosphate crystals are seen, showing positive but weak birefringence, not digested by uricase
  - *Murexide test:* Few drops of nitric acid are added to a suspected substance. Mixture is evaporated to dryness and is then moistened with ammonium hydroxide. If uric acid is present, a purple color (due to murexide) comes.

X-ray Findings

- Earlier, joint appears normal
- Later, replacement of bony structure by urate crystals, gives the characteristic punched out appearance
- Cartilage is destroyed, joint becomes narrowed
- Degenerative arthritic changes are seen.

FACTORS INFLUENCING URIC ACID LEVELS

- Endogenous uric acid arises from destroyed nuclei, particularly extruded nuclei of normoblasts, during process of maturation of erythrocytes.
- Certain diseases such as polycythemia and drugs, such as liver extract, can precipitate arthritis.
- High fat diet decreases its excretion.
- Uric acid is an end product of purine metabolism.

TREATMENT

Prophylaxis demands, avoiding provocative factors.

Acute Attack

- Absolute bed-rest
- Affected extremity immobilized in a splint
- Ice pack reduces the pain
- Colchicine (colchicum) specific for gout, acts as both analgesic and diuretic
- Salicylates, also valuable for their uricosuric effect
- High carbohydrate diet
- Phenylbutazone given, as enteric coated tablets (200 mg three times a day) and oral predinosolone (20–40 mg/day) is effective
- Since colchicines have no uricosuric effect, it should be combined with allopurinol
- Allopurinol is an inhibitor of the enzyme xanthine oxidase, thereby preventing final step in production of uric acid
- Principal side effects of allopurinol are gastrointestinal irritation and dermatitis
- Fever, blood dyscrasia, and hepatic damage can occur rarely
- 300 mg/day is the starting dose of allopurinol.

Surgical Procedure

- During acute attack, immobilization of affected joint will lessen the degree of joint destruction
- A bursa may become distended by urate deposits and the overlying skin is thinned and penetrated or the tendon may be invaded
- A fusiform, nodular enlargement develops within the tendon, which interferes with tendon motion and may predispose to tendon rupture
- Invasion of joint destroys articular cartilage, and capsular structures
- Severe disintegration of joint structure, leads to fibrous ankylosis, which ultimately leads to bony ankylosis
- Surgical stabilization of the joint, in functional position is indicated
- Large bony lesion adjacent to a joint, removal of focus may preserve joint function
- Surgery of gouty lesions, demands observance of following principles:
  - Avoid local anesthesia, as it might impair local blood supply
  - Incision should be made parallel, with course of blood vessels
  - Sharp dissection
  - Loose suturing, to allow escape of liquefied deposits
  - Pressure dressing
  - Avoidance of prolonged splinting, which encourages ankylosis.

PSEUDOGOUT (CHONDROCALCINOSIS)

- Pseudogout arthritis occurs due to deposition of crystals of calcium pyrophosphate dihydrate deposits (CPPD) in synovium or articular cartilage or menisci.
- Clinically it resembles gout, but serum uric acid is normal.
- Most commonly affected joint is knee.

Investigation

X-ray

Calcified spots in menisci and articular cartilage.

Synovial Fluid Analysis

Rhomboid shaped crystals, under microscope.

Treatment

Respond to indomethacin.

HYDROXYAPATITE CRYSTALS DEPOSITION DISEASE

Clinical Presentation

- It may present as primary crystal induced arthopathy or secondary to trauma or degenerative joint disease.
- Hydroxyapatite crystals are deposited in soft tissue of joint space, rotator cuff tendons or bursa.
- Shoulder and knee are commonly involved.
- Hydroxyapatite crystals are nonbirefringent.
- Radiologically, the disease appears as radiopaque calcification, in a local tumor mass like fashion.

Treatment

- Treatment is with nonsteroidal anti-inflammatory drugs (NSAIDs), colchicine and oral, and intra-articular corticosteroids, and physiotherapy.
- Large tumor mass-like deposits may sometime need excision.

CHAPTER

9 Degenerative and Inflammatory Disorders

OBJECTIVES

- Osteoarthritis
- Rheumatoid Arthritis
- Seronegative Arthropathies

OSTEOARTHRITIS

Introduction

It is characterized by degenerative changes in articular cartilage of diarthrodial joints and subsequent new bone formation at the articular margins.

Incidence

- By the age of 40 years, about 40% of population has radiological sign of osteoarthritis of major weight-bearing joints (knee, hip).
- 50% of these will be symptomatic.

Types of Osteoarthritis

Predisposing Factors

- Trauma
- Metabolic disorders
- Infection
- Hemophilia
- Congenital and developing disorders, rheumatoid arthritis (RA), etc.

Etiology

Age

Process begins in second decade of life and by that age 80% have radiological evidence of disease.

Sex

Females, affected more than males.

Hereditary

Articular expression of generalized constitutional condition from inherited metabolic abnormalities.

Obesity

Osteoarthritis is prevalent in obese.

Biomechanical Factors

- Structural abnormalities, like articular, dislocation, acetabular dysplasia, slipped epiphysis, and Perthe's disease will cause abnormally high pressure over the articular surfaces and predispose it for early degeneration.
- Similarly malalignment of joints, like genu varum, genu valgum, and meniscal tears, leads to abnormal stresses, predisposing the joint to early degeneration.

Hormonal Effects

- Acromegaly notably effects articular cartilage.
- Diabetics are often prone for degenerative arthritis.

Chemical Injury

Corticosteroids injected in joint or given systemically, are known to reduce synthesis and loss of prostaglandins (PG).

Repeated Intrasynovial Hemorrhage

Iron and blood pigments, alters physical and chemical properties of cartilage, causing early degeneration, e.g. hemophilic arthritis.

Areas of Involvement

- Varies from person to person and from joint to joint.
- In females, distal interphalangeal (DIP) and first metacarpophalangeal (MCP) joints are most commonly involved.
- In males, hips are most commonly involved.
- In females, knees are most commonly involved.
- Any synovial joint may be affected, but those under compression are more prone.
- Inflammatory process, like rheumatoid arthritis destroys articular cartilage.
- Metabolic disorders, like gouty deposits of urates and alkaptonuric ochronosis deposits, makes cartilage susceptible to destruction.

Changes with Age (Primary Osteoarthritis)

Fibrillation of articular cartilage is age-related and is peculiar to certain locations (e.g. hip, inferiomedial to fovea, and beneath femoral head; patellar medial facet), can lead to osteoarthritis.

Cellular Changes

- In growing epiphyseal cartilage, mitotic activity is present, but in adults there is no change in cell count in superficial zone of cartilage, but increased cellularity is evident in transitional zone, marking the beginning of osteoarthritis.
- *Collagen aging*: With increasing maturity of collagen fibers.

- *Protein and glycosaminoglycan (GAG) synthesis*: Balance between rate of synthesis and rate of degradation is altered with aging.
- *Chemical composition*: Chondrotin-6-sulfate forms the principal GAG, which with advancing age decreases to the level of less than 5% in elderly.

Physical Alterations

- Permeability of articular cartilage decrease, with advancing age up to 40 years, then a variable increase in permeability takes place.
- Elastic properties of articular cartilage also suffer, with advancing age.
- Tensile stiffness of cartilage refers to forces parallel to articular surface, produced as a secondary effect of compression and ability to resist such force is the function of articular cartilage, which decreases with advancing age.

Pathophysiology

- Degeneration of hyaline cartilage is the first lesion.
- Spotty degeneration of hyaline cartilage exposing subchondral bone, with healthy areas intervening.
- Normal areas of cartilage at periphery along with perichondrium, stimulates to overcome losses.
- As a result, nonarticular area elevates above remainder and projects circumferentially known as "lipping".

Formation of Osteophytes

- The cartilaginous outgrowths are ossified to form osteophytes.
- Local periosteal new bone formation, particularly around capsular attachment, also leads to osteophyte formation.

Synovitis and Capsulitis

- Detached cartilaginous flakes lies freely in joint. Cavity readily absorbs the synovial membrane and leads to synovitis, followed by fibrosis.
- Proteoglycans leaks from damaged articular cartilage, leads to irritation of synovial membrane and capsule, which undergoes hyperplasia.

Subchondral Sclerosis

- Proliferation of blood vessels along subchondral bone leads to osteoporosis initially, followed by invasion of larger blood vessels, leading to subchondral sclerosis.
- Formation of subchondral cyst.
- Edema of subchodral bone marrow, followed by formation of mucinous fatty marrow, with dilatation of surrounding sinusoids leads to cyst formation, which increases in size by osteoclastic activity and finally sclerosis around margins of cyst appears due to osteoblastic activity.
- Another theory regarding formation of cyst is from herniation of synovial fluid through denuded subchondral bone.
- An osteoarthritic joint rarely gets completely ankylosed, but gross proliferation with presence of osteophytes out growths and dense capsular fibrosis, may impede free movement of joint, which may simulate some degree of fusion, which in fact does not exist.

Formation of Loose Bodies

Cartilaginous tags occasionally get detached and form loose bodies.

Eburnation

- Exposed bone ends of articular surface are subjected to considerable friction, which leads to bone trabeculae in immediate neighborhood fracture, leading to obliterated marrow spaces.
- Changes involved in only a thin layer abutting on joint and this layer gradually becomes more smooth and polished, as a result of continuous rubbing. This process is known as eburnation.

Stages of Osteoarthritis (As Seen Under Light Microscopy)

Early Stage

- Surface irregularities or fibrillation with small clefts not extending beyond superficial zone.
- Slight hypercellularity.
- Minimal loss of mucopolysaccharides.

Moderately Advanced

- More extensive loss of surface.
- Clefts extending into middle zone and occasionally into calcified zone.
- Loss of mucopolysaccharides, extending into middle zone.
- Hypercellularity in clusters of cells or chondrocyte clones.

Advanced Changes

- Thickness of cartilage is reduced.
- Clefts may extend down to subchondral bone.
- Mucopolysaccharides markedly reduced through entire thickness of cartilage.
- In some areas, complete loss of cartilage with exposure of thick, eburnated subchondral bone.

Clinical Features

Joint Involvement

- Primary generalized osteoarthrosis.
- Distal interphalangeal (DIP) joints of hand with Heberden's nodes.
- More or less symmetrical involvement of other joints, like knee, metatarsophalangeal (MTP) joints of foot, posterior spinal joints, and elbow joint.

Primary Osteoarthritis

Most commonly affected joints are:

- Knee joint
- Hip joint
- Metacarpophalangeal (MCP) joint of thumb
- MTP joint of great toe
- Posterior spinal joint
- Elbow joint.

Radiological Appearance

Stage I

Hyperemia with periarticular osteoporosis.

Stage II

Reduction in joint space.

Stage III

Osteophytes formation with subchondral sclerocystic changes.

Stage IV

Complete loss of joint space with or without subluxation.

Signs and Symptoms

Joint Pain

- Stiffness
- Difficulty in movement.

Deformities

Deformities of limb presentation in osteoarthritis are seen in Figure 1.

Investigations

- Routine investigations in primary OA are usually in normal limits.
- Other investigations are dependent upon the predisposing factors, if present.

Management

Conservative

- Rest
- Range of motion exercises
- Abstinence from weight-bearing
- Vertical load reduction
- Traction
- Physical therapy
- Orthotics
- Heat therapy
- Graduated exercise.

Drug Therapy

- NSAIDs, such as diclofenac and aceclofenac, produce their anti-inflammatory and analgesic effect, by inhibiting cyclo-oxygenase and thus preventing production of prostaglandins from arachidonic acid.
- In addition, aceclofenac has shown some stimulatory effects on cartilage matrix synthesis that may be linked to ability of drug, to inhibit IL-1 activity.
- Chondrosynthesis drugs, i.e. glucosamine and amino monosaccharide.
- Contains component of all human connective tissues.
- Used in body to synthesize GAGs and glycoproteins.
- Proteoglycan and hyaluronic acid (HA) synthesis.
- Imparts high electronegativity in cartilage resulting in water retentions.
- Maintains viscosity of synovial fluid—hyaluronate formation.
- Anti-inflammatory property.
- Active principle, e.g. chondroitin 4 and 6 sulfate.
- Chondroitin.
- Nonspecific slow acting chondro-protective, but helps in chondro synthesis.
- Supplement action of glucosamine.
- Inhibits proinflammatory prostaglandin/leukotrienes.
- Inhibit hyaluronidase enzyme.
- Breakdown HA molecule.
- Viscosity of synovial fluid.
- Chondroprotective and disease modifying drugs.
- Inhibit pain, by inhibiting synthesis of cytokines.
- Improves mobility, by stimulating the production of collagen II and proteoglycan.
- Reduces stiffness, by stimulating the production of hyaluronic acid.
- Antioxidant vitamins, e.g. vitamins C, E and beta-carotene.
- Antioxidant minerals are selenium, manganese, zinc and their properties are:
  - Chondroprotective
  - Given with glucosamine and chondroitin
  - Building blocks in GAGs synthesis
  - *Efficacy:* Well tested
  - No side effects.

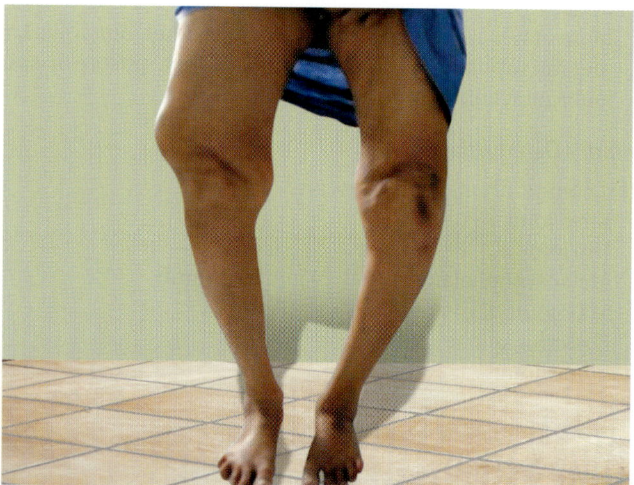

Fig. 1: Deformity of limb present in osteoarthritis.

Semi-invasive Treatment Corticosteroids

Intra-articular Cortisone

- Temporary relief
- Satisfying and lasting in mild and moderate cases
- No response to conservative treatment in acute inflammatory phase
- Severe OA.

Local Steroid

Shows good result, for pain in pericapsular site (outside joint), e.g. pes anserinus and biceps (repeated long-acting depot preparation)
- Risk of joint infection
- Hypopigmentation
- Subcutaneous atrophy
- Osteonecrosis.

Repeated Long-acting Depot Preparation

Intra-articular Injection of Hyaluronic Acid or Visco-Supplementation Therapy

- Safe and effective
- Pain, improves joints function for months

- Five injections, weekly
- Shock absorber. Joint capable of withstanding mechanical stress
- Molecular weight
- Greater viscoelasticity
- Better response.

Other Methods of Treatment

- Surgery
- Synovectomy
- Arthrodesis
- Osteotomies
- Arthroscopic lavage with debridement
- Arthroplasties.

Osteotomies

Features of Osteotomies

- Correction of mechanical malalignment.
- Brings into contact nondamaged articular surface, hence reducing friction and pain.
- Alters weight-bearing and joint reaction forces.
- Decongests venous stasis and venous hypertension in metaphyseal trabecular bone.

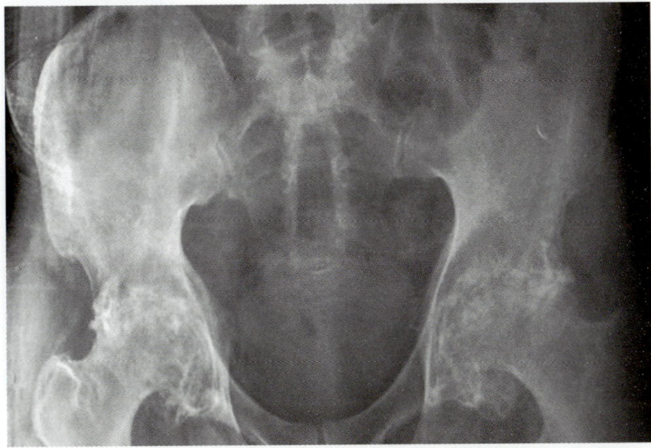

Fig. 2: X-ray showing hip osteoarthritis.

Hip Osteoarthritis (Fig. 2)

- Valgus osteotomy (Figs. 3A to C)
- Varus osteotomy (Figs. 4A to D)
- Total hip replacement (Figs. 5 and 6).

Osteoarthritis of Knee

- High tibial osteotomy (Figs. 7 and 8)
- Total knee replacement (Fig. 9)
- OA elbow (Figs. 10A and B).

RHEUMATOID ARTHRITIS

Introduction

It is a systemic disease of young and middle aged adults, characterized by:

- Proliferation and destructive changes in synovial membrane
- Periarticular structure
- Skeletal muscles and perineural sheaths
- Eventually, the joints are fused and ankylosed.

Etiology

- *Sex:* 80% affected are women; male to female ratio is 1:3.
- *Age:* No age is exempted, mean age is 40 years.
- The exact cause is unknown, theoretical causes include the following:
  - *Infectious:* Hemolytic and nonhemolytic types of streptococci, had been isolated from joint and regional lymph nodes.
  - *Endocrines:* This is suggested by response to adrenocortical steroids.
  - *Allergic:* Rheumatoid arthritis, frequently exhibits various allergic manifestations, eosinophilia is frequently present.
  - *Genetic influence:* Increasing evidence, which suggest that the disease is triggered by T-lymphocytes activation in a genetically predisposed individual, with defined HLA-class II haplotypes (HLA DR4, HLA DR1).
  - *Immune over reactivity:* RA is characterized by persistent cellular activation, autoimmunity, and the presence of

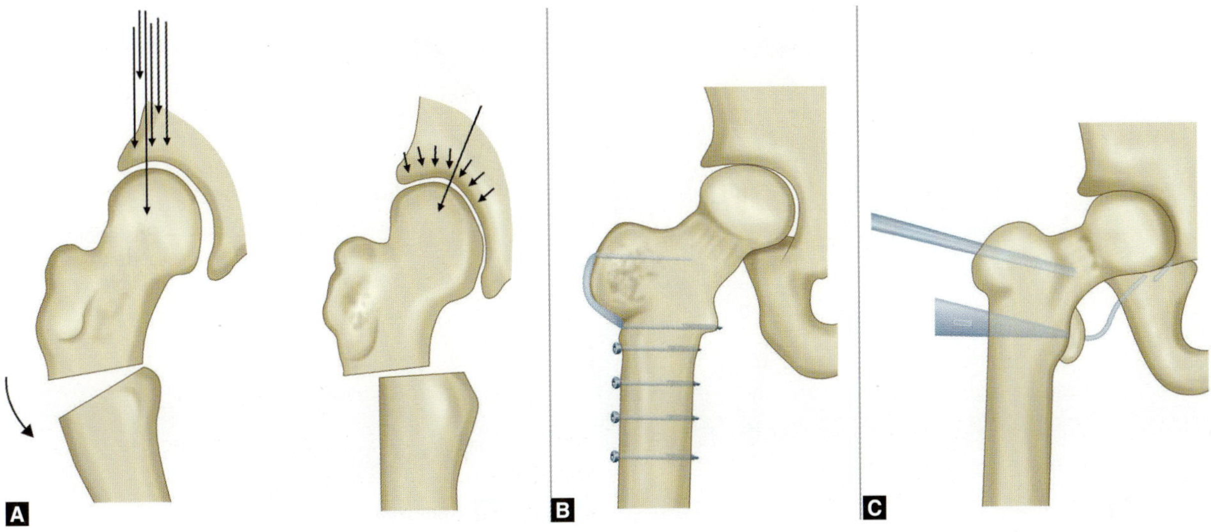

Figs. 3A to C: Valgus osteotomy.

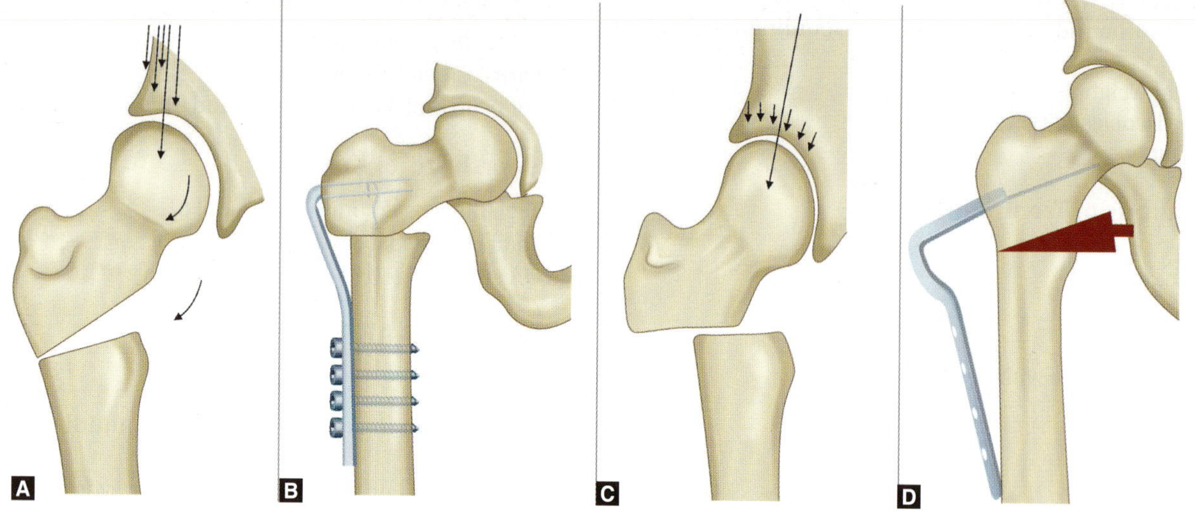

Figs. 4A to D: Varus osteotomy.

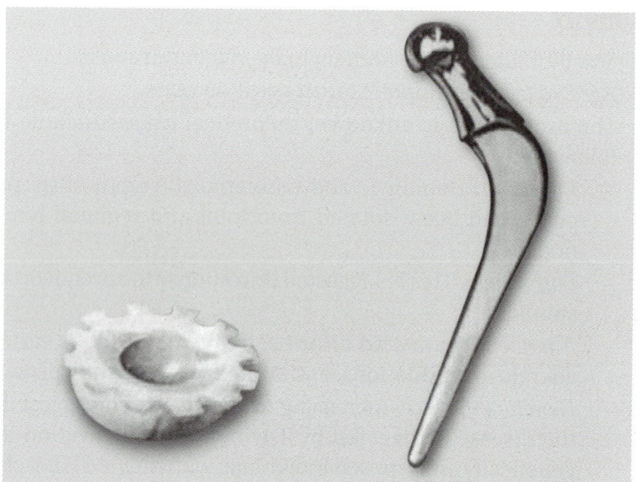

Fig. 5: Total hip replacement implant.

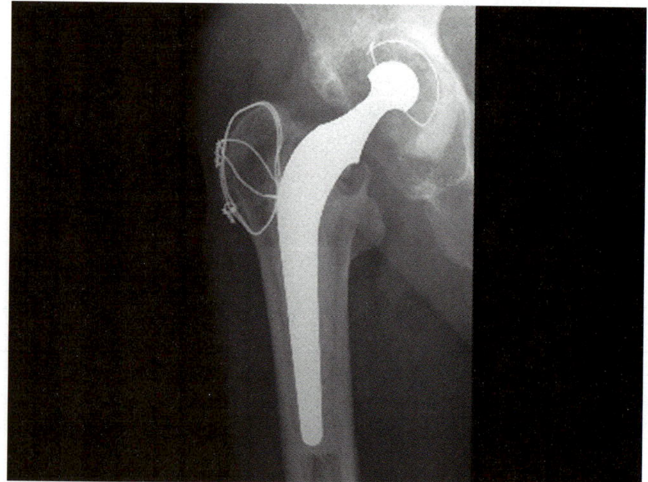

Fig. 6: Image taken after total hip replacement.

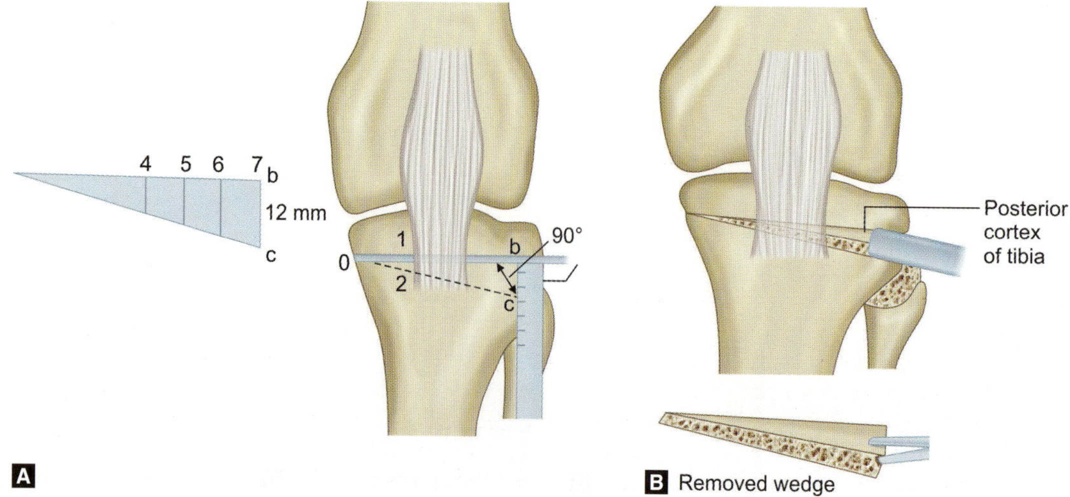

Figs. 7A and B: Steps for high tibial osteotomy.

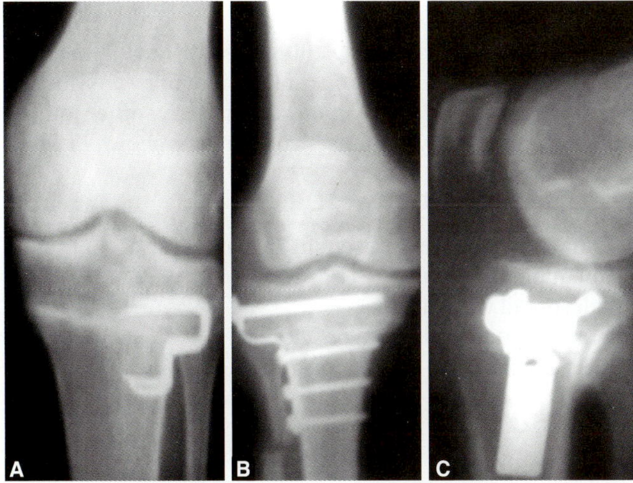

Figs. 8A to C: High tibial osteotomy.

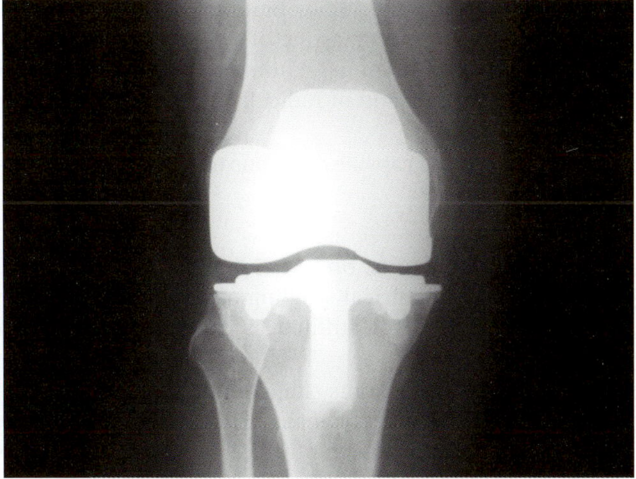

Fig. 9: Total knee replacement.

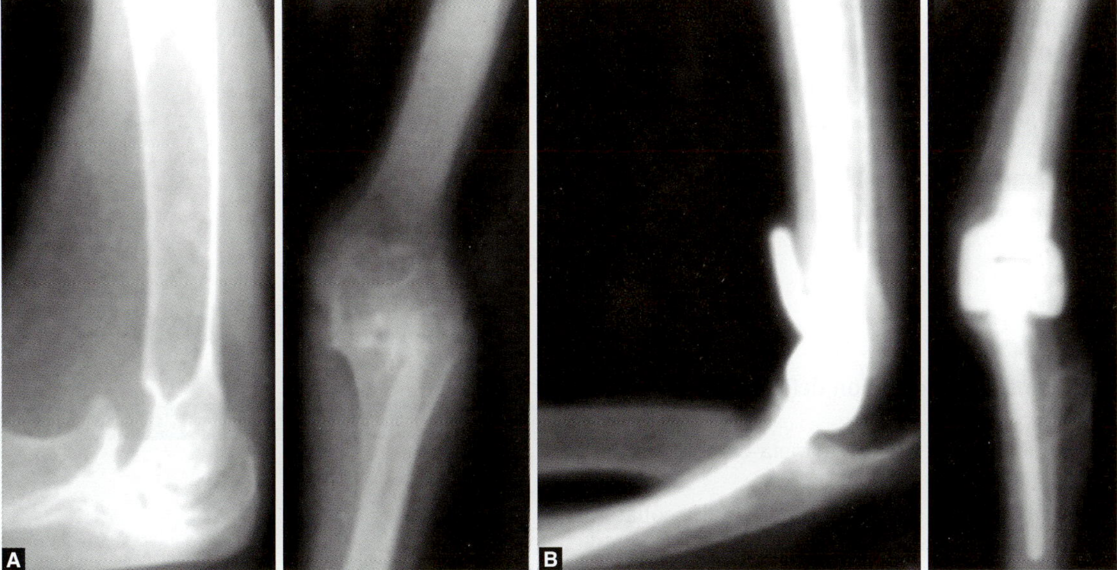

Figs. 10A and B: X-ray film showing OA elbow.

immune complexes, at site of articular and extra-articular lesions.

Pathogenesis

- Most accepted theory is of immunogenic response, taking place in the synovium.
- An unknown exogenous antigen encounters the defender cells, the lymphocytes, which are transformed into plasma cells.
- The plasma cells manufacture antibodies.
- Antibodies, antigen, and complement combine to form complex.
- Scavenger phagocytic cell, engulf the complex, as these phagocytes contain small enzyme sac (lysosomes), that destroys the complex.
- Some of the lysosomes escapes the phagocyte cells and their protease attack the cartilage and synovium.
- Destruction of tissue produces debris that calls for more phagocyte activity to remove the debris.
- Consequently, more phagocyte activity cell pour out more enzymes, which create more destruction and further inflammation and the arthritic changes become self perpetuating.
- The inflammed synovium forms pannus, a granulomatous mass that grows over the destroyed cartilage, tendon, and ligaments.

Pathology

- The earliest changes are swelling and congestion of synovial membrane and the underlying connective tissue, which becomes infiltrated with lymphocytes, plasma cells, and macrophages.
- Effusion of the synovial fluid into joint space, takes place during active phase of the disease.
- Hypertrophy of synovial membrane occurs with formation of lymphoid follicles, resembling active lymph node changes.
- Inflammatory granulation tissue (pannus) is formed, spreading over and under the articular cartilage, which is progressively eroded and destroyed.
- Later, fibrous adhesion takes place between the layers of pannus across the joint space and fibrous ankylosis may occur.

- Microscopically, the subcutaneous nodules shows central area of fibrinoid necrosis, consisting of swollen and fragmented collagen fibers, fibrinous exudates and cellular debris, surrounded by palisade of radically arranged proliferating mononuclear cells.
- Nodules have loose capsule of fibrous tissues.

Clinical Features

- In majority of patients, onset is insidious with joint pain, stiffness and symmetrical swelling of peripheral joints, but rest pain and morning stiffness is characteristic of active inflammatory arthritis.
- In typical cases, small joints of fingers and toes are the first to be affected. Swelling of proximal, but not distal joints of fingers gives a spindled appearance.
- Swelling of MTP joints, resulting in broadening of toes.
- As the disease progresses, involvement of elbow, wrist, shoulder, knee, ankle joints, etc. can occur.
- The hip joint is involved late in the disease.
- Cervical spine affection is common.
- As the disease progresses muscle atrophy, tendon sheath, and joint destruction, results in limitation of joint motion, joint instability occurs.
- Characteristic deformities, like flexion contracture of small joints of hand and feet, besides other joints, i.e. knee, hip, and elbow occurs.

Deformities

Rheumatoid Hand

The following are some of the common deformities seen in the hand:

- Symmetrical peripheral joint swelling of meta-carpophalangeal and interphalangeal joints.
- Ulnar deviation of the hand is due to rupture of the collateral ligaments at the metacarpophalangeal joints, which enable the extensor tendons to slip from their grooves towards the ulnar side.
- Boutonniere's deformity is due to the rupture of central extensor expansion of the fingers, resulting in flexion at the proximal interphalangeal (PIP) joint, which is nearest the knuckle.
- Swan neck deformity is due to the rupture of volar plate of PIP joint, which enables the tendons to slip towards the dorsal side. There is hyperextension of PIP joint and flexion of DIP joint.
- Trigger fingers and trigger thumb, these deformities are due to the nodule over the tendon.
- Z-deformity of the hand.
- Subluxation and dislocation of MCP joints.

Rheumatoid Foot

- Callosity under PIP joint
- Plantar callosity
- Claw toes
- Hammer toe
- Rheumatoid nodules
- Flattening of longitudinal arch
- Hallus valgus.

Other Joints

In knee, initially there is gross swelling due to synovitis, but in later stages patient may develop fibrous ankylosis or bony ankylosis, due to destruction of cartilage by pannus. Similarly, other joints are involved and frequency of joints involvement is shown in Table 1.

Extra-articular Features

Two or more features are present in 75% of cases:

- Subcutaneous nodules
- Widespread vasculitis
- Keratoconjunctivitis sicca or scleritis
- Heart affection like arrhythmias and heart block.

Investigations

- Hemoglobin is low
- White blood cell (WBC) is decreased
- Erythrocyte sedimentation rate (ESR) raised
- Increased C-reactive protein
- Increased alkaline phosphatase
- Increased platelets
- Decreased serum albumin
- Synovial fluid analysis
- Serological tests
  - Latex fixation test
  - Inhibition test.

X-ray (Fig. 11)

- Juxta-articular osteoporosis
- Erosion of joint margin

TABLE 1: Frequency of involvement of joints.

MCP/MTP/PIP joints	90%
Knee, ankle, wrist	80%
Shoulder	60%
Hip, acromion process and elbow joint	50%
Cervical spine	40%
Temporomandibular joint and sternomastoid joint	30%
Cricoarytenoid joint	10%

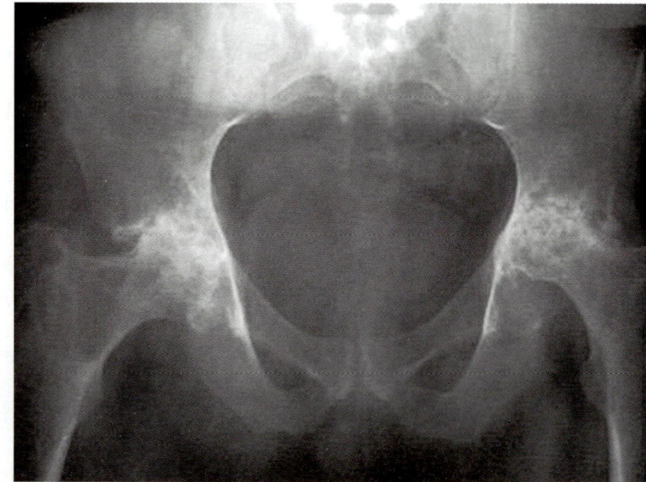

Fig. 11: X-ray showing rheumatoid arthritis.

- Joint space is decreased
- Deformities of joints
- Subcondral erosion and cyst formation
- Fibrous and bony ankylosis, develop in late stages.

Criteria for Diagnosis

- Morning stiffness
- Pain on motion or tenderness in at least one joint
- Swelling (soft tissue thickening or fluid, not bony outgrowth alone) in at least one joint continuously for not less than 6 weeks
- Symmetrical joint swelling
- Subcutaneous nodules
- X-ray changes, typical of rheumatoid arthritis
- Positive latex fixation test
- Poor mucin clot
- Characteristic histological changes in synovial membrane
- Characteristic histological changes in nodules.

Classic case of RA: Any seven criteria for at least 6 weeks

Definite case of RA: Any five criteria for at least 6 weeks

Probable case of RA: Any three criteria for at least 4 weeks.

American College of Rheumatology, Clinical Classification Criteria for Rheumatoid Arthritis

The American College of Rheumatology (ACR) clinical classification criteria for rheumatoid arthritis, using findings of history, physical examination, laboratory, and radiographic findings is described in Table 2 and Flowchart 1. For making the diagnosis of rheumatoid arthritis, four of the below enumerated criteria must be present out of which at least one must be present for a minimum of 6 weeks.

TABLE 2: ACR clinical classification criteria for rheumatoid arthritis.

Morning stiffness 1 hour
Arthritis of 3 or more of the following joints: right or left PIP, MCP, wrist, elbow, knee, ankle, and MTP joints
Arthritis of wrist, MCP, or PIP joint
Symmetric involvement of joints
Rheumatoid nodules over bony prominences, or extensor surfaces, or in juxta-articular regions
Positive serum rheumatoid factor
Radiographic changes including erosions or bony decalcification localized in or adjacent to the involved joints

Flowchart 1: ACR clinical classification criteria for rheumatoid arthritis.

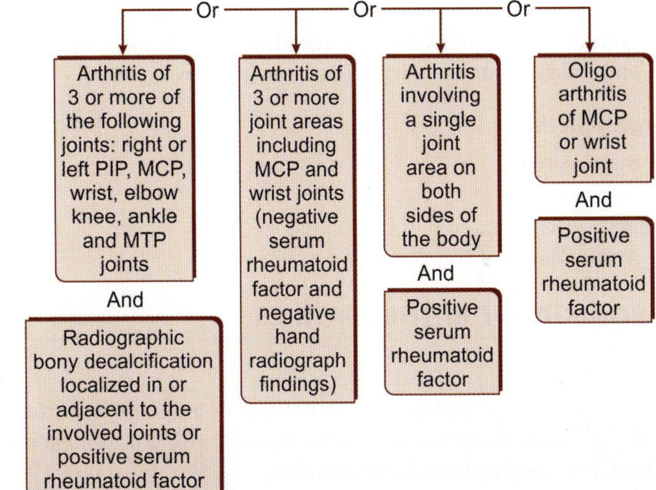

American College of Rheumatology Classification Criteria for Determining Progression of Rheumatoid Arthritis

It is listed in Table 3.

TABLE 3: ACR classification criteria for determining progression of RA.

Stage I	*Early*
	• No destructive changes on roentgenographic examination
	• Radiographic evidence of osteoporosis may be present
Stage II	*Moderate*
	• Radiographic evidence of osteoporosis, with or without slight slub
	• No joint deformities; slight cartilage destruction may be present
	• Adjacent muscle atrophy
	• Extra-articular soft tissue lesions, such as nodules and tenosynovitis may be present
Stage III	*Severe*
	• Radiographic evidence of cartilage and bone destruction, in addition to osteoporosis
	• Joint deformity, such as subluxation, ulnar deviation, or hyperextension, without fibrous or bony ankylosis
	• Extensive muscle atrophy
	• Extra-articular soft tissue lesions, such as nodules and tenosynovitis may be present
Stage IV	*Terminal*
	Fibrous or bony ankylosis
	Stage III criteria

American College of Rheumatology Classification Criteria for Determining Clinical Remission in Rheumatoid Arthritis

Five or more of the following are present for at least two consecutive months:

1. Morning stiffness <15 minutes
2. No fatigue
3. No joint pain
4. No joint tenderness or pain on motion
5. No soft tissue swelling in joints or tendon sheaths
6. ESR (Westergren's method) <30 mm/hour for a female or 20 mm/hour for a male.

American College of Rheumatology Classification Criteria of Functional Status in Rheumatoid Arthritis

Class I: Completely able to perform usual activities of daily living (selfcare, vocational and avocational).

Class II: Able to perform usual selfcare and vocational activities, but limited in avocational activities.

Class III: Able to perform usual selfcare activities, but limited in vocational and avocational activities.

Class IV: Limited ability to perform usual selfcare, vocational and avocational activities.

Management

Aims of Treatment

- To keep inflammatory treatment to minimum
- To keep constitutional symptoms to minimum
- Appropriate splinting to prevent deformities
- Surgical measures to correct deformity.

Drug Therapy

- *Analgesics and anti-inflammatory:* NSAIDs, e.g. aspirin, ibuprofen, and diclofenac sodium.
- *Disease modifying antirheumatic drugs (DMARDs):* Injectable gold and oral gold (sodium aurothiomalate), penicillamine, sulfasalazine, antimalarials (dapsone and levamisole).

Surgery Methods

- Synovectomy
- Osteotomy
- Arthrodesis
- Arthoplasty.

SERONEGATIVE ARTHROPATHIES

Introduction

Seronegative arthropathies can be defined as an acute or chronic condition with characteristic involvement of axial joints, absence of RA factor, and with HLA abnormality.

Clinical Entities

- Ankylosing spondylitis
- Reiter's disease
- Psoriatic arthritis
- Enteropathic arthritis
- Ulcerative colitis
- Crohn's disease
- Whipples disease
- Behcet's syndrome.

Etiology

- Exact pathological mechanism is not known.
- Genetic factors play an important role (the most complete evidence for familial aggregation is that for ankylosing spondylitis, children of a person with HLA-B27 have 50% chance of carrying the same antigen).
- *Salmonella, Shigella, Chlamydia,* and *Yersinia* play an important role in the pathogenesis of this group of arthritis.
- Virus.

Signs and Symptoms

Articular Features

- Low backache
- Morning stiffness
- Decreasing lumbar lordosis
- Diffuse swelling of fingers and toes
- Enthesopathy.

Common Features of Spondyloarthropathies

- Familial clustering
- Association with HLA-B27
- Axial joint involvement
- Asymmetrical peripheral joint involvement
- Enthesitis
- Extra-articular signs
- Negative rheumatoid factor
- Diagnosis of spondyloarthropathies is shown in Table 1.

Extra-articular Features

- *Skin lesions:* These include:
  - Psoriasis
  - Pitting of nails
  - Penile ulcer
- *Eye lesions:*
  - Conjunctivitis
- Bowel disorders and gastrointestinal tract (GIT) disturbance
- Dysuria
- Urethral discharge.

Diagnosis

Radiological Diagnosis

- Affected joint will show punched out areas, exceeding deep into subchondral bone.
- CT scan is indicated, when plane X-ray is normal. Used to see early changes of bone erosion and sclerosis.

Hematological Diagnosis

- HLA-B27 positive in 16–100%
- RA factor negative.

Reactive Arthritis (Reiter's Arthritis)

Introduction

- 15–30% patients progress from acute to chronic arthritis.
- Acute arthritis occurs after genitourinary *(Chlamydia)* or gastrointestinal *(Shigella, Campylobacter, Salmonella,* and *Yersinia)* infection.
- It is a clinical triad of urethritis, arthritis, and conjunctivitis.

Clinical Features

- Mono/oligoarthritis
- Conjunctivitis
- Urethritis
- Keratodermititis (Fig. 12)
- Balanitis (Fig. 13)
- Enthesitis (Fig. 14)
- Circinate balanitis
- Dactylitis
- Recurrent attacks common in *Chlamydia*-induced arthritis (Figs. 12 to 15)
- Prognostic signs for chronicity
  - Hip/heel pain
  - High ESR
  - Family history and HLA-B27 positive.

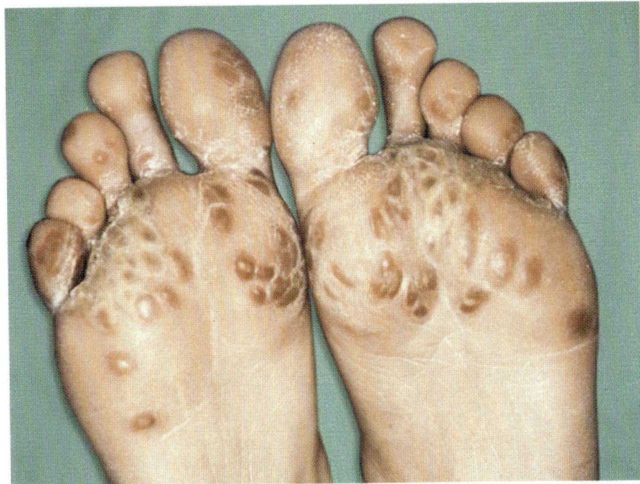

Fig. 12: Keratoderma blennorrhagica in Reiter's syndrome—keratoderma blennorrhagica on the soles of a patient with Reiter's syndrome. These lesions, which are indistinguishable from pustular psoriasis, begin as clear vesicles on erythematous bases and progress to macules, papules and nodules.

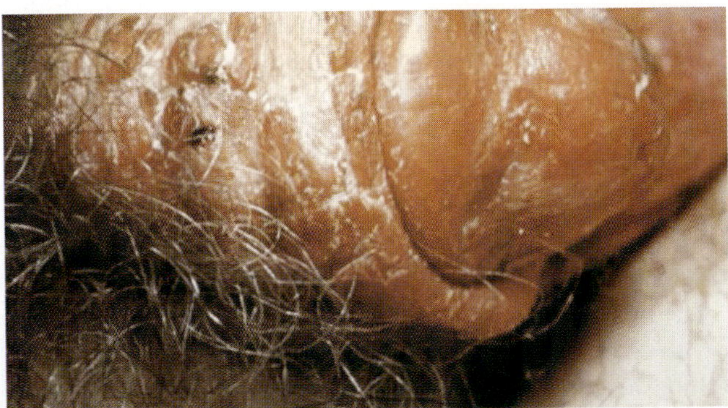

Fig. 13: Circinate balanitis in Reiter's syndrome—circinate balanitis characterized by shallow ulcers on the glans penis and the shaft of the penis. The lesions are generally asymptomatic.

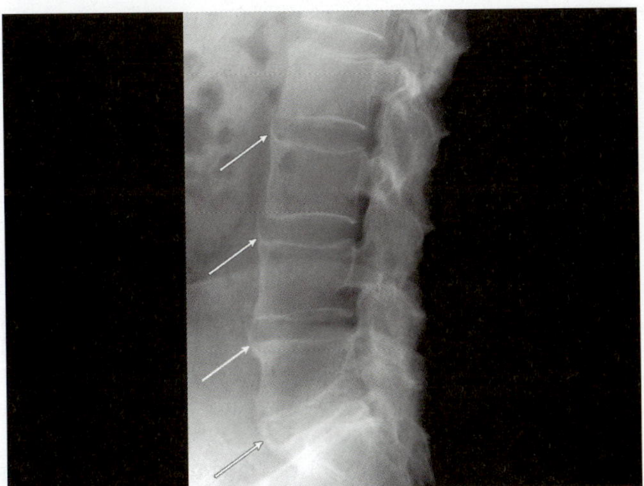

Fig. 14: Syndesmophytes in Reiter's syndrome—anterior syndesmophytes of the spine (arrows) in a patient with Reiter's syndrome. Syndesmophytes are bony out-growths that are induced by an enthesopathy of the spine. The syndesmophytes in Reiter's syndrome and psoriasis are asymmetric, in contrast to their symmetric occurrence in ankylosing spondylitis.

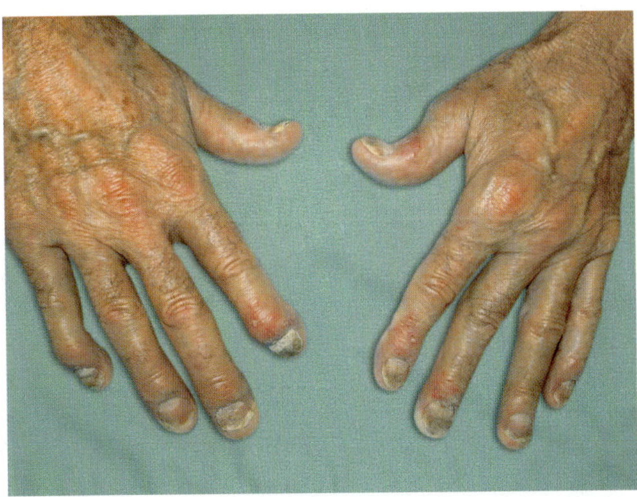

Fig. 15: Distal interphalangeal joint involvement in psoriatic arthritis—psoriatic arthritis with distal joint involvement in the third and fifth digits. Onycholysis is also seen in most of the fingernails.

Therapy for Reactive Arthritis

Acute

- NSAID
- Joint injection (if infection excluded)
- Tetracycline for 3 months in *Chlamydia* infection.

Chronic

- NSAID
- DMARD (e.g. sulfasalazine, methotrexate).

Psoriatic Arthritis

Clinical patterns may include one or more of:

- Symmetrical inflammatory arthritis
- Distal interphalangeal involvement
- Axial disease (often involving cervical spine)
- Monoarthritis
- Oligoarthritis
- Skin lesions.

Other Features (Figs. 15 to 17)

- Dactylitis, enthesistis, nail pitting
- *Psoriasis:* It may be very mild or extensive and it precedes joint disease (Fig. 18)
- Colitis related arthritis.

Pathogenesis

It is an immune mediated disease, with inflamed synovium, and infiltrated with T-cells, B-cells, and macrophages. Synovium produces cytokines.

Arthritis Mutilans

Widespread shortening of digits (telescoping) occur along with coexisting ankylosis and contractures in other digits. This typical pencil-in-cup position is called "opera glass hand".

Investigations

- ESR and CRP often elevated
- Mostly seronegative

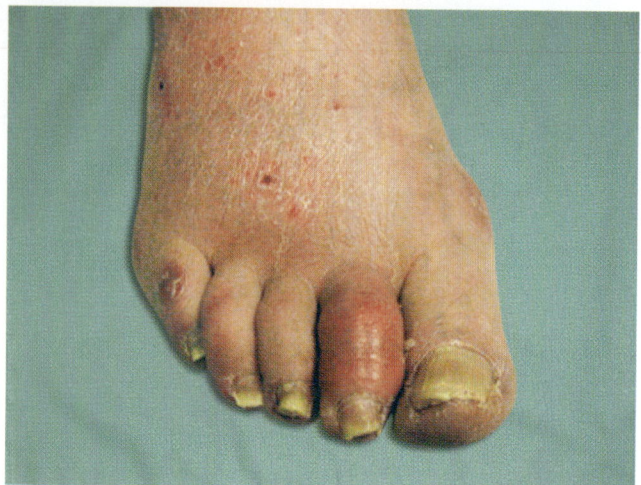

Fig. 16: Psoriatic arthritis—this photograph of the foot of a patient with psoriatic arthritis shows an early separation of the nails (onycholysis), swelling of the entire second toe (dactylitis) and some psoriatic skin lesions.

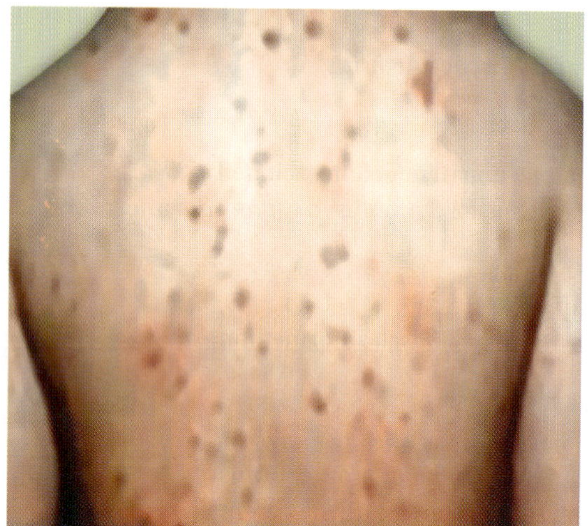

Fig. 17: Skin lesions, seen in psoriatic arthritis.

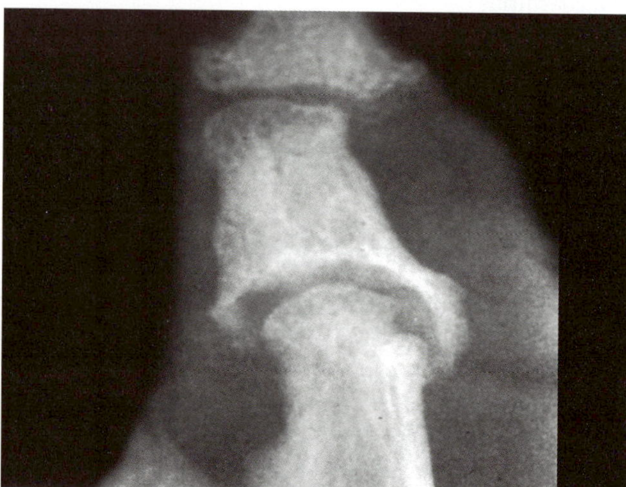

Fig. 18: X-ray showing telescoping of phalanges.

- Uric acid may be elevated in presence of extensive psoriasis
- HLA-B27 positive in 50–70%, with axial involvement. Positive in less than 15–20% with peripheral joint involvement.

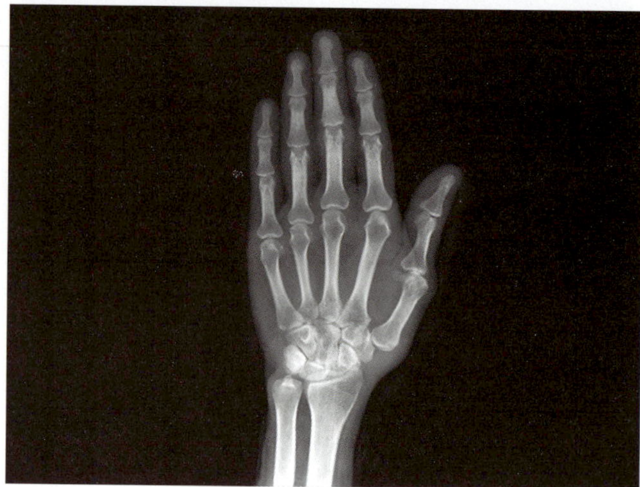

Fig. 19: X-ray showing periostitis of bones.

X-ray (Peripheral)

Distal interphalangeal (DIP) joint involvement with pencil-in-cup deformity. Marginal erosion with adjacent bony proliferation (whiskering), small joint ankylosis is seen with osteolysis of phalanges and metacarpals and telescoping of digits, periostitis of bones (Figs. 18 and 19).

Colitis Related Arthritis

- Can occur in association with Crohn's or ulcerative colitis.
- Peripheral arthritis (often a mono or oligoarthritis) improves with colectomy, axial disease does not improve.
- Sulfasalazine is helpful.

Differential Diagnosis

- Septic arthritis
- Gout
- Acute onset of other seronegative spondyloarthritis.

Investigations

- Raised ESR/CRP
- Aspirate joint to exclude infection/crystals
- Urethral swab, stool culture
- Contact tracing if necessary (Flowchart 2).

Behcet's Disease

- Behcet's syndrome is classically characterized as a triad of symptoms that include recurring crops of mouth ulcers (aphthous ulcers), genital ulcers, and inflammation of a specialized area around the pupil of the eye (uvea). The inflammation of the area of the eye that is around the pupil is called uveitis (Fig. 20). Behcet's syndrome is also sometimes referred to as Behcet's disease.
- Joint inflammation (arthritis) can lead to swelling, stiffness, warmth, pain, and tenderness of joints in patients with Behcet's syndrome.

  This occurs in about half of patients with Behcet's syndrome at some time during their lives. Knees, wrists, ankles, and elbows are the most common joints affected.

Flowchart 2: Diagnosis of spondyloarthropathies.

Inflammatory arthritis that is asymmetric or predominantly lower extermity? and/or Back pain of insidious onset of > 3 months duration associated with morning stiffness and improvement with activity?

No → Unlikely to be a spondyloarthropathy

Yes → Evidence of psoriasis or inflammatory bowel disease?

Yes → Consider enteropathic or psoriatic arthritis

No → One or more of the following?
- Radiographic evidence of sacroiliitis
- Enthesopathy
- Dactylitis
- Buttock pain (unilateral or alternating)
- Urethritis or cervicitis
- Family history
- Iritis
- Acute diarrhea or nongonococcal urethritis within 1 month of onset

No → Unlikely to be a spondyloarthropathy

Yes → Likely to be a spondyloarthropathy → Evidence of spondylitis? (Inflammatory spinal pain and limitation of movement)

Yes → Probably ankylosing spondylitis

No → Probably reactive arthritis/Reiter's syndrome → Evidence of chlamydial infection? (i.e. elevated antichlamydial antibody titers)

No → Reactive arthritis/ Reiter's syndrome

Yes → Chlamydial associated reactive arthritis

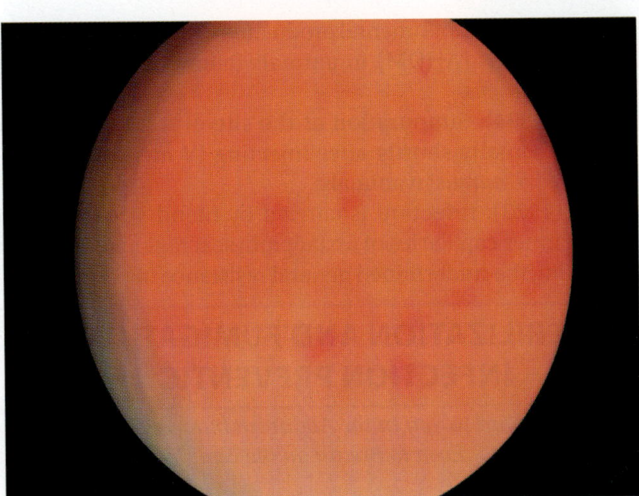

Fig. 20: Uveitis.

- The symptoms of Behcet's syndrome depend on the area of the body affected. Behcet's syndrome can involve inflammation of many areas of the body. These areas include the arteries that supply blood to the body's tissues. Behcet's syndrome can also affect the veins that take the blood back to the lungs to replenish the oxygen content. Other areas of body that can be affected by the inflammation of Behcet's syndrome include the back of the eyes (retina), brain, joints, skin, and bowels.

Marie Stumpell Disease/Bekhterev Disease (Ankylosing Spondylitis)

Definition

It is a chronic progressive inflammatory disease of the sacroiliac joint and the axial skeleton.

For ankylosing spondylitis, please refer to spine section.

CHAPTER

10 Infections in Orthopedics

OBJECTIVES

Sterilization and Fumigation in Infection Prevention
- Basic Definitions
- Instruments: Three Categories
- Cleaning
- Disinfection
- Sterilization
- OT Fumigation Instrumentation and Techniques
- Fumigation
- Several Chemicals are Available but the Economic Limitations are Great Hurdle in Exploring the Utility in Developing Countries

Biocompatibility of Implants
- Early Definition
- Contemporary Definition
- Nuclear Scans
- Positron Emission Tomography
- Management
- Management of Incisional Surgical Site Infection
- Management of Postoperative Joint Infection
- Antibiotic Spacer

Prevention of Surgical Site Infection in Orthopedic Surgery
- Background
- Surface Cleaning and Disinfection
- Work Related Issues
- Preoperative Preparation of the Patient and the Surgical Site
- HIV and Hepatitis B Infected Cases
- Water Supply
- Reprocessing of Single Use Items
- Surgical Attire and Drapes
- Microbiological Sampling
- Staff Health, Infected and Colonized Personnel
- Implementation Aspects
- Investigation of a Case of Surgical Site Infection
- Pyogenic Osteomyelitis
- Acute Hematogenous Osteomyelitis
- Subacute Osteomyelitis
- Chronic Osteomyelitis
- Diseases of Joints (Arthritis)
- Septic Arthritis
- Tuberculosis of Musculoskeletal System
- Tuberculosis of Spine

Skeletal Tuberculosis of Hip, Knee, Shoulder, Ankle, Elbow and Wrist
- Tuberculosis of Hip
- Tuberculosis of Knee
- Tuberculosis of Shoulder
- Tuberculosis of Ankle
- Tuberculosis of Elbow
- Tuberculosis of Wrist
- Actinomycosis
- Mycetoma (Maduromycosis)

INTRODUCTION

The term indicates inflammation of bone caused by infective organisms.

Common Causative Organisms

- Nonspecific pyogenic organisms, such as *Staphylococcus, Streptococcus*
- Specific organisms, such as syphilis, tuberculous, typhoid, paratyphoid, causing organism
- Mycetomal (fungal) organisms
- Parasitic infection, e.g. hydatid cyst.

History

- Recognized as an old disease in Egyptian mummies
- Nelaton (1844): Coined the term osteomyelitis
- Hartmann (1855): Hypothesis of thrombosis of main trunk of nutrient artery
- Lennelongue (1879): Metaphyseal infection
- Rodet (1884): Experimental production of acute hematogenous osteomyelitis (AHOM) in animals following IV injection of *Staphylococcus.*
- Lexer (1894): Suppuration at the site of trauma, produced experimentally shortly after injecting IV measured dose of cultured *S. aureus* in animals.
- Starr (1922): Infection is carried by blood stream till they reach inner capillaries of juxtaepiphyseal region of long bone, lowering the undermined general resistance of patient.

STERILIZATION AND FUMIGATION IN INFECTION PREVENTION

"You can Afford to Spit in the Abdomen but you cannot Afford Even to Breath on the Bone"

BASIC DEFINITIONS

- *Sterilization*—a process that destroys or eliminates all forms of microbial life (Fig. 1).

- *Disinfection*—a process that eliminates many or all pathogenic microorganisms, except bacterial spores, on inanimate objects.
- *Cleaning*—removal of visible soil (e.g. organic and inorganic material) from objects and surfaces.
- *Decontamination*—removes pathogenic microorganisms from objects so they are safe to handle, use, or discard.
- *Antiseptic*—germicides applied to living tissue and skin.
- *Disinfectant*—antimicrobials applied only to inanimate objects.

INSTRUMENTS: THREE CATEGORIES

1. *Low risk (noncritical items)*—come into contact with normal and intact skin as stethoscopes. Cleaning with a detergent and drying is usually adequate.
2. *Intermediate risk (semi critical items)*—do not penetrate skin or enter sterile areas of the body but that are in close contact with mucous membranes or with nonintact skin. Cleaning followed by high level disinfectant (HLD) is usually adequate. For example, respiratory equipment, flexible endoscopes, laryngoscopes, specula, endotracheal tubes, and thermometers.
3. *High risk (critical items)*—penetrate sterile tissues such as body cavities and the vascular system. Cleaning followed by sterilization is required instruments, intra-uterine devices, vascular catheters, implants, etc. (Fig. 2).

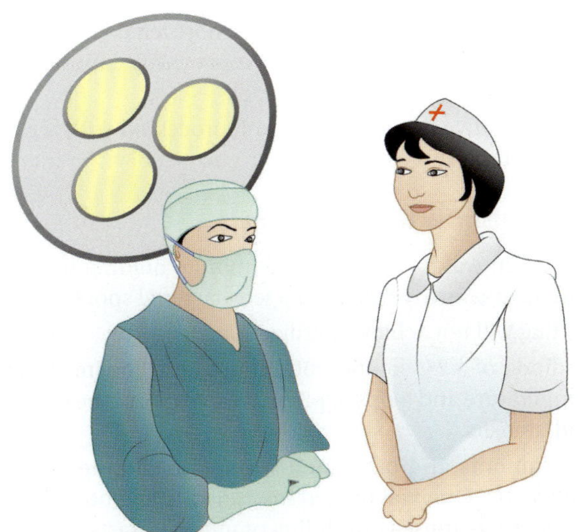

Fig. 1: Surgeon following proper sterile precautions by wearing cap, mask, gown and gloves. Whereas the sister is not following any of these precautions. This is a primary step of sterility in OT.

CLEANING

- Though sterilization is the aim, one cannot directly proceed to sterilization.
- Thorough and meticulous cleaning is the essential primary step.
- Removal of all foreign material (dirt and organic matter)
- Should always precede disinfection and sterilization procedures
- Accomplished by the use of water, detergents, and mechanical actions
- Solution used most often to clean is an enzymatic presoak (protease formula that dissolves protein). Alternatively a detergent can be used (Fig. 3).
- Studies show that thorough cleaning alone can provide a 10,000 fold reduction in contaminant microbes from endoscopes.

Types of Cleaning

- *Mechanical cleaning:*
  - Washing machine
  - Washer/disinfector
  - Ultrasonicator (Fig. 4)
- *Manual cleaning:* Necessary when:
  - Mechanical cleaning facilities are not available
  - Delicate instruments have to be cleaned
  - Items with narrow lumens need to be cleaned (endoscopes).

Steps for Cleaning

- Wear heavy duty rubber gloves, a plastic apron, eye protection, and mask during cleaning (Fig. 5).
- Soak the instrument in normal tap water containing a detergent.

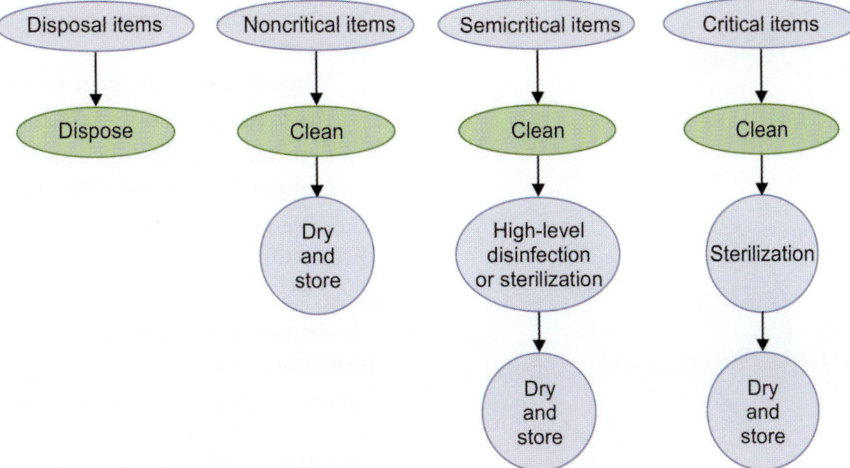

Fig. 2: Types of instrument and its decontamination.

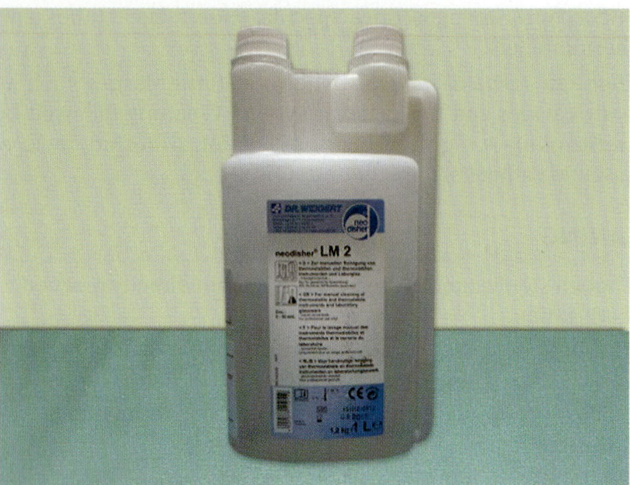

Fig. 3: Presoak for cleaning: Neodisher.

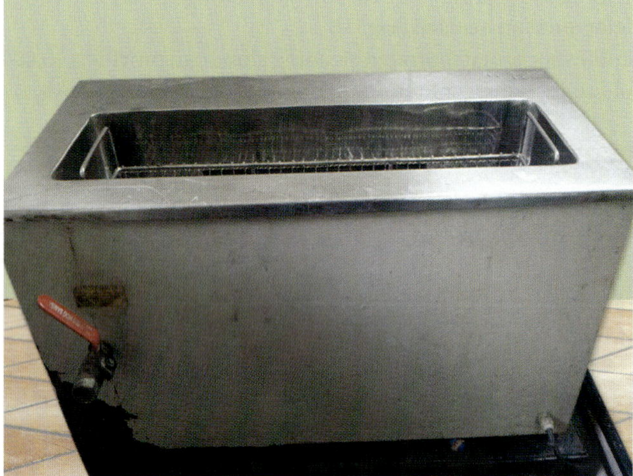

Fig. 4: Ultrasonicator.

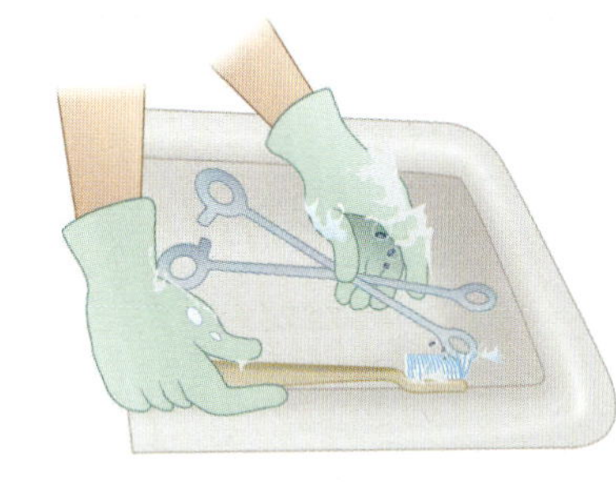

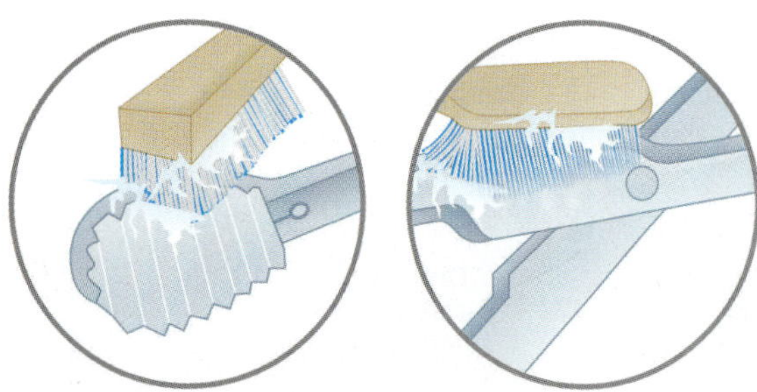

Fig. 5: Steps for cleaning.

- Scrub instrument and other items vigorously lo completely remove all foreign material using a soft brush or old toothbrush, detergent, and water. Hold items under the surface of the water while scrubbing and cleaning to avoid splashing. Disassemble instruments and other item with multiple parts, and be sure to brush in the grooves, teeth and joints to, items here organic material can collect and stick (Figs. 6 and 7).
- Flush through lumens with an adapted water jet (Fig. 8).
- Rinse items thoroughly with clean water to remove all detergent. Any detergent left on the items can reduce the effectiveness of further processing.
- Inspect items to confirm that they are clean.
- Allow items to air dry or dry them with a clean towel if chemical disinfection is going to be used. This is to avoid diluting the chemical solution sued after cleaning. Items that will be high-level disinfected by boiling or steaming do not need to be dried (Fig. 9).

DISINFECTION

- Thermal or chemical
- Thermal disinfection is preferred—more reliable than chemical processes, leaves no residues, is more easily controlled, and is nontoxic
- Heat sensitive items have to be reprocessed with a chemical disinfectant.

Thermal Disinfection—Boiling

- Boiling in water (100°C for one minute holding time), which kills all organisms except for a few bacterial spores.
- Boiling will not achieve sterilization.
- Addition of a 2% solution of sodium bicarbonate elevates the temperature and helps to prevent corrosion of the instruments and utensils.
- Instruments and other items must be completely covered with water. Open all hinged instruments and other items and disassemble those with sliding or multiple parts.

Chemical Disinfection

- Used most commonly for heat-labile equipment (e.g. endoscopes)
- Number of disinfectants can be used for this purpose. For example:
  - Glutaraldehyde 2% for 20 min: CIDEX
  - Hydrogen peroxide 6–7.5% for 20–30 minutes
  - Peracetic acid 0.2–0.35% for 5 minutes
  - Orthophthalaldehyde (OPA) for 5–12 minutes.
- The object must be thoroughly rinsed with sterile water after disinfection (Fig. 10).

Note:

- Concentration of used disinfectant and contact time should be revised.
- Different companies provide different concentrations for a single disinfectant.
- Manufacturer's instructions should be carefully read before use of any disinfectant.

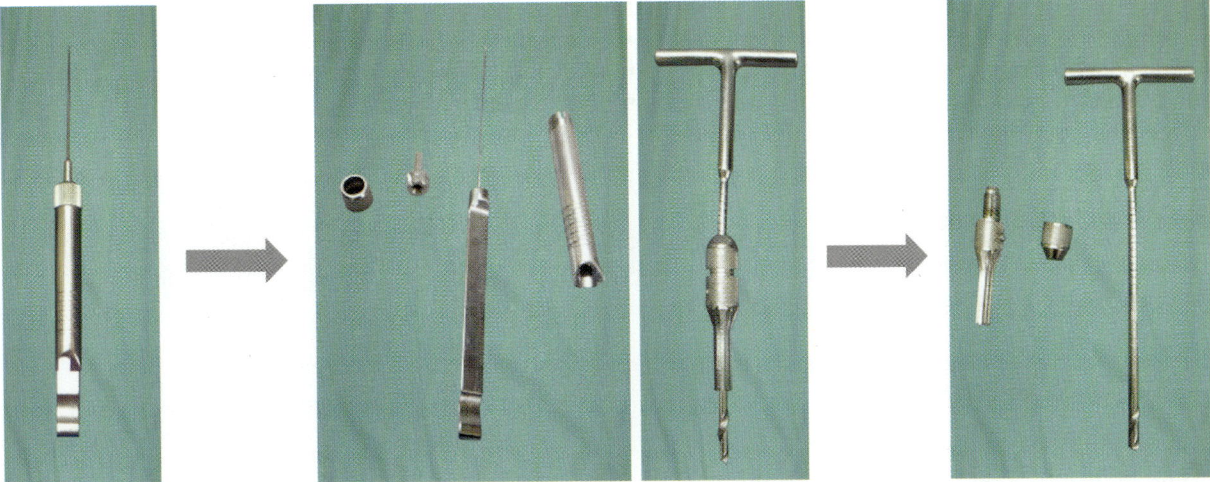

Fig. 6: Disassemble instruments before cleaning.

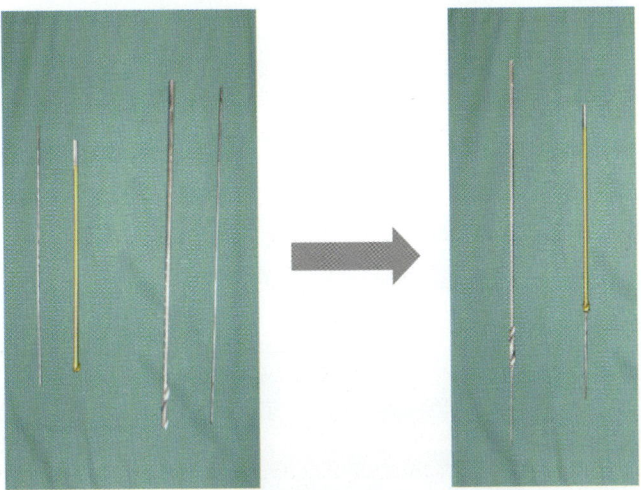

Fig. 7: Disassemble instruments before cleaning.

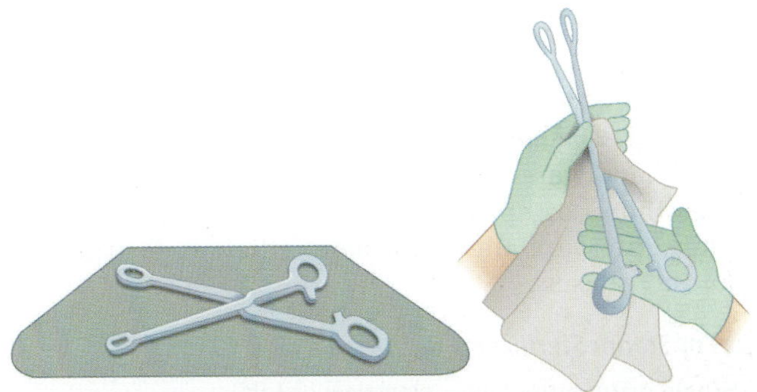

Fig. 9: Allow items to air dry or dry them with a clean towel if chemical disinfection is going to be used.

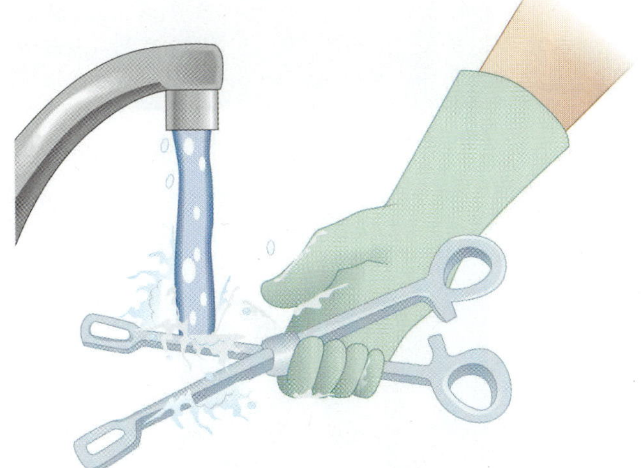

Fig. 8: Flush through lumens with an adapted water jet.

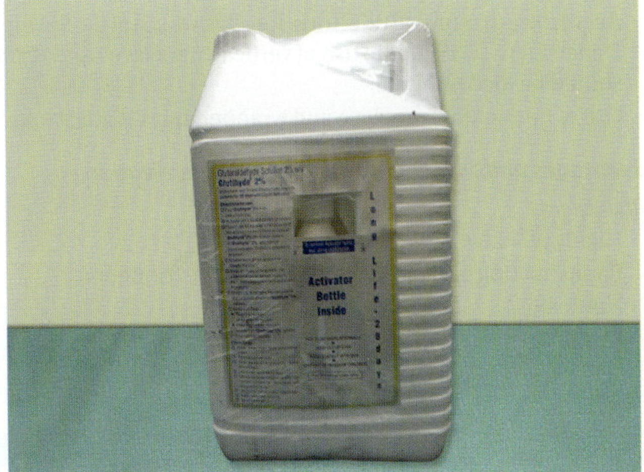

Fig. 10: Glutaraldehyde.

STERILIZATION

- Sterilization is a process which achieves the complete destruction or killing of all microorganisms, including bacterial spores.
- *Sterilization is principally accomplished by:*
  - Steam under pressure (autoclaving)
  - Dry-heat sterilization (hot air oven)
  - The use of chemicals such as ethylene oxide gas (which is mainly used in industry) or other low temperature methods (e.g. hydrogen peroxide gas plasma).
  - Gamma irradiation (usually for implants).

High temp Low temp Gamma irradiation

Autoclave or hot air oven ETO hydrogen peroxide

Note:
- Boiling and flaming are not effective sterilization techniques because they do not effectively kill all microorganisms.
- Large healthcare facilities should have more than one type of sterilization system in case of power outage, equipment failure, or shortage of supplies.

Pressure Steam Sterilization (Autoclaving)

- The most common and most preferred.
- All items that penetrate the skin and mucosa if they are heat stable.
- Dependable, nontoxic, inexpensive, sporicidal, and has rapid heating and good penetration of fabrics.

Method

The steam must be applied for a specified time so that the items reach a specified temperature.

Different temperature and time settings for wrapped and unwrapped instruments (Table 1).

Note:
- Sterilization time does not include the time it takes to reach the required temperature or the time for exhaust and drying; therefore, it is shorter than the total cycle time.
- The temperatures required for steam sterilization are lower than those for dry-heat sterilization because moist heat under pressure allows for more efficient destruction of microorganisms.

Types of Steam Sterilizers

- Single drum autoclave—electrical or LPG
- Double drum vertical autoclaves
- Horizontal autoclaves with automatic cycles—electrically or LPG operated
- Emergency (flash) autoclave
- High-speed vacuum autoclave (Figs. 11 to 13).
- According to new guidelines for Central Sterile Services Department (CSSD), the use of vertical autoclaves and drums should be discontinued.
- Use of horizontal autoclave and wrapped trays is advisable.

Advantages and Disadvantages of Steam Sterilization

Advantages
- Highly effective
- Rapid heating and rapid penetration of instruments
- Nontoxic
- Inexpensive
- Can be used to sterilize liquids.

TABLE 1: Sterilization times.

Type of instrument	*Sterilization time*
Unwrapped 121 C (1.036 Bar)	20 min
Unwrapped 134 C (2.026) (metal and glass only)	3 min
Unwrapped 134 C (2.026 Bar)	10 min
Wrapped 121 C (1.036 Bar)	30 min
Wrapped 134 C (2.026 Bar)	15 min

Disadvantages
- Items must be heat and moisture resistant
- Will not sterilize powders, ointments or oils
- Needs good maintenance

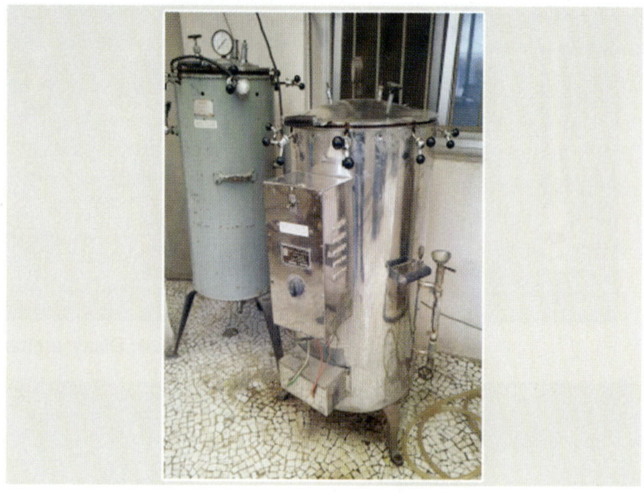

Fig. 11: Vertical autoclave (electrical).

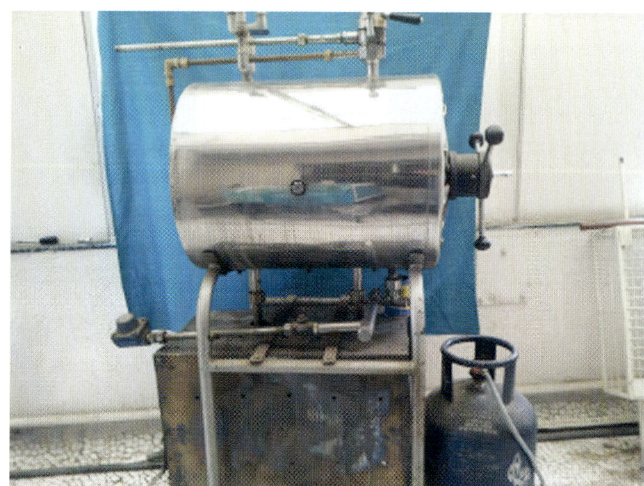

Fig. 12: Horizontal autoclave (LPG).

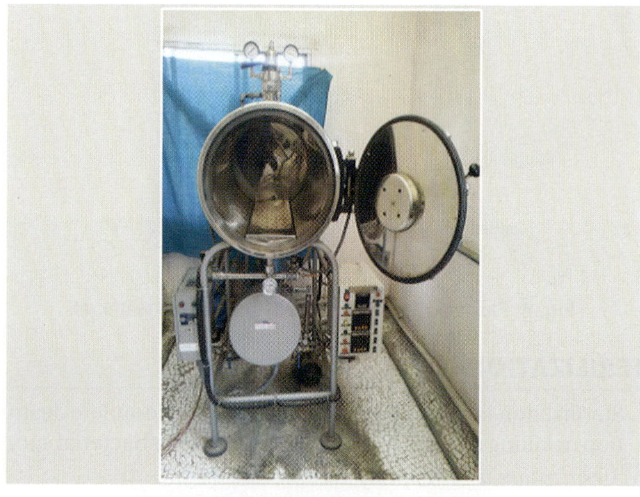

Fig. 13: Horizontal autoclave (electrical).

- To reduce the encrustation of salts over the instruments during autoclaving, distilled water can be used for autoclaving
- Distilled water plant can be setup in the autoclaving room (Fig. 14).

Autoclave Maintenance

- The autoclave should be checked each time it is used.
- An equipment log should be used to monitor performance including temperature, timing, and cycle.
- Routine maintenance should become standard procedure. Someone should be assigned to be responsible for this task.
- Follow the manufacturer's instructions whenever possible since autoclave maintenance varies depending on the type of autoclave.

Dry-Heat Sterilization (Hot Air Oven)

- Preferred for reusable glass, metal instruments, oil, ointments, and powders.
- Do not use this method of sterilization for other items, which may melt or burn (Table 2).

Note:
- The oven must have a thermometer or temperature gauge to make sure that the designated temperature is reached.
- Do not begin timing until the oven reaches the desired temperature.
- If the timing process is forgotten, start it when the oversight is realized.

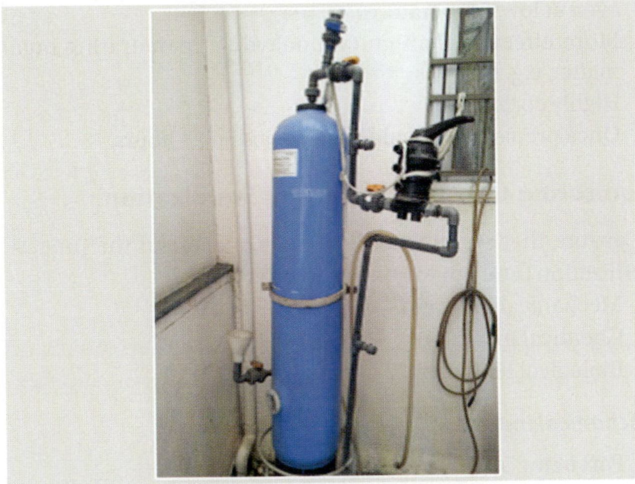

Fig. 14: Distilled water plant.

TABLE 2: Dry-heat sterilization temperatures and times.

Holding temperature	*Sterilization time (after reaching the holding temperature)*
180°C	30 min
170°C	1 hour
160°C	2 hours
149°C	2.5 hours
141°C	3 hours

Advantages and Disadvantages of Dry-Heat Sterilization

Advantages:
- Can be used for powders, anhydrous oils, and glass
- Reaches surfaces of instruments that cannot be disassembled
- No corrosive or rusting effect on instruments
- Low cost.

Disadvantages:
- Penetrates materials slowly and unevenly
- Long exposure times necessary
- High temperatures damage rubber goods and some fabrics
- Limited package materials.

Low Temperature Sterilization

- For heat- and moisture-sensitive medical devices
- Ethylene oxide has been the most common method
- *Other methods:* hydrogen peroxide + gas plasma and immersion in a dilute liquid peracetic acid.

Ethylene Oxide Gas

- Sterilize most articles that can withstand temperatures of 50–60°C—heat-labile equipment, fluids, and rubber, etc.
- Extremely toxic and explosive
- A long period of aeration (to remove all traces of the gas) is required before the equipment can be distributed
- Operating cycle ranges from 2 to 24 hours and it is a relatively expensive process (Figs. 15 to 17).

Hydrogen Peroxide Gas Plasma

- Plasma is the fourth state of matter. It is gas in ionized form
- Generated in a chamber under deep vacuum and acted on by radiofrequency radiation
- Free radical particles disrupt microbial cellular components
- The plasma is combined with hydrogen peroxide
- Cycle time is approximately 75 minutes.

Gamma Irradiation

- Though a highly effective mode of sterilization, not widely used due to radiation norms.
- Presently, limited to sterilization of implants especially those used for arthroplasty.

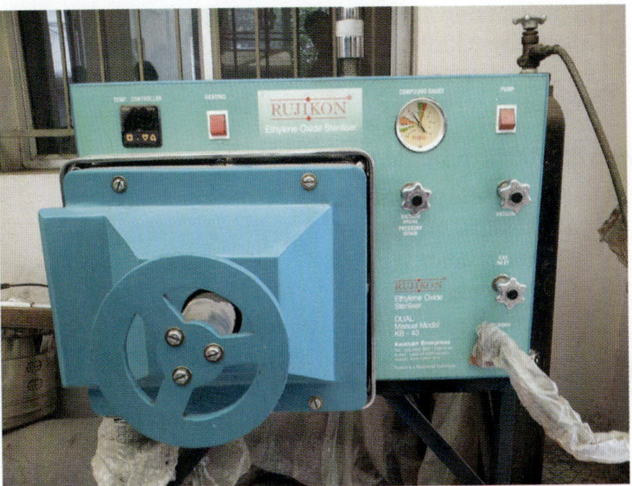

Fig. 15: Ethylene oxide (ETO) sterilizer.

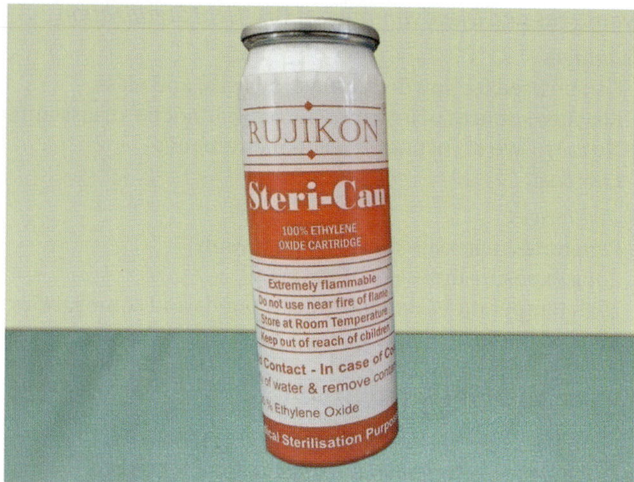

Fig. 16: Disposable ETO cartridge.

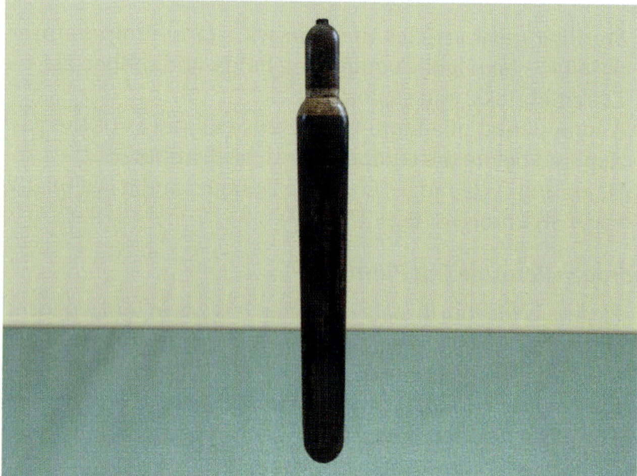

Fig. 17: ETO cylinder.

Chemical Sterilization

- Primarily used for heat-labile equipment (scopes).
- Soaking in a chemical solution followed by rinsing in sterile water.
- The immersion time to achieve sterilization or sporicidal activity is specific for each type of chemical sterilant.
- Item is sterilized chemically; it should be used immediately after sterilization, to be sure that it is sterile.

Types of Chemical Sterilants

- Glutaraldehyde is a commonly available solution.
- *Other chemical sterilants:*
  - Peracetic acid;
  - 7.5% hydrogen peroxide;
  - Hydrogen peroxide (1%) plus peracetic acid (0.08%).

Glutaraldehyde Cidex

- 2% glutaraldehyde solution for at least 10 hours to sterilize heat labile items;
- Irritating to the skin, to the eyes, and to the respiratory tract;
- May cause respiratory illness (asthma) and allergic dermatitis;

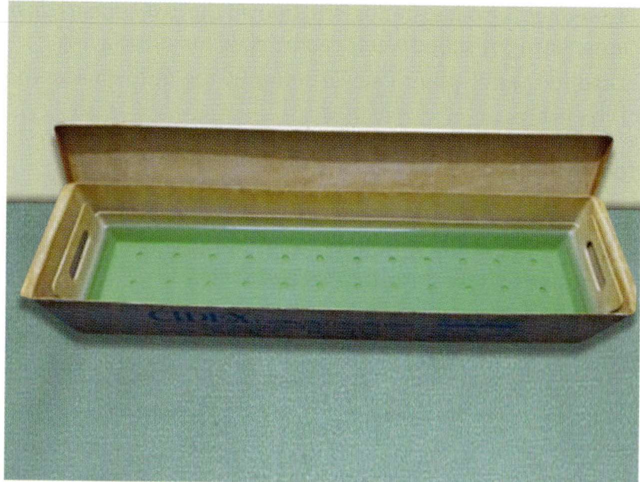

Fig. 18: Glutaraldehyde: Cidex.

- Eye protection, a plastic apron, and gloves must be worn when glutaraldehyde liquid is made up, disposed of, and used for sterilization.
- The length of time that glutaraldehyde solutions can be used varies but they are usually good for up to 14 days. Solutions should be replaced any time they become cloudy (Fig. 18).

Peracetic Acid: Nu-Cidex

- Used to sterilize heat-labile items (e.g. arthroscopes, dental instruments).
- 0.2–0.35% peracetic solution for 10 minutes;
- Effective in the presence of organic matter and is sporicidal even at low temperatures.
- More effective than glutaraldehyde at penetrating organic matter, e.g. biofilms;
- Highly corrosive;
- Once prepared—should be used within 24 hours.

Monitoring the Effectiveness of Sterilization

To ensure that sterilization has been successful the process of sterilization (and not the end product) is tested:

- Mechanical indicators
- Chemical indicators
- Biological indicators.

Mechanical Indicators

- Part of the autoclave or dry-heat oven itself
- Record and allow you to observe time, temperature, and/or pressure readings during the sterilization cycle.

Chemical Indicators

- Tape with lines that change color when the intended temperature has been reached.
- Pellets in glass tubes that melt, indicating that the intended temperature and time have been reached.
- Indicator strips that show that the intended combination of temperature, time, and pressure has been achieved.
- Indicator strips that show that the chemicals and/or gas are still effective.

- Chemical indicators are available for testing ethylene oxide, dry-heat, and steam processes. These indicators are used internally, placed where steam or temperature takes longest to reach, or put on the outside of the wrapped packs to distinguish processed from nonprocessed packages (Figs. 19 to 22).

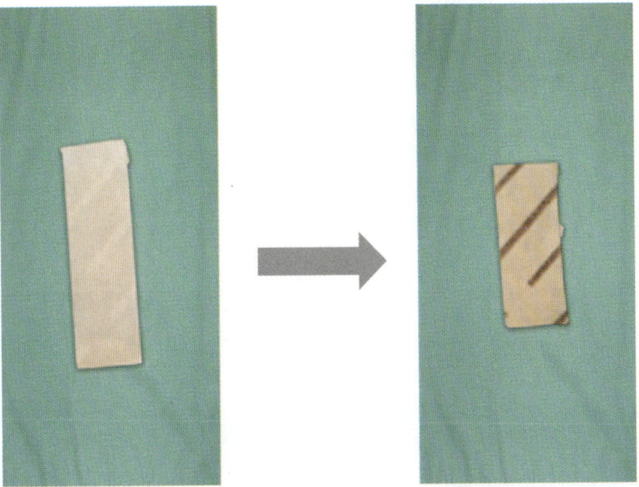

Fig. 19: Chemical indicators (for autoclave).

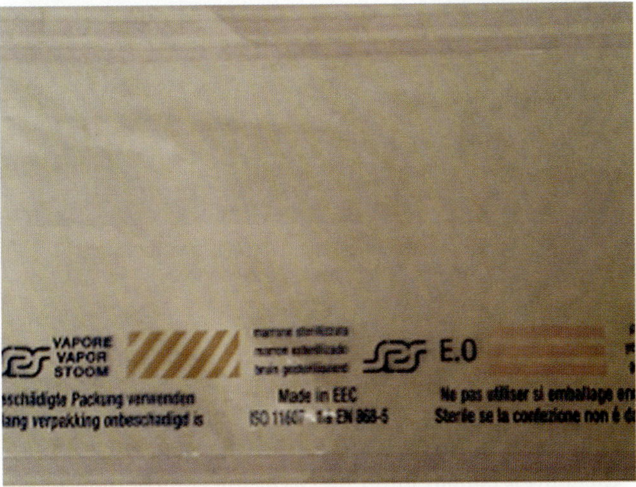

Fig. 20: Chemical indicators (for ETO sterilizer).

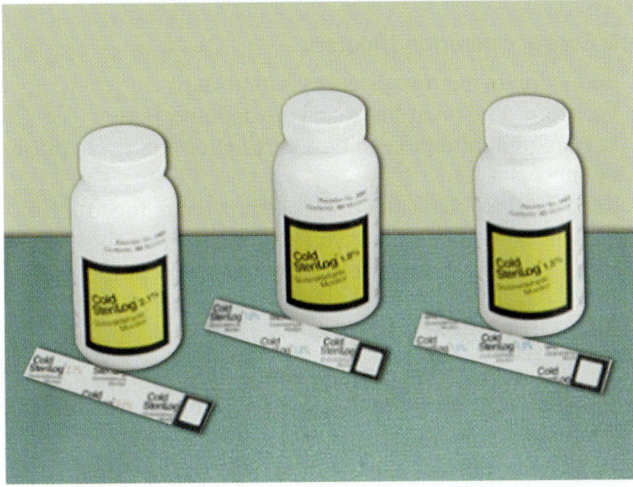

Fig. 21: Chemical indicator strips to monitor effectiveness of glutaraldehyde solutions.

Biological Indicators

- Use heat-resistant bacterial endospores.
- If the bacterial endospores have been killed after sterilization, you can assume that all microorganisms have been killed as well.
- After the sterilization process, the strips are placed in a broth that supports aerobic growth and incubated for 7 days.
- *Advantage:* It directly measures the effectiveness of sterilization.
- *Disadvantage:* Indicator is not immediate, as are mechanical and chemical indicators.

Correcting Sterilization Failure

- If monitoring indicates a failure in sterilization, attempt to determine the cause of the failure and arrange for corrective steps, as follows:
  - Immediately check that the autoclave or dry-heat oven is being used correctly or replace the chemical solution.
  - If correct use of the unit has been documented and monitoring still indicates a failure in sterilization, discontinue using the unit and have it serviced.
  - Any instruments or other items that have been processed in the faulty autoclave or dry-heat oven must be considered nonsterile and must be processed again when the unit is functioning properly.

OT FUMIGATION INSTRUMENTATION AND TECHNIQUES

Role of Cleaning in Theater Asepsis

- Cleaning of the OT is the basic primary and essential step before fumigation
- Only fumigation is ineffective if proper cleaning protocol not followed.

Cleaning Protocol in OT (Fig. 23)

- Continuous process
- At the beginning of the day, between two procedures, by the end of the day, and at the end of the week
- Floor cleaned with 1% sodium hypochlorite. All other surfaces to be cleaned with a disinfectant using a lint-free cloth (Figs. 24 to 26).

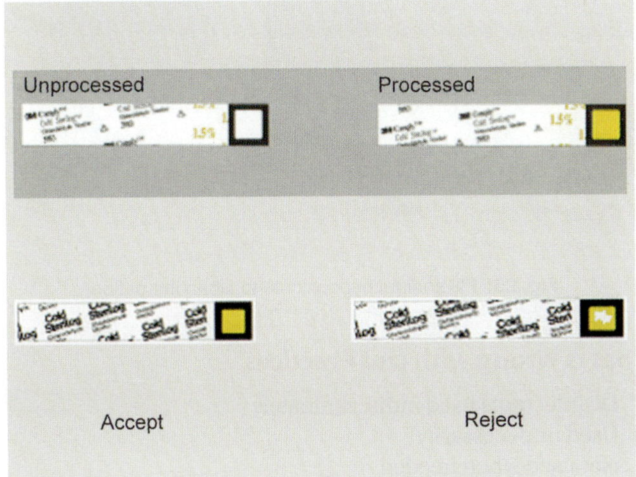

Fig. 22: Changes from white to yellow.

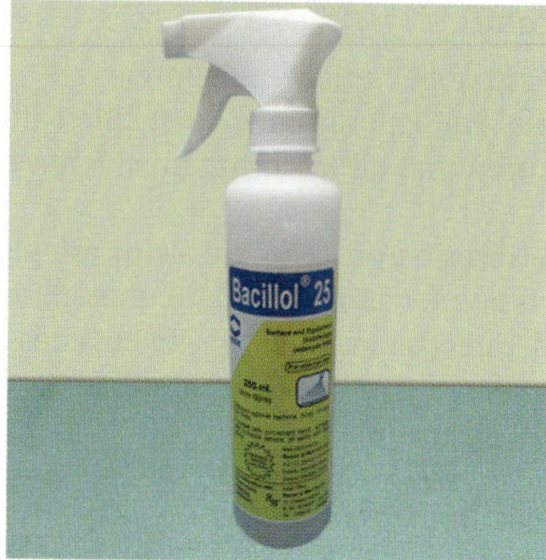

Fig. 23: 1% sodium hypochlorite to clean the ot floor.

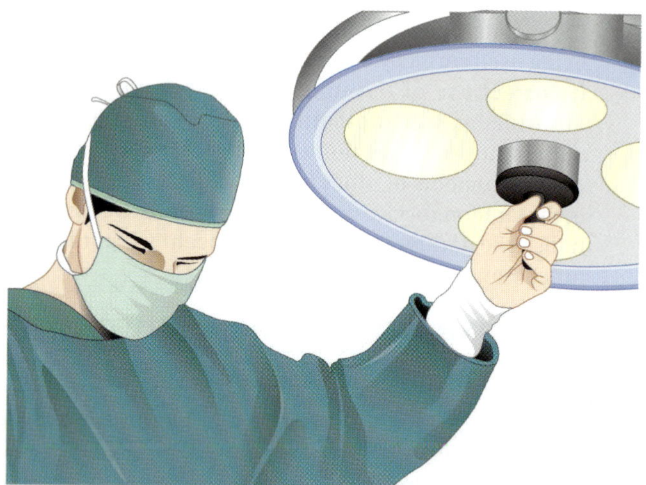

Fig. 24: A disinfectant is used along with lint free cloth to clean surfaces other than the floor.

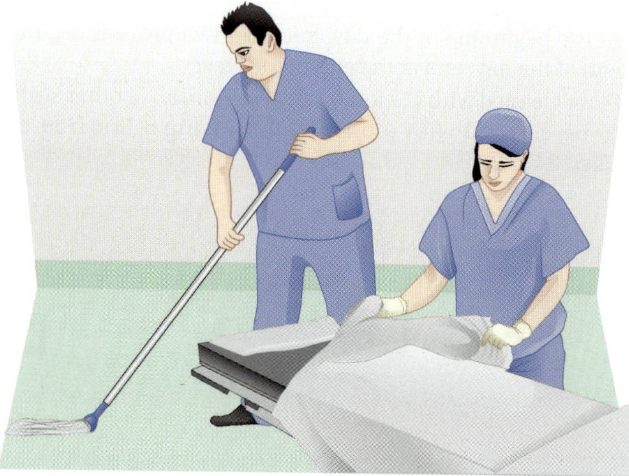

Fig. 25: 1% sodium hypochlorite to clean the ot floor.

What is Wrong with Our Practices

- Disinfectants used indiscriminately
- Used unnecessarily
- Not used when needed
- Concentration not adequate
- Economic consideration

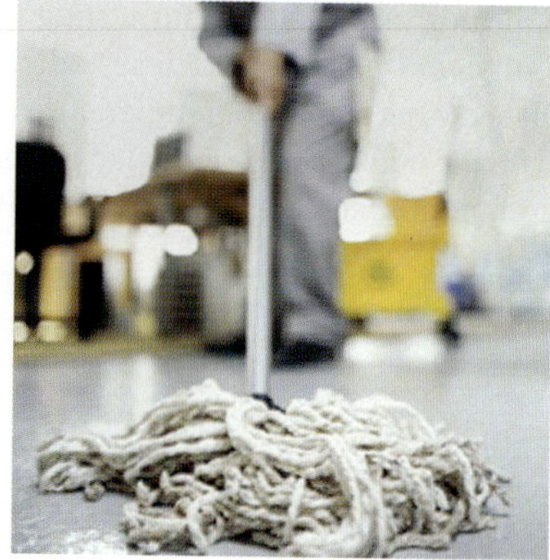

Fig. 26: 1% sodium hypochlorite to clean the ot floor.

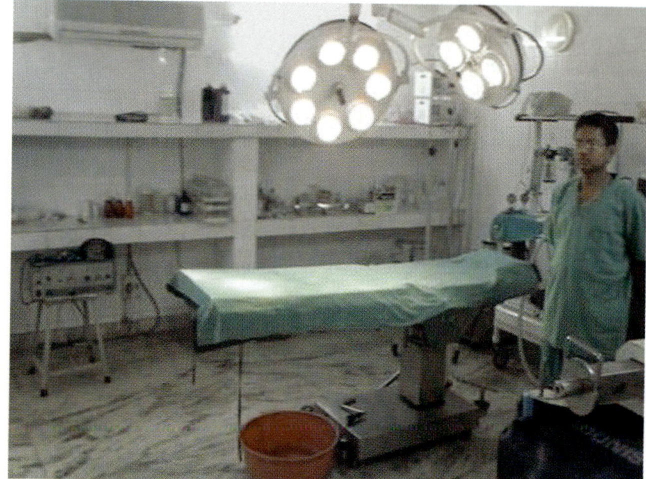

Fig. 27: Frequent cleaning of walls and roof of operation theater is not needed.

- Business promotions
- Laboratory testing and hospital conditions may not correlate.

Basic Principles

- Cleaning is equally important as disinfection and sterilization.
- Cleaning—removes contaminants, dust, and organic matter.
- Disinfection—reduces number of microbes.

Basic Care of Operation Theaters

- Reduction of microbial counts is important
- Very rarely the microbes reach the operation site
- Paying great attention to floors using too many chemicals is not necessary
- Keep the floor clean and dry—bacteria are reduced
- Presence of water and moisture is necessary for the bacteria
- Drying leads to natural death of bacteria except spores.

Disinfection and Sterilization

- Sterilization is absolute, removes microbes and spores too.
- To achieve sterilization is expensive, not sustainable, many times not needed.
- An effective disinfection reduces the infections drastically.
- Frequent cleaning has little effect (Fig. 27).
- Do not disturb these areas unnecessarily.

- *Floors get contaminated quickly (Fig. 28). Contamination depends on:*
  - Number of persons present in the theater
  - Movements they make, has direct relation to increase of bacterial counts.

So, number of OT personnel and their movement should be restricted (Fig. 29).

Do Not Disturb the Roof

- Do not disturb it unnecessarily
- Do not use ceiling fans as they cause aerosol spread.

Care of Floors (Fig. 30)

- Do remember only 1% of the microbes present on the floors are pathogenic
- Floor should be decontaminated with vacuum cleaner and wet cleaning techniques
- Keep the mops dry when not in use
- Use only vacuum cleaners (Fig. 31)
- Do not broom as it increases the bacterial flora in the environment
- A simple detergent reduces flora by 80%
- Addition of disinfectant reduces to 95%
- In busy hospitals, counts increase every 2 hours.

  So, floor cleaning is necessary every 2 hours (Fig. 32).

Environmental Cleaning of Operation Theaters

- Do not waste chemicals
- Only remove the dust with cloth wetted with clean water

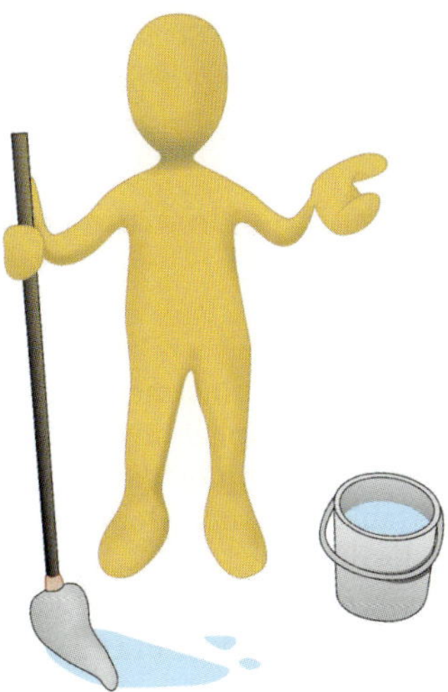

Fig. 30: How you care for floors?

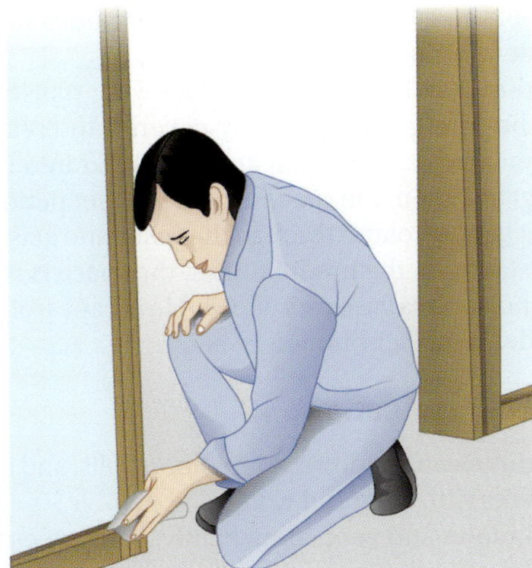

Fig. 28: Proper cleaning of the corner and crevices.

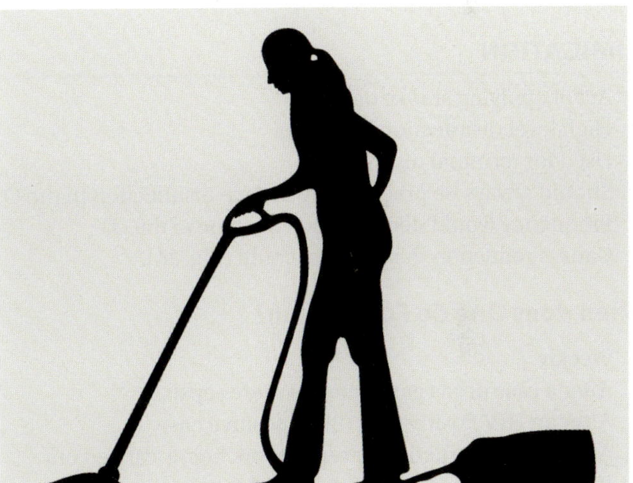

Fig. 31: Cleaning the Floor.

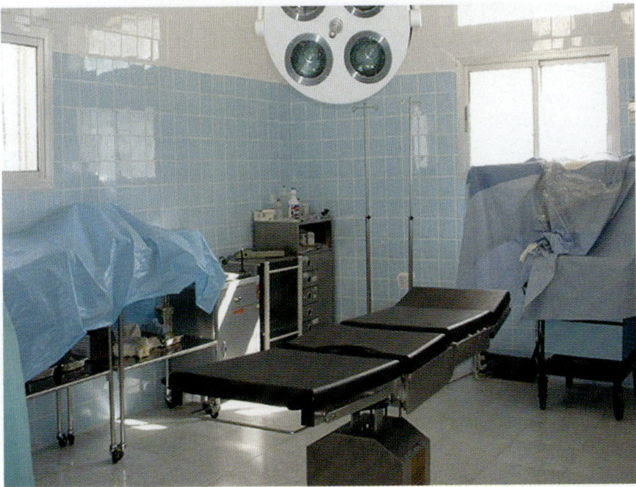

Fig. 29: Proper sterile precautions.

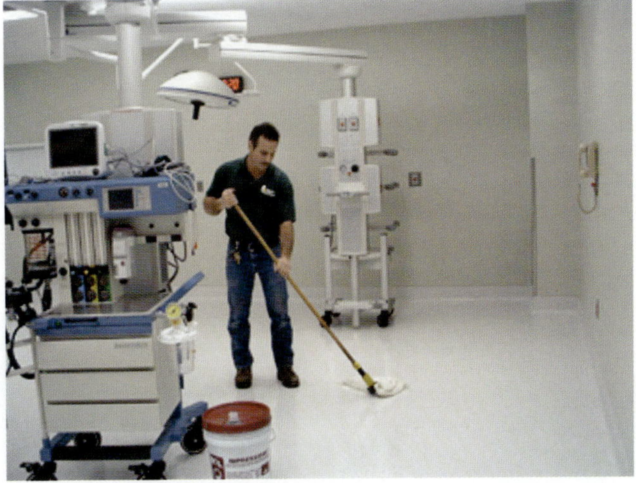

Fig. 32: Floor cleaning necessary every 2 hours.

- Do not use chemicals/disinfectants as a habit
- Use only when contaminated with blood or body fluids.

Environmental Cleaning of Hospital with Chlorinated Compounds

Disinfectant	Purpose
Sodium hypochlorite	Contaminated with Blood and body fluids
Bleaching powder	Toilets, bathrooms 9 grams/lit

Environmental Cleaning of Instruments and Equipment in OT

Disinfectant (Fig. 33)

- Alcohol 70% used in cleaning metal surfaces and trolleys. However, expensive for hospitals in developing countries.
- *At the end of the day in operation theater:*
  - Clean all the table tops, sinks, door handles with detergent/low level of disinfectant
  - Clean the floors with detergents mixed with warm water
  - Finally mop with disinfectant like phenol in the concentration of 1:10
  - Low concentration of phenol serves as perfume and not as disinfectant.

FUMIGATION

- Act of applying smoke or vapor
- High level disinfection of an area
- Used for terminal disinfection
- Should always be preceded by surface disinfection in the OT
- Frequency would depend upon the type of the OT
- Causes reduction in microbial count (Fig. 34).

When does One do Fumigation?

- Weekly
- After a case of gas gangrene or severe sepsis
- After an HIV Positive or HBsAg positive case
- After any construction or repair work being carried out
- Before every joint replacement and transplant case.

Formaldehyde

- Formaldehyde: an age-old compound
- Low-temperature heating produce vapor
- Vapor phase decontaminates the air/environment
- Kills vegetative bacteria/spore
- When formaldehyde mixed with water and exposed to elevated temperature gaseous formaldehyde is generated dependent on time and temperature.

Age-old Method

- Formaldehyde (gaseous form) which is available as formalin (liquid form)
- Three methods of using: (1) Formalin + Potassium Permanganate, (2) Formalin + Water heated on an electric stove, and (3) Formalin + Water dispersed with a fogger
- Effective only when humidity is 60%.

Phases of Fumigation

- To sterilize the operation theater formaldehyde gas (bactericidal and sporicidal, viricidal) is widely employed as it is cheaper for sterilization of huge areas like operation theaters. Formaldehyde kills the microbes by alkylating the amino acids and sulfhydryl group of proteins and purine bases.
- In spite of the gas being hazardous continues to be used in several developing countries.
- Fumigation usually involves the following phases: First, the area to be fumigated is usually covered to create a sealed environment; next, the fumigant is released into the space to be fumigated; then, the space is held for a set period while the fumigant gas percolates through the space and acts on and kills any infestation in the product; next, the space is ventilated so that the poisonous gases are allowed to escape from the space, and render it safe for humans to enter.

Procedure of Fumigation

- Thoroughly clean windows, doors, floor, walls, and all washable equipments with soap and water.
- Close windows and ventilators tightly. If any openings found, seal it with cellophane tape or other material.

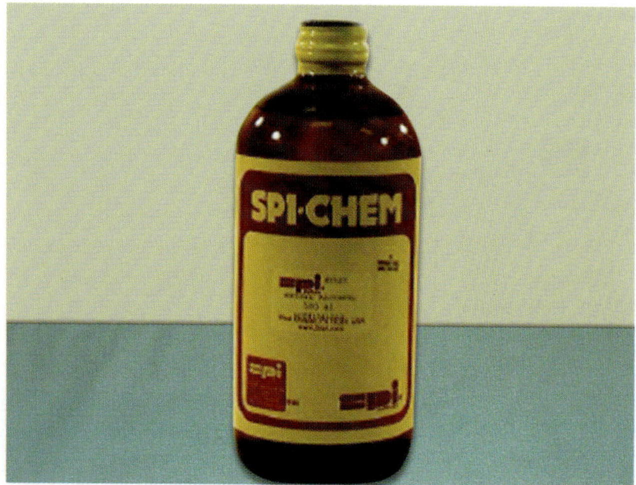

Fig. 33: Disinfectant.

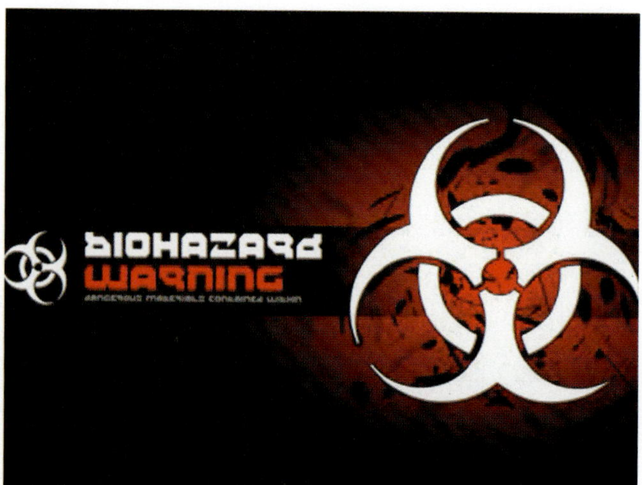

Fig. 34: Fumigation a biohazard procedure?

- Switch off all lights, AC, and other electrical and electronic items.
- Calculate the room size in cubic feet (L × B × H) and calculate the required amount of formaldehyde as given as 500 mL for 1000 cubic feet.

Personal Care during Fumigation

- Adequate care must be taken by wearing cap, mask, foot cover, and spectacle.
- Formaldehyde is irritant to eye and nose; and it has been recognized as a potential carcinogen.
- So, the fumigating employee must be provided with the personal protective equipment.

Creating the Formaldehyde Gas

- *Electric Boiler Fumigation Method*: For each 1,000 cubic feet of the volume of the operation theater 500 mL of formaldehyde (40% solution) added in 1,000 mL of water in an electric boiler. Switch on the boiler, leave the room, and seal the door. After 45 minutes (variable depending to volume present in the boiler) switch off the boiler without entering into the room.

Methods on Fumigation

- In principle, we have to generate formaldehyde gas.
- It can be done by easiest way to mix the needed quantity of formalin to water and heating at lower temperatures at 80–90°C.
- It can also be done with addition of formalin to potassium permanganate.
  Adding potassium permanganate to formaldehyde (Fig. 35).
- *Potassium Permanganate Method*: For every 1,000 cubic feet add 450 g of potassium permanganate ($KMnO_4$) to 500 mL of formaldehyde (40% solution). Take about 5-8 bowls (heat resistant); place it in various locations with equally divided parts of formaldehyde and add equally divided $KMnO_4$ to each bowl. This will cause auto boiling and generate fume.
- After the initiation of formaldehyde vapor, immediately leave the room and seal it for at least 48 hours.
- Avoid switching on exhaust fan when the fumigation is done.
- Exhaust fans drive the sterile air out and brings environmental air.
- Use of neutralizing agent like ammonia is useful.

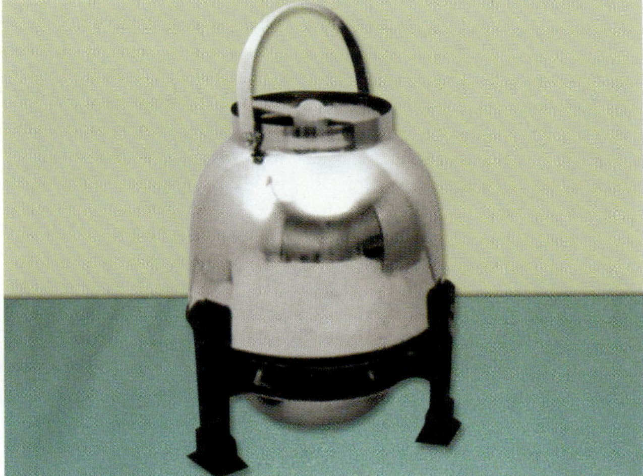

Fig. 35: Adding potassium permanganate to formaldehyde..

Fumigation to be Neutralized

- Neutralize residual formalin gas with ammonia by exposing 250 mL of ammonia per liter of formaldehyde used.
- Place the ammonia solution in the center of the room and leave it for 3 hours to neutralize the formalin vapor (Fig. 36).

An example is set as:

- Operation Theater Volume = L × B × H = 20 × 15 × 10 = 3,000 cubic feet.
- Formaldehyde required for fumigation = 500 mL for 1,000 cubic feet.
- So 1500 mL of formaldehyde required.
- Ammonia required for neutralization = 150 mL of 10% ammonia for 500 mL of formaldehyde
- So, 450 mL of 10% ammonia required.

Ideal Fumigation Agent

- Nontoxic and noncarcinogenic
- Nonirritant and noncorrosive
- Ecofriendly and economical
- Short reaction time with long residual effect
- Sustained release capacity
- Fragrance.

Products Available

- Hydrogen peroxide + Silver nitrate.
- H_2O_2 is the oxidizing agent combined with silver ions. Combination gives a synergistic effect as the H_2O_2 oxidizes the biofilm and the silver penetrates and attacks the microbe.
- Good coverage against bacteria, viruses, mycobacteria, protozoa, and biofilms.

H_2O_2 + Silver Nitrate Continued

- Droplet size of 7–20 microns. These very minute droplets trap the suspended particulate matter and kill the microbes.
- Theater ready in 2 hours.
- *Products available*: Ecoshield from J&J, Envodil from Mil Lab, Virosil from Sanosil.

Products Continued

- Combination of aldehyde, quaternary ammonium compounds, and alcohols.

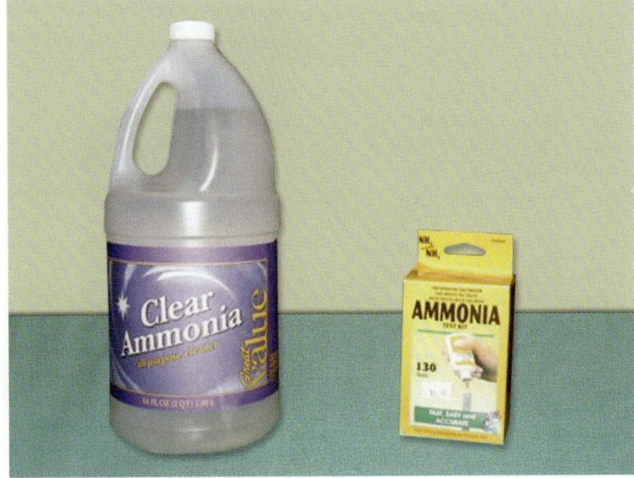

Fig. 36: Ammonia solution to neutralize the formalin vapor.

- Here formaldehyde use is avoided.
- Products available are incidur from Ecolab/Henkel. Available as spray also.
- Aldasan.
- Can be used as a surface cleaning agent as well as for fogging.

Need for Newer Chemical Agents in Hospital Use (Fig. 37)

- A need for Nonaldehyde based chemicals is a growing concern.
- Need for quicker sterilization methods with ever increasing workloads.
- Need for nontoxic safe agents (Fig. 38).

SEVERAL CHEMICALS ARE AVAILABLE BUT THE ECONOMIC LIMITATIONS ARE GREAT HURDLE IN EXPLORING THE UTILITY IN DEVELOPING COUNTRIES

Bacillocid® Rasant (Fig. 39)

- Formaldehyde-free disinfectant cleaner with low use concentration
- Very good cost/benefit ratio
- Good material compatibility
- Excellent cleaning properties
- Virtually no residue
- *Active ingredients*: Glutaral 100 mg/g, benzyl-C12-18-alkyldimethylammonium chlorides 60 mg/g, didecyl-dimethylammonium chloride 60 mg/g
- Bacillocid® rasant is suitable for the disinfectant cleaning of washable surfaces using the wet-wipe-procedure
- Especially suitable for economic short-term disinfection in risk areas that are likely sources of infection.

Use of Incidur with Defogger (Fig. 40)

- Contents of incidur 8.8 g of glyoxal/100 mL solution
- 4.5 g of glutaral/100 mL solution
- Theater can be used in 1 hour

Fumigation Continued

- Fogger machine used
- Kept at a height of 1½–2 ft. from the floor, the angle being 45°
- Agent used to be diluted with water as per manufacturers' instructions
- Quality of water which is used is important.

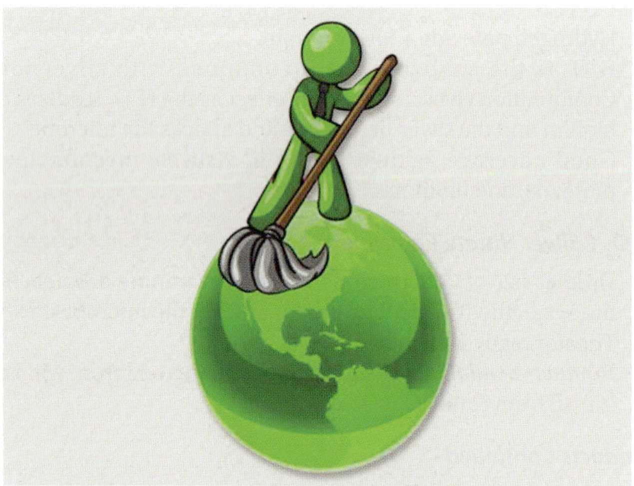

Fig. 37: Need for newer chemical agents in hospital use.

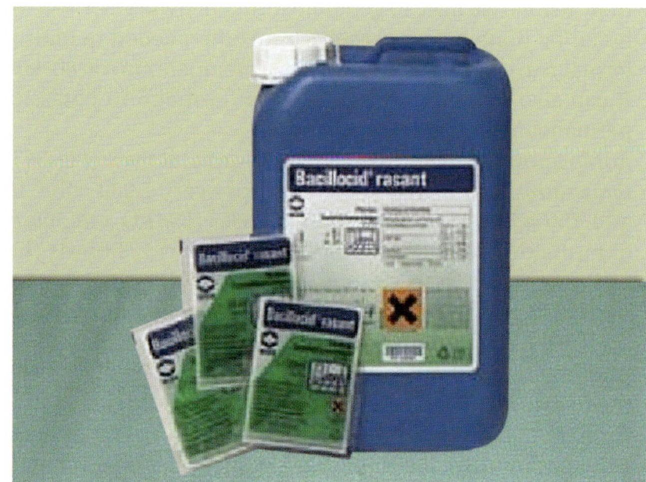

Fig. 39: Bacillocid® rasant.

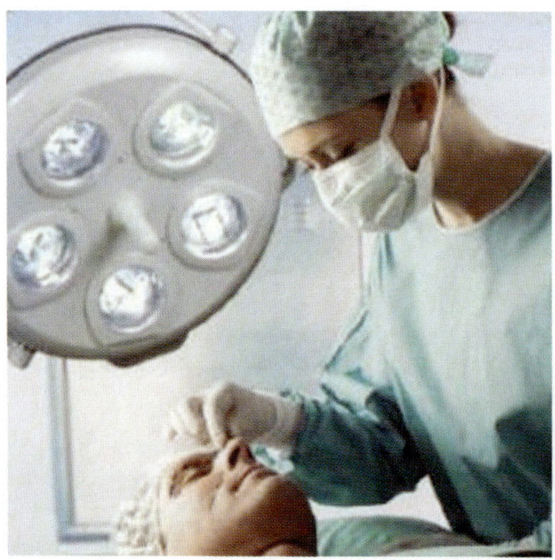

Fig. 38: Need for non-toxic safe agents.

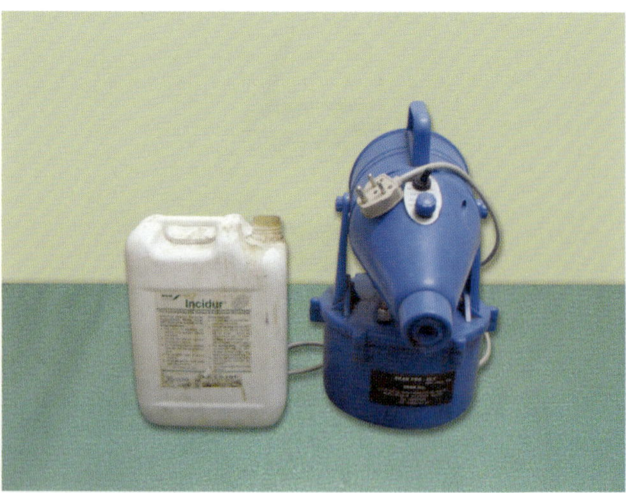

Fig. 40: Use of incidur with defogger.

Newer and Nontoxic Compounds

- A chemical compound VIRKON gaining importance as nonaldehyde compound
- Virkon proved to be safe:
  - Virucidal
  - Bactericidal
  - Fungicidal
  - Mycobactericidal.

VIRKON

- A chemical disinfectant
- Disinfecting medical devices
- Disinfecting laboratory equipment
- Decontaminating spillages with blood and body fluids
- Finding usefulness in replacing autoclaving and saving time.

Postfumigation

- Air sampling done
- In OT's with Laminar flow. The flow is switched on before air sampling and the air in the vicinity of the operating table is sampled
- No traffic in the OT when the sampling is being done.

Take home message

- OT is a sacred place (Figs. 41 and 42);

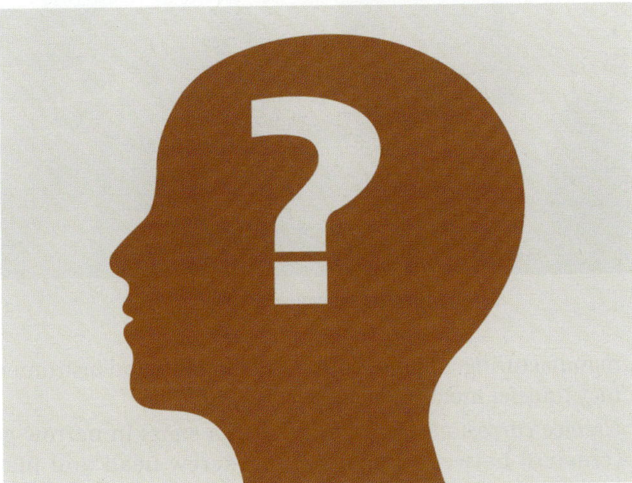

Fig. 41: Operation theater safety is responsibility of everyone.

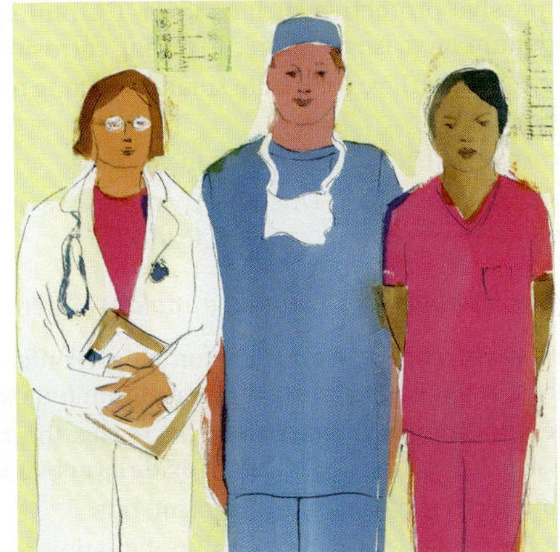

Fig. 42: Everyone plays active role in maintaining operation theater safety.

- Rigid rituals should be followed in sterilization of instruments and OT to get best possible results.

BIOCOMPATIBILITY OF IMPLANTS

EARLY DEFINITION

- Lack of interaction between material and tissue.
- Implies inert, nontoxic, noncarcinogenic, nonallergenic, noninflammatory, nondegradable.
- Thus, material has zero influence.

CONTEMPORARY DEFINITION

- "Ability of a material to perform with an appropriate host response, in a specific application" (Williams 1987).
  - Refers to a collection of processes and interdependent mechanisms of interaction between material and tissue
  - "Ability of material to perform" and not just reside in the body
  - "Appropriate host response" must be acceptable given the desired function
  - "Specific application" must be defined
- Specific application must also consider the time scale over which the host is exposed to the material (Table 3)
- In prelisterian days many surgeons were using hooks, pins, and wires made up of various metals like gold, silver, platinum, or iron to hold fracture fragments.
- But they noted corrosion in them.
- Lavert after many animal experiments found in 1829 that platinum was the most inert material.
- Then came the use of stout steel, a high carbon steel. But still corrosion was the problem.
- It was L Guillet of France who was the first to make alloy systems close to what we now call stainless steel, an alloy of chromium and iron.
- The 18-8 SMo was the first stainless steel to perform satisfactorily as implant.
- This was later modified to what is now called as 316L stainless steel, having an extra low carbon content of 0.03% insuring against the occurrence of carbide precipitates which make it susceptible to intergranular corrosion.
- Biocompatibility is primarily a surface phenomenon (Figs. 43 and 44).

Host Response

- The response of the host organism (local and systemic) to the implanted material or device.

Types of Reactions

- Normal wound healing response
  Protein absorption → Acute Inflammation → Resolution

TABLE 3: Life of the implants and prosthesis to which the host is exposed.

Material	*Time scale*
Bone screw/plate	3–12 months (or more)
Total hip replacement	10–15 years

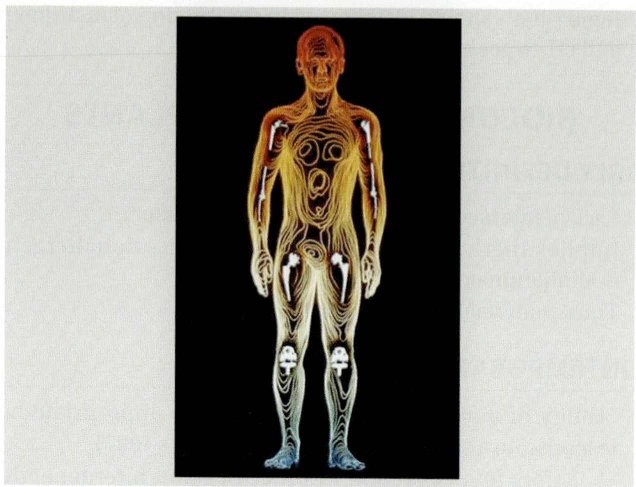

Fig. 43: Biocompatibility of implants.

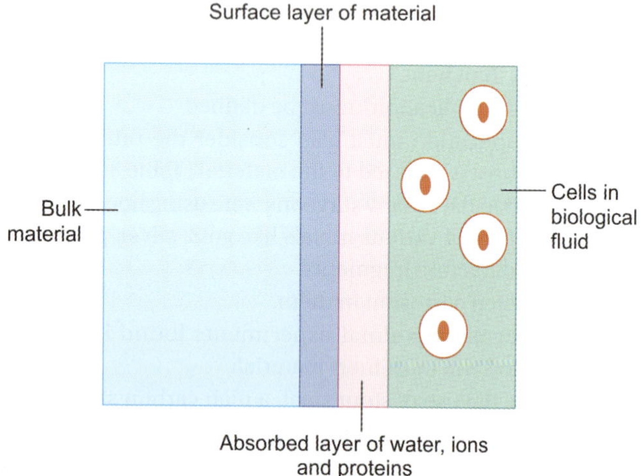

Fig. 44: Process of biocompatibility.

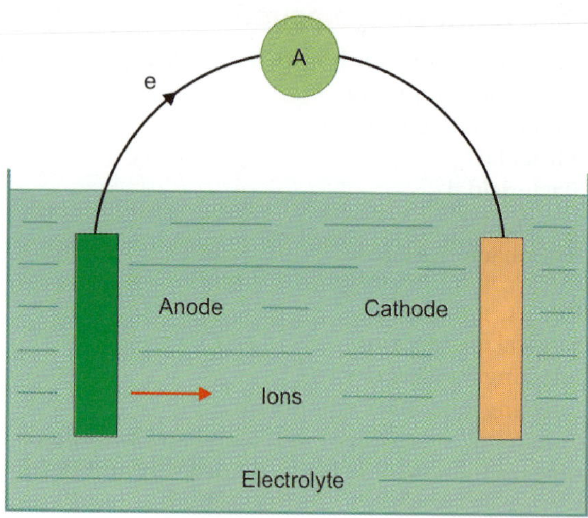

Fig. 45: Process of corrosion.

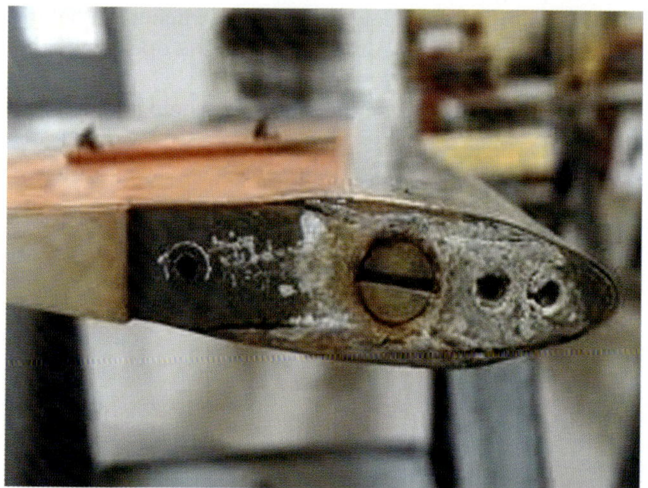

Fig. 46: Galvanic corrosion.

- Persistent inflammation
  Acute → Chronic
- Possibility of remote or systemic effects (transient or chronic) if reaction products are transported away from implant site.
- Effect of relatively reactive tissue environment on material, i.e. corrosion.

Corrosion

- Biocompatibility of an implant is directly related to its corrosion resistance.
- Corrosion is the gradual degradation of metals by electrochemical attack, and is therefore of concern when a metallic implant is placed in electrolytic environment of body (Fig. 45).
- Metals used for orthopedic implants depend on the existence of inert protective layer to prevent corrosion.
- Initiation of corrosion depends on O_2 tension and pH at implantation site.
- Acidic pH with infection may damage the oxide layer and produce corrosion.

Types of Corrosion

- *Galvanic corrosion*: This can occur at the surface of an implant in which an impurity was accidentally introduced during manufacturing. At times rubbing of implants and instruments may transfer metal and lead to corrosion.
- *Crevice corrosion*: Here the corrosion starts in narrow gap (crevice) between implants, e.g. screw head and plate. Molybdenum tends to limit it.
- *Pitting corrosion*: It is similar to crevice corrosion starting in the passive protective surface layer. Chromium, nickel, molybdenum increase resistance to pitting corrosion.
- *Fretting corrosion*: Resulting from small oscillating movements and vibrations.
- *Stress corrosion*: Due to high mechanical stress.
- *Intergranular corrosion*: Due to any impurities aggregating between relatively pure alloys (Figs. 46 to 49).

Corrosion Susceptibility of Orthopedic Implant Materials

- *Stainless steel:* It contains enough chromium to confer corrosion resistance by generating the protective chromium oxide layer.
  - The addition of molybdenum decreases the rate slow, passive dissolution of chromium oxide layer by 1,000 times.
  - It thus has a slow but finite corrosion rate.
  - It is best suited for short-term implantation in the body (Table 4).

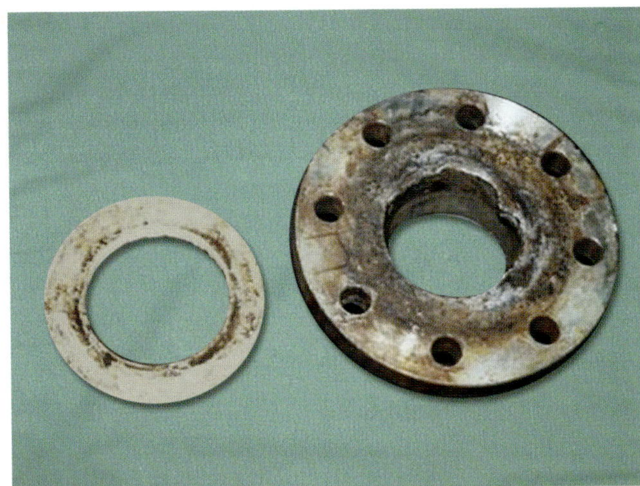

Fig. 47: Crevice corrosion.

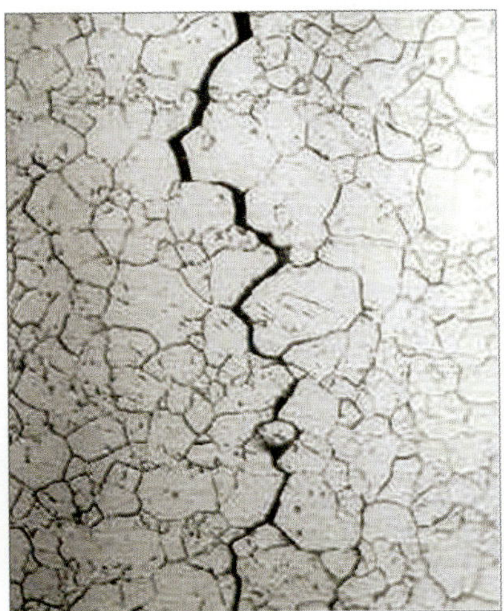

Fig. 48: Stress-corrosion cracking.

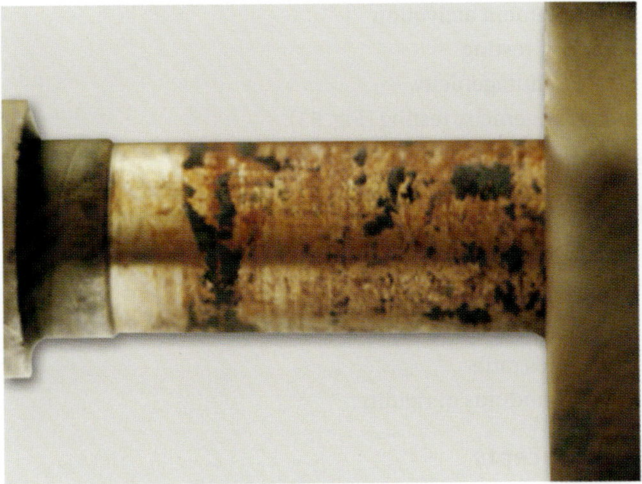

Fig. 49: Fretting corrosion.

- *Cobalt chromium alloy*: Both the cast and wrought varieties are passive in the human body and do not exhibit pitting, though moderate susceptibility to crevice corrosion may be observed.
- *Titanium*: It is a base metal (easily corroded) in context of the electrochemical series. However, it forms an adherent porous layer (TiO_2) and remains passive under physiological conditions. The passive protective layer even if destroyed is restored spontaneously, rapidly and effectively. Titanium implants remain virtually unchanged in appearance and offer superior corrosion resistance.

TABLE 4: The chemical composition of an AISI 316 stainless steel used as a substrate.

		Chemical composition (wt.%)				
Substrate	C	Mn	P	Cr	Ni	Fe
AISI 316	0.08	1.0	1.0	19	11	Bal

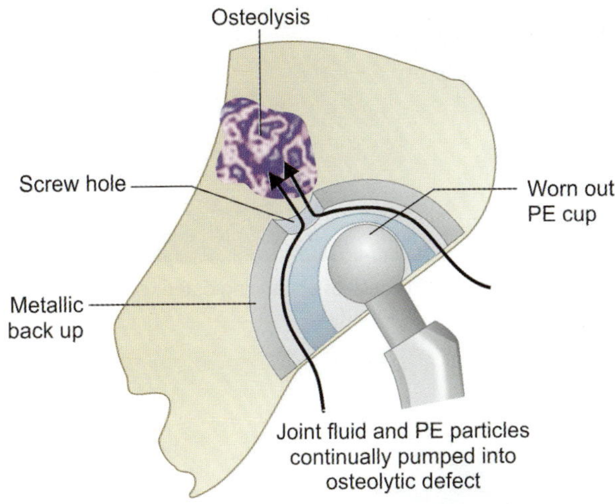

Fig. 50: Process of aseptic loosening and periprosthetic osteolysis.

Osteolysis (Fig. 50)

Aseptic loosening and periprosthetic osteolysis are major problems in artificial hip joint surgery, for which a solution is yet to be found. Biological host response to wear debris combined with cyclic mechanical loading onto the bon bed around hip prosthetic implants has been considered as mechanism responsible for implant-mediated periprosthetic osteolysis. Any type of artificial joint gliding surface continuously produces wear debris, which are derived from implant materials, i.e. ultra-high molecular weight polyethylene, ceramics and metals.

- Fragmented bone cement between the bone and implants is also a source of debris. Currently, generation of debris is still inevitable, although modern technology provides better biocompatible implants to lessen the debris. Debris induces foreign body reaction in periprosthetic connective tissues. The main loci are synovial regenerating capsular tissues and interface tissues between the bone and implants, where macrophages play an important role. Various cellular mediators and proteinases are produced in the process. The reaction affects periprosthetic bone remodeling and can provoke imbalanced bone metabolism around implants. It weakens the bone and causes periprosthetic osteolysis. In addition, the joint fluid, which is released from the inflamed connective tissues, has osteolytic potential. Pumping effect on gait and poor integration of bone implant interface allow penetration of the fluid into intact interface, thus enhancing osteolytic reactions around implants (Fig. 51).

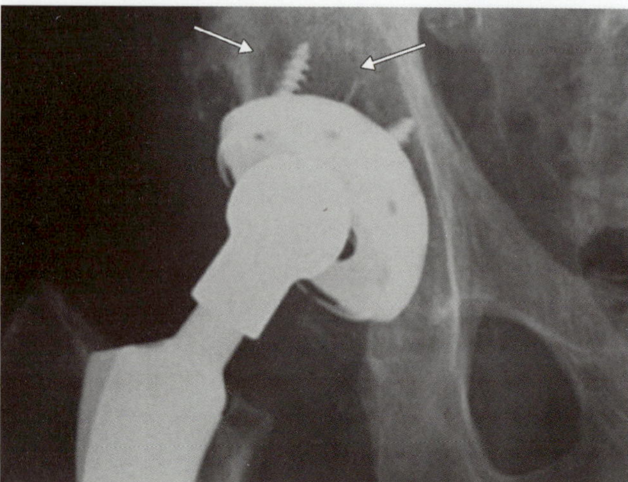

Fig. 51: Process of enhancing osteolysis.

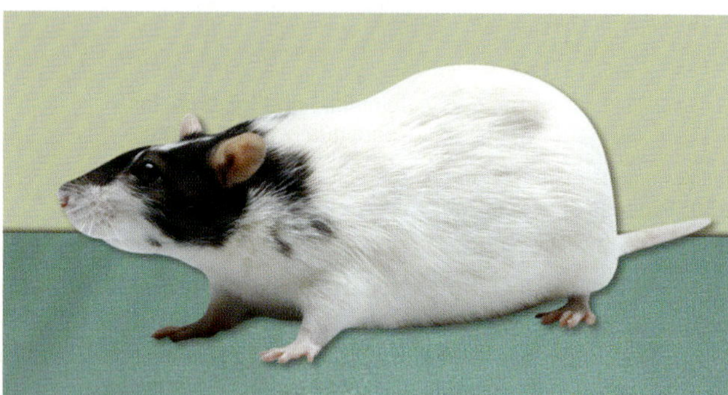

Fig. 52: Irritation testing.

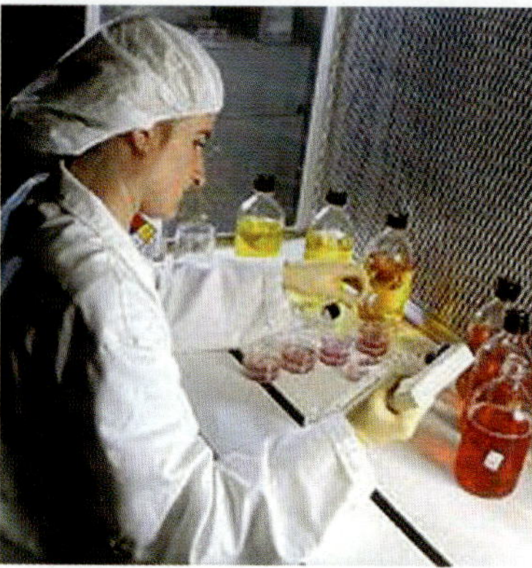

Fig. 53: Carcinogenicity testing.

Neoplasia

- A large number of very small metallic particles are released from metal-on-metal couples. These may cause mutagenic damage (chromatid breaks, chromosome translocations, aneuploidy, etc.). In defining implant biocompatibility it is therefore essential to consider the biological response both to an altered mechanical environment and to the liberation of particulate debris.
- For a material to be deemed biocompatible, any adverse reactions which may ensue at the blood/material or tissue/material interface must be minimal, while resistance to biodegeneration must be high. This requires a biomaterial to interact as a natural material would in the presence of blood and tissue. Ideal implantable materials should not:
    - Destroy or sensitize the cellular elements of blood
    - Alter plasma proteins (including enzymes) so as to trigger undesirable reactions
    - Cause adverse immune responses
    - Cause cancer
    - Cause teratological effects
    - Produce toxic and allergic responses
    - Deplete electrolytes
    - Be affected by sterilization.

Biocompatibility Testing

Considerations

- Type of device
- Principle tissue(s) in contact
- Period of implantation.

Tests for Chronically Implanted Devices

- *In vitro:* Cytotoxicity, carcinogenicity, mutagenicity
- *In vivo:* Pyrogenicity, systemic/acute toxicity
- Chronic animal implantation studies (3 species for 6, 12 and 24 months)
- Human clinical trials.

In vivo services:

- Pyrogen testing
- Sensitization
- Subchronic/chronic toxicity
- Intracutaneous reactivity
- Irritation testing (Fig. 52).

In-vitro services:

- Cytotoxicity
- Hemolysis
- Complement activation
- PT/PTT testing
- AMES mutagenicity
- Carcinogenicity testing (Fig. 53).

Note: No material is universally biocompatible.

Mechanical Properties of implant Materials (Fig. 54)

- Young's modulus of elasticity
- Yield strength
- Ultimate tensile strength
- Poisson's ratio
- Shear modulus of rigidity.

Basic Concepts

- *Normal stress:* The intensity of the internal forces normal to a plane passing through a point in the body.
- *Shear stress:* The intensity of the internal forces parallel to a plane passing through a point in the body.
- *Ductility:* It is a mechanical property that describes the extent in which solid materials can be plastically deformed without fracture.

Young's Modulus of Elasticity (Table 5)

- Also called as elastic modulus.
- It is the ratio of stress to strain; slope of the elastic region of stress–strain curve of a metal (Fig. 55).
- It is the measure of stiffness of an isotropic elastic material.
- Young's modulus of Co-Cr-Mo > stainless steel-316L > Ti-6Al-4V > bone.

Yield Strength

- Stress beyond the elastic limit that results in permanent deformation, i.e. a metal goes from pure elastic behavior to a combination of elastic-plastic behavior.

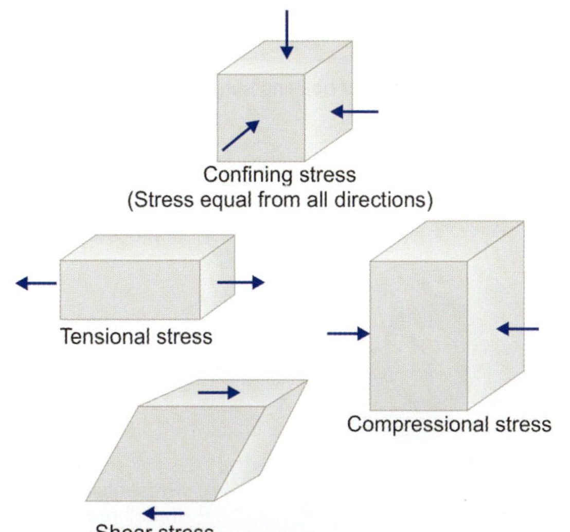

Fig. 54: Pictorial representation of effect of different types of stress on different materials.

TABLE 5: Young's modulus of elasticity.

Material	*Young's modulus (GPa)*
Bone	17
Titanium	105
Stainless steel 316	200
Co-Cr-Mo	210

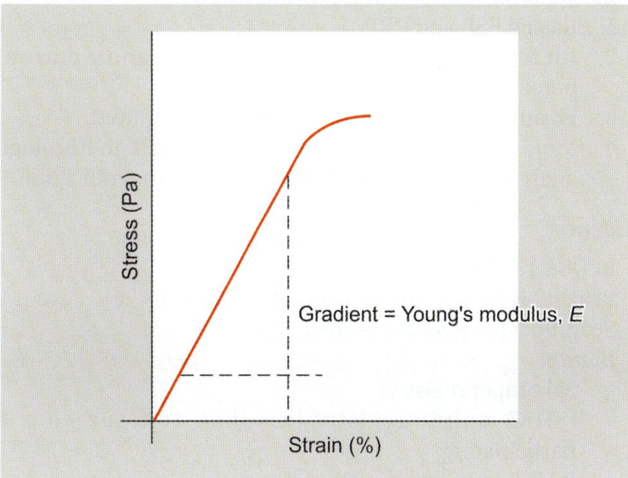

Fig. 55: Line diagram of study of elasticity of different materials.

- Yield strength of Co-Cr-Mo > Ti-6Al-4V > stainless steel 316L > bone.

Ultimate Tensile Strength (Table 6)

- It is the maximum attainable stress of a material after which fracture will occur (Fig. 56).
- It indicates toughness of material.

Poisson's Ratio (Tables 7 and 8)

- It is defined as a ratio of transverse strain to longitudinal strain of a loaded specimen.
- It varies from 0 to 0.5.
- Stiffer materials have lower ratios than softer materials.

TABLE 6: Ultimate tensile strength.

Material	*Ultimate tensile strength (MPa)*
Bone	132
316L	965
Ti	1,173
Co	1,450

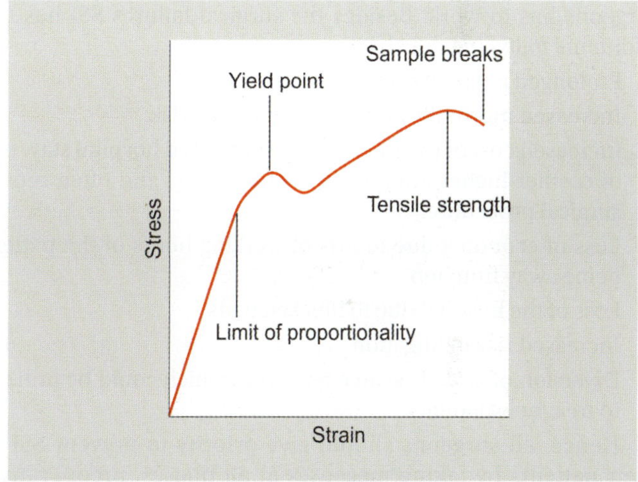

Fig. 56: Line diagram of study of the effect of stress and strain.

TABLE 7: Poisson's ratio of different materials.

Material	*Poisson's ratio*
SS 316L	0.27–0.30
Co-Cr-Mo	0.30
Bone	0.30
Titanium	0.33

TABLE 8: Analytic study of different materials.

Material	*Young's modules (GPa)*	*Yield strength (MPa)*	*Ultimate tensile strength (MPa)*	*Poisson's ratio*
Bone	17		132	0.30
S S 316L	200	795	965	0.27–0.30
Co-Cr-Mo	210	950	1,450	0.30
Titanium	105	895	1,173	0.33

Comparison of Stainless Steel and Titanium

- Both have relative benefits and deficiencies.
- Stainless steel can be produced with a higher elastic modulus and ductility than titanium alloys.
- Stainless steel implants are relatively cheaper.
- The more significant advantage of titanium alloy is their resistance to corrosion and lack of potentially toxic ions.
- Another benefit is its nonallergenicity.
- These properties make it possible to leave titanium implants *in situ* for longer period.
- Cobalt chrome seems to be better than stainless steel 316 L, but it has the disadvantages of it price and the facility to find it.

Microbial contamination that occurs in the wound created by an invasive surgical procedure is generally referred to as surgical site infection (SSI) within 30 days of an operation or within 1 year after surgery if an implant is used. Postoperative infection of surgical site is unpleasant and undesirable. It can destroy the results of the most beautifully executed surgery. It is the third most common hospital acquired infection (HAI) even in the developed countries and as it is preventable, it is identified as a target of many national infection prevention programs. The situation in India is bound to be worse given the operating conditions under which surgeons has to work. Besides the surgical failures SSI has the additional following drawbacks:

- Prolonged hospital stay.
- Increased morbidity and higher mortality risk.
- Increased cost of treatment due to increased hospital stay, use of costlier higher antibiotics, and dressing, and often repeat surgical procedure.
- Loss of economy due to loss of working hours of the patient being away from job.
- Loss of the hospital due to blocked beds.
- Increased risk of litigation.
- Diversion of already scarce resources which could be utilized to treat new patients.

Hence, all surgeons should give priority to prevent SSI in their patients by taking measures at all phases, preoperative, intraoperative, postoperative, and postdischarge phase of the care.

Surgical site infection level can be superficial incisional, deep incisional, or organ/space SSI (Fig. 57). Superficial incisional SSI usually occur within 30 days of procedure involving skin or subcutaneous tissue presenting with symptoms and signs of infection—pain, local redness, heat, swelling, and tenderness with or without purulent discharge. Deep incisional SSI occur within 30 days of procedure (or one year in case of implants used) involving deep soft tissue like facia and muscles presenting signs of infection; pain, fever, locally redness, heat, tenderness of wound, purulent drainage, abscess, separation of the edges of the wound exposing deeper structures. Organ or space SSI usually occurs within 30 days with no implant or 1 year with implant involving any part other than the incision that is opened or manipulated during the surgical procedure, e.g. joint presenting with purulent discharge from a drain, abscess, or other evidence of infection, isolation of organism in bacteriological culture.

SSI at any level can present as early (within 30 days), intermediate (between 1 and 3 months) or late (more than 3 months after surgery) (Fig. 58).

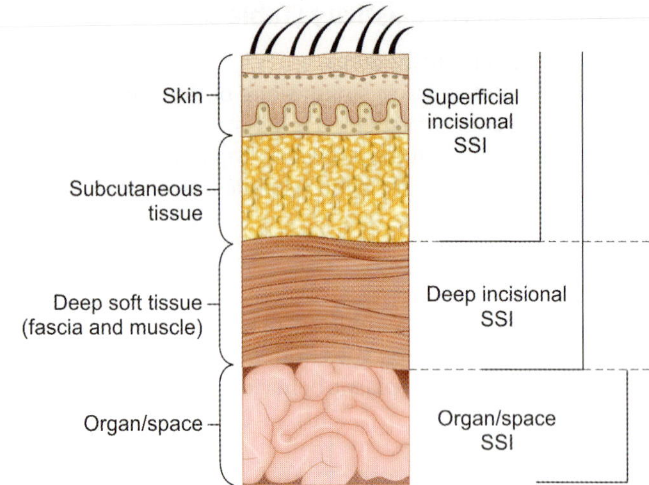

Fig. 57: Criteria for defining surgical site infections.

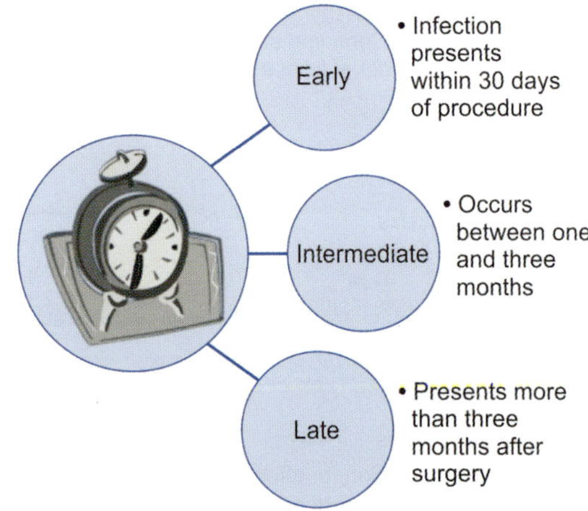

Fig. 58: Pictorial representation showing relationship between grade of infection and duration.

Periprosthetic joint infection following joint replacement (partial or total) according to Musculoskeletal Infection Society (Accepted by AAOS) is another type of SSI presenting as:

- Sinus tract communicating with the prosthesis.
- Positive culture from at least two separate tissue or fluid samples.
- Existence of at least four following criteria:
  1. Raised ESR and CRP.
  2. Increased synovial leukocyte count and neutrophil percentage.
  3. Positive culture of periprosthetic tissue or fluid.
  4. More than 5 neutrophils per HPF in 5 HPF in histological analysis of periprosthetic tissue at X400 magnification.

Incidence

- In USA 1.07% (4%)
- British Medical Research Council 0.3% (5%)
- Scandinavian Registry 7–16%.
- *Indian:*
  - No proper registry;
  - ISHKS online registry less than 10% surgeons are participating.
  - ISHKS states knee > hip.
- Incidence increases in revisions (Figs. 59 and 60).

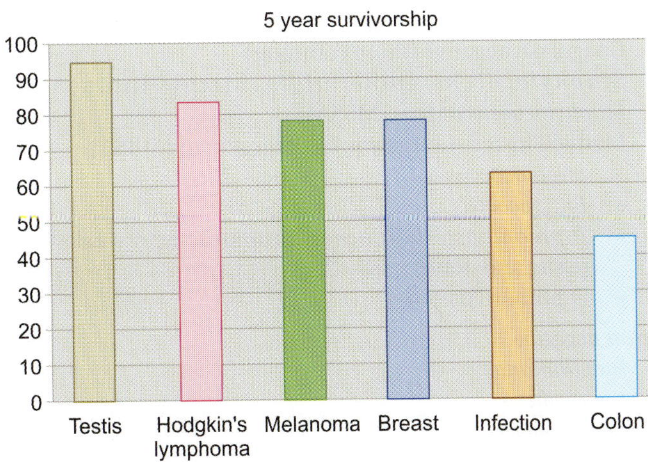

Fig. 59: Mortality is worse than some of malignancies.

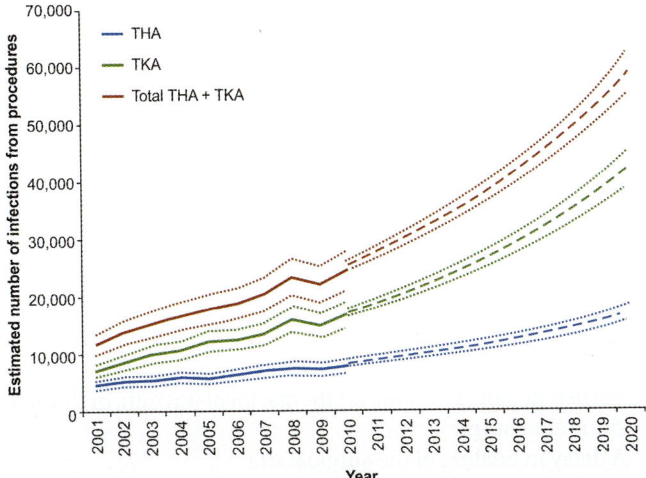

Fig. 60: Economic burden of periprosthetic joint (26,000 infected joints).

Pathogenesis of Surgical Site Infection

Development of SSI depends on contamination of the wound site at the end of surgical procedure and specifically related to the pathogenicity and inoculums of microorganisms present and balance against the host immune response.

Microorganisms that cause SSI are usually derived from the patient (endogenous infection), being present on the skin or from an open viscus.

Exogenous infection occurs when microorganisms from the instrument or the theater environment contaminate the site of operation, when microorganisms from the environment contaminate a traumatic wound or when microorganisms gain access to the wound after surgery before the skin has sealed.

Figure 61 and Table 9 show the influence of the type of wounds like clean, dirty, and contaminated, to the severity and extent of damage of the tissue structure.

Risk Factor for Development of Surgical Site Infection (Fig. 62)

Laminar air flow does not alter infection rate. It is the quality of air circulation and prophylactic antibiotics which are important.

Operative environment and surgeon:

- Poor operating atmosphere
- Increased operating room traffic
- Washing of hands and maintaining basic hygiene of nurse, assistants, and surgeons contamination by surgical team while preparation and draping
- Instrumentation

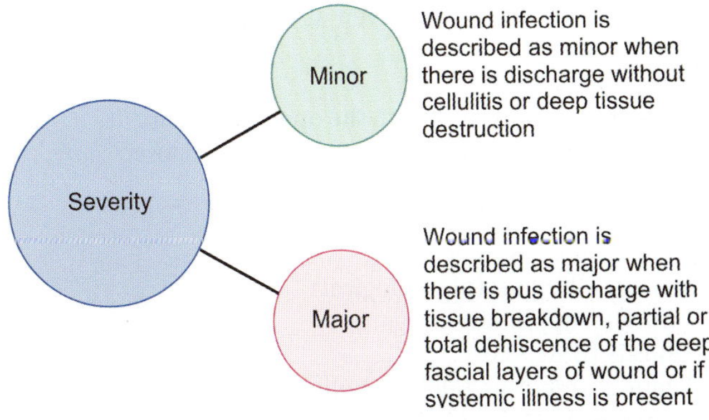

Fig. 61: Severity of infection depends on extent of destruction of the tissue.

TABLE 9: Classification of surgical wounds.

Category	*Criteria*	*Infection rate %*
Clean	• No hollow viscus entered • Primary wound closure • No inflammation • No breaks in aseptic technique • Elective procedure	1–3
Clean-contaminated	• Hollow viscus entered but controlled • No inflammation • Primary wound closure • Minor break in aseptic technique • Mechanical drain used • Bowel preparation preoperatively	5–8
Contaminated	• Uncontrolled spillage from viscus • Open traumatic wound • Major break in aseptic technique	20–25
Dirty	• Untreated, uncontrolled spillage from viscus • Pus in operative wound • Open suppurative wound • Severe inflammation	30–40

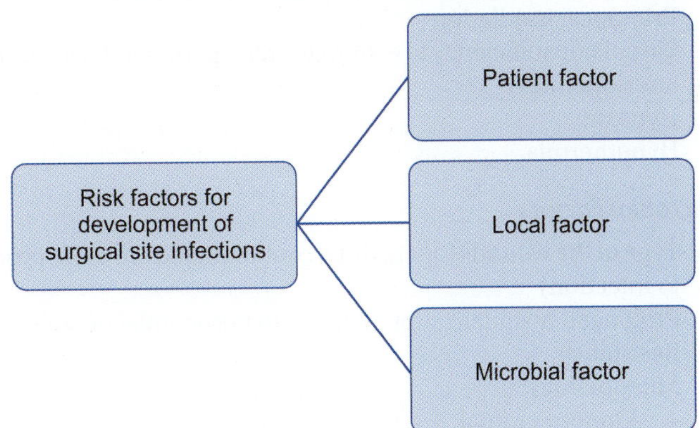

Fig. 62: Risk factors for infection.

- Prophylactic antibiotics given at the proper time and at the correct strength
- Surgical clothing
- Reducing the flow of staff in the operating room
- Surgical time, surgical technique, and blood loss.

Patient-related Factors

- General and systemic
- Old age >80 years (physiological)
- Immunosuppressive drugs
- Obesity (BMI >35)
- Diabetes mellitus (elevated glucose level increases biofilm formation)
- Chronic systemic inflammatory disease
- Malignancy
- Chronic active dermatitis or cellulitis
- Renal failure (multiple dialysis)
- Pulmonary insufficiency
- Hepatic insufficiency
- Chronic indwelling catheter, UTI
- Chronic malnutrition (BMI <25), lack of protein diet, anemia
- Smoking (current status)
- Alcoholism
- Use of steroids
- Radiation.

Local Factors

- Poor skin preparation
- Contamination of instruments
- Inadequate antibiotic prophylaxis
- Prolonged procedures
- Site and complexity of procedures
- Local tissue necrosis
- Multiple incision with skin bridges
- Soft tissue loss from prior trauma
- Prior active infection present >3–4 months
- Thin and fragile dermis and epidermis
- Bursae, Baker's cyst
- Subcutaneous abscess >8 cm^2
- Synovial cutaneous fistula
- Prior periarticular fracture or trauma about a joint
- Prior local irradiation
- Vascular insufficiency to extremity (TAO, peripheral neuro, and arteriopathies)
- Hypoxia
- Hypothermia.

Microbial Factors

- Type of the wounds (open, dirty, contaminated are more prone to infection)
- Prolonged hospitalization (leading to nosocomial organisms)
- Resistance
- Microbiology:
  - Monomicrobial
  - Polymicrobial, anaerobes, mycobacteria
  - Fungal
  - Only small number of microorganisms are needed to seed the implant at the time of surgery
  - Further presence of foreign body can reduce the number of bacteria required.

Gram positive bacteria—Staphylococcus:
- Coagulase negative (more common)
- *Staphylococcus epidermidis,* Methicillin-sensitive *Staphylococcus aureus* (MSSA)
- Methicillin-resistant *staphylococcus aureus* (MRSA)
  - *Streptococcus*
  - *Enterococcus*
  - *Propionibacterium acnes* (propionic acid weakens soft tissue and bone)
  - Diphtheroids.

Gram negative
- *Pseudomonas*
- *Klebsiella*
- *Citrobacter*
- *Corynebacterium*
- *Acinetobacter.*

Biofilm:
- Extracellular pyomeric substance (EPS) produced by bacteria
- It helps bacteria to adhere to each other, tissues and implants and catheter and get embedded
- Antibiotics and macrophages cannot reach the targets and flourish.

Staphylococcus aureus is the microorganism most commonly cultured from SSIs. Operations on site that are normally sterile (clean) thus have relatively low rates of SSI (generally < 2%), whereas after operation in contaminated or dirty sites, rates may exceed 10%.

Clinical Features

- Persistent pain, swelling, erythema, local warmth, or drainage/sinus after surgery
- A delay in healing of the surgical site
- The tissue around the surgical site may be discolored
- A foul odor coming from the incision site
- Examination findings:
  - Tenderness and limitation of range of motion.
  - Painful range of motion of the joint that is disproportionate to the expected recovery from the surgery.
- Wound discharge with no other complications leads to life-threatening condition
- *Other clinical outcomes of SSIs:* Poor scars that are cosmetically unacceptable, (spreading, hypertrophic or keloid, persistent pain and itching, restriction of movement particularly when over the joint)
- Sometimes features are masked due to medications.

Diagnosis

- The presentation of SSIs and PJIs can be varied and the diagnosis challenging.
- The diagnosis is typically based on a combination of clinical, laboratory, and imaging findings.

Clinical examinations reveal the features of the stages and the severity of the SSIs.

In addition to routine laboratory investigations like urine analysis, CBC, ESR, CRP, hemoglobin, blood culture, and sensitivity, one has to carry out other serological test also.

- Total leukocyte count is frequently normal and is of little diagnostic help.

- *ESR:* It is nonspecific indicator of inflammation that peaks 5–7 days after surgery and usually returns to baseline in 3 months to 1 year. Continued elevation of ESR postoperatively is suggestive of infection.
- *CRP:* It is an acute phase reactant produced by hepatocytes in response to infection, inflammation, or acute injury. CRP level peaks 2–3 days after surgery and returns to baseline in 14–21 days. With an abnormal level, 14–21 days after surgery, CRP has sensitivity of 93% and specificity of 83%.
- Serum interleukin-6 (IL-6) level-IL-6 cytokine that stimulate the liver cells to produce acute phase reactants like CRP. Serum IL-6 level can be measured by a simple ELISA test. IL-level peaks 6–12 hours after surgery and returns to baseline after 48–72 hours after surgery. Normal value is <10 pg/mL. IL-6 level has sensitivity of 100% and specificity of 95% in diagnosis of SSIs.
- Calorimetric strip test for leukocyte esterase in the synovial fluid has specificity and positive predictive value in the diagnosis. This is graded as '–', '+', and '++'.

Bacteriological: Culture and Sensitivity

- Gram's staining is of little importance.
- Culture swabs—inadequate specimen, ignorance, and transport medium.
- Synovial fluid culture is gold standard in PJI.
  Always request for transport medium from lab.

In postoperative joint infection (PJI) Joint fluid analysis is very helpful with:

- Cell count, total and differential count, culture and crystals.
- Use of antibiotics prior to aspiration can lead to false-negative results.
- In the setting of 2-stage exchange arthroplasty, delaying knee aspiration at least 4 weeks from the discontinuation of antibiotic therapy can significantly lower the false negative rate.

Molecular Diagnostic Tests

Polymerase Chain Reaction (PCR)

- Amplifies strains of bacterial DNA to allow detection of infectious bacteria.
- PCR can detect nonviable bacteria that do not grow on culture as well as bacteria lysed by ultrasonification with results within 12–13 hours.
- Results of the PCR are unaffected by the administration of antibiotics.
- Comparing DNA sequences of organism can be helpful identifying virulence and antibiotic resistant strains.

Fluorescent In Situ Hybridization (FISH)

- Utilizes fluorescent-labeled oligonucleotide probes that hybridize to their intracellular targets permitting single cell identification and quantification by either epifluorescence microscopy or flow cytometry.

Immunofluorescence Microscopy

- Can give results within 2–3 hours. The technique is relatively inexpensive.
- Immunofluorescence microscopy can distinguish between biofilm. Organism (large aggregates) and contaminants (single dispersed cells/small aggregates) by direct visualization.

Imaging Modalities (Fig. 63)

- *Radiographs show:*
  - Periosteal new bone formation
  - Scattered foci of osteolysis
  - Subchondral bone resorption.

  Are highly suggestive of infection, but are typically late findings.
- Sinogram is very helpful in presence of discharging sinus (Fig. 64).
- USG identifies pockets and guides aspiration.
- CT quantifies Osteolysis.
- MRI—MARS sequence.

NUCLEAR SCANS

- Nuclear scans (results are not impacted by the presence of metallic implants).
- Triple-phase technetium-99 bone scan (TPBS).
- Sensitive in detecting bone remodeling changes round metallic components.
- It cannot distinguish between aseptic loosening and septic loosening.
- TPBS have a high negative predictive value.
- WBC imaging with indium-111 is more sensitive than TPBS but has low specificity.
- Combining an indium-111 WBC scan with a Technetium-99m bone scan improves the accuracy for detecting deep infection up to 95% (Fig. 65).

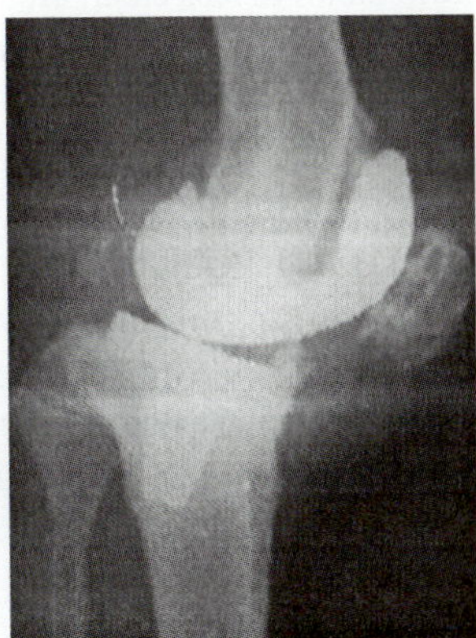
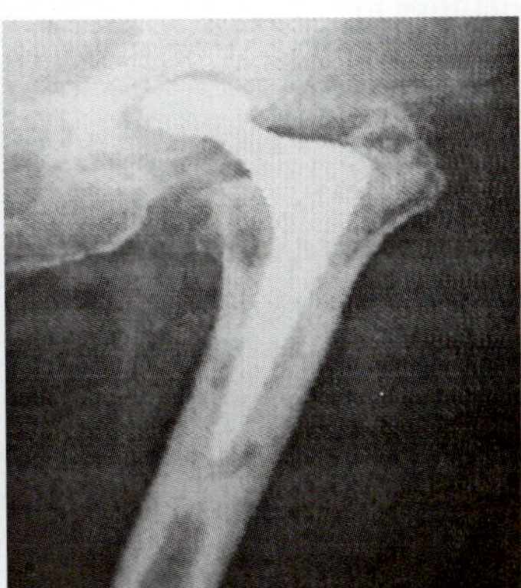
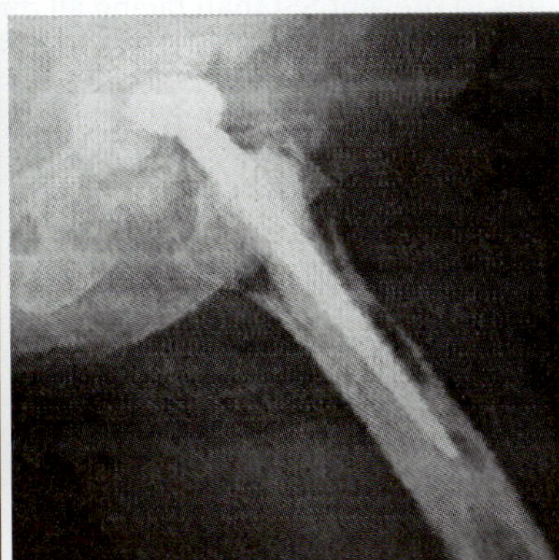

Fig. 63: Imaging modalities.

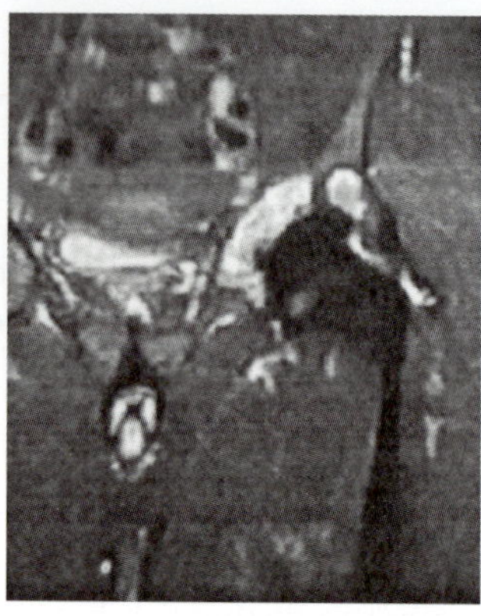
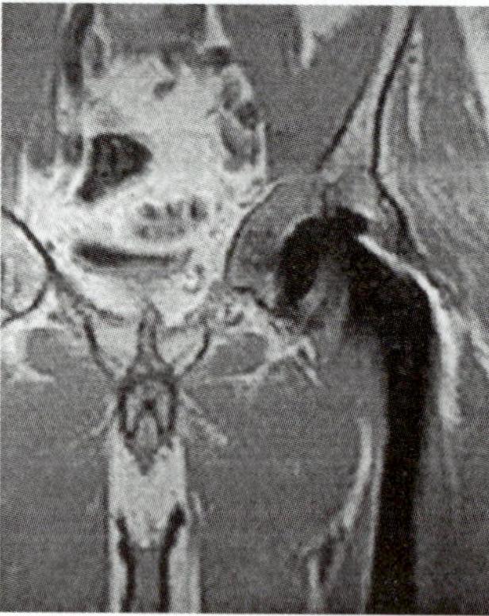

Fig. 64: Image showing sinogram.

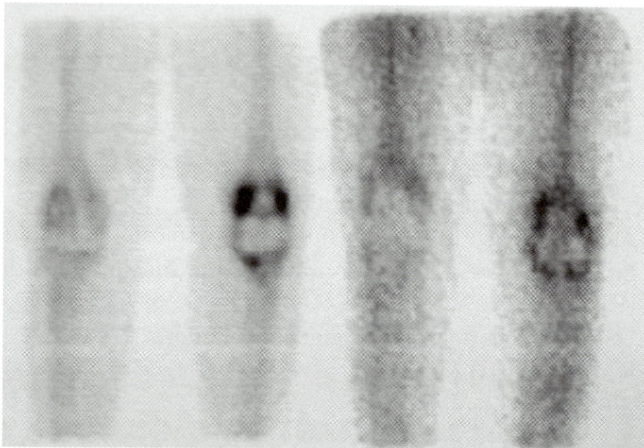

Fig. 65: Figure showing nuclear scan.

POSITRON EMISSION TOMOGRAPHY

- Fluorodeoxyglucose positron emission tomography (FDG-PET).
- Inflammatory cells express more glucose transporters, resulting in intracellular accumulation of deoxyglucose which cannot be metabolized by the cell and can be identified by PET imaging.
- The advantage of PET scan is that only one injection is required and results are available within 4 hours.
- Can produce false positive.

MANAGEMENT

Prevention is better than cure. Hence, we should all insist on planning all measures to prevent SSI than facing all difficulties to cure it.

Guidelines for Prevention of Surgical Site Infection

- Preoperative phase
- Intraoperative phase
- Postoperative phase.

Preoperative Phase

- Preoperative showering (chlorhexidine or soap)
- Hair removal
- Patient theater-wear
- Staff theater-wear
- Staff leaving the operative area
- Remove hand jewelry, artificial nails, and nail polish
- Antibiotic prophylaxis.

Operative Antibiotic Prophylaxis

- Given within 30–120 minutes prior to surgery decreases bacterial counts at surgical site.
- Consider giving a single dose of prophylactic antibiotic.
- In case of infected and dirty wound the patient should be given antibiotics at least 48 hours prior to surgery.
- To give a repeat dose of antibiotic prophylaxis when the operation is longer than the half-life of antibiotic given, usually if the surgery extends more than 2 hours the antibiotic should be repeated.

Intraoperative Phase

- Hand decontamination
- Incise drapes (iodophor impregnated drapes)
- Use of sterile gowns
- Gloves
- Antiseptic skin preparation (providione iodine or chlorhexidine)
- Maintaining patients homeostasis (temp, oxygen, glucose)
- Wound irrigation and intracavity lavage
- Antiseptic and antimicrobial agents before wound closure
- Wound dressing.

Postoperative Phase

- Changing dressing (usually 2nd, 5th and 8th postoperative day) and postoperative cleansing.
- Use sterile saline for wound cleaning up to 48 hours after surgery.
- Topical antimicrobial agents for wound healing by primary intention (some surgeon recommends).

In case of wet wound due to discharge extra precautions are as follows:

- Antiseptic and antimicrobial dressing for wound healing by secondary intention
- Debridement
- Antibiotic according to culture and sensitivity of the discharge.

Parameters for Operating Room Ventilation

- *Temperature:* 73°F, depending on normal ambient temperature
- *Relative humidity:* 30–60%
- *Air movement:* From clean to less clean areas
- *Air changes:* >15 total per hour and > 3 outdoor air per hour.

Practices to Prevent SSI are Therefore Aimed at

- Minimizing the number of microorganisms introduced into the operative site.
- Removing the microorganisms that normally colonize the skin.
- Preventing the multiplication of microorganisms at the operative site, e.g. by using prophylactic antimicrobial therapy.
- Enhancing the patient's defense against infection, e.g. by minimizing the tissue damage and the maintaining the normothermia with local homeostasis.
- Preventing access of microorganisms into the incision postoperatively.

MANAGEMENT OF INCISIONAL SURGICAL SITE INFECTION

Most SSI responds to the removal of sutures with drainage of pus if any and occasionally there is a need of debridement with or without removal of implant after fracture united and open wound care.

Many complications of postoperative wounds do not represent infection but exudation of tissue fluid or an early failure to heal, which is common in patients with a high body mass index (BMI).

Incomplete sealing of the wound edges can often be managed by using a delayed primary or secondary suture or closure with adhesive tape, but in larger open wounds the granulation tissue must be healthy with a low bio-burden of colonizing or contaminating organisms if healing is to occur (Table 10).

MANAGEMENT OF POSTOPERATIVE JOINT INFECTION

- Treatment of infected TKA/THA is complex, expensive.
- Requires more surgical and inpatient time than noninfected revision TKA/THA and is more prone to failure.
- The goal of treatment is eradication of the infection and maintenance of a pain-free, functional joint with recovery and return to job.

Treatment Options

- Irrigation and debridement with component retention (with or without polyethylene exchange in case of joint prosthesis).
- One stage or two stage exchanges.
- Antibiotic suppression in addition to systemic IV/oral sensitive antibiotics local application of antibiotic with continuous IV irrigation, local application of chain of antibiotic loaded cemented bead/IM cemented nail.
- Resection arthroplasty.
- And rarely arthrodesis and amputation.

Irrigation and Debridement

- Irrigation and debridement with component retention (with or without polyethylene exchange).
- It is suitable for selective cases where infection occurs within the first 4–6 weeks of primary surgery or in the setting of acute hematogenous. Gram positive infection with stable implant.
- Polyethylene liner (in TKA) exchange is preferred as it allows better debridement of the posterior synovium and eliminates biofilm on the polyethylene.
- Success of open debridement with polyethylene exchange is limited (23–28% success rate) by persistent of organism on retained implants, cement, and dead bone.

Factor Associated with Success Include

- Early debridement
- Absence of sinus formation
- Multiple debridement rather than a single debridement
- Gram positive infection
- Use of 4–6 weeks of sensitive systemic antibiotics.

Two-stage Exchange Arthroplasty

- First described by Insall, has been the most successful alternative treatment for infected total knee arthroplasty (91% success rate).
- The first stage involves removal of all total knee components and cement, thorough debridement and irrigation.
- Followed by implantation of an antibiotic cement depot in the joint. The antibiotic cement depot releases antibiotics locally at high concentration to eradicate the infection.
- This is supplemented by intravenous antibiotic as per sensitivity for 6–8 weeks.
- If there are no clinical signs of infection and ESR and CRP levels are declining, a decision for second stage implantation is made.

ANTIBIOTIC SPACER

- Static spacer described by Cohen.
- *Problems with static spacers include (Fig. 66):*
  - Contracture of the extensor mechanism
  - Collateral ligament shortening
  - Arthrofibrosis
  - Tibial and femoral bone loss (incidence 60%)
  - Potential difficulty with secondary exposure for reimplantation.

Dynamic/Articulating Spacer

- Maintain joint motion between stages and cause less periarticular scarring resulting in easier surgical exposure at reimplantation.
- The result is marginally better, postoperative ROM and function as compared to static spacers.

Articulating Spacers

- Metal on polyethylene (new components or recycled components)
- Or cement on cement (PROSTALAC)

Problems with articulating spacers (Fig. 67)

- Risk of cement fracture
- Spacers dislocation
- Formation of cement debris
- Potential problem with wound healing.

TABLE 10: Classification based on mode of presentation by Tsukayama, Estrada, and Gustilo.

Type	*Presentation*	*Definition*	*Treatment*
1	Positive intraoperative cultures	>2 positive intraoperative cultures	Appropriate antibiotic therapy
2	Acute postoperative infection	Acute infection within first month	Attempt at debridement and prosthetic retention
3	Acute hematogenous infection	Acute onset of symptom in a previously well-functioning joint replacement	Attempt debridement and prosthetic retention or prosthetic removal
4	Late chronic	Chronic indolent infection presenting >1 month after surgery	Prosthetic removal

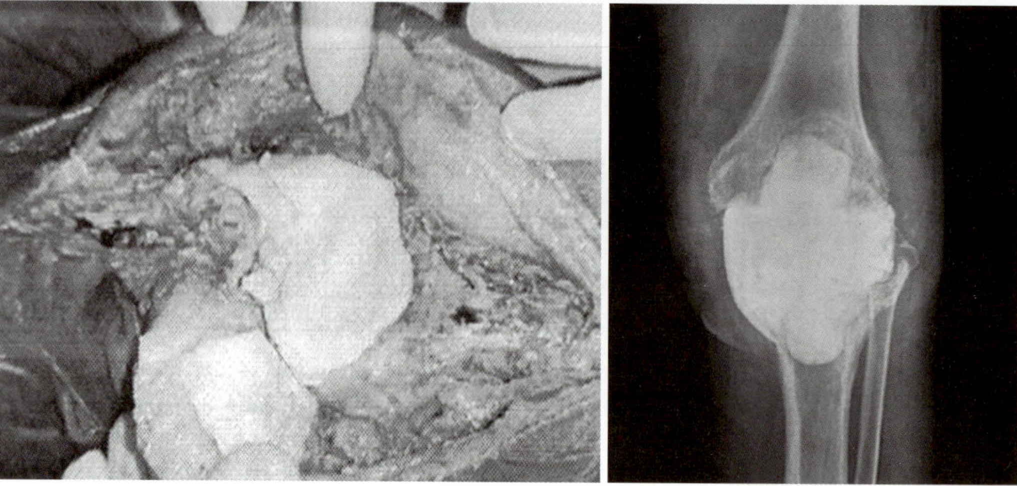

Fig. 66: Figure showing infection of the cement and prosthesis involvement.

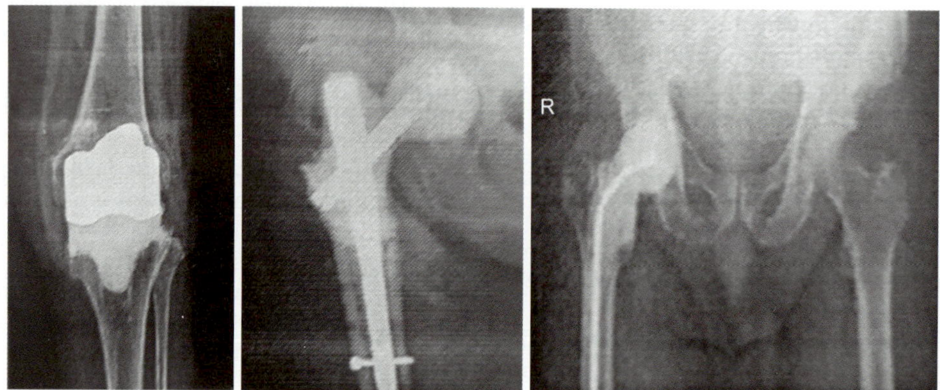

Fig. 67: Figure showing infection of the cement and prosthesis involvement.

One Stage Exchange

- Involves removal of all total joint components, thorough debridement, copious irrigation and reimplantation of new appropriate components with antibiotic impregnated cement.
- Followed by 6–12 weeks systemic antibiotic therapy.
- This is primarily indicated in high morbidity patients unsuitable for multiple operations who are infected with susceptible organisms.
- Advantage of one-stage exchange includes abbreviated recovery and decreased cost and morbidity due to avoidance of second operation.

Antibiotic Suppression Alone

- It is considered only under special circumstances because the prognosis for infection eradication is poor with only 6% success rate.
- It may be considered if the implant is stable.
- The microorganism has low virulence and is susceptible to oral antibiotics.
- The patient has a high anesthesia risk.
- Long-term antibiotic suppression has a risk of antibiotic related adverse effects and emergence of resistant bacteria.

Resection Arthroplasty

- It is suitable for low-demand patients after failure of other treatments in patients with polyarticular rheumatoid arthritis.
- This eradicates infection at the cost of stability and function of the joint.

Arthrodesis

It is indicated for infected TKA with deficient extensor mechanism and in cases with highly resistant organisms or salvage after failed treatments.

Amputation

- Prognosis is poor; most of the patient becomes wheel chair bound
- It is considered for life-threatening systemic sepsis
- Persistent local infection combined with massive bone loss
- Intractable pain.

Other Modalities

- Arthroscopic debridement
- Femorotomy and debridement
- Illizarov.

PREVENTION OF SURGICAL SITE INFECTION IN ORTHOPEDIC SURGERY

INTRODUCTION

Postoperative infection (SSI) of the surgical site can destroy the results of even the most beautifully executed surgery. It is one of the most common hospital acquired infections (HAI) in the developed countries and identified as a target of many national infection prevention programs. The situation in India is bound to be worse given the operating conditions under which our surgeons need to work. In addition to surgical failure, SSI has the following additional effects:

- Increased hospital stay
- Increased morbidity and higher mortality risk
- Increased cost of the treatment due to need for costlier antibiotics, more investigations, and repeat surgical procedures
- Loss to the hospital due to blocked beds
- Increased risk of litigation
- Diversion of already scarce resources, which could be used to treat new patients.

Hence, all surgeons should give priority to prevention of SSI in their patients. Infection can be acquired in any of the phases of hospital stay. Therefore, prevention of SSI includes measures to be taken in preoperative, intraoperative, postoperative, and postdischarge phases of care.

An attempt is made in this chapter to present the ideal infection prevention measures and also customizations that can be done when limited space is available.

BACKGROUND

Sources and Transmission of Infection in the OT (Fig. 68)

- Multiple sources and routes of transmission are present in every OT. Hence, multiple infection control measures are required.
- The sources and transmission routes and therefore the infection risk is always present. Hence, infection prevention measures have to be in place all the time for every patient—it is a permanent program.
- The types of organisms, their prevalence in a given setting, knowledge about infection prevention, technologies used,

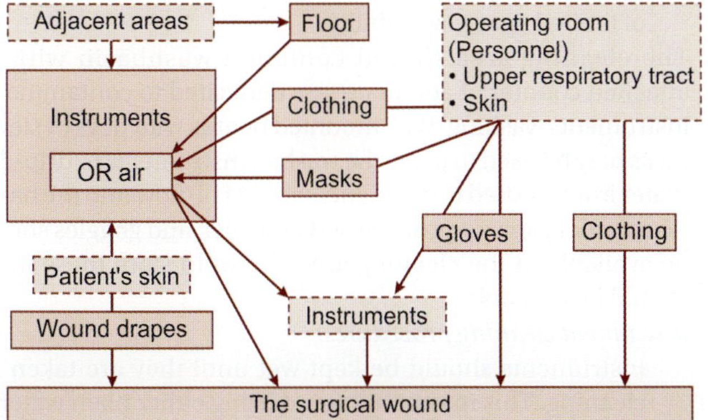

Fig. 68: Sources of infection and common routes of transmission to the surgical wound. Dashed borders indicate sources. Additional sources can be present, e.g. contaminated IV fluids, etc.

etc. change over time with research and development. Hence, a periodic review (at least once a year) of all the infection prevention measures followed should be undertaken to keep the program up to date and effective. This also helps in eliminating measures that are no longer effective thus streamlining the program and making it cost-effective.

The preoperative phase measures include the following:

Design of the Operating Room Complex

- Prepare a workflow diagram of the OT first. This will display exactly how the patient will move through the OT and what care activities are done at each step.
- This will help develop the estimate of the space, numbers of staff required, equipment required etc. at each step.
- After make the first drawing of the OT complex.
- Locate the OT room and the scrub first on the plan and then the other areas.
- *Points to remember:*
  - The OT complex should be located away from common traffic areas. If possible, it can be on a different floor than the OPD area.
  - The complex should have three zones:
    1. *Sterile zone*: It comprises the OT room and scrub basin. Only persons taking part in the surgery are allowed here. OT dress, footwear, caps use is mandatory. Masks should be worn whenever surgery is in progress or sterile equipment is exposed.
    2. *Semisterile zone:* It comprises of all the support and supply areas for the OT, e.g. CSSD, clean storage, dirty utility (as far away from the OT as possible), equipment stores, etc. Note that this extends from the changing room to the scrub basin. OT dress and footwear should be worn in this area and only OT staff are to be allowed here. Cap should be worn at all times and the mask should be worn when scrubbed persons are present and/or sterile equipment is exposed.
    3. *Unsterile zone:* This includes the main entrance and reception areas and the changing room. No limitation on human traffic (except in the changing room); street clothes and footwear allowed; no need for cap, mask, or OT dress.

    The changing room acts as a junction between the unsterile and semisterile areas.
  - The scrub basin should be as close to the OT door as possible so that the person can enter the OT as soon as possible after scrubbing without passing through other areas.
  - The sterility level increases from unsterile to sterile zones (out to in).
  - Physical separation of clean and dirty/contaminated items and activities should be maintained throughout the complex.
  - Working relationship between various areas should be taken into account to decide the traffic routes and separation methods to be employed (Fig. 69).
  - After finalizing the inclusion of various rooms, internal layouts, and furnishings can be decided based on the activities to be done in these rooms.
  - Keep passages to the minimum. They should be wide enough to allow passage of large equipment, and internal surfaces should be easy to clean.

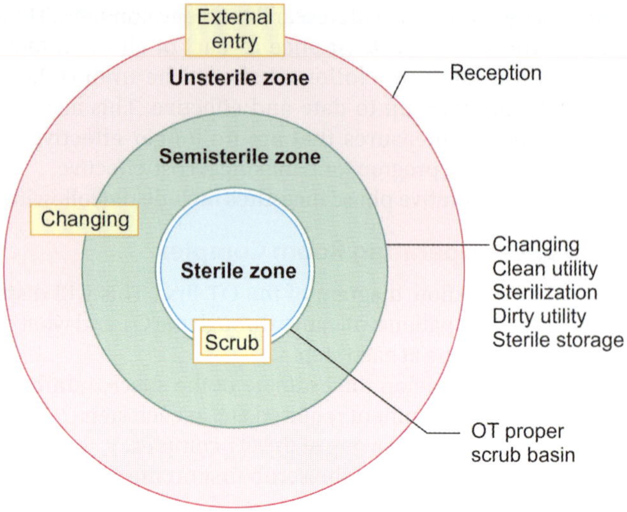

Fig. 69: Diagram showing the three zones of the OT complex with examples of work areas and the junction areas.

- In view of the limited space available in many situations, compromises may need to be done in the form of allotting smaller areas or combining some activities into a single area/room. While doing this, ensure that "clean" and "dirty/contaminated" activities are not combined in one room. If physical separation is not possible, maintain functional separation, e.g. different persons do the "clean" and "dirty" jobs or, the person performs hand hygiene when moving between "dirty" to "clean" jobs. Such compromise should never be done in the actual OT and the scrub area (sterile zone) under any circumstances.
- There should be a separate area for temporary holding of waste and used linen, and a separate area for cleaning and sterilization of surgical instruments.

The Scrub Basin, the Surgical Scrub and Gowning Area

- Place the scrub basin as close as possible to the entrance of the OT.
- All piping joints should be sealed.
- The basin should be broad and deep enough to prevent splashing outside it. Splashguards should be used if necessary.
- Only the antiseptics used for the scrub and the nail-cleaning implement should be there at the scrub.
- The distance between the tap should allow two persons to scrub without their elbows touching each other.
- Keep the area beneath the basin open for daily cleaning and inspection. No storage should be allowed here.
- Put on the cap and mask before scrubbing.
- For the first scrub of the day, clean underneath the fingernails using a nail file or a suitable implement. This step need not be repeated for subsequent scrubs.
- When scrubbing, prefer using soap and water before other antiseptics. A soft soap (total fatty matter (TFM) content ≥70%) should be used. Liquid soaps are preferable. The soap containers should not be topped off (refilled when container is partially empty). If bar soaps are used, the soap holder should be fixed in such a way that residual water from the holder falls into the basin and is drained away.
- An iodine containing preparation may be used after soap. Where surgery is expected to last longer than 2 hours, a chlorhexidine containing preparation may be used instead of iodine or added after it.
- A 3–5 minutes scrub is adequate.
- Ensure the hands are bare (no jewelry) and the nails short to obtain maximal disinfection.
- An alcohol hand rub should be applied to dry hands just before putting on gloves (after gowning) in the OT and it should be dried by rubbing the hands together.
- The gowning area inside the OT should be located away from the entry door.

Cleaning and Sterilization of Surgical Equipment

Layout of the Instrument Cleaning Area

- There should always be a separate area for cleaning and sterilization of used surgical instruments. This should be given top priority. The amount of area allotted will depend upon the expected workload and types of equipment used for the process.
- Ideally the area should consist of the following physically separated rooms: (1) the cleaning area (air exhausted directly outside), (2) the inspection, packaging, and labeling area, (3) the sterilization machine area, and (4) the sterile storage area.
- However, in situations where space is limited, the following can be done:
  - The available room/area should be divided into two by a floor to ceiling partition. One area to be used only for instrument cleaning; and the other for drying, inspection, instrument oiling, packaging of containers, and the actual sterilization and storage of sterilized containers. An exhaust fan should be used in the cleaning area. Ceiling fans should be avoided. The ventilation in the room should be such that air flows from the sterilization area to the cleaning area and is then exhausted outside. Closed cupboards should be used for storing sterilized containers.
  - The same person should perform cleaning of instruments and other activities simultaneously. If separate manpower is not available, the person should perform a handwash and disinfect the hands with an alcohol hand rub after cleaning activities and before beginning other activities like packaging instruments.
  - It must be stated that the above is a reduction of the ideal design and the risk of recontamination of cleaned items and outer surfaces of sterile containers will be higher than desired. However, this would be the best solution in view of limited space availability.
- The cleaning area should contain a washbasin with an attached counter of adequate size dedicated to contaminated instruments washing. Wall mounted boards with pegs or sieved racks may be used to place the washed instruments to drip-dry. Water from washed instruments should fall/flow into the basin.
- Waterproof gloves, apron, closed footwear, and goggles should be available in the cleaning area. Space to store these items should be available.
- *Instrument cleaning procedures:*
  - Instruments should be kept wet until they are taken for cleaning. This may be achieved using either plain water or enzyme cleaner solutions (preferable).
  - Perform a first rinse under flowing water to remove the gross debris and blood.

- Various techniques may be used for cleaning after the first rinse, e.g. brushing in soap water; using an enzymatic/surfactant cleaner; using an ultrasonic cleaner; using a washer disinfector machine, etc. The final combination of methods will depend on the manpower, space, budget, workload, and can vary from one OT to another.
- Choose a combination of cleaning methods that ensures complete removal of organic soiling, is easy for the staff to perform. Cost should be the last consideration here.

- *Some important points:*
  - Brushing should be done underwater (both instrument and brush dipped in water).
  - For small or complicated instruments (e.g. microscopic surgery), use of an ultrasonic cleaner is recommended.
  - Components of each instrument should be opened/disassembled and cleaned in detail.
  - Inspection for damage, residual debris should be carried out at this stage itself.
- If water quality cannot be assured, a final rinse with distilled water/reverse osmosis water should be done.
- Dry the instruments. Prefer wiping with a clean lint-free cloth. If hot air ovens are used (for heavier loads) ensure the water used for cleaning is not excessively hard. Lumened instruments should be dried using forced (compressed) air.
- *Packaging for sterilization*: The arrangement of articles in the sterilization container should allow easy penetration of steam into all parts of the interior. Avoid overfilling the container. Package instruments and linen in the different containers. Joints and hinges of the instruments should be kept open. Linen gowns should be folded loosely in a zigzag manner to allow easier steam penetration.
- *Wrapping of sterile containers*: Avoid using linen as it does not provide a good barrier to microbial and dust penetration after sterilization. Paper wraps are more reliable. If using branded paper (nonwoven) is not possible, ordinary paper of adequate thickness to prevent tearing may also be used. The paper should be dry at the end of the sterilization cycle in the autoclave (a machine with a vacuum cycle is required for this). Do not use paper if the autoclave is of vertical type without a vacuum facility. For sterilization by ETO gas, paper, or paper-plastic packaging material can be used.
- *Monitoring of steam sterilization:*
  - Monitoring of the physical parameters of pressure achieved or temperature achieved or both should be done for every autoclave cycle.
  - Class I chemical indicators (autoclave tape) should be pasted on the outside of every container at the side and in the same location every time. One of these strips should be pasted in the autoclave logbook later. Write the following on the strip: date of sterilization, batch number, initials of the person who packed the container. Another strip may be placed inside the container at the center of the instruments and inside the largest roll of linen to detect steam penetration (optional). Note that this indicator does not indicate sterilization.
  - A Class 6 chemical indicator and biological indicator should be used at least once a week in each type of load (linen, instruments).
  - Newer monitoring devices such as a process challenge devices (PCD), can be used in every cycle. Use of Class 6 chemical indicators can be eliminated if a PCD is used in every cycle.
  - A detailed record of the monitoring of all sterilization processes—logbooks, printouts and lab reports of the biological indicator results—should be meticulously maintained. These documents have legal importance (Tables 11 and 12).
- Use a temperature of 121°C maintained for 30 minutes for routine sterilization. High temperature short time (HTST) cycles (132°C and 134°C) should preferably be avoided as a routine method of sterilization unless cleaning quality can be assured (Table 13).

TABLE 11: Sample schedule for monitoring sterilization (can be adapted to local conditions).

Week day →	*Monday*	*Tuesday*	*Wednesday*	*Thursday*	*Friday*	*Saturday*
Autoclave	Class 1 indicator (Signaloc) for all containers every time.					
	Biological indicator—linen	Class 6 strip in instruments	Class 6 strip in linen	Biological indicator—instruments	Class 6 strip in linen	Class 6 strip in instruments

TABLE 12: Sample format for autoclave logbook.

Date	*Autoclave number* (A, B etc.)	*Cycle number* (Given serially each time the machine is run)	*Load description* (What was autoclaved? —names of containers)	*Pressure* (Noted 15 min after the pressure reaches 15 lbs)	*Class I indicator strip*	*Class 6 indicator*	*Sign/Name* of person operating the machine

TABLE 13: Minimum time and temperature for various steam sterilization cycles.

Type of sterilizer	*Item*	*Exposure time at 250°F (121°C)*	*Exposure time at 270°F (132°C)*	*Drying time*
Gravity displacement	Wrapped instruments	30 min	15 min	15–30 min
	Textile packs	30 min	25 min	15 min
	Wrapped utensils	30 min	15 min	15–30 min
Dynamic-air-removal (e.g. prevacuum)	Wrapped instruments		4 min	20–30 min
	Textile packs		4 min	5–20 min
	Wrapped utensils		4 min	20 min

- *Maximum sterilization (holding) time (time for which the sterilizing temperature is maintained)*; this can be increased up to 45 minutes. Sterilizing beyond that time does not confer any additional advantage.
- "Flash sterilization" in which instruments are autoclaved at high temperature for short time without wrapping should not be used as a routine method of sterilization.
- Use an autoclave machine with facility for prevacuum pulsing.
- Vertical autoclaves are commonly used. These machines do not have proper vacuum generation facility. "Wet loads" (residual water in the sterilization container) are common in these types of machines. The following precautions should be taken when using these machines:
  - Air should be removed at the beginning of the cycle using the method recommended by the manufacturer, if no such recommendation is available, steam should be allowed to escape for at least ten minutes before closing the valve (this process is less effective).
  - The holding time should be calculated from the time the pressure reaches 15 psi. In general, a minimum holding time of 30 minutes for both instruments and linen should be followed.
  - After the holding time is over, the autoclave should be allowed to cool before it is opened. Pressure should not be released manually until it reaches 5 pounds or below.
- The pressure meter and the pressure release valve of the autoclave should be calibrated/replaced periodically, e.g. every 3–6 months.
- Sterilized containers should be stored, protected from dust and spills in a separate dedicated area (sterile storage). If not available store in closed cupboards. These items should be minimally handled and the "first-in, first-out" principle should be followed in their use (containers sterilized first are used first).
- The shelf life of a sterilized container depends on the quality of the wrapping material and storage conditions. Wrapping materials that provide a better barrier to recontamination, e.g. paper, paper-plastic pouches, etc. allow a longer shelf life compared to linen wraps. Containers should be stored protected from liquids, dust, and excessive moisture. A longer shelf-life reduces the need for repeated sterilization and can help reduce the cost. Hence, all efforts should be done to ensure good packaging and storage. The shelf-life can be decided by an individual hospital based on the above.
  - Generally, allot an expiry of 3–4 days if only linen wrapping is used.
  - The expiry can be extended to 1 month if paper wrapping is used.
  - For sealed paper plastic pouches an expiry of 1 year can be allotted.
- Training the staff in cleaning and sterilization methods should be done to ensure quality.

OT Ventilation

- Laminar airflow positive pressure ventilation systems with high efficiency particulate air (HEPA) filters (also called as HVAC system) are recommended and are also mandatory requirements for all hospital accreditations. However, proper system design and maintenance is a must.
- A detailed description of the system design and requirements is beyond the scope of this chapter. However, the salient aspects of the design are as follows:
  - The system should never generate turbulence in any part of the OT room and should minimize dead space (room spaces where there is no airflow). High airflow rates, which will tend to push organisms into the surgical wound should be avoided. Monitoring devices to indicate loss of positive pressure should be installed.
  - Humidity levels should be maintained between 40% and 60% and temperature 18 ± 3°C.
  - A positive pressure of minimum 15 Pascal should be maintained in the OT relative to adjacent areas.
  - Any condensation water generated by the system should drain away from the HEPA filters and the interior of the ducts should always remain dry. Ducting should have cleaning access ports in adequate numbers and at strategic locations.
- *Microbiological monitoring of the system:*
  - Perform weekly air sampling.
  - Maintain a record of the results.
  - Obtain a sample on/over the operating table in an empty OT.
  - Counts should be less than 1 cfu (colony forming unit).
  - A hand-held air sampler or a settle plate method (exposing a culture plate on the OT table) can be used to sample the air.
- Daily temperature and humidity log should be maintained.
- The prefilters in the air handling unit (AHU) should be cleaned every 15 days. The cleaning should be done in an area away from patient care areas.
- Once a year, validation of all system parameters (particle counts, temperature, humidity, positive pressure) and checking of the HEPA filters should be done and records maintained.
- In OTs without such systems, commercially available wall-mounted air purifiers may be used, but their limitations should be kept in mind.
  - They take time to reduce the bioburden and may not be able to deal with excessive levels of bioburden.
- They have to be cleaned and maintained on a regular basis as per the manufacturer's recommendations and the records maintained. The air sampling can be done to evaluate their performance but the above mentioned microbial limits do not apply to these machines.
- Use of air conditioner (AC)—hospitals who use these devices in the OT should consider the following:
  - No AC of any type provides any significant air changes or reduction in bacterial counts.
  - The air from an AC is never sterile. Hence, location of the AC should be such that the air outflow never falls directly onto the operation table or the sterile trolleys.
  - ACs should be cleaned regularly. The air filters should be cleaned at least once a week.
  - Despite all precautions, an AC unit can harbor variety of organisms and is always a potential source in infection.
- Ceiling, stand, or wall fans should not be used in OT.
- A positive pressure ventilation system is not a substitute for other infection control measures such as minimal traffic, minimal movement, and talking, minimal door opening, and these should be followed.

SURFACE CLEANING AND DISINFECTION

- This is one of the most important infection prevention measures and should not be compromised.
- Cleaning and disinfection should always go together and be performed in that order only.

General Aspects

- Never use a broom for OT cleaning. A dry mop may be used for the floor.
- All cleaning should preferably be done by wet mopping. However, a dry mop may be used provided it is cleaned outside the OT complex.
- Use a high level disinfectant (one that kills all viable organisms including *Mycobacterium tuberculosis* and some spores also).
- Ensure proper concentration of the chemical in the working solution. Prepare dilutions by measurement.
- When wet mopping or wiping, use the spray/pour-wipe technique.
  - Prepare the cleaning reagent/disinfectant in a bottle with a hole in the cap.
  - When cleaning the floor, sprinkle the reagent liberally on the floor and wipe with a wet mop. Take clean water in a bucket to rinse the mop and change the water when it appears soiled or when the room is changed.
  - When cleaning equipment, pour the chemical on the mop and then wipe the equipment surface in one direction. Change the fold of the mop when moving from one equipment to another. When all folds are reused, change the mop. The used mop should be kept aside for washing. Do not rinse the mop in water when cleaning equipment.
- After wet wiping/mopping with a disinfectant, the surface should remain wet for at least 1–3 minutes to allow proper action of the disinfectant. Only when plain soap is used, immediate drying can be allowed.
- Prepare cleaning and disinfectant solution in proper concentration by correct measurement as recommended by the manufacturer. Measuring apparatus, such as measuring cylinders/jugs, should be available in the OT. The quantities of various reagents and water to be mixed should be available in written form in the OT for reference.
  - Disinfectants prepared by dilution should always be prepared fresh and the leftover discarded after use.
  - Mops, buckets, and other equipment used in cleaning should be washed with soap and water after use, disinfected using chlorine solution and dried before reuse.
- Use separate mops for the equipment and the environment. Color coding can help differentiate them (useful for untrained staff). Provide enough supply of mops.
- Cleaning and disinfection once begun should not be interrupted. Proper planning can ensure this.
- The OT cleaning and disinfection can be divided into four types:
  1. *Start-of-the-day cleaning and disinfection:* Wipe all horizontal surfaces with disinfectant. Walls may be cleaned as per a fixed schedule (2–3 times/week) and whenever they appear soiled or dusty.
  2. *Between surgeries:* Begin after the patient is shifted out and operating staff has left the OT.
     - Clean blood spills first. Cover large spills with paper and pour 5–10% sodium hypochlorite/a high level disinfectant (diluted as per manufacturer recommendations); small spills (less than 10 mL) may be wiped with a paper soaked in sodium hypochlorite. The paper should be discarded as infected waste and the area wiped again with a disinfectant during the final cleaning step.
     - Then remove all equipment to be reprocessed, used linen and waste.
     - Perform handwashing and wipe all surfaces with a high level disinfectant.
     - The entire floor need not be wiped. The area around the OT table in which the operating team stands can be wiped only.
     - Adequate time should be allowed for proper cleaning.
     - Persons taking part in surgery should not be present in the OT at the time of cleaning.
     - Sterile containers containing materials for the next case should be opened only after the cleaning and disinfection is over.
     - The surgical team and the next patient should come in only after all cleaning is complete.
  3. *The end-of-the-day cleaning:* The between-surgeries cleaning should be repeated after the last case. Wipe all used surfaces with a high level disinfectant and clean the entire floor. Scrubbing the floor with a high level disinfectant twice is recommended.
  4. *Detailed wash-down:* Periodically, the OT and all connected passages and rooms should be wiped liberally with soap and water followed by a high level disinfectant. The frequency should be adjusted according to the dust found in daily inspection of various areas of the OT complex.

Use of Antiseptics

- Iodine-based disinfectants should be dispensed directly from the original container.
- Prepare dilutions by accurate measurement.
- Prepare them in transparent bottles with good seal. Do not use dropping bottles (with tubes/needles pierced through the caps).
- At the minimum, clean tap water of drinking quality should be used for dilution.
- Bottles of diluted disinfectants should be labeled clearly with the reagent name and date of preparation. Prepare just enough solution to last for 2–3 days. Examine the solution for any turbidity or particles daily morning. If present, discard and prepare fresh. Discard any leftover solution at the end of this period and prepare fresh solution in a freshly cleaned and disinfected bottle. This can be done by using a sodium hypochlorite rinse after cleaning.
- Disinfectant bottles used in the OT should not be shared with other locations outside that OT.
- Everyday, at the start of work, these bottles should be inspected carefully for any gross debris and turbidity. If seen, the solution should be discarded and a fresh one prepared in a sterile bottle. The daily inspection is very important and should never be missed.

Fumigation

- "Fumigation" is just high level disinfection of the OT and not "sterilization". Therefore, it is very important that the procedure be carried out as perfectly as possible.
- Fumigation is not required for OTs having a properly designed and working positive pressure airflow system with HEPA filtration. For these OTs the following should be done instead of classical fumigation:
  - Clean and disinfect all surfaces.
  - Close the OT and allow 3–4 air changes to take place. The OT can be used after this.
- Proper cleaning before fumigation is mandatory.
- Adequate quantities and concentrations of the disinfectant should be used as recommended by the manufacturer.
- Proper methods of application should be employed according to the type of disinfectant used. In the case of formalin, the gas has to be liberated from the solution and spread to all parts of the room whereas, in case of glutaraldehyde or hydrogen peroxide or other chemical based reagents, the working solution has to come in contact with all surfaces for it to kill microbes (these reagents have to be applied either by wet mopping, hand spraying or by using a fogging machine). The newer reagents cannot be used in the traditional OT care machine, which is meant for formalin.
- Adequate contact periods (holding time) of the disinfectant with the surfaces are essential for maximal bactericidal activity. For formalin, the usual period is 8 hours whereas for the newer chemicals it is 1 hour.
- Surfaces in the OT should be dry after the contact period. In case of formalin, the irritant fumes should be neutralized by liquor ammonia in proper quantity. Exhaust fans should never be used to evacuate the fumes. Neutralization is not required for other reagents.
- The effect of fumigation is only temporary and recolonization of the OT begins as soon as OT use begins. Therefore, fumigation is just a temporary measure to reduce accumulated bioburden in ORs without ventilation and other IC practices, such as minimization of traffic, physical movement, door opening, vocal activity, etc. are important to minimize the subsequent build-up of bioburden.
- Microbiological testing of various surfaces in the OT after fumigation is important to monitor its adequacy and should be done on a regular basis. A record of the reports should be maintained. This should be a standard practice followed in all ORs.
- Formalin should be phased out as soon as possible. Apart from its carcinogenicity, it is inconvenient to use, has a strong irritant action. More importantly, the conditions of humidity and concentration required for proper bactericidal action of formalin cannot be ensured in the entire room throughout the contact period. Therefore, the results can vary considerably. Additionally, there is no real-time test to assess the efficacy of fumigation.

WORK RELATED ISSUES

- Restrict traffic in the OT complex as much as possible. Movement in the various areas within the complex also should be regulated. During surgery, only persons required for surgery should be present in the actual OT.
- OT equipment and articles should not be shared with other locations outside the complex. If equipment is shared, it should be wiped with a low level disinfectant (if there is soiling with blood/body fluids, use a high level disinfectant) before it is brought inside the OT.
- During surgery, door opening, physical and vocal activity, and movement in and out of the OT should be minimized to the greatest extent possible. Music systems may be used in the OT provided that are kept clean and dust free.
- A cap should be worn by all persons in the semi-restricted and restricted areas at all times. All facial and head hair should be covered whenever cap and mask are worn.
- Sterile equipment should be handled in the sterile field using sterile technique. Scrubbed persons should not handle unsterile items or touch unsterile surfaces.
- Sharps should be passed in a neutral zone, e.g. placed in a kidney tray, not from hand-to-hand.
- Persons assisting in the surgery should not move away from the OT table.
- Doctors should avoid visiting locations outside the OT complex between surgeries. If this is not possible, change the OT dress before reentering the OT. They should avoid examining outpatients between surgeries of the day. Anesthetists should avoid visiting multiple theaters or patients in the intensive care units during an operation. Although a paucity of staff leads to these compromises at times, detailed planning of work reduces such incidences to the minimum.
- Sterile gloved hands should be held clasped together when waiting. They should not be rested on abdomen or folded into the armpits.

PREOPERATIVE PREPARATION OF THE PATIENT AND THE SURGICAL SITE

- Perform a thorough preoperative clinical examination on each patient including an examination of the oral cavity for dental/periodontal disease. Any pre-existing infection should be treated before elective surgery.
- Minimize preoperative stay.
- Hair at the surgical site should not be removed unless it will interfere with the operation or postoperative care. If hair removal is necessary, the following methods should be preferred in the order mentioned: clipping, depilatory creams, shaving.
- The time interval between hair removal and surgery should be as short as possible. The equipment used for hair removal, especially its cutting edges, should be kept clean and all times and be disinfected before each patient. The equipment should be cleaned immediately after use and stored covered.
- If shaving is to be done, perform it within 2 hours before surgery. Do not shave the night before. After shaving, the area should be properly disinfected.
- In patients admitted with soiled wounds, a thorough cleaning of the wounds is extremely important to prevent later infection. No effort should be spared for proper debridement at the initial stage itself.
- Hydrogen peroxide should be used mainly as a debriding agent. The disinfectant action of the reagent in tissues is weak.
- Avoid mixing iodine and hydrogen peroxide as this can reduce the activity of both.

- In cases where the first limb preparation is done on the night before, consider using a 2% chlorhexidine containing antiseptic instead of iodine. Allow to dry naturally after application (do not rub off). A repeat application before surgery can provide a cumulative antiseptic effect.
- The incision site should preferably be cleaned first with soap and water before applying disinfectants. Alternatively, the part may be cleaned with soap and water before the patient is sent to the OT.
- Apply disinfectants in concentric circles or in radial strokes moving outwards from the incision site. Allow the disinfectant to remain wet on the skin for an adequate time to achieve proper bactericidal action (iodine: 1–2 minutes; spirit: 30 seconds; quaternary ammonium compounds: 5–10 min; chlorhexidine: 30 sec to 2 min). Chlorhexidine should be included if the surgery is expected to last for more than 2 hours.
- Do not mix two disinfectants or soap with disinfectants.
- For recommendations on use of surgical site disinfectants, see the section on "use of other chemical disinfectants." Disinfectant bottles used in the OT should not be shared with locations outside it, e.g. the emergency, minor OT, etc.

Antibiotic Prophylaxis

- Perioperative antibiotic prophylaxis should be given. Although recommendations from many guidelines may allow for not using antibiotics for selected procedures, in the author's view, this should not be applied to a hospital in Indian settings without prior appraisal. Only if all infection prevention measures are in place and functioning satisfactorily should elimination of antibiotic coverage be considered.
- In view of the lack of national epidemiological data, it will not be possible to provide clear recommendations on use of specific antibiotics for surgical prophylaxis in clean cases. Many international guidelines are available and in general, second generation cephalosporins are recommended for surgical prophylaxis in all clean cases.
- Since bacterial types and prevalence can vary a lot between hospitals, a detailed analysis of microbiology data should be done to develop a more applicable policy.
- Use of more than one antibiotic in immunocompetent clean cases should be avoided.
- The *most important* aspect of antibiotic prophylaxis is the timing. In clean cases, the first dose should be administered within 30–60 minutes before the surgical incision. Exceptions—vancomycin and quinolones (within 2 hours before the incision). Other aspects of antibiotic prophylaxis are as follows:
  - Take weight into account when calculating the dose.
  - Maintain a gap of 10 minutes between antibiotic administration (first) and tourniquet application (later).
  - If surgery prolongs beyond 3–4 hours, repeat cephalosporin drugs.
  - Giving a "shot" at the end of surgery is not useful in preventing infections.
  - Starting antibiotic one day prior to surgery should be avoided. It is more a risk factor than preventive as resistant organisms can be selected faster.
  - The antibiotic should ideally be stopped within 24–48 hours in the postoperative period. In settings where postoperative care of the wound may be compromised, antibiotics may be continued beyond this period. However, in such settings everything possible should be done to ensure betterment of the postoperative care (e.g. training of staff, education to the patient, provision of clean environment, etc.). Measures, such as handwashing, proper sterilization, storage, and use of materials used in wound dressings, safe injection practices, and proper use of gloves, should be emphasized, rather than relying on antibiotics to prevent infection.
  - In patients with infection in whom surgery cannot be postponed, antibiotics should be used as per the culture-sensitivity report of a proper sample from the infection site.

Surveillance Programs for Surgical Site Infection

- The broad steps of a surveillance program are: Develop definitions to identify infections → case identification, data collection, and processing → analysis of the data → interpretation of the results.
- Document every case of surgical site infection. Diagnose the cases using specific criteria, e.g. the Centers for Disease Control (CDC) criteria to identify various types of SSI. Perform a culture sensitivity test in every case of SSI and document the report. This information is immensely helpful in identification of possible sources of infection, trends of infection, identification of specific infection control measures required, and developing an antibiotic policy.
- The data may be documented using forms specially designed for the purpose or entered directly into an electronic database.
- Calculate the percent SSI rate every month, i.e. number of SSI cases/total number of surgeries × 100.
- Calculate the following types of SSI rates: Overall (all surgeries), procedure-wise, OT-wise and surgeon-wise rates.
- The results should be studied by the surgeon in conjunction with an experienced infection control practitioner. Confidential feedback on a surgeon's infection rates should be given to him.

Disposal of Biomedical Waste

- Government regulations regarding segregation, collection, transport, and disposal of biomedical waste should be followed.
- Segregation of biomedical waste should be done at the point of generation itself, i.e. in the OT itself. Waste should not be pooled in one container and separated later.
- Waste should be removed from the OT as soon as possible after an operation.
- Identify and categorize all types of waste items generated in an OT to minimize confusion among the staff, regarding the segregation and disposal method for a particular item.
- Staff handing waste should wear rubber/heavy duty gloves.
- Put up posters showing the segregation of waste according to the color-coding and train staff at regular intervals on what items to dispose of in each type of container. This training should be given to new staff on joining the hospital.

HIV AND HEPATITIS B INFECTED CASES

- No special measures are required to disinfect and clean surgical instruments and the OT after operating a HIV/Hepatitis B positive patient. The virus is killed by standard disinfectants and disinfection procedures. Lab tests can have false negatives and positives. Hence, it is safer to treat every patient as potentially infected and setup the cleaning and disinfection practices for the instruments, linen, and the environment accordingly.

- Soiled linen need not be discarded unless it is unfit for further use. Linen may be disinfected using freshly prepared 1–2% hypochlorite solutions and then washed in the usual manner.
- There is no need to fumigate an OT after an operation on an HIV infected patient. Proper surface cleaning and disinfection of all surfaces contaminated by blood and body fluids should be emphasized and practiced.
- Proper use of barrier precautions to prevent exposure to blood and body fluids both during the surgery and while cleaning up later is of utmost importance and should NEVER be compromised. Disposable water impermeable fabrics should be preferred for surgical attire wherever available and affordable. Alternatively, water proof aprons (of adequate size) may be worn. OT shoes should be preferred over open footwear (slippers). Goggles/face shields should be worn wherever the possibility of splashing exists.
- Immediate segregation and prompt disposal of sharps after use should be performed.
- Gloves used while cleaning and handling waste should be made of water-proof material and should extend up to the mid-forearms at least. Latex gloves should not be used.
- Education of the staff and doctors is important to ensure correct practices every time.
- During surgery, sharp instruments should be passed in a kidney tray instead of hand-to-hand.

WATER SUPPLY

- Water supply systems should be planned before construction of the OT.
- Tanks and pipelines should be regularly inspected for leakages and repaired immediately whenever found.
- As paucity of municipal supply is a problem at many places, use of borewell water will be inevitable. Hardness and bacteriological quality of this water should be checked regularly and appropriate softening and disinfection procedures (generally chlorination) should be in place as these qualities can vary widely over both region and time.
- As far as possible, borewell water should not be used for cleaning and mopping of equipment and surfaces that come in contact with the patient or sterile equipment/instruments. If it is to be used for this purpose, softening and disinfection should be performed compulsorily. This can be achieved to some degree by boiling it.
- Water storage tanks and containers should have covers/lids that will prevent the entry of dust, insects, and organic debris, such as leaves into them. The tanks/containers should have a smooth finish on the inside. Terrace tanks should be cleaned and disinfected at least once every 3 months or more frequently if contamination by organic debris is found on more than one occasion. Cleaning records should be maintained. Washing with soap and water should be followed by disinfection using hypochlorite solution. The inner surfaces may be liberally mopped with freshly prepared 5% sodium hypochlorite followed by a water rinse.
- *Water testing*: Perform testing of physical parameters, i.e. hardness, etc. once a year and whenever the water source changes. If borewell water is used, this testing may need to be done more frequently, e.g. at change of seasons. Microbiological testing should be done at least once a month and whenever the water source changes or major repairs/replacements are carried out on the supply system.
  - Microbial testing should preferably be done by the membrane filtration method instead of the most probable number (MPN or also called Coliform count) method. The MPN method is suitable for community drinking water supplies and detects fecal contamination only whereas detection of other organisms in the hospital water is also important.
  - The lab should report the number of colonies grown per mL of water and also identify any pathogens, potential pathogens present.

REPROCESSING OF SINGLE USE ITEMS

- Wherever possible, minimize the need to reprocess single-use items. In case single-use disposable items are to be reused, proper methods for reprocessing need to be setup.
- Items that cannot be cleaned properly and those in which penetration of the sterilant/disinfectant agent to all areas cannot be assured, e.g. due to a complicated structure should not be reprocessed.
- All items to be reprocessed should be checked for proper functional and structural integrity first after cleaning them. If it is damaged, do not reprocess.
- The principle of "If it cannot be cleaned, it should not be reprocessed" should be followed.
- In general, all items to be reprocessed should be kept moist/wet until they are taken up for cleaning. This may be done by simply placing them in plain water. Lumens should also be kept wet/moist.
- Adequate cleaning to remove all organic debris is of utmost importance. Enzymatic cleaning solutions should be used for this. The solutions should be used as per the manufacturer's recommendations.
- Traces of the cleaning solution should be flushed away by thoroughly rinsing it with clean plain water before proceeding to the next step.
- Do not reprocess latex gloves. However, if a hospital decides to reuse, the following points should be kept in regarding reprocessing of gloves:
  - Never use reprocessed gloves for any procedure involving handling of sterile materials or where contact with blood/body fluids is likely.
  - If reuse is to be done, reprocessing nitrile gloves would be safer latex.
  - The policy on glove reuse should be clearly known to all persons working in the OT.
- Clean gloves made of waterproof material, e.g. rubber, instead of reprocessed latex/nitrile ones, should be used when performing environmental cleaning, cleaning of surgical instruments, and handling biomedical waste. This is an important occupational safety measure and may have legal and financial implications for the hospital owner in case of accidents.

SURGICAL ATTIRE AND DRAPES

- Surgical attire fabrics should be tightly woven, stain resistant, and durable. Surgical attire should provide comfort in terms of design, fit, breathability, and the weight of the fabric. Pore size should be less than 80 microns. Tightly-woven surgical attire (cotton and polyester [50/50] with 560 × 395 threads/10 cm) reduced the amount of bacteria shed into the air by two to five times. 100% cotton should not be used for surgical attire.

- The OT dress, cap and masks should be stored covered to prevent their contamination.
- The OT dress, cap, and mask need not be sterile.
- A fresh dress should be used each day.
- Wearing street clothing beneath the OT dress should be avoided. If worn, it should be completely covered by the OT dress.
- Jewelry including earrings, necklaces, watches, and bracelets that cannot be covered by the surgical attire should not be worn.
- Dedicated shoes/slippers should be used in the semi-sterile and sterile areas of the OT. Shoes should be made of waterproof material, e.g. rubber and should not have openings through which blood spills/sharps can reach inside. The sole should be thick enough to protect from injuries due to sharps lying on the floor.
- Aprons worn in other areas of the hospital should not be brought into the semisterile and sterile areas of the OT.
- Stethoscopes should be wiped with plain spirit before use in the OT.
- Mobiles should ideally not be brought into the OT. Wipe the cellphone with plain spirit when the person first comes into the OT. Ensure the phone has a screen protector film before wiping with spirit.
- Wearing a cap and mask is mandatory in the following situations: In the OT—whenever an operation is in progress or sterile instruments are exposed; in other parts of the OT complex—whenever sterile equipment is exposed. The cap should be worn at all times in the semirestricted and restricted areas.
- Fresh disposable masks should be worn for each surgery. Avoid linen masks. Disposable masks should be changed every 3–4 hours and whenever they become wet due to any reason.
- The mask should cover as much of the facial skin and hair as possible.
- Masks should be removed as soon their purpose is served and not left hanging around the neck.
- The cap should be worn in a manner that covers all head hair. Female staff and doctors with long hair should use bigger sized caps if required. Long hair should not be accepted as an excuse for incomplete coverage of hair. Linen caps are allowable.
- Surgical attire should be changed as soon as possible, whenever it becomes wet due to any reason, including sweat, and on returning after visiting a location outside the OT complex.
- Ensure availability of a bin/tub to discard used OT dress, caps, and masks in the changing room to prevent them from being spread over the room.

MICROBIOLOGICAL SAMPLING

- Microbiological sampling of air, surfaces, and water should be done at least once a month. A qualified microbiologist should perform the test and report the findings.
- It must be remembered that absence of infection outbreaks in an OT does not mean that the cleaning, fumigation, surface, and water disinfection procedures, and other infection control measures being followed are correct. There are many other factors that affect the patient outcomes.
- Both settle plates and sampling using an air sampler should ideally be done. The plate provides information on the organisms settling on the surfaces (including the surgical wound) whereas the sampler provides information on suspended.
- Intraoperative air sampling should also be done once a month. Intraoperative sampling should be done as close to the surgical site as possible. Intraoperative sampling is useful to detect pathogens that are present only during surgery, e.g. a carrier of *Staphylococcus aureus*, MRSA.
- Surface swabs (popularly referred to as OT swabs) should be sampled to assess the efficacy of surface cleaning and disinfection. More precise tests such as the ATP bioluminescence are now available but are still too costly for most Indian hospitals. Marking with fluorescent ink can be used to assess the cleaning objectively.
- Detailed knowledge of the OT layout and working patterns will be required to judge the source of growth obtained in these samples and the measures to be taken to prevent them.
- Collection, transport, and lab processing of samples should be done in a manner that avoids contamination.
- Records of all microbiological tests of the environment should be maintained by all ORs. Protocols of steps to be taken in case of an unsatisfactory test result should be developed by all ORs. All staff should know the steps in detail.

STAFF HEALTH, INFECTED AND COLONIZED PERSONNEL

- There should be a system for prompt reporting of any illness among the staff to the doctor/OT supervisor.
- Any illness should be immediately investigated and treated.
- Persons with respiratory infections should not work in the OT until cured or at least 2 days of antimicrobial chemotherapy have been completed. If cough is one of the symptoms, he/she should not work in the OT until the symptom has resolved completely irrespective of the days of chemotherapy. If working is unavoidable, he/she should use double masks (one above the other) and change them every 2 hours strictly (please note that is an extreme concession and should be avoided as much as possible).
- Persons with draining skin lesions should not work until the lesions have dried.
- In order to make the above possible in settings with low manpower resources, OT staff should be trained to take over the indisposed person's duties, i.e. multitasking will be required. Training is important as multitasking in the OT may lead to breaches in maintenance of sterility. Details of "who will do what" should be clear.
- Surgeons should lead by example by not operating when they have a respiratory or a skin infection. This may not be possible at all times due to economic or patient load pressures, but every effort should be made to set an example.
- All persons working in an OT should be vaccinated against hepatitis B. The antibody levels (anti-HBs) should be checked 1–2 months after the third dose. If they are less than 10 IU the person should undergo another course of vaccination followed

by rechecking of the antibody levels. If they are still low, then the person cannot be protected by vaccination and should ideally not work in the OT.
- If possible, an annual health checkup should be done for all OT staff and records of the same maintained.

Implementation Aspects

- One of the senior OT staff or if available, the OT incharge should be allotted the responsibility of implementation of infection control practices in the OT.
- Teamwork, coordination, and communication are the most important factors affecting the success of the infection control program in any hospital.
- When deciding the infection control measures, the following criteria should be used—the measures should be based on scientific evidence wherever it is available. If evidence is lacking/insufficient, the measures should be based on microbiological rationale. Measures that are required by local laws will be mandatory. Practicality and feasibility should be considered as resources vary from one hospital to another. Cost effectiveness also should be kept in mind and quality and cost needs to be balanced as much as possible.

INVESTIGATION OF A CASE OF SURGICAL SITE INFECTION (TABLE 14)

First, investigate:
- Perform a culture sensitivity test of the infected wound.
  - The organism grown may give an important clue to the source (endogenous or exogenous source).
  - It will also help to choose the most suitable antibiotic for treatment.

Second, look at the history:
- When did the first sign of infection occur?
  - Within 4 days of surgery—operative factors, OT environment, instrument sterilization faults, break in asepsis during surgery more likely to be responsible.
  - After 4 days of surgery—both, patient factors and operative factors may be responsible.
- Investigate the risk factors one by one and note any gaps.

Third:
- Examine the findings from the above for any correlations that may explain how the infection occurred. The help of an expert in infection prevention should be taken for this analysis.

Fourth:
- Rectify the gaps and continue monitoring the infections.

TABLE 14: Risk factors for SSI.

Patient factors	*Operative factors*

• Age
• Nutritional status
• Diabetes
• Smoking
• Obesity
• Coexistent infections at a remote body site
• Colonization with microorganisms
• Altered immune response
• Length of preoperative stay
	• Duration of surgical scrub
	• Skin antisepsis
	• Preoperative shaving
	• Preoperative skin preparation
	• Duration of operation
	• Antimicrobial prophylaxis
	• Operating room ventilation
	• Inadequate sterilization of instruments
	• Foreign material in the surgical site
	• Surgical drains
	• *Surgical techniques:*
	  – Poor hemostasis
	  – Failure to obliterate dead space
	  – Tissue trauma

PYOGENIC OSTEOMYELITIS

Following are the routes, through which infection may occur:
- *Hematogenous*: Through blood stream from focus of infection elsewhere
- Direct invasion from atmospheric air, e.g. open fractures
- Spread from neighboring focus of infection, e.g. mastoiditis from middle ear infection and osteomyelitis of mandible from dental root infection
- Osteomyelitis associated with vascular insufficiency, mostly involving lower extremity, as in diabetic neuropathy.

Etiology

Patient-dependent Factor

- Nutritional status of the patient
- Immunological status.

Surgeon-dependent Factor

- Skin preparation
- Operating room environment
- Prophylactic antibiotic therapy.

Skillful Surgery

- Proper dissection
- Proper homeostasis
- Proper tissue handling
- Avoid prolonged surgery.

Clinical Features

- Antecedent infection is usually present
- Irritability, restlessness, headache, vomiting, convulsion, chills, fever, etc.
- Pain and swelling
- Local increase of temperature
- Overlying skin becomes shiny, red and edematous
- Discharging sinus may be present
- Sympathetic synovitis of adjacent joint.

Investigations

- *Laboratory studies:* Complete blood count, including differential blood count and erythrocyte sedimentation rate or C-reactive protein
- Synovial fluid analysis
- Plain X-rays
- CT scan
- MRI
- Bone scan
- Leukocyte scanning technique
- Blood culture study
- Pus culture sensitivity
- Ultrasonography
- Polymerase chain reaction.

Treatment

- Appropriate antibiotic
- Surgical debridement, incision and drainage
- Polymethyl methacrylate (PMMA) beads
- Closed suction irrigation
- Splinting and rest to the affected area.

Clinical Types

- Acute hematogenous osteomyelitis (early acute, late acute)
- Subacute osteomyelitis
- Chronic osteomyelitis.

ACUTE HEMATOGENOUS OSTEOMYELITIS

It is defined as a suppurative process of the bone, caused by pyogenic organisms or simply a pyogenic infection of the cancellous portion of bone.

Etiology

Agent Factors

Following myriad of incriminating organisms are responsible for its causation:

- "S" series organisms are *S. aureus* (60–85%) and it is most commonly found. *S. haemolyticus* (8–10%), *Salmonella*, etc.
- "P" series organism: *Pseudomonas, Pneumococcus*, etc.
- "C" series: *Clostridium welchii, Coliforms (E. coli)*, etc.

Host Factors

- *Age:* In children the incidence is 88% and in adults 12%;
- Low socioeconomic groups are more susceptible;
- General factors.

Other Factors

- Anemia
- Debility
- Infection
- Poor nutrition
- Poor immune status
- Trauma.

Local Factors

- Hair pin bend vessels
- Metaphyseal hemorrhage
- Defective phagocytosis
- Rapid growth at metaphysis
- Necrotic tissue act as culture media
- Anoxia
- Vasospasm.

Pathophysiology

- Osteomyelitis is initiated from introduction of bacteria from wound or hematogenous spread from pre-existing focus.
- Infective embolus enters the nutrient artery and trapped in vessel of small caliber and blocks it.
- Small areas of bones become necrotic.
- Active hyperemia develops and polymorphonuclear leukocytes are poured out as exudates, to combat the invader.
- Hyperemia causes decalcification of surrounding bone.
- Proteolytic ferments formed by leukocytes, destroys bacteria, necrotic bone, and medullary elements. Spread of pus takes place along the medullary canal (Fig. 70).
- Along the Haversian and Volkmann's canal superiolaterally, to form subperiosteal abscess, pus penetrates the periosteum and in the soft tissues.
- In the joint, if capsular attachment is up to metaphyseal region, growth plate is resistant to spread of pus, e.g. hip.

Clinical Features

Symptoms

- Fever (95%)
- Sweating
- Chills and rigors
- Local swelling
- Limitation of movement, due to muscle spasm and pain
- Patient may be in shock.

Signs

- Increased temperature
- Increased pulse rate
- Signs of dehydration
- Tenderness
- Local erythema
- Raised temperature
- Joint effusion
- Decreased movement.

Laboratory Investigations

- Hemoglobin is normal or increased;
- ESR, can be normal or increased;
- WBC, neutrophil increased;
- Films are negative within the first week or 10 days;
- Localized area of bone destruction is observed in metaphysic, surrounded by a wide zone of decalcified bone.
- Later, within next few weeks the periosteal shadow is elevated and multiple lamination of bone deposition is present parallel to shaft.
- Eventually more spongy trabeculae are destroyed giving a moth-eaten appearance, extending for varying degree in the diaphysis in 10–20 days (Fig. 71).

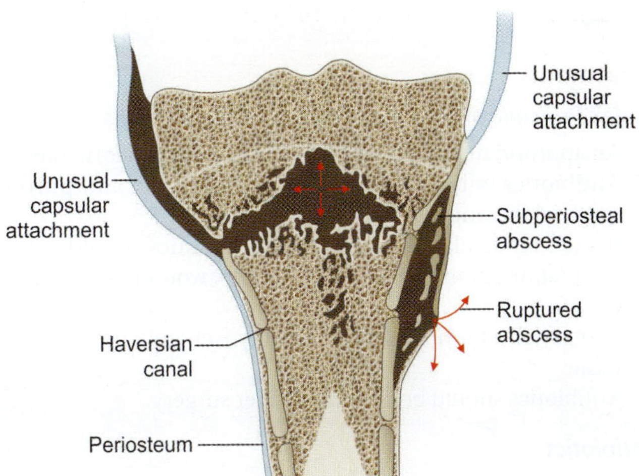

Fig. 70: Spread of pus through various channels.

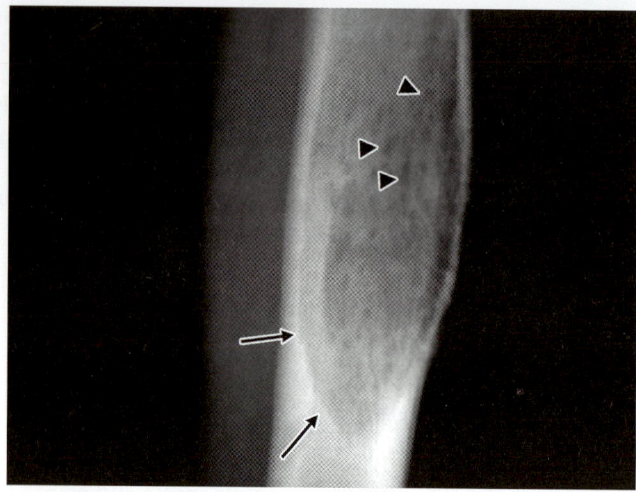

Fig. 71: Trabeculae showing moth-eaten appearance (arrowheads) in X-ray film.

- The external and internal surface of cortex may display multiple scalloped lesion.

Bone Scan

- Confirms diagnosis in 24–48 hours, after the onset in 90–95% of cases
- Focal area of uptake.

Blood Culture

- It is positive in 60% of cases
- Pus culture demonstrates the bacteria.

Ultrasound

- Soft tissue swelling or subperiosteal abscess
- *Leukergy test:* Leukergy is phenomenon, in which WBC agglomerates in the peripheral vessel. This is a sensitive test.

Management

- Easy to remember as "RESTS"
- Rest in bed, protect the affected part with splint, to alleviate pain and spasm
- Elevation of part, warm and moist packs, to reduce swelling
- *Systemic treatment:* Blood transfusion and intravenous fluid, to correct shock and hypovolemia
- Treatment with antibiotics
- Surgery.

Treatment

Nade's Principle of Treatment of Acute Osteomyelitis

- An appropriate antibiotic is effective before pus formation
- Antibiotics will not sterilize avascular tissue and purulent material that must be removed surgically
- If such removal is effective, then antibiotics should prevent their reformation and therefore primary wound closure should be safe
- Surgery should not damage already ischemic bone and soft tissue
- Antibiotics should be continued after surgery.

Antibiotics

- Penicillins
- Lactamase inhibitor
- Cephalosporins
- Ciprofloxacin
- Parental antibiotic for 2 weeks
- Oral antibiotic for 4 weeks
- *Local antibiotics:* Antibiotics impregnated with cemented beads, provide high dose of antibiotics locally.

Surgical Treatment

- *Aspiration:* It helps in decompression and the material so obtained may be used to identify the organism and also check for antibiotic sensitivity
- *Incision and drainage:* To drain the subcutaneous abscess
- Multiple drill holes
- Small bone window.

SUBACUTE OSTEOMYELITIS

Features

- Primary infection of bone
- More insidious onset
- Slow in progress
- Less severe symptoms
- Less virulent organism
- Difficult to diagnose.

Types

- Brodie's abscess
- Salmonella osteomyelitis (Typhoid osteomyelitis)
- Garre's sclerosing osteomyelitis.

Brodie's Abscess

- In medulla of bone
- Low grade infection, by *Staphylococcus*
- Common metaphyseal area, proximal end
- End of tibia or distal end femur.

Clinical features

- Intermittent attacks of pain and swelling
- Local tenderness.

Radiological findings

X-ray shows osteolytic area in the bone with a ring of diffuse sclerosis.

Treatment

Deroofing and curettage.

Salmonella Osteomyelitis

- Ulna, rib and vertebra are commonly affected
- Occurs after some months or years of typhoid or paratyphoid fever attack
- *Infection:* Hematogenous spread from persistent focus of infection in gallbladder
- Also occurs as a complication of sickle cell anemia.

Causative factors

- Local bony tenderness
- Moderate signs of inflammation
- Typhoid spine often mimics caries spine.

Investigations

- *X-ray:* Central or cortical area of rarefication with periosteal reaction

- *Blood:* Widal test
- *Treatment:* Surgery always required along with curettage and local application of chloramphenicol/ciplox.

Garre's Sclerosing Osteomyelitis

- Abscesses and sequestra absent
- Affects children and young adults
- Cause unknown, possibly anaerobic bacteria.

Clinical features

- Intermittent pain of moderate intensity
- Swelling and tenderness over affected bone.

Investigations

- X-ray shows expanded bone with generalized sclerosis (Fig. 72)
- ESR is increased
- *Treatment:* Fenestration of sclerotic bone and antibiotic.

Classification Modified from Roberts

- *Type 1:* Central metaphyseal lesion
- *Type 2*: Eccentric metaphyseal lesion with cortical erosion
- *Type 3:* Diaphyseal cortical lesion
- *Type 4*: Diaphyseal lesion with periosteal new bone
- *Type 5*: Primary subacute epiphyseal osteomyelitis
- *Type 6:* Subacute osteomyelitis, crossing physis, to involve both metaphysis and diaphysis.

CHRONIC OSTEOMYELITIS

Any osteomyelitis lasting for more than 3 weeks is termed as chronic osteomyelitis.

Etiology

Chronic osteomyelitis, can arise from any one of the following:

- Sequel of acute osteomyelitis (5–10%)
- Following compound fractures
- Following surgery in bone and joints
- Chronic from the beginning, (e.g. tuberculosis, syphilis, Brodie's abscess, etc.)
- Anaerobic organisms (Garre's sclerosing osteomyelitis)
- Fungal osteomyelitis.

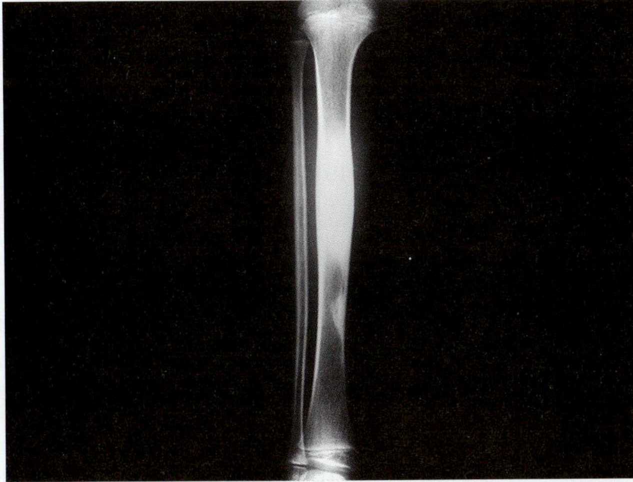

Fig. 72: Thickened and distended bone.

Cierny-Mader Classification

It is based on anatomic and physiologic criteria.

Anatomic Criteria

- Intramedullary (Fig. 73)
- Superficial (Fig. 74)
- Local (Fig. 75)
- Diffuse with segmental bone loss (Fig. 76).

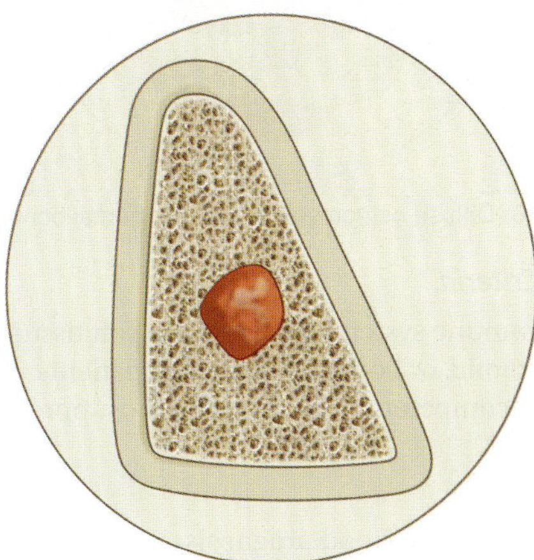

Fig. 73: Intramedullary osteomyelitis.

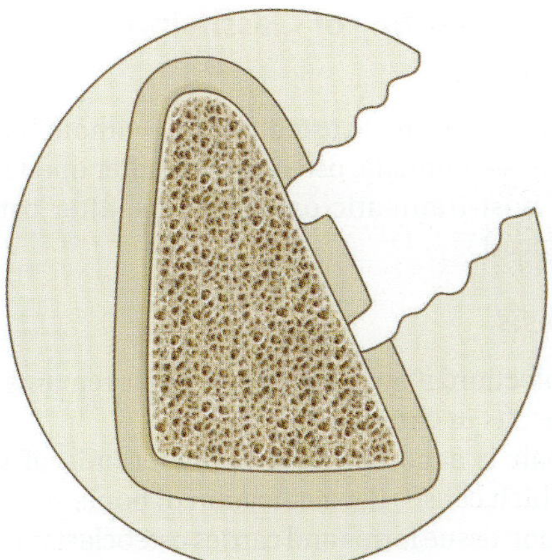

Fig. 74: Superficial osteomyelitis.

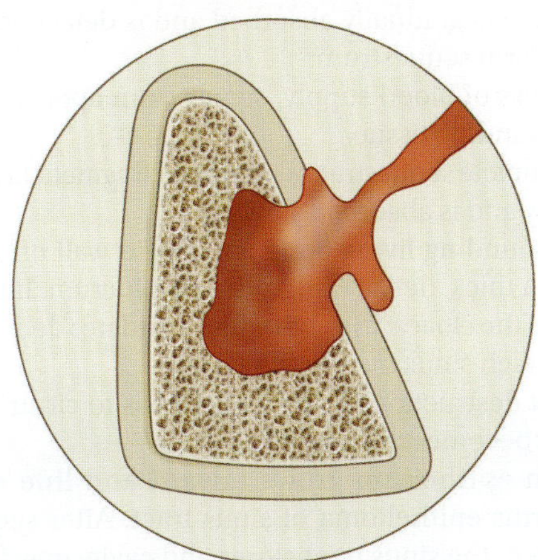

Fig. 75: Local osteomyelitis.

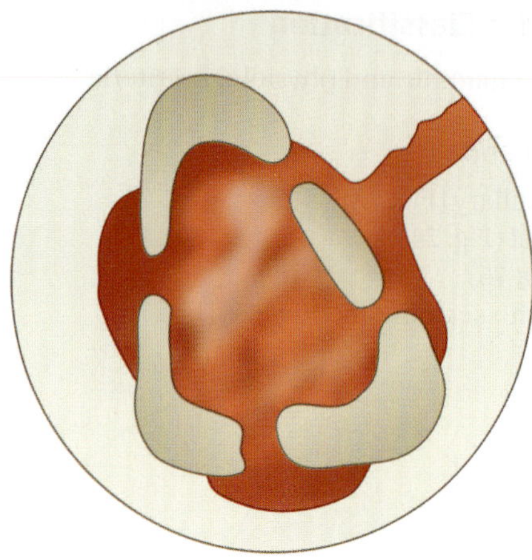

Fig. 76: Diffuse osteomyelitis with segmental bone loss.

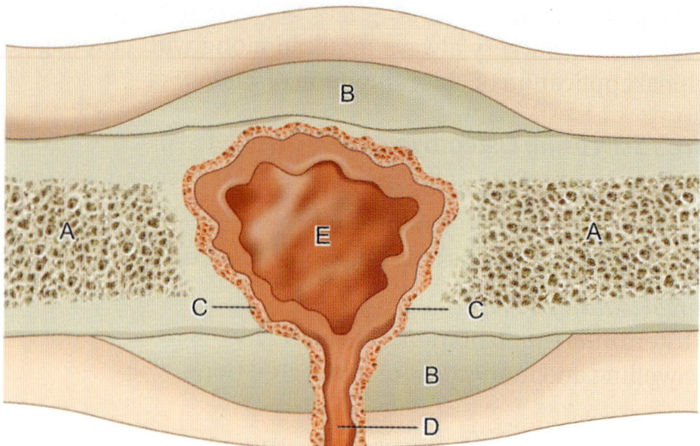

Fig. 77: Formation of sequestrum—A: Sound bone; B: New bone; C: Granulations, lining involucrum; D: Cloaca; E: Sequestrum.

Physiologic Criteria

- Normal immune system and adequate soft tissue envelop
- Local, systemic, or both compromised patients
- Immunoincompetent (requires immunosuppressive therapy).

Prognosis

- *Type I, II, III and A:* Good prognosis
- *Type I, II, III and B:* Guarded
- *Type I, II, III, IV and C:* Poor prognosis.

The Conventional Way of Classifying these Lesions

- Chronic post-traumatic osteomyelitis, without bone injury
- Chronic post-traumatic osteomyelitis, after open fracture
- Chronic post-traumatic osteomyelitis, after osteosynthesis (postsurgical).

Pathogenesis

- In any infection, if any attempt to repair remains incomplete, then it results in chronicity.
- This repair is accomplished by hyperemia of surrounding tissue, which causes decalcification of bone.
- Granulation tissue forms and carries osteoclasts and osteoblasts activity.
- Necrotic cancellous tissue is readily absorbed and new bone is formed.
- Dead bone is gradually absorbed and is detached from living bone to form sequestrum.
- Due to loss of blood supply, sequestrum appears dense than the surrounding tissue.
- After complete sequestration, the dead fragment lies free within the cavity and is absorbed slowly.
- The surrounding living bone attempt to wall off infection by forming a thick, dense wall, called involucrum. It has multiple openings the cloaca, through which exudates debris, sequestra pass through sinus tract to the surface.
- Constant destruction of soft tissue leads to cicatrix formation and skin becomes thin and distorted.
- The skin epithelium grows inward and line sinus tract. Later forms epithelioma of sinus tract. After sequestrum is discharged, the sinus tract closes and cavity may fill with new bone.

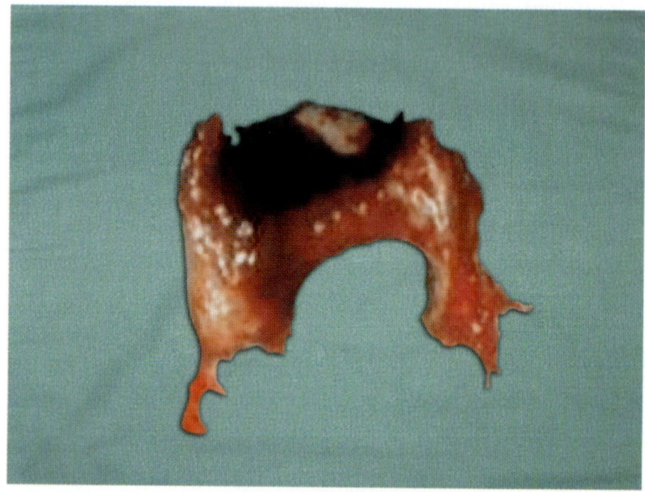

Fig. 78: Isolated sequestrum.

- In adults the cavity may persist and harbors organism and may not correlate with cultures of bone biopsy.

What is Sequestrum?

- It is a piece of dead bone, separated from healthy bone. It has no periosteal covering and outer surface is smooth and shiny. Inner surface is rough and edges are serrated because of osteoclastic absorption.
- Radiologically, sequestrum appears as a dense irregular piece of bone, surrounded by radiolucent area.

Formation of sequestrum

Formation of sequestrum is shown in Figure 77.

Types of Sequestrum

- Feathery sequestrum, e.g. pyogenic infection (Fig. 78)
- Coarse sandy sequestrum, e.g. tuberculosis
- Dense ivory, e.g. syphilis
- Colored sequestrum (black), e.g. ulna and tibia OM
- Ring sequestrum, e.g. amputation stump
- Bombay sequestrum, e.g. phalanx and traumatic amputation
- Coralliform sequestrum, e.g. pyogenic infection
- Button hole, e.g. pin tract infection.

Clinical Features

- *Symptoms*: Fever, pain, and swelling are seen in acute exacerbation of chronic osteomyelitis.

- *Signs*: Irregular thickening develops due to unequal pace of destruction and new bone formation.
- Multiple sinuses develop and their presence indicates unabsorbed sequestra, with presence of secondary infection.
- Scars and muscle contracture develops.
- Shortening or lengthening of bone develops.
- Deformities and decreased movements.
- Pathological fractures.

Investigations

X-ray Findings

- Early stage-moth-eaten appearance
- Elevation of periosteum and subperiosteal new bone formation
- Sharply delineated areas of dense bone with surrounding decalcification
- Gradually necrotic dense bone area is surrounded by white ring of involucrum.

Treatment

- Sequestrectomy and saucerization
- Open bone grafting (papineau technique) is done in three stages:
    1. *Stage I:* Excision of infected tissue, sinus tract, and sequestrum is done. After 4–5 days, daily dressing is done and next stage is delayed until signs of infection are absent and healthy granulation tissue is present.
    2. *Stage II:* Autogenous cancellous bone grafting is done.
    3. *Stage III:* Some cases show spontaneous epithelization, otherwise skin grafting, myocutaneous flap and muscle pedicle flap can be done by either of the following methods:
        - Gentamycin PMMA beads/antibiotic impregnated rod
        - Closed suction drain
        - Soft tissue transfer.

Management of Sequelae of Chronic Osteomyelitis

This is done by Ilizarov technique. Various sequelae of chronic osteomyelitis can be grouped as follows:

- *Group A:* Acute onset, but ends up as chronic osteomyelitis, with persistent infection.
- *Group B:* Post-traumatic chronic osteomyelitis, associated with fractures either united or with nonunion.
- *Group C:* Postoperative iatrogenic osteomyelitis.

Main line of treatment for chronic OM sequelae are:

- Removal of hardware and as per groups A and B
- Hyperbaric oxygen therapy
- Amputation and prosthesis.

Complications

- Growth disturbances
- Pathological fractures
- Muscle contractures
- Secondary septicemia
- Epithelioma
- Joint stiffness
- Amyloidosis.

DISEASES OF JOINTS (ARTHRITIS)

Definition

It is an inflammation of joints. It is characterized by pain, swelling, and limitation of movement and arthralgia is a term used for pain in joints, without inflammation.

Classification

Infectious Arthritis

Acute infection: These include following arthritis:

- Acute pyogenic arthritis
- Acute gonococcal arthritis
- Acute rheumatic arthritis
- Smallpox arthritis.

Chronic infection:

- *Nonspecific:* Pyogenic arthritis
- *Specific:* Tuberculous arthritis, syphilitic arthritis, gonococcal arthritis, etc.
- *Parasitic:* Guinea worm arthritis
- *Rheumatoid arthritis:* Rheumatoid arthritis, juvenile rheumatoid arthritis, etc.
- *Seronegative spondyloarthropathy:* Ankylosing spondylolitis, Reiter's disease, psoriatic arthritis, enteropathic arthritis, etc.

Degenerative Arthritis

- Primary osteoarthritis
- Secondary osteoarthritis.

Neuropathic Arthopathy

- Charcot arthopathy
- Syringomyelia
- Leprosy
- Diabetes mellitus.

Metabolic Arthritis

- Gout
- Pseudogout
- Alkaptonuria.

Arthritis in Systemic Disorder

- Hemophilic arthritis
- Reactive arthritis.

Miscellaneous Condition

- Villonodular synovitis
- Synovial chondromatosis.

SEPTIC ARTHRITIS

Definition

It is defined as a bacterial infection of the joints, which causes an intense inflammatory reaction with migration of polymorphonuclear leukocytes and subsequent release of proteolytic enzymes, causing destruction of articular cartilage and later the joint.

Causative Organisms

Most common organisms are:

- *Staphylococcus aureus* (50%)
- *Streptococcus* (20%)

- *Pneumococcus* (10%)
- *Gonococcus*
- *E. coli*
- *H. influenzae* is common in children less than 2 years of age.

Predisposing Factors

- Trauma
- Diabetes
- Steroid therapy
- Malignancy
- HIV.

Routes of Entry

This includes five P's:

1. Primary focus is in respiratory system, GIT, urinary system, etc.
2. Pyogenic osteomyelitis
3. Punctured wound
4. Pneumonia, typhoid, etc.
5. Primary focus in joint.

Sites of Involvement of the Joints

In adults:

- Knee (53%)
- Hip (20%)
- Elbow (17%)
- Shoulder (10%).

In children:

- Knee (32%)
- Hip (39%).

Pathogenesis

- The presence of bacteria in the joint, incites an intense local reaction.
- The synovial membrane becomes hyperemic, edematous and proliferates, producing purulent fluid containing markedly increased leukocytes.
- As a result, the synovial sac is greatly distended by large amount of fluid.
- The condition is designated as serous arthritis or when precipitation of fibrin is excessive, it is called serofibrinous arthritis.
- Areas of vascular thrombosis and focal necrosis occur.
- Proteolytic enzymes originating from polymorphonuclear leukocytes, dissolve the articular cartilage and may even erode the bone.
- The intense intra-articular pressure, causes necrosis, and destruction of intra-articular soft tissue and capsule.
- The exudates erupt into the surrounding soft tissue and into the skin, forming multiple sinuses.
- This is typical of purulent arthritis characteristic of *Staphylococcus* infection.
- Hemolytic infection is fulminating and quickly destructive.
- The synovial inflammatory signs are intense; vascular thrombosis and necrosis are extreme.
- The exudation in the joint is bloody serous typical of serosanguinous arthritis, the danger of septicemia is greatest.
- In mild cases, healing takes place by resolution.
- In severe cases, healing takes place by resorption of purulent exudates and repair by granulation tissue, which bridges the joint forming fibrous ankylosis.
- The capsule becomes fibrotic, thickened and inelastic. Loss of articular cartilage, exposes the bone to mechanical trauma, resulting in degenerative arthritis.

Clinical Features

Septic arthritis is usually present as monoarticular feature in (90%) and polyarticular in (10%) of cases.

Symptoms

- Constitutional symptoms are chills, fever, sweats, malaise, anorexia, and in infants nausea, vomiting, etc.
- Pain gradually increases in intensity over several hours and becomes excruciating.
- Pain accentuates on movement of joints and thus limits the movement.
- Swelling
- The patient holds the limb in position of maximum capacity to reduce the intraarticular pressure and thus minimizes pain.
- *The position of maximum intra-articular volume are:*
  - *Hip:* 60° flexion, 15° abduction, and 15° of external rotation
  - *Knee:* 30–60° flexion
  - *Ankle:* 15° plantar flexion
  - *Shoulder:* 30–60° abduction
  - *Elbow:* 30–60° flexion
  - *Wrist:* Neutral.

Signs

- The joint is swollen, red, warm, and tender throughout
- Patient holds the limb in position of maximum relief
- Local temperature is increased
- Muscle spasm is seen
- Reduced range of motion
- In case of knee, due to distention of joint, patellar tap is positive due to floating patella.

Laboratory Investigations

- WBC's (polymorphs) are raised to 50,000–100,000 (80%)
- ESR is raised more than 20 mm/hour (50%)
- Hemoglobin is decreased
- Blood culture is positive in 35–50% of cases
- CRP is positive, it should be done 24 hours before presentation. Note, if CRP is less than 10 mg/dL, the probability that the patient does not have septic arthritis is 87%
- *Joint fluid aspirate and synovial fluid aspirate:* It is critical for diagnosing and treatment of septic arthritis. Diagnosis of septic arthritis, is based on the results of analysis of synovial fluid is shown in Table 15.

Radiological Findings

- Films are generally negative in beginning
- Ballooning of synovial sac may be seen from rounded soft tissue swelling
- If infection persists, osteoporosis of adjacent bone is seen
- Destruction of cartilage and narrowing of joint space
- Degenerative arthritis supervenes
- In late cases, fibrous ankylosis and bony ankylosis is seen.

TABLE 15: Diagnosis of septic arthritis, based on the results of synovial fluid analysis.

Analysis	*Nonseptic arthritis*	*Septic arthritis*
Gross appearance		
Color	Straw or clear yellow	Serosanguinous or purulent
Volume	0.13–0.5 mL	Increased
Clarity	Clear	Turbid
Viscosity and mucin		
Clot viscosity	High	Very low
Mucin clot	Good	Poor
Microscopic examination		
Leukocytes	<300	>50,000
Neutrophils	<25%	>80%
Bacteria	Negative	Positive
Biochemistry		
Serum/synovial fluid glucose ratio	0.8–1.0	Low
Protein	2 g/dL	<8 g/dL
Culture	Negative	Positive

Treatment

- *Arthotomy or joint drainage:* The joint is aspirated first, if pus is present
- Arthroscopic drainage
- Antibiotics are given in adequate amount. Cephalosporins or penicillin, which combat gram-positive organisms and aminoglycosides, which combat gram-negative organism are started in combination.
- Broad spectrum antibiotics, like chlortetracycline and oxytetracycline can be given. Appropriate antibiotics can be started after culture sensitivity
- *Immobilization:* It is done by plaster of Paris. Splint in functional position reduces pain.

TUBERCULOSIS OF MUSCULOSKELETAL SYSTEM

Introduction

- Though ubiquitous in distribution, tuberculosis (TB) has firmly entrenched itself with the third world. The main causes are illiteracy, poverty, poor hygienic condition, and other favorable factors.
- Tuberculosis bacilli have lived in symbiosis with mankind, since time immemorial.
- In India *Rigveda*, *Atharvaveda*, *Charaka Samhita* and *Sushruta*, have mentioned the disease by the name *Yakshma* in all its form.
- TB is the oldest disease affecting mankind. It has been found in Egyptian mummies, dating back to 3400 BC.
- Hippocrates (460-370 BC) was the first to suggest relationship between pulmonary and spinal deformity.
- Percival Pott (1714–1788), described the Gibbus deformity and its sequelae.
- Laennec (1781-1826) described the basic microscopic lesion the tubercle.
- Drugs streptomycin was first introduced in 1947, para-aminosalicylic acid (PAS) in 1949 and isoniazid (INH) in 1952:
  - India is infamous for hosting nearly one-fifth of the 30 million people, suffering from tuberculosis throughout the world.
  - There are 6 million radiologically proven cases of tuberculosis in India and perhaps a quarter of these are sputum positive.
  - Skeletal tuberculosis is always secondary, the primary foci being the lungs, lymph nodes, and gastrointestinal tract.
  - Of all the patients, suffering from tuberculosis, nearly 1–3% show, skeletal system involvement.
  - Vertebral tuberculosis is the most common form and it constitutes 50% of skeletal tuberculosis.
  - The major areas of predilection are spine, hip, knee, foot, elbow, hand, shoulder, and others.

Causative Organisms

- *Mycobacterium* tubercle is the main causative organism. In 1882, Robert Koch discovered the tubercle bacillus. Most of the skeletal TB is caused by typical *Mycobacterium. Mycobacterium* tubercle bacilli, varies in size about 3 × 0.3 m.
- They are acid fast bacilli, aerobic and grow at temperatures varying from 30–40°C and can be grown on Löwenstein-Jensen medium.
- They are killed by heat at 60°C in 15–20 minutes and survive for many weeks in moist conditions.

Predisposing Factors

- Malnutrition
- Poor sanitation
- Living in crowded area
- Close contact with TB patient
- Repeated pregnancies
- Exanthematous fever
- Immunodeficiency status.

Pathology and Pathogenesis

- A minimum period of 2-3 years is required between the primary and secondary TB.
- Primary focus may be active or quiescent (lungs, tonsils, mediastinum, mesentery, etc.).
- *Bacillemia:* Through the arteries and veins (e.g. Batson plexuses in spine) reach the skeletal system, tubercle develops.

What is Tubercle?

The tubercle is a microscopic pathological lesion with a central necrosis, surrounded by epitheloid cells, Langerhans giant cells, and round cells.

The future course of tubercle varies.

- *It may resolve completely:* The disease may heal completely with varying degrees of residual deformities and/or loss of function. The lesion may be completely walled off and the caseous tissue may be calcified. A low grade chronic fibromatous granulating and caseating lesion, may persist with a grumbling activity.
- The infection may spread locally by contiguity and systemically by blood stream, as seen in immunocompromised patients.

Clinical Features

- The disease may be insidious in onset
- Monoarticular and monoosseous involvement
- Other visceral lesions
- *Constitutional symptoms:* Low grade fever, especially in evening, anorexia, weight loss, night sweats, night cries, tachycardia, and anemia
- *Local symptoms and signs:* Swelling, synovial involvement, pain, tenderness, muscle spasm, night cries, stiffness, and later, actual limitation of movements, due to fibrous ankylosis, limp, and muscle atrophy.

Types

Granular: Mild, nondestructive, and fibrosing

Caseous and exudative: Destructive abscess forming.

Laboratory Findings

- HMG with ESR is raised
- Total leukocyte count (TLC) and differential leukocyte count (DLC)
- Culture sensitivity
- Ziehl-Neelsen (ZN) staining
- Sputum for acid-fast bacillus (AFB)
- Guinea-pig inoculation
- Mantoux test
- X-rays
- Biopsy of draining lymph nodes
- CT scan
- MRI.

Treatment

General Treatment

This includes rich protein diet, rest, immobilization and braces, hematinics, adequate exposure to sunshine, etc. The aim is to improve the immunity.

Chemotherapy

Drugs used for the treatment of tuberculosis are grouped as follows:

First line of drugs:

P: Pyrazinamide
R: Rifampicin
I: Isonicotinylhydrazide (INH)
S: Streptomycin
E: Ethambutol.

Second line of drugs:

C: Capreomycin/ciprofloxacin/ofloxacin
A: Amikacin
K: Kanamycin
E: Ethionamide
C: Cycloserine
A: Para-aminosalicylic acid (PAS).

Drugs useful for chemotherapy in skeletal system are shown in Table 16.

TABLE 16: Chemotherapeutic drugs in skeletal system.

S. no.	*Drugs*	*Daily adult dose*	*Drug toxicity*
1.	Streptomycin (injection)	20–35 mg/kg	Vestibular damage, deafness, fever, rashes, contact dermatitis, nephrotoxicity
2.	INH	300–400 mg (5 mg/kg of body weight in adult, 10–20 mg/kg of body weight in children)	Peripheral neuropathy, behavior disorders, convulsions, hepatitis, hypersensitivity
3.	Ethambutol	15–25 mg/kg in single or divided doses (not used in children <5 years.)	Retrobulbar neuritis with loss of vision and color blindness
4.	Para-aminosalicylic acid	12 g in single or divided doses	Gastrointestinal disturbances, rashes, fever, lymphadenopathy, hepatotoxicity
5.	Thiacetazone	150 g in single dose	Anorexia, nausea, vomiting, liver damage, marrow depression
6.	Ethionamide	250 mg/BD, 15–20 mg/kg	GIT upsets, abnormal liver test, peripheral neuritis, convulsion
7.	Pyrazinamide	40 mg/kg in single or two divided doses	Hepatotoxicity
8.	Cycloserine	15–20 mg/kg	CNS toxicity
9.	Capreomycin	15–30 mg/kg single dose	Nephrotoxicity
10.	Kanamycin	15 mg/kg single dose	Ototoxicity
11.	Amikacin	15 mg/kg/day	Ototoxicity, nephrotoxicity

GIT: gastrointestinal tract; CNS: central nervous system

Chemotherapy Regime

- *Nine months regime:* Nine months of rifampicin and INH are effective in all forms of disease.
- *Six months regime:* First 2 months INH, rifampicin, and pyrazinamide.
- Next four months INH and rifampicin. When primary resistance to INH is high, therapy is usually initiated with four first line drugs.
- *Eighteen months regime:* Four-drug therapy is done by rifampicin, INH, pyrazinamide, and ethambutol for 3 months. Ethambutol is withdrawn and three drugs are continued for 9 months. Later, rifampicin and INH is continued for 6 months.
- *Tuli's sixteen months regime:* Rifampicin, INH, and ethambutol for first 4 months.
- Pyrazinamide replaces rifampicin in second 4 months.
- In next 4 months, rifampicin is given with INH.
- In last 4 months, INH is only drug given.

Local Treatment

Aim is to prevent, correct, or decrease the deformities. If the disease is osseous, aim at ankylosis in functional position by immobilization. If the disease is synovial, aim at mobility with traction.

Operative Treatment

- Synovectomy
- Curettage
- Osteotomies
- Arthrodesis
- Drainage of abscess.

Recent Advancements in Management of Skeletal TB

- Lab investigations
- Imaging modalities
- Treatment.

Laboratory Investigations

Routine

- *Complete blood count:*
  - Hemoglobin decreased
  - *TLC:* Increased
  - *DLC:* Increased lymphocytes
  - *Lymphocyte:* Monocyte ratio normally is 5:1. If less than 5:1, bad prognosis
  - Blood culture
  - Pus culture
  - *Sputum:* AFB
  - Tissue biopsy
  - FNAC
  - RFT
  - LFT
  - Blood sugar
  - *Skin test:* Mantoux test
  - HIV
  - HBsAg.

Recent

- Twenty-four hours urine for AFB, TB-PCR;
- *Blood TB-PCR:* Here amplification of the nucleic acid is done enzymatically, by polymerase chain reaction and identified, by using nucleic acid probes. It is very beneficial.
- *TB-ELISA:* IgG, IgM assessment by A60 Ag. It has 60–80% specificity.
- *ELISPOT (T-spot ELISA):* It measures the T-cell interferon (secreted by the T-lymphocytes of the affected person).
- *BACTEC:* It is a rapid culturing method. BACTEC radiometric cultural assay, can detect *Mycobacterium tuberculi,* as early as 7 days on the basis of release of radio labeled CO_2, from growth of *Mycobacterium* in a selective liquid medium containing C-14 labeled isotopes. It has 95% sensitivity.
- *HPLC (High performance liquid chromatography):* It measures the mycolic acid, which is present in the cell of *Mycobacterium tuberculosis.* It helps in differentiating various acid fast bacilli.
- *GLC (Gas liquid chromatography):* Mycobacteria are identified on the basis of secretion of cellular fatty acid, by gas liquid chromatography.
- *QTB (Quantiferin gold TB):* It measures the T-lymphocytes secreting-interferons, when the whole blood is attached by antigen. It can be measured by blood sample. Results come in 3–5 days and are not affected by previous BCG vaccination.
- *FTB (Fast plaque TB):* It can be done on anybody fluid, like aspirate, pus, sputum, blood. It gives results in 48–72 hours. It can also infer about the effectiveness of the drug.
- Nucleic acid probe (Radioactive labeled DNA probes).
- Molecular typing.

Imaging

Routine

- *X-ray chest:* PA view
- X-ray spine (cervical, D-L, L-S): AP and lateral views
- USG
- Myelography
- CT myelography
- MRI.

Recent

- *Abreugraphy:* It is also called as miniature chest radiography and is helpful in detection of TB and its differentiation from other respiratory diseases. It is cheaper, comparative to other techniques, and is used for mass screening.
- *Contrast MRI:* It gives accurate idea about intraosseous abscess, ligamentous involvement, and dural involvement. It helps in postoperative imaging add-in doing follow-ups of cases. It can be done in patients with titanium implants.
- *Bone scan:* Technetium-99m, ciprofloxacin scintigraphy is more sensitive. It can be done in patients with stainless steel implants.
- *PET scan:* It gives early diagnosis.
- *MP CT:* Multiplanar CT.
- *3D CT:* Reconstructive CT.

Treatment

- Conservative
- Surgical.

Conservative Treatment

- Anti-tubercular drugs
- High protein diet
- *Braces:* SOMI for cervical spine, Taylor's brace for dorsolumbar spine, etc.
- Early mobilization and rehabilitation
- Adequate exposure to sunlight and fresh air
- Improve hygiene.

Anti-tubercular drugs therapy

First line drugs:

- Isoniazid—5 mg/kg body wt
- Rifampicin—10 mg/kg
- Pyrazinamide—25 mg/kg
- Ethambutol—15 mg/kg
- Streptomycin—15 mg/kg.

Second line drugs:

- Para-aminosalicylic acid
- Thiacetazone
- Ethionamide
- Capreomycin
- Ethambutol
- Kanamycin

- Amikacin
- Ciprofloxacin.

Recent drugs:
- *Rifamycin:* Rifabutin, rifapentin
- Clofazimine
- Beta lactams: Augmentin
- *Macrolides:* Azithromycin, clarithromycin.

Future drugs:
- Immunomodulators
- Gamma interferons
- Interleukins—2 and 12
- Alfa TNF.

Recent Treatment Regimen According to Revised National Tuberculosis Control Program (RNTCP)

Category I (Table 17):
- New (untreated) smear positive pulmonary TB
- New smear negative pulmonary TB with extensive parenchymal involvement
- New cases of severe forms of extrapulmonary TB like meningitis, miliary, pericarditis, peritonitis, bilateral or extensive pleural effusion, spinal, intestinal, genitourinary TB.

Category II (Table 18):
- Smear positive failure cases
- Relapse cases
- Interrupted treatment cases.

Category III (Table 19):
New cases of smear negative pulmonary TB with limited parenchymal involvement or less severe forms of extrapulmonary TB, e.g. lymph node, unilateral pleural effusion, bone (excluding spine), peripheral joint or skin TB. This is shown in Table 19.

TABLE 17: Category I of recent treatment regimen, according to RNTCP.

Category	*Initial phase*	*Continuation phase*	*Total duration in months*
I	2HRZE	$4HR/4H_3R_3$ or 6HE	6 8

RNTCP: Revised National Tuberculosis Control Program

TABLE 18: Category II of recent treatment regimen, according to RNTCP.

Category	*Initial phase*	*Continuation phase*	*Total duration in months*
II	2HRZES + 1HRZE	5HRE or $5H_3R_3E_3$	8 8

RNTCP: Revised National Tuberculosis Control Program

TABLE 19: Category III of recent treatment regimen, according to RNTCP.

Category	*Initial phase*	*Continuation phase*	*Total duration in months*
III	2HRZ	$4HR/4H_3R_3$ or 6HE	6 8

RNTCP: Revised National Tuberculosis Control Program

Category IV:
- Multidrug resistant (MDR) TB cases
- Second-line of drugs is used.

Surgical Treatment

Indications in patients with no neurological deficit:
- No recovery after treatment
- First-line drug resistance or irregular treatment
- *To prevent deformity:*
  - *In adults:* If vertebral height loss (collapse) in dorsolumbar spine is greater than 0.75 and in lumbar spine greater than 1
  - *In children:* If kyphosis is greater than 30°
- Children with "spine at risk signs", explained in Table 20
- *Each sign is allocated one point, to create a spinal instability score:*
  - If score is greater than 2, need surgery and spinal fixation
  - If score is less than 2, no need of fixation, observe following:
    - If CT guided biopsy study is inconclusive
    - If cervical spine abscess is causing compression and difficulties in swallowing
    - If abscess is not healed
  - Indication for patients with neurological deficit:
    - Neurological deficit develops, while patient is under treatment
  - No recovery after 4 weeks of chemotherapy
  - Exaggeration of deficit, while under treatment
  - Recurrence after correction
  - Advanced stage of deficit (bladder involvement, etc.).

Surgical options
- Drainage of abscess
- Costotransversectomy
- Anterolateral decompression
- *Anterior decompression with interbody fixation:*
  - *By using cage with bone graft*: It can be expandable or nonexpendable
  - Using local graft.
- Posterior decompression
- Posterior decompression with fixation (instrumentation):
  - Use of transpedicular screws, e.g. stainless steel, titanium, etc.
  - *Use of Moss-Miami system:* Unidirectional or polydirectional screws
  - Titanium implants are generally used because postoperative MRI, can be done for evaluation, follow-up MRI can be done
  - *Global fixation:* Anterior spinal fusion, posterior spinal fusion, interbody fusion, intertransverse fusion, and instrumentation
  - Recently, endoscopic spine surgery.
- Surgery should be done under antitubercular treatment (ATT) cover.

TABLE 20: Spinal instability scores.

S. no.	*Radiological signs of instability*	*Score*
1.	Separation of facets	1
2.	Posterior retropulsion	1
3.	Lateral translation on AP view	1
4.	Toppling (sign) of superior vertebra	1

Prognosis (Table 21)

"Middle Path Regime", by Tuli.

- Bed rest on hard bed or plaster shell.
  Drug regime: Total duration is 16 months (H: Isoniazid, R: Rifampicin, E: Ethambutol, Z: Pyrazinamide, S: Streptomycin).
  - 4 months: HRE
  - 4 months: HZE
  - 4 months: HR
  - 4 months: H.
- Supportive treatment with vitamins, antioxidants
- X-ray at 3–6 months
- Drainage of abscess
- Decompression
- Fusion for unstable spine
- Postoperative care.

Note: Implants can be used in TB, under ATT cover as no biofilm is produced.

TABLE 21: Prognosis of tuberculosis.		
	Good	*Bad*
Age	Younger	Older
Onset	Early	Late
Duration	Shorter	Longer
Kyphosis	<60°	>60°
Stage	Active	Healed

TUBERCULOSIS OF SPINE

Introduction

- It is the most common type of skeletal TB, constituting of 50% of all cases.
- *Regional distribution of TB are:*
  - *Cervical:* 12%
  - *Cervicodorsal:* 5%
  - *Dorsal:* 42%
  - *Dorsolumbar:* 12%
  - *Lumbar:* 26%
  - *Lumbosacral:* 3%
  - Thus, lower thoracic and lower lumbar accounting for about 80% of all cases.
- *The reasons for this area of predilection are:*
  - Large amount of spongy tissues within the vertebral body
  - Degree of weight-bearing, which is comparatively more
  - More vertebral mobility is seen here.

Sites of Involvement within the Vertebra

Spinal TB can start in any part of vertebrae, but there are mainly four sites, as shown in Figure 79:

1. Paradiscal
2. Central
3. Anterior
4. Appendical (involving pedicles, laminae, spinous process or transverse process):
   - 95%: Anterior element
   - 5%: Posterior element.

Pathogenesis

- Primary foci in lung, lymph nodes or abdomen. Bacillemia develops and the organism reaches the spine through the Batson plexus.
- Tuberculosis endarteritis, which develops following the infection, results in marrow devitalizations. Later on, the tubercular follicle develops. Lamellae are destroyed due to hyperemia, causing osteoporosis. As a result, the vertebral body gets easily compressed.
- In thoracic vertebrae because of normal kyphotic curve, anterior wedging is common. In lordotic, cervical, and lumbar vertebra, wedging is minimal.
- Two types of vertebral reactions, commonly encountered in skeletal TB are shown in Table 22.

Abscess Formation

- It is the most common complication about 20%.
- At first, abscess collects under the anterior longitudinal ligament in front of the vertebral bodies and then it further disseminate along one or several courses.
- It may pass backward and invade the vertebral canal, a serious complication and causes pressure on the spinal cord.
- It may track forwards and become diverted by various anatomical structures, such as blood vessels, nerves, or muscles (Flowchart 1).

Clinical Features

- Constitutional symptoms include weakness, anorexia, weight loss, night sweats and evening rise of temperature, etc.
- Patient gives a history of backache

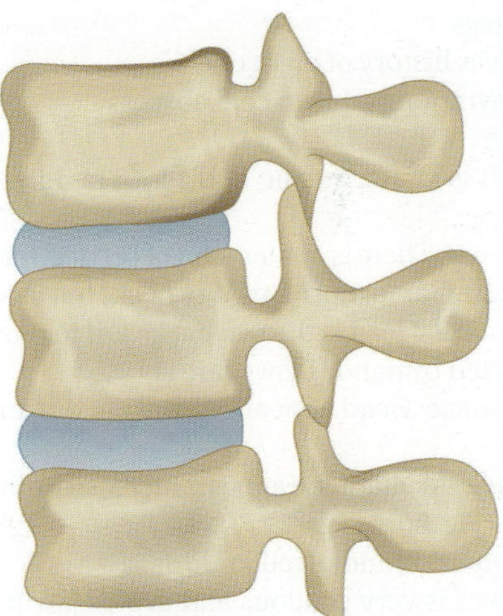

Fig. 79: Major sites of vertebral TB.

TABLE 22: Two types of vertebral reactions commonly encountered in skeletal tuberculosis.	
Exudative reaction	*Caseative reaction*
• Common	• Rarer
• Severe hyperic reaction severe osteoporosis	• Mechanism of formation and spread is similar to exudative type but is slower
• Rapid spread	
• Abscess is formed frequently	
• Constitutional symptoms are more pronounced	

Flowchart 1: Showing spreading of abscess, from different vertebral sections to different anatomical body parts.

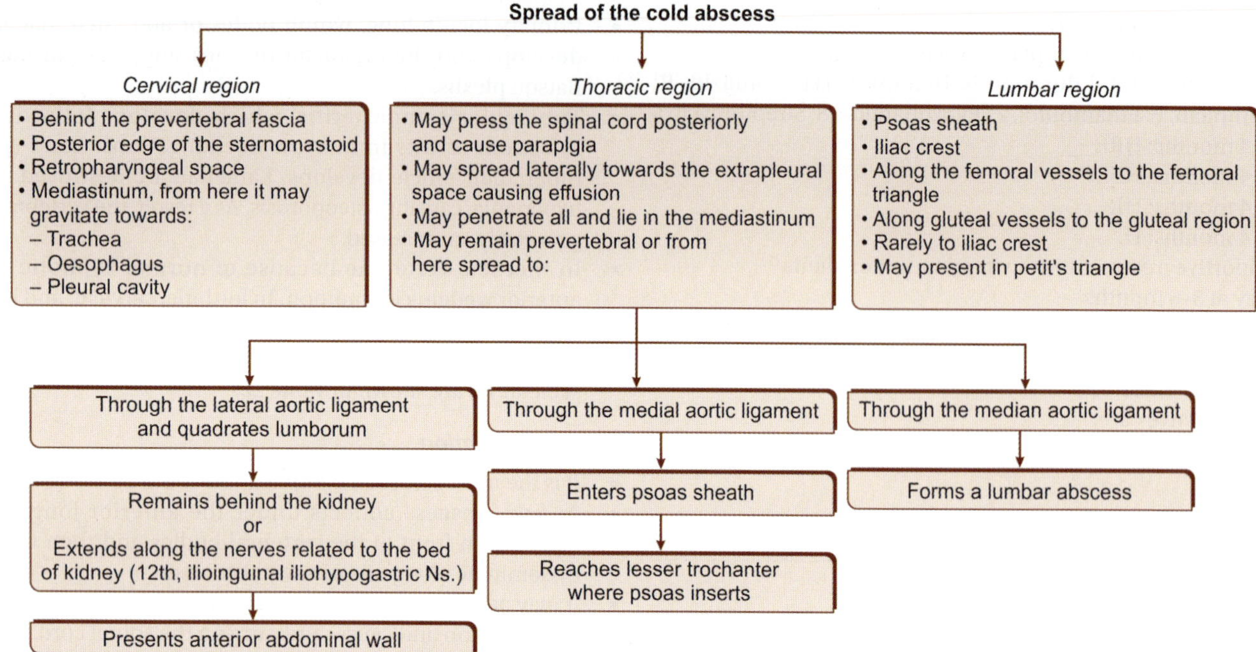

- Slight pain and stiffness are earliest complaints
- Pain is initially localized, dull aching, brought down by jarring, or movement of spine
- Later on, it is referred pain depending on the nerve root involvement, e.g. cervical lesion causing pain over occiput, ear, jaw, upper limb; upper thoracic, intercostals neuralgia, thoracolumbar girdle pain or epigastric pain and lumbar to hips and legs
- Patient gives history of night cries
- Pressure symptoms due to cold abscess
- Paraplegia
- *Attitude:* It is characteristic of disease in different regions of spine
- *Cervical spine:* There is obliteration of cervical lordosis, position of head is similar to that of in "Wry neck", but face is not rotated
- *Lower cervical:* Head is thrown backward to one side and may be supported by hand (Flowchart 1)
- *Upper thoracic:* Head appears shrunken, due to shortening of neck
- *Mid thoracic:* AP diameter appears increased, due to shortening of stature (Fig. 80)
- *Lower lumbar:* Pronounced lordosis
- *Gait:* Patient is very cautious and avoids jarring of spine and walks with legs apart and waddles, so called "Alderman's gait"
- Muscle spasm
- Angular type of kyphosis or gibbus is present
- Tenderness is present over the vertebrae
- Movement of spine are restricted
- Formation of cold abscesses and spread.

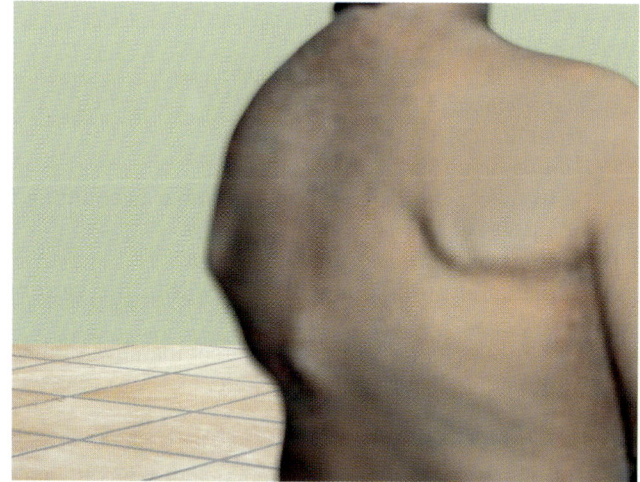

Fig. 80: Mid-thoracic AP diameter increases due to shortening of stature.

Radiological Findings

Earliest Changes (Fig. 81)

- Consists of disk space narrowing. Subsequent loss of disk space is common
- *Paradiscal lesion:* The bones look rarified and osteopenic.

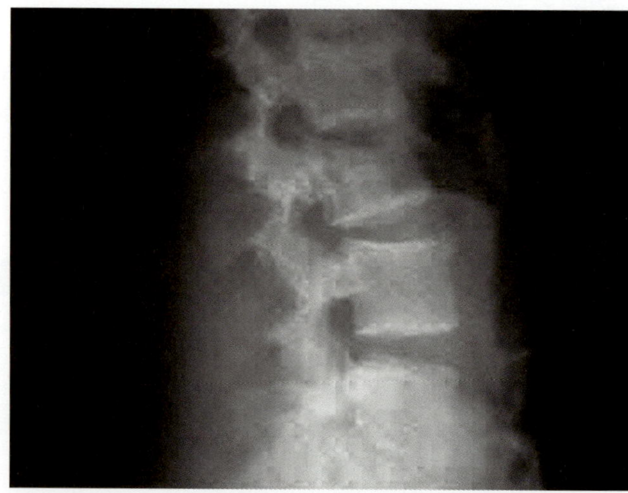

Fig. 81: X-ray showing earliest changes in the vertebrae.

Late Changes (Fig. 82)

- This includes anterior wedge compression in anterior vertebral involvement
- Central vertebral body collapse also called as "concertina collapse" in central involvement
- Destruction of the posterior elements in the posterior affection
- Soft tissue swelling and its calcification are highly predictable of tuberculosis
- In healing stage, the vertebral body and posterior elements may appear more dense due to sclerosis paravertebral shadow, which indicates cold abscesses
- *Cervical region:* Retropharangeal
- *Upper thoracic:* V-shaped shadow and widened mediastinum
- *Below fourth thoracic vertebra:* Fusiform or bird nest appearance
- Bilaterally widened psoas shadow, in lumbar region.

Investigations

- *Hemoglobin:* Reduced hemoglobin. High lymphocytes and low monocytes count, suggest good resistance
- If ratio is 5:1, it is favorable ratio. If it is less than 5:1, then it is poor prognosis
- ESR raised
- Mantoux test positive
- Sputum for AFB
- Biopsy and aspiration of abscesses
- CT scan
- MRI
- Bone scan
- Sonography
- Twenty-four hours urine for PCR and AFB.

Treatment

General treatment: Rest, well-balanced diet, and hygienic surroundings are essential with chemotherapy.

Antitubercular Drugs

- *INH:* 5–10 mg/kg up to 300 mg
- *Rifampicin:* 10 mg/kg up to 600 mg
- *Streptomycin:* 15–20 mg/kg up to 0.75 g
- *Pyrazinamide:* 20–35 mg/kg up to 2.09 g
- *Ethambutol:* 15 mg/kg
- *PAS:* 150–300 mg/kg up to 10 g.

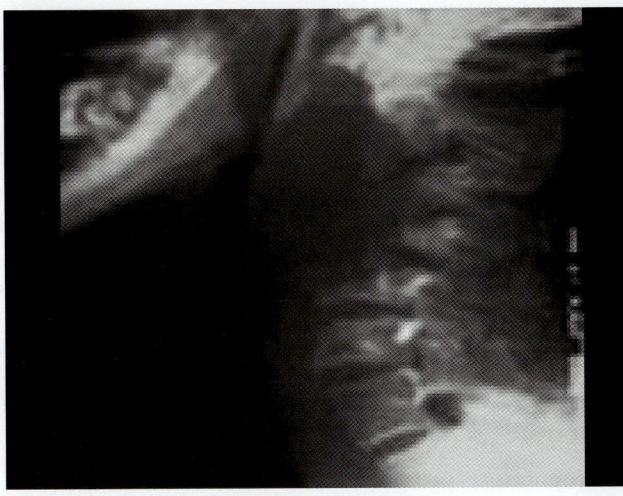

Fig. 82: Late changes.

Drug Recommendation for Tuberculosis of Bones and Joints

Intensive phase:
- SM/EMB
- INH
- Rifampicin daily for 2 months
- Pyrazinamide.

Continuation phase:
- INH
- RMP daily for 7 months.

Tuli's "middle path" regime:
- Rest in hard bed or plaster of Paris bed
- Antitubercular drugs for 16 months
- INH and rifampicin for first 4 months
- INH and pyrazinamide for second 4 months
- INH and rifampicin for next 4 months
- INH alone for last 4 months
- Support should be given, with multivitamins, hematinics, and high protein diet
- Radiographic and ESR are taken at 3–6 months interval
- Gradual mobilization
- Abscesses are aspirated, as they cause pressure effect and complications
- Sinus excision
- Decompression
- Operative debridement.

Complications

- Paraplegia
- Cold abscess
- Sinuses
- Secondary infection
- Amyloid disease.

Pott's Paraplegia

Incidence of this complication is 10% of all cases.

Causes of Paraplegia

- *Inflammatory:* Edema, TB granulation tissue, TB abscesses, TB caseous tissue, etc.
- *Mechanical:* Tubercular debris, sequestra from vertebral body, constriction of vertebral body due to stenosis of vertebral body and localized pressure due to internal gibbus.
- *Intrinsic:* Prolonged stretching of cord over a severe deformity, infective thrombosis, pathological dislocation, tuberculous meningomyelitis, spinal tumor syndrome, etc.

Classification

Depending on the Onset and Duration of Disease (Griffiths and Seddon):
- *Group A:* Early onset paraplegia.
- *Group B:* Late onset paraplegia.

Depending on Motor Power (Tuli and Kumar):

- *Grade 1:* Negligible, patient unaware of neural deficit, physician detects plantar extensor and/or ankle clonus.
- *Grade 2:* Mild, patient aware of deficit, but manages to walk with support. Clinical signs of spastic paresis.
- *Grade 3:* Moderate, nonambulatory because of paralysis (in extension). Sensory deficit less than 50%.
- *Grade 4:* Severe, flexor spasm, sensory deficit more than 50% and sphincter involved.

Treatment

Indications for surgery absolute

- Paraplegia with onset during usual conservative treatment
- Paraplegia getting worse or remaining stationary, despite sufficient conservative treatment
- Complete loss of motor power for 1 month despite sufficient conservative treatment
- Paraplegia accompanied by uncontrolled spasticity
- Severe paraplegia of rapid onset
- Any severe paraplegia.

Relative

- Recurrent paraplegia
- Paraplegia with onset in old age
- Painful paraplegia
- Complication such as UTI and renal stones.

Rare indication

- Posterior spinal disease
- Spinal tumor syndrome
- Severe cauda equina paralysis.

Surgery

- Costotransversectomy
- Anterior decompression
- Laminectomy
- Posterior spinal fusion.

Note: Please also refer "TB Spine in Spine" chapter.

SKELETAL TUBERCULOSIS OF HIP, KNEE, SHOULDER, ANKLE, ELBOW AND WRIST

TUBERCULOSIS OF HIP

Please refer to Hip section, Regional Orthopedics, Chapter 30.

TUBERCULOSIS OF KNEE

Introduction

- Knee is the third most common site and accounts for 10% of skeletal involvement
- Knee involvement more in adults. Tubercles may remain dormant for years
- It is always secondary and may start in any of the following sites:
  - Synovium (common)
  - Subchondral bone (of lower end of femur, upper end of tibia, or patella)
  - Juxta-articular osseous foci.

Pathology

- Typical granular infection, starting in synovial membrane is of two types:
  1. Low grade (hematogenous; more common)
  2. High grade (osseous).

Low-grade Infection

- Synovial membrane becomes congested, edematous, and studded with tubercle
- Caseative destruction is not a common tendency towards resorption of tubercles or healing by fibrosis
- Pannus formation at synovial reflection
- Articular damage with subchondral bone erosion
- Synovial fluid is thin, watery, opalescent, increased in quantity contains flakes of fibrin, and mononuclear cells.

High-grade Infection

- Tuberculous granulation tissue, such as pannus erodes the articular margins, destroys the bones, and involves periarticular tissues, capsule, and ligaments.
- Nutrition is thus interfered and articular cartilage loses its smooth glistening appearance, becoming rough, pitted, and soft.
- Caseating destruction, with marked synovial swelling, sinus formation, effusion, and tuberculous abscess in subchondral bone, epiphyseal, or metaphyseal bone.
- Muscles atrophy of thigh and calf occurs rapidly.
- Knee flexion with posterior subluxation, abduction, and external rotation of knee, due to contracture of biceps femoris and iliotibial band (triple deformity).

Clinical Features

Early Stage

- Joint effusion and evidence of synovial hypertrophy
- Skin may be stretched and blanched, giving an appearance of a white swelling (tumor alba) and is edematous
- Tenderness along the joint line and synovial reflection.

Middle Stage of Arthritis

- Joint movements are grossly restricted, with painful spasms (particularly of hamstrings)
- Quadriceps atrophy
- Lymphadenopathy
- In growing child, transient limb lengthening may be seen due to juxtaepiphyseal hyperemia.

Advanced Stage

Triple deformity (actually is a quadruple deformity): It is characterized as:

- Flexion (to accommodate for increased swelling and is the position of ease as well as maximum capacity)
- External rotation (from the hip) posterior and lateral subluxation (due to action of biceps femoris and ITB contracture)
- Abduction of tibia (above deforming forces further pull the leg into valgus).

Radiology

- Osteoporosis of juxta-articular structure
- Ballooning of capsule

- Enlarged ossification center
- Loss of definition of articular cortex with extreme thinning
- Posterior subluxation and valgus deformity.

Treatment

Synovitis

- Chemotherapy
- Traction
- Joint aspiration.

When Active Symptoms Decrease?

- Active and assisted exercise
- Crutch walking for 6–12 months
- Protected weight-bearing for 18–24 months
- If disease is not responding favorably, arthrotomy, and synovectomy should be done.

Early Arthritis

- Synovectomy
- Joint debridement
- Curettage of juxta-articular foci.

Postoperative Regimen

- Drug therapy
- Traction
- Exercise
- Suitable braces.

Advanced Arthritis

Arthrodesis.

TUBERCULOSIS OF SHOULDER

Introduction

This is very rare constituting nearly 1–2% of skeletal tuberculosis and can start in any of the following sites:

- Synovium (rarely)
- Glenoid
- Head of humerus.

Clinical Features

Early Stage

- Painful limitation of abduction and external rotation occur early
- Marked wasting of the deltoid, supraspinatus, and other muscles
- Common variety is dry type and is called "caries sicca", since there is no effusion in the joint
- *Cold abscess formed could present at:*
  - Supraspinous fossa
  - Deltoid
  - Biceps.

Late Stage

- Destruction of the upper end of the humerus and glenoid cavity
- Fibrous ankylosis is the end result.

Radiology

- Generalized rarefaction (Fig. 83)
- Articular cartilage erosion
- Cavities in the head of humerus
- Periosteal reaction (Fig. 84).

Treatment

- Chemotherapy is the mainstay of the treatment
- Shoulder immobilization by plaster shoulder spica in 70°–90° of abduction, 30° of forward flexion and about 30° of internal rotation (saluting position), to encourage ankylosis in functional position, for 3 months
- Arthrodesis in painful ankylosis, recurrence, etc.

TUBERCULOSIS OF ANKLE

This is very uncommon and the incidence is only 5%. Sites of involvement could be:

- Synovium
- Distal end of tibia
- Malleoli
- Talus
- Calcaneum (rarely).

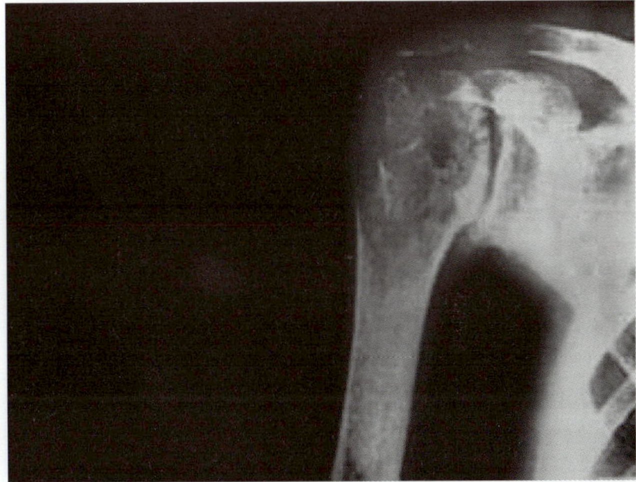

Fig. 83: Generalized rarefaction.

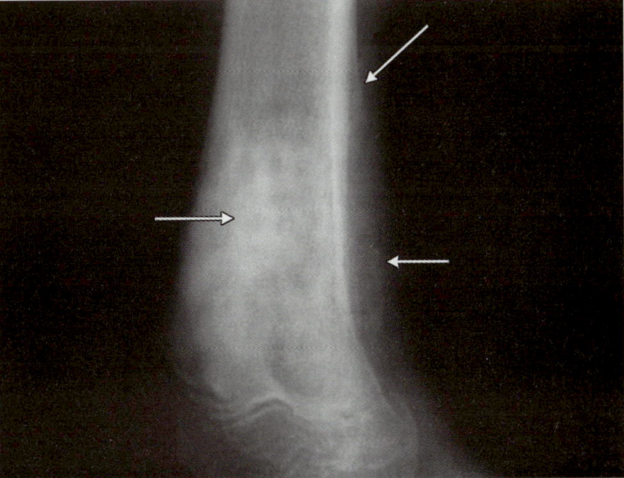

Fig. 84: Periosteal reaction.

Clinical Features

Early Stage

- Pain
- Limp
- Swelling
- Ankle is held in plantar flexion.

Late Stage

- Pathological anterior dislocation of the ankle
- Limitation of movements
- Wasting of calf muscles
- Sinus formation.

Radiology

- Marked osteoporosis (Fig. 85)
- Destruction of ankle joint (Fig. 86).

Treatment

- Chemotherapy is the mainstay of the treatment
- Below knee plaster cast for 8–12 weeks
- Synovectomy and joint debridement, during earlier stages
- Arthrodesis for advanced and persistence disease.

TUBERCULOSIS OF ELBOW

Introduction

Tuberculosis of the elbow is rare and constitutes nearly 2–5% of all skeletal tuberculosis. The sites are:

- Olecranon
- Lower end of humerus
- Synovium
- Upper end of radius.

Clinical Features

- Pain
- Swelling
- Limitation of movements
- Wasting of arm and forearm muscles
- Lymphadenopathy
- Sinus.

Radiology (Figs. 87 and 88)

- Destruction commonly in olecranon or left at the end of humerus
- Generalized demineralization and fuzziness of joint margins
- Subperiosteal new bone formation on the upper end of ulna resembling (spina ventosa) or lower end of humerus
- Pathological posterior dislocation.

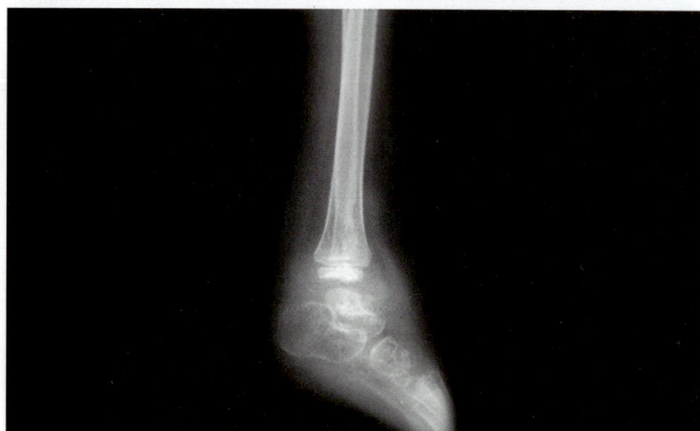

Fig. 85: Marked osteoporosis.

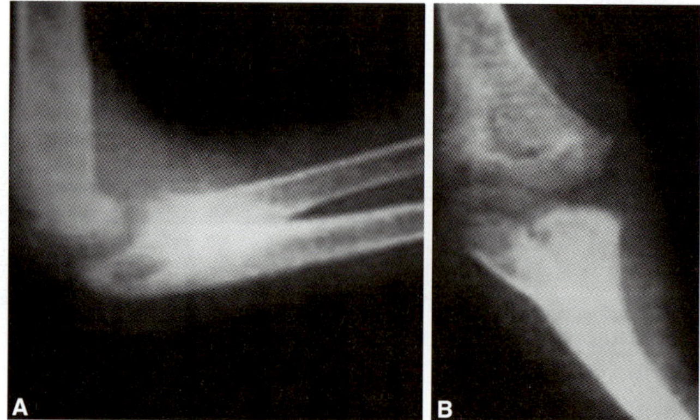

Figs. 87A and B: X-rays showing tuberculosis of the elbow.

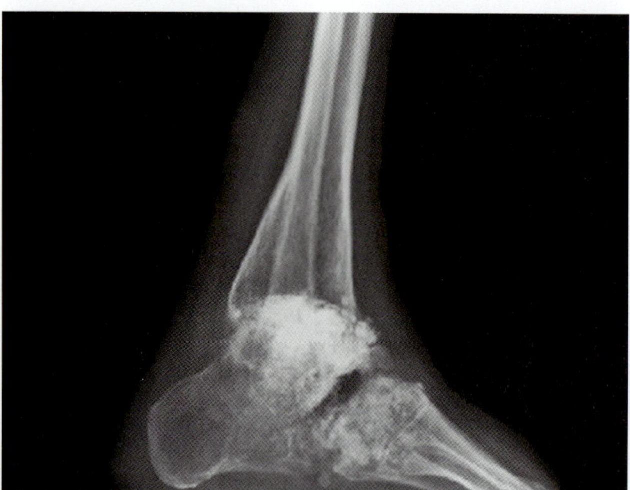

Fig. 86: Destruction of ankle joint.

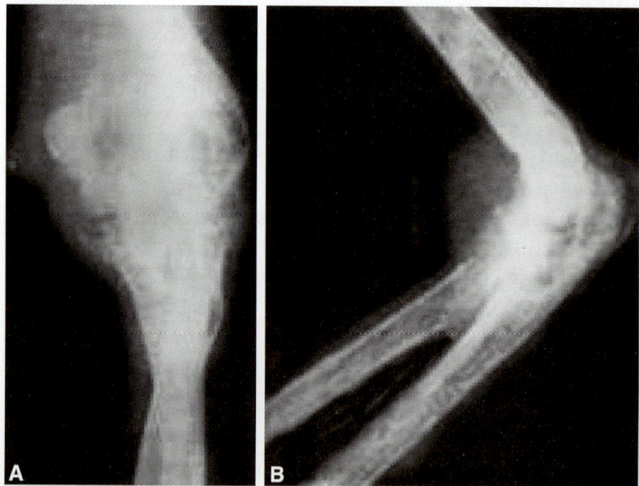

Figs. 88A and B: Pathological posterior dislocation due to TB of elbow joint.

Treatment

- Chemotherapy is the mainstay of treatment
- Plaster in 90° of flexion and midprone position of the forearm is advisable
- As pain reliefs, splint is advisable for 6–9 months
- Synovectomy
- Excision arthroplasty in advanced arthritis/ankylosis
- Rarely arthrodesis of elbow is justified for heavy manual work.

TUBERCULOSIS OF WRIST

Introduction

It is very rare, localized and more frequent in adults. The sites are:

- Synovium
- Whole carpus
- Dorsal end of radius
- Neighboring extensors/flexors tendons.

Clinical Features

Early Stage

- Pain
- Swelling
- Lymphadenopathy
- Limitation of movements
- Palmar flexion deformity.

Late Stage

- Limitation of pronation and supination
- Anterior subluxation/dislocation at the radiocarpal articulation.

Radiology (Figs. 89A and B)

- Demineralization
- Marginal erosion
- Slight diminution of joint space (Fig. 90).

Treatment

- Chemotherapy is the mainstay of treatment
- Splinting of wrist in 10–15° of dorsiflexion and forearm in midprone position for 12–18 months in between exercises
- Synovectomy and curettage
- Arthrodesis in severe ankylosis.

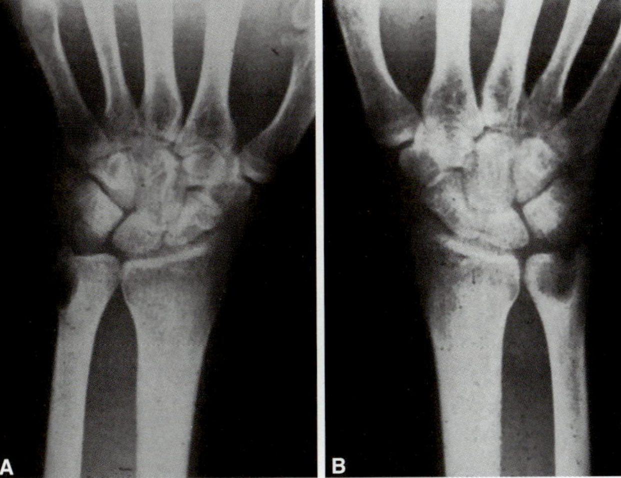

Figs. 89A and B: X-rays showing tuberculosis of wrist.

ACTINOMYCOSIS

Introduction

- The disease is a chronic granulomatous infection, occurring in human beings and animals. It is characterized by the development of indurated swellings, mainly in the connective tissue, suppuration, and discharge of sulfur granules (Figs. 91 and 92).
- The lesion often points towards the skin, leading to multiple sinuses (Fig. 92).
- Actinomycosis in human beings is an endogenous infection.
- The *Actinomyces* species are normally present in the mouth, intestine, and vagina.
- Trauma, foreign bodies, or poor oral hygiene may favor tissue invasion.
- *Actinomyces israelii* is the most common causative agent.
- Actinomycosis is usually a cooperative disease, the *Actinomyces* being accompanied by other associated bacteria, which may enhance the pathogenic effect.

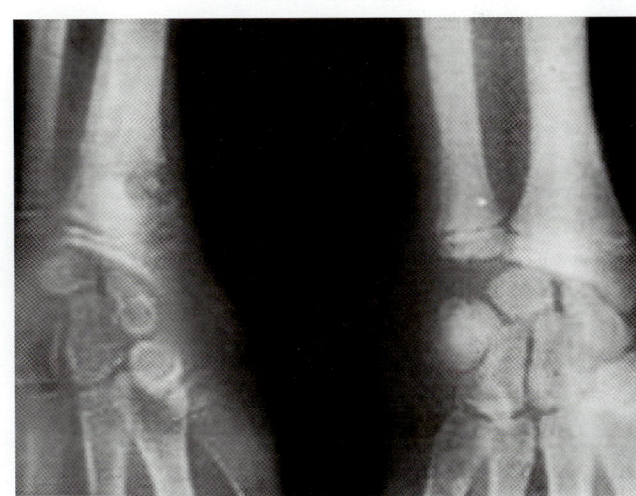

Fig. 90: Slight diminution of joint space.

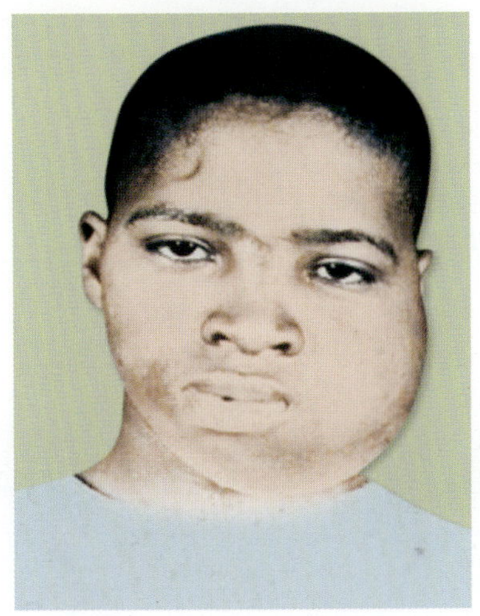

Fig. 91: Actinomycosis of jaw.

- Actinomycosis in human beings occurs in four main clinical forms:
  1. *Cervicofacial:* With indurated lesions on the cheek and submaxillary regions.
  2. *Thoracic:* With lesions in the lung that may involve the pleura, and pericardium, and spread outwards through the chest wall.
  3. *Abdominal:* Where the lesion is usually around the cecum, with involvement of the neighboring tissues, and the abdominal wall. Sometimes, the infection spreads to the liver via portal vein.
  4. *Pelvic:* Many cases of pelvic actinomycosis have been reported in association with the use of intrauterine devices.
- *Actinomyces* has been incriminated in inflammatory diseases of the gums (gingivitis and periodontitis) and with sublingual plaques, leading to root surface caries.
- Actinomycosis may also present as mycetoma.

Laboratory Diagnosis

- The diagnosis is made by demonstrating actinomycetes in the lesion, by microscopy, and by isolation in culture (Figs. 93 and 94).
- The specimen to be collected is pus.
- In pulmonary disease, sputum is collected.
- Sulfur granules may be demonstrated in pus, by shaking it up in a test tube with some saline (Fig. 95).
- On standing, the granules sediment and may be withdrawn with a capillary pipette.
- Granules may also be obtained by applying gauze pads over the discharging sinuses.
- The granules are white or yellowish and ranges in size from minute specks to about 5 mm.
- They are crushed between slides and stained by gram stain and examined. The granules are in fact, bacterial colonies and will be found to consist of dense network of thin gram-positive filaments, surrounded by peripheral zone of swollen radiating club shaped structures, presenting a sun ray appearance (Fig. 96).
- The clubs are believed to be antigen-antibody complexes.
- Sulfur granules or pus containing *Actinomyces* are washed and inoculated into thioglycollate liquid medium or streaked on brain-heart infusion agar and incubated anaerobically at 37°C.
- In thioglycollate, *A. bovis* produces general turbidity, whereas *A. israelii* grows as fluffy balls at the bottom of the tube.
- On solid media, *A. israelii* produces small spidery colonies in 48–72 hours that become heaped up, white, and irregular, or smooth, large colonies in 10 days.

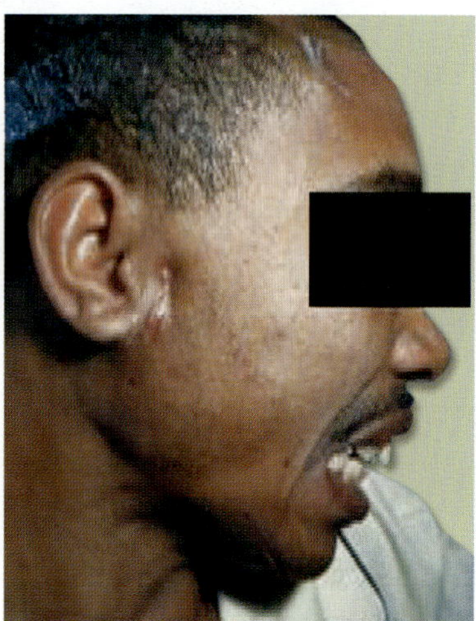

Fig. 92: Actinomycosis with multiple sinuses in the skin.

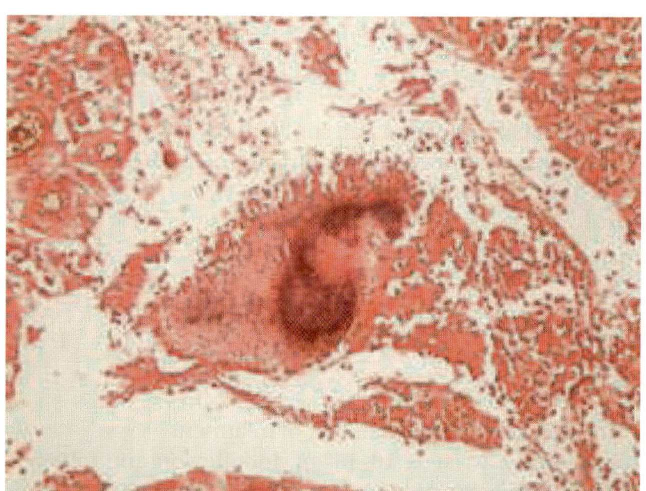

Fig. 94: Demonstration of actinomycetes (High power).

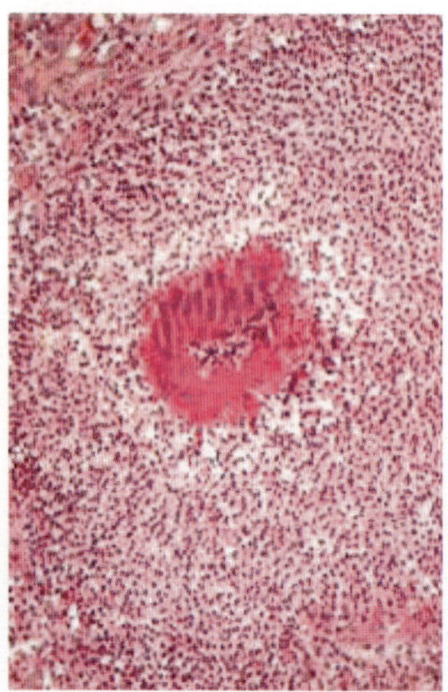

Fig. 93: Demonstration of actinomycetes (Low power).

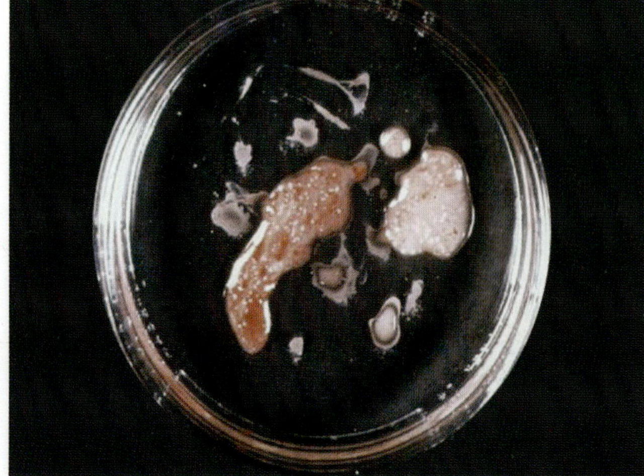

Fig. 95: Demonstration of sulfur granules in pus, by shaking in test tube.

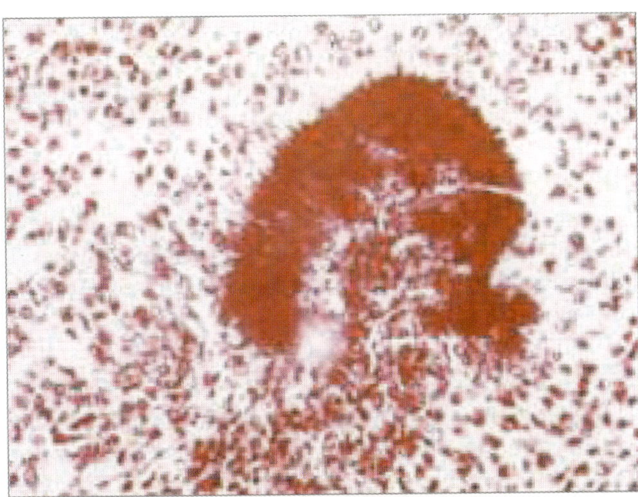

Fig. 96: Granules presenting a sun-ray appearance.

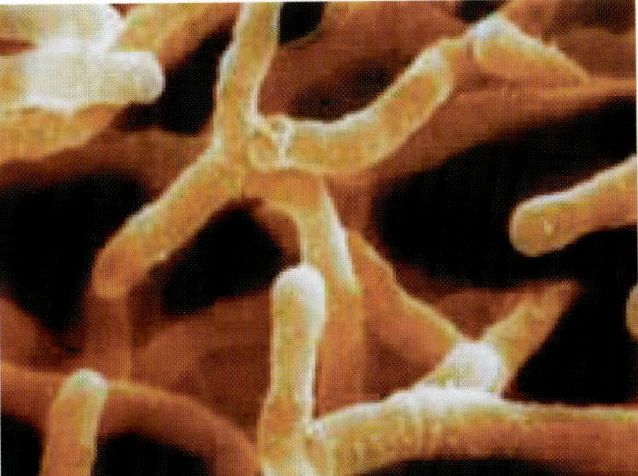

Fig. 97: Differentiating *Actinomyces israelii* from other actinomycetes.

- Other species have different types of colonies.
- The isolate is identified by microscopy, biochemical reactions, and fluorescent antibody methods.
- Gel diffusion and immunofluorescence can differentiate *A. israelii* from other actinomycete species and from other filamentous anaerobes that may produce granules in tissues (Fig. 97).

Epidemiology

- The disease occurs throughout the world, but its incidence in the advanced countries has been declining, probably as a result of the widespread use of antibiotics.
- Actinomycosis is more common in rural areas and in agricultural workers.
- Young male patients are most commonly affected.
- The reason for this predisposition is not known.
- About 60% cases are cervicofascial and 20% are abdominal.
- Pelvic actinomycosis is seen mainly in women, using intrauterine devices.

Treatment

- The bacterial infection is mostly treated with antibiotics, such as penicillin, usually given through a vein in the first instance, followed up by tablets. Depending on the seriousness of the infection, it may be necessary to continue antibiotics for 6–12 months, to prevent relapse.
- In some cases, surgery may also be necessary to drain deep abscesses and to remove the sinuses. Surgery can also be used to remove the large infected lumps and to seal off any sinuses, which have moved into the bone structure.
- *Actinomyces* bacteria can also be treated with other medications, including chloramphenicol, erythromycin, tetracyclines, and clindamycin. However, they almost always respond to the combination of antibiotics and surgery.

MYCETOMA (MADUROMYCOSIS)

Introduction

Mycetoma or maduromycosis is a slow-growing bacterial or fungal infection, focused in one area of the body, usually the foot. For this reason and because the first medical reports were from doctors in Madura India, an alternate name for the disease is Madura foot. The infection is characterized by an abnormal tissue mass beneath the skin, formation of cavities within the mass and a fluid discharge. As the infection progresses, it affects the muscles and bones and at this advanced stage, disability may result.

Description

Although the bacteria and fungi that cause mycetoma are found in soil worldwide, the disease occurs mainly in tropical areas in India, Africa, South America, Central America, and South-east Asia. Mycetoma is an uncommon disease, affecting an unknown number of people annually.

There are more than 30 species of bacteria and fungi that can cause mycetoma. Bacteria or fungi can be introduced into the body, through a relatively minor skin wound. The disease advances slowly over months or years, typically with minimal pain. When pain is experienced, it is usually due to secondary infections or bone involvement. Although it is rarely fatal, mycetoma causes deformities and potential disability at its advanced stage.

Source of Infection

Thorn trees contain the organisms, when it injures the skin and open the wound, it inoculates the organisms into subcutaneous tissues. When conditions are suitable, they grow, and form grains and granuloma will be formed around the grain as a part of the host response to the organisms. The granuloma is firm, but can be cystic, or soft. As the grains grow upwards, they attach to the skin and through it the sinus opens and discharges pus. The color and consistency of the pus depends on the etiological agent.

They may spread downwards affecting muscles and bones. Mycetoma affects many sites of body, but more commonly the foot (Madura foot). It can also infect upper limb, chest, abdomen, perineum, head, and neck. Infection of head and neck is the most serious condition, as it compresses the cranium, and causes abnormal neurological signs and symptoms.

Classification

Eumycete or True Fungi

It is a fungal infection:

- *Madurella mycetomatis:* Form big black grains
- *Madurella grisea:* Form black grains

- *Curvularia lunata:* Also cause black grain
- *Aspergillus nidulans:* Form white soft grains.

Actinomycetoma

It is a bacterial infection:

- *Streptomyces somaliensis:* Causes dirty yellow grains like sand
- *Actinomadura madurae*: Cause white soft grains
- *A. pelletierii:* Small red soft grains
- *Nocardia brasiliensis:* Form very small creamy white or orange colored grains
- *Pseudallescheria boydii (Scedosporium apiospermum).*

History

- The earliest sign of mycetoma is a painless subcutaneous swelling. Some patients have a history of a penetrating injury at that site.
- Several years later, a painless subcutaneous nodule is observed. After some years, massive swelling of the area occurs, with induration, skin rupture, and sinus tract formation.
- As the infection spreads to contiguous body parts, old sinuses close and new ones open.
- Nearly 20% of patients with mycetoma experience associated pain, usually due to secondary bacterial infection or less commonly due to bone invasion.
- Constitutional symptoms and signs of mycetoma are rare.
- Patients may report a deep itching sensation.

Clinical Features

- Irrespective of the causative agent, the appearance of the mycetoma lesion is consistent as follows:
  - Initially, subcutaneous swelling is present
  - In a later phase, a subcutaneous nodule develops
  - Eventually, massive swelling with induration, rupture of the skin, and formation of sinus tracts occur (Fig. 98)
- A chronic, slowly progressing bacterial or fungal infection, usually of the foot or leg, characterized by nodules that discharge an oily pus. Also called "Madura boil"
- In general, eumycetoma is more circumscribed and progresses slower than actinomycetoma
- Regional lymphatic obstruction and fibrosis can cause *lymphedema* and *erythema*
- Pulmonary mycetoma has been found to develop and progress more rapidly in individuals infected with HIV.

Primary Osseous Mycetoma

This results from direct inoculation of the organisms into bones, causing bone lesions especially in tibia and calcaneus bones. The condition is presented with pain and can be diagnosed by radiology or surgical exploration.

Spread of Infection

The organisms spread from one site of body to another site by facia and less commonly by lymphatics. Hematogenous spread is unknown to occur in individuals except in immunocompromised patients.

Microscopic Features (Figs. 99 and 100)

Treatment

Actinomycetoma:

- It is a bacterial infection that can respond to antibiotics if treatment is administered early in the course of the disease.
- A combination of two drugs in 5 weeks cycles is used. If needed, the cycles can be repeated once or twice.
- The following agents have been used in combination:
  - Trimethoprim-sulfamethoxazole (TMP-SMZ)
  - Dapsone (diaminodiphenyl sulfone)
  - Streptomycin sulfate.
- Amikacin can be substituted for streptomycin, but is usually kept as a second-line drug because of its cost;
- Rifampin has been used as a second-line drug in resistant cases;
- An effective and convenient regimen combining a short course of intravenous gentamicin with a 6 months oral course of cotrimoxazole and doxycycline has recently been described.

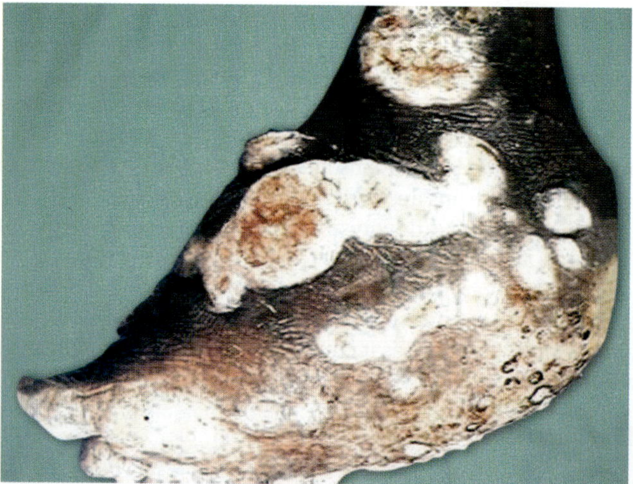

Fig. 98: Formation of sinus tract due to fungal infection.

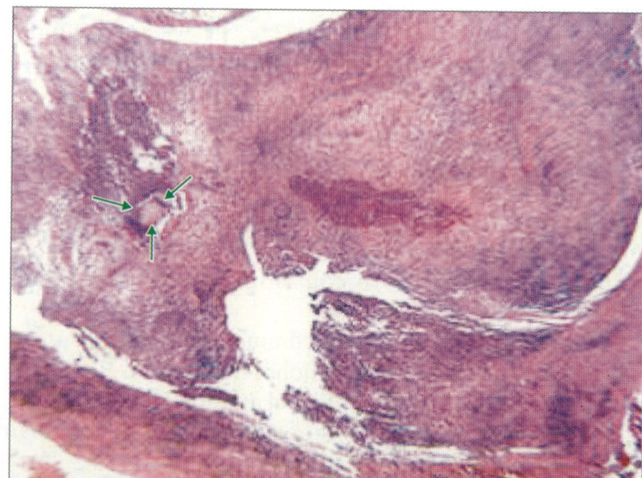

Fig. 99: Microscopic features of mycetoma—the tissue above the lower one-fourth of the field is granulation tissue. The two darker zones in the granulation tissue are areas of suppuration. In the zone of suppuration to the left, green arrows identify a colony of organisms. The colony is a "Grain" (mycetoma).

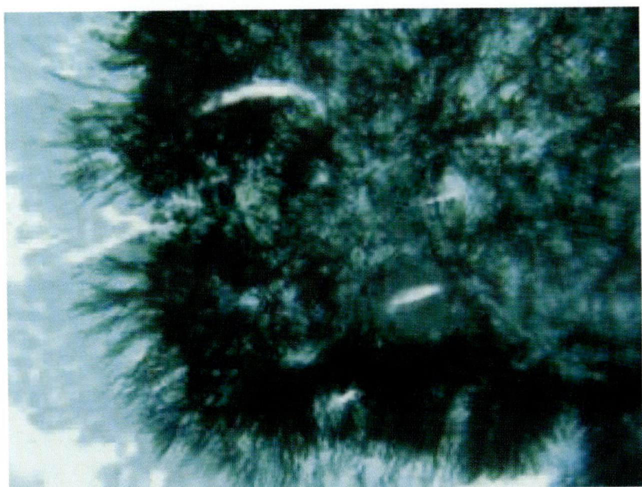

Fig. 100: Microscopic features of mycetoma—with a silver methenamine stain, the organisms are filamentous.

Eumycetoma:

- It may respond partially to antifungal agents, although surgical therapy is preferred for localized disease.
- *Madurella mycetomatis,* mycetoma may respond to ketoconazole (200 mg bid).
- *P. boydii (S. apiospermum)* mycetoma should be treated primarily with voriconazole, although it may also respond to itraconazole.
- Other agents that cause eumycetoma, may respond intermittently to itraconazole (200 mg bid) or amphotericin B.
- The minimum treatment duration is 10 months.
- Voriconazole is the drug of choice for invasive infections, caused by agents of eumycetoma in immunocompromised patients.
- Surgery is recommended for localized mycetoma lesions that can be excised completely without residual disability. Surgical reduction of large lesions can improve the patient's response to medical treatment; however, partial surgical resection without subsequent use of appropriate antimicrobial or antifungal agents is prone to failure.
- Amputation is also done for mycetoma in limb extremities.
- External beam radiotherapy in doses ranging from 3.5 Gy to 14 Gy has been considered successful treatment in a few selected cases.

Prognosis

- Recovery from mycetoma may take months or years and the infection recurs after surgery in at least 20% of cases.
- Drug therapy can reduce the chances of a re-established infection.
- The extent of deformity or disability depends on the severity of infection; the more deeply entrenched the infection, the greater the damage.
- By itself, mycetoma is rarely fatal, but secondary infections can be fatal.

Prevention

Mycetoma is a rare condition that is not contagious, regular aseptic precautions are recommended.

BIBLIOGRAPHY

1. American Academy of Ophthalmology (2012). Information Statement. Minimizing Transmission of Bloodborne Pathogens and Surface Infectious Agents in Ophthalmic Offices and Operating Rooms. [online] Available from: http://www.progressivesurgicalsolutions.com/wp-content/uploads/2016/03/6_AAO.pdf. [Last accessed March, 2019]
2. American Society of Health-System Pharmacists (1999). ASHP Therapeutic Guidelines on Antimicrobial Prophylaxis in Surgery. [online] Available from: https://www.ashp.org/-/media/assets/policy-guidelines/docs/therapeutic-guidelines/therapeutic-guidelines-antimicrobial-prophylaxis-surgery.ashx. [Last accessed March, 2019].
3. AORN Recommended Practices Committee. Recommended practices for surgical attire. AORN J. 2005;81(2):413-20.
4. Boyce JM, Pittet D; Healthcare Infection Control Practices Advisory Committee; HICPAC/SHEA/APIC/IDSA Hand Hygiene Task Force. Guideline for Hand Hygiene in Health-Care Settings. Recommendations of the Healthcare Infection Control Practices Advisory Committee and the HICPAC/SHEA/APIC/IDSA Hand HygieneTask Force. Society for Healthcare Epidemiology of America/ Association for Professionals in Infection Control/Infectious Diseases Society of America. MMWR Recomm Rep. 2002;51(RR-16):1-45, quiz CE1-4.
5. Canada Communicable Disease Report. Vol. 24S8 (1998). Infection Control Guidelines: Handwashing, Cleaning, Disinfection and Sterilization in Health Care. Canada. [online] Available from: http://www.fiocruz.br/biosseguranca/Bis/manuais/descontaminacao/infection_control_guidelines.pdf. [Last accessed Mar., 2019].
6. Efhss.com (European Forum for Hospital Sterile Supply). Questions and Answers. Q000-166 Acrylic Chambers. [online] Available from: http://wfhss.deconidi.ie/html/comm/efhss_training_programme.pdf. [Last accessed March, 2019].
7. Mangram AJ, Horan TC, Pearson ML, et al. Guideline for prevention of surgical site infection, 1999. Hospital Infection Control Practices Advisory Committee. Infect Control Hosp Epidemiol. 1999;20(4):250-78; quiz 279-80.
8. Rutala WA, Weber DJ; Healthcare Infection Control Practices Advisory Committee (HICPAC). Guideline for Disinfection and Sterilization in Healthcare Facilities. Atlanta: Centers for Disease Control and Prevention (CDC); 2003.
9. Rutala WA. APIC guideline for selection and use of disinfectants. 1994, 1995, and 1996 APIC Guidelines Committee. Association for Professionals in Infection Control and Epidemiology, Inc. Am J Infect Control. 1996;24(4):313-42.
10. Sunaric-Mégevand G, Pournaras CJ. Current approach to postoperative endophthalmitis. Br J Ophthalmol. 1997;81(11): 1006-15.
11. The American Institute of Architects Academy of Architecture for Health. The Facility Guidelines Institute with assistance from the US Department of Health and Human Services. Guidelines for Design and Construction of Hospital and Healthcare Facilities, 2001 edition. [online] Available from: https://www.fgiguidelines.org/wp-content/uploads/2015/08/2001guidelines.pdf. [Last accessed March, 2019].
12. The Royal College of Ophthalmologists (2010). Cataract Surgery Guidelines. [online] Available from: https://www.rcophth.ac.uk/wp-content/uploads/2014/12/2010-SCI-069-Cataract-Surgery-Guidelines-2010-SEPTEMBER-2010-1.pdf. [Last accessed Mar., 2019].
13. Woodhead K, Taylor EW, Bannister G, et al. Behaviors and rituals in the operating theatre. A report from the Hospital Infection Society working party on Infection Control in Operating Theatres. J Hosp Infect. 2002;51(4):241-55.
14. World Health Organization. In: Ducel G, Fabry J, Nicolle L (Eds). Prevention of Hospital-Acquired Infections: A Practical Guide, 2nd edition. Geneva, Switzerland: World Health Organization; 2002.

CHAPTER

11 Bone Tumors

OBJECTIVES

- Etiology
- Classification of Bone Tumors
- Principles of Diagnosis
- Diagnostic Parameters of Bone Tumors
- Diagnosing Bone Tumor
- Bone-Biopsy
- Staging of Tumor
- Principles and Methods of Treatment
- Benign Tumors of the Bone
- Giant Cell Tumor
- Osteogenic Sarcoma (Osteosarcoma)
- Biopsy
- Chondrosarcoma
- Ewing's Sarcoma
- Multiple Myeloma
- Metastatic Bone Disease
- Maffucci Syndrome
- Dyschondroplasia (Enchondromatosis or Ollier's Disease)
- Dyschondrosteosis
- Paget's Disease (Osteitis Deformans)
- Fibrous Dysplasia

INTRODUCTION

- Like any other system in the body, musculoskeletal system may also develop tumors either as primary or secondary from a distant primary location.
- In clinical practice true neoplasm of bone has to be differentiated from hamartoma and reactive bone lesions. The group of lesion which shows abnormal proliferation of cells which soon matures and stop proliferation is called hamartoma. These are really benign growth disorder. Examples are osteochondroma, osteoma, and enchondroma.
- Bone also reacts to different type of injury by new bone formation. This reactive or reparative bone can also simulate neoplasia histologically.
- Clinically certain neoplastic lesions of bone present as swelling in the bone simulating tumor, e.g. solitary bone cyst, fibrous dysplasia and brown tumor in hyperparathyroidism.
- Primary bone tumor can be benign or malignant. Incidence of bone tumor is very low (1–1.5%) of total malignancy in body. Since the cells of musculoskeletal system are derived from mesoderm, primary bone tumors are called sarcomas. All these are derived from primitive mesenchymal cells hence containing not only bone cells but also cartilage and fibrous tissue in varying degree. There is also a group of myelogenic tumors arising from derivatives from marrow retinacular tissue. Tumors spreading secondary to bone are called metastatic carcinoma generally from primary carcinoma of breast, thyroid, lung, prostate, and kidney.
- Bone tumors can be broadly divided into true bone tumor and tumor like condition of bone. True bone tumor can be benign or malignant. The differences between benign and malignant are given in Table 1.
- The complexity in presentation of the tumors clinically, radiographically, and histologically presents an enormous challenge to the orthopedic surgeon, radiologist, and the pathologist who deal with these tumors.
- In general, bone tumors can occur from the age of 1–70 years.
- Most benign bone lesions, osteosarcoma, and Ewing's sarcoma occur in the 2nd and 3rd decade of life.
- Giant cell tumor (GCT) usually occurs in 3rd or 4th decade, while multiple myeloma, chondrosarcoma, fibrosarcoma, and metastatic bone tumors are frequent in older ages.
- Most of the tumors except GCT are more common in males.

TABLE 1: Differences between benign and malignant tumor.

Benign	*Malignant*
Slowly growing	Rapidly growing
well-circumscribed	Not well-circumscribed
Noninvading	Invading
No or few symptoms	Associated with pain and disability
Does not metastasize	Metastasizes
X-ray shows lesion confined to the bone	X-ray shows ill-defined bone lesion, mottled appearance, cortex may be broken

ETIOLOGY

- The genetic basis for some tumors has for long been suggested. The genetic basis of these tumors is based on the concept of oncogenes, tumor suppressor genes, and mutation.
- Oncogenes are mutated versions of normal cellular genes. The function of oncogenes varies but is generally related to growth factor stimulation of cells. These oncogenes induce tumors to form.
- On the other hand, tumor suppressor genes prevent tumors from developing. Affected members carry germ line mutations in these tumor suppressor genes.

- Other postulated causes are irradiation, viral etiology, and trauma.

CLASSIFICATION OF BONE TUMORS (TABLES 2 TO 4)

- A general accepted classification system is based on the predominant matrix component and type of cell differentiation within the lesion.
- The classification system divides all lesions into benign and malignant categories but there is little evidence to suggest that the malignant lesions occur as differentiation of their benign counterparts.

TABLE 2: Lichtenstein classification of primary bone tumors.

Histologic types	*Benign*	*Malignant*
Hemopoietic		Myeloma
Chondrogenic	• Osteochondroma • Chondroma • Chondroblastoma • Chondromyxoid fibroma	• Primary chondrosarcoma • Secondary chondrosarcoma • Clear cell chondrosarcoma
Osteogenic	• Osteoid • Osteoma benign • Osteoblastoma	• Osteosarcoma • Parosteal osteosarcoma • Periosteal osteosarcoma
Unknown origin	• Giant cell tumor • Fibrous histocytoma	• Ewing's tumor • Malignant giant cell tumor • Adamantinoma
Fibrogenic	• Fibroma • Desmoplastic fibroma	• Fibrosarcoma • Malignant fibrous histocytoma
Notochordal		Chodroma
Vascular	Hemangioma	• Hemangioendothelioma • Hemangiopericytoma
Lipogenic	Lipoma	
Neurogenic	Neurilemmoma	

TABLE 3: Bristol University classification of bone tumors.

Origin	*Benign*	*Malignant*
Cartilage	• Osteochondroma • Chondroma • Chondroblastoma • Chondromyxoid fibroma	Chondrosarcoma
Bone	• Osteoid osteoma • Osteoblastoma	Osteosarcoma
Bone marrow		• Multiple myeloma • Malignant lymphoma
Fibrous tissue	Desmoplastic fibroma	Fibrosarcoma
Unknown origin	• Giant cell tumor • Fibrous histiocytoma	• Malignant giant cell tumor • Ewing's tumor • Adamantinoma
Vascular tissue	• Aneurysmal bone cyst • Hemangioma	
Synovium	Synovioma	Synovial sarcoma

WHO Classification

Bone Forming Tumors

- *Benign:*
  - Osteoid osteoma and osteoblastoma
  - Intermediate
  - Aggressive (malignant) osteoblastoma.
- *Malignant:*
  - Central (medullary)
  - Surface (peripheral) Parosteal.
- *Periosteal:*
  - High-grade surface.

Cartilage forming Tumors

- Benign
- Chondroma
- *Enchondroma:*
  - Periosteal (juxtacortical)
  - Osteochondroma.
- *Solitary:*
  - Multiple hereditary
  - Chondroblastoma (epiphyseal chondroblastoma)
  - Chondromyxoid fibroma.
- *Malignant:*
  - Chondrosarcoma (primary/secondary)
  - Dedifferentiated chondrosarcoma
  - Juxtacortical chondrosarcoma
  - Mesenchymal chondrosarcoma
  - Clear cell chondrosarcoma.

TABLE 4: ABC classification of bone tumors by Charles Price.

Section	*Benign*	*Malignant*
Section A Angioid tumor	• Angioma • Aneurysmal bone cyst • Glomus tumor	Angiosarcoma
Section B	• Osteoma • Osteoblastoma • Osteoid osteoma	• Osteosarcoma • Periosteal osteosarcoma
Section C Cartilage formanic tumors	• Chondroma • Osteochondroma • Chondroblastoma	Chondrosarcoma
Section D Dental and Allied	• Odontogenic cyst • Ameloblastoma	Malignant odontoma
Section E Embryogenic vestigial tissue		Chondroma
Section F Fibroblastic	Fibroma	Fibrosarcoma
Section H Heterotrophic tissue	Dermoid	Adamantinoma
Section N Nonosseous connective tissue	Lipoma Neurofibroma Neurilemmoma	• Liposarcoma • Ewing's sarcoma • Myeloma
Section S Synovial tissue	Synovioma	Synovial sarcoma
Section U Undifferentiated connective tissue	Osteoclastoma	Malignant osteoclastoma

- *Giant cell tumor:*
  - Osteoclastoma
  - Marrow tumors
  - Ewing's sarcoma of the bone
  - Neuroectodermal tumor of the bone
  - Malignant lymphoma of bone (primary/secondary)
  - Myeloma.
- *Vascular tumors:*
  - *Benign:*
    - Hemangioma
    - Lymphangioma
    - Glomus tumor (glomangioma).
  - *Intermediate:*
    - Hemangioendothelioma
    - Hemangiopericytoma.
  - Malignant
    - Angiosarcoma
    - Malignant hemangiopericytoma.
- *Other connective tissue tumors:*
  - *Benign:*
    - Benign fibrous histocytoma
    - Lipoma.
  - *Intermediate:*
    - Desmoplastic fibroma.
  - *Malignant:*
    - Fibrosarcoma
    - Malignant fibrous histocytoma
    - Liposarcoma
    - Malignant mesenchymoma
    - Leiomyosarcoma
    - Undifferentiated sarcoma.
- *Other tumors:*
  - *Benign:*
    - Neurilemmoma
    - Neurofibroma.
  - *Malignant:*
    - Chordoma
    - Adamantinoma.
- *Secondary malignant tumors:*
  - Thyroid
  - Breast
  - Lungs
  - Kidney
  - Prostrate.

PRINCIPLES OF DIAGNOSIS

- Team work between orthopedicians, radiologists, pathologists, radiotherapists, and medical oncologists is necessary for evaluation and institution of appropriate therapy.
- Much of this depends on the prebiopsy workup which includes detailed history, physical examination, laboratory tests, X-rays of the lesion, chest X-ray and occasionally bone scan.

DIAGNOSTIC PARAMETERS OF BONE TUMOR

Clinical examination eliciting history and physical sign is first essential step.

History

- Pain and mass disability are presenting symptoms.
- Age has important relation to tumor. For example, Ewing's sarcoma (5–15), osteosarcoma (10–20), giant cell tumor (20–40), and secondaries in bone seen in elderly age group. Osteochondroma is seen in adolescent age group.
- *Onset:* Benign tumor is insidious in onset whereas malignant tumors are acute in onset, unexplained pain always precedes onset of swelling.
- *Constitutional symptoms:* Anorexia, weight loss, and fever are more pronounced in malignant tumors whereas absent in benign tumors.
- *Other symptoms:* Pulmonary metastasis may cause respiratory symptoms. Metastasis in spinal column may cause backache and neurological complaints. Thus when a tumor metastases and involve other systems presents with corresponding features of that involved system.
- *Rate of growth:* Rapid growth suggests malignancy and vice-versa. Sudden rapid growth in short time in a tumor of long standing duration suggests malignant transformation of benign lesion

Clinical Examination

- General examination for evidence of anemia, cachexia, and lymphadenopathy.
- Local examination done to know extent of plane of tumor or presence of any pathological fracture.

Look

- *Attitude of limb:* Some amount of immobility of limb is seen in malignant tumors whereas in benign immobility is insignificant. Thus pathological fracture of malignant tumor make limb totally immobile.
- *Changes seen over the skin:* Skin is stretched and shiny in large sized tumor, dilated tortuous vein indicates venous obstruction, and possibility of malignancy, visible pulsation indicates increased vascularity or tumor of vascular origin. Redness over skin indicates inflammation. Any sinus, scar mark or ulcer, fungating growth.

Feel

- Nonpinchable skin indicates that the tumor has infiltrated the skin impending a break, and proceeds toward fungation at site of rapid growth. Presence of signs of inflammation suggests malignancy or secondary infection, e.g. adventitious bursitis in osteochondroma.
- Freely mobile muscles in relation to tumor are usually benign. Immobility of the muscles due to adhesion of tumor is suggestive of infiltration of muscles by the malignant tumors.
- Benign tumor has got a smooth regular surface while in malignant tumor it is irregular and variable.
- Bony hard consistency suggests predominance of bony element, firm with cartilaginous element, soft with fibrous and vascular elements. Variegated consistency is feature of malignant tumor while uniform is of benign tumor. A change in consistency toward soft indicates degeneration from tumor necrosis. Fungation indicates fairly advanced stage of tumor. It is important to know anatomical plane of tumor by palpation, pinching the skin, making the overlying or underlying muscle

to contract and assessing the mobility and size of tumor. Edges of tumor arising from bone will not be felt properly and will be continuous with the bone.
- Local tenderness should be elicited last as patient may refuse for further examination. Tenderness is a sign of malignancy or secondary infection or pathological fracture. Tenderness felt over previous painless tumor suggests malignancy.

Move

- Painful limitation of joint movement is a feature of malignancy. Joint movement usually does not get restricted in benign tumor except a tumor in a vicinity of joint which causes mechanical obstruction, e.g. osteochondroma.
- Enlarged tender firm or hard lymph node and later on which gets attached to underlying structure suggest lymphatic spread.
- Other systems also should be examined for especially thorax and abdomen for abdominal mass, fluid collection and organomegaly.
- In spinal tumor neurological examination is mandatory.

Investigations

- Routine laboratory investigation
- Special Investigation
- Tumor biopsy.

Routine Laboratory Investigation

- Hb% is decreased
- Total WBC count and differential count are increased or decreased
- ESR is increased
- Serum calcium and phosphorous are increased
- Serum alkaline phosphatase is increased in tumors like osteogenic sarcoma
- Serum acid phosphatase is increased in tumors like metastatic tumors
- Urine-analysis
- Tumor markers.

Special Investigation

- Radiological investigations
- Chest X-ray for evidence of secondaries
- CT scan
- Arteriography or angiography
- Ultrasonography
- MRI
- Bone scan.

Radiological Findings in Case of Bone Tumors

- Age of patients; the presence of epiphysis and growth plate in growing skeleton, absence means mature skeleton and osteoporotic means aged skeleton. Middle aged skeleton shows features between porotic and adult skeleton (Tables 5 and 6).

TABLE 5: Age wise distribution of the bone tumors (benign and malignant).

Age (years)	*Benign*	*Malignant tumor*
10–20	• Fibrous dysplasia • Osteochondroma • Aneurysmal bone cyst • Unicameral bone cyst • Benign chondroblastoma • Osteoid osteoma	• Osteosarcoma • Ewing's tumor
20–40	Giant cell tumor	Chondrosarcoma
>40	Rare	• Myeloma • Fibrosarcoma • Secondary sarcomas • Secondaries

TABLE 6: Radiological features suggesting probable diagnosis.

Radiological features	*Probable diagnosis*
"Kissing" bones (lytic lesions in adjacent epiphysis)	GCT, angiosarcomal, pigmented villonodular synovitis, infections
Codman triangle	Osteosarcoma, osteomyelitis, ABC
Complete sclerotic rim, no break	Benign lesion (95% accuracy)
Cumulus cloud appearance	Osteosarcoma, stress fracture
Epiphyseal, solitary, eccentric lytic lesion with sclerotic margin	Chondroblastoma, enchondroma, GCT
Epiphyseal, solitary, lytic lesion without sclerotic margin	GCT
Expansile lesion, poorly demarcated with windblown calcifications	Chondrosarcoma
Expansile lesion nontrabeculated lesion	Benign tumor (majority of cases), Grade I sarcoma, solitary myeloma, metastasis (a small percent of cases)
Expansile, trabeculated lesion	Grade I sarcoma, GCT, myeloma
Fallen fragment sign	Simple bone cyst
Finger-in-the-balloon appearance	ABC
Ground-glass appearance	Fibrous dysplasia Osteoblastoma Grade I osteosarcoma
Onion-skinning	Ewing's sarcoma, subacute osteomyelitis, eosinophilic granuloma
Punched out lesions	Multiple myeloma
Ring-like to popcorn density	Enchondroma and secondary chondrosarcoma

DIAGNOSING BONE TUMOR

Diagnose bone tumor in following orders:
- Clues by appearance of lesion
- Clues by location of lesion
- Clues by density of lesion
- Other clues.

Clues by Appearance of Lesion

- Patterns of bone destruction
- Periosteal reactions
- Tumor matrix
- Expansile lesions of bone.

Patterns of Bone Destruction (Fig. 1)

- Geographic
- Moth-eaten
- Permeative.

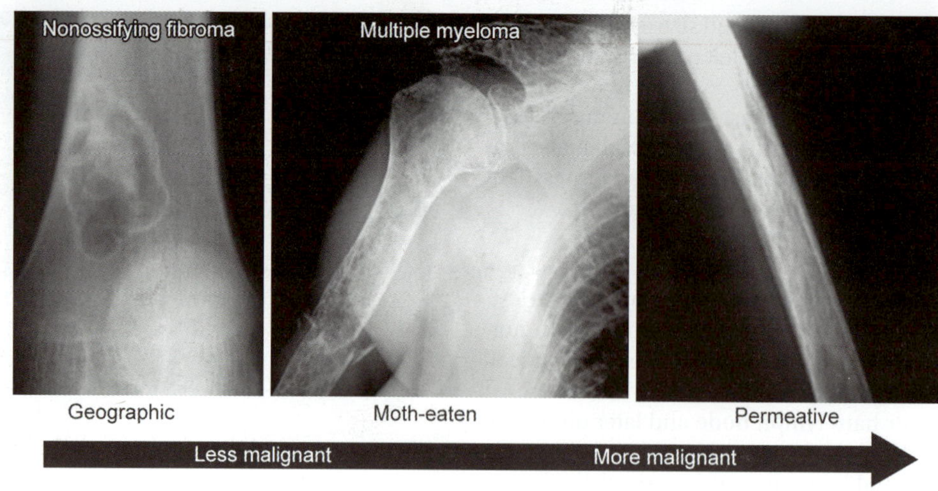

Fig. 1: Patterns of bone destruction.

Geographic bone destruction: Examples
- Nonossifying fibroma
- Chondromyxoid fibroma
- Eosinophilic granuloma.

Moth-eaten bone destruction:
- Areas of destruction with ragged borders
- Implies more rapid growth
  - Probably a malignancy.
- *Examples:*
  - Myeloma
  - Metastases
  - Lymphoma
  - Ewing's sarcoma.

Permeative bone destruction:
- Ill-defined lesion with multiple "worm-holes"
- Spreads through marrow space
- Wide transition zone
- Implies an aggressive malignancy
  - Round-cell lesions.

Periosteal Reactions (Figs. 2 and 3)

- It helps to differentiate benign, malignant, and specific tumor types.
- *Benign:*
  - None
  - Solid
- *More aggressive or malignant:*
  - Lamellated or onion peel
  - Sunburst
  - Codman triangle.

Types of periosteal reaction
- *Solid:* Thin/thick
- *Interrupted:* Codman triangle, lamellated (onion skin), perpendicular or spiculated or sunray (regular), sunburst (irregular)
- *Disorganized or complex:* A combination of both solid and interrupted.

Tumor Matrix (Figs. 4 and 5)

- *Osteoblastic:*
  - Fluffy, cotton-like or cloud-like densities
  - Osteosarcoma

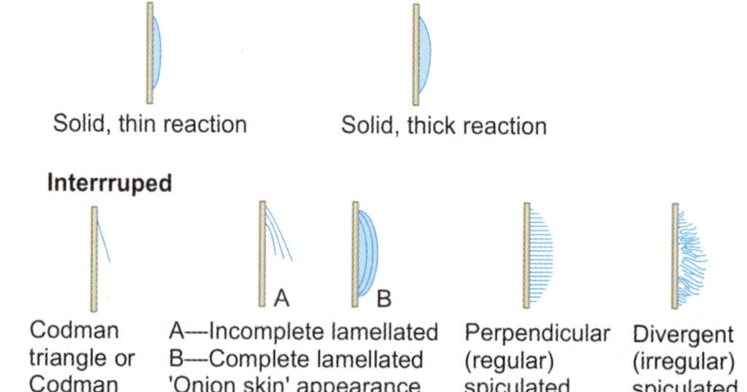

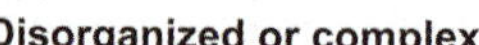

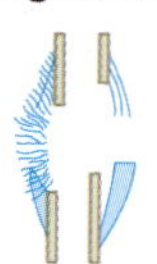

Fig. 2: Periosteal reaction.

- *Cartilaginous:*
  - Comma-shaped, punctate, annular, popcorn-like
  - Enchondroma, chondrosarcoma, chondromyxoid fibroma.

Expansile Lesions of Bone (Figs. 6 to 11)

- Multiple myeloma
- Mets
- Brown tumor
- Enchondroma
- Aneurysmal bone cyst
- Fibrous dysplasia.

Clues by Location of Lesion

- In the transverse plane (Fig. 12)
- In the longitudinal plane
- Characteristic locations by tumors
- Characteristic tumors by body site
  - Pelvic lesions
  - Expansile rib lesions
  - Lesions of the spine.

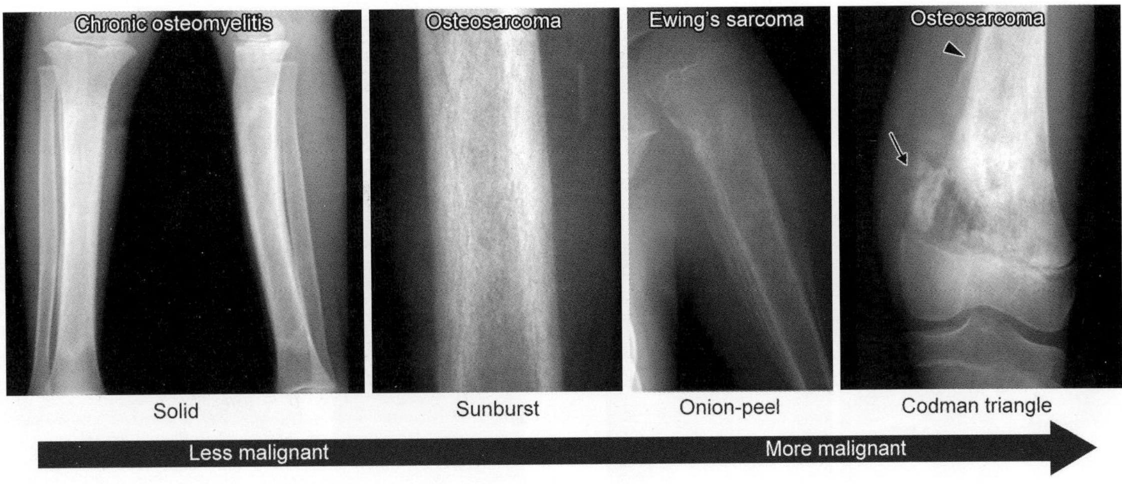

Fig. 3: Types of periosteal reactions.

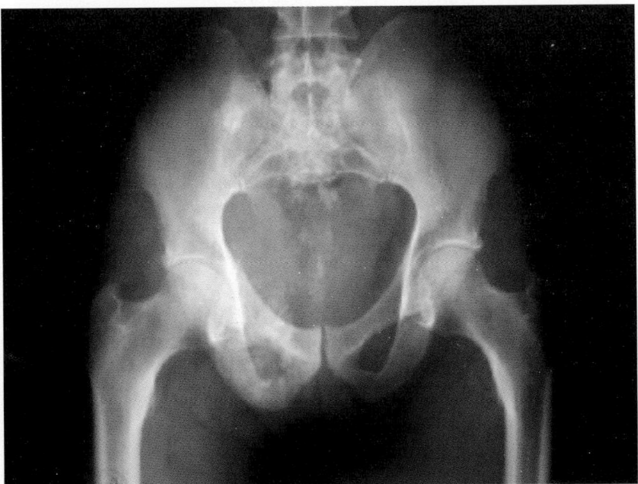

Fig. 4: Osteoblastic type.

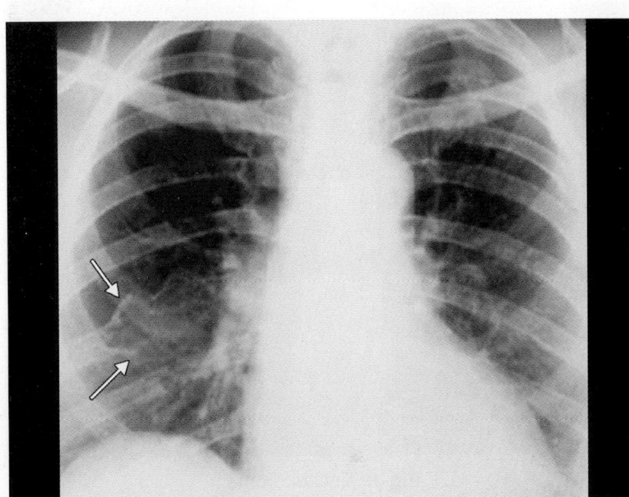

Fig. 6: Multiple myeloma.

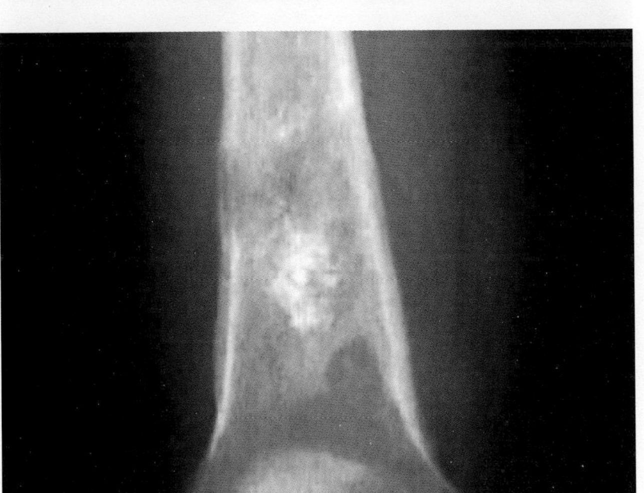

Fig. 5: Cartilaginous—chondrosarcoma.

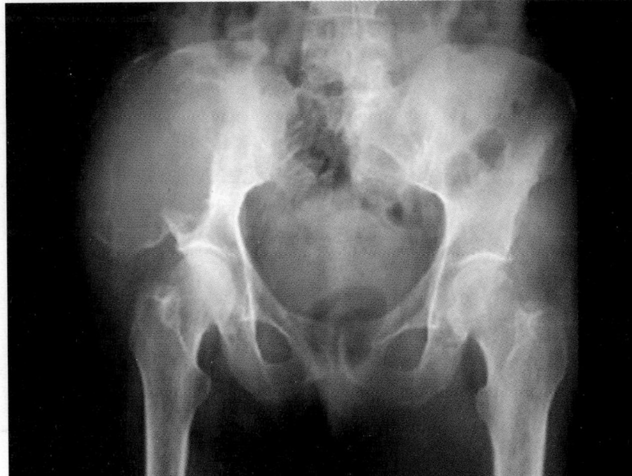

Fig. 7: Mets—renal cell carcinoma.

In the longitudinal plane:
- *Epiphyseal:* GCT, chondroblastoma
- *Metaphyseal:* Osteomyelitis, osteo- and chondrosarcoma
- *Diaphyseal:* Round cell lesions, ABC, enchondroma.

Characteristic locations by tumors (Figs. 13 to 18):
- *Simple bone cyst:* Proximal humerus
- *Chondroblastoma:* Epiphyses
- *Giant cell tumor:* Epiphyses

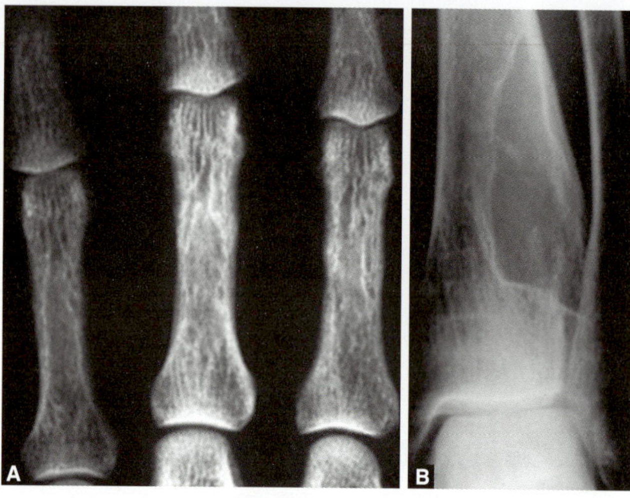

Figs. 8A and B: Brown tumor.

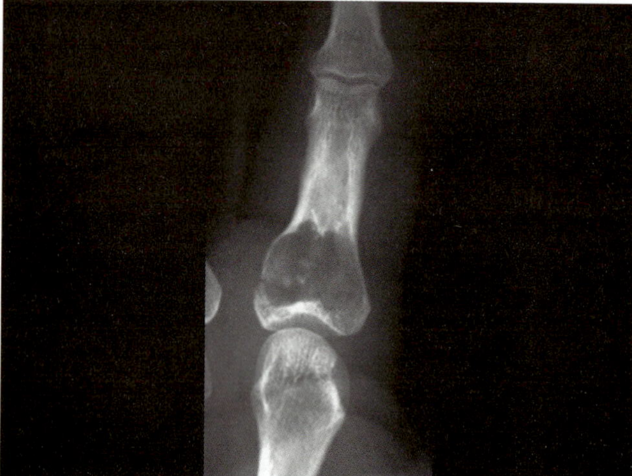
Fig. 9: Enchondroma.

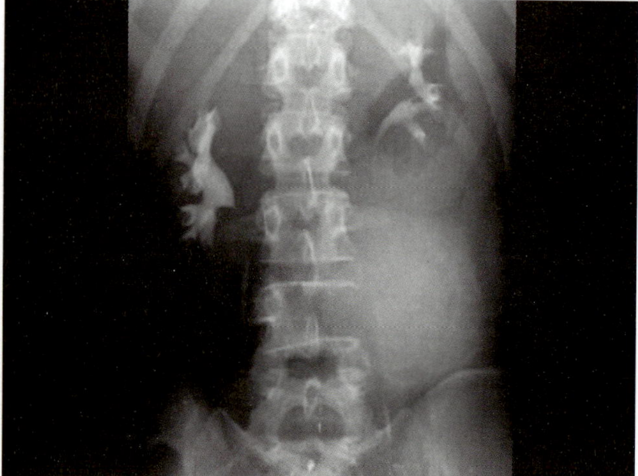
Fig. 10: Aneurysmal bone cyst.

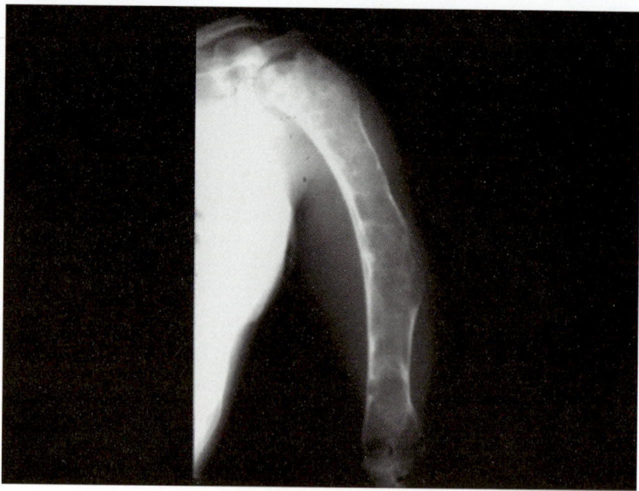
Fig. 11: Fibrous dysplasia.

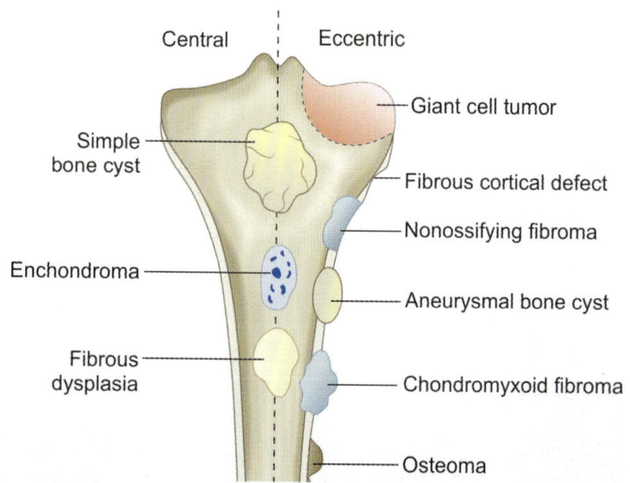

Fig. 12: Transverse plane.

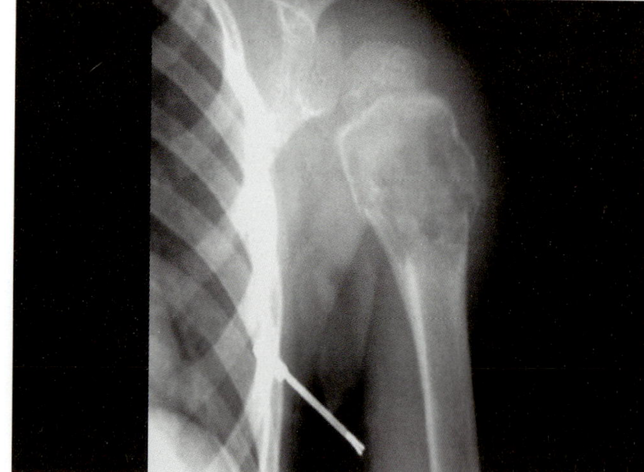
Fig. 13: Simple bone cyst.

- *Adamantinoma:* Tibia
- *Chordoma:* Sacrum, clivus
- *Osteoblastoma:* Spine (posterior).

Clues by Density of Lesion (Figs. 19 to 29)

- *Sclerotic cortical lesions:*
  - Osteoid osteoma
  - Brodie's abscess
- *Lytic lesions in children:*
  - Eosinophilic granuloma
  - Leukemia
- *Lytic lesions in adults:*
  - *Metastatic lesions:*
    - Lung
    - Renal
    - Thyroid

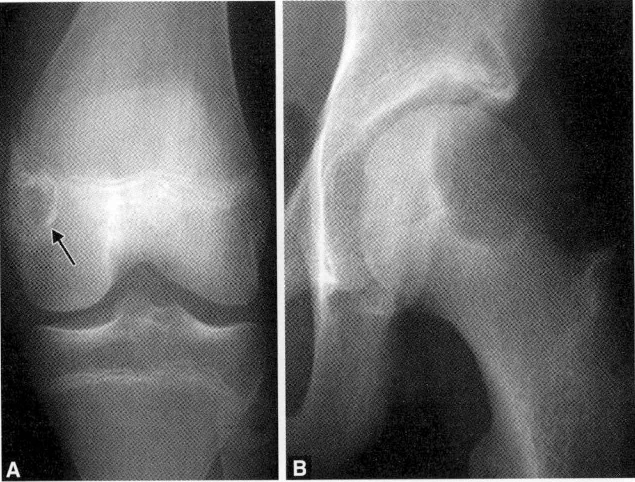

Figs. 14A and B: Chondroblastoma.

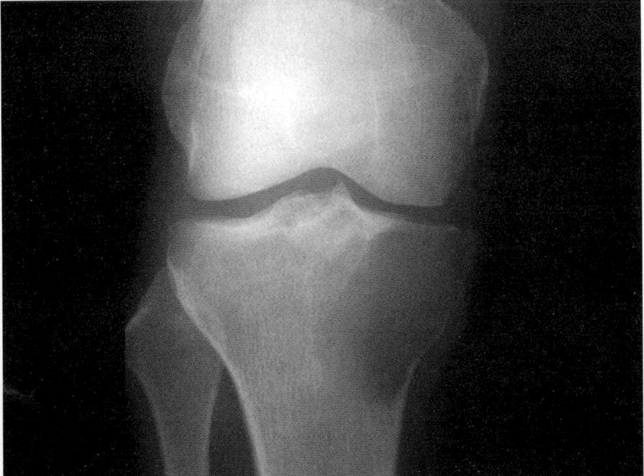

Fig. 15: Giant Cell tumor.

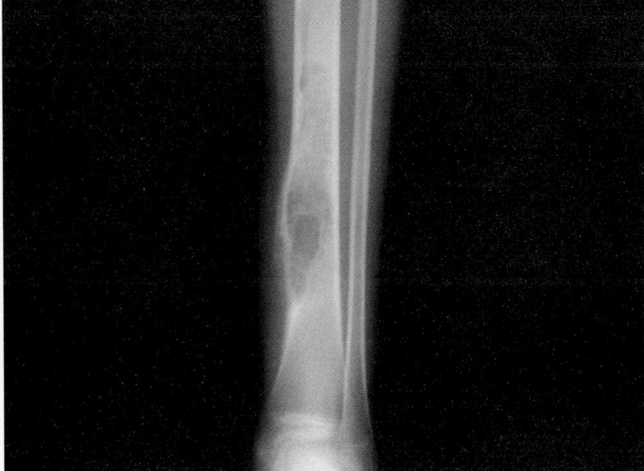

Fig. 16: Adamantinoma.

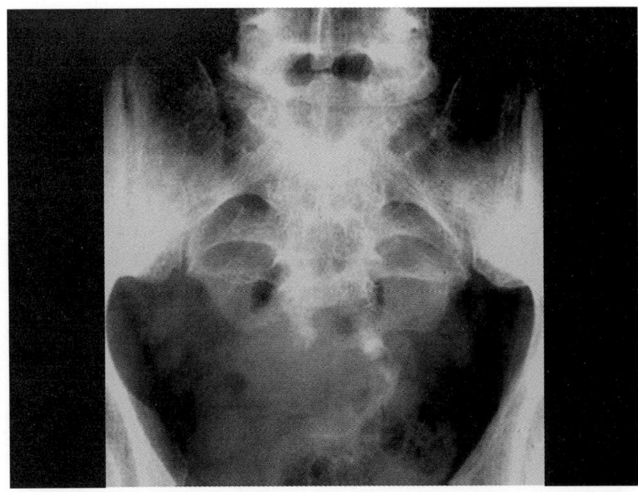

Fig. 17: Chordoma.

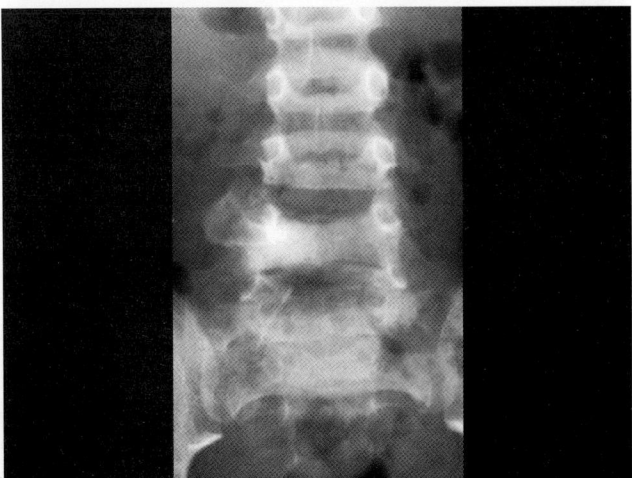

Fig. 18: Osteoblastoma.

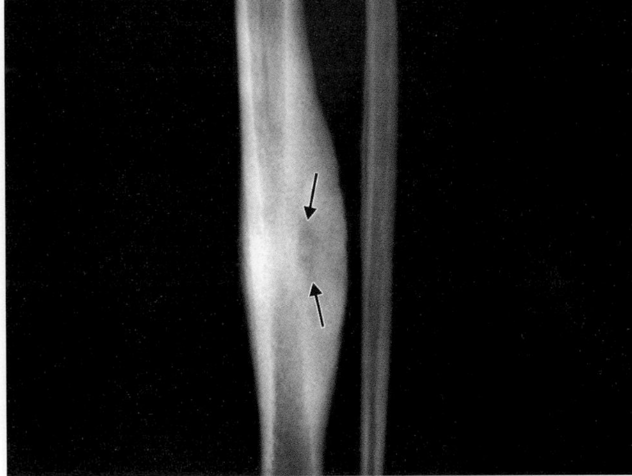

Fig. 19: Osteoid osteoma.

  - Multiple myeloma
  - Primary bone tumor
- *Blastic lesions in children:*
  - Lymphoma
- *Blastic lesions in adults:*
  - *Metastatic disease:*
    - Breast—female
    - Prostate—male
  - Lymphoma
  - Paget's disease
  - Fluorosis.

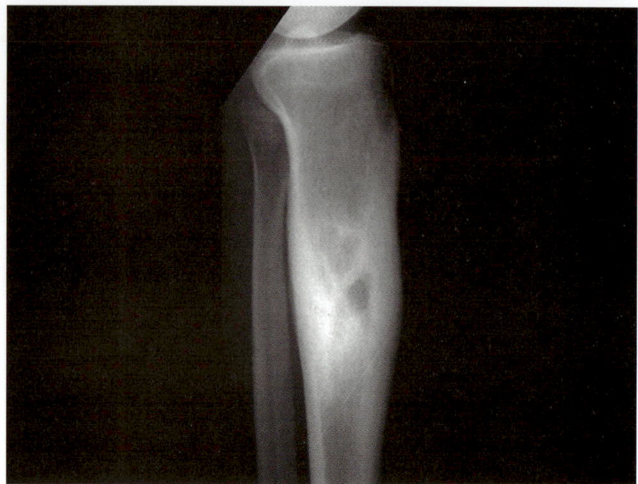

Fig. 20: Brodie's abscess.

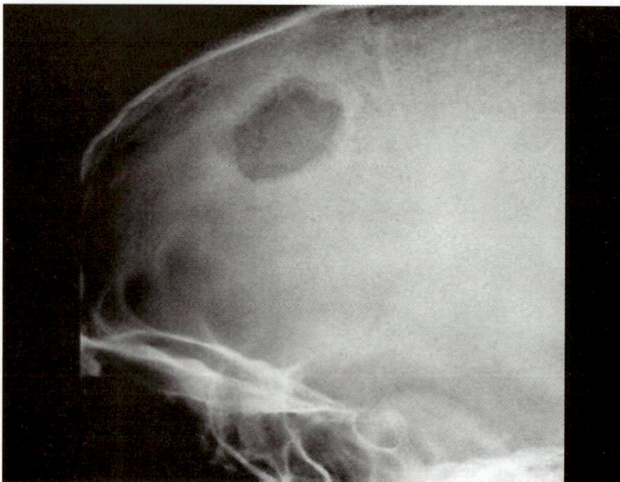

Fig. 21: Eosinophilic granuloma.

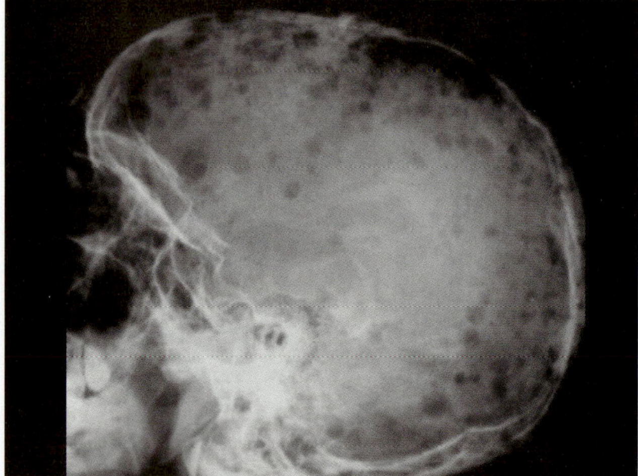

Fig. 22: Leukemia.

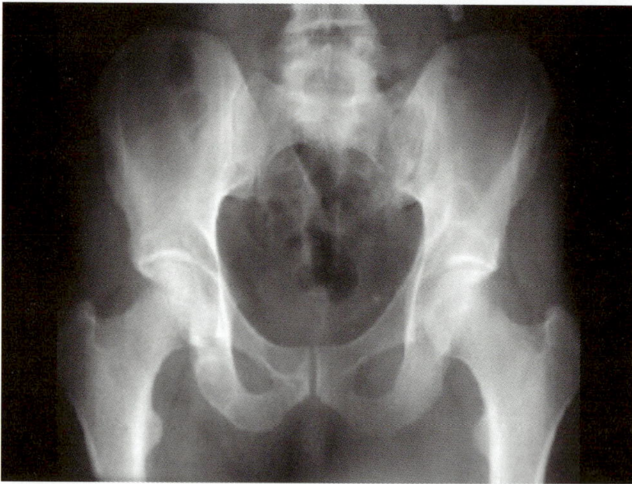

Fig. 23: Metastatic thyroid carcinoma.

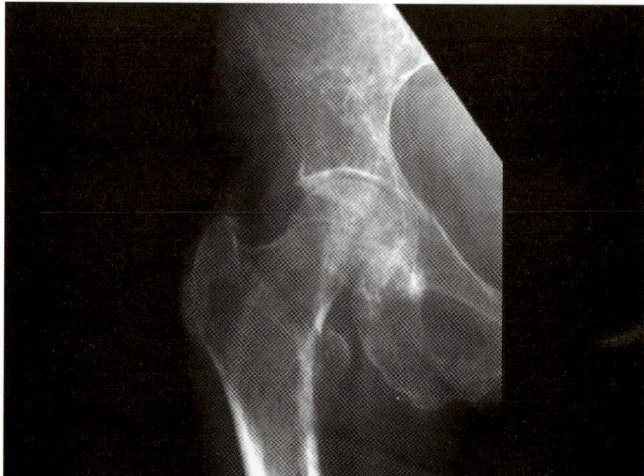

Fig. 24: Multiple myeloma.

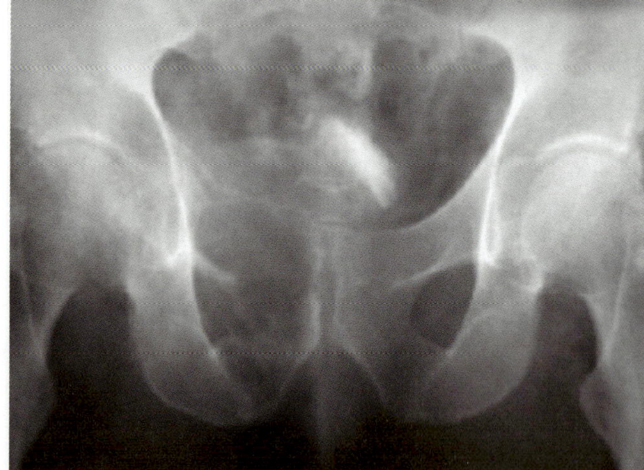

Fig. 25: Primary bone tumor: Chondrosarcoma.

Other Clues (Figs. 30 and 31)

- Soft tissue extension
- Benign versus malignant lesion.

Soft Tissue Extension

- *Usually implies malignancy:*
  - More likely to form discrete soft tissue mass.
- *Benign conditions with soft tissue extension:*
  - Osteomyelitis—usually infiltration of fat.

Angiography

- Useful when there is need to assess the vascularity of the tumor and to localize the vessel when a radical surgical procedure is planned.

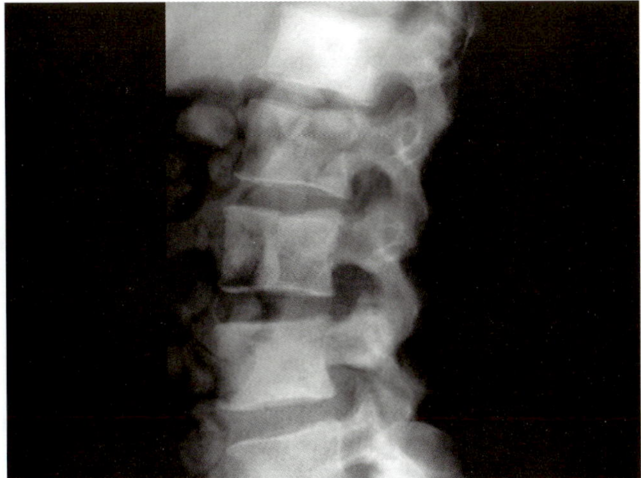
Fig. 26: Blastic lesions in children: Lymphoma.

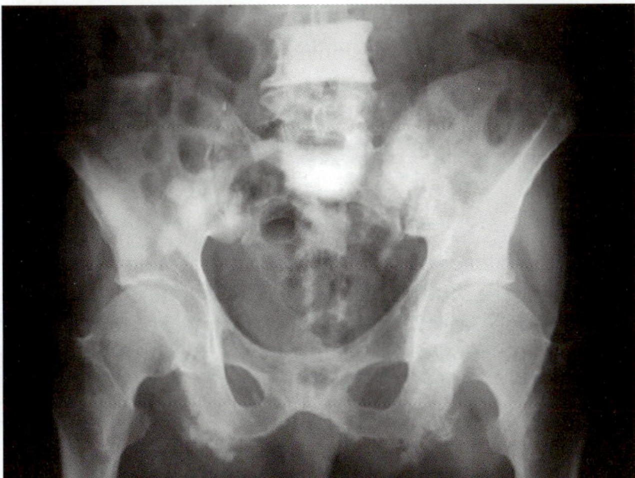
Fig. 27: Prostatic carcinoma.

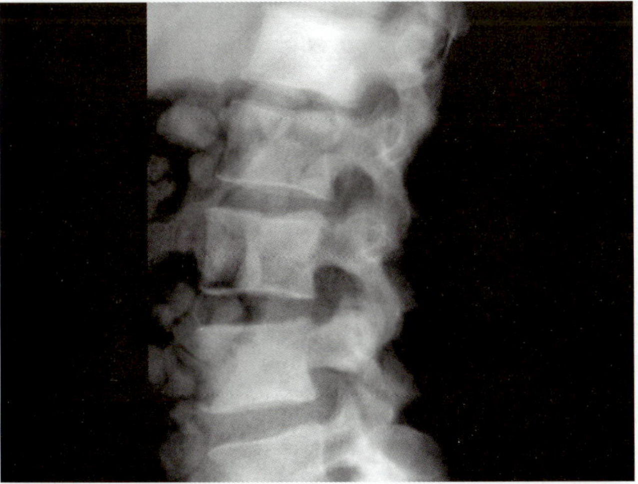
Fig. 28: Blastic lesions in adults: Lymphoma.

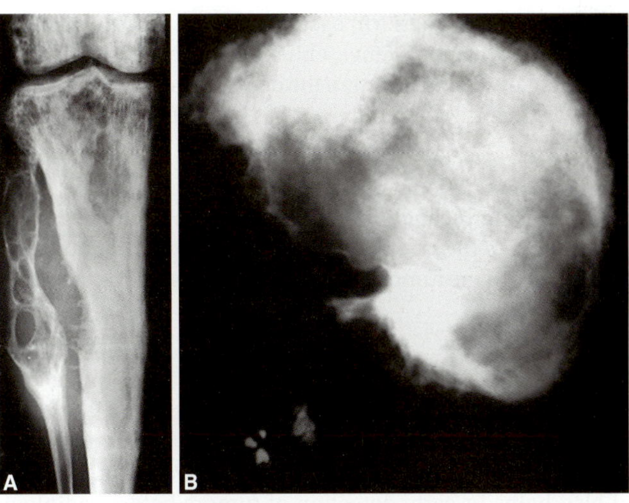

Figs. 29A and B: Paget's disease.

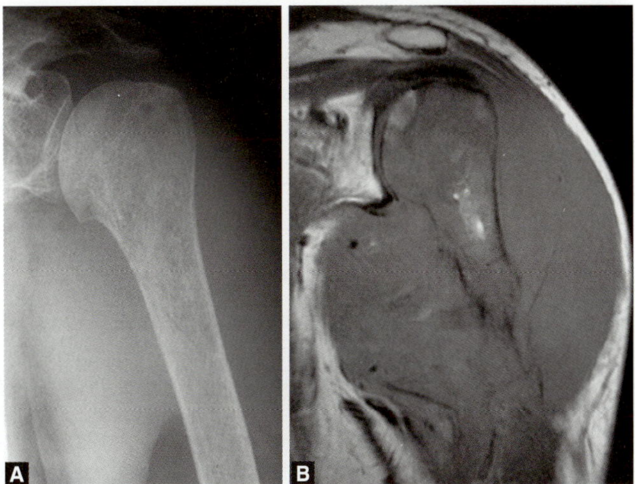

Figs. 30A and B: Soft tissue extension: Lymphoma.

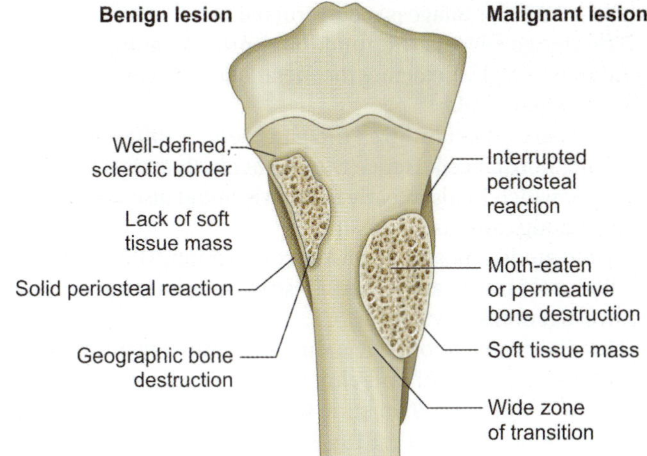

Fig. 31: Benign versus malignant lesion.

- In certain conditions, vessels get involved in the tumor tissue and separation becomes difficult during surgery. Hence, a need arises to sacrifice some of its branches. In such cases preoperative angiography is useful in determining the presence of good and adequate vascular anastomosis which can salvage limb. For example, brachial artery involvement at the elbow and popliteal artery involvement around the knee
- Also useful in identifying skipped lesions when used with other imaging technique, e.g. CT angiography

- *Tumor blush* seen in osteosarcoma which promotes neovascularization. Hence, enhancement of contrast medium. After giving chemotherapy if the neovascularization is not seen, it infers that the chemotherapy has been effective.

Bone Scan

Bone scan using Technetium-99m diphosphonate (99m Tc- HDP) is of immense help as it clearly shows the hot spots in the skeleton. Even smallest of the tumor can be diagnosed as well as the skipped metastasis.

CT Scan

It is not the substitute for radiographs or bone scan but it is adjuvant to these investigations, when there is a need for clear delineation of tissues. It is useful to assess the intra- and extraosseous extension and also helps in early detection of tumors before radiological changes are seen.

Magnetic Resonance Imaging

- It delineates the soft tissue better than CT and useful in visualizing the soft tissue extension and invasion of the tumor into neighboring structures, e.g. muscles, nerve and vessels.
- Also helps in staging of the tumor and planning for the surgery.

Positron Emission Tomography

- It reveals how body parts are functioning unlike CT and MRI which simply gives an image.
- Not only useful in early diagnosis but also useful in evaluating response to treatment.
- A radioactive tracer FDG (fluorodeoxyglucose) is inserted into the human body. This molecule of glucose tagged with radioactive tracer is utilized by the tissues of the body for energy and as it breaks down it emits positrons. The gamma rays emitted indirectly by the positrons, is detected by the machine and a 3D color image is reconstructed.
- The image reveals the functional process going on in the human body by detecting the metabolic changes occurring at the cellular level.
- The diseased cell utilizes the glucose in a different manner than a normal cell. Hence the image obtained is a functional image which helps in early diagnosis of the disease as well as evaluating response to treatment.
- All the modern positron emission tomography (PET) machines allow a CT image along the PET scan, simultaneously. Hence, investigation known as PET CT.
- The disadvantage of PET is that it is almost five times more expensive than MRI and almost eight times more expensive than a Technetium-99m bone scan
- A byproduct of FDG, i.e. F18 is being effectively used for a bone scan. This reduces the cost of bone scan.

BONE-BIOPSY

The following types of tissue are performed to diagnose bone tumor:
- Close biopsy
- Open biopsy.

Close Biopsy

- Fine needle aspiration cytology where 22 gauge needle yields very little tissue for examination, useful only when lesion is soft and homogeneous which is usually not suitable for bone biopsy.
- Core biopsy by a trephine needle and trocar usually taken from multiple sites.
- Image guidance is preferred because it guides sites for biopsy. CT-guided needle biopsy is used in lesion present in inaccessible areas spine and pelvis.

Advantages

- No incision is required.
- Tissue is obtained through a puncture hence minimizes tissue contamination. Nowadays core biopsy is used widely. It cannot be used in an osteosclerotic bone.

Open Biopsy

- It can be incisional, excisional.
- Excisional can be intralesional, marginal, wide marginal, and radical.
- Open biopsy is done only when core biopsy report is inconclusive or ancillary studies is necessary for detail planning.

Advantages

- Provides sufficient amount of tissue for histology.
- Provides adequate tissue material for performing other supportive studies such as immunohistochemistry, cytogenetics, molecular genetics, flow cytometry and electron microscopy.
- These studies are useful in final diagnosis, subclassification of bone tumors and definitive treatment.
- It is always good practice to send the biopsied sample for culture and vice-versa.

Rules of Tumor Biopsy

- In malignant tumors remove tumor "en bloc"
- No transverse incision
- No important neurovascular structures should be exposed
- It should transverse only one compartment
- Collect the sample from periphery of the tumor
- If bone sample has to be taken, make a small oval or circular hole in the bone to prevent pathological fracture.

Diagnostic Evaluation

The diagnostic evaluation of bone-biopsy is shown in Figures 32 to 34.

STAGING OF TUMOR

- TNM staging system advocated by UICC/American Joint Committee.
- Musculoskeletal Tumor Society staging system devised by Enneking.

TNM Staging System

- G—histological grade
- G1—well differentiated

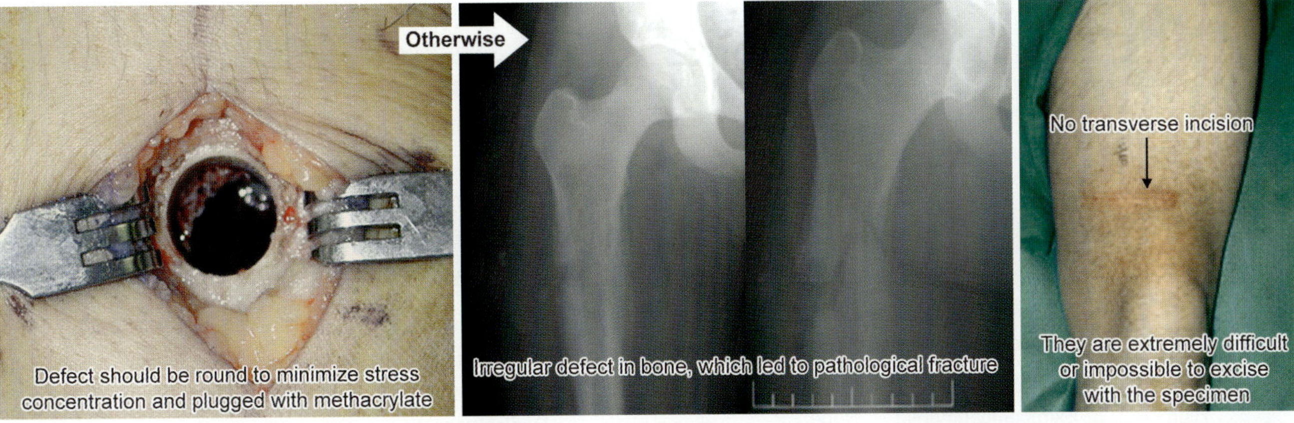

Fig. 32: Bone-biopsy: Open and close.

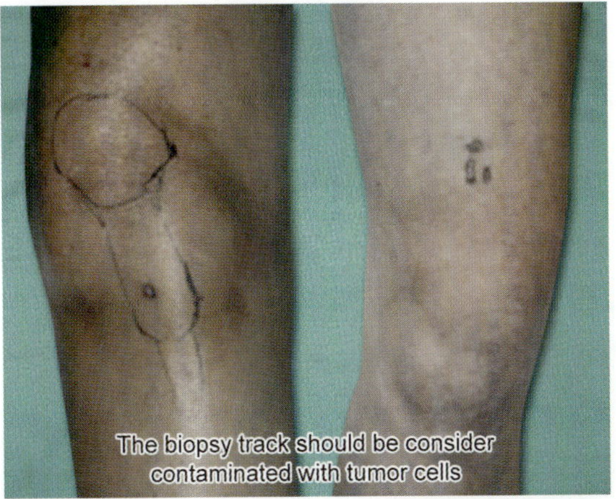

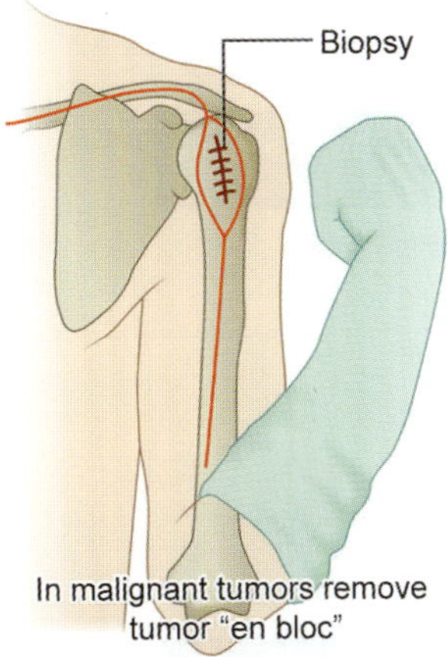

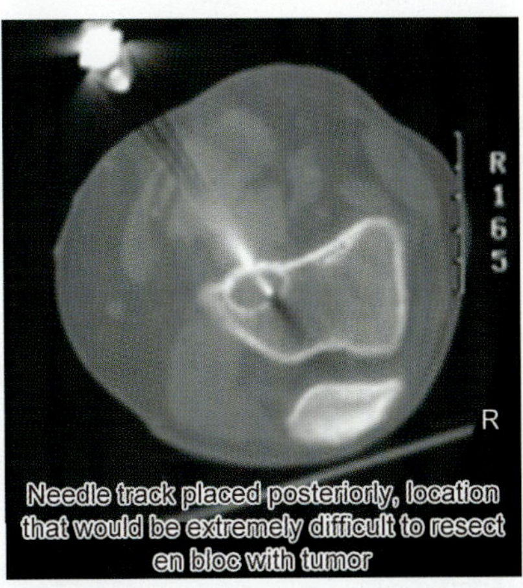

Fig. 33: Biopsy.

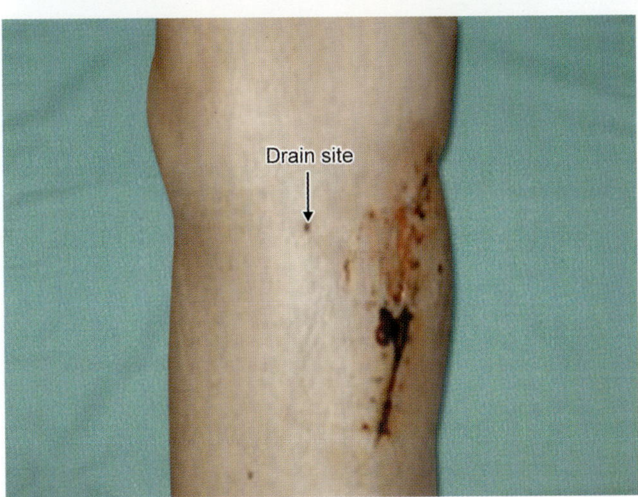

Fig. 34: Drain site was not placed in line with incision (It should be in line with incision).

- G2—moderately differentiated
- G3—poorly differentiated
- G4—undifferentiated
- T—primary tumor
- TX—primary tumor cannot be assessed
- T0—no evidence of primary tumor
- T1—tumor 8 cm or less in greatest dimension
- T2—tumor more than 8 cm in greatest dimension
- T3—discontinous tumors in the primary bone site
- N—regional lymph nodes
- NX—regional lymph nodes cannot be assessed
- N0—no regional lymph node metastasis
- N1—regional lymph node metastasis
- M—distant metastasis
- MX—distant metastasis cannot be assessed
- M0—no distant metastasis
- M1—distant metastasis
- M1a—lung
- M1b—other distant metastasis.

Stage IA	T1	N0	M0	G1, 2 low grade
Stage IB	T2	N0	M0	G1, 2 low grade
Stage IIA	T1	N0	M0	G3, 4 high grade
Stage IIB	T2	N0	M0	G3,4 high grade
Stage III	T3	N0	M0	Any G
Stage IVA	Any T	N0	Any M	Any G
Stage IVB	Any T	N1	Any M	Any G
	Any T	Any N	M1b	Any G

Enneking Staging System

- Designed for sarcomas arising from mesenchymal connective tissue of the musculoskeletal system.
- Lesions derived from the reticuloendothelial tissue and mesenchymal soft tissue are excluded.
- It is based on histological grade, local tumor extent, and presence or absence of metastasis (Tables 7 to 9).

TABLE 7: Enneking system for staging benign and malignant musculoskeletal tumors.

Benign			
1. Latent			
2. Active			
3. Aggressive			
Malignant			
Stage	*Grade*	*Site*	*Metastases*
IA	Low	Intracompartmental	None
IB	Low	Extracompartmental	None
IIA	High	Intracompartmental	None
IIB	High	Extracompartmental	None
III	Any	Any	Regional or distant metastases

TABLE 8: American Joint Committee on Cancer System for staging soft-tissue sarcomas.

Stage	*Grade*	*Size*	*Depth*	*Metastases*
I	Low	Any	Any	None
II	Low	≤5 cm	Any	None
	High	>5 cm	Superficial	None
III	High	>5 cm	Deep	None
IV	Any	Any	Any	Regional or distant

TABLE 9: American Joint Committee on Cancer System for staging bone sarcomas.

Stage	*Grade*	*Size*	*Metastases*
IA	Low	≤8 cm	None
IB	Low	>8 cm	None
IIA	High	≤8 cm	None
IIB	High	>8 cm	None
III	Any	Any	Skip metastasis
IVA	Any	Any	Pulmonary metastases
IVB	Any	Any	Nonpulmonary metastases

PRINCIPLES AND METHODS OF TREATMENT

- Surgical
- Adjuvant.

Adjuvant Therapy

- *Chemotherapy:* Chemotherapy has become normal practice in all bone tumors nowadays. Allow the primary tumor to shrink down and become safer to operate on.
- Radiation therapy.

Surgical Treatment (Table 10)

Choice of surgical procedure can be ascertained by Enneking staging of tumors, as suggested here (Fig. 35 and 36):

- Grade IA—requires local procedure like curettage
- Grade IB—wide excision
- Grade IIA—radical excision
- Grade IIB—radical amputation
- Grade III—multiprolonged approach such as surgery, chemotherapy, and radiotherapy.

Other surgical procedures include:

- Curettage
- Limb-salvage surgeries
- Resection and reconstruction
- Amputation.

Principle of Surgery

- Site of the tumor
- Extend of the tumor

TABLE 10: Enneking System for Staging malignant musculoskeletal tumors.

Stage	*Grade*	*Site*	*Metastases*
IA	Low	Intracompartmental	None
IB	Low	Extracompartmental	None
IIA	High	Intracompartmental	None
IIB	High	Extracompartmental	None
III	Any	Any	Regional or distant metastases

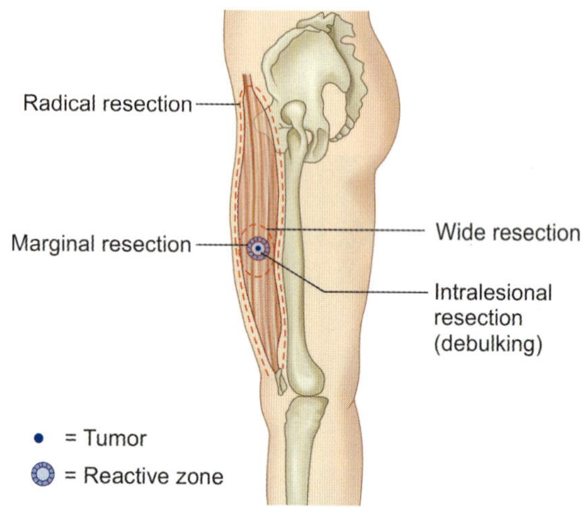

Fig. 35: Enneking classification of local procedures.

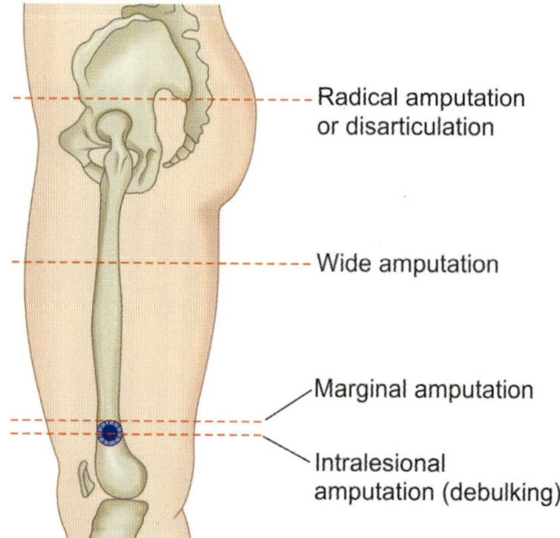

Fig. 36: Enneking classification of amputations.

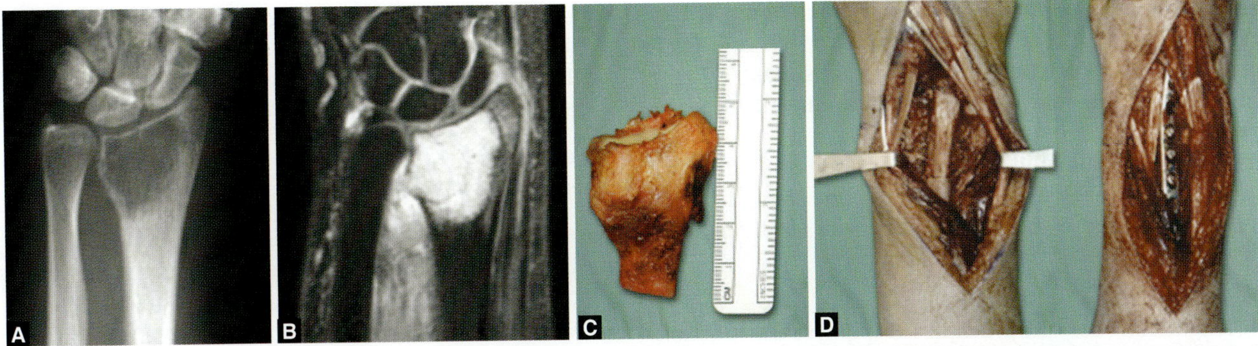

Figs. 37A to D: Autograft. (A) Anteroposterior radiograph of a 56-year-old woman with giant cell tumor of distal radius; (B) MRI shows extent of tumor and soft-tissue mass; (C) Resected specimen; (D) Proximal fibular autograft fashioned to fit defect.

- Response of tumor to the chemotherapy
- Wide or radical margin resection should be achieved in malignant tumor by limb salvage or amputation to avoid chances of recurrence.

Decision Making between Limb Salvage and Amputation

- Resection of an upper extremity lesion with limb salvage, even with the sacrifice of one or two nerves, generally provides better function than amputation and subsequent prosthetic fitting.
- Resection of a proximal femoral or pelvic lesion with local reconstruction generally provides better function than would be possible after a hip disarticulation or hemipelvectomy.
- Around the ankle and foot, however, large sarcomas frequently are treated with amputation followed by prosthetic fitting.
- Osteosarcoma around the knee is treated with wide resection with prosthetic knee replacement or transfemoral amputation.
- In general if the main nerve to the limb has to be sacrificed along with the bone then limb salvage is not going to produce useful limb then amputation should be considered, but this is not true in case of blood vessels.

Types of Limb Salvage

- Autograft
- Allograft
- Bone lengthening
- Endoprosthetic replacement
- Arthrodesis
- Rotationplasty.

Autograft (Figs. 37A to D):

- Use bone from the patient to fill the defect from the tumor.
- For example: Fibula is used for Replace the tumor of distal radius and part of humerus.
- In lower limb isolated autograft is unlikely to be sufficiently strong to allow weight bearing so should be combined with other form of bone graft.
- Recently a lot of interest in using the patient's own tumor bone and replacing it after Radiotherapy, pasteurizing liquid nitrogen or autoclaving.
- Of all available methods, extracorporeal irradiation and reimplantation of the bone is most useful.
- Such a technique is useful in pelvis and ankle region.

Allograft (Figs. 38 and 39):

- Dead piece of bone, harvested from bone donor.

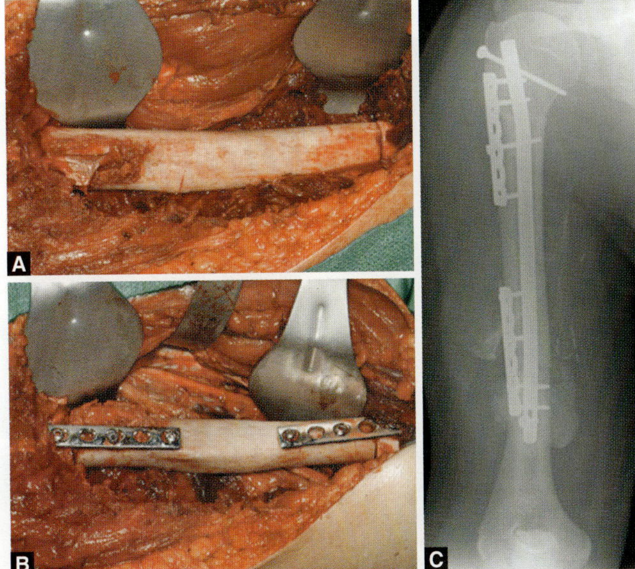

Figs. 38A to C: Allograft: Intercalary humeral allograft in 19-year-old man with Ewing's sarcoma. (A) Allograft is fashioned to fit defect and is fixed with intramedullary nail; (B) Compression plates used to fix proximal and distal junctions; (C) Postoperative radiograph.

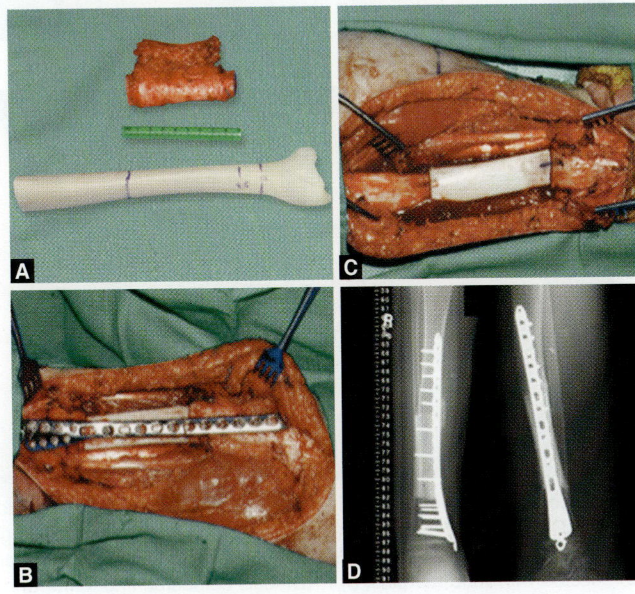

Figs. 39A to D: Allograft in Ewing's sarcoma of tibia.

- Chance of high-risk contamination from bone donor site or storage site.
- Alternative to endoprostheses in limb salvage surgery.
- Complications are delayed union, nonunion, infection, or fracture.
- Can be used with autograft (vascularized fibula graft) and give good results (like early weight bearing or bone strength).
- An allograft prosthesis combination has been used, replacing joint with prosthesis and bone with allograft.

Bone lengthening:

- Bone lengthening uses the principles of epiphyseal distraction.
- In some situation, the bone is stabilized using an external fixator and bone is then transported to fill the defect.
- Time consuming process.
- Only advantage after the surgery patient has a vascularized new bone.
- Time length of the treatment will be approximately 2 month for each centimeter of bone that excised.

Endoprosthetic replacement:

Refer Figures 40A to K.

Arthrodesis:

- Excision and arthrodesis was one of the first types of limb salvage operation carried out for tumor around knee.
- Various methods have been used involving turn up or turn downs of part of the femur or tibia as well as the allograft or fibula graft.
- Advantage is, it is relatively cheap.

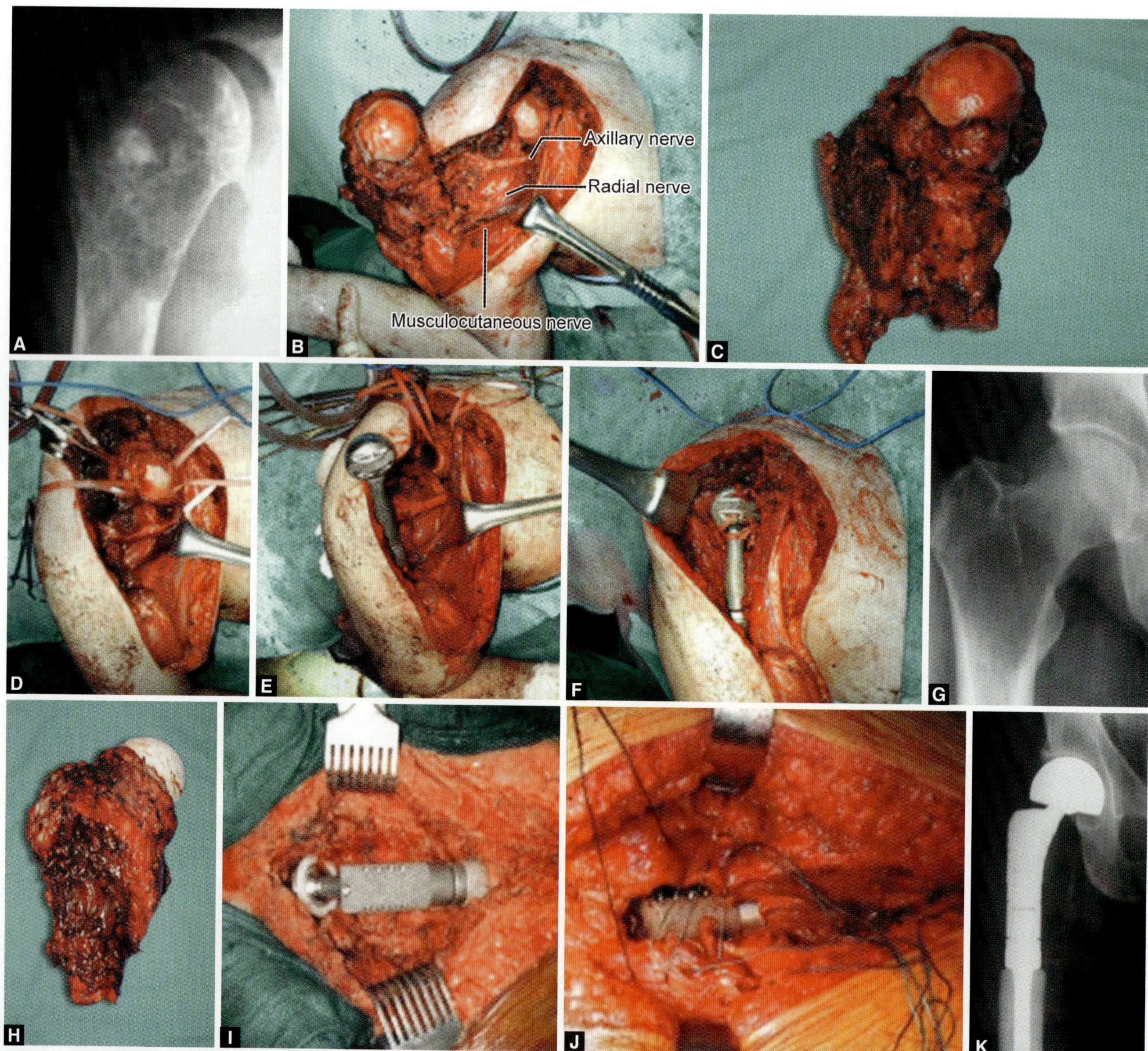

Figs. 40A to K: (A) Radiograph of right proximal humerus of a 47-year-old man with chondrosarcoma; (B) Intraoperative photograph during wide resection of tumor; (C) Resected specimen; (D) Mersilene tapes placed through glenoid labrum; (E) Prosthesis cemented into distal humerus; (F) Humeral head secured by Mersilene tape; (G) Resection of proximal femur with endoprosthetic reconstruction. Malignant tumor in proximal femur; (H) Proximal femur was resected with wide margins; (I) Prosthesis cemented into femur and bipolar component reduced into acetabulum; (J) Abductors and vastus lateralis repaired through holes in prosthesis; (K) Postoperative anteroposterior radiograph.

- Complications are high risk of delayed union or nonunion, fracture, and functional drawbacks like difficulty while sitting.

Rotationplasty

Winkelmann classified rotationplasty into five groups, as follows:

- *Group AI—Lesion in distal femur.* The distal femur, knee joint, and proximal tibia are resected; the lower leg is rotated 180°; and the tibia is joined to the remaining femur (Fig. 41).
- *Group AII—Lesion in the proximal tibia.* The distal most femur, knee joint, and proximal tibia are resected. After rotation of 180°, the distal tibia is joined to the distal femur (Fig. 42).
- *Group BI—Lesion in the proximal femur sparing the hip joint and gluteal muscles.* The upper femur and hip joint are resected, and the leg is rotated 180°. The distal femur is joined to the pelvis so that the knee functions as the hip, and the ankle functions as the knee (Fig. 43).
- *Group BII—Lesion in the proximal femur with involvement of hip joint and contiguous soft tissue.* The upper femur, hip joint, and lower hemipelvis are resected, and the leg is rotated 180°. The remaining femur is joined to the remnant of the ilium so that the knee functions as a hinged hip joint and the ankle functions as the knee (Fig. 44).
- *Group BIII—Lesion in the midfemur.* The entire femur is resected. The tibia is attached to the pelvis using an endoprosthesis (Fig. 45).

Considerations for Pediatric Patients

- The surgical technique for implantation of repiphysis noninvasive expandable prosthesis device is similar to that of other endoprostheses (Figs. 46 and 47).
- The postoperative course, rehabilitation, function, and complications likewise are similar.
- Only Repiphysis noninvasive expandable prosthesis is used in place of normal prosthesis.
- Uses energy stored in a compressed spring to allow for future expansion of the prosthesis as the child grows.

Reepiphysis Lengthening Procedure

- The procedure is done in the fluoroscopy suite with the patient under light sedation (Figs. 48A to F).
- The locking mechanism on the prosthesis is identified using fluoroscopy, and marked.

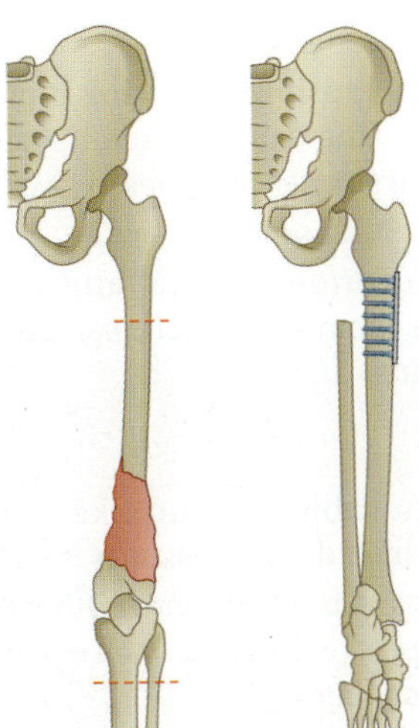

Fig. 41: Rotationplasty Group AI for a lesion in the distal femur.

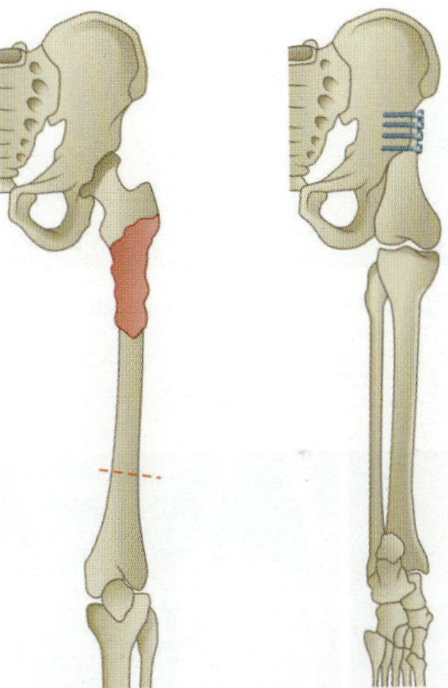

Fig. 43: Rotationplasty Group BI for lesion in proximal femur sparing the hip joint and gluteal muscles.

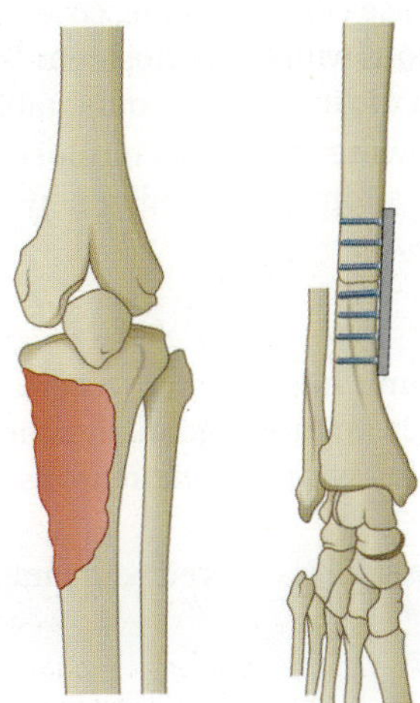

Fig. 42: Rotationplasty Group AII for a lesion in the proximal tibia.

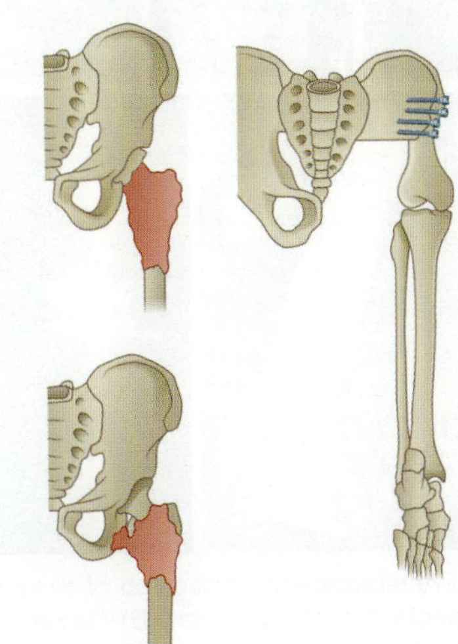

Fig. 44: Rotationplasty Group BII for lesion in proximal femur with involvement of hip joint and contiguous soft tissue.

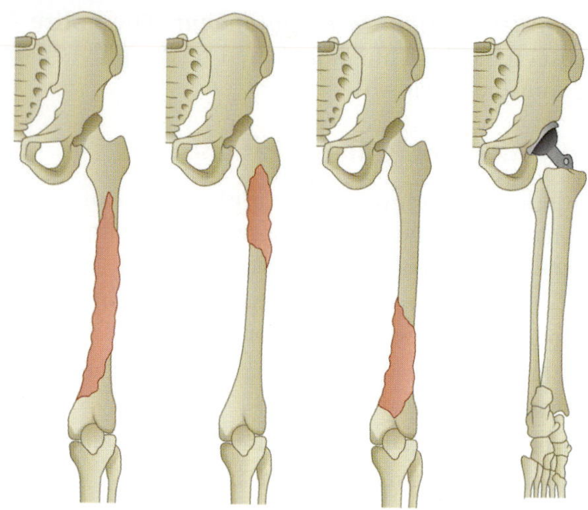

Fig. 45: Rotationplasty Group BIII for lesion in the midfemur.

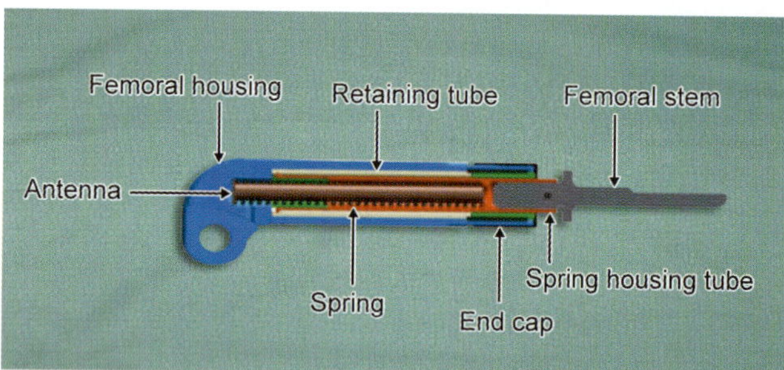

Fig. 46: Repiphysis noninvasive expandable prosthesis.

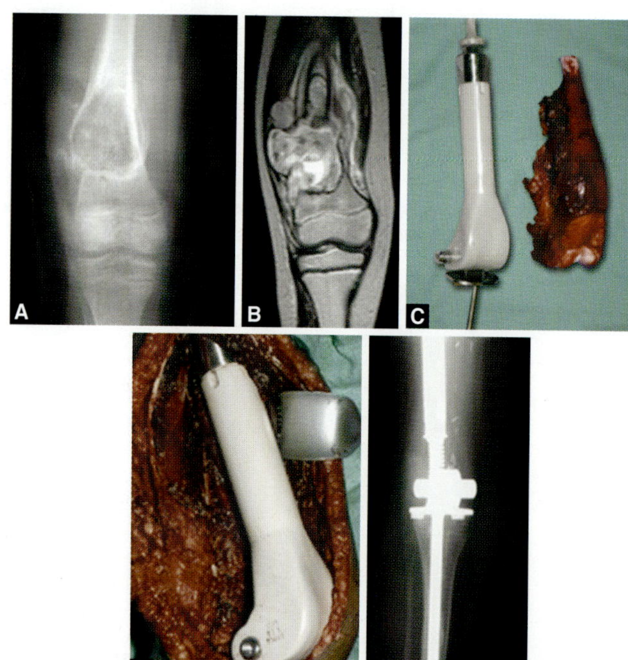

Figs. 47A to E: (A) Anteroposterior radiograph of distal femur of 7-year-old girl with telangiectatic osteosarcoma; (B) Coronal MR image; (C) Intraoperative photograph of resected specimen and custom repiphysis prosthesis; (D) Intraoperative photograph after placement of prosthesis; (E) Anteroposterior radiograph.

- Electromagnetic coil is placed over the patient's leg at that level.
- Electromagnetic coil is activated for 20 seconds, which heats an element in the prosthesis, melting a small segment of polyethylene and allowing controlled expansion of the spring.
- The leg lengths are reevaluated under fluoroscopy, and the procedure is repeated one or two times as necessary.
- Able to gain 0.5–1.5 cm during each scheduled expansion session.
- Patients usually are able to ambulate immediately.

BENIGN TUMORS OF THE BONE

The benign tumors of the bone are:

- Osteoma
- Osteoid osteoma
- Osteoblastoma
- Chondroma
- Chondroblastoma
- Osteochondroma
- Chondromyxoid fibroma
- Aneurysmal bone cyst.

Osteoma

An osteoma is a benign slowly growing tumor, occurring in the membranous bones of the skull and face. Usually it is solitary, found in cranial vault, nasal sinuses or bones of jaw.

- *Age:* Onset is in childhood.
- *Predominant location:* Frontal and facial bones, usually external, but they may be intracranial, intranasal, intraorbital, and within a sinus.

Clinical Features

- It is hard, immovable, mound like or sessile, nontender swelling, over which the soft tissue is freely movable.
- External tumors are asymptomatic. Others produce symptoms referable to the part (e.g. intracranial osteomas cause epileptic seizures and headache).

Pathology

- The most common type of slowly growing osteoma is composed of dense compact bone, covered by a fibrous tissue capsule continuous with the periosteum. The bony structure is continuous with the inner or the outer tables of the skull.
- The rapidly growing tumor is composed of a proliferating vascular fibrous stroma, containing newly formed osteoid or osseous spicules.

Treatment

- Once the osteoma has reached a certain size, it remains stationary. It does not undergo malignant change. Excision is indicated, only for symptomatic reasons, rarely for cosmetic reasons.
- The defect in the skull is covered with tantalum plate.

Osteoid Osteoma

An osteoid osteoma is a benign osteoblastic tumor with a well-demarcated nidus of less than 1 cm, surrounded by a distinct reactive bone.

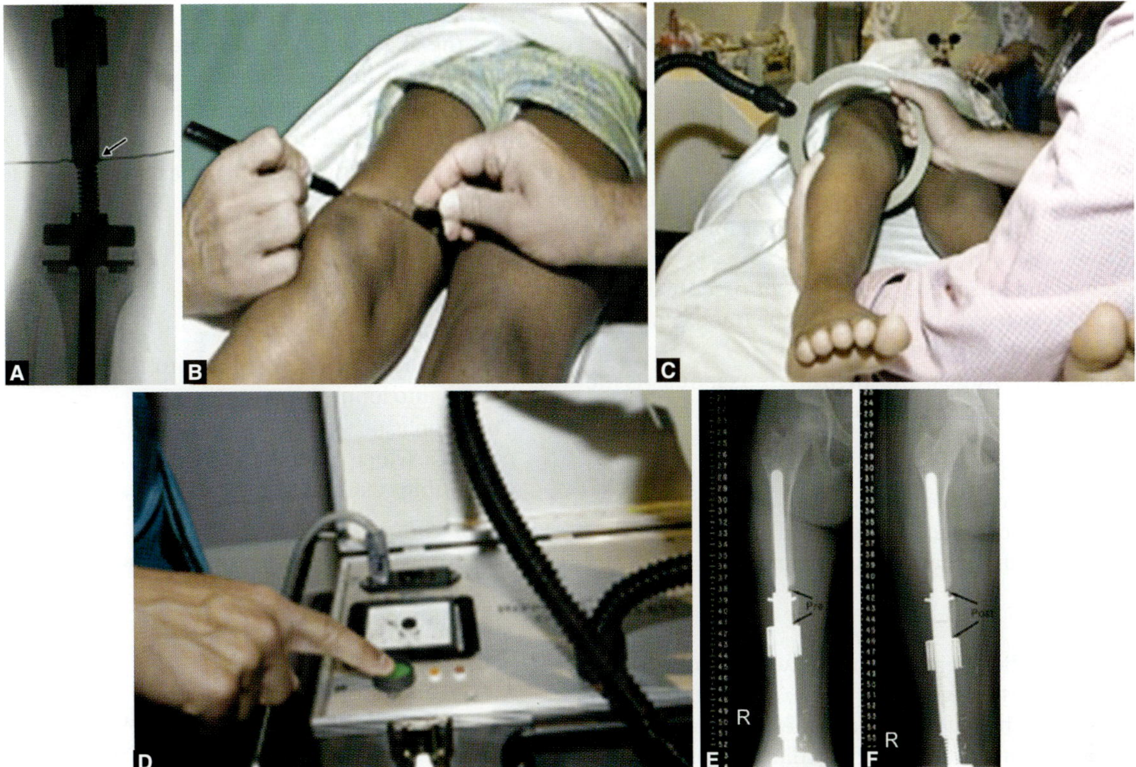

Figs. 48A to F: Lengthening procedure with repiphysis expandable prosthesis.

- *Age:* It is common in young adults between 10 and 25 years of age.
- *Sex:* Male preponderance (male to female ratio is 2:1)
- *Sites:* Long bones usually tibia and femur are more commonly affected.

Clinical Features

- The patient complains of vague and intermittent pain, which is more at night.
- The pain dramatically decreases after giving aspirin, so much so that this is called as the therapeutic test
- Patient complains of limp due to pain.
- There is mild swelling; the local area may be tender; temperature is not raised; and the skin is not stretched, shiny or warm.
- When the lesion occurs in spine, the patient complains of pain.

Radiology

- The classic radiological presentation of an osteoid osteoma is a radiolucent nidus, surrounded by a dramatic reactive sclerosis in the cortex of the bone.
- The center can range from partially mineralized to osteolytic to entirely calcified.
- The lesion can occur only in the cortex, in both the cortex and medulla, or only in the medulla. The reactive sclerosis may be present or absent.

Differential Diagnosis

- Sclerosing nonsuppurative osteomyelitis of Garre
- Brodie's abscess
- Chronic osteomyelitis with annular sequestrum
- Syphilitic ossifying periostitis
- Eosinophilic granulomas.

Treatment

- Complete excision of the nidus immediately and effectively relieves the pain.
- Latest treatments are arthroscopically assisted excision for intra-articular situated lesions, CT-guided endoscopic removal, percutaneous excision, MRI guided cryotreatment, and CT guided biopsy and thermocoagulation.

Osteoblastoma

A benign osteoblastoma also known as osteogenic fibroma of bone or giant osteoid osteoma. It is an uncommon vascular osteoid and bone forming tumor. It is slow growing and causes symptoms by encroachment on neighboring structures.

- *Age:* Young adults, usually less than 20 years of age.
- *Sex:* Male to female ratio is 2:1.
- *Location:* The majority occurs in the spine, affecting the posterior element, the metaphyseal or diaphyseal areas of the long bones of the lower extremities, and the small bones of hand and feet.

Clinical Features

Symptoms

- Dull aching pain, not nocturnal or relieved by aspirin.
- When the tumor involves cervical or thoracic vertebra, the tumor encroaches the spinal cord, so weakness and paresthesia develops.
- Symptoms occur usually from few months to 2 years, before the tumor is discovered.

Signs
- Single tender mass is palpable, when the tumor is superficial.
- Scoliosis and neurological complaints may be present.

Pathology

- Mass is deep red, friable, and gritty. It is richly vascular.
- Microscopically features show a loosely fibrillar and vascular tissue, containing numerous dilated thin walled vascular channels.
- Within the vascular tissue, a profusion of osteoblast lies between sheets of osteoid and primitive bone trabeculae.
- Degree of mineralization of osteoid varies.
- In more advanced stages, the primitive osseous tissue undergoes osteoclastic resorption and replacement by mature lamellar bone.
- Giant cells are prominent; represents osteoclast and macrophages; and are unlike those in giant cell tumors.
- The stromal cells are compact, round, ovoid or spindly, but are distinct, relatively uniform, and mitotic figures are rare.

Radiological Findings

Lesion is essentially radiolucent or mottled, well circumscribed and as it enlarges, the cortex is gradually attenuated, but the tumor is delimited by delicate shell of periosteal bone. Within the tumor, faint stippled densities are noted. Long standing tumors become extremely dense, especially after radiation treatment.

Differential Diagnosis

- Osteoid osteoma
- Osteogenic sarcoma
- Giant cell tumor.

Treatment

- Complete excision results in cure.
- Large defect may be filled with bone grafting.
- Radiotherapy to inaccessible tumors.

Chondroma

It is also known as enchondroma.
- *Age:* 20–30 years of age.
- *Site:* Phalanges of hand and feet, spine, pelvis, and ribs.
- *Location:* About two-thirds of the lesion arise in metaphysic and one third arise in diaphysis.

Clinical Features

- Slight soreness and severe pain occurs, actual from a pathologic or slowly from malignant transformation.
- The phalanges are enlarged as a result of distension of a thinned cortex. In a long bone, no deformity is observed and the tumor remains intramedullary.

Radiological Findings

- X-ray, shows a small translucent loculated or nonloculated area, well demarcated from surrounding bone in a phalanx, the cortex is thinned and expanded. In large long bone cortex is not involved.
- The center may exhibit stippling of calcification and striation of fibrous space. No reactive bone formation is present.
- In small bones of hand and feet the cortex may be perforated and the shadow of the tumor extends into the soft tissues, although the tumor is benign.
- On the other hand, erosion of the cortex in a large tubular bone and spreading externally, strongly suggests malignant change.
- This is particularly true, when the borders of the lesion become mottled and hazy.

Pathology

Macroscopically
- The tumor is surrounded by a fibrous capsule, which on cut section displays extensions into the interior, dividing the growth into lobules.
- The neoplastic tissue is composed of bluish white translucent cartilage, which contains white areas of calcification and cysts containing gelatinous or myxomatous substance.

Microscopically
- The tumor shows stages of formation of cartilage from embryonic tissue.
- The mesenchymal type of tissue is seen only at the periphery of the tumor.
- The most mature cartilage is found in the center of the tumor, where it may undergo the usual degenerative changes of cartilage, namely calcification cystic disintegration and myxomatous change.
- These chondrocytes are normal in appearance.

Treatment

- Tumor is excised or curetted and the wall cauterized.
- The capsule is removed, to reduce the possibility of recurrence.
- Large defect is filled with bone graft.
- Tumors of long bone should be considered as malignant, and radical resection should be done.

Chondromyxoid Fibroma

Chondromyxoid fibroma or fibromyxoid chondroma is a rare tumor of bone, occurring mainly in adolescent and in young adult.
- *Age:* Usually second or third decade and less often in childhood.
- *Sex:* No predominance.
- *Location:* Most commonly, metaphyseal region of large tubular bone of lower limb. May also involve thin tubular bone such as fibula, phalanx, and calcaneum.

Clinical Features

- In adolescent or young adult, the tumor causes mild or no pain.
- Slowly increasing local swelling.
- Palpable tender mass fixed to underlying bone.
- It never metastasizes and sarcomatous degeneration is extremely rare.

Radiological Findings

- The lesion is translucent mass of variable size, usually located eccentrically in the metaphysic.
- On the medullary aspect of the lesion, the margin is scalloped and sclerosed.
- Over the outer aspect, the cortex is expanded and thinned and may appear interrupted.

- In children, at the edge of the tumor, triangular periosteal bone formation, not unlike Codman triangle often forms.
- Within the tumor, a faint trabecular pattern is apparent.
- When the tumor involves the narrow tubular bone or small tubular bone, it generally occupies the entire width of the bone, producing fusiform expansion and thinning of cortex.

Treatment

- Local excision and filling of cavity with autogenous bone graft.
- Curettage is not sufficient because the tumor may recur.
- Wide en bloc excision result in high rate of tumor.

Chondroblastoma

A chondroblastoma is a cellular, vascular, and cartilaginous tumor of young adult, occurring about the epiphyseal line. Destroying cancellous bone and characteristically containing multiple calcium deposits.

- *Age:* Onset occurs before obliteration of epiphyseal line from 10 to 20 years.
- *Sex:* Male predominance.
- *Location:* Ends of long bones, about the knee and humerus.
- *Position:* About one side of epiphyseal line, chiefly in the metaphysic, it may extent to epiphysis.

Clinical Features

- Pain, tenderness, and swelling in most cases
- Occasionally, limp and joint effusion is present.

Radiological Findings

- Lesion begins or is centered within the epiphysis.
- It is oval to round with well-defined borders. The epiphyses are opened at the time of initial presentation.
- They fill less than one half of the epiphyseal end of the bone. The opposite is true for the GCT.
- It is eccentrically positioned.
- Thin ring sclerosis is present around the tumor, with punctated densities in tumor mass.

Treatment

Curettage and obliteration of tumor with bone graft.

Osteochondroma (Exostosis)

It is benign cartilage capped, protuberance of the metaphysis or diaphysis.

- *Age:* With solitary form 75% of the patients are 30 years of age or younger. More than 95% of patients with multiple lesion are younger than 20 years of age.
- *Incidence:* Osteochondroma represents 20% of all benign tumors. Solitary osteochondroma represents 7.9% and multiple variant represents 0.6%.
- *Sex:* Male to female ratio is 1.6:1.

Location

- About 80% of the lesions occur in long bone, particularly around the knee and in upper humerus.
- Pelvis, scapula and ribs are involved in 20% of cases.
- Usually, osteochondromas are metaphyseal for meta-diaphyseal located.

Clinical Features

- Some patients develop pain due to mechanical irritation. Pedunculated osteochondromas can result in irritation of muscle, ligaments or tendons, during motion, nerve compression or fracture through the stalk.
- Lumps can be palpated, which can be painful or painless.
- It can be associated with aneurysm and bursitis.

Hereditary Multiple Exostoses

- Hereditary multiple exostoses (HME) is an autosomal dominant condition, associated with short stature, multiple osteochondromas, and asymmetrical growth at the knees and ankles. It may lead to deformities.
- The leg length inequality is usually about 4 cm and the risk of malignant degeneration is between 1% and 20%.
- The osteochondromas are located close to the metaphyses and they may be sessile or pedunculated.
- The cortex of the lesion is continuous with the cortex of the bone, with a homogeneous continuation of the medulla.

Dysplasia Epiphysealis Hemimelica

- Dysplasia epiphysealis hemimelica (DEH) or Trevor disease is characterized by osteochondromas, arising in the epiphyses and thus involving the joint.
- The lesions are usually restricted to one side of the body, either left or right. Hence, the name hemimelica is used to reflect involvement of one side of the body.
- There may be multiple lesions in a single limb.
- DEH usually occurs in infants or young children.
- DEH primarily involves one side of an epiphysis, the medial side is affected twice as often as the lateral side.
- On macroscopic inspection, the bony lesion is found to be a pedunculated mass closely connected to the epiphysis with a cartilaginous cap.
- The histologic appearances are similar to those of an osteochondroma.

Multiple Epiphyseal Dysplasia

- Multiple epiphyseal dysplasia is another autosomal dominant condition characterized by the presence of irregular epiphyseal ossification, with intracapsular or periarticular chondromas of the knees and ankles.
- This condition is usually present in late childhood.
- The spine is usually normal.

Dominant Carpotarsal Osteochondromatosis

- Dominant carpotarsal osteochondromatosis is another autosomal dominant entity, which Maroteaux and colleagues described in a mother and son.
- The osteochondromas are confined to carpotarsal bones.
- Maroteaux suggested that dominant carpotarsal osteo-chondromatosis is a condition distinct from DEH.
- Dominant carpotarsal osteochondromatosis is usually sporadic.

Pathogenesis

- Osteochondromas develop due to a beaked failure of constriction, with cortical overgrowth adjacent to the growth

plate and subsequent eccentric bony growth from this beak, usually away from the joint.
- The excrescence that forms, then continues to grow until the growth plate closes. Growth ceases at puberty
- Malignant degeneration occurs in 1–25% of cases and should be suspected, if an exostosis rapidly increases in size, especially in an adult.
- Spontaneous resolution of osteochondromas has been described.
- Osteochondromas that continue to grow after puberty, should raise the possibility of chondrosarcomatous transformation.
- The pathogenesis of HME is poorly understood, but many theories have been put forward to explain its development.
- The isolation of islets of cartilaginous tissues from the diaphyseal surface of growing cartilage had been hypothesized to cause abnormal osteogenesis.
- Further theories postulate that osteochondroma formation is related to a defect in the anchoring of germinal cartilage cells to the physes or to the failure of a thin, cortical sleeve of bone, acting as a structural constraint, with this failure, allowing a spillover of physeal cells onto the metaphysis.
- The physical stress theory postulates that focal accumulations of embryonic connective tissue at sites of tendon attachments are converted to hyaline cartilage.

Theories

- Müller supports a clonal etiology and theorizes that osteochondromas result from a primary defect in periosteal differentiation, in which ectopic collections of cartilage cells arise from the proliferative layer of the metaphyseal periosteum. Multipotent mesenchymal cells in the region of the perichondral groove of Ranvier have also been implicated in the development of osteochondromas.
- Langenskiöld believes that proliferative interstitial physeal chondrocytes persist in chondrogenesis, as they are transformed into the proliferative layer of the metaphyseal periosteum.
- Clonal karyotypic abnormalities have been documented in osteochondromas. Studies indicate that the cartilaginous portion of the osteochondroma has a clonal or neoplastic origin.
- Porter and Simpson believe that the osteal portion of the osteochondroma provides only a supportive stroma, an idea that is supported by the fact that ablation of the cartilage cap alone is followed by cessation of growth of the osteochondroma. Currently, however, no molecular or immunohistochemical data supports this observation.
- *The physical-stress theory:* This theory is postulated by Geschickter and Copeland, states that focal accumulations of embryonic connective tissue at sites of tendon attachments are converted to hyaline cartilage.
- *Theory of histogenesis:* Throughout the life, the deep layer of the periosteum retains the potential for forming cartilage or bone, the cambium layer produces an embryonic tissue that is the common forerunner for bone and cartilage, the tumor may represent a perverted activity of the periosteum, which reverts to its role as perichondrium.
- *Neoplastic theory:* Research has shown loss of heterozygosity at the EXT loci in the cartilaginous cap of osteochondromas and in tissue from chondrosarcomas. Further, clonal karyotypic anomalies have been documented in osteochondromas. These studies indicate that the cartilaginous portion of the osteochondroma has a clonal or neoplastic origin.

Radiological Features

- All osteochondromas solitary or multiple are bony protruberance, showing as a pedunculated stalk or sessile. They typically point away from joint.
- The cortical and medullary portion of the tumor is continuous with cortex and medulla of the bone.
- The cartilage covering is invisible, unless it is calcified.

Pathology

- An osteochondroma is composed of two basic parts, a cartilage-capped protruberance, and its bony stalk.
- Bony stalk may be pedunculated or sessile.
- The shape of the cap is usually mushroom like and rounded to irregularly bosselated.
- On cut section large osteochondroma may demonstrate irregular conglomeration of hard, gritty whitish to yellowish areas that contain variably sized fragments of translucent to whitish calcified cartilage.

Treatment

Total excision of the tumor.

Aneurysmal Bone Cyst

- It is a benign, solitary, expansile, and erosive lesion of bone.
- One percent of benign bone lesion.
- *Age:* Most frequent in children (85% cases are less than 20 years old).
- *Sex:* Female to male ratio is 2:1.
- *Location:* Aneurysmal bone cyst (ABC) can be found in any bone of the body. The most common location is metaphysic of the lower extremity long bones, more so than the upper extremity. Approximately one half of the lesions in flat bones occur in pelvis.

Etiology

- Unknown, but ABCs are thought to be a reactive process secondary to trauma or vascular disturbances.
- One theory of primary ABC is that these lesions are secondary to increased venous pressure that leads to hemorrhage, which causes osteolysis. Osteolysis can in turn promote more hemorrhage, causing amplification of cyst.
- Aneurysmal bone cyst can be secondary to underlying disease.
- The most common precursor lesion was giant cell tumor (19–39% of cases), followed by osteoblastoma, angioma, and chondroblastoma.

Pathology

- Macroscopically, an ABC is like a blood filled sponge, with a thin periosteal membrane. Soft fibrous walls separate spaces filled with friable blood clot.
- Microscopically, the ABC has cystic spaces filled with blood. The fibrous septa have immature woven bone trabeculae as well as macrophages, filled with hemosiderin, fibroblast, capillaries, and giant cells.

Clinical Features

- Swelling, tenderness and pain.
- Occasionally, there is a limited range of motion due to joint obstruction.
- Spinal lesion can cause neurological symptoms secondary to cord compression.
- Pathological fractures are rare due to the eccentric location of the lesion.

Differential Diagnosis

- Unicameral bone cyst
- Chondromyxoid fibroma
- Giant cell tumor
- Osteoblastoma
- Telangiectatic osteosarcoma.

Radiographic Features

- ABC is placed eccentrically in the metaphysic and appears osteolytic.
- The periosteum is elevated and the cortex is eroded to a thin margin.
- The expansile nature of the lesion is often reflected by a "blow-out" or soap bubble appearance.
- Pencil-in-cup appearance.

Radiological Classification of Aneurysmal Bone Cyst (Companacci's Classification)

- *Type I:* Cyst in middle with little or no expansion.
- *Type II:* Lesion substitutes the whole bone segment.
- *Type III:* Eccentric interosseous lesion with little or no expansion.
- *Type IV:* Subperosteal cyst and superficial erosion of cortex.
- *Type V:* Periosteum eroded and expansion into soft tissue.

Treatment

- Curettage with bone grafting
- Curettage with cementing
- Cryosurgery
- En bloc excision with or without reconstruction of skeletal defect.

GIANT CELL TUMOR

- Giant cell tumor (GCT) is a benign but aggressive lesion consisting of osteoclast-like giant cells, fibroblast-like stromal cells, and blood vessels. This originates within epiphysis of adult bones.
- This is histologically composed of proliferating mononuclear cells and osteoclast-like multinucleated giant cells.

To be differentiated from other giant cell containing lesions: (Giant Cell Variance)

- Chondroblastoma (Codman tumor)
- Osteochondroma and osteoblastoma
- Chondromyxoid fibroma
- GCT of Paget's disease
- Brown tumor of hyperparathyroidism
- Nonossifying fibroma
- Aneurysmal bone cyst and unicameral bone cyst
- Fibrous dysplasia
- Admantinoma
- Metastatic carcinoma with Giant cell
- Pigmented villonodular synovitis of bone
- Secondary sarcomatous changes can occur especially after previous surgery or irradiation, usually an osteosarcoma, malignant fibrous histiocytoma, or a fibrosarcoma.
- *Incidence:* 5% of all skeletal tumors and 21% of benign ones.
- *Age:* Skeletally mature individuals. Peak incidence in third decade of life (20–50 years) and 10% are from 15 to 20 years age. About 98% in epiphyseal plate.
  - 30 and 45 years of age with a female predominance
- *Sex:* Slight predominance in females, 1.3:1.
- *Sites:* Ends of long bone.
  - Epiphysis of long bones and may extend into the metaphysis.
  - Most GCTs occur after physeal closure in the involved bone.
  - *Common sites:* Knee, tibial plateau, femoral condyle, distal radius.
  - *Uncommon sites:* Sacrum, distal tibia, proximal femur and proximal fibula.
  - *Rare Sites:* Bone of hand, vertebra, and ribs.

Pathology

- Grossly the tumor consists of ragged, friable, and bleeding tissue filled with old or fresh blood clot with various sized cysts and cavities.
- Eccentric or central tumor, expanded cortex which is undergone resorption.
- Gray to reddish brown in color, soft vascular friable tissue.
- Epiphyseal end of the bone is distorted.
- Tumor extension in the joint cavity is usually not seen and there is no evidence of periosteal reaction.
- Tumor covered by thin sheet of new subperiosteal bone.
- Areas of necrosis and hemorrhage resulting in cystification mimics aneurysmal bone cyst.
- Microscopically the tumor is encompassed by a fibrous capsule at the periphery.
- Presence of abundant tumor giant cells is quite characteristic.
- These cells are characteristic by their larger size, multiple nuclei more than 150 in number which are distributed throughout the cell.
- Appearance of spindle cell indicates malignant potential.

Histology

- Vascularized network with two types of cells.
- *Stromal cells:* Round, oval or spindle shaped cells.
- Single large nucleus surrounded by indistinct cytoplasm.

Multinucleated Giant Cells

- Nuclei similar to stromal cells, variable in numbers.
- Mitosis and intravascular invasion does not necessarily represent malignant nature.
- Osteoid production and ossification are in small foci particularly at periphery.
- Correlation between histologic appearance and biologic behavior proved unreliable.

Histological Grading (Jaffe's Criterion)

- *Grade 1:*
  - Presence of characteristic stromal cells <30%
  - Little intercellular collagen
  - Spindle cells are adjacent to the necrotic tissue.

- *Grade II:* Random distribution of giant cell are seen among the stromal cell >30% to <50%.
- *Grade III:* Nuclei of giant Cell are identical to those of the stromal cells >50%.

Enneking Staging of Benign GCT

Stage 1 (Latent)
- Incidence is 10–15%
- Discovered accidentally, no symptoms
- Pathological fractures may be present.

Stage 2 (Active)
- Incidence is 70%
- Symptomatic, pathological fracture may be present
- Benign

Stage 3 (Aggressive)
- Incidence is 10–15%
- Symptomatic rapidly growing
- Benign, cortex is perforated.

Clinical Presentation

- The course of the tumor is chronic.
- Unlike osteogenic sarcoma, pain is not the presenting feature but history of trauma is there, the patient complains of swelling which is situated on one side of the bone.
- Skin over the tumor is stretched but there are no dilated veins.
- Tenderness is moderate or absent.
- Egg shell crackling sensation may be present or absent.
- Invasion in the joint is rare and joint effusion is rare.
- Pathological fracture is a late feature.
- Local tissue seeding or may spread to lungs.

Diagnosis

Radiography (Figs. 49A and B)

- Lytic lesion in epiphyseal region involving metaphysis.
- Expansile growth with thin shell of subperiosteal new bone.
- No gross periosteal reaction unless pathological fracture.
- Tumor matrix shows no mineralization.
- Multiple septa may give rise to "soap bubble" appearance.

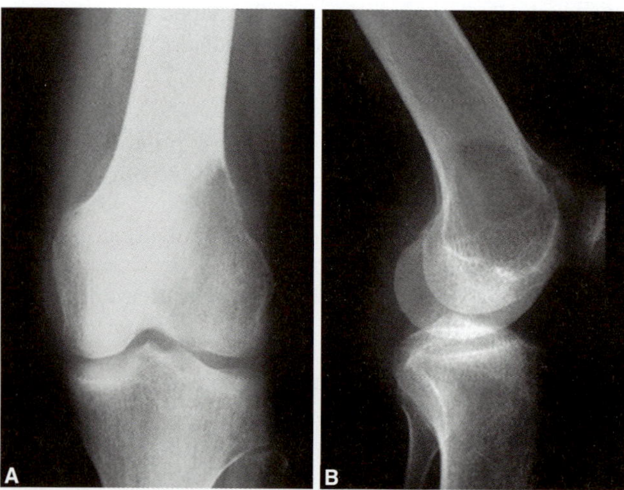

Figs. 49A and B: Radiological features of giant cell tumor.

Radionuclide Scintigraphy

- Increased uptake of Technetium-99m
- False uptake in adjacent areas may occur
- Hence nonspecific and unreliable in defining the extent of tumor
- May be useful in rare multiple lesions.

Angiography

- Seldom used as diagnostic modality
- Useful in determining the relationship with major vessel preoperatively
- Effect of embolization.

Computed Tomography

- Useful in determining cortical integrity, extraosseous extension, and its relation to adjacent structures and tumor recurrence.
- Distinction between tumor and muscle tissue is difficult.

Magnetic Resonance Imaging

- Best imaging modality due to superior contrast resolution.
- Intramedullary tumor best seen in T1-weighted images.
- Extraosseous portion best seen in T2-weighted images.
- Useful in determining joint involvement.
- Cortical integrity and recurrence are best seen on CT than MRI.

Biopsy
- Needle biopsy (Tru Cut) under fluoroscopic visualization is preferred to surgical
- Accuracy is almost up to 90%.

Treatment

The most accepted form of treatment is surgical excision by various ways.

Intralesional Excision

- Curettage is usually supplemented by bonegrafts (autografts or allografts).
- Even careful and through curettage can leave behind microscopic disease especially in walls.
- Recurrence rate has been as high as 40–60%.
- Complete deroofing the tumor, total exteriorization of contents and extensive irrigation are important steps.
- Sequential use of sharp instruments or high-speed burr is desirable.

Intralesional excision with adjuvant therapy
- Addition of adjuvants can extend the margin of excision.
- Commonly used adjuvants are phenol, liquid nitrogen or methylmethacrylate (cement).
  - *Phenol:* Chemical agent applied to wall after curettage (recurrence is 25%)
  - *Liquid nitrogen:* Physical means (cryosurgery) (recurrence is 10% but more complications compared to PMMA and on lay bone grafts)
  - *Methylmethacrylate:* (PMMA) more accepted mode.
- Exothermic reaction generating local heat induces necrosis of remaining neoplastic tissue.
- Polymerization of methylmethacrylate may produce local cytotoxic effect.
- Prevents diffusion of nutrients and lowers local oxygen tension.

- Local relapse as low as 10%.
- CO_2 *laser:* As adjuvant—limited experience.

Wide Local or Marginal Excision

- Most desired form of treatment especially in aggressive lesions.
- It is advisable to go beyond the tumor margin and reactive zone.
- Extra-articular excision and even local synovectomy should be done if any doubt.

Enneking System

- IA—local wide resection
- IB—wide amputation
- IIA—local radical resection
- IIB—radical amputation

Reconstruction:

- Defect after resection of large mass at the end of long needs reconstruction
- Can be achieved in following ways:
  - *Reconstruction with prosthesis:* Using custom made prosthesis.
  - Young age, in which this disease is common, restricts these indications.
  - *Biologic reconstruction:* Arthrodesis using autograft (turn-up or turn-down)
  - Using fibula as substitute or radius.
  - Using massive allografts.
  - Bone transport using Ilizarov technique.

Resection-arthrodesis for malignant and potentially malignant lesions about the knee using an intramedullary rod and local bone grafts—Enneking and Shirley (Figs. 50A to J).

Resection and Reconstruction

Refer Figures 51A to L.

Amputation

As a last resort if growth is extensive or intramedullary spread or a recurrence or the malignant changes.

Chemotherapy

There are no effective chemotherapeutic agents available.

Radiotherapy

- Close association with secondary sarcomatous changes.
- With new super voltage therapy with different particle or secondary tumor.
- Should also be considered in sites like spine or sacrum.
- Tumor dose of 1,500–5,000 rads given in divided doses in 5–6 weeks is considered adequate.

Tumor Embolization

Preoperative

- Done in large vascular growths to reduce the tumor mass and vascularity.
- Selective injection of Gelfoam or polyvinyl alcohol into arteries supplying the tumor.
- Done 1–5 days prior.

Therapeutic

- Done in unresectable tumors of sacrum or spine.
- Done at month interval till pain occurs (three or four times)
- *Risk:* Ischemic injury to nerves and spinal cord.

OSTEOGENIC SARCOMA (OSTEOSARCOMA)

- It is the most common malignant primary bone tumor arising from multipotent mesenchymal tissue of bone.
- It is characterized by direct formation of immature bone or osteoid by proliferating tumor cells.
- *Incidence:* 1/75,000 of the population.
  - Common primary malignant bone tumor next to multiple myeloma.
  - The peak incidence is in the adolescent years, but a second peak is seen in advanced age.
  - Occurs in young, between 10 and 20 years, mostly second decade. Rare before 10 years.
  - Male predominance, when seen in females starts at early age.
  - Male to Female ratio is 3:2 *(with the exception that parosteal osteosarcoma is more common in females).*

Pathology

- Grossly, it is hard, immovable, mound like or sessile, nontender swelling, over which the soft tissue is freely movable.
- It is a large tumor with areas of destruction and gives an appearance of "leg of mutton".
- At the areas of rapid growth, there are areas of cavitation, necrotic foci, and hemorrhages.
- Sunray appearance seen is due to the bone deposition along the vessels (Figs. 52A and B).
- Consistency range from hard to soft.
- Color of tumor could be white, if fibroblastic, yellowish- white, if osteoblastic, and bluish, if cartilaginous (Figs. 53A to C).
- Codman triangle is the subperiosteal reactive new bone formation parallel to the bone.
- Thus there are two types of new bone formation—(1) tumor new osteoid or bone formation along blood vessels (sunray/ sunburst appearance); (2) Codman triangle reactive new bone formation (Figs. 54A and B).

History

- English Surgeon John Abernathy in 1804 introduced the term "Sarcoma" derived from Greek roots meaning "fleshy excrescence" (Peltier, 1993).
- In 1805, the French Surgeon Alexis Boyer (personal surgeon to Napoleon) first used the term "Osteosarcoma" (Rutkow, 1993; Peltier, 1993).
- Ernest Amory Codman (along with James Ewing and Joseph Bloodgood) created the Registry of Bone Sarcoma in 1921in USA to study these tumors (Mallon, 2000).
- By the mid-1900s, Henry L Jaffe and Lichtenstein established virtually all of the key histologic criteria that are used to diagnose most of the bone tumors.
- A different Dr Jaffe (Norman Jaffe), used chemotherapeutic agents in the 1970s and 1980s. For example, Adriamycin and methotrexate (Link 1986, Jaffe N 1998)
- An Orthopedic Surgeon William F Enneking introduced his surgical staging system for musculoskeletal sarcomas (Enneking, 1980).

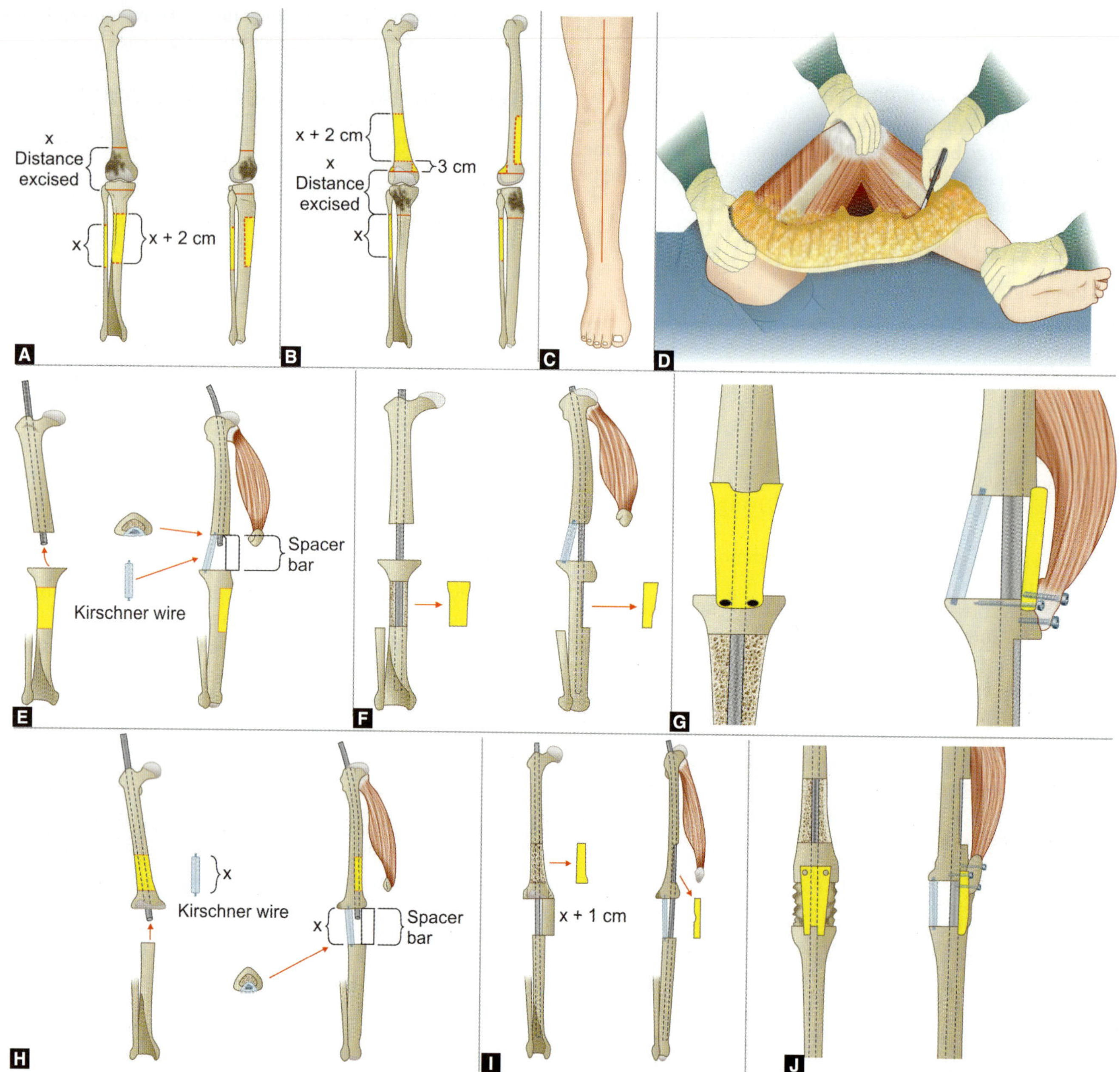

Figs. 50A to J: (A and B) General plan for resection-arthrodesis of femoral and tibial areas showing resection sites (broken lines) and grafts (yellow areas): (A) Femoral lesion and (B) Tibial lesion; (C) Midline incision for exposure; (D) Development of medial and lateral flaps; (E) Rod has been inserted retrograde into femur; posterior fibular graft with medullary pin in place is advanced 1 cm into cancellous bone of tibia, and spacer block is inserted before driving rod down tibia; (F) Rod is in place, and the tibial cortical graft has been removed, leaving a tibial metaphyseal bridge; (G) Anterior graft from tibia is inserted into slot in femur proximally, countersunk into tibial bridge distally, and fixed with two screws. In a through-the-knee resection, posteriorly decorticated patella also is fixed over distal end of graft with two screws. (H to J) Technique for arthrodesis after resection of tibial lesion: (H) Rod has been inserted retrograde into femur; posterior fibular graft, x cm in length (x being length of gap), is pushed into cancellous bone of femur. Spacer block, x – 1 cm long, is placed in gap, and rod is driven distally down tibia; (I) Rod is in place, and femoral cortical graft has been removed, leaving femoral metaphyseal cortical bridge; (J) Anterior graft from femur is inserted into slot in tibia distally, countersunk in femoral bridge proximally, and fixed with two screws. In through-the-joint resection, decorticated patella also is fixed over distal end of graft with two screws.

Etiology

- The exact cause of osteosarcoma is unknown.
- Risk factors are rapid bone growth,
- Environmental factors, e.g. exposure to radiation and genetic predisposition (Clark, 2008)
- Known causative agents are divided into chemicals, viruses, radiation, and miscellaneous (Fuchs and Pritchard, 2002)
- Chemical factors, e.g. beryllium compounds and 20 methyl cholanthrene act by leading to genetic alterations.
- *Virus:*
  - RNA: Harvey and Moloney mouse virus
  - DNA: Polyomavirus and SV40
- *Radiation:* A dose of 2,000 rads if given to osteoprogenitor cells situated in the area of active growth at the metaphysis, malignancy sets in.

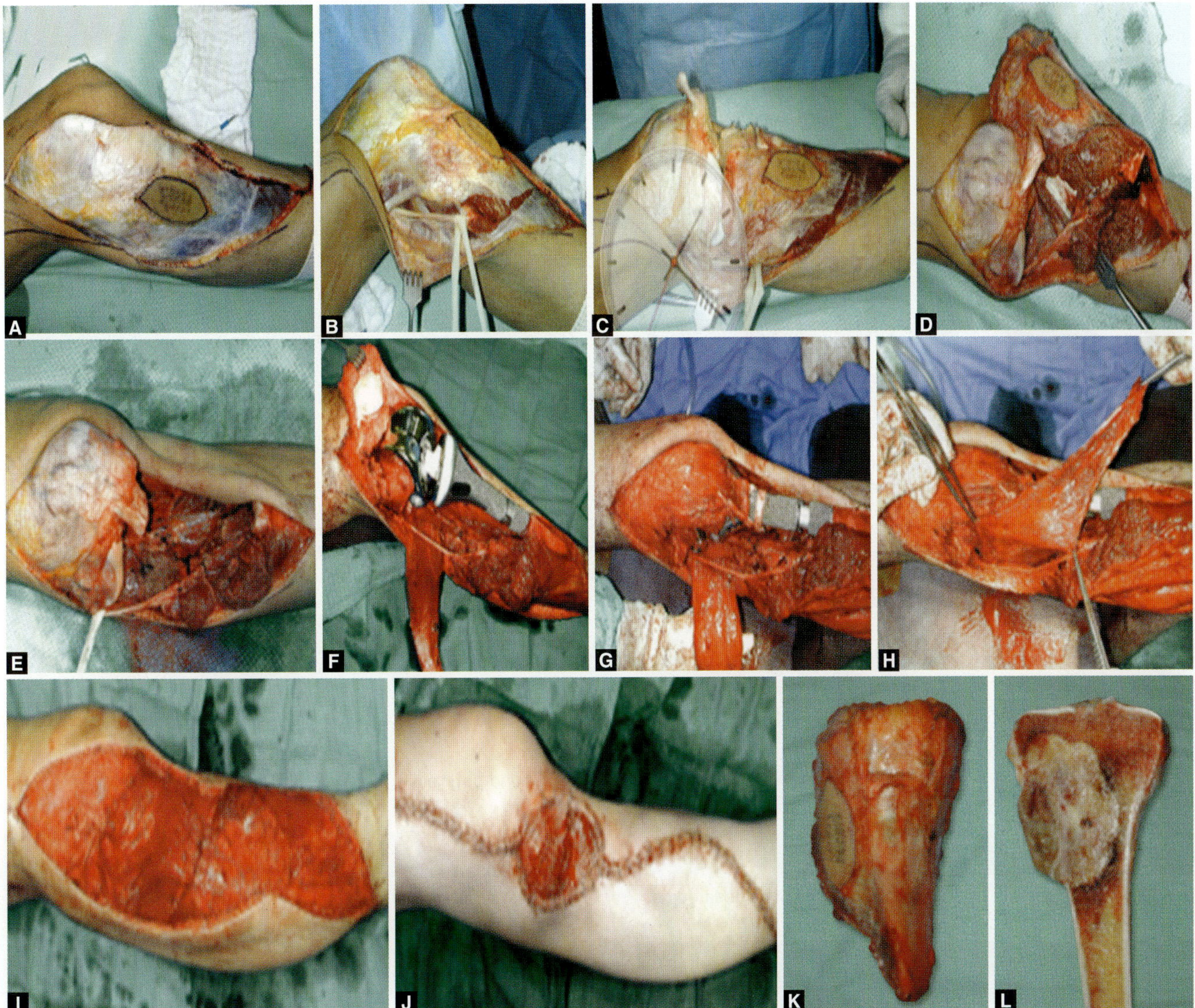

Figs. 51A to L: (A) Incision made, taking care to remove biopsy track en bloc with tumor; (B) Common peroneal nerve isolated and protected; (C) Joint capsule incised and patellar tendon reflected proximally; (D) Distal tibial cut made and tumor rotated so that posterior tibial neurovascular bundle can be dissected free; (E) Specimen removed; (F) Knee reconstructed with modular proximal tibial prosthesis with rotating hinge; (G) Patellar tendon secured to porous-coated surface of prosthesis; (H and I) Lateral gastrocnemius flap raised and sutured over repaired extensor mechanism. This creates secure soft-tissue sleeve that increases strength of knee extension and decreases problems with wound heal; (J) Split-thickness skin graft placed over gastrocnemius flapping; (K) Resected proximal tibia with biopsy track intact; (L) Cut specimen after removal of soft tissue.

- Role of radiation in osteosarcoma is best delineated by its association with formation of secondary sarcomas occurring years after radiation treatment (Enzinger, 1995)
- Genetic alteration includes mutation of retinoblastoma (RB) gene and *p53* gene (tumor suppressor). Loss of function of this gene allows cells to grow unregulated, leading to formation of certain cancers, including osteosarcoma (Ladanyi, 2003)
- Human epidermal growth factor receptor (HER-2 or ERB-2) is another molecular alteration associated with osteosarcoma. Its overexpression is associated with a more clinically aggressive tumor, increased metastatic potential, shorter recurrence-free intervals and worse overall survival rates (Ferrari, 2004).
- *Sites:*
  - It tends to be a disease of the metaphysis (91%) or diaphysis (<9%).
  - Distal end of femur.
  - Proximal end of tibia.
  - Proximal end of humerus.
  - May affect the jaws in the aged.
  - *Location:* About 58% in femur, 9% in greater trochanter, 8% in tibia and 14% in humerus. It is common in the upper aspect but rare below deltoid tuberosity (Fig. 55).

Differential Diagnosis (Fig. 56)

- Giant cell tumor
- Osteomyelitis
- Ewing's sarcoma
- Chondroblastoma
- Osteoblastoma
- Stress fracture
- Post-traumatic callus.

Other to be considered:

- Osteochondroma (parosteal osteosarcoma)

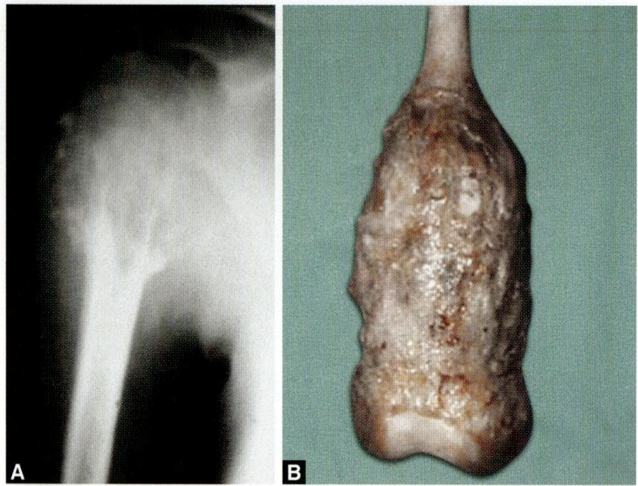

Figs. 52A and B: Sunray appearance seen is due to the bone deposition along the vessels.

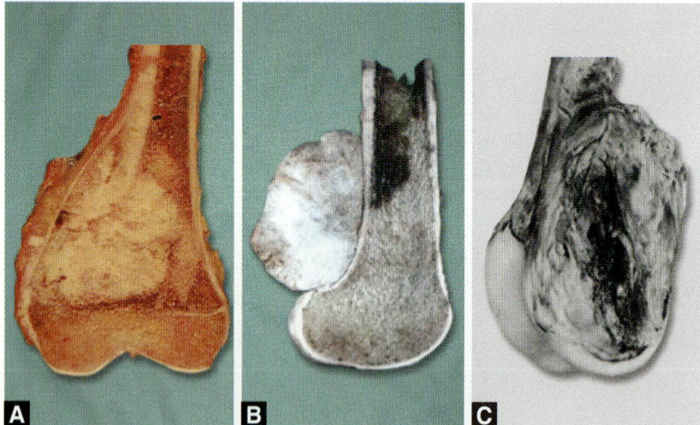

Figs. 53A to C: Different colors in different types of osteosarcoma.

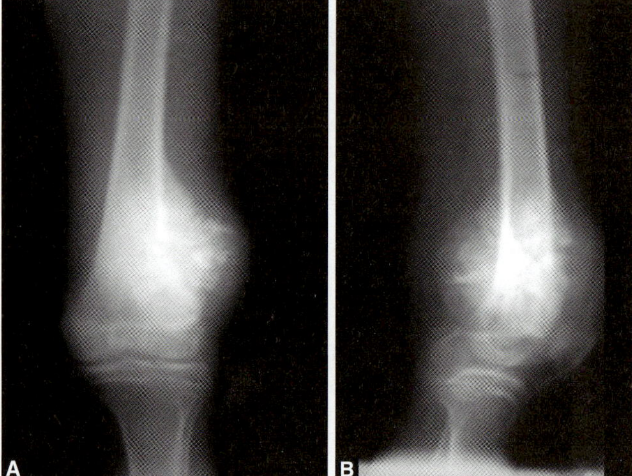

Figs. 54A and B: Radiological features of osteogenic sarcoma.

- Myositis ossificans (parosteal osteosarcoma)
- Aneurysmal bone cyst (telangiectatic osteosarcoma).

Classification of Osteosarcoma

Primary Osteosarcomas

- Conventional osteosarcoma
- Low-grade intramedullary osteosarcoma

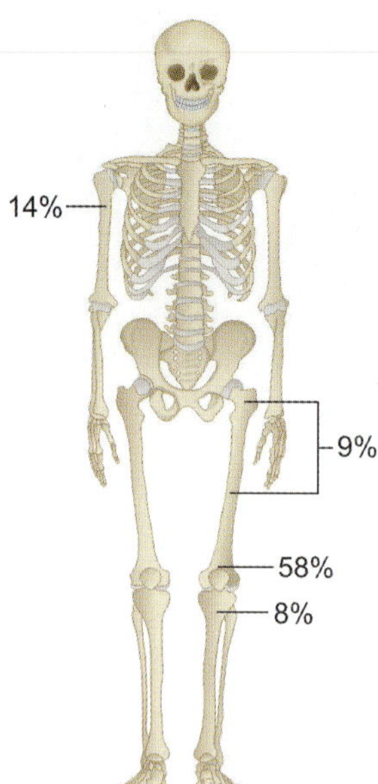

Fig. 55: Percentage of distribution of the tumor according to the location.

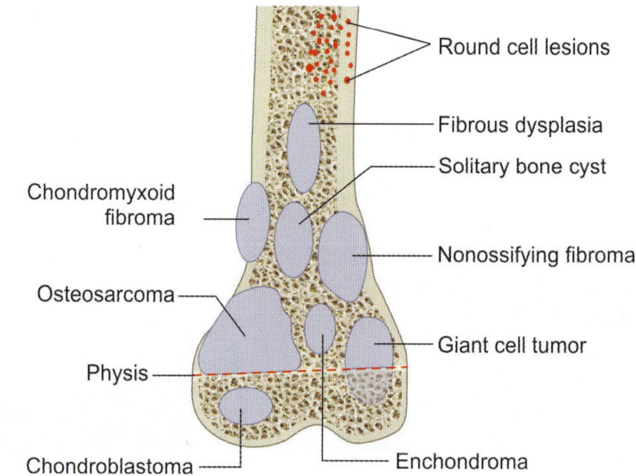

Fig. 56: Differential diagnosis according to location of tumor in the bone.

- Parosteal osteosarcoma
- Periosteal osteosarcoma
- High-grade surface osteosarcoma
- Telangiectatic osteosarcoma
- Small cell osteosarcoma
- Surface (juxtacortical) osteosarcoma.

Secondary Osteosarcoma

- Postirradiation
- Paget's sarcoma
- Solitary/multiple osteochondromatosis
- Bone infarction
- Chronic osteomyelitis
- *Miscellaneous*—GCT, fibrous dysplasia, chondroblastoma, osteoblastoma
- *Rare osteosarcoma:*
  - Li-Fraumeni syndrome (p53 mutation in association with retinoblastoma)
  - Osteosarcoma of the jaw
  - Multicentric osteosarcoma.

Other Classifications

Dahlin's (prognostic) Classification

- Osteoblastic—poor 5 years survival rate
- Chondroblastic—5 years survival rate is 3 times more than osteoblastic variety.
- Fibroblastic—5 years survival rate, 2 times more than osteoblastic variety.

Geschickter and Copeland Classification

- Sclerosing type
- Osteolytic type
- Mixed type with both osteoblastic and osteolytic varieties
- Telangiectatic type.

Lichtenstein Criteria

It is to identify osteogenic sarcoma, includes the following:

- Sarcomatous stroma
- Spindle cells
- Direct formation of neoplastic osteoid and bone.

Staging

- The staging system devised and introduced by Enneking in 1980s is applied to all musculoskeletal tumors.
- The key components to the staging system are the histologic grade of the tumor (low grade vs. high grade), the anatomic location of the tumor (intracompartmental vs. extracompartmental), and the absence or presence of metastatic disease.
- A compartment may be defined as any individual bone, intra-articular space and clearly identified fascially enclosed space (*see* Table 10).

Clinical Presentation (Figs. 57 and 58)

Pain

- The pain may be progressive for many months, and initially be confused with more common sources such as muscle soreness, overuse injury or "growing pains."
- Night pain is an important clue to the true diagnosis (25%).
- The primary reason for delay in the diagnosis is failure to obtain radiographs at the initial visit.
- *Pain that fails to resolve or is present at rest or wakes the patient from sleep should alert the clinician that further evaluation is needed.*

Swelling

- Palpable mass is noted in up to one-third of patients at the first visit.
- Bony swelling appears after some weeks.
- Swelling progressively increases in size.

Limp

In smaller children, a limp may be the only symptom. And also *restriction* of movement of the adjacent joint.

Pathological Fracture

This can increase the rate of local recurrence of the tumor after surgery and decrease the patient's overall survival.

Fever, malaise or other constitutional symptoms are not typical features of osteosarcoma.

General Examination

- General health deteriorates with anemia, loss of weight, and cachexia.
- Patient develops pulmonary symptoms due to secondaries.

On examination:

- Swelling is fusiform
- Skin is stretched, shiny, and vascular, with prominent veins
- Swelling is warm to touch and show pulsation if tumor is highly vascular
- It is firm to hard in consistency
- In late stages tumor fungates.

Workup

Important laboratory studies include the following:

- *Full blood count:* Anemia
- *ESR, CRP:* Infections
- *Lactate dehydrogenase (LDH):* A high rate of turnover with destroyed cells leading to an elevated LDH activity; elevated level is associated with poor prognosis.

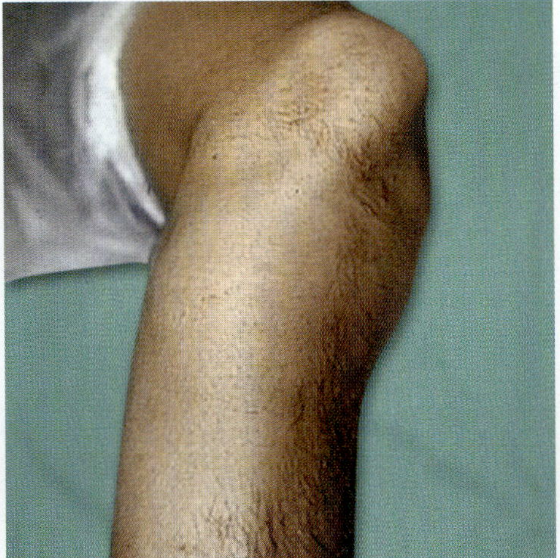

Fig. 57: Photographic representation of the clinical appearance of the upper part of leg medial side affected.

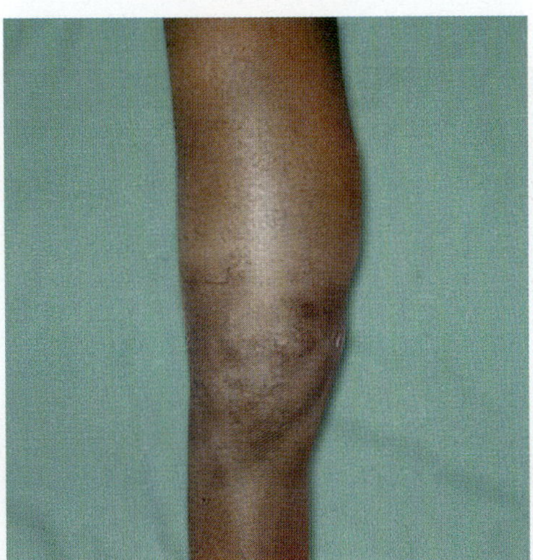

Fig. 58: Photographic representation of the clinical appearance of the lower part of the thigh front and medial side affected.

- *Serum alkaline phosphatase (ALP)* signifies increased activity of bone cells—postoperative, post-amputation, post-chemotherapy, follow-up, if levels are elevated at diagnosis signify increased risk of pulmonary metastasis.
- *Serum acid phosphatase* is increased in tumors, like metastatic tumors.
- *Osteocalcin A*—may be of value in diagnosing osteosarcoma.
- Platelet count
- Electrolyte levels—serum calcium and phosphorous are increased.
- Liver function tests
- Renal function tests
- Urinalysis.

Imagining Studies

- Plain X-rays
- Obtain plain films of the suspected lesions in two views. With joint above and joint below.
- Lesions are usually permeative, associated with destruction of the cancellous and cortical elements of the bone, and show ossification within the soft tissue component.
- Chest X-ray to rule out secondaries is a must.

Radiological Features (see Figs. 54A and B)

- Tumor arises from metaphyseal region of the bone either centrally or from cortex.
- Mottled area of rarefaction with areas of osteosclerosis.
- The classic radiological presentation of a well demarcated nidus of less than 1 cm, surrounded by a distinct reactive bone.
- When it extends beyond the cortex, the periosteum is raised and there is new bone formation in lines at right angle to the cortex this cause sunray appearance on X-ray (approximately 60% of cases) (Fig. 59).
- Codman triangle is seen at the junction of normal bone and tumor area; it is a reactive new bone formation subperiosteally (Fig. 60).
- Telangiectatic osteosarcomas are often very cystic and can be mistaken for an aneurysmal bone cyst (hence biopsy is needed) (Figs. 61A to F).
- Chest X-ray may show secondaries in chest.
- Osteosarcoma lesions can be purely osteolytic (30%), purely osteoblastic (45%), or a mixture of both (Figs. 62A to C).
- *CT scanning:* CT scan of the chest is more sensitive than plain film radiography for assessing pulmonary metastases (Fig. 63A).
- *MRI:* MRI of the primary lesion is the best method to assess the extent of intramedullary disease as well as associated soft tissue masses and skip lesions (Fig. 63B).
- *Bone scan:* A bone scan should be obtained to look for skeletal metastases or multifocal disease (Fig. 63C).
- *Thallium scan:*
  - Monitor effects of chemotherapy
  - Detect local recurrence of tumor.
- *Angiography:*
  - Determine vascularity of the tumor
  - Detect vascular displacement and determine relationship of vessels to the tumor.
- Identify vascular anomalies
- Estimate effects of chemotherapy.

Once all the initial imaging and laboratory examination have been done biopsy is performed to confirm the diagnosis (Figs. 64A and B).

BIOPSY

Principles of Biopsy

- A biopsy should be planned as carefully as the definitive procedure.
- Biopsy should be done only after complete clinical, laboratory, and radiographic examinations.
- The biopsy track should be considered contaminated with tumor cells and should be excised en bloc with the tumor.
- If a tourniquet is used, the limb may be elevated before inflation but should not be exsanguinated by compression.
- Transverse incisions should be avoided.
- The deep incision should go through a single muscle compartment.
- Soft-tissue extension of a bone lesion should be sampled, if possible.
- No important neurovascular structures should be exposed
- If a hole must be made in the bone, it should be round or oval to minimize stress concentration and prevent a subsequent fracture.
- The hole should be plugged with methylmethacrylate to limit hematoma formation.
- Biopsy should be taken from the periphery of a lesion as it usually contains the most viable tissue.
- A frozen section should be sent intraoperatively to ensure that diagnostic tissue has been obtained.

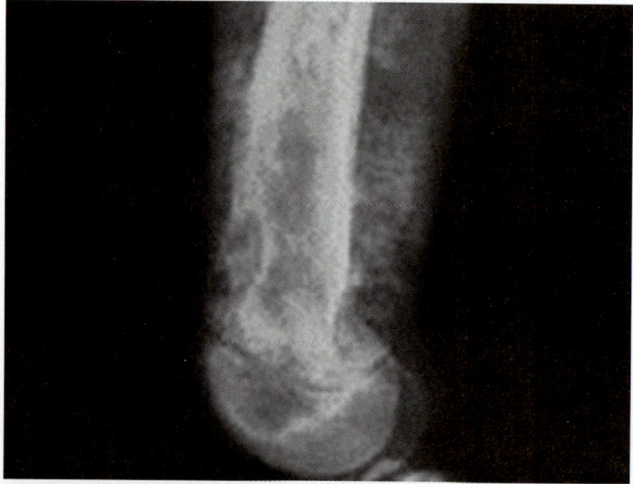

Fig. 59: Sunburst appearance.

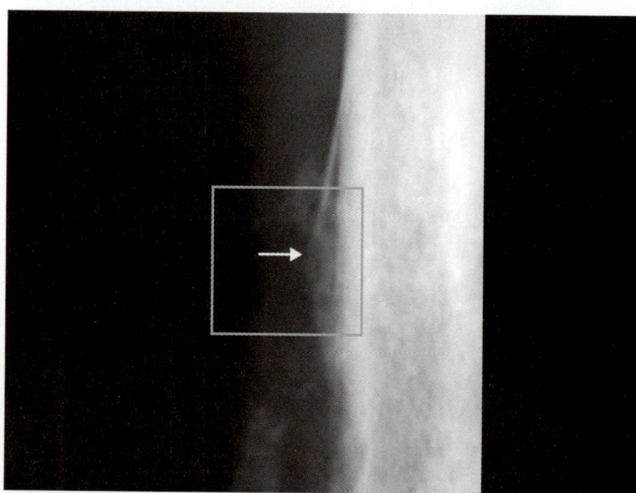

Fig. 60: Codman triangle.

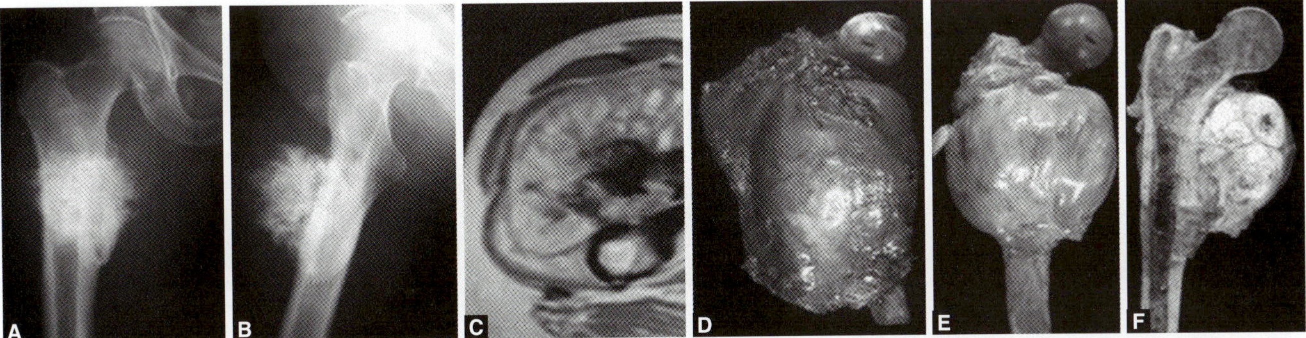

Figs. 61A to F: Telangiectatic osteosarcomas which require biopsy to confirm the diagnosis and differentiate from aneurysmal bone cyst.

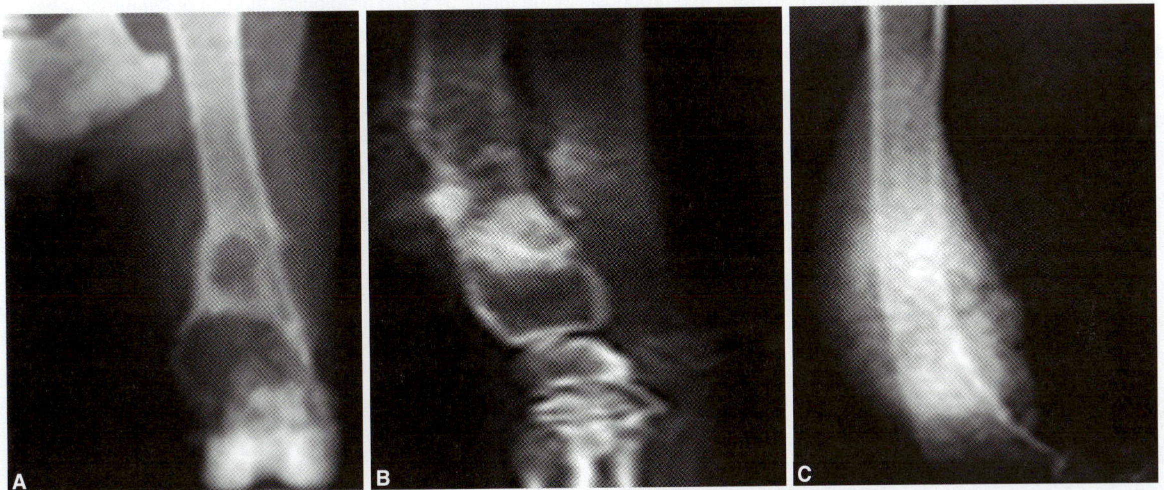

Figs. 62A to C: Osteosarcoma. (A) Purely osteolytic; (B) Purely osteoblastic; (C) Mixture of both.

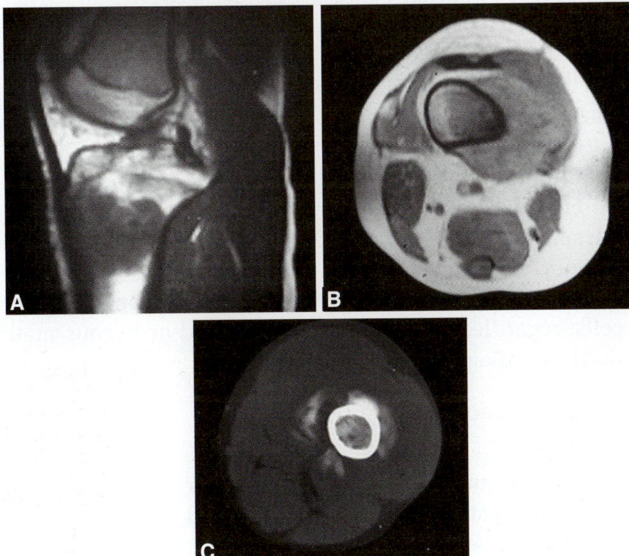

Fig. 63A to C: (A) CT scan; (B) MRI; (C) Bone scan.

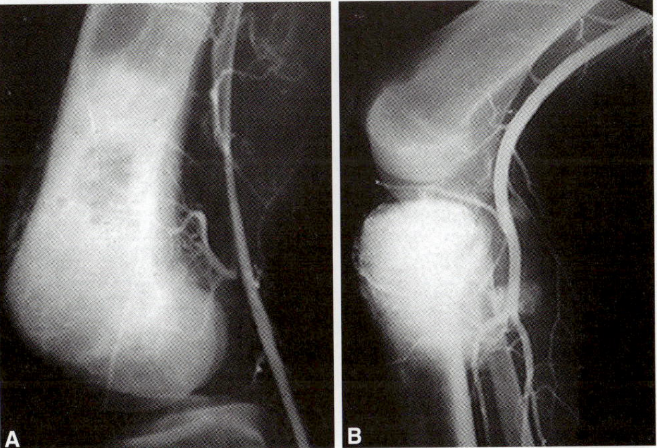

Figs. 64A and B: To confirm the diagnosis and effect of chemotherapy, biopsy is required.

- Meticulous hemostasis should be ensured before closure.
- The wound should be closed tightly in layers.

Types of Biopsy

- Fine needle aspiration
- Core needle biopsy (Trephine)
- Open incisional biopsy.

Histology (Figs. 65 to 67)

- Small spindle cells with hyperchromatic nuclei.
- Shape may be round, cuboidal, columnar.
- Cells are pleomorphic in nature.
- Giant cells are often present.
- Matrix may be myxomatous, cartilaginous or osseous.
- Areas of hemorrhages may be present.

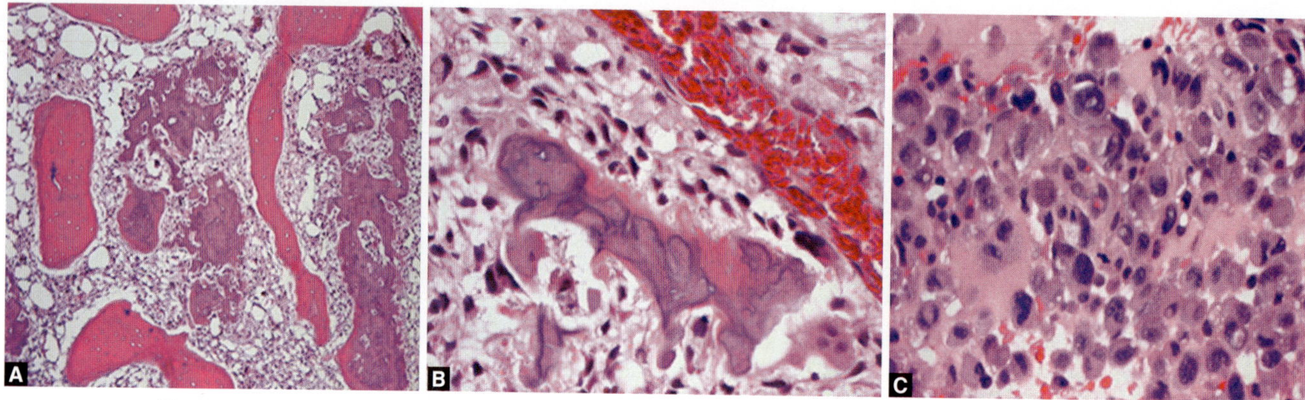

Figs. 65A to C: Effect of chemotherapy and prognosis of the tumor by serial histological studies of the tumor.

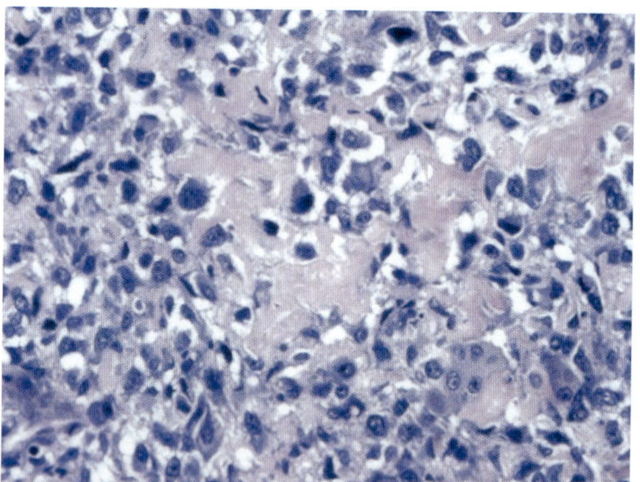

Fig. 66: Osteosarcoma histology. Sheets of pleomorphic osteoblasts associated with lace-like pink osteoid deposition.

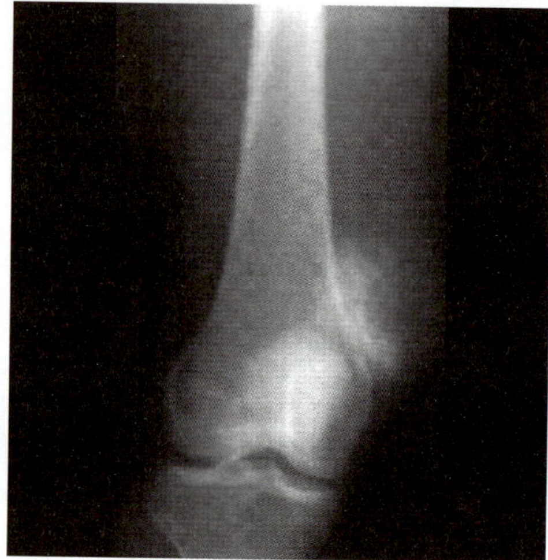

Fig. 68: Parosteal osteosarcoma.

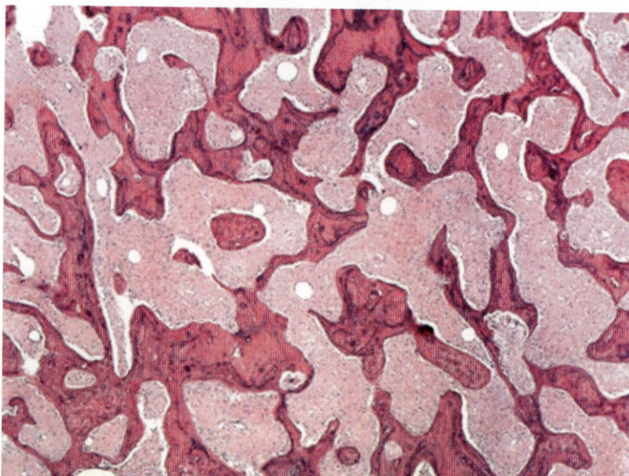

Fig. 67: Parosteal osteosarcoma, low-powered photomicrograph. Anastamosing strands of bone separated by fibrous tissue.

Conventional Osteosarcoma

- These high-grade tumors begin in an intramedullary location, but may break through the cortex and form a soft-tissue mass.
- The histologic hallmark of conventional osteosarcoma is the presence malignant osteoblastic spindle cells producing osteoid. Currently WHO recognizes three distinct subtypes of conventional osteosarcoma:
  1. Osteoblastic
  2. Chondroblastic
  3. Fibroblastic (Raymond, 2002).
- Mistaken diagnoses of chondrosarcoma or malignant fibrous histiocytoma may occur.
- The presence of woven bone with malignant appearing stromal cells, regardless of associated chondroid or fibrous matrix, makes the diagnosis of osteosarcoma.

Parosteal Osteosarcoma (Fig. 68)

- *Incidence:*
  - 1% of primary malignant bone tumors
  - Usually patient more than 20 years old
  - *Peak incidence:* 30–50 years
  - Male to female ratio is 2:3.
- *Clinically:*
  - Present with a constant ache or lump
  - Usually a long bone juxtametaphyseal
  - Usually presents as a Stage 1A lesion (low grade).
- Most common site—posterior aspect of distal femur.

Investigations—X-rays (Fig. 69)

- Well-circumscribed mass
- May be separated from cortex by a lucent line (30%)

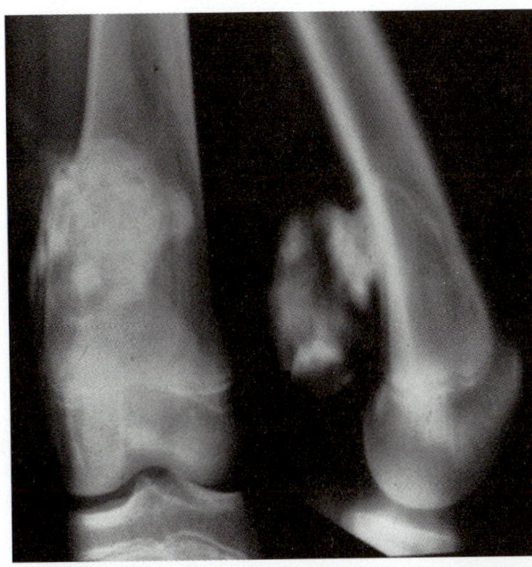

Fig. 69: X-ray of parosteal osteosarcoma.

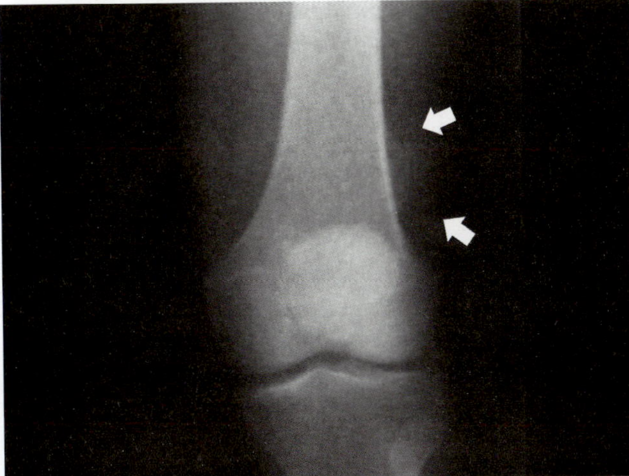

Fig. 70: Periosteal osteosarcoma.

- Broad based tumor with mottled calcification
- Cortex not eroded
- Does not invade medullary cavity
- Tends to encircle bone.

Differential Diagnosis

- Osteochondroma
- Myositis ossificans.

Treatment

- Chemotherapy or radiotherapy not effective
- Wide surgical resection.

Prognosis

- Better than classical osteosarcoma
- About 70–80% survival at 5 years.

Periosteal Osteosarcoma (Fig. 70)

- Arises from surface of diaphysis
- Characterized by bony spicule formation perpendicular to shaft
- Sunburst
- Low grade
- Wide excision.

Telangiectatic Osteosarcoma

- Aggressive
- Presents with pathological fracture
- 5% of all osteosarcomas
- Arises within the diaphysis.

Radiology

- Often entirely osteolytic
- Bone and cortex destruction
- Periosteal reaction
- Codman triangles.

Pathology

- Gross appearance is multicystic similar to an aneurysmal bone cyst.
- Microscopically it has large blood filled spaces and thin septation. Within the septa there is scanty osteoid production by the pleomorphic malignant cells of this high-grade tumor.

Secondary Osteosarcoma

- Secondary osteosarcomas occur at the site of another disease process.
- They constitute almost half of the osteosarcomas in patients older than 50 years.
- The most common type of secondary osteosarcomas are:
  - Paget's disease
  - Previous radiation treatment.

Treatment

- *Current standard of care:*
  - Radiological staging
  - Biopsy to confirm diagnosis
  - Preoperative chemotherapy
  - Repeat radiological staging (access chemo response, finalize surgical treatment plan)
  - Surgical resection with wide margin
  - Reconstruction using one of many techniques
  - Postoperative chemotherapy based on preoperative response.
- The aim of treatment is to confirm the diagnosis and to evaluate the spread and to execute adequate treatment.
- Confirmation of diagnosis is done clinically, histologically, radiologically and laboratory findings.
- Evaluation of the spread of the tumors is done. Lung is common area of metastasis CXR should be done. CT and MRI will detect the extent of tumor and soft tissue involvement.
- Bone scan will detect skip lesions (Fig. 71).

Prognostic Factors

- Extent of the disease—patients with pulmonary, nonpulmonary (bone) or skip metastasis have poor prognosis.
- Grade of the tumor—high-grade tumor have poor prognosis.
- Size of the primary lesion—large size tumors have worse prognosis then small size tumors.
- Skeletal location—proximal tumors do worse than distal tumors.
- Secondary osteosarcoma—poor prognosis.

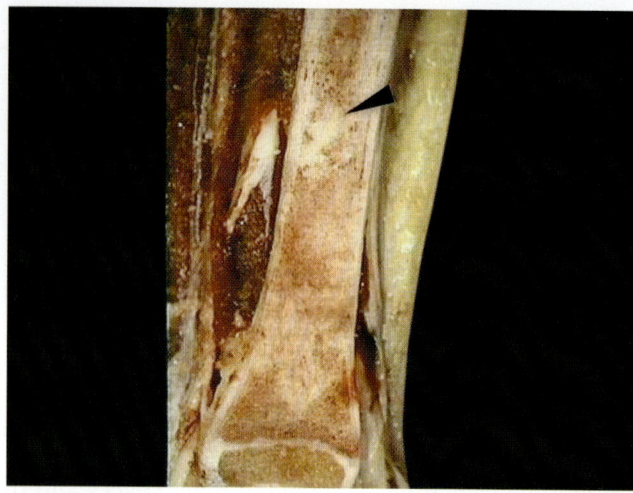

Fig. 71: Micrometastasis.

Chemotherapy

- Before the era of chemotherapy, osteosarcoma was usually treated with immediate wide or radical amputation on diagnosis.
- This usually treated the local disease adequately. However, 80% of patients eventually died of micrometastatic disease.
- With the use of modern chemotherapy protocols, the current 5-year survival rate for osteosarcoma is approximately 70%.
- It is given pre- and postoperatively to control the micro metastasis.
- Chemotherapy given preoperatively is known as neoadjuvant and that given postoperatively is known as adjuvant chemotherapy.
- Theoretical advantages of neoadjuvant chemotherapy include:
  - It causes regression of the primary tumor, making a successful limb salvage operation easier.
  - It allows for histological evaluation of the effectiveness of treatment.
  - It may decrease the spread of tumor cells at the time of surgery.
  - It usually can be started immediately, effectively treating micrometastasis at the earliest time possible.
  - It avoids tumor progression, which may occur during any delay before surgery.
  - It allows time to plan the operation properly, including the possible manufacturing of a custom implant.
  - It also allows time for the patient and the family to consider fully the options of limb salvage surgery versus amputation.
- Neoadjuvant chemotherapy is given for about 3–4 weeks before definitive procedure.
- After ablation of the primary tumor, it produces a disease-free state for many months.
- If given before the metastasis is apparent, it improves the 5-year survival rate by 60%.
- Chemotherapy started early after the diagnosis destroys the microscopic foci at a stage when they are most susceptible to the action of drugs.
- It prevents metastasis in 60% of the cases; the remaining 40% become disease free due to aggressive attack on the metastasis. After metastasis has occurred, chemotherapy decreases the tumor size and enables easy removal.

The drugs used most often to treat osteosarcoma are:

- Methotrexate with leucovorin (folinic acid)
- Doxorubicin (adriamycin)
- Cisplatin or carboplatin
- Etoposide
- Ifosfamide
- Cyclophosphamide
- Actinomycin D (dactinomycin)
- Bleomycin.

  (American Cancer Society www.cancer.org 2009)
- *CA regimen:*
  - *Cisplatin:* 90 mg/m^2 IV over 6 hours on day 1.
  - *Adriamycin:* 75 mg/m^2 IV 48 hours after cisplatin on day 3.
  - Frequency—repeat cycle every 21 days.
  - *VML-A regimen:*
  - *Vincristine:* 2.0 mg/m^2 IV on day 1.
  - *Methotrexate:* 7,500 mg/m^2 IV over 6 hours beginning 30 minutes after vincristine.
  - *Leucovorin:* 15 mg IV every 3 hours, 8 times, then 15 mg orally every 6 hours, 8 times, beginning 2 hours after methotrexate administration is completed.
  - *Adriamycin:* 75 mg/m^2 IV every 3 weeks, 6 times, beginning with the fifth course of VML.

Side Effects

General side effects:

- Nausea and vomiting
- Loss of appetite
- Hair loss
- Mouth sores.

Chemotherapy can damage the blood-producing cells resulting in:

- Increased chance of infection (↓ WBC)
- Bleeding or bruising (↓ Platelets)
- Fatigue or shortness of breath (↓ RBCs)

Most of these side effects are short-term and tend to go away after treatment is finished.

Side effects of specific drugs:

- Ifosfamide and cyclophosphamide—hemorrhagic cystitis.
- Cisplatin—neuropathy, nephropathy, ototoxicity.
- High-dose methotrexate—leukoencephalopathy and liver or kidney damage.
- Doxorubicin (Adriamycin)—can cause heart damage over time.

Long-term side effects:

- Infertility
- Heart damage
- Developing a second cancer.

Surgical Options

Surgical procedures fall into three basic categories:

1. Amputation
2. Limb salvage
3. Rotationplasty.

While differences between amputation and limb-sparing procedures do exist, long-term outcomes with regards to patient function and satisfaction appear to be similar (DiCaprio, 2003; Refaat, 2002; Nagarajan, 2002).

- With Multimodal treatment including surgery and chemotherapy, long-term survival has improved from 20 to 70% in most series.

- For osteosarcoma of the distal femur, the rate of local recurrence after wide resection as well as transfemoral amputation is approximately 5–10%.
- Attainment of a wide margin is the most important technical aspect of the surgical procedure with regard to overall patient survival.
- With regard to function, location of the tumor is the most important issue.
- Surgery—early and radical ablation is the surgery of choice. The main goal of surgery is to safely and completely remove the tumor.
- Historically, most patients had an amputation. Over the past 30 years, limb-sparing procedures have become the standard, mainly due to advances in chemotherapy and sophisticated imaging techniques (Scully, 2002).
- Limb salvage procedures now can provide rates of local control and long-term survival equal to amputation.
- Level of amputation:
  - Upper extremity (u/e) of humerus—forequarter amputation.
  - u/e tibia—mid thigh amputation.
  - u/e femur—hind quarter amputation and hip disarticulation.
  - lower extremity of femur—mid-thigh amputation and hip disarticulation
- *Newer techniques:*
  - Limb salvage with tumor endoprosthesis.
  - In juxtaarticular—intraepiphyseal resection and biological reconstruction is done.

Amputation versus Limb Salvage (Fig. 72)

- If the tumor can be removed safely while retaining a viable extremity, a limb sparing procedure may be appropriate.
- If major nerves or blood vessels are involved, or if complete tumor removal results in significant loss of function, amputation may be a better choice.
- Patient's age, desired level of function, cosmetic preference and long-term prognosis must also be considered.

Indications for Amputation

- Grossly displaced pathologic fracture
- Encasement of neurovascular bundle

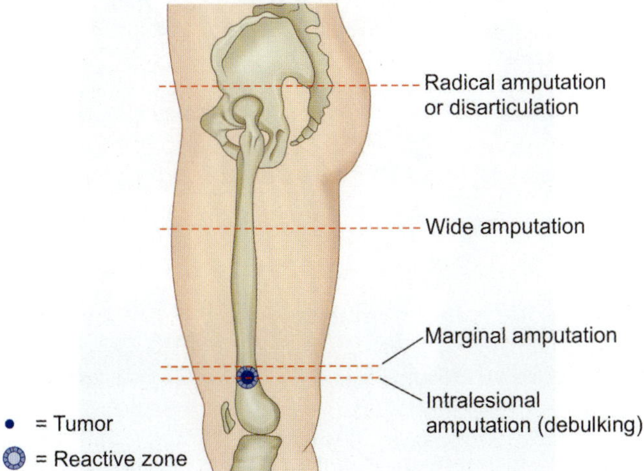

Fig. 72: Enneking classification of surgical options.

- Tumor that enlarges during preoperative chemotherapy and is adjacent to neurovascular bundle
- Palliative measure in metastatic disease
- If the tumor has caused massive necrosis, fungation, infection, or vascular compromise.

Although cure is not the goal, amputation dramatically improves the functional status and pain relief for the remaining months.

Enneking Staging of Tumors

- Grade IA—requires local procedure like curettage
- Grade IB—wide excision
- Grade IIA—radical excision
- Grade IIB—radical amputation
- Grade III—multiprolonged approach, like surgery, chemotherapy and radiotherapy.

Surgical Margins (*see* Fig. 35)

In orthopedic oncology, the surgical margin is described by one of four terms—intralesional, marginal, wide, or radical. Amputations and limb-sparing resections may be associated with any of the four types of margins.

1. *Intralesional margin* is one in which the plane of surgical dissection is within the tumor. Also known as debulking. It is appropriate for some symptomatic benign lesions or as a palliative procedure in metastatic disease.
2. *Marginal margin* is achieved when the closest plane of dissection passes through the pseudocapsule. It is used for most benign lesions and some low-grade malignancies.
3. *Wide margins* are achieved when the plane of dissection is in normal tissue. Although no specific distance is defined, the entire tumor remains completely surrounded by a cuff of normal tissue. If the plane of dissection touches the pseudocapsule at any point, the margin should be defined as being marginal and not wide.
4. *Radical margins* are achieved when all the compartments that contain tumor are removed en bloc. For bone tumors, this involves removing the entire bone and the compartments of any involved muscles. Radical operations were previously the procedures of choice for most high-grade neoplasms.

Postoperative Care

- Team approach is needed including the surgeon, physical medicine specialist, a physical therapist, an occupational therapist, a psychologist, and a social worker. Pain management includes the brief use of intravenous narcotics followed by oral pain medicine that is tapered as soon as tolerated.
- Rigid dressing is preferable over "conventional" soft dressings.
- Prevent edema at the surgical site, protect the wound from bed trauma, enhance wound healing and early maturation of the stump, decrease postoperative pain, allowing earlier mobilization from bed to chair prevent the formation of knee flexion contractures.
- Drains usually are removed at 48 hours.
- The stump is elevated by raising the foot of the bed, which helps manage edema and postoperative pain. The patient is cautioned against leaving the stump in a dependent position. Patients should be mobilized from bed to chair on the first postoperative day.

- The rigid dressing should be removed and the wound inspected in 7–10 days. Any systemic symptoms of wound infection are indications for earlier cast removal. If the wound is healing well, a new rigid dressing is applied; the cast should be changed weekly until the wound has healed.

Complications

- Hematoma
- Infection
- Wound necrosis
- Contracture
- Pain
- Phantom leg pain
- Residual limb pain
- Radiculopathy.

Dermatological Problems

- Endoprosthetic reconstruction has gained wide popularity for limb-sparing surgery. This involves replacing the removed bone with a metal implant
- Complications with this type of reconstruction include component loosening and wound problems.
- Even if catastrophic complications are avoided, multiple revision/lengthening procedures may be needed.
- LEAP—Lewis Expandable Adjustable Prosthesis
- Rotationplasty is a compromise between amputation and limb salvage most commonly used for osteosarcomas of the distal femur.
- It is a procedure where the neurovascular structures and distal aspect of the limb (leg) are retained, and re-attached to the proximal portion after the tumor has been removed.
- For functional purposes, the distal segment is turned 180° so that the ankle joint functions as a knee joint, thus converting an above-knee to a below-knee amputation in order for prosthetic use to be maximized.
- Rotationplasty is best suited for skeletally immature patients (less than 12 years old) with tumors about the knee (Figs. 73 and 74). The main disadvantage to this form of reconstruction is the cosmetic appearance.

Winkelmann classified rotationplasty into five groups:

- *Group AI:* Lesion of distal femur
- *Group AII:* Lesion of proximal tibia
- *Group BI:* Lesion of proximal femur sparing the hip joint
- *Group BII:* Lesion of proximal femur involving the hip joint
- *Group BIII:* Lesion of the mid femur.

Radiotherapy

- Radiation therapy has no major role in osteosarcoma.
- Radiation therapy may be useful in some cases where the tumor cannot be completely removed by surgery. For example, in pelvic bones or in the bones of the face. In these situations, as much tumor as possible is removed, and then radiation is given to try to kill the remaining cancer cells. Chemotherapy may be used after radiation.
- Radiation can also be helpful in controlling symptoms like pain and swelling if the cancer has come back or surgery is not possible.
- Bone-seeking radioactive drugs, such as samarium-153, are sometimes used to treat symptoms such as pain in people with advanced osteosarcoma. They are injected into a vein and collect in bones. The radiation they give off kills the cancer cells and relieves some of the pain caused by bone metastases.
- These drugs are especially helpful in metastatic disease
- The major side effect of these drugs is a lowering of blood cell counts, which could increase the risk for infections or bleeding, especially if the blood counts are already low.

Megavoltage Radiotherapy

- Radiation is given preoperatively to decrease the viable cells that get disseminated into bloodstream.
- Useful adjuvant in the treatment of resectable tumors.
- Radiation destroys tumor cells with minimal effect on uninvolved parts.
- Total dose is 6,000–8,000 rads or 230 rads/day or 1,000 rads/week.
- Preliminaries before irradiation therapy are:
  - Bone scan are done to detect the skip lesion
  - Biopsy scar is limited to <2 cm size to avoid skin necrosis.
  - Chemotherapy is given to increase the susceptibility of tissue to irradiation.
- *Immunotherapy:* New concept, the sensitized lymphocytes from the survivors are infused in the patient.
- *Coley's toxin:* Combination of heat killed mixture of *Streptococcus pyogenes* and *Serratia marcescens.*

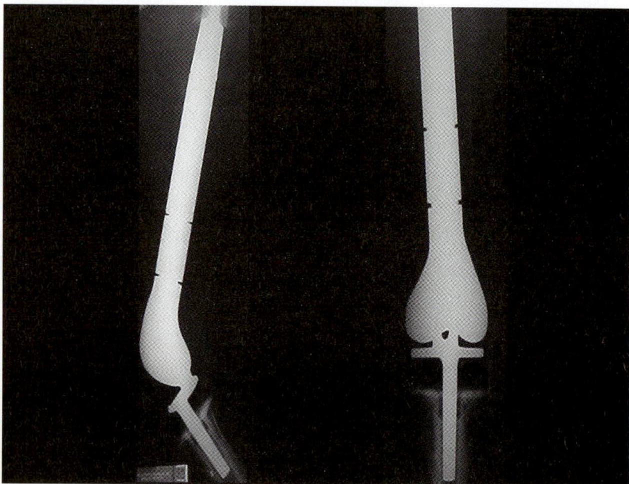

Fig. 73: Radiological picture of rotationplasty.

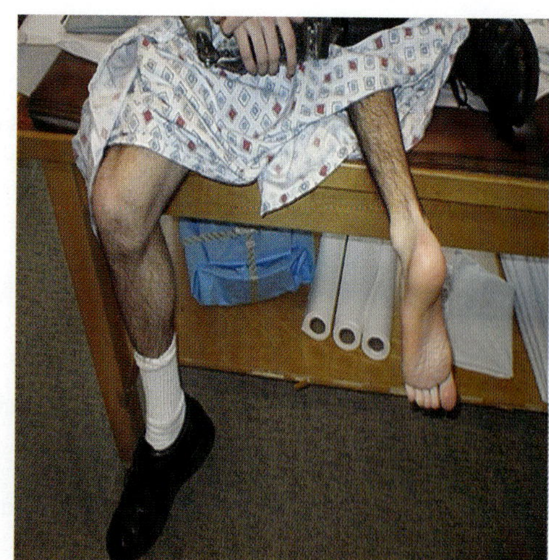

Fig. 74: Clinical picture of rotationplasty.

- The immunological status is increased by giving specific antibiotics, BCG vaccine, interferon, etc.
- Allogenic sarcoma tumor cell vaccine for 2 years
- A new agent that targets ERK pathway, PD98 059, has been developed which targets inflammatory kinase in osteosarcoma.
- *Follow-up:* Every 6–8 weeks for recurrence and metastasis.
- *Prognosis:* Without therapy death occurs in 2 years to 6 months and with surgery and chemotherapy 5 years disease-free life seen in 70% of patients.

CHONDROSARCOMA

- Chondrosarcoma is a malignant tumor of cartilage producing cells (Fig. 75).
- Cartilaginous tumors most often are found in bones arising from endochondral ossification.
- Chondrosarcoma is the most common sarcoma of the bone in patients over 20 years of age.
- It represents around 25% of all sarcomas and typically occurs in adults aged between 30 and 60 years.

Classification of Chondrosarcoma

- *Primary:*
  - Central (medullary) type
  - Juxtacortical (peri-/parosteal)
  - Clear cell chondrosarcoma
  - Mesenchymal chondrosarcoma
  - Dedifferentiated chondrosarcoma
- *Secondary:*
  - Arising from pre-existing benign condition, such as exostosis or multiple enchondromas.
- *Conventional (primary) chondrosarcoma:*
  - Borderline can be low grade or high grade
- *Secondary chondrosarcoma:*
  - Solitary/multiple exostosis
  - Solitary/multiple enchondromatosis
- Peripheral chondrosarcoma
- Dedifferentiated chondrosarcoma.

Primary Chondrosarcoma

- A malignant cartilage tumor arising centrally in a previously normal bone is known as primary chondrosarcoma.

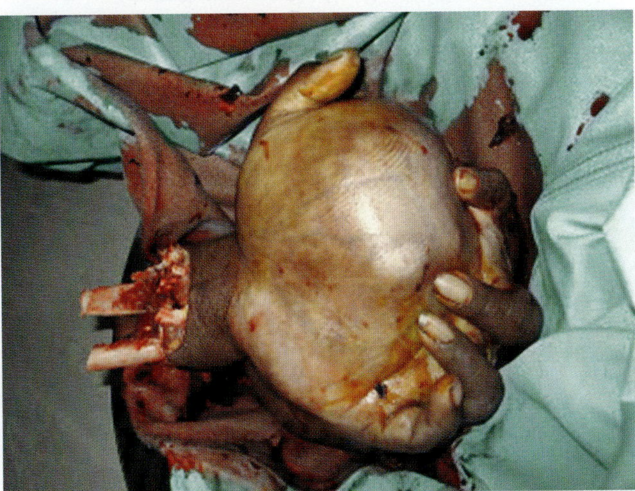

Fig. 75: Chondrosarcoma.

- It is also known as central or conventional sarcoma.
- After myeloma and osteosarcoma, it is the third most common primary malignancy of the bone.
- Of the chondrosarcomas, more than 90% are of primary (conventional) type.

Age and Sex Distribution

Age:

- This is a tumor of adulthood and old age; usually beyond the 3rd decade of life.
- Peak incidence is in the 5th–7th decades of life.

Sex:

- Male are affected twice as often as females.

Sites of Involvement (Figs. 76 and 77)

- Pelvis is the most common site of skeletal involvement (the ilium is the most frequently involved bone) followed by proximal femur, proximal humerus, distal femur (Fig. 78) and ribs.
- Primary chondrosarcoma is uncommon in the small bones of the hands and feet.
- The spine and craniofacial bones are very rare sites for chondrosarcoma.

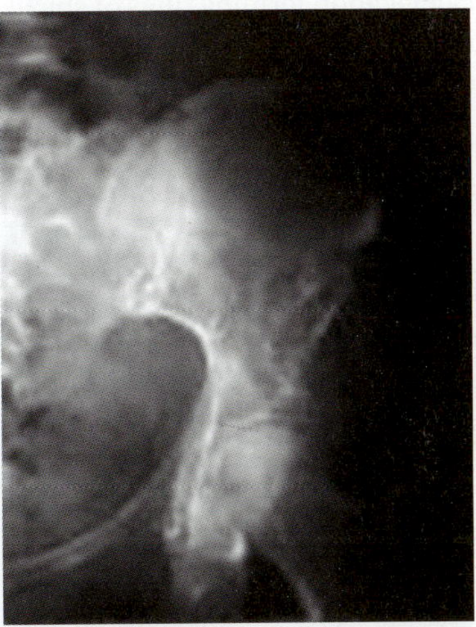

Fig. 76: X-ray findings of chondrosaroma of the pelvis and proximal femur.

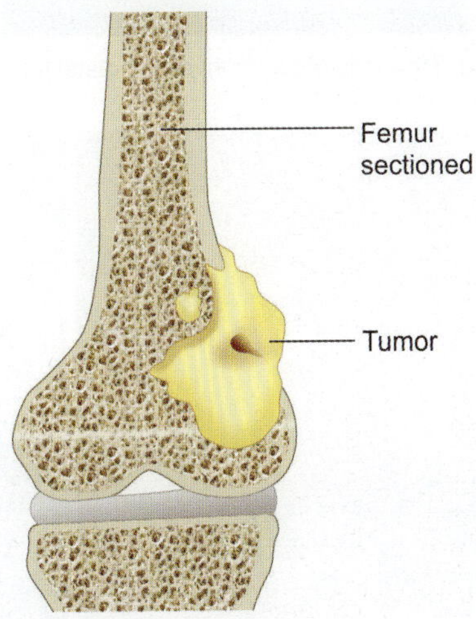

Fig. 77: Tumor showing involvement of distal femur.

Clinical Features

- Pain is the most common and often the only presentation in these patients.
- More than 50% of patients have rest or night pain.
- Nearly 80% of patients with intermediate or high-grade chondrosarcoma have pain.
- Pathologic fractures through the tumor are rare and occur in about 3–8% patients with chondrosarcoma.

Radiologic Findings

- On plain radiographs, the typical findings are expansion of the medullary portion of the bone and thickening of the cortex, but periosteal reaction is scant or absent.
- Chondrosarcomas can show adaptive and aggressive radiologic signs.
- Cortical expansion and thickening are adaptive changes and cortical disruption and soft tissue masses are aggressive radiological changes.
- *Central tumors:*
  - Central lytic lesion with calcification gives fluffy, cotton wool, popcorn or bread-crumb appearance.
  - It invades the soft tissue little or no periosteal reaction.
- *Peripheral tumors:* Very large tumors and central part is calcified.
- *Low-grade features:*
  - Dense calcification forming rings or spicules.
  - Widespread or uniformly distributed calcifications.
  - Eccentric lobular growth of a soft tissue mass.

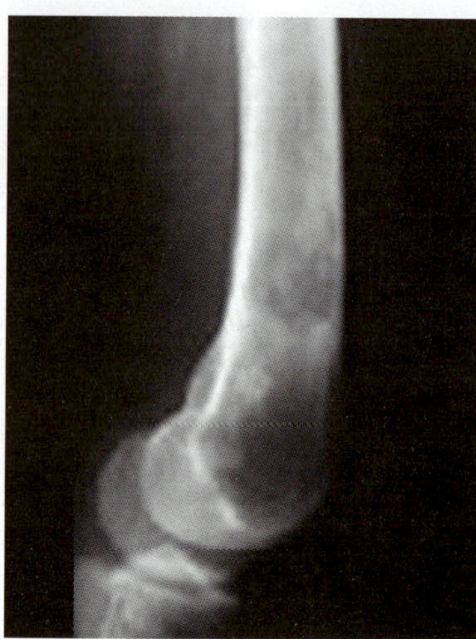

Fig. 78: X-ray of tumor involving distal femur.

- *High-grade features:*
  - Faint amorphous calcification.
  - Large noncalcified areas.
  - Concentric growth of a soft tissue mass.
- Symptomatic intramedullary cartilaginous tumors that display neither adaptive nor aggressive radiologic changes are likely to be enchondromas or low-grade chondrosarcomas.

Pathology

Macroscopically

- Tumor is lobulated, appears as white or bluish mass.
- Firm in consistency.
- Areas of myxomatous degeneration and softening.
- Irregular patchy areas of calcification seen.

Microscopically

- Masses of cartilage cells with more than one nucleus and are hyperchromatic.

Histologically

Tumor is based on cellularity, pleomorphism and mitosis (Figs. 79A to C).

- *Grade 1:* Low grade
- *Grade 2:* Intermediate grade
- *Grade 3:* High grade.

Treatment

- If tumor does not respond to radiotherapy and chemotherapy, then surgery is the treatment of choice.
- *Low and medium grade:* En bloc excision and reconstruction of skeletal defects, endoprosthesis, etc.
- *High-grade lesion:* Radical excision and chemotherapy or amputation at appropriate level.
- *Palliative radiotherapy:* If tumor is present in inaccessible area.

Prognosis

Prognosis is poor in following cases:

- Axial skeleton and proximal bone tumors
- Childhood and young adults
- Cytologically suggesting high-grade malignancy
- Secondary chondrosarcoma
- Survival time after treatment is 10 years.

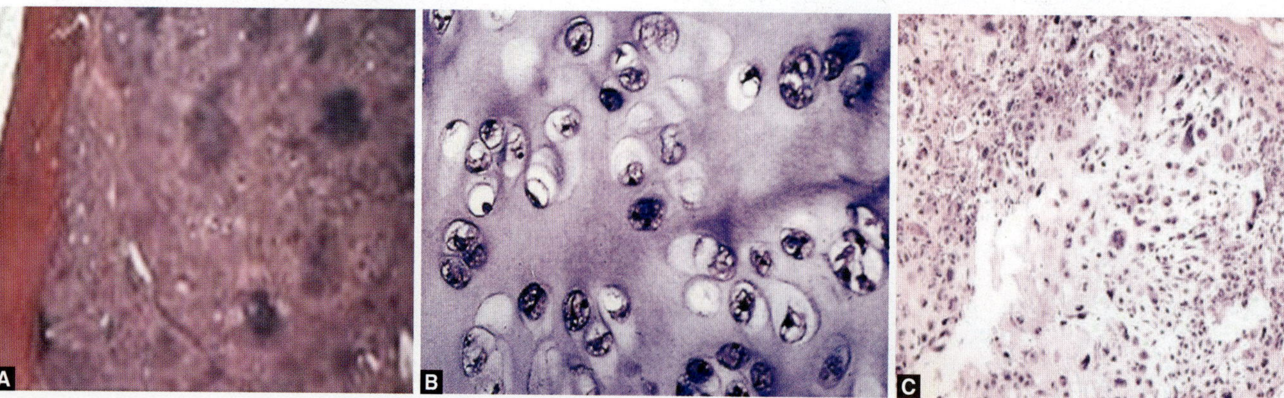

Figs. 79A to C: (A) Grade 1; (B) Grade 2; (C) Grade 3.

Dedifferentiated Chondrosarcoma

- Most malignant variety of chondrosarcoma
- Accounts for 10% of all chondrosarcoma
- It is second mutation with the pre-existing chondrosarcoma, with the second sarcoma taking on microscopic features of high-grade fibrosarcoma or osteosarcoma.

Age and Sex

- *Age:* The average age of presentation is between 50 and 60 years.
- *Sex:* Males and females are equally affected.

Sites of Involvement

- The most common sites of involvement are pelvis, the proximal femur, proximal humerus, distal femur, and ribs (Fig. 80).

Clinical Features

- Pain is the most common presenting symptom.
- However, swelling, paresthesia, and pathological fractures are also common presentations.

Imaging

- Radiographic presentation is variable.
- On plain roentgenograms, the tumor usually shows a poorly defined, lytic, intraosseous lesion with associated cortical perforation and extraosseous extension into the soft tissues producing a large mass.
- The cartilaginous portion of the disease is sharply distinct from the lytic, permeative and destructive component.
- The large size of the tissue mass and the presence of metastases at presentation are useful clues to the possible diagnosis.

Gross

- On the cut surface of the tumor, both tumor components are grossly apparent in varying proportions.
- The lobulated low-grade cartilaginous component is blue-gray in color, and is usually central in location, while the hemorrhagic high-grade component is predominantly extraosseous.

Histopathology

- The hallmark of this lesion is the appearance of an aggressive sarcoma engrafted on an indolent appearing chondrosarcoma.
- The cartilaginous component is usually a low-grade chondrosarcoma (Fig. 81).

Prognostic Factors

- Dedifferentiated chondrosarcomas are aggressive tumors and have a very poor prognosis.
- Despite aggressive treatment, approximately 90% of the patients die with distant metastases within 2 years.
- Distant metastases usually consist solely of the high-grade anaplastic component.
- Certain reports advocate the use of chemotherapy (similar to that used in osteosarcoma) in improving outcomes but the efficacy is debatable.

Mesenchymal Chondrosarcoma

- Mesenchymal chondrosarcoma is a malignant tumor characterized by a bimorphic pattern that is composed of highly undifferentiated small round cells and islands of well differentiated hyaline cartilage.
- It is a rare lesion representing less than 1% of all malignant bone tumors.
- It accounts for <3–10% of all primary chondrosarcomas and may occur at any age.

Age and Sex

- *Age:* The tumors affect all ages (5–74 years) with a peak occurrence in the 2nd and 3rd decades.
- *Sex:* Males and females are equally affected.

Sites of Involvement

- The craniofacial bones (especially the jaw bones), the ribs, the ilium, and the vertebrae are the most common sites.
- The meninges are the most common sites of extraskeletal involvement followed by the leg or thigh.
- Metastases to regional and distant lymph nodes and to other bones are common; unlike conventional chondrosarcoma.

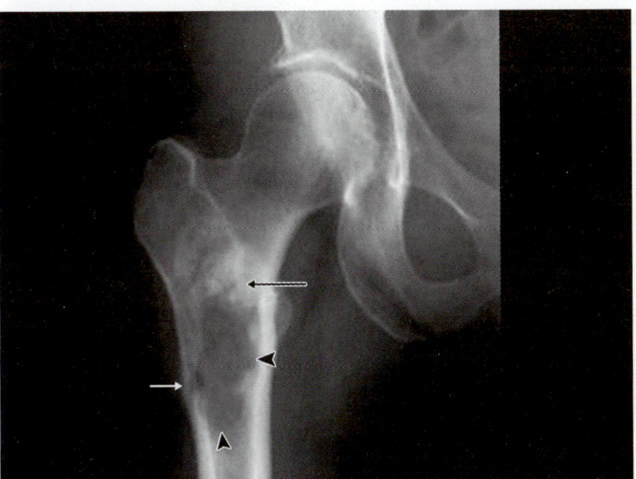

Fig. 80: X-ray showing tumor involving proximal femur.

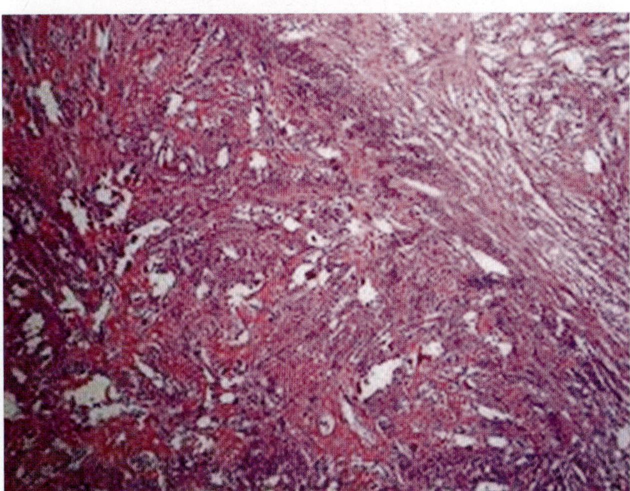

Fig. 81: Histological finding of the tumor.

Clinical Features

- The chief presenting symptoms are pain and swelling which range in duration from a few days to several years.
- Often these symptoms are present for more than a year in duration.

Imaging

- Radiologically, in most cases it resembles conventional chondrosarcoma (Fig. 82).
- The bony lesions are primarily lytic and destructive with mottled calcification and indistinct margins.
- Cortical destruction or cortical breakthrough with extra-osseous extension of soft tissue is a common finding.

Prognostic Factors

- Mesenchymal chondrosarcoma is a rare but highly malignant tumor with a strong tendency for local recurrence and distant metastasis.
- It may manifest even after a delay of more than 20 years.
- This makes long term follow-up mandatory.
- Mesenchymal chondrosarcoma has a poor 10-years survival of 28%.

Clear Cell Chondrosarcoma

- This is a rare low-grade type of chondrosarcoma.
- It is a highly uncommon sarcoma, comprising less than 4% of all chondrosarcomas.

Age and Sex

Age:
- The reported age range is from 12 to 84 years.
- Most patients are between 25 and 50 years.

Sex:
- The male to female ratio of occurrence of this disease is around 3:1.

Sites of Involvement

- Clear cell chondrosarcoma has been reported in most of the bones.
- The most commonly affected sites are the proximal part of the femur, humerus or tibia.

Clinical Features

- Pain is the most common presenting symptom.
- Half the patients have pain longer than a year.

Treatment

- Recurrence after intralesional curettage is common.
- Wide resection is the treatment of choice.
- Marginal excision or curettage has an 86% recurrence rate.

Imaging

- Radiologically clear cell chondrosarcoma usually presents as a well defined, slightly expansile, lytic lesion, often with a sharp margin, in the epiphysis of a long bone (Fig. 83).
- It may occasionally have a sclerotic rim.

Prognostic Factors

- Metastasis is rare.
- Approximately 15% of the patients, however, die due to their tumors.
- In the incompletely excised cases, metastases, usually to the lungs and other bones may develop.
- Dedifferentiation to high-grade sarcoma has been reported.

Secondary Chondrosarcoma

- Chondrosarcoma arising in a known benign precursor lesion is known as a secondary chondrosarcoma.
- This precursor lesion may either be an osteochondroma or an enchondroma.
- The risk of chondrosarcoma arising in a solitary osteochondroma has been reported to be <1%.
- However, in osteochondromatosis, this risk increases to 1–5%.
- Secondary chondrosarcoma develops at a somewhat earlier age than primary chondrosarcoma.
- They are usually of low-grade malignancy and have a favorable prognosis.
- Chondrosarcoma developing on the surface of a bone as a result of malignant transformation within the cartilage cap of a pre-existent osteochondroma is also called as a peripheral chondrosarcoma.

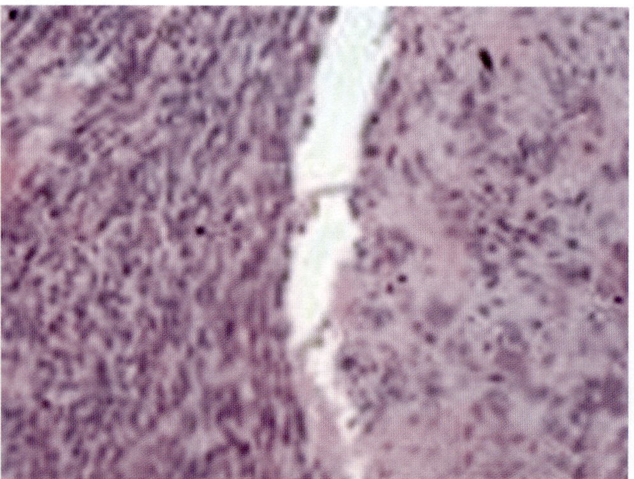

Fig. 82: Histological finding of chondrosarcoma.

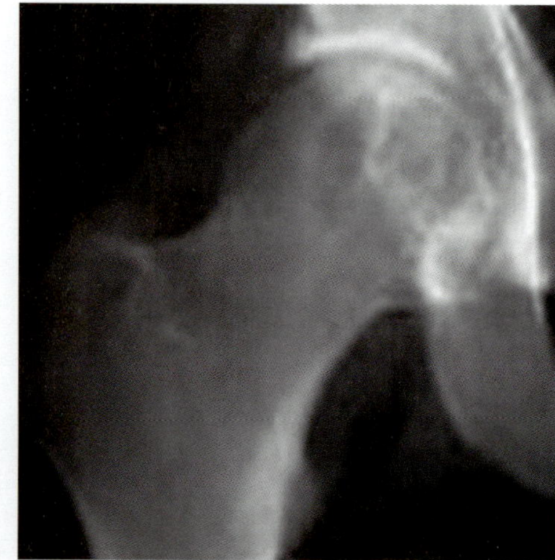

Fig. 83: X-ray showing chondrosarcoma of proximal femur.

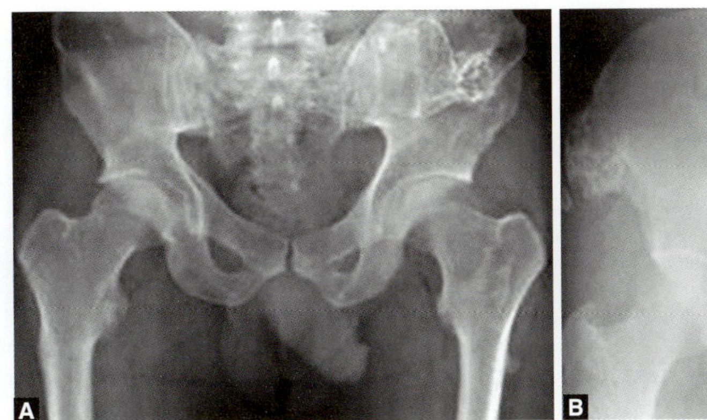
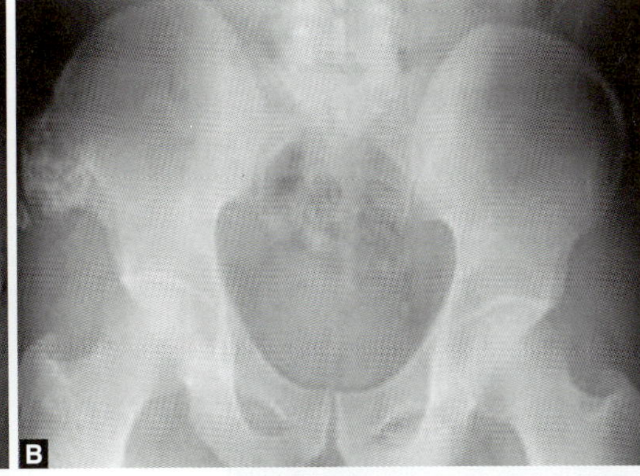

Figs. 84A and B: X-rays showing involvement of pelvic bones.

Sites of Involvement (Figs. 84A and B)

- Any part of the skeleton may be involved.
- However, pelvic and shoulder girdle bones are more commonly affected.

Clinical Features

- A change or onset of clinical symptoms in a patient with a known precursor lesion (osteochondroma or enchondroma) is the usual clinical presentation of secondary chondrosarcoma.
- Sudden onset of pain or increase in size of the swelling is frequent complaints.

Imaging

- Plain roentgenograms show irregular mineralization and increased thickness of the cartilage cap in osteochondromas.
- In pre-existing enchondromas, plain roentgenograms show destructive permeation of bone and development of soft tissue mass.

Gross

Secondary chondrosarcoma arising in enchondromas are usually very myxoid; unlike the solid blue areas of enchondroma.

Histopathology

- Secondary chondrosarcomas are usually grade 1 tumors though higher grades can occur.
- Invasion of the surroundings tissues and marked myxoid changes in the matrix are features useful in making the diagnosis.

Treatment

- Treatment of choice is complete wide surgical excision of the lesion.
- The cartilaginous cap should not be violated during resection of a chondrosarcoma arising in osteochondroma as it will increase the risk of local recurrence.

Prognostic Factors

Patients with secondary chondrosarcoma in osteochondroma have excellent prognosis.

EWING'S SARCOMA

- Ewing's sarcoma was first described by Ewing in 1928.
- It arises from primitive mesenchymal cells of the medullary cavity.

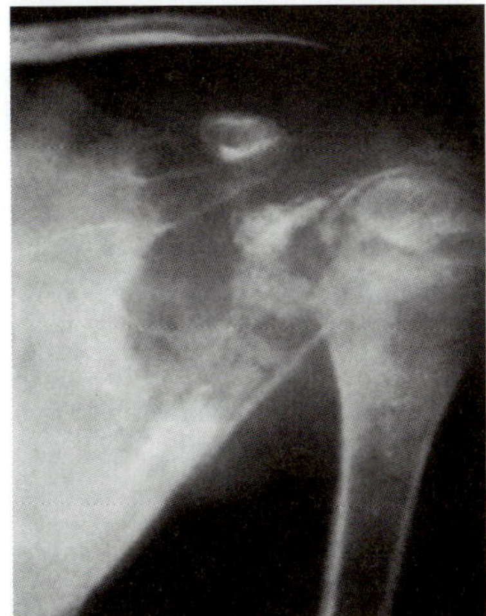

Fig. 85: Ewing's sarcoma.

- This is a rare primary malignant bone tumor (10–14%) of all malignant bone tumors, affecting children.
- It is a lethal tumor with poor survival rate of 5 years (Fig. 85).

Age and Sex

- *Age:* Common between 4 and 25 years of age group (80%).
- *Sex:* More common in males.

Sites of Involvement

- Diaphysis of long bones, i.e. femur, tibia, fibula, humerus.
- About 20% of bone tumors are seen in flat bones (Fig. 86).

Clinical Features

General Examination

- Patient has moderate fever; anemia, pain, and swelling are the common symptoms.

Local Examination

- Visible or palpable tender swelling
- Rapidly increasing in size
- Rise of local temperature with dilated veins
- Location in rib, may be associated with pleural effusion
- Constitutional symptoms, such as fever, sweating, chills, anemia, and leukocytosis creates confusion, as it mimics acute osteomyelitis.

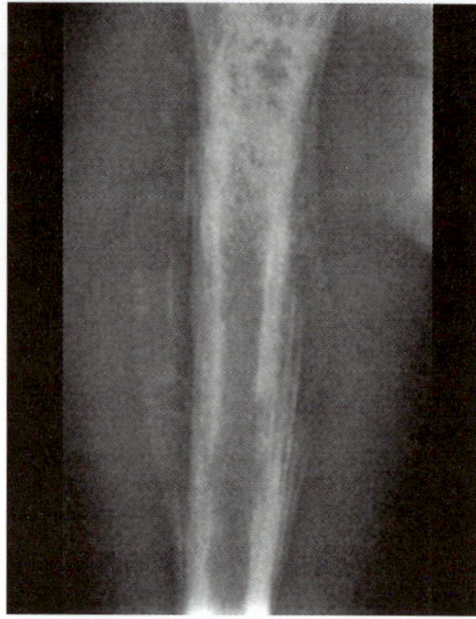

Fig. 86: Ewing's sarcoma involving the proximal humerus in a 15-year-old boy pronounced periosteal new borne formation produces "onion steel" appearance.

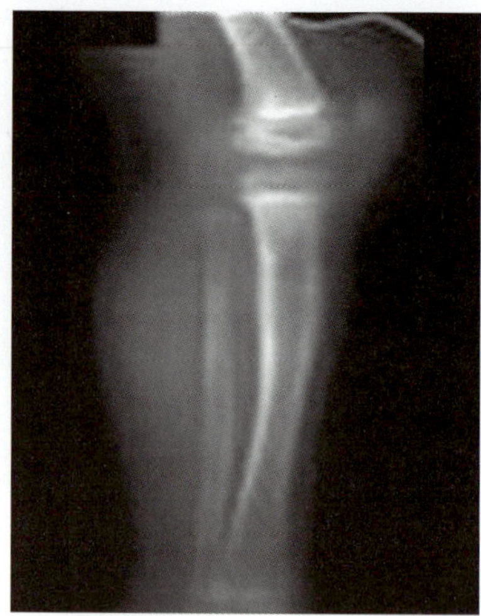

Fig. 87: Radiograph showing Ewing's sarcoma.

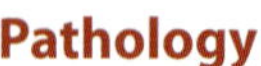

Pathology

Macroscopically

- Tumor is pale soft mass, with minimal bone tissue.
- Areas of cystic degeneration and hemorrhages.
- There is simulation of osteomyelitis by the presence of milky pus, like fluid due to degeneration.
- From the medulla, it reaches to the surface through the haversian canals.

Microscopically

- Tumor is very cellular with minimal stromal tissue.
- Characteristic cells are small polyhedral, with pale cytoplasm and large nucleus.
- Appearance is monotonously uniform.
- In some areas, there was pseudorosette formation, simulating rosette formation by neuroblastoma.
- Tumor can be differentiated from reticulum cell sarcoma, as it stains for glycogen positively by periodic acid-Schiff (PAS) stain and in reticulum cell sarcoma, silver stain is positive.

Radiographic Features

- Lesion can be lytic, sclerotic or mixed.
- Diaphyseal lesion, with irregular destruction ("moth-eaten" appearance or "cracked ice" appearance) (Fig. 87).
- Periosteal new bone formation is in layers giving an "onion peel" appearance.
- Permeative margin.
- Biopsy is necessary for diagnosis.

Investigations

Laboratory Tests

- Increased ESR
- Leukocytosis
- Anemia
- Urine for vanillylmandelic acid
- Immunohistochemical markers
- Electron microscopy study
- Tissue for glycogen stain
- Special staining with HBA-71, which recognizes a product of *MIC 2* gene, has been suggested to be specific for Ewing's sarcoma and neuroectodermal tumors.
- Ewing's sarcoma is associated with chromosomal transformation (11 and 22). The tumor markers include neuron specific enolase, myeloperoxidase.

Differential Diagnosis

- Osteomyelitis
- Osteosarcoma
- Malignant lymphoma.

Treatment

- Tumor is highly sensitive to radiation; it melts like snow.
- Combination of radiotherapy and chemotherapy is used.
- Even after chemotherapy, recurrence rate is 20–30%, because of radiation induced sarcomas.
- Therefore, surgical resection for the control of primary lesion is used.
- *Effective chemotherapy:* Drugs, such as ifosfamide, cisplatinum, epipodophyllin toxin for short period of time.
- *Radiation:* Highly sensitive; it is mainstay of treatment and dose is 4,000 rads, for entire limb and 1,000 rads, as boost to tumor.
- *Surgery:* Amputation, conservative surgery, like debulking or limb salving surgery.

Prognosis

- *Unfavorable prognostic factors:*
  - Male patient
  - Humerus, if involved
  - Pelvic bone, if involved
  - Distant metastasis
- Primary irradiation with amputation, has 2-year survival rate of 15%.
- A combination of chemotherapy, radiotherapy with surgery improves the survival rate of 50–75% for 3–5 years.

MULTIPLE MYELOMA

Introduction

- Multiple myeloma is the most common primary malignancy of bone, representing more than 40% of primary bone cancers.
- Its peak incidence is in the 5th to 7th decades with a 2:1 male predominance.
- Multiple myeloma and metastatic carcinoma should be included in the differential diagnosis for any patient older than age 40 with a new bone tumor.
- The disease rarely occurs before the fifth decade of life. In many patients the malignant cells extend throughout the bone marrow (BM), so a BM aspiration provides diagnostic tissue.
- Most patients have moderate-to-severe anemia, an elevated ESR, and an abnormal serum protein electrophoresis and immunoelectrophoresis.
- Occasionally, patients present with a solitary focus of plasma cells referred to as a plasmacytoma. These individuals usually develop diffuse disease after a latent period of up to 5–10 years.

Definition

Malignant tumor arising from plasma cells of reticuloendothelial cells of bone marrow.

It can occur as:

- *Solitary plasmocytoma:* It constitutes less than 10% of the myelomas. It is a low-grade lesion, which involves the younger age group. In about 30% of the patients, systemic evidence of multiple myeloma develops.
- *Multiple myeloma*
- *Osteosclerotic myelomas:* It is a rare variant, characterized by sclerotic or mixed sclerotic/lytic lesion, involving spine, pelvis, and ribs.
- *Site:* Flat bones, such as vertebra, skull, ribs, and pelvis where red marrow is present.

Pathological Features

Grossly

- Tumor is dark red in color
- Soft in consistency and lies within medulla
- The cortex is thin and broken.

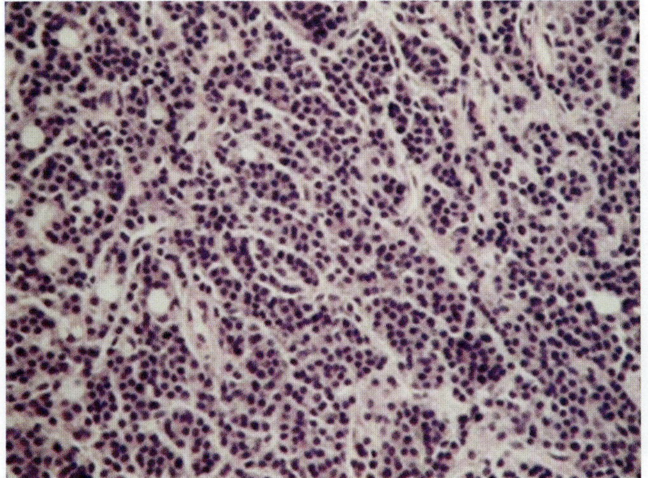

Fig. 88: Typical microscopic appearance—sheets of plasma cells.

Microscopically

- Consist of round cells, with eccentrically placed nucleus with nucleolus (Fig. 88)
- Chromatin is sparse and is arranged in spokes of wheel fashion
- Perinuclear halo, typical of plasma cell not seen in multiple myeloma.

Associated Pathology

- Interstitial fibrosis in the kidney
- Nodules in the lungs.

Clinical Features

- Most patients with multiple myeloma have bone pain that is diffused or localized to regions of bone destruction. Because the disease often involves the vertebral bodies, patients can develop back pain and vertebral compression fractures.
- In addition, many affected individuals have systemic symptoms including weakness, fatigability, and weight loss.
- Most patients have moderate-to-severe anemia, an elevated ESR, and an abnormal serum protein electrophoresis and immunoelectrophoresis.
- *General examination:*
  - Patient becomes severely anemic, loses weight and becomes cachexic.
  - In the late stages, patient develops hyperazotemia, uremic syndrome, hypercalcemia, hyperuricemic syndrome and hemorrhagic diasthesis.

Signs and Symptoms

- Generalized bone pain and pain in back—pain may be intermittent, but later become intense.
- In the early stages, there are hardly any clinical symptoms. In late stages, patient complaint of soft tissue swelling and sign of pathological fracture.
- The sternum and ribs may be tender and sign of vertebral collapse present.

Staging of Multiple Myeloma

Patients of myeloma are staged on the basis of hemoglobin, quantity of M-protein, and hypercalcemia.

- *Stage I:* Hb >10 g/dL, S. ca <8.5 mg%, M-protein Ig G <5 g/dL and IgA <3 g/dL.
- *Stage II:* Hb 8.5–10 g/dL, S. ca 8.5–12 mg%, M-protein Ig G 5–7 g/dL and IgA 3–5 g/dL
- *Stage III:* Hb <8.5 g/dL, S. ca >12 mg%, M-protein Ig G >7 g/dL and IgA >5 g/dL.

Laboratory Findings

- Low hemoglobin
- High ESR
- Increased total protein, A/G ratio reversed
- Increased serum calcium
- Low to normal alkaline phosphatase, but is raised in pathological fracture
- Urine Bence-Jones proteins are found in 30% of patients
- *Serum electrophoresis:* M spike of gamma globulin in 90% of cases, e.g. G-60%, A-25% and others 15%
- *Sternal puncture:* Myeloma cell may be seen
- Bone marrow shows 5–100% plasma cells

- Bone scan
- Open biopsy
- Serum alpha-2 microglobulin is increased (tumor marker).

Diagnostic Criteria (Salmon and Durie)

Major Criteria

1. Bone marrow plasmacytosis of greater than 30%.
2. Biopsy confirmation of plasmacytoma.
3. M protein Ig G > 3 g% and Ig A > 2 g%.
4. 24 hours urine excretion >1 g of kappa or lambda light chains.

Minor Criteria

a. Bone marrow plasmacytosis of 10–30%.
b. M protein less than the levels of major criteria.
c. Discrete lytic bone lesions.
d. Reduction of normal serum Igs like IgM <50 mg%, IgA <100 mg%, IgG <600 mg%.

Following combinations of major and minor criteria are diagnostic:
1 + (b or c or d)
2 + (a or b) or (c or d)
3 + a
4 + a
a + b + c

Radiological Features (Figs. 89A to C)

- The radiographic features of multiple myeloma vary from multiple "punched out" areas of bone destruction often in the skull and pelvis, to diffuse osteopenia.
- Radiographically, multiple myeloma appears as multiple, "punched-out," sharply demarcated, purely lytic lesions without any surrounding reactive sclerosis.

Complications

- Pathological fractures of rib
- Spinal cord or nerve root compression
- Renal failure
- Severe infection
- Amyloidosis.

Treatment

- Radiation alone can effectively treat a plasmacytoma.
- Chemotherapy with radiation is the treatment of choice for disseminated disease.
- Recently, stem cell transplant has been used with success in many patients.

Management of Multiple Myeloma

Patients with stage I myeloma can be followed without treatment.

Indications of Treatment

- All patients with stage II and stage III myeloma
- Stage I patients with Bence-Jones protenuria
- Refractory hypercalcemia
- Vertebral compression fractures
- Progressive lytic bone lesions
- Severe bone pains
- Rising of M component level or doubling of M component levels in one year.

Chemotherapy

- Chemotherapy includes administration of cytotoxic drugs either singly or in combination with or without glucocorticoids.
- Alkylating agents melphalan and cyclophosphamide have shown significant activity in multiple myeloma, used in standard as well as high doses in the management of this disease.
- Multiagent combination chemotherapy regimens have also been used routinely. Two most used regimens are
  1. Melphalan + Prednisolone (MP regimen)
  2. Vincristine + Doxorubicin + Dexamethasone (VAD regimen)
- Patients are typically treated for six or more cycles of chemotherapy to attain the plateau state, which is defined as stable urine and M protein level with no other evidence of progression of disease.

MP Regimen

- It has advantage of oral administration.
- Stem cell toxic, hence cannot be used in patients with renal impairment.
- Commonly preferred in older patients who are not able for autologous stem cell transplantation.

VAD Regimen

- It is to be given continuous intravenous administration over 96 hours necessitating an infusion pump and central venous line.

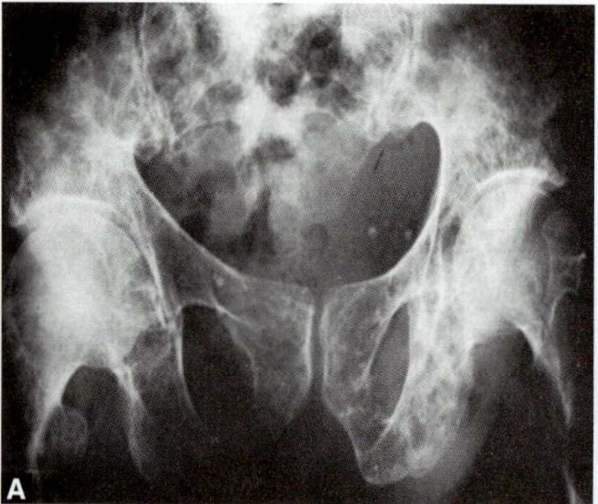

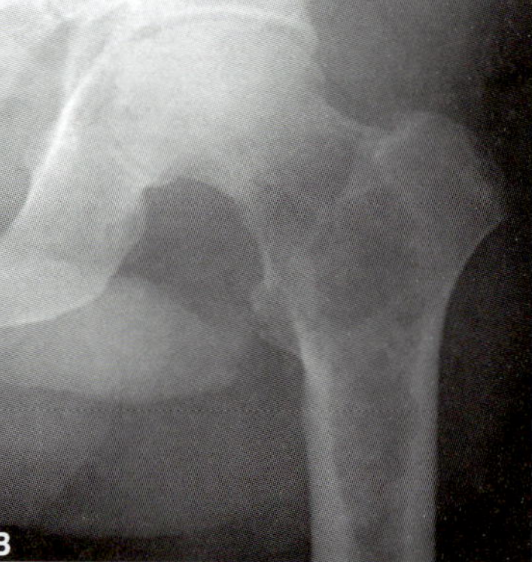

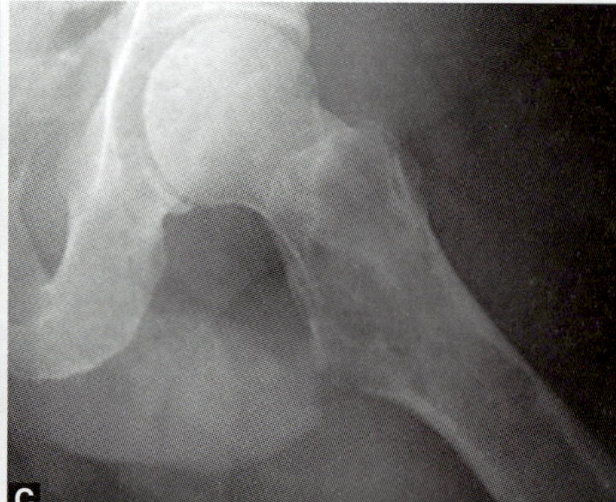

Figs. 89A to C: (A) Radiographs showing the multiple punctate lucent defects in the pelvis of a patient with multiple myeloma; (B and C) Anteroposterior and lateral radiographs of proximal femur of a 61-year-old man with multiple myeloma show multiple lytic lesions.

- It has the advantage of faster onset of action.
- Being nonstem cell toxic, it can be used in renal failure patients.
- It is preferred in young patients who are able to undergo autologous stem cell transplantation in future.
- All patients are at risk of tumor lysis syndrome after the start of chemotherapy.
- Syndrome characterized by hyperuricemia, renal failure, various dyselectrolytemias.
- Standard preventive measures like hydration, alkalinization of urine and administration of Allopurinol should be implemented in all patients to prevent this complication.

Supportive Care

- High fluid intake throughout their lives which prevents many hyperviscosity syndrome and other complications.
- Recombinant human erythropoietin has been effective in correcting anemia in 80% of patients. Coexisting deficiency of iron, folic acid, and cobalamin should be corrected before using erythropoietin.
- Monthly infusions of IV immunoglobulins of 0.4 g/kg to be given to reduce risk of serious infections.
- Bisphosphonates to reduce bone pain and to reduce frequency of pathologic fractures and prevent hypercalcemia.
- Commonly used are pamidronate 90 mg per month over 3 hours and zoledronic acid 4 mg per month over 15 minutes.

Radiotherapy

- Palliative irradiation (20–30 Gy in 5–7 fractions over 1–2 weeks) should be considered only in patients with localized disease who are not responding.
- Concurrent chemo-radiotherapy to be avoided as it causes severe myelocompression, interval of 3 weeks to be maintained.
- Patients who are at risk of fracture can also be given local radiotherapy to osseous lesions.
- Other indications are sphenoid and orbital bone involvement, compressive lesions.

Surgical Treatment

- The primary treatment of multiple myeloma is chemotherapy.
- Symptomatic bone lesions usually respond rapidly to radiation treatment.
- The orthopedic surgeon most commonly is consulted to treat impending or actual pathological fractures of the spine, acetabulum, proximal femur, or proximal humerus.
- Because most of these patients have a short life expectancy, every effort should be made to perform the operation that would allow the earliest resumption of full activity. This may include debulking the tumor and using internal fixation augmented with methacrylate.
- If this method would not allow immediate full weight bearing, cemented total joint arthroplasty or hemiarthroplasty should be considered.
- In most patients, local radiation treatment should be instituted approximately 3 weeks after surgery or when the wound appears to be healed.

Prognosis

- Despite aggressive treatment, the prognosis for multiple myeloma continues to be poor.
- Most patients die as a result of their disease within 3 years after diagnosis. Long-term survival is exceedingly rare.
- Patients who present with a solitary plasmacytoma without evidence of systemic involvement (i.e. negative bone marrow biopsy and negative skeletal survey) have a better prognosis.
- Although more than half of patients who present with a solitary plasmacytoma eventually go on to develop.

Conclusion

- Multiple myeloma remains as incurable disease.
- Alkylating agents, steroids either alone or in combination remain the standard initial treatment.
- Autologous transplantation has improved the outcome and is currently offered to all eligible patients.
- Supportive treatment like bisphosphonates have improved the quality of life of these patients and perhaps also improved survival.

METASTATIC BONE DISEASE

Introduction

- Metastatic bone disease is a painful condition that develops in conjunction with malignancies of breast, prostate, lung and other organs.
- Skeleton is the third most common site of metastasis after lung and liver.
- Besides myelomas and lymphomas the common tumors metastasize to skeleton are mostly from breast, prostate, lung, kidney, and thyroid.
- Soft tissue sarcomas and primary bone tumors can metastasize to bone, but this is extremely rare.
- Prevalence of skeletal disease is highest in breast and prostate carcinoma which accounts for more than 80% cases of metastatic bone disease.
- Most carcinomas metastatic to bone are from the breast and prostate, followed by the lung, kidney, thyroid, and gastrointestinal tract in order of decreasing frequency.
- For patients who have suspected metastases of unknown origin, however, the most common primary malignancies are in the lung or kidney.
- Breast and prostate are uncommon sites of primary disease for this group of patients. This phenomenon has several possible explanations.
- First, the primary lesions in patients with breast cancer or prostate cancer may be detected more easily early in the disease course.
- Secondly, breast cancer and prostate cancer may not metastasize to bone until relatively late. Finally, lung and kidney cancer may escape detection until very late in the disease course and may metastasize to bone relatively earlier.

Metastatic Bone Lesion

- Metastatic bone lesions are painful and frequently cause pathologic fractures.
- They occur most commonly in the vertebrae, pelvis, ribs, and proximal appendicular skeleton .
- Although bone metastases occur primarily in adults over 45 years of age, neuroblastomas can metastasize to bone in children.

- Most patients with bone pain or a pathologic fracture from skeletal metastases have a known primary malignant tumor, but occasionally the skeletal metastasis is the first indication of a primary malignancy.
- For this reason, the possibility of metastatic carcinoma should be investigated in middle-aged and older patients with a destructive bone lesion.
- In patients with metastatic bone disease, the tumor must destroy 30–50% of the bone before a plain radiograph reveals the lesion.
- A technetium bone scan offers a more sensitive method of detecting metastatic disease, although it may not be reliable for rapidly destructive lesions such as multiple myeloma or renal cell carcinoma.
- Most metastases destroy bone, but those from prostate and breast cancers can stimulate bone formation and appear as regions of increased bone density on plain radiographs.
- If plain radiographs or bone scans fail to demonstrate suspected bone metastasis, an MRI scan may provide more detailed information.

Clinical Features

- Bone pain
- Hypercalcemia
- Pathological fractures
- Spinal cord or nerve root involvement
- Bone marrow infiltration/leukoerythroblastic anemia
- Bone pain is the most feared clinical manifestation of metastatic bone disease, which is described as continuous deep boring type of pain accompanied by episodes of stabbing discomfort.
- *Likely mechanisms of bone pain are:*
  - Direct pressure and destruction of mechano and nociceptors in bone due to invasion of bone by tumor.
  - Release of various pain mediator chemicals such as prostaglandins, histamine and bradykinin.
  - Hormonal influence.
- *Control of bone pain by:*
  - Drug therapy by analgesics and bisphosphonates
  - Physical therapy by splints
  - Radiotherapy
  - Anesthetic methods like blocks
  - Neurosurgical methods like hypophysectomy.
  - Relaxation techniques.

Histology (Figs. 90A to C)

- The microscopic appearance of metastatic carcinoma usually is similar to the primary lesion. In well-differentiated cases, the biopsy easily yields the correct diagnosis. In some cases, such as a sarcomatoid kidney cancer, immunohistochemistry may be required to reveal epithelial markers.

Radiological Features (Figs. 91 to 96 and Table 11)

- The radiographic appearance of metastatic carcinoma varies. The appearance usually is aggressive, suggesting malignancy. The lesions may be lytic, blastic or mixed.
- Breast cancer and prostate cancer typically produce blastic lesions. Kidney cancer and thyroid cancer usually are purely lytic.
- Lung cancer may produce a mixed appearance. If the lesion is distal to the elbow or knee, lung cancer is the most likely primary lesion.
- Additionally, metastatic lung cancer may have the distinct appearance of a "bite" taken out of the cortex.

Treatment

- The treatment of carcinoma metastatic to bone is multimodal. Systemic treatment with cytotoxic agents is directed by the medical oncologist.
- Hormone manipulation may be beneficial for patients with breast or prostate cancer. Radioactive iodine may be beneficial for some patients with metastatic thyroid cancer.
- New evidence suggests that bisphosphonates may have a role in preventing new metastatic bone lesions and may slow the growth of existing lesions by inhibiting osteoclast resorption of bone.
- Most symptomatic bone metastases are responsive to radiation. Some carcinomas, especially kidney cancer, are typically radioresistant.
- Surgery is required for treatment of impending or actual pathological fractures.

Nonoperative Treatment

- Radiotherapy is effective method and its primary aim is relief of pain, restoration of function, and arrest of tumor.
- Additional treatment with bisphosphonates has improved to prevent fractures or the necessity of additional radiotherapy.

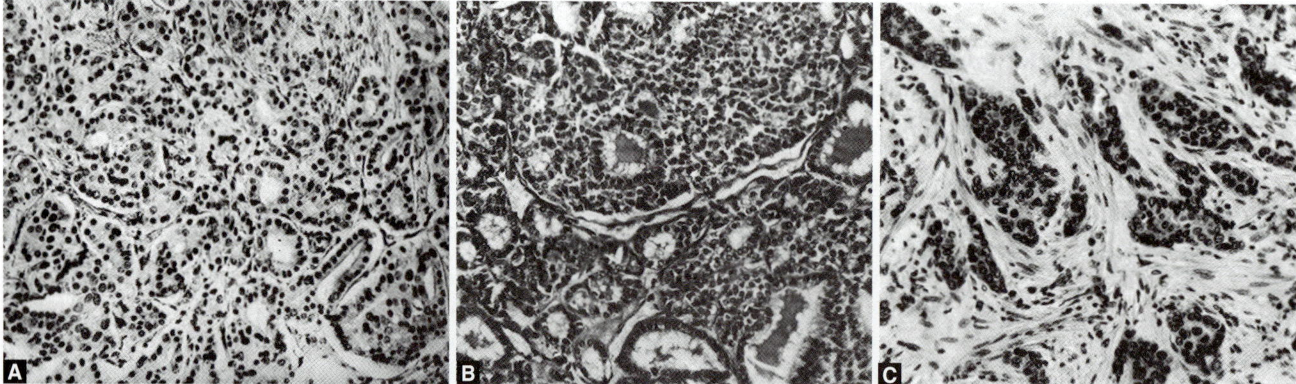

Figs. 90A to C: (A) A histologic section showing metastatic prostate carcinoma. The lesion consists of gland-forming epithelial cells; (B) A histologic section of metastatic carcinoma of the thyroid gland. Note the filled spaces with a similar appearance to native thyroid tissue; (C) A histologic section showing a metastatic carcinoma of the breast. The lesion consists of islands of neoplastic epithelial cells surrounded by reactive fibrous tissue.

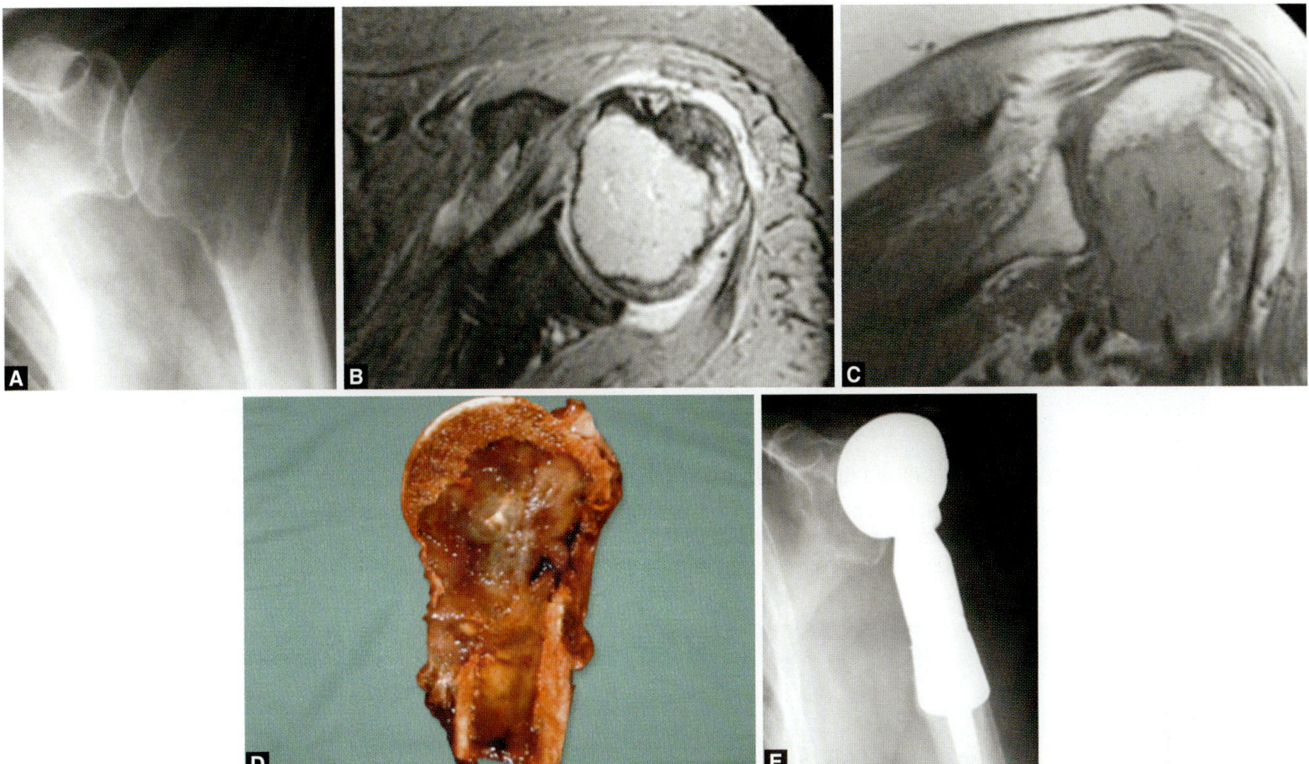

Figs. 91A to E: (A) Anteroposterior radiograph of 77-year-old woman with renal cancer metastatic to left proximal humerus; (B and C) MRI show extent of lesion. This was only site of metastatic disease, so patient was treated with wide resection and endoprosthetic reconstruction; (D) Photograph of resected specimen; (E) Anteroposterior view of left shoulder after endoprosthetic reconstruction.

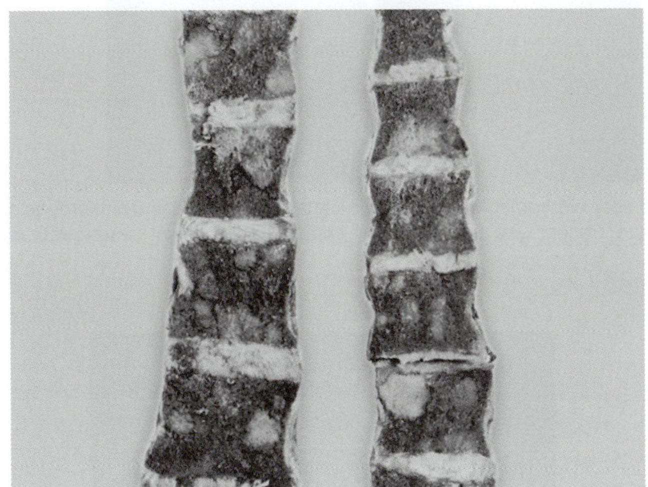

Fig. 92: Thoracic and lumbar vertebra with multiple metastasis from breast carcinoma. The roughly spherical metastatic lesions have replaced bone marrow in part of every vertebral body.

- In some cases radioactive isotopes are used to palliate pain. I-131 provides pain relief due to thyroid metastasis.

Surgical Treatment (Table 12)

- Operative treatment of metastatic bone disease can preserve musculoskeletal function and relieve pain.
- Options include prophylactic internal fixation or prosthetic reconstruction of involved bones to prevent pathologic fractures. New implants and techniques are available to provide durable reconstructions.
- Methyl methacrylate is often used as a local adjuvant to add strength to the metal construct. Postoperatively, radiation is often effective in maintaining local control.
- Bisphosphonates are now used routinely in patients with lytic bone metastasis and inhibit osteoclast-mediated bone destruction.
- Tumor resection and replacement with endoprosthesis.
- Tumor curettage + cemented osteosynthesis.
- Use of local adjuvants (phenol) to improve margins of sterilization and polymethyl methacrylate to enhance structural strength.

MAFFUCCI SYNDROME

This rare disorder is characterized by the development of multiple enchondromas and soft-tissue hemangiomas of the skin and viscera.

- Lesions appear during childhood.
- Boys and girls are affected with equal frequency.
- There is a strong tendency for malignant change to occur, in both soft-tissue and bone lesions.
- The incidence of sarcomatous transformation in one of the enchondromas is probably greater than 50%, but fortunately these tumors are not highly malignant.
- Patients with Maffucci syndrome should be monitored regularly throughout life for any changes in either the bone or the visceral lesions.

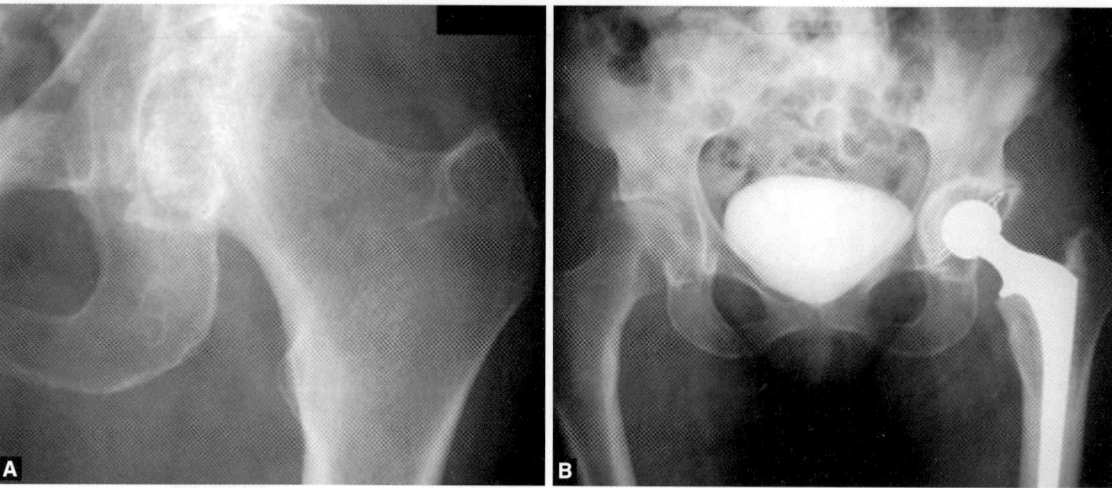

Figs. 93A and B: (A) Anteroposterior view of left hip of patient treated with radiation for metastatic breast cancer. She subsequently developed osteonecrosis of femoral head; (B) AP view of pelvis after treatment with cemented total hip arthroplasty. Because bone had been irradiated, femoral and acetabular components were cemented.

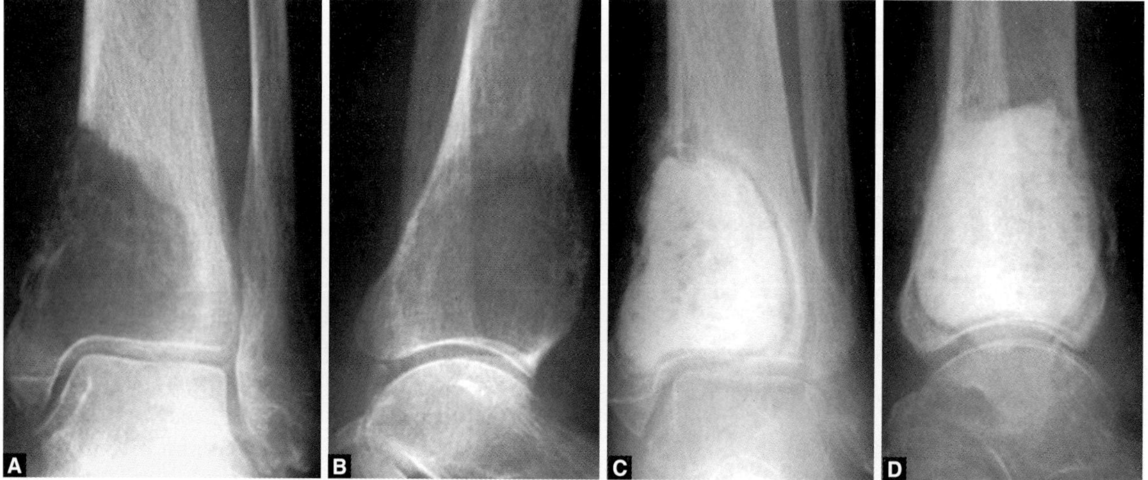

Figs. 94A to D: (A and B) Anteroposterior and lateral radiographs of left ankle of 78-year-old woman with metastatic kidney cancer; (C and D) Anteroposterior and lateral views after extended curettage and packing of defect with methacrylate. Patient was able to resume immediate full weight bearing with relief of her pain.

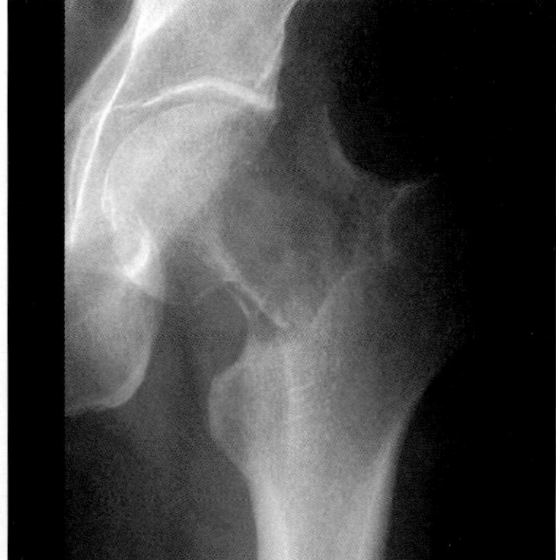

Fig. 95: Radiograph of the hip showing a pathologic fracture from metastatic renal cell carcinoma.

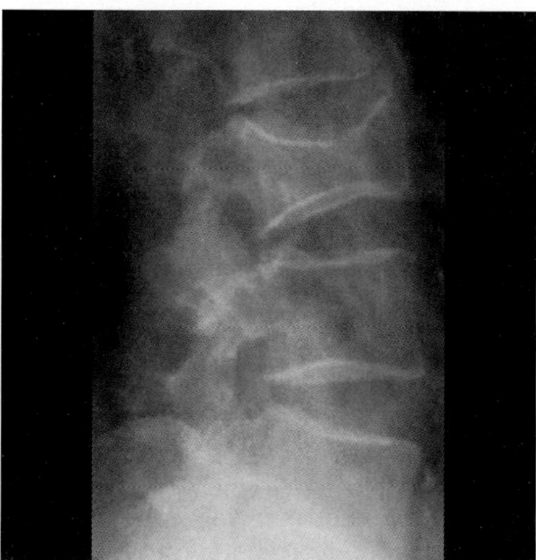

Fig. 96: Radiograph showing a pathologic compression fracture of a vertebral body caused by metastatic breast carcinoma.

TABLE 11: Typical radiographic features of metastasis from various primary tumors.

Commonly lytic	*Commonly blastic*	*Commonly mixed*
Lung	Prostate	Breast
Kidney	Bladder with prostate	Lung
Thyroid	Bronchial carcinoid	Ovary
Adrenal		Testis
Uterus		Cervix

TABLE 12: Mirel's Scoring System*.

Variable	*Risk score 1*	*2*	*3*
Site	Upper limb	Lower limb	Peritrochanter
Pain	Mild	Moderate	Weight bearing
Lesion	Blastic	Mixed	Lytic
Size w.r.t. bone diameter	<1/3	1/3–2/3	>2/3

*Mirels suggested that a
- Score of ≤7 out of 12 is indicative of minimal risk of fracture.
- Score of 8 out of 12 is associated of 15% risk.
- Score of 9 is of 33% risk of fracture.
- Score of 9 or >9 is indicative of prophylactic fixation.

DYSCHONDROPLASIA (ENCHONDROMATOSIS OR OLLIER'S DISEASE)

This is a rare, but easily recognized disorder, in which there is defective transformation of physeal cartilage columns into bone.

Clinical Features

Typically, the disorder is unilateral, indeed only one limb or even one bone may be involved. An affected limb is short and if the growth plate is asymmetrically involved, the bone grows in a bent fashion. Bowing of the distal end of the femur or tibia is not uncommon and the patient may present with valgus or varus deformity at the knee and ankle. Shortening of the ulna may lead to bowing of the radius and sometimes dislocation of the radial head. The fingers or toes frequently contain multiple enchondromata, which are characteristic of the disease and may be so numerous that the hand is crippled. A rare variety of dyschondroplasia is associated with multiple hemangiomata (Maffucci syndrome), this is described here. The condition is not inherited. Indeed, it is probably an embryonal rather than a genetic disorder.

Radiological Features

The characteristic change in the long bones is radiolucent streaking, extending from the physis into the metaphysic, the appearance of persistent, incompletely ossified cartilage columns trapped in bone. If only half of the physis is affected, growth is asymmetrically retarded and the bone becomes curved. With maturation the radiolucent columns eventually ossify, but the deformities remain. In the hands and feet, the cartilage islands characteristically produce multiple enchondromata. Beware of any change in the appearance of the lesions after the end of normal growth, as this may be a sign of malignant change, which occurs in 5–10% of cases.

Treatment

Bone deformity may need correction, but this should be deferred until growth is complete, otherwise it is likely to recur.

DYSCHONDROSTEOSIS

In this disorder, there is also disproportionate shortening of the limbs, but it is mainly the middle segments (forearms and legs), which are affected. It is the most common of the mesomelic dysplasias and is transmitted as an autosomal dominant defect. Stature is reduced, but not as markedly as in achondroplasia. The most characteristic X-rays changes are shortening of the forearms and leg bones, bowing of the radius and Madelung's deformity of the wrist, which may require operative treatment.

PAGET'S DISEASE (OSTEITIS DEFORMANS)

Paget's disease is characterized by enlargement and thickening of the bone, but the internal architecture is abnormal and the bone is unusually brittle. The condition has a curious ethnic and geographic distribution, being relatively common in North America, Britain, Germany, and Australia (more than 3% of people aged over 40 years), but rare in Asia, Africa, and the Middle East. There is a tendency to familial aggregation. The cause is unknown, although the discovery of inclusion bodies in the osteoclasts has suggested a viral infection (Rebel et al. 1980).

Pathology

The disease may appear in one or several sites. In the tubular bones, it starts at one end and progresses slowly toward the diaphysis, leaving a trail of altered architecture behind. The characteristic cellular change is a marked increase in osteoclastic and osteoblastic activity. Bone turnover is accelerated, plasma alkaline phosphatase is raised (a sign of osteoblastic activity) and there is increased excretion of hydroxyproline in the urine (due to osteoclastic activity).

In the osteolytic (or vascular) stage, there is avid resorption of existing bone by large osteoclasts, the excavations being filled with vascular fibrous tissue. In adjacent areas, osteoblastic activity produces new woven and lamellar bone, which in turn is attacked by osteoclasts. This alternating activity extends on both endosteal and periosteal surfaces, so the bone increases in thickness, but is structurally weak and easily deformed. Gradually, osteoclastic activity abates and the eroded areas fill with new lamellar bone, leaving an irregular pattern of cement lines that mark the limits of the old resorption cavities. These "tidemarks" produce a marbled or mosaic appearance on microscopy. In the late, osteoblastic stage the thickened bone becomes increasingly sclerotic and brittle.

Clinical Features

Paget's disease affects men and women equally. Only occasionally does it present in patients under 50 years, but from that age onwards, it becomes increasingly common. The disease may be present for many years remain localized to part or the whole of one bone, e.g. the pelvis and tibia being the most common sites and the femur, skull, spine and clavicle the next common ones.

Most people with Paget's disease are asymptomatic, the disorder being diagnosed when an X-ray is taken for some unrelated condition or after the incidental discovery of a raised serum alkaline phosphatase level. When patients do present, it is usually because of pain or deformity or some complication of the disease.

The pain is a dull constant ache, worse in bed, when the patient warms up, but rarely severe, unless a fracture occurs or sarcoma supervenes. Deformities are seen mainly in the lower limbs. Long bones bend across the trajectories of mechanical stress, thus the tibia bows anteriorly and the femur anterolaterally. The limb looks bent and feels thick and the skin is unduly warm, hence the term "osteitis deformans". If the skull is affected, it enlarges. The patient may complain that old hats no longer fit. The skull base may become flattened (platybasia), giving the appearance of a short neck. In generalized Paget's disease, there may also be considerable kyphosis, so the patient becomes shorter and ape-like, with bent legs and arms hanging in front of him.

Cranial nerve compression may lead to impaired vision, facial palsy, trigeminal neuralgia or deafness. Another cause of deafness is otosclerosis. Vertebral thickening may cause spinal cord or nerve root compression.

Steal syndromes, in which blood is diverted from internal organs to the surrounding skeletal circulation, may cause cerebral impairment and spinal cord ischemia. If there is also spinal stenosis, the patient develops typical symptoms of spinal claudication and lower limb weakness.

X-ray Findings

The appearances are so characteristic that the diagnosis is seldom in doubt. During the resorptive phase, there may be localized areas of osteolysis, most typical is the flame-shaped lesion, extending along the shaft of the bone or a circumscribed patch of osteoporosis in the skull (osteoporosis circumscripta). Later, the bone becomes thick and sclerotic, with coarse trabeculation. The femur or tibia sometimes develops fine cracks on the convex surface stress fractures that heal with increasing deformity of the bone. Occasionally, the diagnosis is made only when the patient presents with a pathological fracture. Silent lesions are revealed by increased activity in the radio nuclide scan.

Biochemistry

Serum calcium and phosphate levels are usually normal. The most useful test is measurement of the serum alkaline phosphatase level, which correlates with the activity and extent of disease. Twenty-four hours urinary excretion of pyridinoline cross-links is a good indicator of disease activity and bone resorption. However, the test is expensive and is, therefore, not used routinely. Patients who are immobilized may develop hypercalcemia.

Complications

- *Fractures:* They are common, especially in the weight-bearing long bones. In the femoral neck, they are often vertical. Elsewhere, the fracture line is usually partly transverse and partly oblique, like the line of section of a felled tree. In the femur, there is a high rate of nonunion, for femoral neck fractures prosthetic replacement and for shaft fractures early internal fixation is recommended. Small stress fractures may be a very painful and they resemble "looser's zones" on X- ray, except that they occur on convex surfaces.
- *Osteoarthritis:* Osteoarthritis of the hip or knee is not merely a consequence of abnormal loading due to bone deformity, in the hip it seldom occurs, unless the innominate bone is involved. The X-ray appearances suggest an atrophic arthritis, with sparse remodeling and at operated joint, vascularity is increased.
- *Nerve compression and spinal stenosis:* Occasionally, this is the first abnormality to be detected and may call for definitive surgical treatment.
- *Bone sarcoma:* Osteosarcoma arising in an elderly patient is almost always due to malignant transformation in Paget's disease. The frequency of malignant change is probably around 1%. It should always be suspected, if a previously diseased bone becomes more painful, swollen and tender. Occasionally, it presents as the first evidence of Paget's disease. The prognosis is extremely grave.
- *High-output cardiac failure:* Though rare, this is an important general complication. It is due to prolonged increased bone blood flow.
- *Hypercalcemia:* Hypercalcemia may occur, if the patient is immobilized for long. In spite of all these complications, patients with Paget's disease usually come to terms with the condition and live to a ripe old age.

Treatment

Most patients with Paget's disease never have any symptom and require no treatment. Sometimes pain is due to an associated arthritis, rather than bone disease and this may respond to nonsteroidal anti-inflammatory therapy. Patients should be examined and the alkaline phosphatase level should be measured, at least once a year. Any change in symptoms or a rise in alkaline phosphatase, calls for further investigation and if necessary, more active treatment.

The indications for specific treatment are:

- Persistent bone pain
- Repeated fractures
- Neurological complications
- High-output cardiac failure
- Hypercalcemia, due to immobilization
- For some months before and after, major bone surgery, where there is a risk of excessive hemorrhage. Drugs that suppress bone turnover, notably calcitonin and bisphosphonates, are most effective, when the disease is active and bone turnover is high.

Calcitonin is most widely used. It reduces bone resorption, by decreasing both the activity and the number of osteoclasts, serum alkaline phosphatase and urinary pyridinoline cross-link levels are lowered. Salmon calcitonin is more effective than the porcine variety, subcutaneous injections of 50–100 MRC units are given daily, until pain is relieved and the alkaline phosphatase levels are reduced and stabilized. Maintenance injections once or twice weekly may have to be continued indefinitely, but some authorities advocate stopping the drug and resuming treatment, if symptoms recur. Drug resistance, due to antibody formation may occur, but this will be avoided, when human calcitonin is more generally available.

Bisphosphonates, bind to hydroxyapatite crystals, inhibiting their rate of growth and dissolution. It is claimed that the reduction in bone turnover following their use, is associated with the formation of lamellar rather than woven bone and that, even after treatment is stopped, there may be prolonged remission of disease

(Bickerstaff et al. 1990). Etidronate can be given orally (always on an empty stomach), but dosage should be kept low (e.g. 5 mg/kg per day for up to 6 months), lest impaired bone mineralization results in osteomalacia.

The newer bisphosphonates, such as pamidronate and alendronate are more effective and produce remissions, even with short courses of 1 or 2 weeks. They do not impair bone mineralization and can be repeated if necessary.

Surgery

The main indication for operation is a pathological fracture, which (in a long bone) usually requires internal fixation. When the fracture is treated, the opportunity should be taken to straighten the bone. Other indications for surgery are painful osteoarthritis (total joint replacement), nerve entrapment (decompression) and severe spinal stenosis (decompression). Beware, blood loss is likely to be excessive in these cases. An osteosarcoma, if detected early, may be resectable, but generally the prognosis is grave.

FIBROUS DYSPLASIA

Fibrous dysplasia or (fibro-osseous dysplasia) is a skeletal developmental anomaly of the bone-forming mesenchyme that manifests as a defect in osteoblastic differentiation and maturation. Thus, leading to replacement of normal marrow and cancellous bone, by immature bone and fibrous stroma.

- It is a benign condition, in which normal bone is replaced by fibrous connective tissue, due to a defect in osteoblast differentiation and maturation.
- Relatively common disorder of bone, involving the proliferation and maturation of fibroblasts.
- Etiology is unknown.
- Recognized most frequent during 2nd and 3rd decade of life.
- Females affected more than males.
- Possible developmental dysplasia.
- "Great imitator of bone disease".
- May affect one or more bones.
- Less than 1% transformation to malignancy.

Three Basic Forms

1. Monostotic (70%)
2. Polyostotic (27%)
3. Polyostotic, with endocrine dysfunction (3%)

Pathological Features

- Normal bone undergoes physiologic resorption and is replaced by irregular shaped woven bone, which is dispersed haphazardly into a predominately fibrous collagenous matrix.
- The variable amount of bone, accounts for the range of roentgen density. Radiolucent to ground glass.

Clinical Manifestations

- Signs and symptoms depend on the size, location, and number of lesions.
- Asymptomatic to intermittent pain
- Local swelling
- Deformity and fracture
- Spontaneous scalp hemorrhage
- *Café-au-lait spots:*
  - Tanned to dark brown skin lesions and is not raised
  - Fibrous dysplasia "Coast of Maine"
  - Neurofibromatosis "Coast of California"
  - Most common extraskeletal manifestation.
- *McCune-Albright syndrome:*
  - Predominantly in females
  - *Consists of:*
    - Polyostotic fibrous dysplasia
    - Café-au-lait spots
    - Endocrine dysfunction (hyperthyroidism, premature puberty, acromegaly, hyperpara- thyroidism, Cushing's syndrome and vitamin D resistant rickets).

Laboratory Features

- Normal calcium and phosphorus levels
- Occasional elevations of alkaline phosphatase.

Plain Radiography (Figs. 97A to C)

First-line of imaging modality.

Advanced Imaging

- Bone scintigraphy, helps to determine activity and areas of skeletal involvement (Fig. 98)
- *CT scan (Fig. 99):*

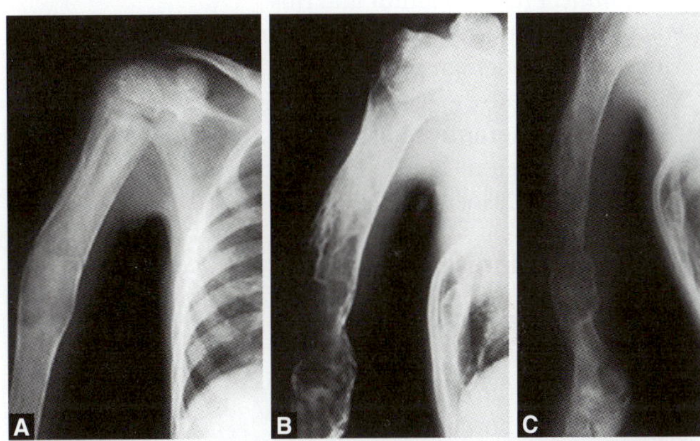

Figs. 97A to C: Fibrous dysplasia of humerus: The medullary cavity is replaced by fibrous tissue showing ground-glass appearance.

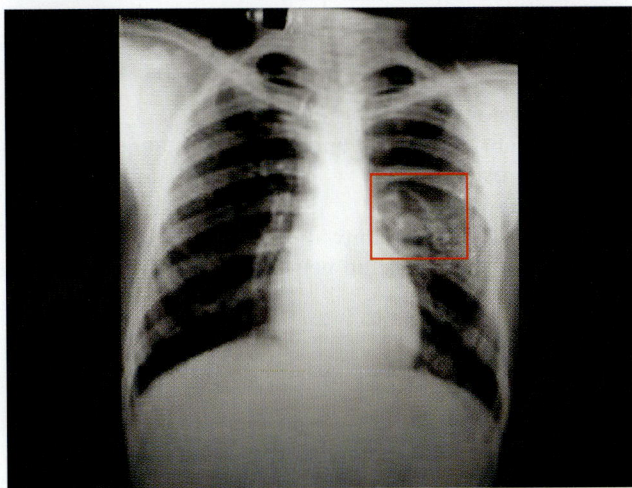

Fig. 98: Bone scintigraphy helps to determine activity and areas of skeletal involvement.

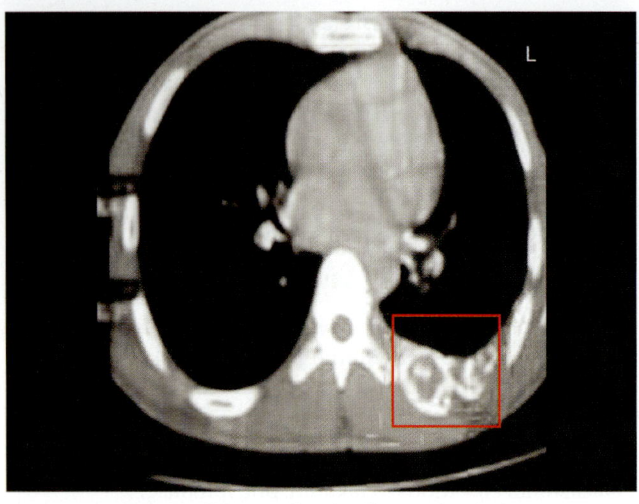

Fig. 99: CT scan showing fibrous dysplasia.

  - Cystic area
  - Well-defined thick sharp border
  - Useful to define extent of craniofacial disease
- *MRI:* Typically moderately low signal T1 and bright or mixed signal on T2.

Skeletal Locations

- *Monostotic:* Proximal femur and ribs
- *Polyostotic:* Femur, skull, tibia, humerus, ribs, etc.
- Most common benign rib lesion
- May demonstrate the "extrapleural sign"
- Diaphyseal-metaphyseal location, typically sparring the subarticular region
- Usually centrally located.

Radiographic Manifestations

Monostotic

- Geographic
- Lucent, smoky (ground glass) (Fig. 99)
- Thick sclerotic border (Rind sign)
- Occasionally septated or trabeculated
- Expansile lesion
- Cortical thinning and scalloping
- Elongated lesion.

Polyostotic

- Pseudofractures and deformities
- Involvement of the skull and facial bones, tends to produce more sclerosis
- Pseudoarthrosis:
  - Usually lower extremity
  - Fibrous dysplasia and neurofibromatosis most common causes.

Craniofacial Type

- 10–25% in monostotic
- 50% in polyostotic form
- Occurs in an isolated craniofacial form
- *Sites of involvement:* Frontal region, these include following sites:
  - Sphenoid (vestibular dysfunction, tinnitus, hearing loss)
  - Maxillary hypertelorism, cranial asymmetry, facial deformity (i.e. leontiasis ossea)
  - Orbital and periorbital bones, visual impairment, exophthalmos and blindness
  - Ethmoidal bones
  - Cribriform plate, hyposmia or anosmia may result.

Treatment

- Splints and casts
- Curettage and bone grafting
- Bone grafting and stabilization
- En bloc resection
- Osteotomy.

Complications

- Pathological fractures are most common.
- Bowing deformities, e.g.
  - Shepherd's crook
  - Leontiasis ossea.
- Sarcomatous transformation in 0.5–1%
  - Fibrosarcoma most common
  - Femur and skull (most common sites).

Prognosis

- Depends on extent and degree of initial skeletal involvement and extraskeletal features
- Size and shape of lesions may change
- Generally becomes quiescent at puberty and remains so
- *Monostotic:*
  - Excellent prognosis, if the bone can be strengthened
  - Usually, it does not change to polyostotic
- *Polyostotic:*
  - Several operative procedures, to achieve bone strength and correct deformity
- Malignant degeneration is rare.

Associated Disorders

Cherubism

- Familial fibrous dysplasia of the jaws (autosomal dominant)
- Begins during 18 months to 2 years and regresses during puberty
- Swelling of the lower face
- "Eyes-raised-to-heaven" sign
- Multilocular cystic lesions, with asymmetric distribution.

Differential Diagnosis

- Eosinophilic granuloma
- Nonossifying fibroma
- Bone hemangioma
- Hyperparathyroidism
- Paget's disease
- Brown tumor
- Aneurysmal bone cyst.

Mazabraud Syndrome

It is a fibrous dysplasia and soft-tissue myxomas.

CHAPTER

Gait Analysis

12

OBJECTIVES

- Gait
- Gait Cycle
- Gait Measurement Technique
- Gait Energy
- Gait Abnormalities

GAIT

Continuous rhythmic alternative movements of lower limbs, in order to propulse the body forward, by moving center of gravity in forward direction with minimal expenditure of energy.

GAIT CYCLE

It is the duration that occurs from the time, when the heel of one foot strikes the ground to the time at which the same foot contacts the ground again. Normally, the gait cycle is of 1–2 seconds.

Two phases of gait cycle are shown in Figure 1.

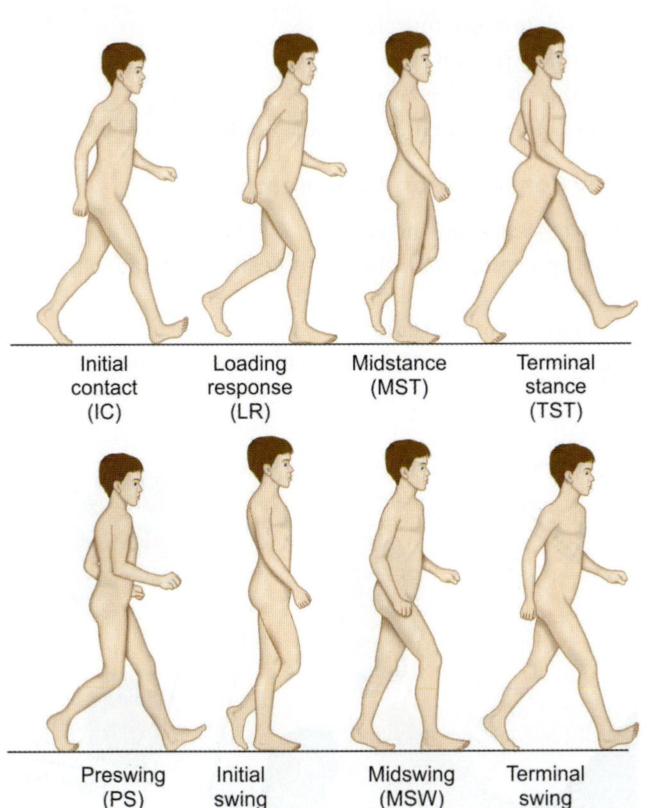

Fig. 1: The descriptive phases of a normal gait cycle.

Phases of Gait Cycle

- Stance phase (60% of a gait cycle)
- Swing phase (40% of a gait cycle).

Stance Phase

It is the time during which the limb is in contact with the ground and supporting the weight of the body from heel strike, to toe off.

It comprises 60% of the gait cycle and is divided into following five phases:

1. *Initial contact or heel strike:*
   - Knee is extended and ankle is in neutral position
   - Normally, heel contacts the ground first.
2. *Loading response or flat foot:*
   - Corresponds to the gait cycle's first period of double limb support and ends with a contralateral toe off, when the opposite extremities leaves the ground
   - During loading, knee flexes 15°, while ankle plantar flexes 15°, which is an energy conserving mechanism
   - Throughout the first phase of stance, hamstrings and ankle dorsiflexors remain active
   - Quadriceps and gluteal muscles act during loading and through the early midstance to maintain hip and knee stability.
3. *Midstance:*
   - Begin with contralateral toe off. The center of gravity is directly over the reference foot (stance foot)
   - By midstance, the knee is extended and ankle is neutral again
   - The triceps surae acts to control tibial advancement (preventing tendency of ankle to dorsiflex, due to body weight and inertia).
4. *Terminal stance or heel off:*
   - Begins when center of gravity is over the supporting foot and ends when contralateral foot contacts the ground
   - Terminal stance and midstance are only phases when center of gravity truly lies over the base of support.
5. *Preswing (toe off):*
   - Begins at contralateral initial contact and ends at toe off

- Preswing corresponds to the gait cycle seconds period of double limb support
- At preswing, knee flexes 35° and ankle plantar flexes at 20°
- In these last phases of stance, the toes, which have been neutral, dorsiflex at the metatarsophalangeal joint.

Swing Phase

It is the time period during which the limb is off the ground and advancing forward, the body weight is supported by contralateral limb, i.e. acceleration to deceleration. It comprises of 40% of gait cycle (Fig. 2) and is divided into three phases:

1. *Initial swing or acceleration:*
   - Begins at toe off and continues until maximum knee flexion (60°) occurs
   - Contraction of quadriceps initiated before toe off and serves two purposes:
     - It prevents heel from rising too high in a posterior direction
     - It helps to initiate forward swing of leg.
2. *Mid swing:*
   From maximum knee flexion, until the tibia is vertical or perpendicular to the ground.
3. *Terminal swing or deceleration:*
   - Begins, where tibia is vertical and ends at initial contact
   - Hamstrings muscles become active, to decelerate forward swing of the leg.

GAIT MEASUREMENT TECHNIQUE

- Force
- Motion
- Electromyography
- Energy consumption.

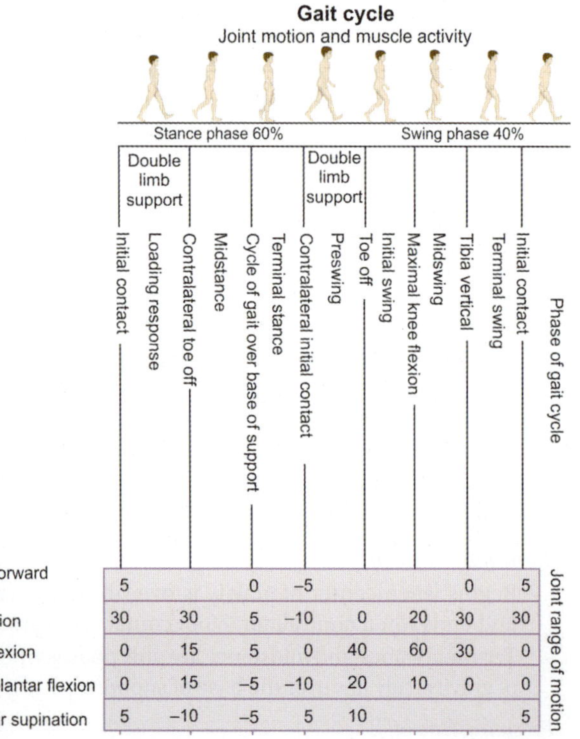

Fig. 2: Gait cycle, with different phases and range of motion at various joints.

Force or Pressure Measurements

- Glass plate views
- Pressure distribution
- Pressure plates
- Pressure distribution inside a shoe
- Pressure in the soles is seen in Figure 3.

Motion Measurements

- *Goniometers* is used for measuring range of motion
- *Electrogoniometers* for joint angle at successive instants
- Conductive walkway, stride length, cadence, velocity, etc.
- Dynamic base, etc.
- *Video cameras* is used for measuring stride length, cadence, velocity, dynamic base, etc.
- *High speed video:* Stop motion measurements
- *Accelerometers:* It is used for measuring accelerations and is comparatively cheaper than other instruments
- *Gyroscopes* is used for measuring change in orientation
- *3D marker system* for all possible kinematic measures.

Electromyography (EMG) Measurement

- Noisy and qualitative
- Indicator of when the muscle is active
- *Surface EMG (most common):*
  - Cheap, easy
  - Difficult to interpret because of cross talk and noise
- *Fine wire and needle EMG:*
  - Penetrate skin
  - Isolate single muscle
  - Mildly painful
  - May change behavior
- Parameters of gait measurement are shown in Figure 4.

Energy Consumption Measurement

- *Heart rate:* Cheap and easy
- *Oxygen consumption:* Better indication of relative metabolic state
- Indicator of overall effort
- Often difficult to detect change because of variability.

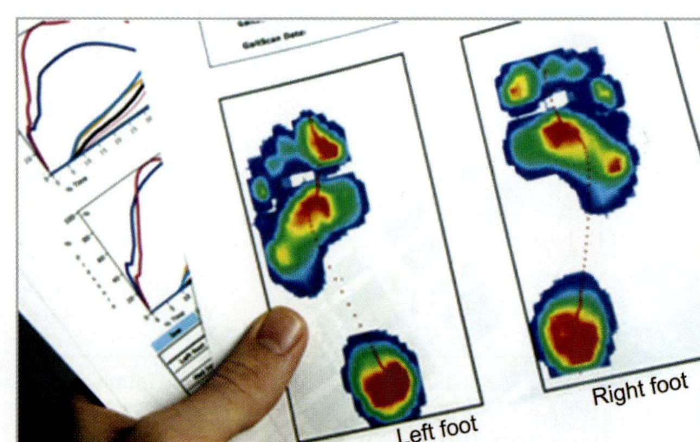

Fig. 3: Pressures in the soles of left and right feet.

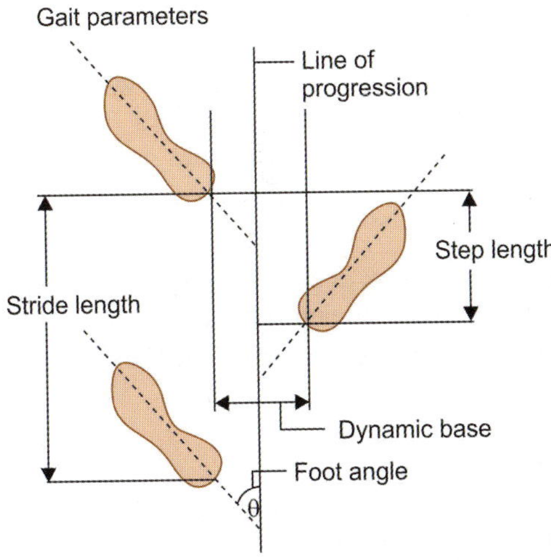

Fig. 4: Parameters for gait measurement.

GAIT ENERGY

- Bipedal gait is inherently unstable and inefficient
- To conserve energy, the movement of joint minimizes the rise and fall of center of gravity, located just anterior to S2 vertebra
- Muscular activities are coordinated
- Inertia is used to its fullest advantage, to lessen the work of walking.

Kinematics

It is defined as the study of the angular rotation of each joint during movement. Kinematics can be observed in three planes:

1. *Sagittal plane:* Flexion and extension
2. *Coronal plane:* Hip abduction and adduction
3. *Transverse plane:* Rotation of hip, tibia or feet.

Approach to Analysis

- Analysis of motion plus measurement of muscle activating plus reaction force between the patient's foot and ground provides a comprehensive assessment of biomechanics of locomotion.
- Quantitative gait analysis still does not replace observational gait analysis done in clinical examination.

Measurable Determinants (by Inman)

- Width of the base from heel-to-heel should be less than 2–4 inches
- Body's cog lies 2 inches in front of S2, in a normal condition
- Gait oscillates less than 2 inches in vertical direction
- Pelvis and trunk shifts laterally, approximately 1 inch to weight-bearing side
- Average length of step approximately 15 inches
- Average adult approximately walks 90–120 steps/min, with average energy cost of only 100 calorie/mile
- During swing phase, pelvis rotates 40° forward, while hip joint on the opposite side acts as the fulcrum for rotation.

GAIT ABNORMALITIES

Antalgic Gait or Painful Gait

- Due to pain anywhere from foot-to-hip to spine
- The patient avoids to bear weight on the affected limb (avoid stance phase). Quick, short steps on affected limb, thereby reducing the stance phase and increasing stance phase of unaffected limb
- *Hip abnormality:* The patient leans toward the affected side during stance phase
- *Spine abnormality:* Patient may not walk or walks slowly to avoid pain.

Trendelenburg Gait

- It may be unilateral or bilateral
- When unilateral, the patient leans on the affected side with swaying of the pelvis and shoulder of the unaffected side, as the pelvis drops on the opposite side of the hip and to keep cog over the stance leg. Any condition, in which there is a deficit in the abduction mechanism of the hip joint, medial deviation of the mechanical axis of lower limb and costopelvic impingement, causes this abnormal gait pattern.
- Abduction mechanism can be deficit in fulcrum (hip joint), lever arm (neck of femur), power (gluteus medius), e.g. congenital dislocation of hip, fracture of the neck of femur and polio paralysis.

Stiff Hip Gait

- Patient walks without flexing the hip (about 20° of flexing of hip is essential for normal gait)
- To compensate patient raises pelvis and semicircumducts the limb to propel forward
- Increase motion of pelvis on lumbar spine during swing.

Stiff Knee Gait

Pelvis is raised during swing phase, so that heel clears the floor.

Gluteus Maximus Weakness Gait

- In normal gait gluteus maximus, provides for stability in sagittal plane and for restrain of forward progression. This muscle helps to counteract flexion moment at the hip in early part of stance and restrains the forward movement of femur in late swing in normal gait
- In gluteus maximus, weak trunk must be thrown posteriorly at heel strike, to prevent trunk from falling forward, when there is flexion moment at hip
- Hip in hyperextension, so the center of gravity is behind the joint
- The backward lean is typical of a gluteus maximus weakness gait.

Quadriceps Weakness Gait

- In very weak or paralyzed quadriceps, patient stabilizes his knees for weight-bearing by little leaning on effected side and pressing over the lower thigh by his ipsilateral hand
- Walking on level surface may appear to be normal
- At speed, limb behaves as pendulum, due to full extension of knee joint. This is a preparatory step to heel strike
- At full extension, action of quads is not necessary for stability of knee joint
- If line of gravity is maintained anteriorly to the axis of motion of knee joint, full extension persists through stance phase
- Such a patient, however, will be unable to run and may have difficulty in walking on rough or inclined surface and stairs because in those full extensions is not attained and knee tends to buckle into flexion.

Spastic Gait

- Spastic muscles does not allow hip and knee to be flexed enough for foot to clear the ground
- Therefore, patient partially drags his weight on the spastic leg. In this attempt, there is some circumduction effect on the lower limb, e.g. hemiplegia, diplegia, cerebral palsy, etc.

High Stepping Gait

Patient flexes the hip and knee excessively, to clear the ground, e.g. foot drop.

Short Limb Gait

- Less than 3.5–5.5% compensation, by walking on toes on the short limb, flexes the hip and knee of opposite side during stance phase
- Greater than 3.5–5.5% gait manifests and there is no compensation.

Ataxic Gait

Gait in which foot is raised higher than normal and brought down suddenly in a flapping manner.

Knock Knee Gait

While walking, patient flexes hip slightly, knees points and appose each other, ankles and feet are kept apart with tendency of toeing.

Stamping Gait

Patient raises his feet abnormally high and jerks them forward to strike ground, with a "stamp", e.g. sensory ataxia (tabes dorsalis).

Short Shuffling Gait

The patient with stooping body, is propelled forward quickly in successions, as if trying to catch-up with center of gravity, e.g. Parkinsonism.

Gluteus Medius Gait

More or less like Trendelenburg gait occurs in paralysis of gluteus medius.

Cerebellar Gait

Staggering gait often with tendency to fall to one or other side, forward or backward.

Hysterical Gait

- Diagnosed by exclusion, bizarre and inconsistency. Does not fits with available clinical signs
- History of emotional upset is present.

Wobbling Gait or Chorus Girl Swing

- In bilateral weakness of gluteus medius muscle, gait shows accentuated side-to-side movement
- This gait is also being seen in congenital dislocation of the hip (CDH) and coxa vara.

Calcaneal Gait

Patient walks on his broadened heel with a tendency of rotating the foot outwards, tendency of genu recurvatum, with no calcaneal pick up, no push off and is due to weakness of triceps surae.

Scissors Gait

- One leg crosses directly over other with each steps, like crossing of the blade of scissors due to adductor tightness
- Knee may also be flexed resulting in couching, which lead to couch gait
- During the swing phase, one lower extremity crosses the other leg which is in stance phase
- Seen in cerebral diplegia.

Lathyriatic Gait

Combination of spasticity, hyperabduction and dragging of lower limb elements in the gait.

Helicopod Gait

Legs and feet are thrown in half circles as in hemiplegia.

Drunken or Reeling Gait

Patient walks irregularly on wide base, swinging side way without stability and balance, with tendency of falling with each step.

Genu Recurvatum Gait

- In paralysis of hamstring muscle the knee goes for hyperextension, while transmitting weight in mid stance phase
- Seen in poliomyelitis.

SECTION

2

General Surgery Related to Orthopedics

- Tetanus
- Deep Vein Thrombosis
- Fat Embolism Syndrome
- Peripheral Nerve Injuries
- Peripheral Vascular Disease
- An Overview of Diabetes Mellitus
- Shock
- Gas Gangrene
- Head Injury
- Chest Trauma
- Abdominal Trauma
- Polytrauma and Management of Polytrauma Patient
- Soft Tissue Coverage in Orthopedics
- Amputation Surgery

CHAPTER

13

Tetanus

OBJECTIVES

- *Clostridium tetani*
- Types
- Treatment
- Classification of the Patients: Depending upon their Immune Status
- Course (Manifestation of Disease)
- Prevention

INTRODUCTION

Tetanus is a neurological disorder, characterized by increased muscle tone and spasms. It is caused by tetanospasmin, a powerful protein toxin elaborated by *Clostridium tetani.*

It occurs in several clinical forms, including generalized, neonatal, and localized disease. Mortality in developing countries like India is approximately 90% and 50% in developed countries like USA.

CLOSTRIDIUM TETANI

The important features of Clostridium tetani are:

- Anaerobic, motile, gram-positive, and rod like
- Forms an oval and colorless, terminal spores
- Assumes a shape resembling a tennis racket or drum-stick (Fig. 1)
- Found worldwide in soil, in the inanimate environment, in animal feces and occasionally in human feces
- Spores may survive for years in some environments and are resistant to various disinfectants and to boiling for 20 minutes
- Vegetative cells are easily inactivated and several antibiotics, including metronidazole and penicillin are effective against it. (*Note:* Round terminal spores give cells a "drumstick" or "tennis racket" appearance.)
- Tetanus occurs sporadically and almost always affects unimmunized persons, partially immunized persons, and fully immunized individuals, who fail to maintain adequate immunity with booster doses of vaccine, may be affected as well
- Not contagious from person-to-person
- It is an only vaccine-preventable disease that is infectious but not contagious
- *Temporal pattern:* Peak in winter and summer season
- *Incubation period:* 8 days (3–21 days).

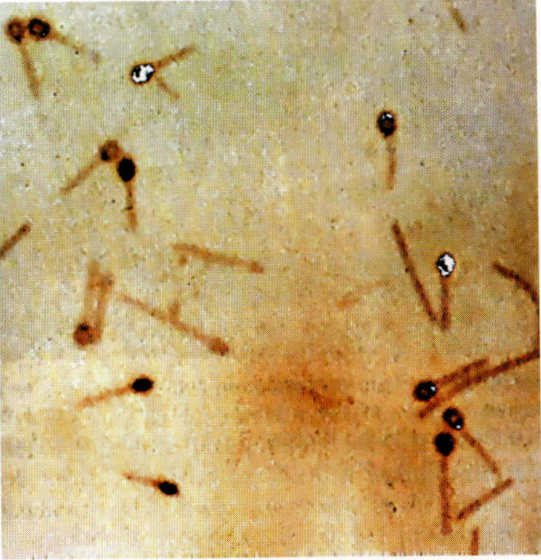

Fig. 1: *Clostridium tetani*—shape resembling a tennis racket or drumstick.

Host Factors

- *Age:* It is a disease of active age (5–40 years), newborn baby, female during delivery, or abortion
- *Sex:* Higher incidence in males than females
- *Occupation:* Agricultural workers are at higher risk
- *Rural and urban difference:* Incidence of tetanus in urban areas is much lower than in rural areas
- *Immunity:* Herd immunity does not protect the individual
- *Environmental and social factors:* Unhygienic custom habits and unhygienic delivery practices
- Most cases follow an acute injury (puncture wound, laceration, abrasion, or other trauma)
- Abdominal surgeries, anterior/anterolateral approach of spine, foot surgeries, rarely contaminated hand surgeries
- Complicated chronic conditions such as skin ulcers, abscesses, and gangrene
- Tetanus has also been associated with burns, frost-bite, middle-ear infection, abortion, childbirth, body piercing, and drug abuse (notably "skin popping")
- Tetanus is a notifiable disease in many countries.

Pathogenesis

- Entry of *C. tetani* into the body usually involves implantation of spores into a wound (Fig. 2). It multiplies and produces a powerful toxin in any deep, contused wound in the presence

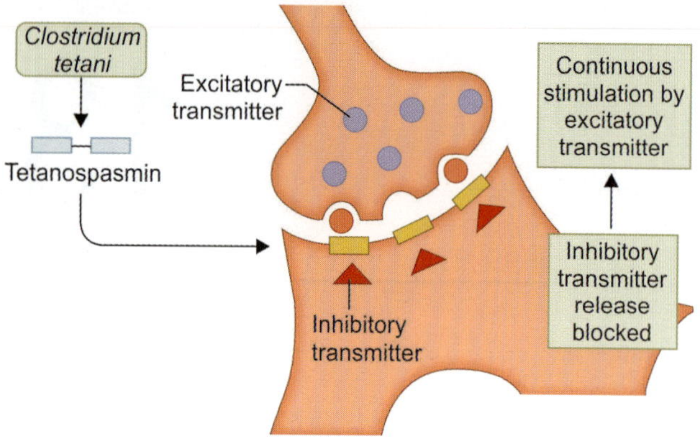

Fig. 2: Pathogenesis of *Clostridium tetani.*

of dead tissue, foreign bodies, and other bacteria. When the oxygen levels of the surrounding tissue is sufficiently low, the implanted *C. tetani* spore then germinates into a new, active vegetative cell that grows and multiplies and most importantly produces toxins.

- Cardiotoxin (endotoxin) acts on hematopoietic cells and cardiac tissue.
- *Tetanospasmin (exotoxin) acts on CNS:* The effects of this toxin are so severe that the effects of the cardiotoxin are completely masked by it. As growing cells produce tetanospasmin at the wound site, the toxin starts to migrate along nerves and acts mainly on four areas of nervous system. These areas are:
  1. Motor end plate
  2. Spinal cord
  3. Brain
  4. Sympathetic system.
- The exotoxin produced in the inoculation site inhibits cholinesterase at the motor end plates, resulting in an excess of acetylcholine locally and therefore, a sustained state of tonic muscle spasm.
- The exotoxin also travels along the nerves to the central nervous system (CNS) and causes extreme hyper-excitability of motor neurons in the anterior horn cells, thereby evoking explosive and widespread reflex spasms of muscle in response to sensory stimuli.
- Once fixed in the nerve tissue, the toxin can no longer be neutralized by antitoxin.
- The shorter the interval between the first symptom and the first reflex spasm, the poorer is the prognosis.
- If the interval is < 48 hours, death is likely.
- Wounds containing tetanus organisms may have healed and been forgotten for months or years before some (unknown) change produces the right conditions for the organism to multiply and produce toxin (latent tetanus).

TYPES

Generalized Tetanus

- Also called descending tetanus
- The most common form of the disease
- Toxin released in the wound enters the lymphatics and bloodstream and is spread widely to distant nerve terminals
- The blood-brain barrier blocks direct entry into the CNS
- Characterized by increased muscle tone and generalized spasms

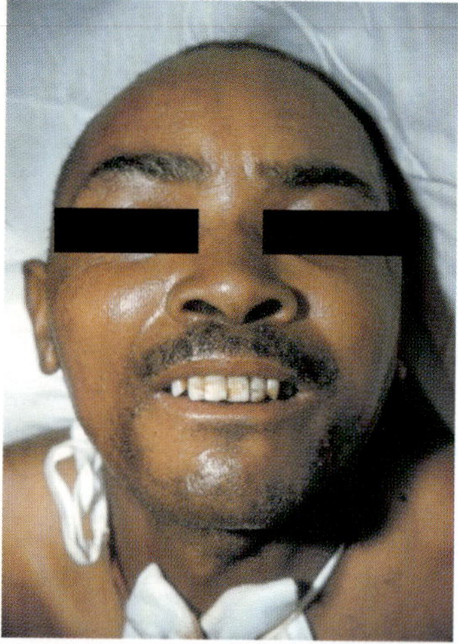

Fig. 3: Increased tone in masseter muscle.

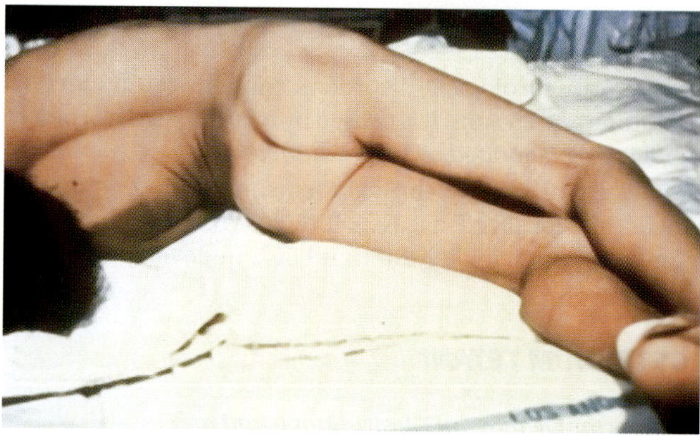

Fig. 4: Opisthotonic position after contraction of back muscles (seen from back).

- Median time of onset after injury is 7 days (15% of cases occur within 3 days and 10% after 14 days)
- Short nerves are affected before long nerves; this fact explains the sequential involvement of nerves of the head, trunk, and extremities in generalized tetanus.

Signs and Symptoms

- Increased tone in the masseter muscles (trismus or lockjaw) (Fig. 3)
- Dysphagia, stiffness, or pain in the neck, shoulder, and back
- Involvement of other muscles produces a rigid abdomen and stiff proximal limb muscles (the hands and feet are relatively spared)
- *Opisthotonus:* Contraction of the back muscles produces an arched back (Figs. 4 and 5)
- *Risus sardonicus*: Sustained contraction of the facial muscles results in a grimace or sneer (Fig. 6)
- Some patients develop paroxysmal, violent, painful, generalized muscle spasms that may cause cyanosis and threaten ventilation
- Spasms occur repetitively and may be spontaneous or provoked by even the slightest stimulation
- A constant threat is reduced ventilation or laryngospasm causing apnea
- The patient may be febrile, although many patients have no fever

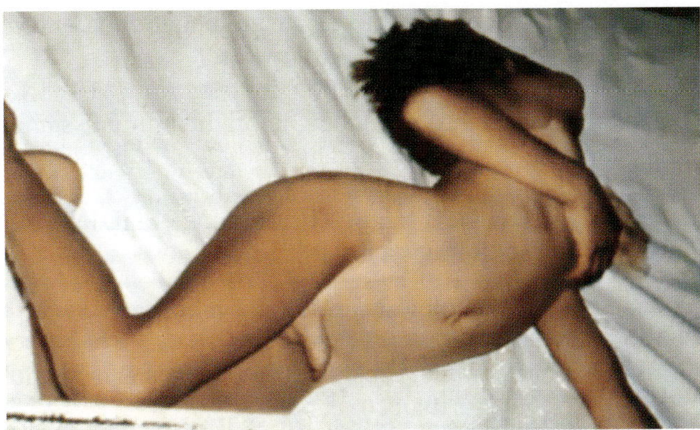

Fig. 5: Opisthotonic position (seen from front).

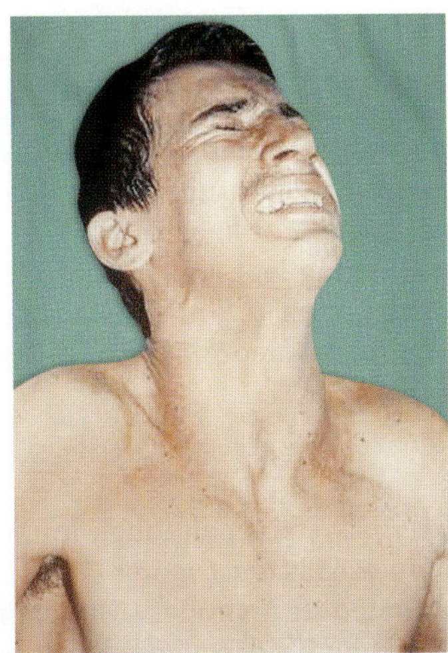

Fig. 6: Risus sardonicus, due to sustained facial muscles contraction.

- Mentation is unimpaired
- Deep tendon reflexes may be increased
- Dysphagia or ileus may preclude oral feeding
- *The severity of illness may be:*
  - Mild (muscle rigidity and few or no spasms)
  - Moderate (trismus, dysphagia, rigidity, and spasms)
  - Severe (frequent explosive paroxysms).
- *Autonomic dysfunction:* This can occur due to following factors:
  - Labile or sustained hypertension
  - Tachycardia
  - Dysrhythmia
  - Hyperpyrexia, profuse sweating, and peripheral vasoconstriction
  - Increased plasma and urinary catecholamine levels
  - Periods of bradycardia and hypotension may also be documented.

Localized Tetanus

- Also called ascending tetanus
- Uncommon form
- Toxins travel along the peripheral nerves
- Disease confined to the extremities
- Seen most often in inadequately immunized persons
- May last for months, but usually resolves spontaneously.

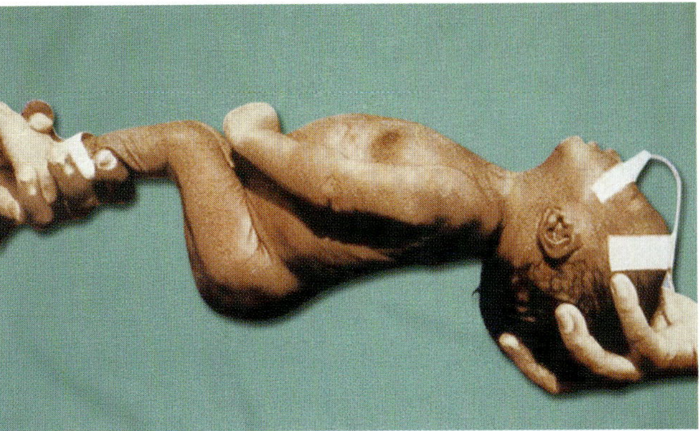

Fig. 7: Neonatal tetanus.

Cephalic Tetanus

- Rare form of localized tetanus
- Results from head wounds and affects the face
- Most commonly the muscles are innervated by lower cranial nerves
- Can occur in fully-immunized persons
- The incubation period is a few days and mortality is high
- The outcome is typically poor
- Mild cases (often associated with otitis media) have more favorable outcomes.

Neonatal Tetanus

- Seen in newborns, when the mother lacks immunity and the umbilical stump becomes contaminated with *C. tetani* spores.
- Detected at an early stage, by the refusal of feeds and absence of suckling reflex (Fig. 7).

Diagnosis

- Suspected upon exposure to a bite or puncture wound
- Based entirely on clinical findings
- Unlikely, if a reliable history indicates the completion of a primary vaccination series and the receipt of appropriate booster doses
- Wounds should be cultured in suspected cases
- *C. tetani* can be isolated from wounds of patients, without tetanus and frequently cannot be recovered from wounds of those with tetanus
- The leukocyte count may be elevated
- Cerebrospinal fluid examination yields normal results
- Electromyograms may show continuous discharge of motor units and shortening or absence of the silent interval normally seen after an action potential
- Muscle enzymes levels may be raised
- Serum antitoxin levels of 0.1 IU/mL (as measured by enzyme-linked immunosorbent assay) are considered protective and make tetanus unlikely, although cases in patients with protective antitoxin levels have been reported.

TREATMENT

The goals of therapy are:

- Eliminate the source of toxin
- Neutralize unbound toxin

- Prevent muscle spasms, while monitoring the patient's condition and providing support, especially respiratory support, until recovery
- Patients should be admitted to a quiet room in an intensive care unit, where observation and cardiopulmonary monitoring can be maintained continuously, but stimulation can be minimized
- Protection of the airway is vital
- Wounds should be explored, carefully cleansed, and thoroughly debrided
- Antibiotic therapy is administered to eradicate vegetative cells, i.e. the source of toxin
- The use of penicillin G (10–12 million units IV, given daily for 10 days) has been recommended, but metronidazole (500 mg every 6 hours or 1 g every 12 hours) is preferred by some experts. On the basis of this drug's excellent antimicrobial activity and the absence of the GABA-antagonistic activity seen with penicillin
- Clindamycin and erythromycin are alternatives for the treatment of penicillin-allergic patients
- Additional specific antimicrobial therapy should be given for active infection with other organisms.

Control of Muscle Spasms

- Can be painful and can threaten ventilation, by causing laryngospasm or sustained contraction of ventilatory muscles
- The ideal therapeutic regimen would be to abolish spasmodic activity, without causing over sedation and hypoventilation
- Diazepam, a benzodiazepine, and GABA agonist is in wide use
- Barbiturates and chlorpromazine are considered second-line agents
- Therapeutic paralysis with a nondepolarizing neuro-muscular blocking agent and mechanical ventilation may be used for spasms unresponsive to medication or spasms that threaten ventilation.

Respiratory Care

- Intubation or tracheostomy, with or without mechanical ventilation, may be required for hypoventilation due to over sedation or laryngospasm or for the avoidance of aspiration by patients with trismus, disordered swallowing or dysphagia.
- The need for these procedures should be anticipated and they should be undertaken electively and as early as possible.

Wound Management

- Proper wound management requires consideration of the need for:
  - Active immunization with tetanus toxoid vaccine
  - Passive immunization with tetanus immune globulin (TIG)
- The dose of TIG for passive immunization of wounds with average severity produces a protective serum antibody level for at least 4–6 weeks
- Vaccine and antibody should be administered at separate sites with separate syringes
- In established cases, intrathecal injection of TIG has shown better results than intramuscular injections
- All wounds receive surgical toilet
- Wounds less than 6 hours old, clean, nonpenetrating, and with negligible tissue damage
- Dose of tetanus toxoid and antitetanus serum (ATS), which must be administered depending upon the immune status of the patient has been described in Tables 1 and 2 respectively.

CLASSIFICATION OF THE PATIENTS: DEPENDING UPON THEIR IMMUNE STATUS

- *Class A* has had complete dose of toxoid or booster dose within past 5 years.
- *Class B* has had complete dose of toxoid or booster dose within past 5 years, but less than 10 years.
- *Class C* has had complete dose of toxoid or booster dose more than 10 years ago.
- *Class D* has not had a complete dose or immunity status unknown.

COURSE (MANIFESTATION OF DISEASE)

- The course of tetanus extends over 4–6 weeks and patients may require prolonged ventilator support.
- Increased tone and minor spasms can last for months, but recovery is usually complete.
- Death may occur from tetanus, often from cardiac and respiratory effects or secondary complications from the infection.

PREVENTION

- Spores are extremely stable, although immersion in boiling water for 15 minutes kills most spores
- Exposure to saturated steam under 15 lbs of pressure for 15–20 minutes at 121°C is highly effective against spores
- Sterilization by dry heat is slower than by moist heat (1–3 hours at 160°C), but it is also effective against spores
- Ethylene oxide sterilization is also sporicidal
- Sterilization of operation theater with 500 mL of formalin, 200 g of potassium permanganate/30 cubic meter of space
- All windows and doors are closed except one
- Fissures between the panels of the doors and windows are closed with adhesive tape

TABLE 1: Dose of tetanus toxoid, depending upon the immunity category.

Immunity category	*Treatment*
A	Nothing more required
B	Toxoid 1 dose
C	Toxoid 1 dose
D	Toxoid complete dose

TABLE 2: Dose of tetanus toxoid and antitetanus serum (ATS), depending upon the immunity category.

Immunity category	*Treatment*
A	Nothing more required
B	Toxoid 1 dose
C	Toxoid 1 dose + human ATS
D	Toxoid complete dose + human ATS

- After 12 hours, the doors and windows are opened and the theater is aired for 24 hours before commissioning it.

Active Immunization

- All partially immunized and unimmunized adults should receive vaccine
- The primary series for adults of tetanus toxoid consists of three doses:
  - The first and second doses are given 4–8 weeks apart
  - The third dose is given 6–12 months after the second.
- A booster dose is required every 10 years.

Passive Immunization

- ATS *(equine)* 1500 IU (SC) after sensitivity test
- *ATS (human) 250–500 IU:* No anaphylactic shock, very safe but costly.

CHAPTER

14 Deep Vein Thrombosis

OBJECTIVES

- Venous Anatomy
- Venous Thromboembolism

VENOUS ANATOMY

Venous anatomy is divided into the superficial, deep, and perforator components. In the lower extremity, the major superficial veins are (Fig. 1):

- The greater saphenous vein (located anterior to the medial malleolus and travelling medially to the fossa ovalis in the groin).
- The lesser saphenous vein (posterior to the lateral malleolus, coursing posterolaterally to the popliteal fossa).
- The posterior arch vein, also called Leonardo's vein (beginning in the medial ankle and joining the greater saphenous vein below the knee).
- The deep veins of the calf typically are duplicated as venae comitantes with numerous communicating branches.
- The posterior tibial and peroneal veins also communicate with the soleal sinusoids.
- In the thigh, the deep venous system includes the superficial and deep femoral veins that join about 4 cm below the inguinal ligament.
- The superficial and deep systems are connected by perforating veins (direct and indirect).
- Most blood flows from the superficial to the deep system via the direct perforators, but indirect perforators (small superficial veins draining into muscles that connect to the deep system via intramuscular veins).
- Blood is propelled toward the heart by compression of the deep veins by calf muscle contractions during walking and flow is unidirectional due to a series of one-way valves (also called as peripheral heart).

ETIOLOGY

- Congenital (although it may present later in life)
- Primary (cause undetermined)

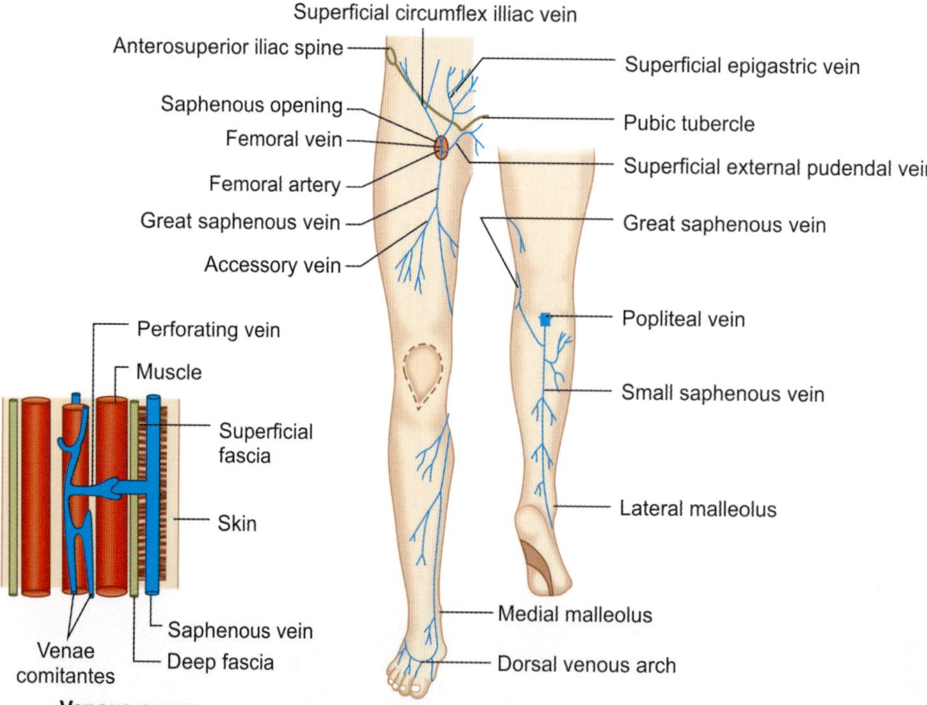

Fig. 1: Venous distribution of lower limb.

- Secondary (post-thrombotic, post-traumatic, or other)
- Deep venous thrombosis (DVT) accounts for most of the secondary cases and may be responsible for a significant number of other cases because many deep vein thrombi are asymptomatic
- Diagnosis is made by history, physical examination, and noninvasive studies.

HISTORY

- A history of any DVT or trauma should be sought, as well as any family history of varicose veins.
- Patients may complain of lower-extremity edema, aching, skin irritation, or varicose veins. Leg pain is described as a dull ache, worsening at the end of the day, and often relieved with exercise or elevation.
- In severe cases, individuals can experience acute and bursting pain with ambulation (venous claudication). Prolonged rest and leg elevation (20 minutes) are needed to obtain relief.

PHYSICAL EXAMINATION

Physical examination reveals following findings:

- Ankle edema (Fig. 2)
- Subcutaneous fibrosis and hyperpigmentation (brownish discoloration secondary to hemosiderin deposition)
- Lipodermatosclerosis
- Venous eczema and dilatation of subcutaneous veins, including telangiectasias (0.1–1.0 mm), reticular veins (1–4 mm), and varicose veins (> 4 mm).
- Ultimately, ulcers develop typically proximal to the medial malleolus. Any signs of infection should be noted. Arterial pulses should be examined and are usually adequate.

VENOUS THROMBOEMBOLISM

Epidemiology

Venous thromboembolism, which includes DVT and pulmonary embolism (PE), is a common cause of death. The true incidence of DVT is difficult to determine because its clinical diagnosis can be inaccurate and it often occurs in the setting of other critical illnesses.

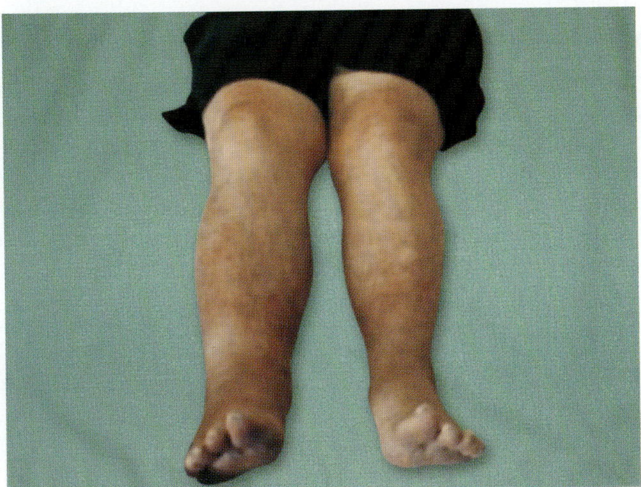

Fig. 2: Ankle edema.

- Deep vein thrombosis commonly affects the leg veins (such as the femoral vein or the popliteal vein) or the deep veins of the pelvis.
- Occasionally, the veins of the arm are affected (if spontaneous, this is known as Paget–Schroetter disease)
- Virchow's triad (Fig. 3).

Mechanism

Venous thrombosis occurs via three mechanisms:

1. Decreased flow rate of the blood
2. Damage to the blood vessel wall
3. An increased tendency of the blood to clot (hypercoagulability).

Pathophysiology (Fig. 4)

- The DVT starts as a platelet nidus, usually in the venous valves of the calf. The thrombogenic nature of the nidus activates the clotting cascade, leading to a thrombus that grows by accumulating more platelets and fibrin (Fig. 5).
- The fibrinolytic system is also activated, and thrombogenesis and thrombolysis compete for dominance.
- The thrombus grows, if thrombogenesis predominates. A thrombus can detach from the endothelium and migrate into the pulmonary system, becoming a PE (Fig. 6).
- A thrombus can also organize and grow into the endothelium, resulting in venous valve incompetency and phlebitis.

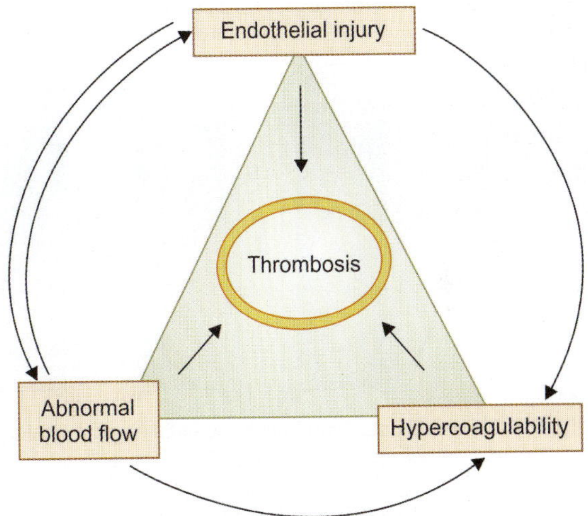

Fig. 3: Virchow's triad.

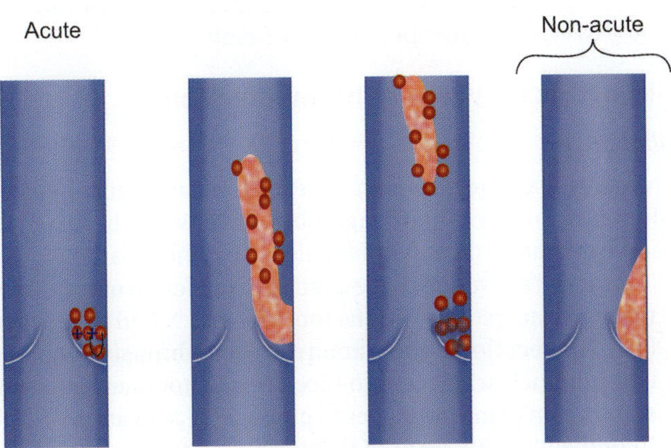

Fig. 4: Pathophysiology of DVT.

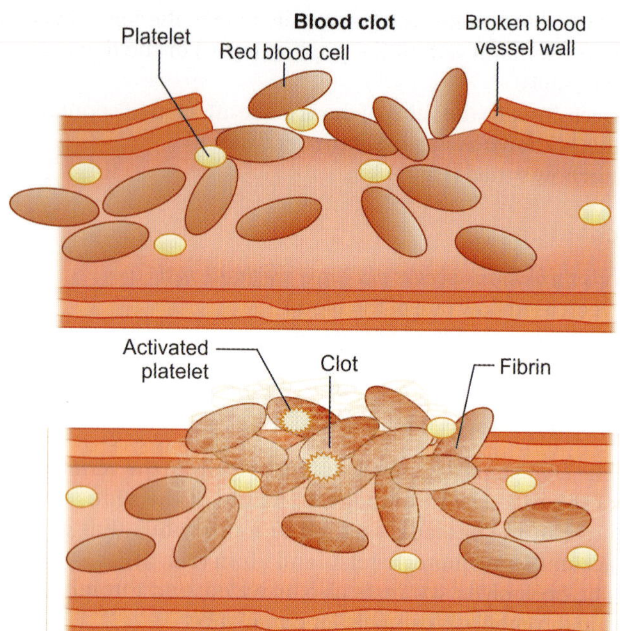

Fig. 5: Deep vein thrombosis (DVT) starts as a platelet nidus in the venous valves of the calf. The thrombogenic nature of the nidus activates the clotting cascade, leading to a thrombus that grows by accumulating more platelets and fibrin.

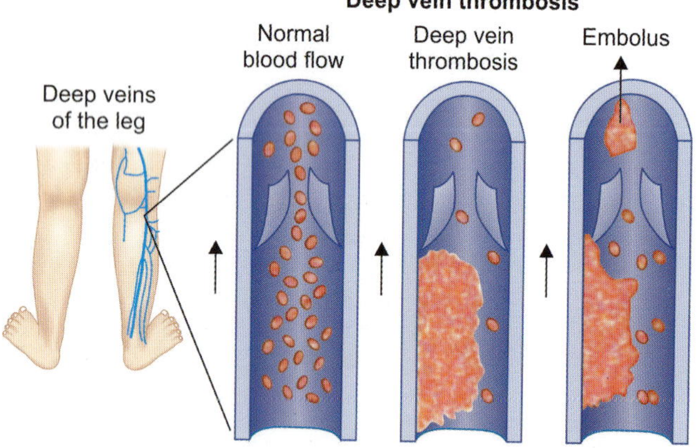

Fig. 6: A thrombus detaching from endothelium and migrating to become a pulmonary embolism.

- Thrombi localized to the calf have less tendency to embolize than thrombi that extend to the thigh veins.
- Approximately 20% cases of calf DVT propagate to the thigh and 50% cases of thigh or proximal DVT embolize.

Risk Factors for Venous Thromboembolism

Malignancy

Trousseau was the first to suggest an association between malignancy and a hypercoagulable state when he observed episodic migratory thrombophlebitis in his cancer patients.

- Tumor cell activation of the clotting cascade can occur directly through interactions with factors VIIa and X and tissue factor (TF). Indirect clotting activation can occur through stimulation of mononuclear cells to produce TF or factor X activators and stimulation of macrophages to produce TF activators.
- *Endothelial injury*: Another mechanism for the association of malignancy and thrombus formation is endothelial injury. Adhesion of tumor cells to endothelium can lead to disruption of endothelial intracellular junctions and expose the highly thrombogenic subendothelial surface.

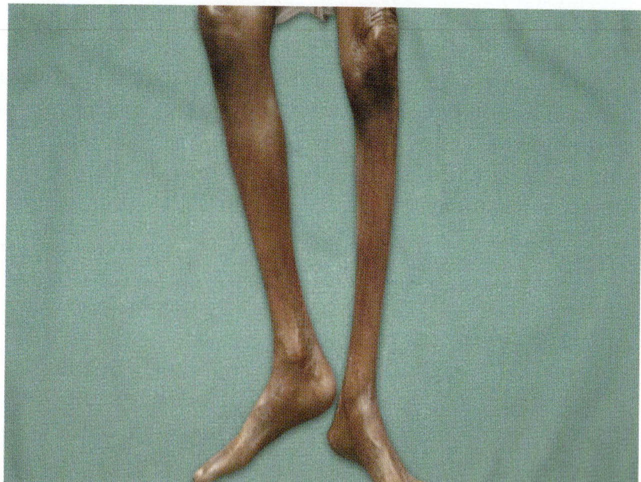

Fig. 7: Deep vein thrombosis due to prolonged nonambulatory state.

- *Chemotherapeutic drugs*: These include drugs such as bleomycin, carmustine, vincristine, and adriamycin, which can also cause vascular endothelial cell damage.
- Recent surgery or hospitalization.
- Advanced age.
- Obesity.
- Infection.
- Immobilization.
- Tobacco usage.
- Air travel ("economy class syndrome"—a combination of immobility and relative dehydration) is one of the better known causes.
- A prolonged nonambulatory state, such as fracture of the hip, pelvis, or leg; multisystem trauma, neurologic injury, or other critical injury requiring bed rest can increase DVT risk (Fig. 7).
- The use of oral contraceptives (OCPs) and estrogen hormone replacement therapy has been linked to increased risk of venous thrombus formation.

Hypercoagulable States

Hypercoagulable states can also lead to DVT formation. Primary hypercoagulable states are inherited conditions that can lead to abnormal endothelial cell thromboregulation (e.g. decreased thrombomodulin—dependent activation of protein C, impaired heparin binding of antithrombin III, down-regulation of membrane-associated plasmin production) or decreased thrombogenic inhibitors (e.g. antithrombin III, protein C, protein S).

- *Factor V*: Leiden mutation
- Prothrombin gene mutation
- Protein C deficiency
- Protein S deficiency
- Antithrombin III deficiency
- Homocysteine
- Antiphospholipid syndrome.

Clinical Presentation

- Pain/swelling of the extremity
- Increased circumference of affected extremity, with respect to the contralateral extremity
- Dilation of superficial veins of the suspected extremity only
- Calf pain on dorsiflexion of the ankle. Positive "Homans' sign" (pain on dorsiflexion of foot in the calf muscles)
- *Moses' sign*: Squeezing of posterior calf elicits pain
- Palpable "cord" indicates superficial thrombophlebitis
- A more severe presentation of DVT is "phlegmasia cerulea dolens" in which pain and swelling are accompanied by cyanosis, a sign of arterial ischemia.

Procedure for Predicting the Pretest Probability of Deep Venous Thrombosis (Wells Scoring System)

This has been illustrated in the Table 1.

Diagnostic Methods for DVT (Flowchart 1)

- Clinical findings
- D-dimer
- Blood tests
- Conventional X-ray contrast venogram
- Duplex Doppler ultrasound
- Magnetic resonance imaging (MRI)
- Radionuclide methods.

Blood Tests

- The quantitative plasma D-dimer enzyme-linked immunosorbent assay (ELISA) rises in the presence of DVT or PE because of plasmin breakdown of fibrin
- The D-dimer assay is not specific. Levels increase in patients with myocardial infarction, pneumonia, sepsis, cancer, during postoperative state, and second or third trimester of pregnancy
- *D-dimer:* Blood testing for acute thrombosis
- Degradation product of circulating cross-linked fibrin
- Elevated levels in acute thrombosis
- This cross-linked fibrin degradation product is an indication that thrombosis is occurring and that the blood clot is being dissolved by plasmin
- Various assays are not standardized (ELISA, latex, and immunofiltration)
- Studies have not looked for presence or absence of both DVT and PE
- Complete blood count
- Primary coagulation studies
- Prothrombin time (PT)
- Activated plasma thromboplastin time (aPTT)
- Fibrinogen
- Liver enzymes
- Renal function
- Electrolytes.

Ultrasonography of the Deep Leg Veins

Criteria for establishing the diagnosis of acute DVT are:

- Lack of vein compressibility (the principal criterion). Vein does not "wink" when it is gently compressed in cross-section.
- Failure to appose the walls of the vein due to passive distension. Direct visualization of thrombus homogeneous low echogenicity and abnormal Doppler flow.
- *Dynamics normal response*: Calf compression augments, Doppler flow signal, and confirms vein patency proximal.
- *Distal to Doppler abnormal response:* Flow blunted rather than augmented with calf compression.

Ultrasound Examination (Fig. 8)

- The vein is not compressible and thrombus (far left arrow, as seen in Figure 8) is visualized directly in the deep venous system.

TABLE 1: Procedure for predicting the pretest probability of deep venous thrombosis (DVT).

Clinical characteristics	*Score*
Active cancer (patient receiving treatment for cancer within the previous 6 months or currently receiving palliative treatment)	1
Paralysis, paresis, or recent plaster immobilization of the lower extremities	1
Recently bedridden for 3 days or more, or major surgery within the previous 12 weeks requiring general or regional anesthesia	1
Localized tenderness along the distribution of the deep venous system	1
Entire leg swollen	1
Calf swelling at least 3 cm larger than that on the asymptomatic side (measured 10 cm below tibial tuberosity)	1
Pitting edema confined to symptomatic leg	1
Collateral superficial veins (nonvaricose)	1
Previously documented DVT	1
Alternative diagnosis at least as likely as DVT	2
Clinical probability	*Total Score*
DVT unlikely	<2
DVT likely	2

Flowchart 1: Diagnostic methods for deep vein thrombosis (DVT).

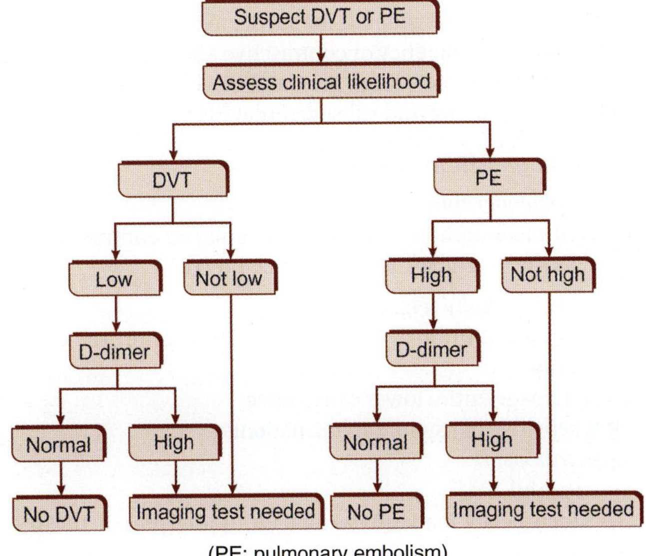

(PE: pulmonary embolism)

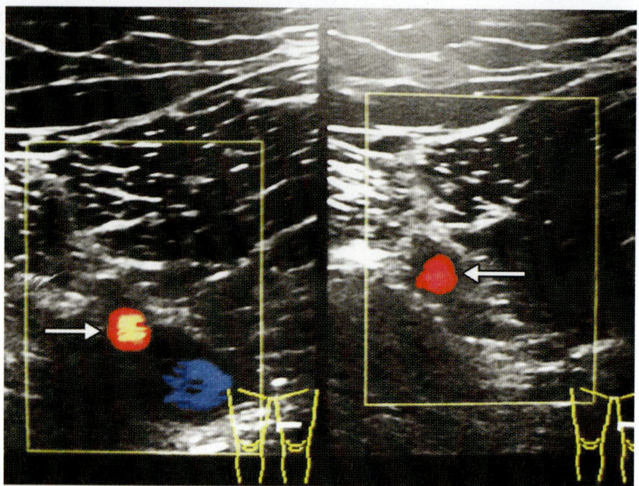

Fig. 8: Color Doppler for detecting thrombus.

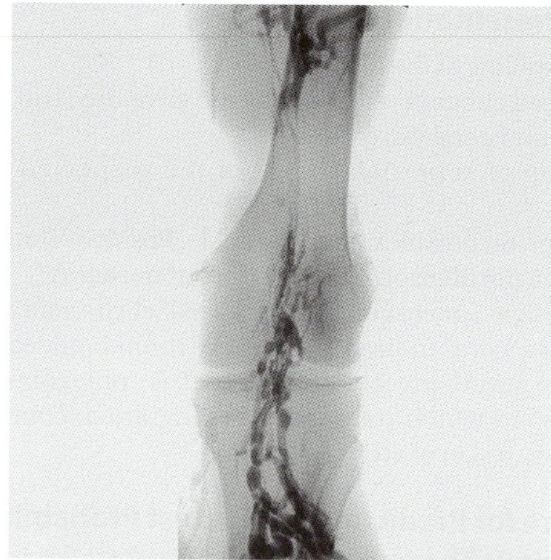

Fig. 9: Contrast venography detecting the block in the flow.

- Superficial femoral vein (SFV)
- Deep femoral vein (DFV).

Venous Doppler

Advantages:

- High sensitivity (82–100%) for proximal DVT (thighs and knees) in patients with localizing signs and symptoms.
- Fast
- Low cost per procedure.

Drawbacks:

- Heavily operator dependent
- Some segments may be "blind" to sampling
- Calf veins are usually not studied, but with new generation equipment, calf veins can be reliably seen in 60–90%, if seen Doppler 90% sensitive and specific for clot in them.

Magnetic Resonance (Contrast Enhanced)

- When ultrasound is equivocal, magnetic resonance (MR) venography is an excellent imaging modality to diagnose DVT.
- Magnetic resonance utilizes gadolinium-contrast agent, which, unlike iodinated contrast agents used in venography or CT angiography, is not nephrotoxic.
- MRI should be considered for suspected DVT or PE patients, with renal insufficiency or contrast dye allergy. MR pulmonary angiography detects large proximal PE, but is not reliable for smaller segmental and subsegmental PE.

Invasive Diagnostic Modalities

Contrast phlebography:

Venous ultrasonography has virtually replaced contrast phlebography, as the diagnostic test for suspected DVT.

Contrast venography (Fig. 9):

- It is "gold standard" for imaging DVT when technically adequate
- It can image entire lower extremities
- It is sensitive in asymptomatic patients
- *Limitations:*
  - Painful
  - Technically inadequate/difficult to interpret in 10–30% of cases.

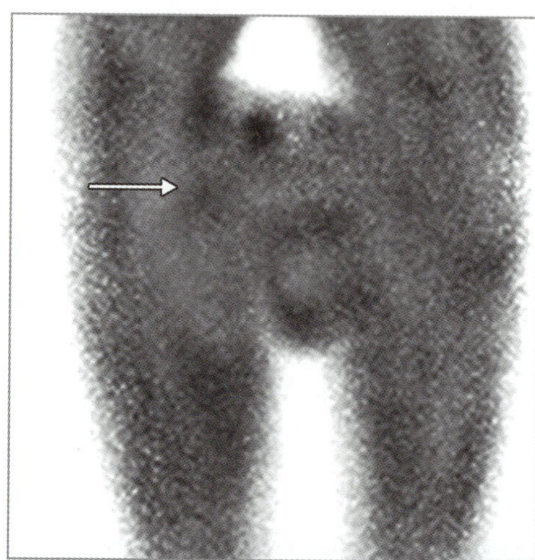

Fig. 10: Nuclear venographic image.

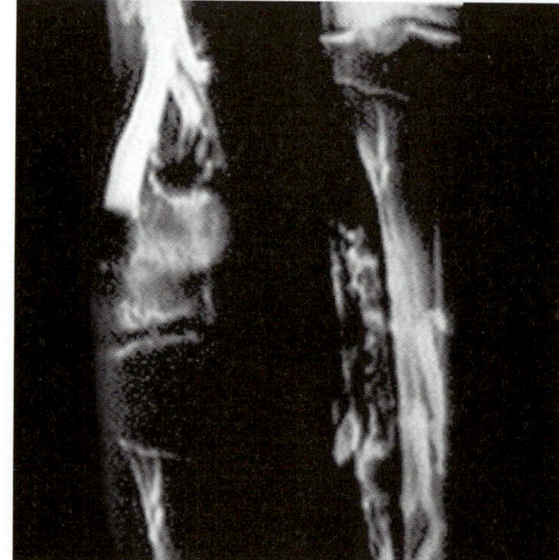

Fig. 11: Nuclear scan diagnosing deep vein thrombosis.

Nuclear Venography (Figs. 10 and 11)

- Technetium-99m (Tc-MAA)
- Sensitivity (94%)
- Specificity (92%)

- *Pros*:
  - Lung perfusion
  - Iliac/inferior vena cava (IVC)
- *Cons*:
  - Calf veins
  - Nonobstructing clot without collaterals
- Tc-99m apcitide scintigraphy specific for acute DVT (Figs. 12A and B)
- Binding to platelet (Fig. 13) glycoprotein (GPIIb/IIIa)
- *Tc-99m apcitide*: Normal biodistribution
- *Tc-99m apcitide*: Positive cases.

For suspected DVT, compression ultrasonography of the femoral, popliteal, and calf trifurcation veins is highly sensitive (> 90%) in detecting thrombosis of the proximal veins (femoral and popliteal), but less sensitive (50%) in detecting calf vein thrombosis.

- Chest CT can be combined with CT angiography of pelvic and deep thigh veins to detect DVT as well as PE.

Prophylaxis

- Prophylaxis is achieved by either altering the blood coagulation state, preventing venous stasis, or preventing embolization.
- Low-dose unfractionated heparin is given subcutaneously at 5,000 units, 2 hours before surgery, and every 8 or 12 hours postoperatively. Low-dose heparin reduces the risk of venous thromboembolism by 50–70%.

Prevention of Venous Thromboembolism

Preventive measures of venous thromboembolism are discussed in Table 2.

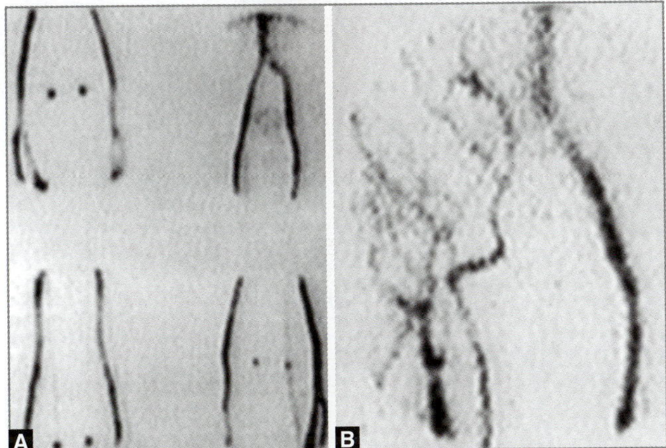

Figs. 12A and B: Technetium-99m (Tc-99m) apcitide scintigraphy specific for acute deep vein thrombosis.

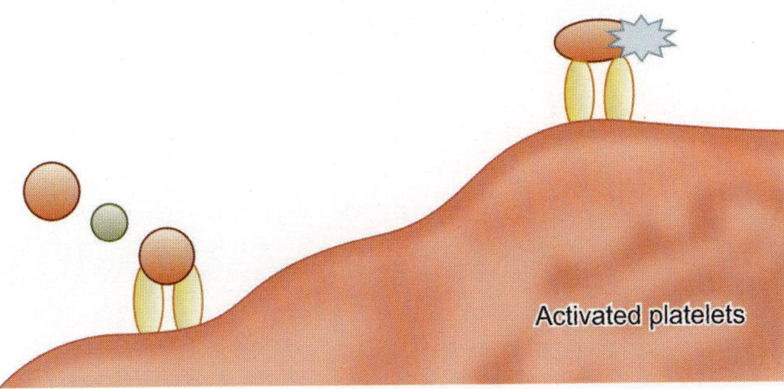

Fig. 13: Receptors binding to activated platelets.

Treatment

Hospitalization should be considered in patients with more than two of the following risk factors, as these patients may have more risk of complications during treatment:

- Bilateral DVT
- Renal insufficiency
- Body weight > 70 kg/154 lbs
- Recent immobility
- Chronic heart failure
- Cancer
- Anticoagulation is the usual treatment for DVT
- In general, patients are initiated on a brief course (i.e. less than a week) of heparin treatment, while they start on a 3–6 months course of warfarin (or related vitamin K inhibitors). Low-molecular-weight heparin (LMWH) is preferred, though unfractionated heparin is given in patients who have a contraindication to LMWH (renal failure or imminent need for invasive procedure).
- *LMWH displayed the following:*
  - Reduced antifactor IIa activity, relative to antifactor Xa activity
  - More favorable benefit-risk ratio in experimental animals
  - Superior pharmacokinetic properties.
- LMWHs are derived from heparin by chemical or enzymatic depolymerization, yielding fragments approximately one-third the size of heparin.
- LMWHs have a mean molecular weight of 4,500–5,000 Da with a distribution of 1,000–10,000 Da.
- Low-binding properties of LMWH, to circulating and cellular protein.
- Cleared by renal route.
- LMWH therapy was started postoperatively, the first dose administered 12–24 hours after surgery, which increased the acceptability of prophylaxis.

TABLE 2: Preventive measures of venous thromboembolism in different conditions.

Condition	*Prophylaxis strategy*
High-risk general surgery	Mini-UFH + GCS or LMWH + GCS
Thoracic surgery	Mini-UFH + IPC
Cancer surgery, including gynecologic cancer surgery	LMWH, consider 1 month of prophylaxis
Total hip replacement, total knee replacement, hip fracture surgery	LMWH, fondaparinux (a pentasaccharide) 2.5 mg SC, once daily or warfarin (target INR 2.5) (except for total knee replacement)
Neurosurgery	GCS + IPC
Neurosurgery for brain tumor	Mini-UFH or LMWH + IPC + predischarge venous ultrasonography
Anticoagulation contraindicated	GCS + IPC
Minidose unfractionated heparin (Mini-UFH)	IPC: Intermittent pneumatic compression devices
Graduated compression stockings (GCS)	LMWH: Low-molecular-weight heparin

(INR: international normalized ratio; IPC: intermittent pneumatic compression; LMWH: low-molecular-weight heparin)

- This approach is particularly appealing in view of concerns about the risk of spinal cord hematoma, when anticoagulant prophylaxis is used in conjunction with spinal anesthesia.
- The first dose of LMWH should be delayed, until after the epidural catheter has been removed. When this is not possible, the catheter should be removed at least 8 hours after the last dose of LMWH.
- Under these circumstances, other drugs that impair hemostasis (such as nonsteroidal anti-inflammatory agents) should be avoided.

Multiple Trauma

- LMWH (enoxaparin sodium 30 mg SC 12 hourly) is the treatment started within 36 hours of multiple trauma.
- LMWH (tinzaparin, 175 U/kg SC 6 hourly) or heparin (50 U/kg IV bolus followed by an infusion of 500 U/kg/day) adjusted to an aPTT ratio of 2.0–3.0 for prevention of recurrent thromboembolism, major bleeding, and death.
- Thrombolysis is generally reserved for extensive clot, e.g. an iliofemoral thrombosis.
- In the case of known bilateral lower-extremity DVT, the compression device can be placed on the upper extremity.
- Pedal compression devices are also effective in patients, whose body habits do not allow conventionally sized devices to fit around their thighs or calves.
- Graduated compression stockings are effective in preventing DVT formation, by reducing venous stasis. However, this efficacy has been shown just for calf DVT (Fig. 14).
- "Beginning within 1 month of diagnosis of proximal DVT and continuing for a minimum of 1 year after diagnosis".
- Intermittent pneumatic compression of the extremities enhances blood flow in the deep veins and increases blood fibrinolytic activity (Fig. 15).
- For patients with significant bleeding risk with anticoagulation, pneumatic compression is an effective alternative.

Interventional Techniques

- Caval interruption with intracaval filters
- Inferior vena cava filter reduces PE and is an option for patients with an absolute contraindication to anticoagulant treatment (e.g. cerebral hemorrhage) or those rare patients who have objectively documented recurrent PE, while on anticoagulation, an inferior vena cava filter (also referred to as

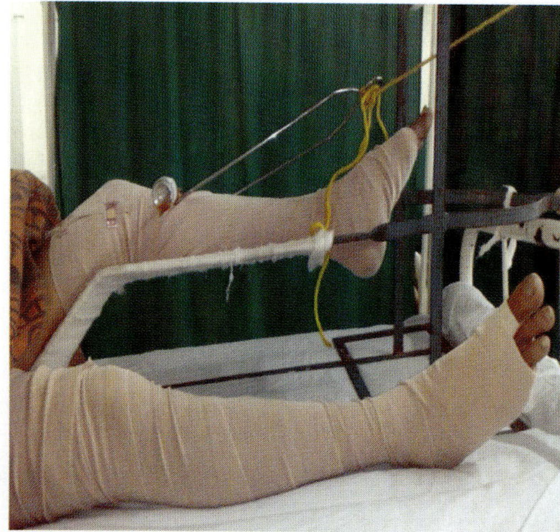

Fig. 14: Graduated compression stockings are effective in preventing deep vein thrombosis formation.

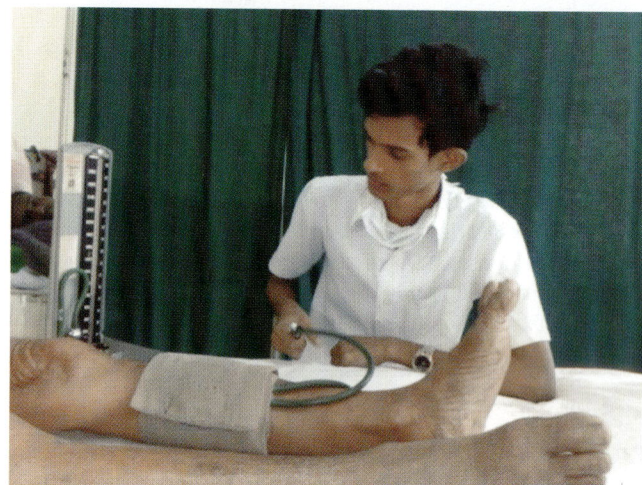

Fig. 15: Intermittent pneumatic compression given on extremities.

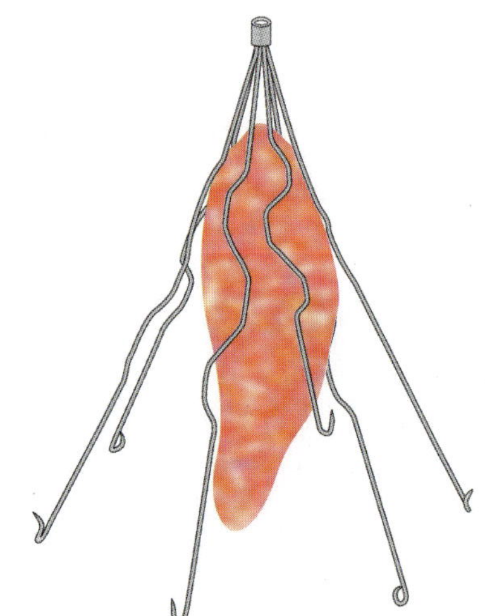

Fig. 16: Greenfield filter.

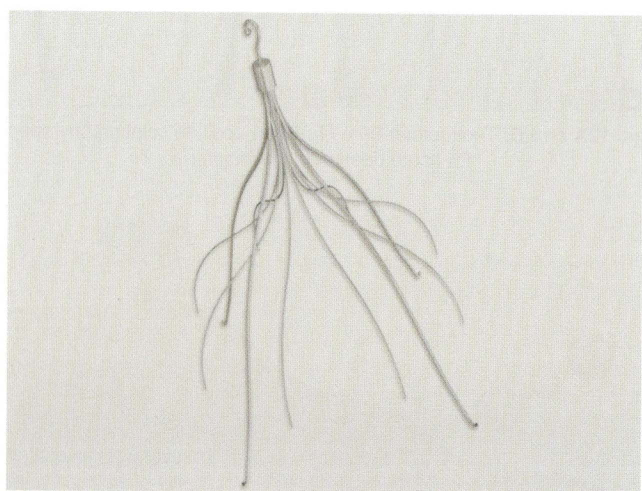

Fig. 17: Tulip filters.

a greenfield filter) may prevent pulmonary embolization of the leg clot (Fig. 16).

- These filters are themselves potential foci of thrombosis, IVC filters are viewed as a temporizing measure for preventing life-threatening PE.
- The procedure for insertion of intracaval filters is known as sieve procedure.

Types of filter:

- Tulip filter (Fig. 17)
- Catheter-directed thrombolysis of acute DVT with or without mechanical thrombectomy devices has been advocated in order to avoid sequelae of DVT.

The goals are to restore venous flow, preserve venous valve function, and eliminate the possibility of thromboembolism.

- Thromboembolectomy.

Differential Diagnosis

- Ruptured Baker's cyst
- Cellulitis
- *Postphlebitic syndrome/venous insufficiency*: It presents with leg edema, pain, nocturnal cramping, venous claudication, skin pigmentation, dermatitis, and ulceration (usually on the medial aspect of the lower leg)
- Hematoma.

CHAPTER

15 Fat Embolism Syndrome

OBJECTIVES

- History
- Fat Embolism versus Fat Embolism Syndrome
- Pathogenesis of ARDS in Fat Embolism
- Treatment

HISTORY

- Fat embolism syndrome was first diagnosed by Dr Von Bergmann in 1873.
- In 1879, Fenger and Salisbury published description of fat embolism syndrome (FES).

FAT EMBOLISM VERSUS FAT EMBOLISM SYNDROME

Fat Embolism

It is fat in the vascular circulation which can cause embolic phenomenon. It is more common, i.e. 90% of patients with traumatic injury suffer from it (reports have shown high incidence of fat embolism after fractures and orthopedic surgery).

Fat Embolism Syndrome

- Fat embolism occurs with pattern of symptoms.
- *Incidence:* 1–3% femur fractures and 5–10% if bilateral or multiple fractures.
- *Mortality:* 5–15%
- *Clinical diagnosis*: No specific laboratory test is diagnostic. Mostly associated with long bone and pelvic fractures and more frequent in closed fractures. Single long bone fracture has 1–3% chance of developing FES and it increases with number of fractures.
- *Onset:* 24–72 hours from initial insult.
- *Causes:* Nontrauma related factors. These include:
  - Pancreatitis
  - Diabetes mellitus
  - Osteomyelitis and panniculitis
  - Bone tumor lysis
  - Steroid therapy
  - Sickle cell hemoglobinopathy
  - Alcoholic liver disease
  - Lipid infusion
  - Cyclosporine A solvent.

Diagnostic Criteria

Gurd's criteria (Table 1):

- Gurd's criteria is most commonly used
- One major and four minor.

Schonfeld's criteria: Schonfeld's criteria for diagnosis of fat embolism (Table 2).

Pathogenesis (Fat Embolism)

Direct entry of fat globules (fat enters torn venules) predisposed by:

- Torn vessels
- Free fat present
- Temporary rise in marrow pressure above venous pressure
- In orthopedic surgery, echogenic material can be seen in right heart circulation
- *Paradoxical embolism:* Fat embolism in arterial system, e.g. patent foramen ovale.

TABLE 1: Gurd's criteria for diagnosing features of fat embolism.

Major criteria	• Petechial rash • Respiratory symptoms—tachypnea, dyspnea, bilateral inspiratory crepitations, hemoptysis, bilateral diffuse patchy shadowing on chest X-ray • Neurological signs—confusion, drowsiness, coma
Minor criteria	• Tachycardia >120 beats/min • Pyrexia >34.9°C • Retinal changes—fat or petechiae • Jaundice • Renal changes–anuria or oliguria
Laboratory features	• Thrombocytopenia >50% decrease on admission value • Sudden decrease in hemoglobin level >20% of admission value • High erythrocyte sedimentation rate >71 mm/h • Fat macroglobulinemia

TABLE 2: Schonfeld's criteria for diagnosis of fat embolism.

	Score
Petechiae	5
X-ray chest diffuse infiltrates	4
Hypoxemia	3
Fever	1
Tachycardia	1
Tachypnea	1
Confusion	1

Pathogenesis (Fat Embolism Syndrome)

- Production of toxic byproducts from triglyceride (TG)/ chylomicrons (lipase).
- Fat embolism syndrome results from degradation of fat from FE to free fatty acids [these have been shown in animal models to cause vasculitis/acute respiratory distress syndrome (ARDS)].
- Probably phospholipase A2 (PLA2) and C-reactive protein (CRP)-mediated (inflammatory mediated).
- C-reactive protein is also shown to be elevated in FE and causes fat agglutination (Fig. 1).

PATHOGENESIS OF ARDS IN FAT EMBOLISM

- Fat emboli obstruct lung vessel (20 μ). Platelets and fibrin adhere there (Fig. 2)
- Lipase creases free fatty acid
- Inflammatory changes lead to endothelial damage, which are contributing factors for ARDS.

Triad of Fat Embolism Syndrome

- Hypoxemia (Pulmonary)
- Neurological abnormalities (Cerebral)
- Petechial rash (Cutaneous).

Early Signs

- Dyspnea
- Tachypnea
- Hypoxemia
- Pulmonary
- Hypoxia, rales, pleural friction rub, etc.
- ARDS may develop.
- Half of the patients with FES require mechanical ventilation
- Chest X-ray usually normal early, later may show "snow storm" pattern with diffuse bilateral infiltrates (Fig. 3)
- *CT chest:* Ground-glass opacification with interlobular septal thickening.

Neurological Findings

- Usually occur after respiratory symptoms
- *Incidence:* 80% patients with FES
- Minor global dysfunction most common, but ranges from mild delirium to coma
- Seizures/focal deficits not common, but can occur
- Transient and reversible in most cases
- *CT head:* General edema, usually nonspecific
- *MRI brain:* Low density on T1 and high intensity T2 signal correlates to degree of impairment.

Cutaneous Findings

- Rash
- Petechial
- Usually on conjunctiva, mucous membrane, neck, and axillae
- Result from occlusion of dermal capillaries, by fat globules and then extravasations of RBC
- Resolve in 5–7 days
- Pathognomonic, but only present in 20–50% of patients.

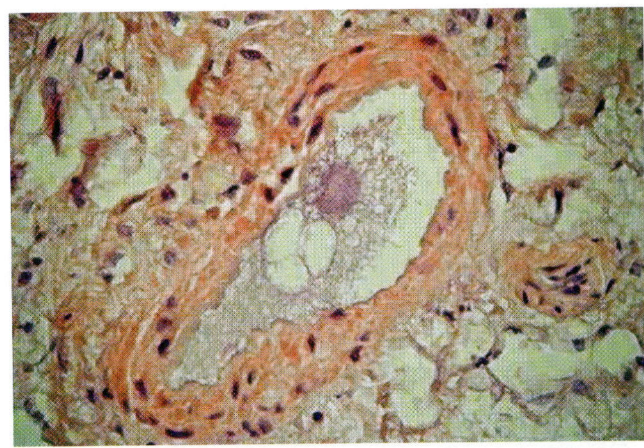

Fig. 1: Hematoxylin and eosin stain of a section of the lungs showing a blood vessel with fibrinoid material and an optical empty space indicative of the presence of lipid dissolved during the staining process. This 55-year-old woman died of massive fat embolism after developing pancreatitis due to endoscopic retrograde cholangiopancreatography.
Source: Pancreatitis with an unusual fatal complication following endoscopic retrograde cholangiopancreatography.

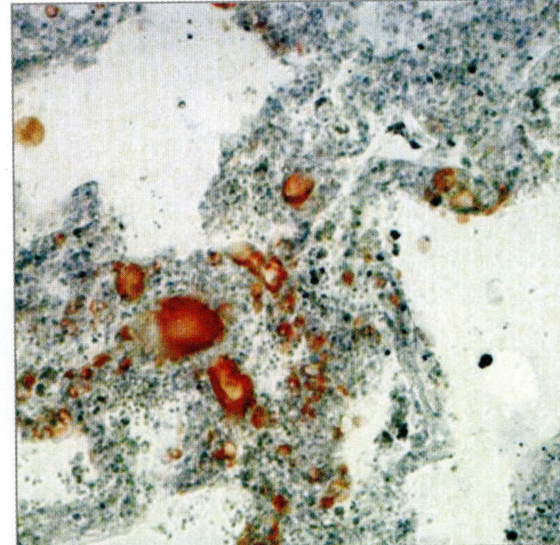

Fig. 2: Fat emboli obstruct lung vessel.

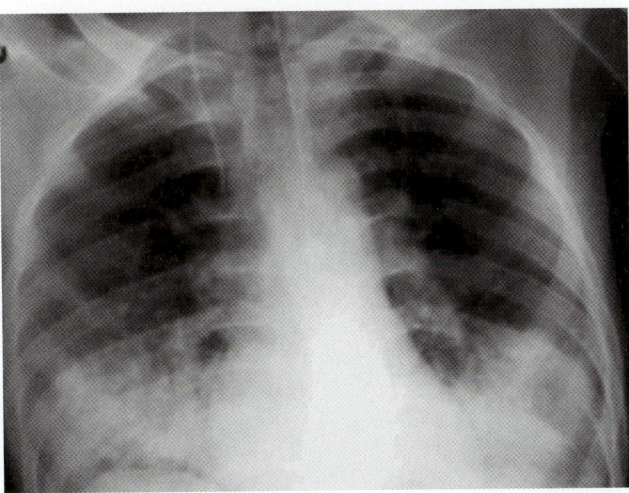

Fig. 3: Snow storm pattern, with diffuse bilateral infiltrates.

Other Findings

- Retinopathy (exudates, cotton wool spots, hemorrhage, etc.)
- Lipiduria
- Fever
- Disseminated intravascular coagulation (DIC)
- Myocardial depression (Right heart strain)
- Thrombocytopenia/anemia
- Hypocalcemia.

Laboratory Findings

- Laboratory tests are mostly nonspecific
- Serum lipase level increases in bone trauma, which is often misleading
- Cytologic examination of urine, blood, and sputum with Sudan or oil red O staining, may detect fat globules that are either free or in macrophages
- Blood lipid level is not helpful for diagnosis
- Decreased hematocrit occurs within 24–48 hours and is attributed to intra-alveolar hemorrhage
- Alteration in coagulation and thrombocytopenia.

  In summary, the diagnosis of FES may be difficult, as except petechiae, there are no pathognomic signs.

TREATMENT

- Supportive care
- Early immobilization of fractures reduces incidents of FES
- Open reduction internal fixation (ORIF) over conservative treatment also reduces risk
- Higher incidence rate occurs, when fixation is delayed for more than 24 hours
- External fixation or fixation with plate and screw produces lesser lung injury than nailing the medullary cavity.

Supportive Care

- Maintenance of intravascular volume, as shock can exacerbate the lung injury caused by FES.
- Albumin has been recommended for volume resuscitation in addition to balanced electrolyte solution, as it also binds fatty acids and may decrease the extent of lung injury.
- Mechanical ventilation and positive end-expiratory pressure (PEEP) may be required to maintain arterial oxygenation.

Steroids

- Steroid prophylaxis is controversial to prevent FES.
- Theorized to cause blunting of inflammatory response and complement activation.
- Prospective studies suggest that prophylactic steroids benefit high-risk patients.
- Few studies and small study size, hence remains controversial.
- Once FES is established, steroids have not shown to improve outcomes.
- Heparin and acetyl salicylic acids have also been proposed for treatment, as they activate lipase and block thromboxane respectively, but no evidence exists for either use in FES.

CHAPTER

16

Peripheral Nerve Injuries

OBJECTIVES

- Anatomy
- Etiology
- Classification
- Motor Effect of Peripheral Nerve Injuries
- Diagnostic Tests
- Management of Nerve Injuries

ANATOMY

- Each segmental spinal nerve is formed at or near its intervertebral foramen by the union of its dorsal or sensory root, with its ventral or motor root. In most of the thoracic segments, these mixed spinal nerves retain their autonomy and supply one intercostal dermatomal and myotomal segment.
- Other segments of the spinal axis, the spinal nerves join with others to form a plexus that innervates a limb or a special body segment that no longer retains the primitive myomeric pattern.
- A total of 31 mixed spinal nerves leave their respective foramina on each side of the spine, to innervate the homolateral trunk and extremities. They are, 8—cervical; 12—thoracic; 5—lumbar; 5—sacral; and 1—coccygeal.

Components of Mixed Spinal Nerve (Fig. 1)

Motor

- Several rootlets leave the anterolateral sulcus of the spinal cord and unite to form each motor root.
- The fibers traversing these roots arise from the anterior horn cells and innervate the skeletal muscles.

Sensory

- The sensory fibers arise from pain, thermal, tactile, and stretch receptors.
- Cell bodies for these fibers are located within the dorsal root ganglia, with axons entering the posterolateral sulcus of the cord via several rootlets.

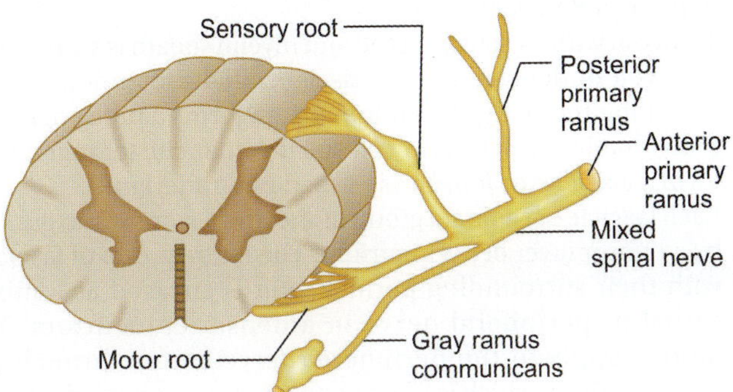

Fig. 1: Components of mixed spinal nerve.

- The fibers conveying joint or position sensibility and some tactile fibers turn cephalad in the dorsal columns and do not synapse before reaching the gracile and cuneate nuclei at the cervicomedullary junction.
- Pain and temperature fibers synapse in the substantia gelatinosa and cross to ascend in the dorsal spinothalamic tract.
- Tactile fibers enter synapse and cross to ascend in the ventral spinothalamic tract.

Sympathetic

- The sympathetic component of all 31 mixed spinal nerves leaves the spinal cord along with only 14 motor roots.
- The fibers exit from the cord with the 12 thoracic and first 2 lumbar motor roots enter the respective mixed spinal nerve and promptly emerge from it as white rami. The white rami pass anteriorly to the corresponding sympathetic ganglion.
- Synapse may occur within the ganglion, with which the ramus is associated and postganglionic fibers pass back to the mixed spinal nerve as a gray ramus.
- More often, however, the fibers entering the ganglion via the white rami pass for variable distances up or down the paravertebral chain, to synapse at higher or lower levels.
- The postganglionic fibers pass along gray rami to cervical, lower lumbar, or sacrococcygeal mixed spinal nerves having no white rami.
- Sweat glands, blood vessels, and erector pili are innervated also in a segmental pattern.
- Mixed spinal nerves, having left the intervertebral foramina, receive their sympathetic component and promptly branch into anterior and posterior primary rami.

Posterior primary rami

- Directed posteriorly and supply the paraspinal musculature and the skin along the posterior aspect of the trunk, neck, and head.
- The upper three cervical posterior rami are larger than their corresponding anterior rami, supplying relatively large areas of the scalp posteriorly and the musculature around the craniocervical junction.
- With these exceptions, posterior primary rami are small and the major part of each spinal nerve continues laterally in an anterior primary ramus, to enter a plexus or to become an intercostal nerve.

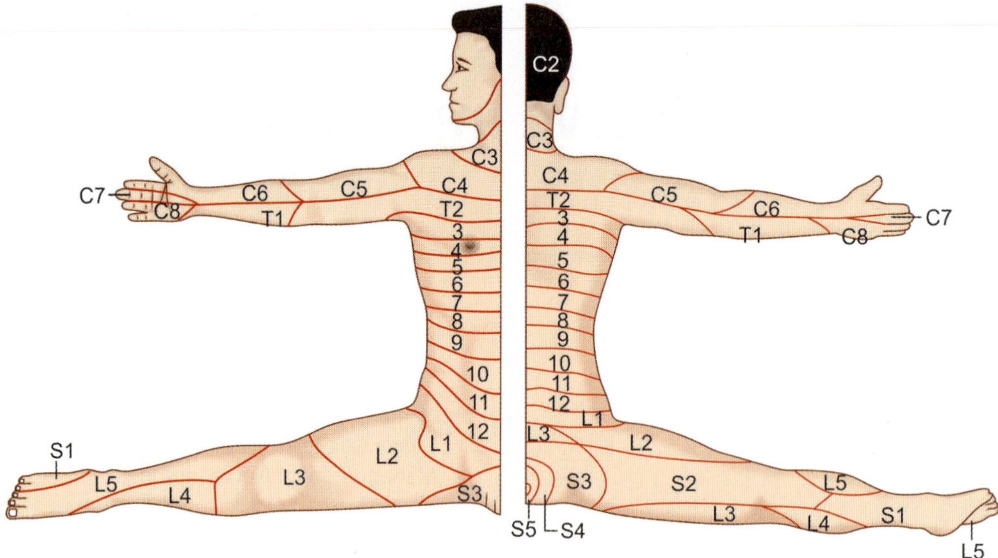

Fig. 2: Dermatomal patterns.

Anterior primary rami

- The cervical, the first thoracic, and all the lumbosacral nerves join in the formation of plexuses.
- The upper four cervical anterior rami form the cervical plexus.
- The lower four cervical and first thoracic anterior rami form the brachial plexus.
- The first three and a part of the fourth lumbar anterior rami form the lumbar plexus.
- The sacral anterior rami along with the fifth lumbar and a part of the fourth join to form the lumbosacral plexus.
- The area of skin supplied by the fibers of a single spinal root is called a dermatome.
- Segmental dermatomal patterns are well preserved in the thoracic region, but not in the limbs (Fig. 2).
- Migration of the limb buds accounts for the displacement of midcervical dermatomes along the lateral aspect of the arm and radial aspect of the forearm and of the lower cervical and upper thoracic dermatomes along the medial aspect of the arm and the ulnar aspect of the forearm.
- Lumbar and sacral dermatomal alignment along the various aspects of the lower extremity is similarly explained.
- The line separating the more rostral segmental dermatomes from the more caudal ones is called the axial line and may be followed into the spinal axis.

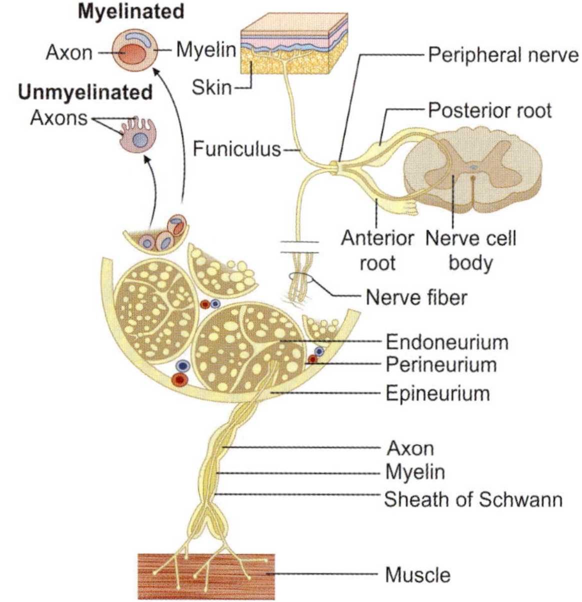

Fig. 3: Microscopic anatomy.

Microscopic Anatomy (Fig. 3)

- Each nerve fiber or axon is a direct extension of a dorsal root ganglion cell (sensory), an anterior horn cell (motor) or a postganglionic sympathetic nerve cell and it is either myelinated or unmyelinated. Sensory and motor nerves contain unmyelinated and myelinated fibers in a ratio of 4:1.
- In the unmyelinated or sparsely myelinated fibers, several axons are wrapped by a single Schwann cell. In the more heavily myelinated fibers, the Schwann cell, by rotation forms a multilaminated structure that encloses a myelin sheath around a single axon.
- The segment of myelinated nerve fiber enclosed by a single Schwann cell is referred to as an internode with the more heavily myelinated fibers, having the longer internodes (Fig. 4). The point at which one Schwann cell ends and the next begins is relatively sparse in myelin and is called the nodal gap or node of Ranvier.
- The axon with its Schwann cell and myelin sheath is surrounded by a veil of delicate fibrous tissue called the endoneurium. Seen longitudinally, the endoneurium forms a tube encircling individually the Schwann cell sheaths that cluster together to form a fascicle (or *funicle* as termed by Sunderland).
- Each fascicle or separate group of sheathed axons is surrounded by a denser layer of perineurium. The entire group of fascicles with their surrounding perineurium is encased as a mixed spinal or peripheral nerve in a denser epineurium. The blood supply to the peripheral nerve enters through the mesoneurium, which is loose connective tissue extending from the epineurium to the surrounding tissues.

- There is an extrinsic (segmental) and an intrinsic (longitudinal) blood supply to each nerve.
- The intrinsic blood supply that runs longitudinally within the epineurium, perineurium, and endoneurium is fairly extensive and allows surgical mobilization without complete devascularization over variable lengths of nerves.

ETIOLOGY

Peripheral nerves can be injured by metabolic or collagen diseases, malignancies, endogenous, or exogenous toxins, thermal, chemical, or mechanical trauma. Every patient, who has injured a limb or limb girdle should be evaluated for possible musculoskeletal, vascular, and peripheral nerve damage.

CLASSIFICATION

Seddon in 1943 divided nerve injuries into three categories:

1. *Neurapraxia:* Designating minor contusion or compression of a peripheral nerve with preservation of the axis cylinder, but with possibly minor edema or breakdown of a localized segment of myelin sheath. Transmission of impulses is physiologically interrupted for a time, but recovery is complete in a few days or weeks.
2. *Axonotmesis:* Designating more significant injury with breakdown of the axon and distal Wallerian degeneration, but with preservation of the Schwann cell and endoneurial tubes. Spontaneous regeneration with good functional recovery can be expected.

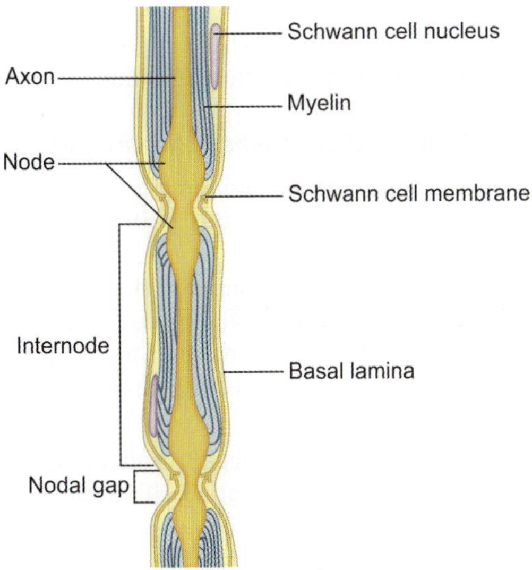

Fig. 4: Myelinated nerve fiber.

3. *Neurotmesis:* Designating a more severe injury, with complete anatomical severance of the nerve or extensive avulsing or crushing injury. The axon, the Schwann cell, and endoneurial tubes are completely disrupted. The perineurium and epineurium also are disrupted to varying degrees. Segments of the latter two may bridge the gap, if complete severance is not apparent. In this group, significant spontaneous recovery cannot be expected.

The Sunderland 1951, Classification

- It is more readily applicable clinically, each degree of injury suggesting a greater anatomical disruption with its correspondingly altered prognosis. In this classification, peripheral nerve injuries are arranged in ascending order of severity from the first to the fifth degree (Table 1).
- In first-degree injury, conduction along the axon is physiologically interrupted at the site of injury, but the axon is not disrupted. No Wallerian degeneration occurs and recovery is spontaneous and usually complete within a few days or weeks. This injury coincides with the neurapraxia of Seddon.
- The loss of function varies. Usually, motor function is more profoundly affected than sensory function. Sensory modalities are affected in order of decreasing frequency as follows—proprioception, touch, temperature, and pain. A characteristic of this injury is the simultaneous return of motor function in the proximal and distal musculature.
- In second-degree injury, disruption of the axon is evident, with Wallerian degeneration distal to the point of injury and degeneration proximal for one or more nodal segments. The integrity of the endoneurial tube (Schwann cell basal lamina) is maintained, providing a perfect anatomical course for regeneration. Any permanent deficit is related to the number of neural somas that die, such death being more common in injuries at the more proximal levels. Clinically, the neurological deficit is complete with loss of motor, sensory, and sympathetic function. Motor reinnervation is accomplished in a progressive manner from proximal to distal.
- In third-degree injury, the axons and endoneurial tubes are disrupted, but the perineurium is preserved. The result is disorganization resulting from disruption of the endoneurial tubes. Scar tissue within the endoneurium can obstruct certain tubes and divert sprouts to paths other than their own. Clinically, the neurological loss is complete in most instances and because of the additional time required for the regenerating axon tips to penetrate the fibrous barrier, the duration of loss is

TABLE 1: The Sunderland 1951, classification.

Degree of injury		*Histopathological changes*					*Tinel sign*	
Sunderland	*Seddon*	*Myelin*	*Axon*	*Endoneurium*	*Perineurium*	*Epineurium*	*Present*	*Progresses distally*
I	Neurapraxia	±					–	–
II	Axonotmesis	+	+				+	+
III	Neurotmesis	+	+	+			+	+
IV	Neurotmesis	+	+	+	+		+	–
V	Neurotmesis	+	+	+	+	+	+	–

more prolonged than in second-degree injury. Returning motor function is evident from proximal to distal, but with varying degrees of permanent motor or sensory deficit.

- In fourth-degree injury, the axon and endoneurium are disrupted, but some of the epineurium and possibly some of the perineurium are preserved, so complete severance of the entire trunk does not occur. Retrograde degeneration is more severe after this degree of injury and the mortality among neuronal soma is higher, sometimes resulting in a significant reduction in the number of surviving axons. Essentially, nerve continuity is maintained only by scar tissue, preventing proximal axons from entering the distal endoneurial tubes.
- In fifth-degree injury, the nerve is completely transected, resulting in a variable distance between the neural stumps. These injuries occur only in open wounds and usually are identified at the time of early surgical exploration. The likelihood of any significant bridging by axonal sprouts is remote and the possibility of any significant return of function without appropriate surgery is equally remote.
- Sixth-degree (Mackinnon) or mixed injuries occur, in which a nerve trunk is partially severed and the remaining part of the trunk sustains fourth-degree, third-degree, second-degree or rarely even first-degree injury. A neuroma in continuity is present and the recovery pattern is mixed depending on the degree of injury to each portion of the nerve. Surgical intervention to correct the fourth-degree and fifth-degree components may sacrifice the function of lesser injured fascicles.

MOTOR EFFECT OF PERIPHERAL NERVE INJURIES

- When a peripheral nerve is severed at a given level, all motor functions of the nerve distal to that level are abolished. All muscles supplied by branches of the nerve distal to that level are paralyzed and become atonic.
- Significant electromyography (EMG) changes are not apparent for 8–14 days, at which time transient fibrillation potentials on needle insertion may become apparent. Spontaneous fibrillations may become evident after 2–4 weeks, coinciding with the onset of atrophic change within the muscle fibers. Atrophy of muscle bulk progresses rapidly to 50–70% at the end of about 2 months (Sunderland, 1952).
- Atrophy continues at a much slower rate and the connective tissue component of the muscles increases. Striations and motor end plate configurations are retained for longer than 12 months, whereas the empty endoneurial tubes shrink to about one-third of their normal diameter (Sunderland and Bradley, 1950). Complete disruption and replacement of muscle fibers may not become complete, until after 3 years.

Muscle Function Assessment after Peripheral Nerve Injuries (Table 2)

Sensory

- Sensory loss usually follows a definite anatomical pattern, although the factor of overlap from adjacent nerves may confuse inexperienced surgeons. After severance of a peripheral nerve, only a small area of complete sensory loss is found. This area is supplied exclusively by the severed nerve and is called the autonomous zone or isolated zone of supply for that nerve.

TABLE 2: Muscle function assessment.

M0	No contraction
M1	Return of perceptible contraction in proximal muscles
M2	Return of perceptible contraction in proximal and distal muscles
M3	Return of function in proximal and distal muscles of such a degree that all important muscles are sufficiently powerful to act against resistance
M4	Return of function as in stage 3; in addition, all synergistic and independent movements are possible
M5	Complete recovery

- A larger area of tactile and thermal anesthesia is readily delineated and corresponds more closely to the gross anatomical distribution of the nerve. This larger area is known as the intermediate zone.
- When a nerve is intact and the adjacent nerves are blocked or sectioned, an area of sensibility exceeds the gross anatomical distribution of the nerve, then this area is known as the maximal zone.

Sensibility Recovery Sequence

- Myelinated and unmyelinated fibers (restore perception of pain and temperature) and pseudomotor function
- *Touch perception:*
  - Perception of 30 cps of vibratory stimulus
  - Perception of moving touch
  - Perception of constant touch
  - Perception of 256 cps vibratory stimulus.

Sensation Assessment after Peripheral Nerve Injury

- *S0:* Absence of sensibility in autonomous area.
- *S1:* Recovery of deep cutaneous pain sensibility within autonomous area of the nerve.
- *S2:* Return of some degree of superficial cutaneous pain and tactile sensibility within autonomous area of the nerve.
- *S3:* Return of superficial cutaneous pain and tactile sensibility throughout autonomous area, with disappearance of any previous over response.
- *S3+:* Return of sensibility as in stage 3, in addition, there is some recovery of two-point discrimination within autonomous area.
- *S4:* Complete recovery.

Reflex

Complete severance of a peripheral nerve abolishes all reflex activity transmitted by that nerve. This is true in severance of the afferent or the efferent arc. Commonly, however, reflex activity is abolished in partial nerve injuries, when neither arc is completely interrupted and is not a reliable guide to the severity of injury.

Autonomic

- Interruption of a peripheral nerve is followed by loss of sweating and of pilomotor response and by vasomotor paralysis in the autonomous zone. The area of anhidrosis usually corresponds to, but may be slightly larger than the sensory deficit.

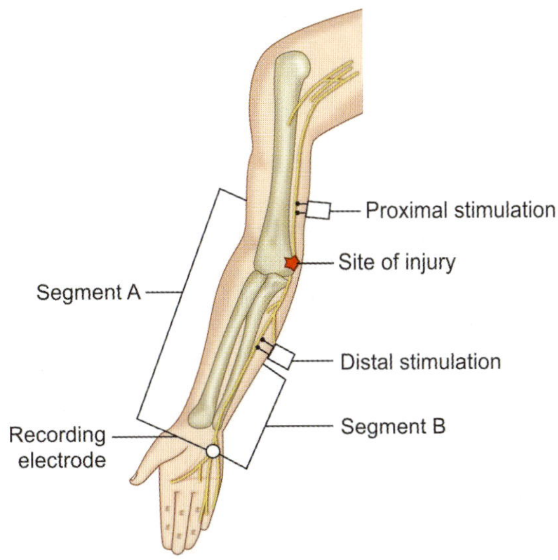

Fig. 5: Nerve conduction velocity.

TABLE 3: Nerve conduction velocity.

Injury pattern	*Proximal stimulation (Segment A)*	*Immediately after injury distal stimulation (Segment B)*	*Ten days after injury distal stimulation (Segment B)*
Neuropraxia	No response	[waveform]	[waveform]
Axonotmosis or neurotmesis	No response	[waveform]	No response

- If the injury is incomplete and especially, if it is associated with causalgia, sweating may be excessive, and may involve areas beyond the intermediate zone of the nerve. Vasodilation occurs in complete lesions and the area affected is at first warmer and pinker than the rest of the limb. After 2–3 weeks, however, the affected area becomes colder than the adjacent normal areas and the skin may be pale, cyanotic, or mottled in an area often extending beyond the maximal zone of the injured nerve. Trophic changes occur commonly and are most evident in the hands and feet. The skin becomes thin and glistening and when subjected to trauma that ordinarily does little harm, it breaks down to form ulcers that heal slowly. The fingernails become distorted, often ridged, or brittle, and may be lost entirely.

DIAGNOSTIC TESTS

Diagnostic tests majorly include electrodiagnostic tests. These are explained below.

Nerve Conduction Velocity (Fig. 5)

Stimulation of a peripheral nerve by an electrode placed on the skin overlying the nerve readily evokes a response from the muscle innervated by that nerve. This response can be seen, palpated, and measured. The nerve is stimulated proximal to distal and across the level of injury, with subsequent distal evoked potential recording, achieved using a needle or surface pick-up electrode (Table 3).

Electromyography

- Muscle activity observed with a needle pick-up electrode (e.g. monopolar, concentric, single fiber) placed in myotomes, innervated by an injured nerve provides crucial information.
- At approximately 10–14 days after neural injury, abnormal spontaneous rest potentials (positive sharp waves) appear in innervated myotomes, where axonal injury has occurred. At 14–18 days, fibrillations appear. At approximately 3 months after injury, some peripheral neural sprouting has occurred and the motor unit potential amplitude has progressively increased. This is preceded at times by polyphasic configuration potentials. After 2–6 months of injury, larger potentials are established and remain so, until the reinnervation is completed, at which time the motor unit potential configuration returns to a more normal appearing pattern.

Tinel Sign

The Tinel sign is elicited by gentle percussion, by a finger or percussion hammer along the course of an injured nerve. A transient tingling sensation should be felt by the patient in the distribution of the injured nerve, rather than in the area percussed and the sensation should persist for several seconds after stimulation. It should be tested for in a distal to proximal direction. A positive Tinel sign is presumptive evidence that regenerating axonal sprouts that have not obtained complete myelinization and progressing along the endoneurial tube.

Sweat Test

The time-honored sweat test (iodine starch test) consists of dusting the extremity with quinizarin powder. Sweating is induced by various means. The powder remains dry and light gray throughout the denervated area and assumes a deep purple color throughout the area of normal sweating.

Skin Resistance Test

The skin resistance test is another method of evaluating autonomic interruption. In it, a Richter dermometer is used. The autonomous zone with absence of sweating shows an increased resistance to the passage of electrical current. The adjacent innervated areas have a normal resistance and further decreased resistance in these areas can be elicited by high external temperatures that do not affect the denervated area.

MANAGEMENT OF NERVE INJURIES

Factors that influence regeneration after neurorrhaphy are illustrated below:

- Age of the patient
- Gap between the nerve ends
- Delay between the time of injury and repair
- Level of injury
- Condition of the nerve ends
- Experience and techniques of the surgeon.

Technique of Nerve Repair

Endoneurolysis

The epineurium is incised longitudinally proximal to the lesion, beginning not more than 0.5 cm from the level of gross changes in the nerve, as determined by palpation. The flaps of epineurium on each side may be retracted laterally by nylon sutures and are undermined widely. The funiculi are separated, if possible with a pointed or diamond-bladed knife, using sharp or blunt dissection as necessary. Spring-loaded microscissors also are helpful in this dissection. The surgeon constantly should be aware of the possibility of plexus formation between fascicles and protect these.

Partial Neurorrhaphy

When the decision has been made to perform partial neurorrhaphy, the incision is extended longitudinally in the epineurium proximally and distally several centimeters, as necessary. The intact funiculi are dissected out for the same distance. The ends of the injured part of the nerve are resected to normal tissue. At the cut ends, an end-to-end neurorrhaphy is performed.

Complete Neurorrhaphy and Nerve Grafting

Technique of Neurorrhaphy

- Epineurial
- Perineurial
- Interfascicular nerve grafting.

Methods of Closing Gaps between the Nerve Ends

- Mobilization
- Positioning of extremity
- Transposition
- Bone resection
- Nerve grafting
- Nerve stretching and bulb suture
- Nerve crossing (pedicle grafting).

CHAPTER

Peripheral Vascular Disease

17

OBJECTIVES

- Peripheral Arterial Disease
- Arterial Disorders
- Vasospastic Conditions
- Frostbite
- Peripheral Venous Disease

INTRODUCTION

Peripheral vascular disease refers to any disease or disorder of the circulatory system outside of the brain and heart.

It is divided into two disorders:

1. Arterial disorders
2. Venous disorders.

Arterial Disorders

- *Pain:* Aching to sharp brought on by exercise and is relieved by rest
- *Pulses:* Diminished or absent
- *Edema:* None
- *Skin changes:* Skin becomes cold, dry, shiny, and hairless. Pallor, when elevated, and red, when dangling.

Venous Disorders

- *Pain:* Aching to cramp like and relieved by activity or elevating the extremity
- *Pulses:* Usually present
- *Edema:* Present, increases at the end of the day
- *Skin changes:* Warm, thick, tough, darkened, and stasis ulcers.

PERIPHERAL ARTERIAL DISEASE

Definition

Decreased patency of the arterial supply to the lower extremities leading to claudication, ischemia, and potentially limb loss as well as narrowing of the arteries of the extremities due to atherosclerosis.

Risk Factors

- Positive family history of premature heart attacks or strokes
- Older than 50 years
- Obesity
- Inactive (sedentary) lifestyle
- Smoking
- Diabetes
- High blood pressure
- High cholesterol or LDL (bad cholesterol), plus high triglycerides and low HDL (the good cholesterol)
- Men are slightly more likely affected than women.

ARTERIAL DISORDERS

Arterial disorders include:

- Arterial stenosis
- Acute arterial occlusion
- Gangrene
- Arteritis.

Arterial Stenosis

- The most common cause of peripheral artery disease is due to atherosclerosis.
- This is a gradual process in which a fatty material builds up inside the arteries.
- The fatty material mixes with calcium, scar tissues, and other substances and then hardens slightly, forming plaques of arteriosclerosis.
- These plaques block, narrow, or weaken the vessel walls. Blood flow through the arteries can be restricted or blocked totally.

Symptoms and Signs of Arterial Occlusion

Claudication pain:

- It is an intermittent cramp-like pain felt in the muscles that is brought on, by walking, not present on taking the first step and relieved by standing still.
- Claudication is the muscle pain due to accumulation of excessive P substance, owing to inadequate blood flow.
- The pain develops only when the muscles are working and disappears when exercise stops. Claudication pain is most commonly felt in calf, but can affect thigh or buttock.
- Pain in the buttock, occurring on exercise (walking) and associated sexual impotence, which result from arterial ischemia are given the eponymous title "Leriche's syndrome". Distance walked is called claudication distance.
- *Boyd's classification of claudication pain:*
  - *Grade 1:* Claudication pain appears, but as the patient continues the exercise, claudication pain disappears.
  - *Grade 2:* Pain continues and the patient can still walk with effort.
  - *Grade 3:* Pain compels the patient to take rest.
  - *Grade 4:* Rest pain.

- Spinal claudication/neurogenic claudication is not due to lack of blood supply, but rather it is caused by nerve root compression and/or stenosis of the spinal canal, usually from a degenerative spine.
- This may result from many factors, such as bulging disk, herniated disk, or fragments from previously herniated disks (postoperative), scar tissue from previous surgeries, osteophytes, or other causes.
- *Vascular claudication:*
  - Arterial pulses are diminished
  - Relieved by rest
  - Typically occurs after activities/ambulation for a distance with resultant vascular insufficiency
  - Not associated with weakness.
- *Neuro claudication:*
  - Arterial pulses are normal
  - Symptoms may be relieved by sitting down (flexing the spine)
  - Typically, occurs after standing erect or standing and walking
  - Generally associated with weakness.

Rest pain:

It is severe pain felt in the foot at rest, made worse by lying down, or elevation of the foot. The pain is worse at night and relieved by hanging the foot out of bed or by sleeping in a chair. It is described "cry of dying nerves".

Coldness, numbness, and paresthesia:

These are common in moderate and severe ischemia, but in the absence of color changes, it is essential to exclude neurological cause (Fig. 1).

Color changes:

- Severely ischemic limbs develop purple discoloration on dependency. Bright red color is due to extravasation of RBC through capillary walls.
  Buerger's postural test: The limb is raised for a minute or two. With a normal peripheral circulation, the toes should remain pink at 90°. In an ischemic limb because arterial pressure is unable to overcome gravity, the elevated leg becomes waxy, cadaveric, white color, best seen on the sole of the foot. The angle to which the leg must be raised before it becomes white, is the vascular angle or Buerger's angle, usually less than 30° in an ischemic limb. When the limb is hung down, it gradually becomes a bluish-red color due to reactive hyperemia.
- *Capillary filling*: The time will be longer in case of ischemic limb.
- *Cross legged test*: This is to detect popliteal pulsations. The patient is asked to sit with legs crossed one above the other so that popliteal fossa of one leg will lie against the knee of the other leg. Patient's attention is diverted. Crossed leg will show oscillatory movements of the foot, which occur synchronously with the pulse of the popliteal artery.
- *Allen's test*: Instruct the patient to clench his/her fist. Using your fingers, apply occlusive pressure to both the ulnar and radial arteries. This maneuver obstructs blood flow to the hand. While applying occlusive pressure to both the arteries, patient should relax his/her hand. Blanching of the palm and fingers should occur. If it does not, you have not completely occluded the arteries with your fingers. Release the occlusive pressure on the ulnar artery. You should notice a flushing of the hand within 5–15 seconds. This denotes that the ulnar artery is patent and has good blood flow.

Ulceration and gangrene:

- Ulceration occurs with severe arterial insufficiency and is often present as painful superficial erosion between toes (Figs. 2 and 3).
- *Sensation and movement:* Severe chronic ischemia produces hyperesthesia especially on the borderline skin of gangrene.
- *Arterial pulsations:* Arterial pulsation below occlusion is usually absent or diminished in the presence of good collaterals. Expansile arterial pulsation with a mass may indicate an aneurysm.
- Other physical findings include loss of hair, nail changes (brittle nails), pallor on elevation, and dependent rubor of the affected extremities.

Symptoms:

Symptoms are related to the organ supplied by the artery:

- *Lower limb:* Claudication, rest pain, and gangrene
- *Brain:* Transient ischemic attacks and hemiplegia

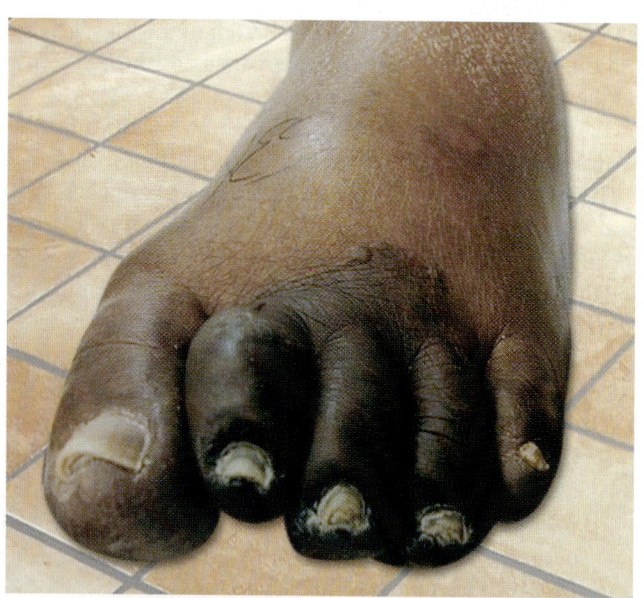

Fig. 1: Severe ischemia of the foot.

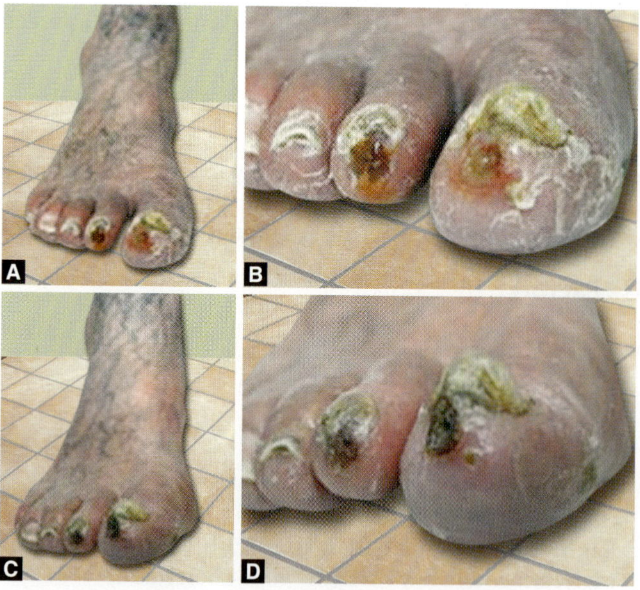

Figs. 2A to D: Ulceration of the toes.

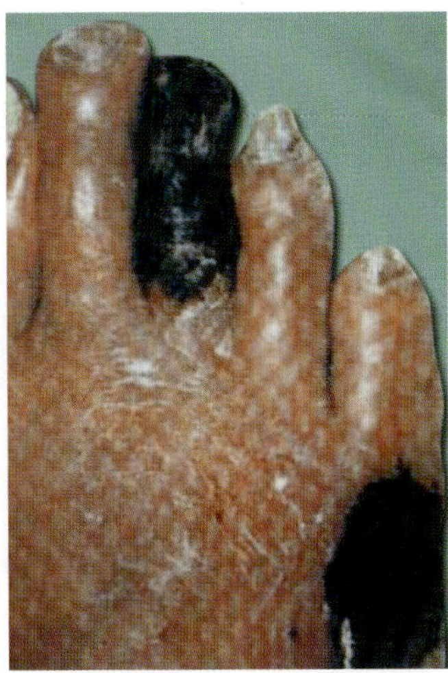

Fig. 3: Severe chronic ischemia with dry gangrene.

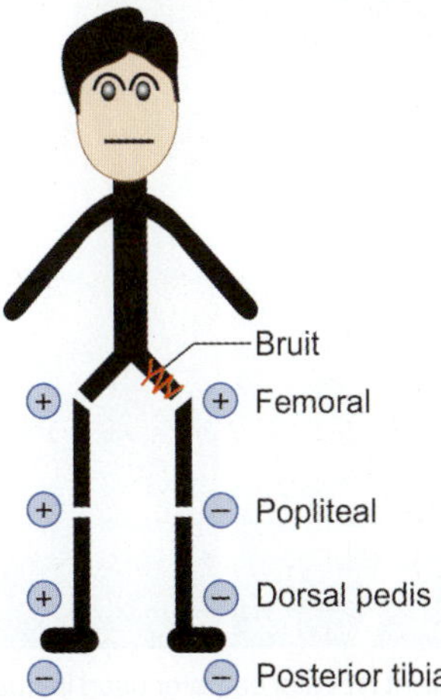

Fig. 4: Physical signs, in case of arterial occlusion.

- *Myocardium:* Angina and myocardial infarction
- *Kidney:* Hypertension or infarction
- *Intestine:* Abdominal pain and infarction.

Physical signs:

- In case of arterial occlusion with normal distal pulses and highly developed collateral circulation (Fig. 4).
- *Disappearing pulse:* On exercising till claudication, palpable pulse disappears. Then after 1–2 minutes of rest the disappearing pulse reappears.
- *Arterial bruits:* Auscultation of subclavian arteries and systolic bruits.
- Bruit in neck at the level of mandibular angle, without supraclavicular bruit means carotid artery stenosis.

Diagnosis and Investigations

Routine investigation:

- Hemoglobin, full blood count, ESR, plasma fibrinogen, protein electrophoresis, blood and urine glucose, blood lipid profile, and exercise ECG.

Noninvasive tests:

- *Doppler ultrasound:* Use a stethoscope with sphygmomanometer to assess the systolic blood pressure in relatively small vessels (Fig. 5).
  Ankle brachial index (ABI): It is the ratio of systolic pressure at ankle artery to that in brachial artery. Numerator is systolic pressure in dorsalis pedis and posterior tibial arteries and denominator is taken as systolic pressure of brachial arteries. ABI values for different conditions are illustrated in Table 1.
  Duplex imaging: It provides an image of vessels, which can give detailed knowledge of vessel blood flow and turbulence (Figs. 6 and 7).
- *Color duplex:* Visualization of blood flow indicates change in direction and velocity of blood flow; increased flow depicts stenosis.
- *Treadmill:* It is useful in the assessment of walking distance in claudicants.

Invasive tests:

- *Arterial digital subtraction angiography (DSA):* This technique, which is in widespread use, employs a computer system to digitize the angiographic information (Fig. 8).
- Conventional arteriography (Fig. 9).

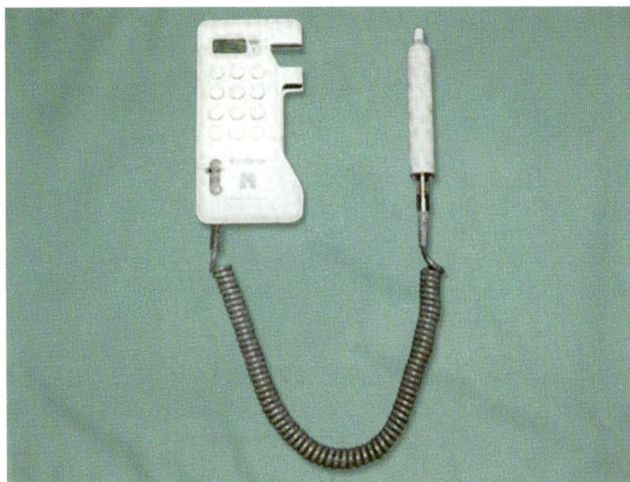

Fig. 5: Doppler ultrasound.

TABLE 1: Ankle brachial index (ABI) values and associated conditions.

ABI	*Interpretation*
1 or slightly greater	Normal
<0.8	Arterial obstruction
<0.5	Rest pain
<0.3	Imminent necrosis

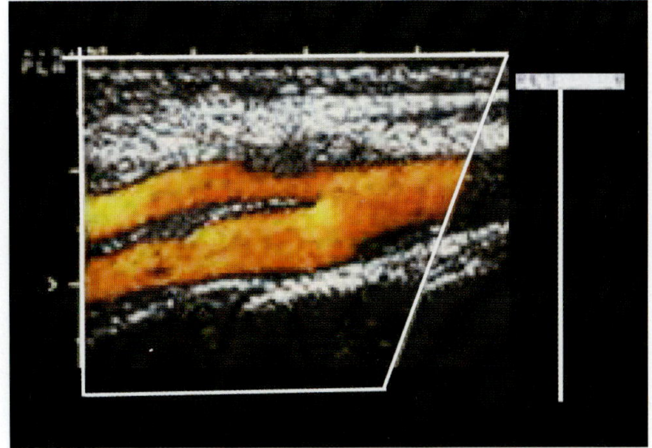

Fig. 6: Duplex imaging.

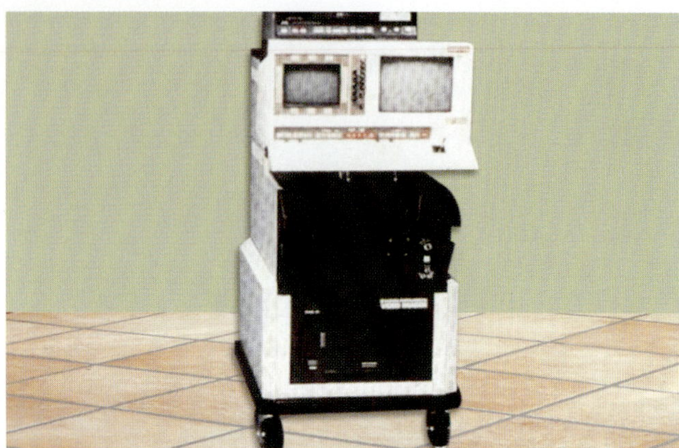

Fig. 7: Duplex imaging machine.

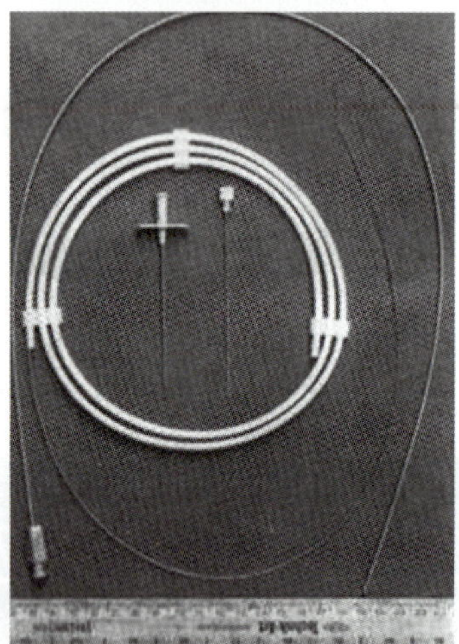

Fig. 8: Arterial digital subtraction angiography.

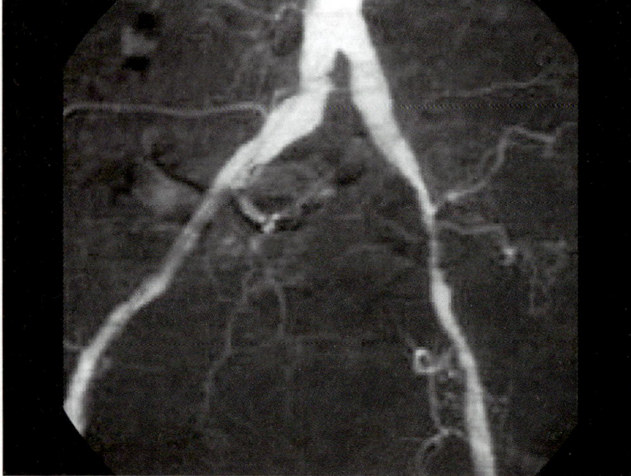

Fig. 9: Conventional arteriography.

- *Plethysmography:* It assesses change in volume of a limb or digit over the cardiac cycle.

Management (Arterial Stenosis)

Conservative treatment:

- Stop smoking
- Taking regular exercise within the limits of the pain

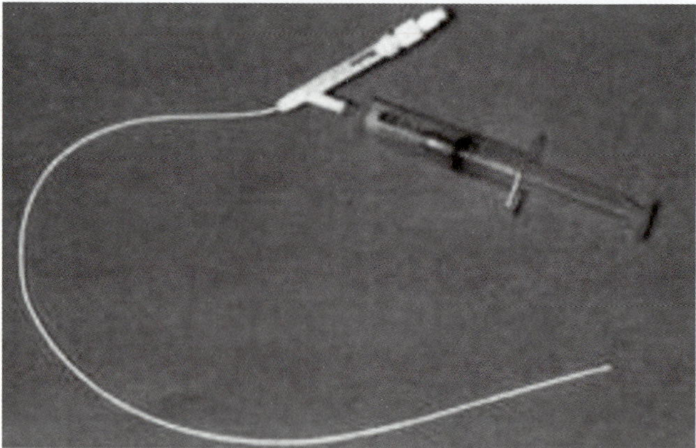

Fig. 10: Balloon catheter; used for transluminal angioplasty.

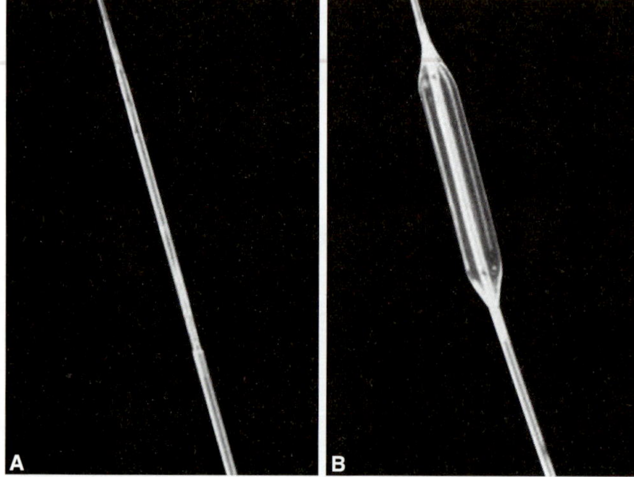

Figs. 11A and B: Different types of catheter used in transluminal angioplasty.

- Suitable diet to reduce weight in obese and hyperlipidemics
- *Heel raise:* Claudication distance may be increased by raising the heels of shoes by 1 cm. The work of the calf muscles is reduced.

Drugs:

- Rest pain can be relieved by analgesics and elevation of the head of bed (Buerger's position), pentoxifylline for treatment of intermittent claudication, aspirin in small dose of 150 mg/day to prevent thrombosis.
- Two medications have been approved by the United States Food and Drug Administration (FDA) for direct treatment of the symptoms of intermittent claudication.
- *Pentoxifylline (Trental):* How this drug helps in intermittent claudication is not completely understood. It is believed to improve blood flow, by decreasing the viscosity of blood and making red blood cells more flexible. With these alterations, the blood can move more easily past obstructions in the blood vessel.
- *Cilostazol (Pletal):* This drug keeps platelets from clumping together. This clumping promotes formation of clots and slows down blood flow. The drug also helps to dilate or expand the blood vessels, encouraging the flow of blood.

Nonoperative procedures to improve arterial flow:

- *Transluminal angioplasty:* Inserting a balloon catheter into an artery and inflating it within a narrowed area (Figs. 10 and 11).

- *Percutaneous transluminal angioplasty (PTA):* In this inflatable balloon may be used for stenosis or short occlusions.
- *Intraluminal stents:* After balloon dilatation, the vessel may fail to stay dilated then it is possible to keep open lumen by a metal stent (Figs. 12A and B).
- *Lasers and atherectomy catheters:* Lasers can be used to open occluded arteries, so that a balloon angioplasty catheter can be inserted. Atherectomy catheters actually remove atherosclerotic plaque from arterial wall, either by cutting or extracting.

Operations for arterial occlusion:
- *Sympathectomy:* Relieves pain.
- *Aortoiliac occlusion:* Good caliber vessels below the site of disease respond well to aortofemoral bypass. If not, an iliac endarterectomy might be considered, but PTA with or without a stent is probably a better alternative.
- *Superficial femoral and profunda femoris artery occlusion (with unilateral symptoms):* For severe disease, angioplasty or bypass may be used. A femoropopliteal bypass graft is the most usual operation (to overcome a blocked superficial femoral artery). Patient's own saphenous vein is the best graft (Figs. 13A and B). *Occlusive disease below the popliteal artery (usually unreconstructable):* Bypass to tibial vessels (down ankle level) can be successful. Long saphenous vein used in the in situ fashion, after disrupting the valves with a valvulotome. If the saphenous vein is not available, a polytetrafluoroethylene (PTFE) graft is used.

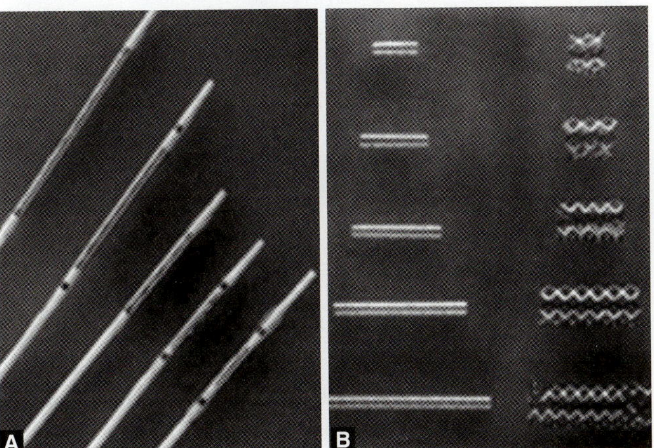

Figs. 12A and B: Different intraluminal stents.

Acute Arterial Occlusion

Definition

Sudden occlusion of an artery is commonly due to either emboli or trauma.

Clinical Picture

Six P's (Fig. 14):
1. Pain
2. Pallor
3. Pulselessness
4. Paresthesia
5. Paralysis
6. Progressive coldness.

Embolic Occlusion

Definition:

An embolus is a body, which is foreign to the bloodstream and which may become lodged in a vessel and cause obstruction.

Simple emboli:
- Simple emboli are due to blood thrombus. The sources are most commonly mural thrombus, following a myocardial infarct (a third of cases), mitral stenosis, cardiac arrhythmias (particularly atrial fibrillation), and aneurysms.
- Emboli may lodge in any organ including brain, mesentric vessels, spleen, kidneys, lungs, lower limbs, etc. with resultant ischemia (Fig. 15).
- The diagnosis can be made clinically in the majority of cases. The patient, who has no previous symptoms of claudication or limb pain and has a source of emboli, suddenly develops severe pain or numbness of the limb, which becomes cold with mottled blue and white discoloration. Movement of the toes becomes progressively more difficult and sensation to touch is lost. Pulses are absent distally.

Treatment:
- The immediate administration of heparin, 5,000 units intravenously, can reduce this extension and maintain patency

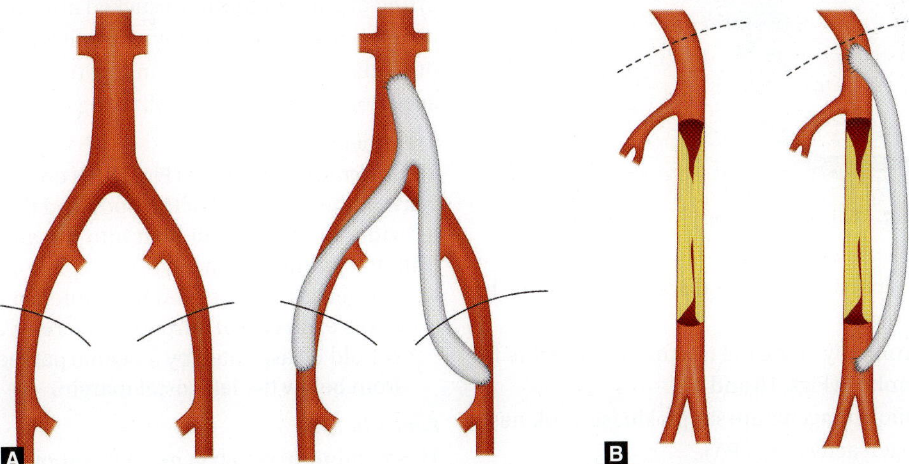

Figs. 13A and B: (A) Atherosclerotic narrowing of the aortic bifurcation, aortobifemoral graft to bypass stenosis; (B) Superficial femoral and profunda femoris stenosis providing poor collateral circulation, femoropopliteal graft used to bypass the occluded area into good "runoff" below.

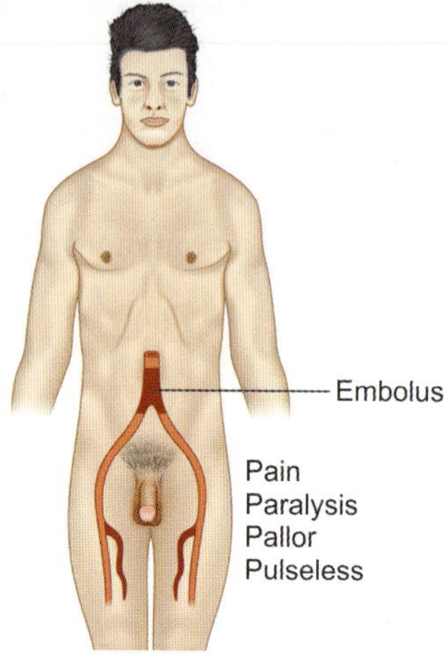

Fig. 14: Clinical picture of an acute arterial occlusion.

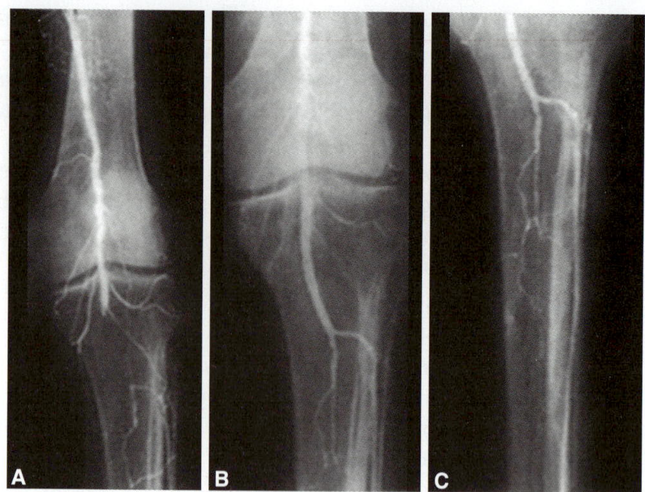

Figs. 17A to C: (A) Angiography showing blockade; (B and C) Reflow after embolectomy.

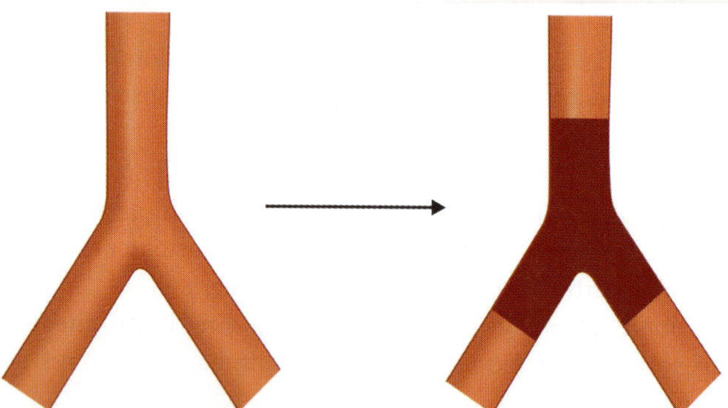

Fig. 15: Aortic bifurcation embolus.

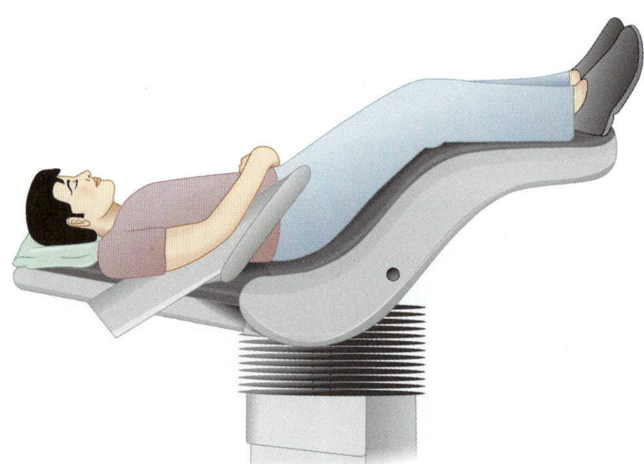

Fig. 18: Trendelenburg's position.

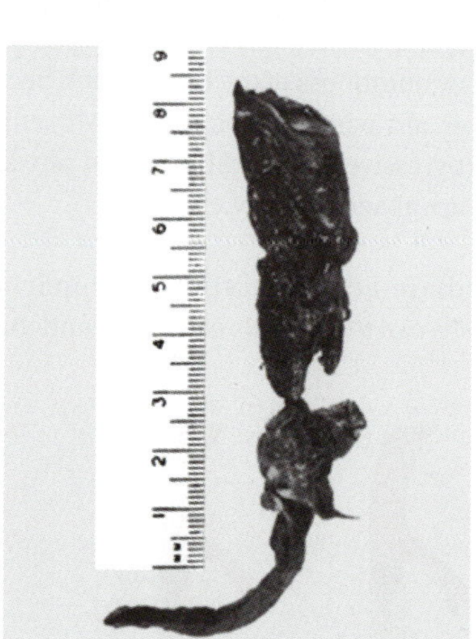

Fig. 16: Limb embolus.

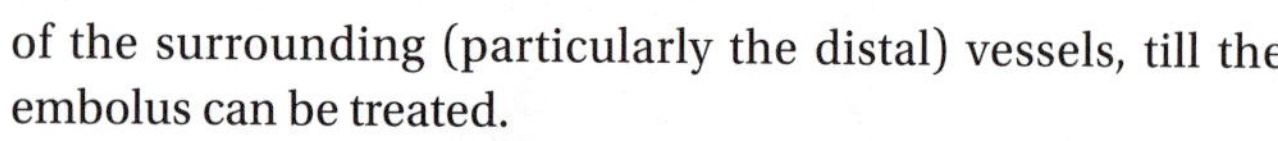

of the surrounding (particularly the distal) vessels, till the embolus can be treated.

- Embolectomy or thrombolysis are the treatments available for patients with limb emboli (Figs. 16 and 17).
- The common thrombolytic agents are streptokinase, urokinase, and tissue plasminogen activator (TPA).
- Whichever drug is used, regular angiograms are carried out to check the extent of lysis. Using streptokinase, lysis was usually complete within 48 hours. TPA may achieve lysis within 24 hours and pulse spray TPA may take less than 6 hours.

Air embolism:
Air may be accidentally injected into the venous circulation, e.g. artificial pneumothorax or sucked into an open vein. Thus, venous air embolism occasionally complicates operations on the neck or axilla, if a large vein is inadvertently opened or it may be an accessory cause of death following a cut throat.

Treatment:
Trendelenburg's position (Fig. 18): It encourages air to pass into the veins of the lower half of the body and the patient is placed on the left side, so that air will float into the apex of the ventricle, away from the pulmonary artery.

- Oxygen is administered to counteract hypoxemia and to assist in the excretion of nitrogen. In serious cases, the right ventricle should be aspirated by a needle passed upward and backward from below the left costal margin.

Fat embolism:
This condition, which is more common than generally supposed, usually follows severe injuries with multiple or major fractures. Cases have also been recorded following electroconvulsive therapy.

The fat may be derived from bone marrow or adipose tissue, but recent work suggests that it is metabolic in origin, perhaps by aggregation of chylomicrons.

- Symptoms are evident a day or so after injury and two more or less distinct types, cerebral and pulmonary are recognized.
- In the cerebral type, the patient becomes drowsy, restless, and disorientated (delirium tremens may be suspected). Subsequently, the patient is comatose, the pupils become small and pyrexia ensues.
- The pulmonary type is ushered in with cyanosis, which increases in intensity and signs of right heart failure. White froth may occur at the mouth and nostrils.
- The sputum should be examined for fat droplets and fat may be excreted in the urine. A fall in the hemoglobin value of the blood is a constant sign. Petechial hemorrhages often occur.
- Treatment consists of oxygen, early heparinization, and intravenous low molecular weight dextran.

Gangrene

Gangrene implies death with putrefaction of macroscopic portions of tissue. It is commonly seen affecting the distal part of a limb, the appendix or a loop of small intestine, and sometimes organs such as the gallbladder, the pancreas, or the testis.

Types of Gangrene (Based upon the Cause)

- *Secondary to arterial obstruction*: It can be from disease, for example:
  - Thrombosis of an atherosclerotic artery
  - Embolus from the heart in atrial fibrillation or after coronary thrombosis
  - Arteritis with neuropathy in diabetes
  - Buerger's disease
  - Arterial shutdown in Raynaud's disease or ergotism
  - Effect of intra-arterial injections, i.e. thiopentone and cytotoxic substances.
- *Infective:* Boils and carbuncles, gas gangrene, gangrene of the scrotum (Fournier's gangrene), etc.
- *Traumatic:* Due to direct trauma, such as crushes, pressure sores, and the constriction groove of strangulated bowel or indirect, due to injury of vessels at some distance from the site of gangrene, e.g. pressure on the popliteal artery, by the lower end of a fractured femur.
- *Physical:* For example, burns, scalds, frostbite, chemicals, irradiation, and electricity.
- Venous gangrene.

Clinical Features of Gangrene

- A gangrenous part lacks arterial pulsation, venous return, capillary response to pressure (color returns), sensation, warmth, and function.
- The color of the part changes through a variety of shades, according to circumstances (pallor, dusky gray, mottled, purple), until finally taking on the characteristic dark brown, greenish black, or black appearance, which is due to the disintegration of hemoglobin and the formation of iron sulfide (Fig. 3).
  Clinical types: These include following types of gangrene, with their different clinical presentation.
- *Dry gangrene:* Dry gangrene occurs when the tissues are desiccated by gradual slowing of the bloodstream. It is typically the result of atherosclerosis. The affected part becomes dry and wrinkled, discolored from disintegration of hemoglobin and greasy to the touch (Fig. 19).
- *Moist gangrene:* This occurs when venous as well as arterial obstruction is present, when the artery is suddenly occluded, as by a ligature, or embolus, and in diabetes.
  Infection and putrefaction are always present, the affected part becomes swollen and discolored and the epidermis may be raised in blebs. Crepitus may be palpated, owing to infection by gas forming organisms (Fig. 20).

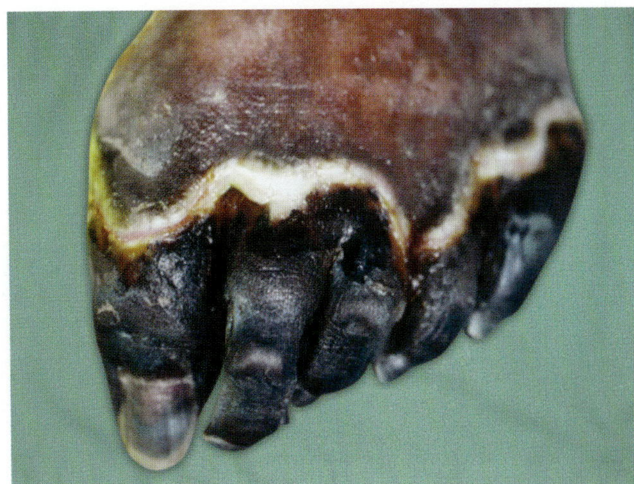

Fig. 19: Dry gangrene of the toes.

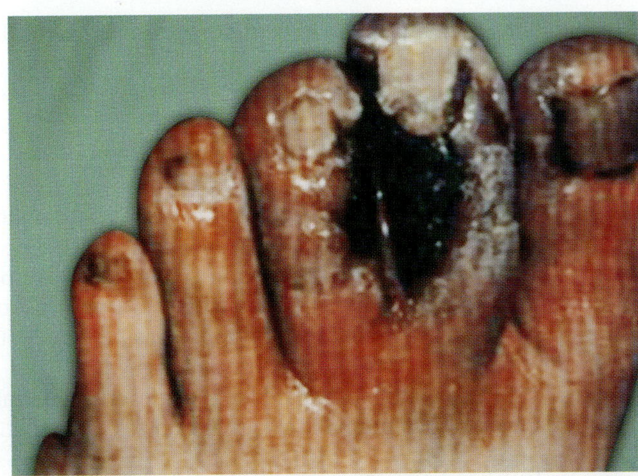

Fig. 20: Moist gangrene.

Separation of Gangrene

Separation by demarcation:

- A zone of demarcation between the truly viable and the dead or dying tissue appears first. It is indicated on the surface, by a band of hyperemia and hyperesthesia. Separation is achieved by the development of a layer of granulation tissue, which forms between the dead and the living parts.
- In dry gangrene, if the blood supply of the proximal tissues is adequate, the final line of demarcation appears in a matter of days and separation begins to take place neatly and with the minimum of infection (so-called separation by aseptic ulceration).
- In moist gangrene, there is more infection and suppuration extends into the neighboring living tissue, thereby causing

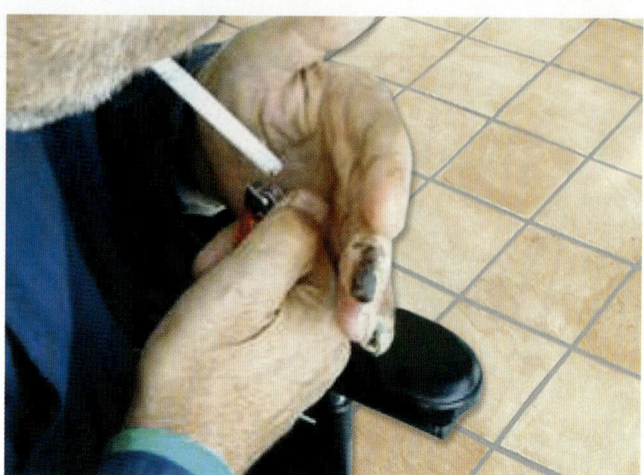
Fig. 21: Discolored nails depicting Buerger's disease.

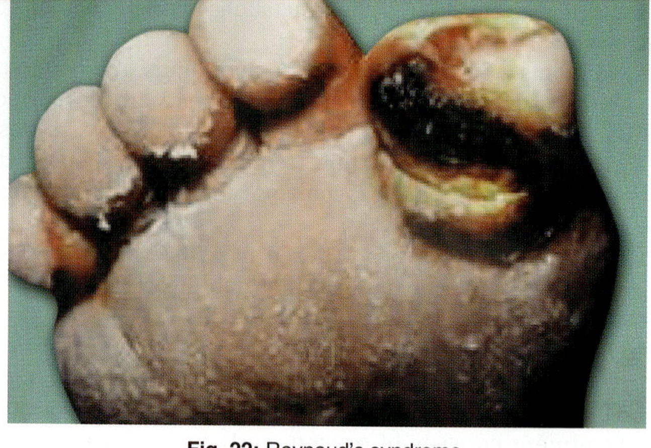
Fig. 22: Raynaud's syndrome.

the final line of demarcation to be more proximal than in dry gangrene.
- Separation by septic ulceration.

Treatment of Gangrene

General principles of treatment include:
- A limb-saving attitude is needed in most cases of symptomatic gangrene affecting hands and feet.
- With arterial disease all depends upon a good blood supply to the limb above the gangrene or whether a poor blood supply can be improved by such measures, as percutaneous transluminal angioplasty or direct arterial surgery.
- A life-saving amputation is required for a badly crushed limb, rapidly spreading symptomatic gangrene and gas gangrene.

General treatment includes:
- Treatment of cardiac failure, atrial fibrillation, and anemia to improve the tissue oxygenation.
- A nutritious diet is essential in all forms of gangrene and the control of diabetes, when present, are additional items of care.

Local treatment includes:
- Care of the affected part includes keeping it absolutely dry. Exposure and the use of a fan may assist in the desiccation and may relieve pain. The limb must not be heated.
- A bed-cradle, padded rings, foam blocks, and air beds are useful preventive aids.
- The release of pus assists in relief of pain.

Arteritis

Thromboangiitis Obliterans (Buerger's Disease) (Fig. 21)

- This is a condition characterized by occlusive disease of the small and medium-sized arteries (plantars, tibials, radial, etc.), thrombophlebitis of superficial or deep veins and Raynaud's syndrome, occurring in male patients in a young age group (usually under the age of 30 years) (Fig. 22).
- The condition does not occur in women or nonsmokers. It is not as used to be stated more common in Russian and Jews, but cases are seen in different races all over the world.

Histology:

Localized inflammatory changes occur in the walls of arteries and veins, leading to thrombosis. The usual symptoms and signs of arterial occlusive disease are present. Gangrene of the toes and fingers is common and progressive (Figs. 23A to C).

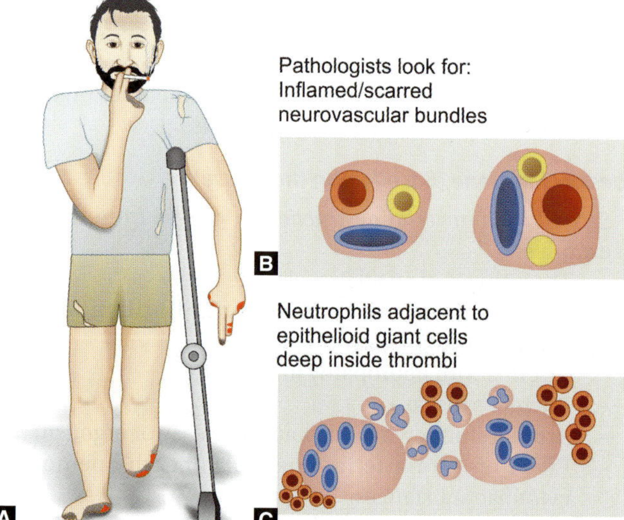

Figs. 23A to C: Histological changes seen in Buerger's thromboangiitis obliterans.

Investigations:
- A formal vascular assessment should be undertaken, e.g. ESR, autoantibodies, coagulation screening, and lipid profile.
- Arteriography sometimes shows a characteristic "corrugation" of the femoral arteries as well as the distal arterial occlusions and helps to distinguish the condition from presenile atherosclerosis.

Treatment:
- The treatment is total abstinence from smoking. While this will arrest the disease, it will not reverse established arterial occlusions.
- Use of vascular growth factor and stem cell injections has been showing promise in clinical studies.
- Streptokinase has been proposed as adjuvant therapy in some cases.
- Established arterial occlusions may be treated along the usual lines and sympathectomy may be a useful adjunctive procedure. Nevertheless, amputations, conservative, if possible, may eventually be required.

Takayasu's Arteritis (Fig. 24)

- Takayasu's arteritis (also known as "aortic arch syndrome" and "pulseless disease") is an inflammatory disease with an unknown cause.
- It affects the aorta, the main blood vessel from the heart, as well as the blood vessels that attach to it.
- Females are about 8–9 times more likely to get it than males. People usually get the disease between 15 years and 30 years of age.
- It is also known as "pulseless disease" because pulses on the upper extremities, such as the wrist pulse may not be felt.
- Although, its etiology is unknown, the condition is characterized by segmental and patchy granulomatous inflammation of the aorta and major derivative branches. This inflammation leads to arterial stenosis, thrombosis, and aneurysms.

Symptoms:
- About half of all patients develop an initial systemic illness, with symptoms of malaise, fever, night sweats, weight loss, arthralgia, and fatigue. There is often an anemia and marked elevation of the ESR.
- This is followed by a more chronic stage characterized by inflammatory and obliterative changes in the aorta and its branches.
- In the late stage, weakness of the arterial walls may give rise to localized aneurysms.
- Raynaud's phenomenon is commonly found in this disease.

Treatment:
- The great majority of patients with Takayasu's arteritis respond to prednisolone. The usual starting dose is approximately 1 mg per kg of body weight per day.
- Surgical options may need to be explored for patients, who do not respond to steroids. Reperfusion of tissues can be achieved by large vessel reconstructive surgery, such as bypass grafting.

Other Types of Arteritis

Other types of arteritis are encountered in rheumatoid arthritis, diffuse lupus erythematosus, and polyarteritis. Treatment is similar.

VASOSPASTIC CONDITIONS

Raynaud's Syndrome

Raynaud's syndrome may be:
- Primary
- Secondary.

Primary Raynaud's Syndrome

- The primary idiopathic form usually occurs in young women and affects the upper extremities more than the lower. The peripheral pulses are normal.
- The condition is attributable to abnormal sensitivity in the direct response of the arterioles to cold.
- When cooled, these vessels constrict and as a result, the part (usually the fingers) becomes blanched and incapable of finer movements.
- The capillaries then dilate and fill with slowly flowing deoxygenated blood, the digits therefore becoming swollen and dusky. As the attack passes off, the arterioles relax, oxygenated blood returns into the dilated capillaries, and the digits become red (Figs. 25A to C).

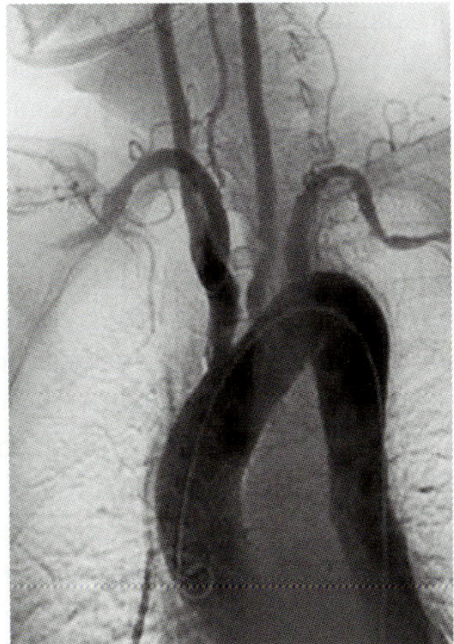

Fig. 24: Takayasu's arteritis.

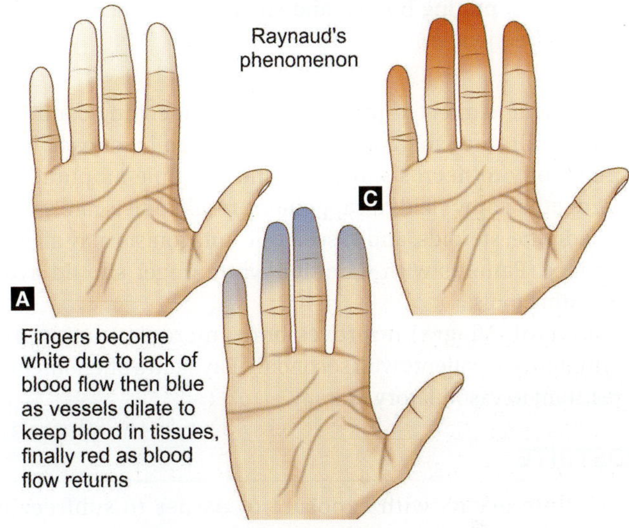

Figs. 25A to C: Raynaud's syndrome.

- Thus, the condition is recognized by the characteristic sequence of blanching, dusky cyanosis, and red engorgement, often accompanied by pain.
- Raynaud's disease or "Primary Raynaud's" is diagnosed, if the symptoms are idiopathic, that is, they occur by themselves and not in association with other diseases. Some refer to primary Raynaud's disease as being allergic to coldness.

Conservative treatment:
- Avoid environmental triggers, e.g. cold, vibration, etc. Emotional stress is another recognized trigger
- Quit smoking
- Avoid caffeine, other stimulants, and vasoconstrictors.

Treatment:
- Treatment for Raynaud's phenomenon may include prescription medicines that dilate blood vessels, such as calcium channel blockers—nifedipine or diltiazem.
- There is some evidence that angiotensin II receptor antagonists (Losartan) reduce frequency and severity of attacks.
- Fluoxetine, a selective serotonin reuptake inhibitor, and other antidepressant medications may reduce the frequency and severity of episodes.

- Infusions of prostaglandins, e.g. prostacyclin, may be tried.
- In severe cases, a sympathectomy procedure can be performed. Here, the nerves that signal the blood vessels of the fingertips to constrict are surgically cut.

Secondary Raynaud's Syndrome

- Raynaud's syndrome or "Secondary Raynaud's" occurs secondary to a wide variety of other conditions. This was previously called Raynaud's disease (a term to be avoided).
- Although peripheral vasospasm may be noted in atherosclerosis, thoracic outlet syndrome, carpal tunnel, etc. The term secondary Raynaud's syndrome is most often used for a peripheral arterial manifestation of the collagen diseases, especially progressive systemic sclerosis (scleroderma) and systemic lupus erythromatosis.
- It may also follow the use of vibrating tools (when it is commonly known as "vibration white finger"), e.g. pneumatic road drills, mining borers, and chain saws, which vibrate at certain frequencies.

Treatment:

- Treatment is directed primarily at the underlying condition. The syndrome when secondary to the collagenoses leads frequently to necrosis of digits and multiple amputations. Sympathectomy yields disappointing results and is rarely used.
- Nifedipine, steroids, and vasospastic antagonists may all have a place. Patients with vibration white finger should avoid vibrating tools.
- Sildenafil (Viagra) improves both microcirculation and symptoms in patients with secondary Raynaud's phenomenon, resistant to vasodilatory therapy.

FROSTBITE

- Frostbite occurs with exposure of tissues to subfreezing temperatures for a period of several hours.
- Short-term exposure to sub-zero temperatures, results in a different form of frostbite, commonly occurring in airplanes at high altitudes and characterized by the term "high-altitude" frostbite.
- It has been demonstrated experimentally that cold-induced injury to mammalian tissues begins when the tissue temperature reaches 10°C. At 5°C, cells lose the ability to recover from the freezing process.
- The pathophysiologic features of frostbite depend on the degree of cold-induced injury. Initially, vasoconstriction occurs on exposure to the cold. The histologic findings in mild frostbite consist of a low-grade vasculitis.
- The process progresses to an intense inflammatory reaction of the intima with severe frostbite.
- The capillary endothelium becomes permeable and the resultant extravascular fluid accumulation produces soft-tissue edema.
- Thrombi form in the terminal arterioles and capillaries and irreversible tissue necrosis develops.
- It is not known, whether the fundamental cold injury occurs as a result of direct freezing with disruption of cell membranes or from ischemic necrosis, secondary to widespread thrombosis of the arterioles and capillaries.

Classification of Frostbite

- First degree injury, consists of edema and redness without necrosis.
- In second degree injury, blistering becomes evident.
- Third degree injury constitutes of necrosis of skin.
- Fourth degree injury; gangrene develops in fourth degree injury, necessitating amputation of the affected extremity.
- A simpler categorization of frostbite divides injuries into superficial and deep classifications. Superficial frostbite involves the skin and superficial subcutaneous tissue, deep frostbite involves the deeper subcutaneous tissue, muscle, and even bone.

Treatment

- The treatment of frostbite begins with rapid warming of the injured tissue. The involved body part should be immersed in warm water with a temperature in the range of 40°–44°C.
- Complete rewarming generally requires about 20 minutes. Once warm, the injured extremity should be elevated to minimize the formation of edema and antibiotics with antitetanus therapy are instituted.
- The extent of gangrene is difficult to assess early in the course of frostbite. The degree of irreversible injury is often much less than initially feared because the skin may be involved to a much greater extent than the subcutaneous tissue.
- For this reason, amputation should be delayed for several weeks, until the precise extent of gangrene can be accurately determined.
- If the injury is severe enough to produce tissue necrosis, operative sympathectomy should be performed within the first few days.
- Sympathectomy is also useful in alleviating the late sequelae of cold injury, including hyperhidrosis, cold sensitivity, and pain.

PERIPHERAL VENOUS DISEASE

Venous Incompetence (Varicose Veins)

One of the most common problems with the veins of the leg is failure of their valves. This occurs frequently in the superficial venous system, resulting in varicose veins (Fig. 26).

Incidence

In developing countries, where a primitive way of life is maintained, there is a very low incidence of varicose veins. The reasons for this difference are unclear, but are probably related to differences in diet.

Causative Factors

- It is common in people, who have long standing jobs.
- *A further major factor is inheritance:* Women in whom neither parent has varicose veins, have a 10% risk of developing varices, but when both parents are affected, there is an 80% chance. Men are affected less frequently than women.

Mechanism (Figs. 27A and B)

- The mechanisms that cause the superficial vein valves to fail have not been fully established. What appears to happen, is that first a small gap appears between the valve cusps at the commissure.

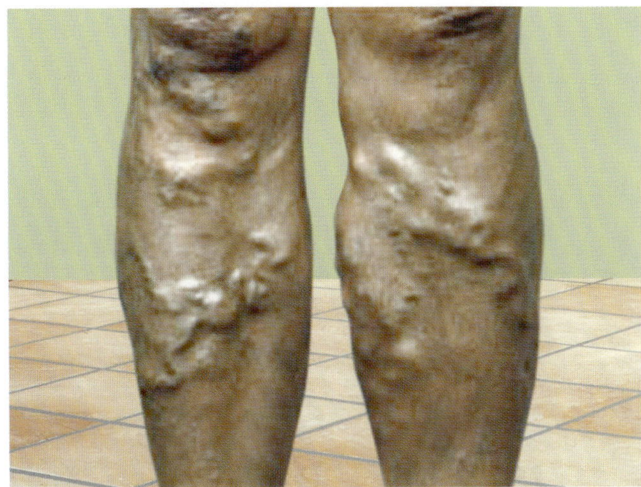

Fig. 26: Varicose veins.

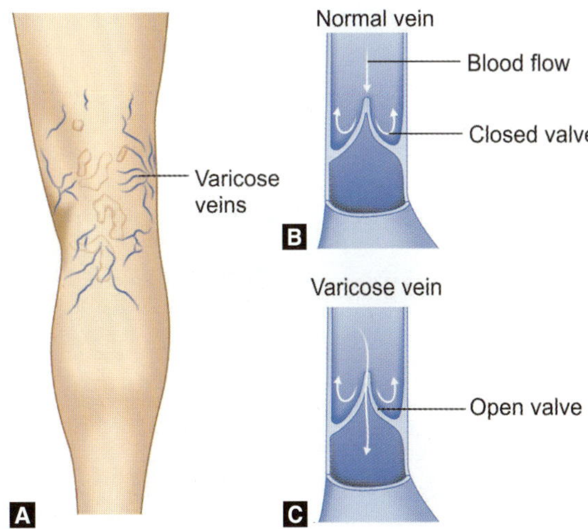

Figs. 28A to C: Diagrammatic comparison of normal vein and varicose vein.

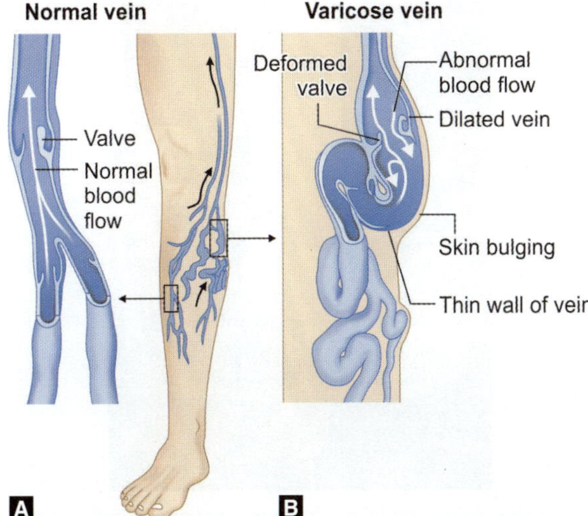

Figs. 27A and B: Mechanism causing varicose veins.

- This gap widens and more reverse flow (venous reflux) is allowed. The valve cusps degenerate and holes develop in them. Eventually, they disappear completely. The vein below the valve responds by dilating.
- Varicose veins are thought to develop more often in people, who stand during their work. People who sit or walk are at less risk of developing varices.
- They often develop during pregnancy, under the influence of estrogen and progesterone, which cause the smooth muscles in the vein wall to relax.

Clinical Features

- Varices are recognized as tortuous dilated veins in the leg, but physiologically speaking a varicose vein is one, which permits reverse flow through its faulty valves (Figs. 28A to C).
- Varices of the major tributaries of the saphenous veins or the saphenous veins themselves are large (5–15 mm diameter) and usually start in the calf. Later varices of the long saphenous system may also appear in the thigh.
- Patients may develop much smaller varices. These range from 0.5 mm to 2 mm diameter vessels in the skin, which are commonly referred to as thread veins.
- Slightly larger veins (1–3 mm diameter), lying immediately beneath the skin may also be present as small varicosities. These are usually referred to as reticular varices.
- Patients may also report aching, especially on standing, itching, "restless legs", and ankle swelling. The severity of the symptoms is unrelated to the size of the veins, and is often more severe during the early stages of development of varices.

Complications

- Thrombosis, referred to as superficial thrombophlebitis
- Spectacular hemorrhage can occur, when large superficial varices are damaged
- The most serious problem is venous ulceration, which complicates varicose veins in less than 5% of patients.

Venous Incompetence (Deep Vein Incompetence)

Valvular incompetence of the deep veins may develop in the same way as in the superficial venous system, with the degeneration of the valve cusps, resulting in reverse flow in these veins. In other patients, it may develop following a deep vein thrombosis.

Clinical Features

- In patients with venous valvular incompetence, the calf muscle increases in size, apparently in response to the greater work in returning blood from the leg.
- Ankle edema.
- Skin complications, like eczema to severe ulceration.
- An early sign of skin injury is brown pigmentation, due to hemosiderin deposition in the skin.
- A later and more serious stage is lipodermatosclerosis, in which palpable induration develops in the skin and subcutaneous tissues. This particularly affects the greater area of the leg, just above the malleoli and may be the precursor of leg ulceration.
- Contraction of the skin and subcutaneous tissues is seen and the ankle becomes narrower. The combination of a narrow ankle and prominent calf is often referred to as a (Fig. 29) "Champagne bottle leg".
- *Ambulatory venous hypertension:* Incompetence of the deep veins usually has a more severe effect on the venous physiology than the superficial venous incompetence, as the deep veins

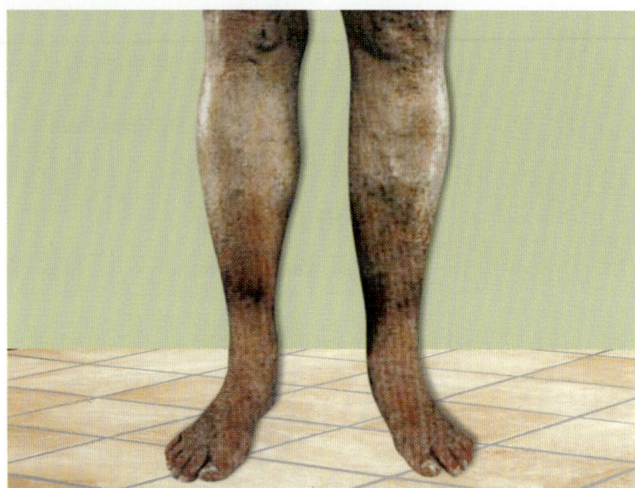

Fig. 29: Champagne bottle legs, seen in venous incompetence.

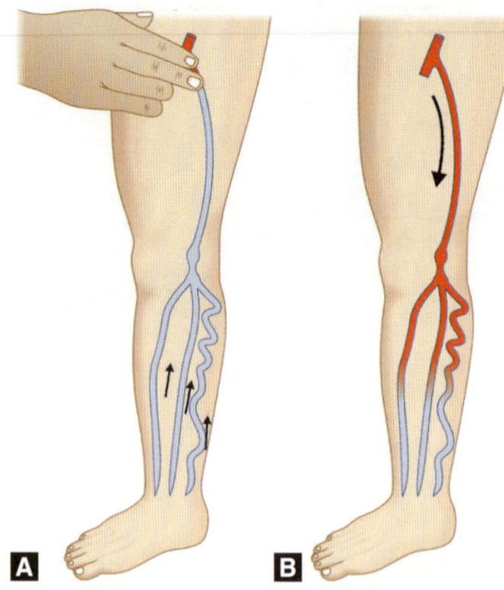

Figs. 30A and B: Tourniquet test, done for checking venous sufficiencies.

are much larger than the superficial veins. The effect of reverse flow in the deep or superficial veins is to prevent the superficial venous pressure from falling during exercise. This is referred to as ambulatory venous hypertension and is the main cause of venous leg ulceration.

- Persistently raised venous pressure tracks back to the microcirculation of the skin and causes skin damage that eventually may result in venous ulceration.

Investigation of Venous Disease

A full history should always be taken, enquiring about any injury to the leg or swelling, which may suggest a previous episode of deep vein thrombosis.

Clinical Symptoms

- These include tiredness, aching, tingling, and ankle swelling, which get progressively worse toward the end of the day and are relieved by elevating the leg.
- Sometimes patients report cramps in the legs, which are usually worse at night.
- Patients with severe deep vein obstruction may also develop bursting pain in the calf on walking, due to the very high venous pressures that may occur under these conditions.
- *Venous refilling:* The limb should be elevated for 30 seconds and then laid flat on the bed. Normal refilling occurs within seconds. Reduced venous filling is often present in the severer forms of arterial insufficiency.
- *Harvey's sign:* If the two index fingers are placed firmly, side by side on a vein and the finger nearer the heart is moved, so as to empty a short length of vein, the release of the distal finger will allow the speed of venous refilling to be observed. Increased venous return and varicosities of veins are associated with arteriovenous fistulas.
- *Tourniquet test (Figs. 30A and B):* The patient lies and the leg is elevated to empty the veins. The tourniquet is applied high on the thigh and the patient stands again. The speed at which the varices fill is observed. In the case of varices from the long saphenous vein, these fill within a few seconds without a tourniquet, but with the trunk of the long saphenous vein compressed in the thigh, much slower filling takes place over 15–20 seconds. The tourniquet is often replaced by the hand of the examiner, used to compress the long or short saphenous vein.

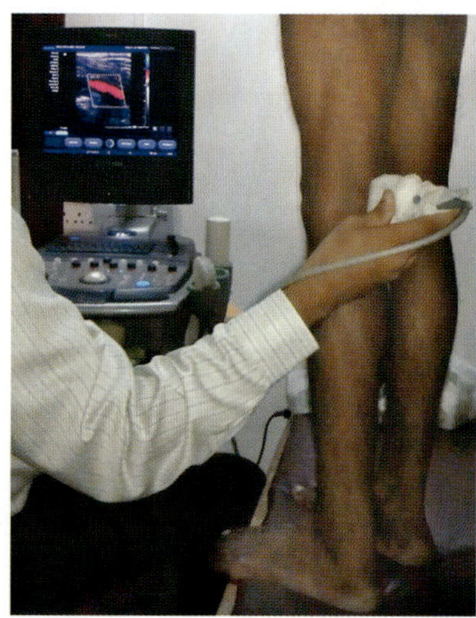

Fig. 31: Doppler ultrasound taken, for checking venous sufficiency.

Other Investigations

- Doppler ultrasound (Fig. 31)
- Duplex ultrasound imaging (Fig. 32)
- Venography (Fig. 33).

Management

- Elevating the legs often provides temporary symptomatic relief.
- *Compression stockings:* The wearing of graduated compression stockings, with a pressure of 30–40 mm Hg has been shown to correct the swelling, nutritional exchange, and improve the microcirculation in legs, affected by varicose veins (Fig. 34).
- Avoid prolonged standing.
- *Injection sclerotherapy (Fig. 35):* Injection sclerotherapy is best used in the management of small varices and those where the main long and short saphenous veins and their major tributaries are competent. This type of treatment is also effective, where the larger varices have been removed surgically and only small varices remain.
- The basis of sclerotherapy is that a solution which destroys the endothelial lining of the veins is injected.

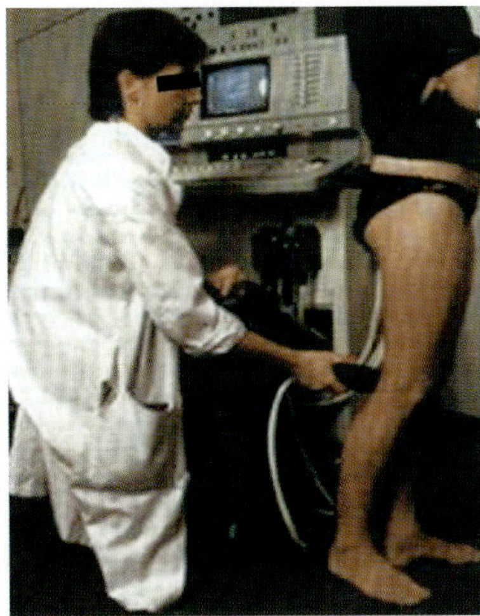

Fig. 32: Duplex ultrasound imaging.

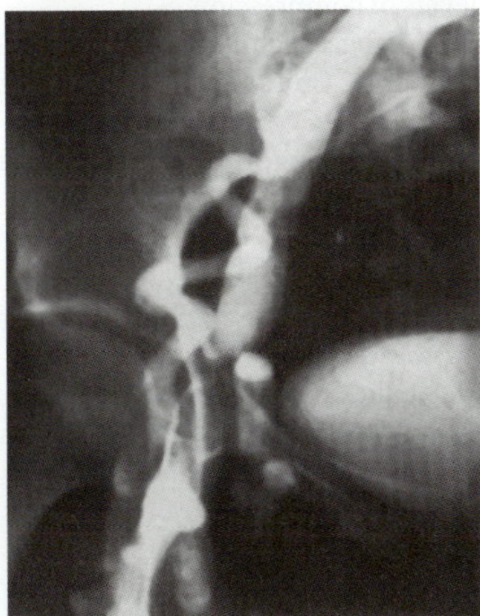

Fig. 33: Venograph, showing diseased veins.

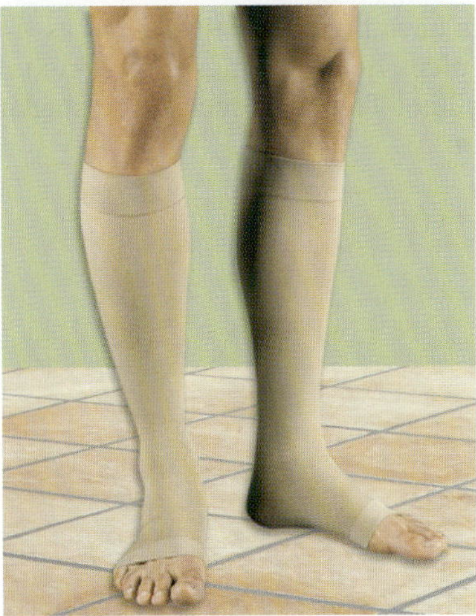

Fig. 34: Compression stockings.

- In UK, the most widely employed drug is sodium tetradecyl (STD), which is chemically a soap.
- To be effective, the sclerosant has to be given into an empty vein that is compressed immediately after the injection has been given, to avoid the development of thrombosis within the vein.

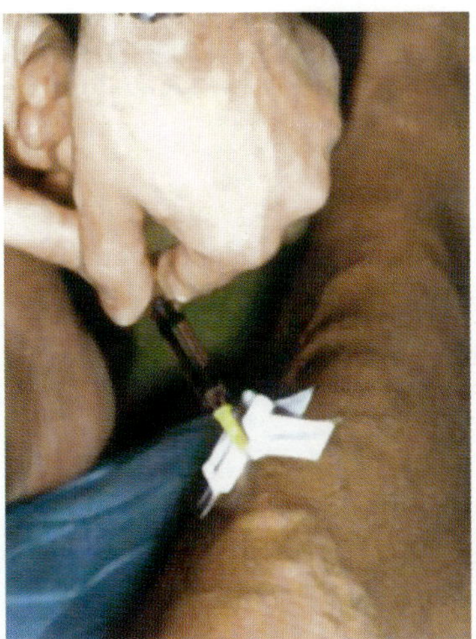

Fig. 35: Injection sclerotherapy.

The complications of this treatment include skin pigmentation and ulceration, if the sclerosant is not injected within a vein.

Surgical treatment of varicose veins:

- The main principles of surgical treatment are to ligate the source of the venous reflux, usually the saphenous femoral junction (SFJ), or the saphenous popliteal junction (SPJ), and to remove the incompetent saphenous trunks and the associated varices.
- Saphenofemoral ligation alone, sometimes referred to as a Trendelenburg procedure, is associated with a high rate of recurrence of varices.
- Recent research has shown that it is necessary to remove the long saphenous vein, to ensure that as much venous reflux as possible is eliminated.
- Similarly, communications between the many deep veins in the popliteal fossa and the short saphenous vein means that some patients develop recurrences in the short saphenous vein, due to the re-establishment of reflux from these veins. This problem may be eliminated by removing the short saphenous vein.
- Complications of varicose vein surgery, include:
  - Sensory nerve injury
  - Motor nerve injury
  - Deep vein thrombosis.
- *Recurrence:* In recurrence, venous reconstructive surgery can be considered.

Leg Ulcers

The most common cause of leg ulceration in western countries is venous disease of the lower limb. However, many patients have other causes for their leg ulcer. Some common causes of leg ulcers are listed in Box 1.

Examination and Investigation

- Venous ulcers usually lie just proximal to the medial or lateral malleolus, although they may extend to the ankle and dorsum of the foot (Fig. 36).
- Venous ulcers are accompanied by lipodermatosclerosis and hemosiderosis. The presence of obvious varicose veins should be recorded, although these are often not present or not visible in patients with venous ulcers.
- The peripheral pulses should be palpated to assess the peripheral arteries.

Box 1: Common causes of leg ulcers.

- Venous disease of the lower limb
- Peripheral arterial disease
- Diabetes
- Neuropathy
- Rheumatoid disease
- Autoimmune disease (systemic sclerosis, systemic lupus erythematosus)
- Trauma
- Malignant ulcers (basal cell carcinoma, squamous cell carcinoma, malignant melanoma)
- Infective

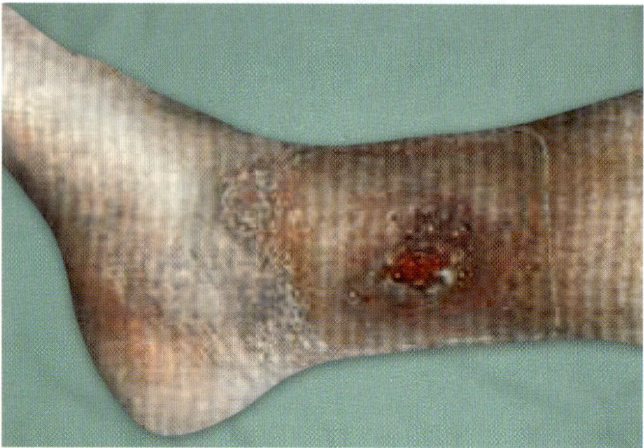

Fig. 36: Venous ulcers.

- The presence of loss of sensation in the foot or area of ulceration should be assessed, especially in a diabetic patient. Diabetic leg ulceration usually affects the foot and is almost always associated with peripheral neuropathy.

Management of Venous Leg Ulcers

- In patients who have venous ulceration due to superficial venous incompetence alone, varicose vein surgery is effective in producing ulcer healing.
- The ulcer is covered by a dressing during surgery and prophylactic antibiotics are given, to prevent infection of the surgical wounds with any bacteria present in the ulcer.
- Ulcers managed in this way usually heal rapidly (within 4 weeks) following surgery.
- In patients with deep venous insufficiency or who are unfit or unwilling to undergo surgery, standard ulcer management should be used. The mainstay of this is local ulcer management combined with the application of compression. The ulcer is cleaned by soaking in tap water (the use of sterile water is unnecessary) and debriding the ulcer to remove any slough.
- The skin of the leg often becomes very scaly beneath compression dressings and should be treated with emulsifying ointment. Topical antibiotics are ineffective in healing leg ulcers and are particularly likely to produce skin sensitization. They should never be used in the management of venous ulceration.
- The most important factor in achieving healing is the use of high levels of compression. The use of dressings alone leads to a very slow rate of ulcer healing. It has been found that pressures of 30–45 mm Hg applied to the ulcer are much more effective than lower levels of compression.
- The best known of these techniques is the "four-layer bandage" developed at Charing Cross Hospital in London. This method achieves pressures of 45 mm Hg at the ankle and has been shown to produce healing of 70% of venous ulcers within 12 weeks.

Prevention of Recurrence

- Even when healing has been achieved, there is a risk that further ulcers may develop.
- Patients with healed ulcers should be encouraged to wear support stockings and rest with their feet elevated, whenever possible.
- Drug treatment for leg ulcers.
- No drugs have been found, which are more effective than compression bandaging in the management of venous leg ulceration.
- Antibiotics have no effect on ulcer healing, but are required if infection develops around an ulcer.
- A few drugs have been investigated, to assess their efficacy in venous ulcer healing. These have included aspirin, to pentoxyphylline (Trental, Hoechst), prostaglandin El analog, and diosmin.

CHAPTER

An Overview of Diabetes Mellitus 18

OBJECTIVES

- Types of Diabetes Mellitus
- Diagnosis
- Diabetic Foot
- Diabetic Ulcer

INTRODUCTION

- Diabetes mellitus comprises of a group of common metabolic disorders that share the phenotype of hyperglycemia.
- Several distinct types of diabetes exist and are caused by complex interaction of genetics, environmental factors, and lifestyle choices.
- Depending on the etiology of diabetes mellitus, factors contributing to hyperglycemia may include reduced insulin secretion, decreased glucose usage, and increased glucose production.
- Diabetes mellitus is the leading cause of nontraumatic lower extremity amputation in United States.
- Foot ulcers and infections are also a major source of morbidity in individuals with diabetes mellitus.
- The reasons for the increased incidence of these disorders in diabetes mellitus are complex and involve the interaction of several pathogenic factors, like neuropathy, abnormal foot biomechanics, peripheral vascular disease, and poor wound healing. The peripheral sensory neuropathy interferes with normal protective mechanisms and allows the patient to sustain major or repeated minor trauma to the foot, often without knowledge of the injury.
- Disordered proprioception causes abnormal weight bearing while walking and subsequent callus formation or ulceration.
- Motor or sensory neuropathy leads to abnormal foot mechanics and structural changes in the foot (hammer toe, claw toe deformity, prominent metatarsal heads, etc.)
- Autonomic neuropathy results in anhidrosis and altered superficial blood flow in the foot, which promotes drying of the skin and fissure formation.
- Peripheral vascular disease and poor wound healing impede resolution of minor breaks in the skin, allowing them to enlarge and to become infected.
- Approximately 15% of individuals with diabetes mellitus develop foot ulcer and a significant number of these individuals will sometimes undergo foot amputation.
- Risk factors for foot ulcers or amputation include:
  - Male sex
  - Diabetes more than 10 years duration
  - Peripheral neuropathy
  - Abnormal structure of foot (bony abnormalities, callus, thickened nails)
  - Peripheral vascular disease
  - Smoking
  - History of previous ulcer or amputation
  - Glycemic control is also a risk factor, each 2% increase in the HbA1c increases the risk of a lower extremity ulcer by 1.6 times and the risk of lower extremity amputation by 1.5 times.

TYPES OF DIABETES MELLITUS

Two broad categories of diabetes mellitus are—type I and type II.

Type I

- Type IA results from autoimmune beta cell destruction, which usually leads to insulin deficiency.
- Type IB diabetes mellitus is also characterized by insulin deficiency as well as tendency to develop ketosis, however, immunologic markers indicative of an autoimmune destructive process of beta cells are absent.

Type II

It is a heterogeneous group of disorders, usually characterized by variable degrees of insulin resistance, impaired insulin secretion, and increased glucose production.

DIAGNOSIS

Revised criteria for diagnosing diabetes mellitus have been issued by panel of experts from National Diabetes Data Group and World Health Organization. These are:

- Either symptoms of diabetes plus random blood glucose concentration greater than 200 mg%
- Fasting plasma glucose greater than 126 mg% (fasting is defined as no caloric intake for 8 hours)
- Two hours plasma glucose greater than 200 mg%, during an oral glucose tolerance test
- Insulin resistance associated with obesity augments the genetically determined insulin resistance of type 2 diabetes mellitus. Adipocytes secrete a number of biologic products (leptin, tumor necrosis factor, free fatty acids, etc.) that contribute to insulin resistance.

DIABETIC FOOT

Introduction

- In the diabetic foot, ischemia and infection are serious and sometimes life-threatening conditions, however neuropathy is the most difficult condition to treat.
- Neuropathy, angiopathy, retinopathy, and nephropathy alone or in combination and in varying degrees of severity may influence the treatment of the diabetic foot.
- Neuropathy may be mild with minimal somatic sensory changes and no autonomic nervous system changes.
- In its severest form, total anesthesia from the midtibia distally (somatic loss) and complete absence of sweating (autonomic loss), result in a dry, scaly, swollen, clumsy limb that the patient dissociates from the rest of the body because of the loss of the sensory feedback.
- Vibratory and position senses are lost early and the patient does not know, where in space the foot is located at a given time. This is especially catastrophic, if the patient also cannot see the foot.
- Feet show most severe complications of diabetes, i.e. dry-scaly skin, swelling, and venous shunting from autosympathectomy.
- Deformity from neuropathic arthopathy in mid foot, with collapse of archon left foot with prominent bony protrusions medially and plantar ward and further deformity from amputation of left fourth toe.

DIABETIC ULCER

- Diabetic ulcers are most common in the fore foot, beneath one of the metatarsal heads or in the interphalangeal joint of the hallux (Figs. 1 and 2).
- If the ulcer is associated with fixed clawing of the toes as a result of intrinsic muscle paralysis of diabetic, somatic, or peripheral neuropathy, successful treatment is difficult.
- This is especially true if the ulcer is beneath the first metatarsal head (Fig. 3), where the sesamoid bones are beneath the skin.
- Patient with diabetes mellitus and neuropathy had severe claw toes and shear forces across plantar surface of first metatarsal head, causing recurrent ulceration (Fig. 3).
  In approximately 30% of the patients with diabetic fore foot, plantar ulcerations, atherosclerosis of the tibial and peroneal arteries contributes to the prolonged healing time.

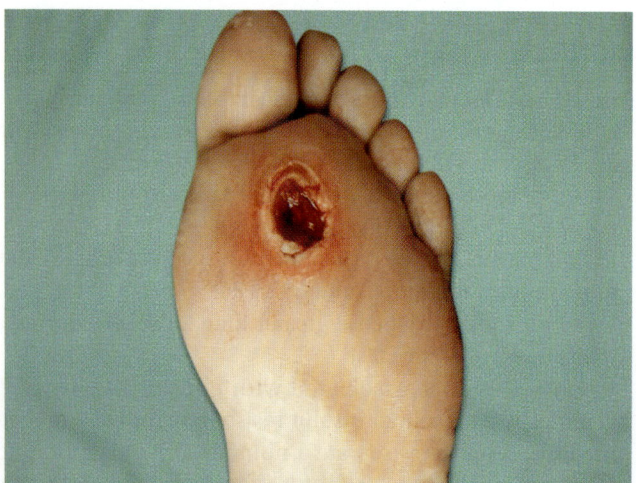

Fig. 1: Diabetic ulcer beneath metatarsal heads.

- Patient with diabetes had arteriosclerotic and neuropathic involvement of foot.
- Because of recurrent infections and deformities in multiple toes, patient had multiple toes on left amputated and transmetatarsal amputation on right with primary healing.
- You can also see the shoe box filler in right shoe and ulcerated claw toes that duplicate forerunners of previously amputated toes (Fig. 4).

Classification of Diabetic Ulcers and Diagnostic Aids

- Wagner developed a classification system for diabetic plantar ulcers and a treatment algorithm for each grade of ulcer.
- He asserted that the ischemic index derived from Doppler flow pressures is an essential baseline test, to predict ulcer healing and to predict healing of a limited foot amputation, if it becomes necessary.
- The ischemic index is the ratio of ankle to brachial pressure (Fig. 5). Normal condition on right side of the body with ankle systolic pressure equal to brachial systolic pressure.
- Ankle pressure divided by arm pressure determines ankle/arm index, in this case 1 (Fig. 5).
- On left side ankle/arm index is 0.6, indicating only 60% of expected normal flow at rest.

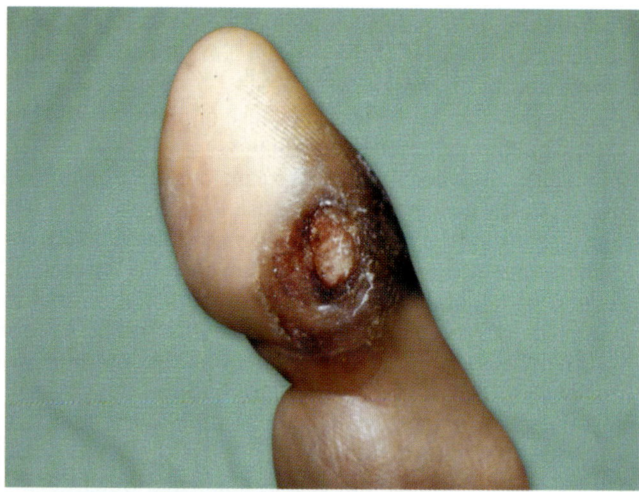

Fig. 2: Diabetic ulcer in the interphalangeal joint of the hallux.

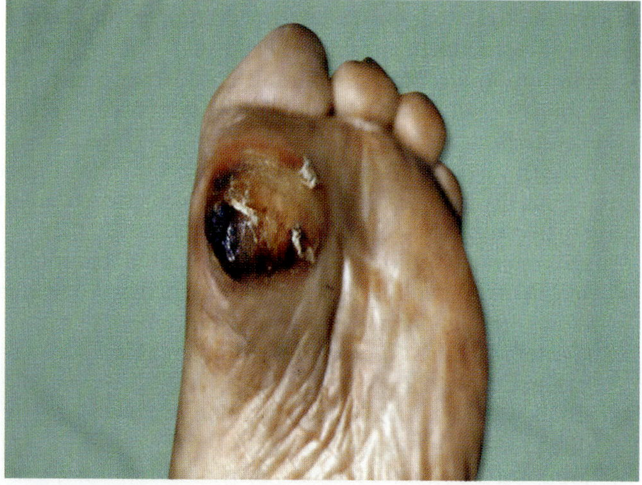

Fig. 3: Diabetic ulcer beneath first metatarsal heads and claw toes.

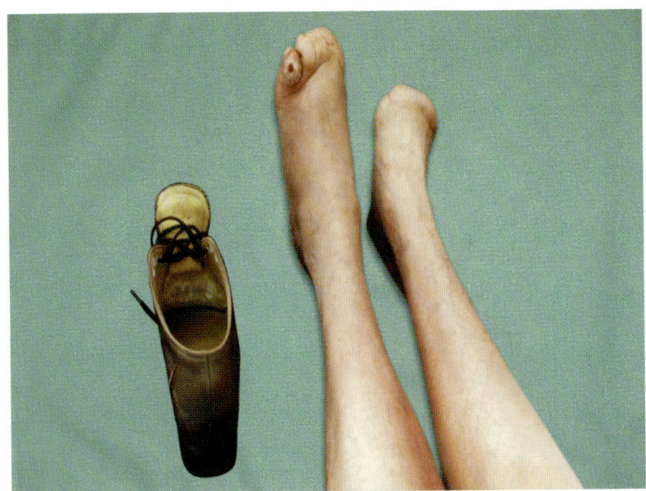

Fig. 4: Shoe box filler in right shoe and ulcerated claw toes that duplicate forerunners of previously amputated toes.

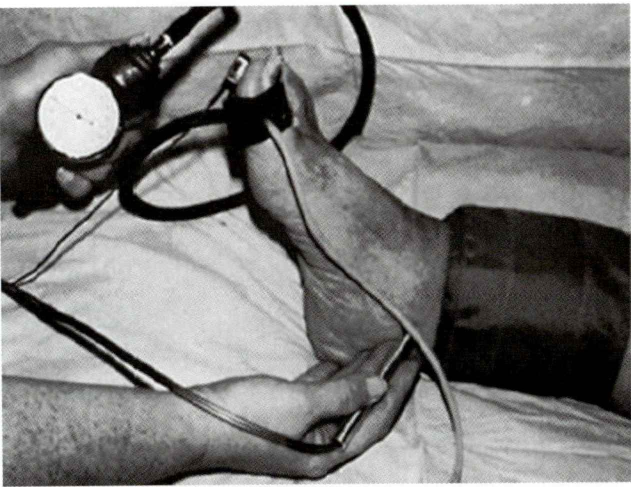

Fig. 6: Measurement of posterior tibial ankle pressure and great toe pressure is shown by using Doppler ultrasound device and photoplethysmography.

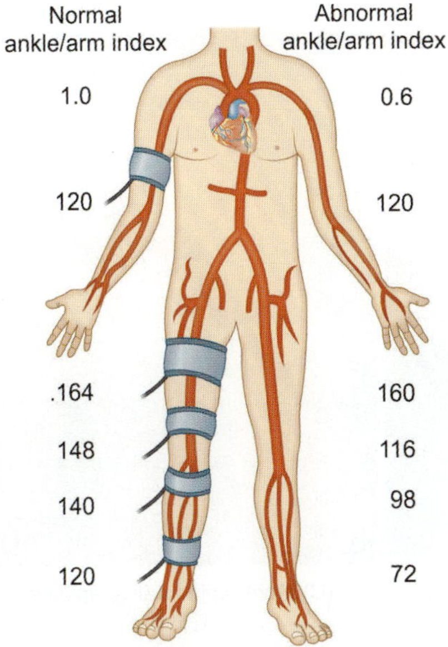

Fig. 5: Ischemic indices (both normal and abnormal for different areas) derived from Doppler flow pressures.

- In addition, any gradient greater than 30 mm Hg between two successive cuffs indicates high grade stenosis or occlusion.
- In this case, 44 mm Hg high gradient localizes diseased segment to superficial femoral artery.
- An ankle to brachial pressure ratio of 0.6, an absolute ankle pressure of 70 mm Hg or more, an absolute toe pressure of 40 mm Hg or more, and a transcutaneous oxygen measurement of 30 mm Hg or more are strong indicators that a limited foot amputation should heal.
- Measurement of posterior tibial ankle pressure and great toe pressure is shown using Doppler ultrasound device and photoplethysmography (Fig. 6).

Wagner Classification of Diabetic Ulcer

- *Grade 0:* Skin intact, but bony deformities produce a "foot at risk" (Fig. 7)
- *Grade 1:* Localized superficial ulcer (Figs. 8A and B)
- *Grade 2:* Deep ulcer to tendon, bone, ligament, or joint

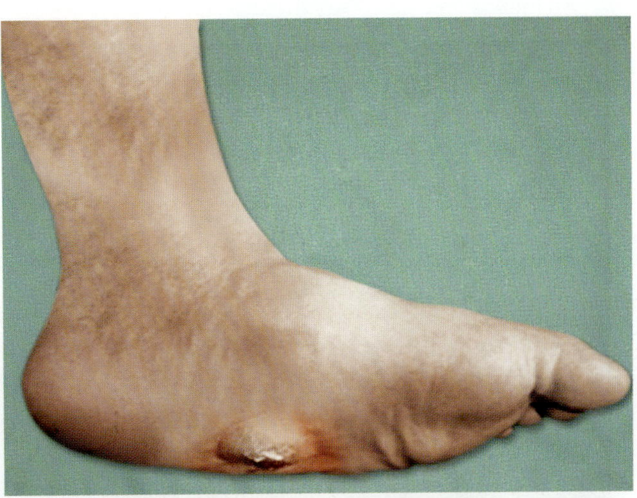

Fig. 7: Collapsed midfoot shown in the figure due to diabetic neuroarthropathy and preulcerative lesion.

- Metatarsophalangeal joint can be dislocated, plantar plate disrupted, and bone with tendon is exposed (Figs. 9A to C)
- *Grade 3:* Deep abscess, osteomyelitis. Diabetic abscess is shown in Figures 10A and B
- *Grade 4:* Gangrene of toes or forefoot (Fig. 11)
- *Grade 5:* Gangrene of entire foot
- The purpose of this classification is to clarify the prognosis and treatment plan
- In caring for an ulcerated diabetic foot, it is necessary to determine, if the ulcer is primarily neurotrophic or ischemic. If the ulcer is localized or has a deep abscess with multiple tissue plane involvement and if osteomyelitis or pyarthrosisis present, it would allow a reasonable treatment plan.

Brodsky's Classification of Diabetic Ulcer

This does not include gangrene:

- *Grade 0:* Intact skin, but represents a preulcerative lesion with erythema, call us formation, and intradermal hemorrhage over a bony prominence.
- *Grade 1:* It is a superficial, but full thickness skin ulcer down but not through the subcutaneous tissue.

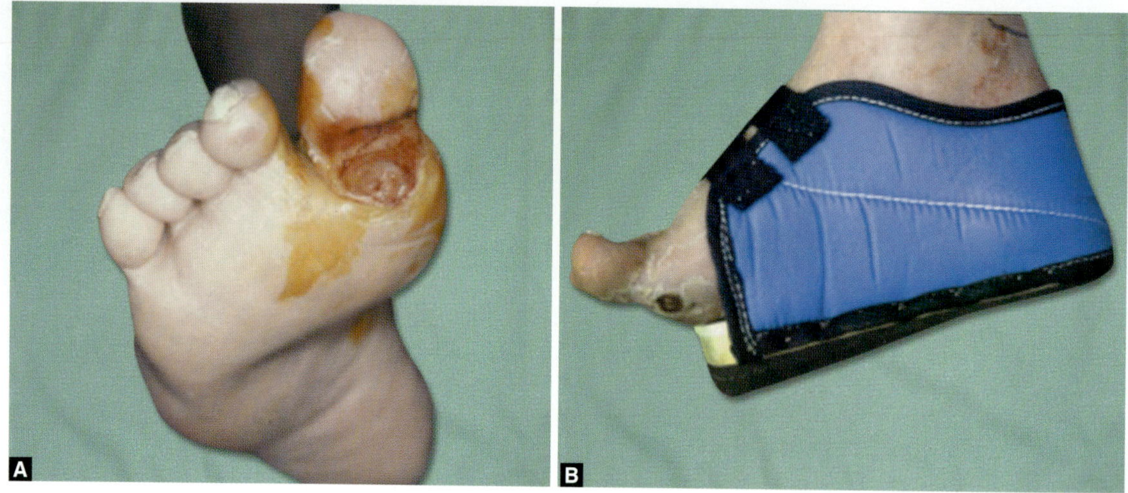

Figs. 8A and B: (A) Localized superficial ulcer treated in cut-off postoperative shoe; (B) Six weeks in shoe.

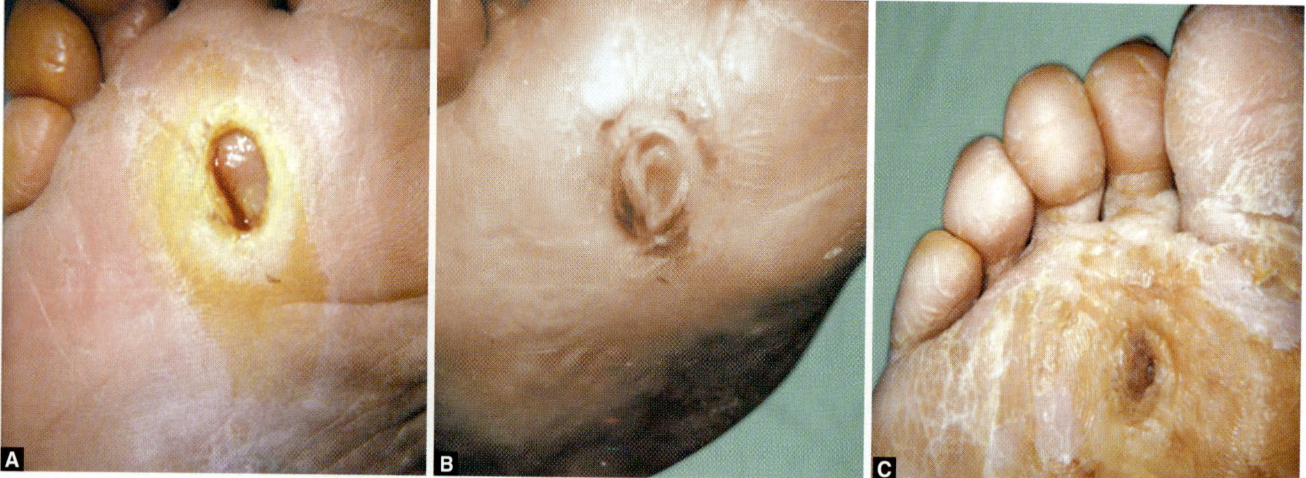

Figs. 9A to C: (A) Fibrinous bed to deep ulcer over metatarsal head; (B) Shows ulcer has started healing; (C) More rapid healing ensues in occlusive cast.

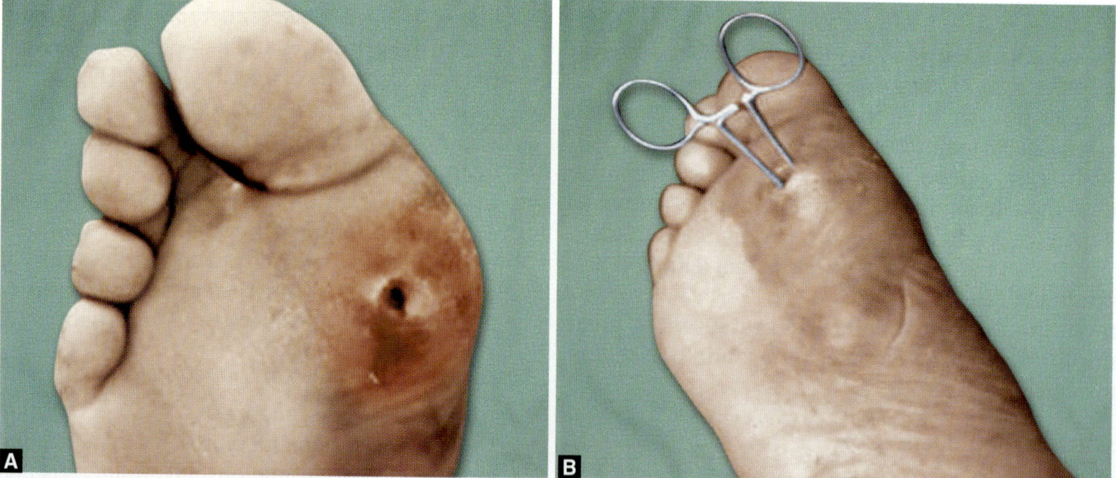

Figs. 10A and B: Diabetic abscess—(A) Note discoloration proximal to abscess beneath first metatarsal head; (B) Picture showing depth of abscess.

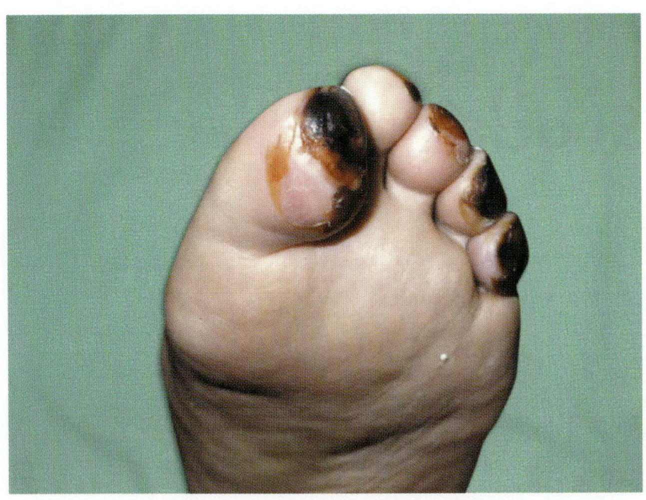

Fig. 11: Gangrene of toes due to diabetes.

- *Grade 2:* Ulceration is down to the tendon and joint capsule, but neither the joint nor the bone is visible.
- *Grade 3:* Ulceration implies exposed bone or joint and osteomyelitis orpyarthrosis.
- The ulcerated foot, with no palpable pedal pulses needs at least Doppler pressures.
- The ischemic index is helpful.
- In general, an occlusive cast is not used, if no pedal pulses are present.
- Occasionally in limbs, unsuitable for vascular reconstruction with reliable ischemic index of 0.6 or greater and wound margins that bleed when debrided, an occlusive cast can be used. The risk of loss of avascularity deficient foot in an occlusive cast must be weighed against the risk of leaving the ulcer.
- Treatment with hyperbaric oxygen may help to heal an ischemic ulcer.

Neuropathic Ulcer

- If the ulcer is primarily neurotrophic, local debridement, and occlusive casts are helpful.
- Removal of bony prominences followed by casting may be required.
- Any localized fore foot ulcer, 3 cm or less in diameter with good pedal pulses, can be treated inocclusive healing cast.
- Even osteomyelitis, if localized to a small area of bone adjacent to the ulcer, can be treated by cast technique.
- Many off-the-shelf products are available to unload the diabetic foot.
- Total contact casts have been shown to be more effective in healing ulcers and in a shorter time than these products.
- The key is localized ulceration with good vascularity.

CHAPTER

19 Shock

OBJECTIVES

- Types
- Pathophysiology
- Different Stages of Shock
- Signs and Symptoms
- Signs of Severity
- Treatment
- Complications
- Prognosis

INTRODUCTION

Definition

Shock is a serious, life-threatening medical condition, characterized by a decrease in tissue perfusion to a point, at which it is inadequate to meet cellular metabolic needs.

TYPES

Hinshaw and Cox Classification

In 1972, Hinshaw and Cox suggested the following classification, which is still used today.

It names four types of shock; these are enumerated below:

1. Hypovolemic shock
2. Cardiogenic shock
3. Distributive shock
4. Obstructive shock.

In many patients, shock is a combination of two or more of these four types of shock.

Hypovolemic Shock

- This is the most common type of shock and based on insufficient circulating volume.
- Primary cause is loss of fluid from the circulation (most often "hemorrhagic shock").

Causes

- Blood loss following trauma (intra-abdominal, intra-thoracic)
- Blood loss during surgery
- Burns
- Dehydration (vomiting and diarrhea).

Cardiogenic Shock

- This type of shock is caused by the failure of the heart to pump effectively.
- This can be due to damage to the heart muscle, most often from a large myocardial infarction.
- Other causes of cardiogenic shock include:
  - Arrhythmias
  - Cardiomyopathy
  - Congestive heart failure
  - Commotio cordis
  - Cardiac valve defects.

Distributive Shock

- There is an insufficient intravascular volume of blood.
- This form of "relative" hypovolemia is the result of dilation of blood vessels, which diminishes systemic vascular resistance.
- Examples of this form of shock are:
  - Septic shock
  - Anaphylactic shock
  - Neurogenic shock.

Septic Shock

- It is caused by an overwhelming systemic infection, resulting in vasodilation leading to hypotension.
- Two stages are recognized:
  1. Hyperdynamic (warm) septic shock
  2. Hypovolemic hypodynamic (cold) septic shock.

Hyperdynamic septic shock

- This occurs in patients with serious Gram-negative infections.
- In this stage, patient has increased cardiac output, with tachycardia and warm dry skin.
- The tissue cells get damaged, by anaerobic metabolism (lactic acidosis).
- The capillary membranes start to leak and endotoxins enter the bloodstream leading to generalized inflammatory state.

Hypovolemic hypodynamic septic shock

- This stage follows if severe endotoxemia or sepsis is allowed to persist.
- Generalized capillary leakage and fluid loss lead to severe hypovolemia, with reduced cardiac output, tachycardia, and vasoconstriction.
- The systemic infection induces cardiac depression, pulmonary hypertension, pulmonary edema, and hypoxia, which in turn reduces cardiac output further.

Anaphylactic Shock

It is caused by a severe anaphylactic reaction to an allergen, antigen, drug or foreign protein, causing the release of histamine, which causes widespread vasodilation, leading to hypotension, and increased capillary permeability.

Neurogenic Shock

- Neurogenic shock is the rarest form of shock. It is caused by trauma to the spinal cord, resulting in the sudden loss of autonomic and motor reflexes below the injury level.
- Without stimulation by sympathetic nervous system, the vessel walls relax uncontrollably, resulting in a sudden decrease in peripheral vascular resistance, leading to vasodilation and hypotension.
- This term can be confused with spinal shock, which is a recoverable loss of function of the spinal cord after injury and does not refer to the hemodynamic instability.

Obstructive Shock

- In this situation, the flow of blood is obstructed, which impedes circulation and can result in circulatory arrest. Several conditions result in this form of shock, e.g. cardiac tamponade, tension pneumothorax, pulmonary embolism, aortic stenosis, etc.
- *Cardiac tamponade:* In this, fluid in the pericardium prevents inflow of blood into the heart (venous return). Constrictive pericarditis, in which the pericardium shrinks and hardens, is similar in presentation.
- *Tension pneumothorax:* Due to increased intrathoracic pressure, blood flow to the heart is prevented (venous return).
- *Massive pulmonary embolism:* It is the result of a thromboembolic incident in the blood vessels of the lungs and hinders the return of blood to the heart.
- *Aortic stenosis:* Hinders circulation by obstructing the ventricular outflow tract.

Transient Shock

- Transitory, i.e. lasts for few seconds to minutes.
- Characterized by loss of consciousness, weakness, and sinking sensation.
- On examination, rapid pulse, low blood pressure, and clammy extremities are observed.
- Occurs as a result of sudden reduction of venous return, with peripheral pooling of blood, leading to decreased cardiac output.
- Rapidly followed by compensation with regulation of blood pressure.
- Causes include—trauma, severe pain, and emotional overexertion.

PATHOPHYSIOLOGY

Flowchart 1 shows pathophysiology of shock.

DIFFERENT STAGES OF SHOCK

There are four stages of shock. As it is a complex and continuous condition, there is no sudden transition from one stage to the next.

- *Stage 1:* Initial
- *Stage 2:* Compensatory (Compensating)
- *Stage 3:* Progressive (Decompensating)
- *Stage 4:* Refractory (Irreversible).

Flowchart 1: Pathophysiology of shock.

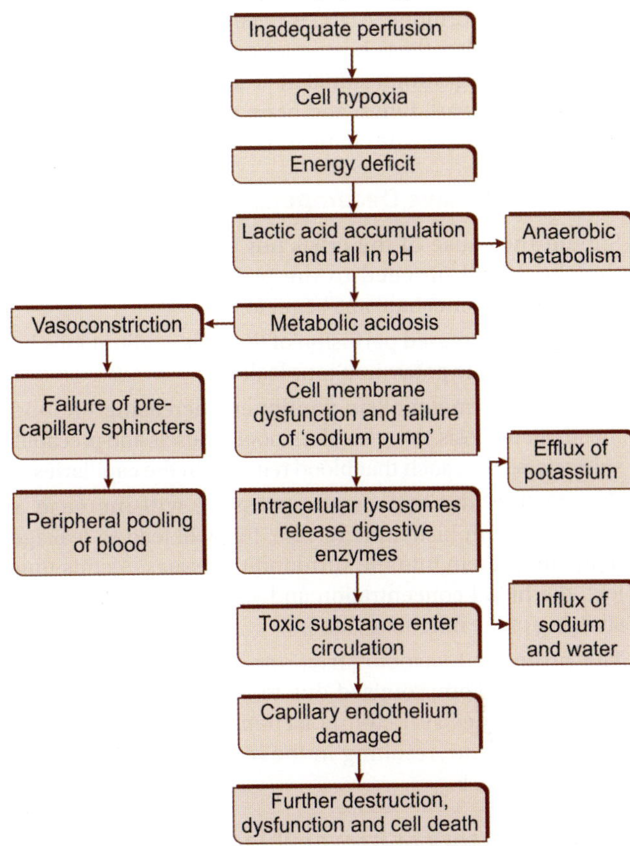

Stage 1: Initial Stage

- During this stage, the hypoperfusional state causes hypoxia, leading to the mitochondria being unable to produce adenosine triphosphate (ATP).
- Due to this lack of oxygen, the cell membranes become damaged, they become leaky to extracellular fluid and the cells perform anaerobic respiration.
- This causes a build-up of lactic and pyruvic acid, which results in systemic metabolic acidosis.
- The process of removing these compounds from the cells, by the liver requires oxygen, which is absent.

Stage 2: Compensatory Stage

- This stage is characterized by the body employing physiological mechanisms, including neural, hormonal, and biochemical mechanisms in an attempt to reverse the condition.
- As a result of the acidosis, the person will begin to hyperventilate, in order to rid the body of carbon dioxide (CO_2). CO_2 indirectly acts to acidify the blood and by removing it, the body is attempting to raise the pH of the blood.
- The baroreceptors in the arteries detect the resulting hypotension and cause the release of adrenaline and noradrenaline.
- Noradrenaline causes predominately vasoconstriction with a mild increase in heart rate, whereas adrenaline predominately causes an increase in heart rate with a small effect on the vascular tone. The combined effect results in an increase in blood pressure. This is known as Cushing's reflex and its triad is the subjective identifying characteristic of this stage.

- Renin-angiotensin axis is activated and arginine vasopressin (antidiuretic hormone, ADH) is released to conserve fluid via the kidneys. Also, these hormones cause the vasoconstriction of the kidneys, gastrointestinal tract and other organs, to divert blood to the heart, lungs, and brain. The lack of blood to the renal system causes the characteristic low urine production.

Stage 3: Progressive Decompensating

- Should the cause of the crisis not be successfully treated, the shock will proceed to the progressive stage and the compensatory mechanisms begin to fail.
- Due to the decreased perfusion of the cells, sodium ions build up within, while potassium ions leak out.
- As anaerobic metabolism continues, increasing the body's metabolic acidosis, the arteriolar smooth muscle and precapillary sphincters relax, such that blood remains in the capillaries.
- Due to this, the hydrostatic pressure will increase and combined with histamine release, this will lead to leakage of fluid and protein into the surrounding tissues. As this fluid is lost, the blood concentration and viscosity increase, causing sludging of the microcirculation.
- The prolonged vasoconstriction will also cause the vital organs to be compromised due to reduced perfusion. If the bowel becomes sufficiently ischemic, bacteria may enter the bloodstream, resulting in the increased complication of endotoxic shock.

Stage 4: Refractory or Irreversible

At this stage, the vital organs have failed and the shock can no longer be reversed. Brain damage and cell death have occurred. Death will occur immediately.

SIGNS AND SYMPTOMS

- The essential signs of shock are seen as tachycardia/tachypnea (compensatory mechanisms), hypotension, and signs of poor end-organ perfusion (such as low urine output, confusion, or loss of consciousness, or failure to compensate).
- Other signs should be looked for, to establish the underlying cause for the shock to guide effective treatment.

SIGNS OF SEVERITY

The severity of shock can be graded 1 to 4, based on the physical signs. This approximates to the effective loss of blood volume. The blood volume does not have to actually be lost from the circulation, as an expansion in the volume of the circulatory system (e.g. in septic shock) will render the patient proportionally hypovolemic.

Grade I

- Up to about 15% loss of effective blood volume (~750 mL in an average adult, who is assumed to have a blood volume of 5 liters).
- This leads to a mild resting tachycardia and can be well tolerated in otherwise healthy individuals. In the elderly or those with underlying conditions, such as ischemic heart disease the additional myocardial oxygen demands may not be tolerated so well.

Grade II

Between 15% and 30% loss of blood volume (750–1,500 mL) will provoke a moderate tachycardia and begin to narrow the pulse pressure. The time taken for the capillaries to refill after 5 seconds of pressure (capillary refill time) will be extended.

Grade III

At 30–40% loss of effective blood volume (1,500–2,000 mL) the compensatory mechanisms begin to fail and hypotension, tachycardia, and low urine output (less than 0.5 mL/kg/hr in adults) are seen.

Grade IV

At 40–50% loss of blood volume (2,000–2,500 mL) profound hypotension will develop and if prolonged, will cause end-organ damage and death.

Signs Relating to Different Causes

Hypovolemic Shock

- Anxiety, restlessness, and altered mental state due to decreased cerebral perfusion and subsequent hypoxia
- Hypotension due to decrease in circulatory volume
- A rapid, thready pulse due to decreased blood flow combined with tachycardia
- Rapid and shallow respirations due to sympathetic nervous system stimulation and acidosis
- Hypothermia due to decreased perfusion and evaporation of sweat
- Thirst and dry mouth due to fluid depletion
- Fatigue due to inadequate oxygenation
- Cold and mottled skin (cutis marmorata), especially extremities, due to insufficient perfusion of the skin
- Distracted look in the eyes or staring into space, often with pupils dilated.

Cardiogenic Shock

- Similar to hypovolemic shock, but in addition, distended jugular veins due to increased jugular venous pressure.
- Weak or absent pulse.
- Arrhythmia, often tachycardic.

Obstructive Shock

- Similar to hypovolemic shock but in addition shows other clinical features, like distended jugular veins, due to increased jugular venous pressure.
- Pulsus paradoxus, in case of tamponade.

Septic Shock

- Similar to hypovolemic shock except, pyrexia due to increased level of cytokines.
- Hypotension, due to systemic vasodilatation.
- Warm and sweaty skin, due to vasodilatation.

Neurogenic Shock

- As with hypovolemic shock, but in high spinal injuries may also be accompanied by other signs and symptoms, like profound bradycardia, due to loss of the cardiac accelerating nerve fibers from the sympathetic nervous system at T1-T4.

- The skin is warm and dry or a clear sweat line exists, above which the skin is diaphoretic.
- Priapism, due to peripheral nervous system stimulation.

Anaphylactic Shock

- Skin eruptions and large welts.
- Localized edema, especially around the face.
- Weak and rapid pulse.
- Breathlessness and cough, due to narrowing of airways and swelling of the throat.

TREATMENT

- Shock requires immediate interventions to preserve life. Therefore, the early recognition and treatment is essential, even before a specific diagnosis is made.
- As a general rule, you should treat for a sustained wound and shock.
- Most forms of shock seen in trauma or sepsis respond initially to aggressive intravenous fluids (e.g. 1 liter normal saline bolus, over 10 minutes or 20 mL/kg in a child). Therefore, this treatment is usually instituted as the person is being further evaluated.
- Re-establishing perfusion to the organs is the primary goal, by restoring and maintaining the blood circulating volume ensuring oxygenation and blood pressure are adequate, achieving and maintaining effective cardiac function, and preventing complications.
- Patients attending with the symptoms of shock should have, regardless of the type of shock, their airway managed and oxygen therapy initiated. In case of respiratory insufficiency (i.e. diminished levels of consciousness, hyperventilation due to acid-base disturbances or pneumonia) intubation and mechanical ventilation may be necessary.

Treatment (Hypovolemic Shock)

- Limbs should be freed from any tight clothing.
- Head in low position, with foot end elevation.
- Maintenance of airway. This can be done by:
  - Removing any debris from mouth
  - Suction
  - Endotracheal intubation, if patient is unconscious.
- Maintaining breathing.
- After monitoring respiratory rate, administration of 100% O_2, if there is any sign of respiratory failure (cyanosis, pallor, etc.).
- Endotracheal intubation with assisted ventilation, if necessary.
- Tracheostomy.
- Maintaining circulation.
- Monitoring blood pressure and starting on intravenous fluids immediately.
- IV cannula (16–18G) to be passed.
- If veins are not visible, venesection in antecubital fossa to be done.
- In children, intraosseous transfusion can be done (less than 6 years in tibia).

Fluid Selection in Shock

Crystalloids

- Normal saline (0.9%) and Ringer lactate solution
- They expand the interstitial space and not intravascular space
- Dextrose can potentiate ischemia to organs particularly brain, by increasing lactic acid production through anaerobic glycolysis
- Hence, IV fluids containing dextrose are contraindicated in shock (DNS, 5D, 10D, 25D, etc.).

Colloids

- *Albumin* (5–25% solution in isotonic saline):
  - Responsible for 80% of osmotic pressure of plasma and is an effective colloid
  - Increases intravenous volume, by an excess of what is transfused (e.g. transfusion of 100 mL of 25% albumin increases the intravenous volume of 500 mL)
  - Effect lasts for about 36 hours
  - Adverse effects include allergic reaction and dilutional coagulopathies.
- *Dextran* (10% solution):
  - Polysaccharide obtained from sugar beets
  - Expands intravenous volume, by twice the volume transfused
  - Effect lasts for about 6 hours
  - Adverse effects include, anaphylaxis, bleeding risks, acute renal failure, interference with cross matching of blood, as it coats RBC.
- *Hetastarch:*
  - Synthetic starch available as 6% solution
  - Will expand the intravascular volume, by twice the amount transfused
  - Duration of action is around 24 hours
  - Starch is degraded by amylase to small particles and is excreted in urine
  - Adverse effects include allergic reactions and hyperamylasemia.

Whole Blood Transfusion

- Contains 350 mL blood and 50 mL anticoagulants (citrate/phosphate/dextrose)
- Stored at 1–6°C temperature
- Shelf-life is 21 days
- Should be used after warming to normal body temperature
- Rate is 8–15 drops per minute
- Adverse effects include anaphylactic reactions, thrombocytopenia, hypocalcemia, hypothermia, metabolic acidosis, etc.

Drugs Used in Shock

- Dopamine, 5–15 µg/kg/min
- Dobutamine, 2–3 µg/kg/min
- Norepinephrine, 15–20 µg/kg/min
- Corticosteroids, 100–500 mg
- Antibiotics.

Treatment (Cardiogenic Shock)

- Depending on the type of myocardial infarction, one can infuse fluids.
- *Inotropic agents:* Inotropic agents, which enhance the heart's pumping capabilities, are used to improve the contractility and correct the hypotension. Should that not suffice, an intra-aortic balloon pump can be considered (which reduces the workload

for the heart and improves perfusion of the coronary arteries) or a left ventricular assist device (which augments the pump function of the heart).
- Use of vasopressing drugs (to induce vasoconstriction).
- Use of pneumatic antishock garment (PASG), which compresses the legs and concentrate the blood in the vital organs (lungs, heart, brain, etc.).
- Use of blankets to keep the patient warm, e.g. metallic PET film emergency blankets are used to reflect the patient's body heat back to the patient.

Treatment (Distributive Shock)

- In distributive shock caused by sepsis, the infection is treated with antibiotics and supportive care is given (i.e. inotropic, mechanical ventilation, renal function replacement).
- Anaphylaxis is treated with epinephrine "adrenaline", to stimulate cardiac performance and corticosteroids, and to reduce the inflammatory response.
- More suitable would be the use of vasopressors, such as norepinephrine, to decrease vasodilatation.

Treatment (Obstructive Shock)

- In obstructive shock, the only therapy consists of removing the obstruction.
- Pneumothorax or hemothorax is treated by inserting a chest tube.
- Pulmonary embolism requires thrombolysis or embolectomy.
- Cardiac tamponade is treated by draining fluid from the pericardial space through pericardiocentesis.

Treatment (Endocrine Shock)

- The major and generally accepted modalities for treatment of hyperthyroidism, involve initial temporary use of suppressive thyrostatics medication and possibly later use of permanent surgical or radioisotope therapy.
- All approaches may cause underactive thyroid function (hypothyroidism), which is easily managed with levothyroxine supplementation.
- Adrenal deficiencies are often treated with use of corticosteroids.

COMPLICATIONS

- Disseminated intravascular coagulation
- Acute renal failure
- Adult respiratory distress syndrome
- Damage to brain, heart, adrenals, and GIT.

PROGNOSIS

- The prognosis of shock depends on the underlying cause and the nature and extent of concurrent problems.
- Hypovolemic, anaphylactic, and neurogenic shocks are readily treatable and respond well to medical therapy.
- Septic shock, however, is a grave condition and with a mortality rate between 30% and 50%.
- Prolonged hypovolemia and hypotension carry a risk of respiratory and then cardiac arrest. Perfusion of the brain may be the greatest danger during shock. Therefore, urgent treatment (cessation of bleeding, rapid restoration of circulating blood volume, and ready respiratory support) is essential for a good prognosis in hypovolemic shock.

CHAPTER

20

Gas Gangrene

OBJECTIVES

- Background
- Etiology
- Pathophysiology
- Clinical Features
- Differential Diagnosis
- Treatment
- Prognosis
- Complications

INTRODUCTION

- Gas gangrene (Fig. 1) is a type of clostridial infection, characterized by rapid and extensive necrosis of muscle, accompanied by gas formation and systemic toxicity and occurs when bacteria invade healthy muscle.
- Gas gangrene and clostridial myonecrosis are interchangeable terms used to describe an infection of muscle tissue, by toxin-producing clostridia.

BACKGROUND

- Louis Pasteur identified the first clostridial species, *Clostridium butyricum* in 1861.
- In 1892 and later, Welch, Nuttall and other scientists isolated a Gram-positive anaerobic bacillus from gangrenous wounds.
- The organism was later renamed *Bacillus perfringens* and then *Clostridium welchii*. The organism is now named *Clostridium perfringens.*

ETIOLOGY

- Organisms in the formation of gas gangrene include spore-forming clostridial species, including *Clostridium perfringens, Clostridium septicum,* and *Clostridium novyi,* which constitute most of the cases.
- Less pathogenic species include *C. histolyticum, C. fallax, C. bifermentans,* and *C. sporogenes.*
- A nonclostridial form also occurs, which is caused by a mixed infection of aerobic and anaerobic organisms.
- These organisms are true saprophytes and are ubiquitous in soil and dust.
- Clostridia have been isolated from the mucous membranes of humans, including the gastrointestinal (GI) tract and the female genital tract.
- Clostridia are obligate anaerobes, but some species are relatively aerotolerant.
- A recent clinical series on gas gangrene demonstrated a predominance (83.3%) of aerobic Gram-negative bacilli in wound cultures compared with anaerobic Gram-positive bacilli.
- The most frequently identified aerobic Gram-negative bacteria were *Escherichia coli, Proteus, Pseudomonas aeruginosa* and *Klebsiella pneumoniae.*
- Genus *Clostridium* are Gram-positive, spore-forming, obligate anaerobes, that are arranged in pairs and short chains with rounded or pointed ends that are ubiquitous and pleomorphic in nature (Fig. 2).
- Some species of clostridia, such as *C. novyi* type A are strict anaerobes.
- *C. perfringens,* is the most commonly isolated *Clostridium* species and causes around 80% of the cases of gas gangrene, usually may be divided into 5 types (A–E), depending on the toxins they produce.
- The other 20% cases are constituted by *C. novyi* and *C. septicum.*

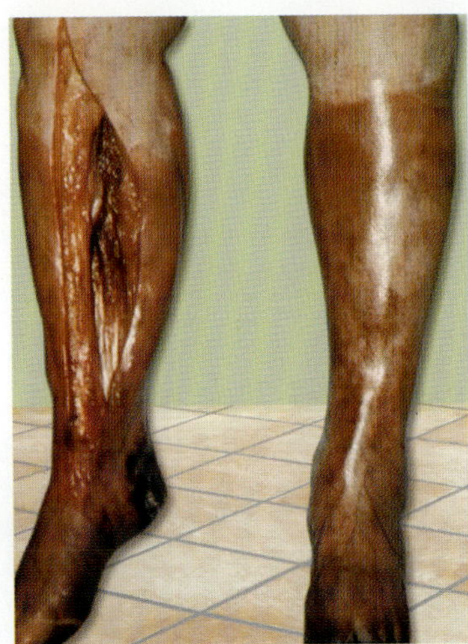

Fig. 1: Gas gangrene of lower extremities, due to toxin producing clostridium.

PATHOPHYSIOLOGY (FIGS. 3A AND B)

- Contamination with clostridial spores, in post-traumatic or postoperative lesions establishes the initial stage of infection.
- Local wound conditions are more important than the degree of clostridial contamination in the development of gas gangrene.
- Disrupted or necrotic tissue provides the necessary enzymes and a low oxidation/reduction potential, allowing for spore germination.

- Foreign bodies, premature wound closure, and devitalized muscle, reduce the spore inoculum necessary to cause infection in laboratory animals.
- The typical incubation period for gas gangrene is frequently short (i.e. less than 24 hours).
- Self-perpetuating destruction of tissue occurs via a rapidly multiplying microbial population and the production of locally and systemically acting exotoxins.
- Local effects include necrosis of muscle and subcutaneous fat as well as thrombosis of blood vessels.
- Marked edema may further compromise blood supply to the region. Fermentation of glucose is probably the main mechanism of gas production in gas gangrene. In spontaneous gas gangrene, nitrogen is the predominant gas component followed by oxygen, hydrogen, and carbon dioxide.
- Production of gas begins late and dissects along muscle bellies and fascial planes. These local effects create an environment, which facilitates rapid spread of the infection.
- Systemically, exotoxins may cause severe hemolysis. Hemoglobin levels may drop to very low levels and when occurring with hypotension, may cause acute tubular necrosis and renal failure.
- A rapidly progressive infection can quickly result in shock. The mechanism of shock is poorly understood.
- Spontaneous gas gangrene is most often caused by hematogenous spread of *C. septicum* from the GI tract in patients with colon cancer or other portals of entry.
- With *C. perfringens,* the local and systemic manifestations of infection are due to the production of potent extracellular protein toxins by the bacteria.

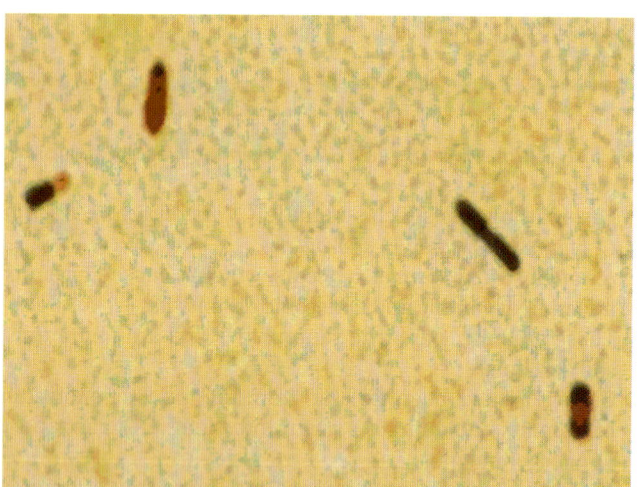

Fig. 2: Genus *Clostridium* organisms.

Exotoxins

Different exotoxins and the biological effects of *C. perfringens* are illustrated here:

- *Alpha toxin:* Lethal, lecithinase, necrotizing, hemolytic, and cardiotoxic
- *Beta toxin:* Lethal and necrotizing
- *Epsilon toxin:* Lethal, permease
- *Iota toxin* : Lethal and necrotizing
- *Delta toxin:* Lethal, hemolysin
- *Phi toxin:* Hemolysin, cytolysin
- *Kappa toxin*: Lethal, collagenase, gelatinase, necrotizing
- *Lambda toxin*: Protease
- *Mu toxin*: Hyaluronidase
- *Nu toxin*: Lethal, deoxyribonuclease, hemolytic, necrotizing

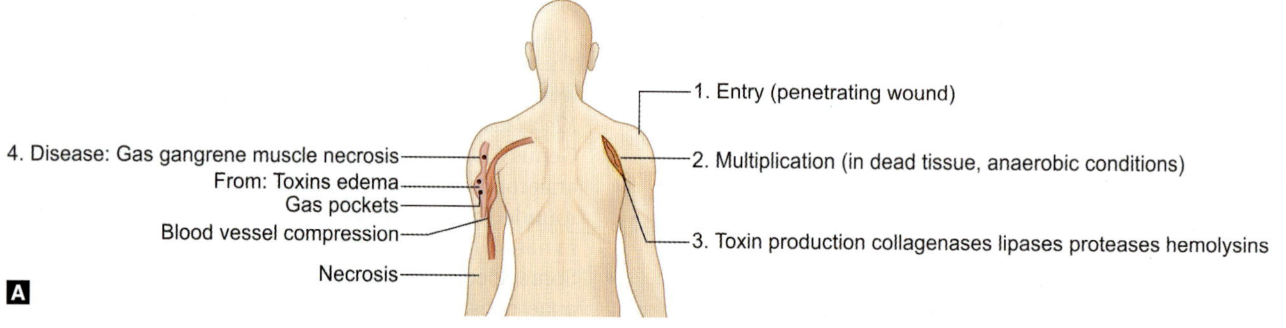

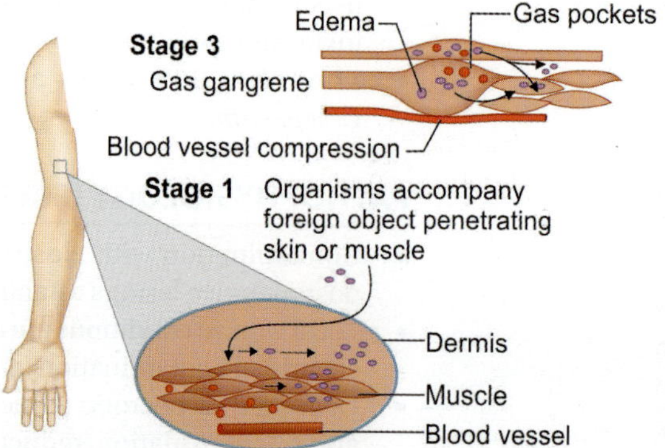

Figs. 3A and B: Diagrammatic representation of manifestations and stages of gas gangrene.

- These toxins are lethal, as tested by injection in mice
- Alpha toxin is apparently of utmost importance. The alpha toxin is a zinc metalloenzyme that has phospholipase-C activity (i.e. lecithinase) and causes cell destruction by hydrolysis of key cell membrane components. This toxin can cause lysis of erythrocytes, leukocytes, platelets, fibroblasts, and muscle cells
- These toxins hydrolyze cell membranes, cause abnormal coagulation, leading to microvascular thrombosis (further extending the borders of devascularized and thus anaerobic tissue) and have direct cardiodepressive effects
- The products of tissue breakdown, including creatine phosphokinase, myoglobin and potassium, may cause secondary toxicity and renal impairment
- Significant and refractory anemia may also be present, which may be a direct consequence of toxin-mediated hemolysis of RBC, when significant amounts of alpha toxin are released into the bloodstream
- Alpha toxin has negative inotropic effects on cardiac myocytes, contributing to the severe, refractory hypotension seen in some cases of gas gangrene
- Theta toxin causes a cytokine cascade, which results in peripheral vasodilation, similar to that seen in septic shock.

Causes

- Gas gangrene can be classified as post-traumatic, postoperative, or spontaneous.
- Post-traumatic gas gangrene accounts for 60% of all gas gangrene cases. Most of these cases involve automobile collisions.
- Other complications of trauma arise from crush injuries, compound fractures, gunshot wounds, thermal or electrical burns, and frostbite.
- Farm or industrial injuries contaminated with soil are especially prone to developing gas gangrene.
- Intramuscular or subcutaneous injections with insulin, epinephrine, quinine, or cocaine are rare antecedent events leading to gas gangrene (Fig. 4).
- Postoperative clostridial infections follow cases of colon resection, ruptured appendix, bowel perforation, and biliary or other GI surgery, including laparoscopic cholecystectomy and colonoscopy.
- Septic backstreet abortions are the main cause of uterine gas gangrene.
- Spontaneous gas gangrene without external wound or injury occurs frequently in patients, who have serious underlying conditions.
- Colorectal adenocarcinoma is the most prevalent risk factor in this group. Hematologic malignancy is also a major premorbid condition.
- In children, neutropenia, either induced by chemotherapy or cyclic in nature, represents the single most important risk factor for spontaneous *C. septicum* infections.
- The remaining cases are associated with diabetes or neutropenic colitis.
- Patients with *C. septicum* infections have overt or occult malignancies approximately 5 times more often, than patients with other clostridial infections.

Risk Factors

- Atherosclerosis
- Burns
- Corticosteroid use
- Diabetes
- GI malignancy
- HIV/AIDS
- Hypoalbuminemia
- Intravenous (IV) drug abuse
- Chronic alcoholism (Fig. 5)
- Obesity
- Open fractures
- Peripheral vascular disease
- Surgery
- Trauma.

CLINICAL FEATURES

History

- Most patients with post-traumatic gas gangrene have sustained serious injury on the skin or soft tissues, or have experienced open fractures. Patients with postoperative gas gangrene have frequently undergone recent surgery of the GI or biliary tract.

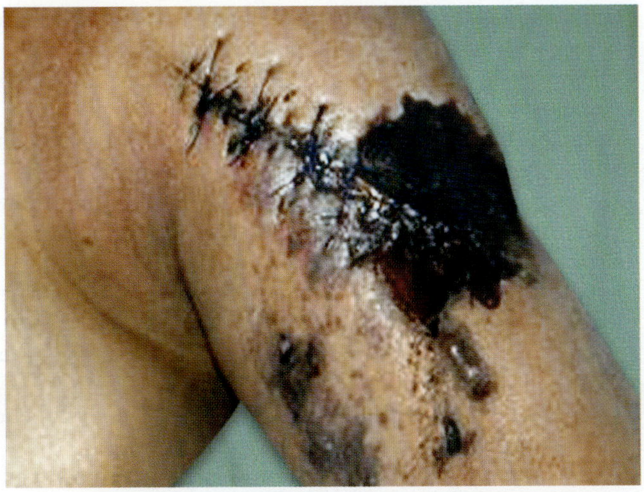

Fig. 4: Patient developed gas gangrene after injecting cocaine. *C. septicum* was isolated in both blood and wound cultures.

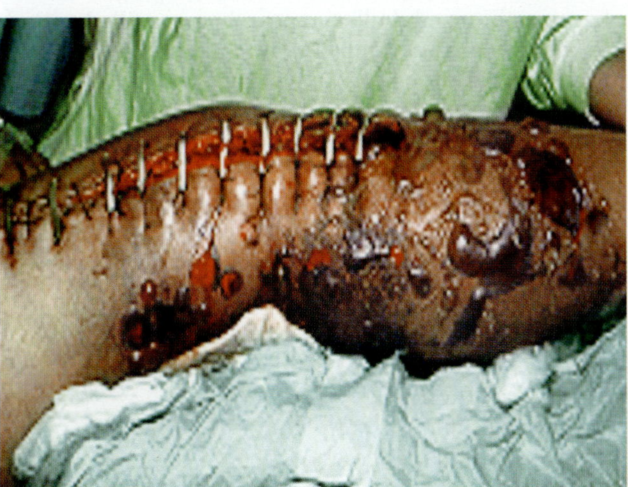

Fig. 5: Gas gangrene formed with chronic alcoholism.

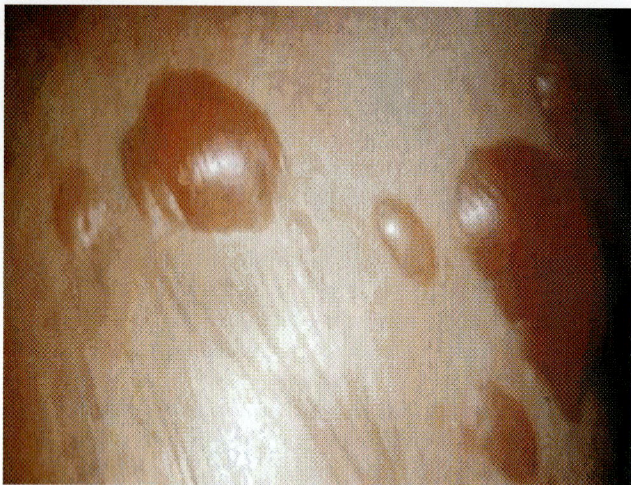

Fig. 6: Cutaneous gangrene.

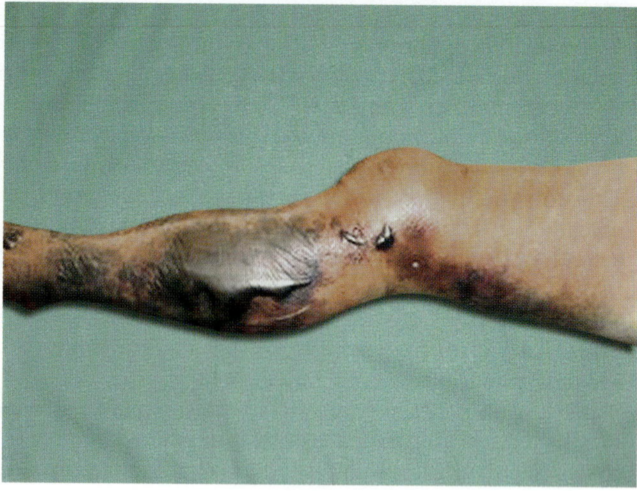

Fig. 7: Myonecrosis of extremities.

Signs and Symptoms

- Typically, gas gangrene begins with the sudden onset of pain in the region of the wound, which helps to differentiate it from spreading cellulitis.
- Following pain, local swelling, and edema accompanied by a thin often hemorrhagic exudate appear.
- Patients frequently develop marked tachycardia.
- Elevation in temperature may be only minimal.
- Gas usually is not obvious at early stages and may be completely absent.
- Frothiness of the wound exudate may be noted.
- The skin is tense, white, often marbled with blue, and may be cooler than normal.
- The symptoms progress rapidly. Swelling, edema, and toxemia increase and a profuse serous discharge appears, having a peculiar sweetish smell.
- Gram's staining of the wound exudate shows many Gram-positive rods with relatively few inflammatory cells.
- Despite hypotension, renal failure, and (often) body crepitation, patients with myonecrosis frequently have a heightened awareness of their surroundings until just before death, when they lapse into toxic delirium and coma.
- In untreated cases, as the local wounds progress, the skin becomes bronzed, bullae appear, become filled with dark red fluid, and are accompanied by dark patches of cutaneous gangrene (Fig. 6).
- Gas appears in later phases, but may not be as obvious as in anaerobic cellulitis. Jaundice is rare in wound gas gangrene (in contrast to uterine infections).
- Cases of clostridial myonecrosis without a history of trauma have bullous lesions and crepitation of the skin; they present with a rapidly worsening course that includes myonecrosis, especially of the extremities (Fig. 7).

DIFFERENTIAL DIAGNOSIS

- Abdominable abscess
- Anthrax infection
- Pyomyositis (muscle abscess)
- Cellulitis
- Rhabdomyolysis
- Deep venous thrombosis and thrombophlebitis
- Streptococcal (pyogenes) myositis
- Necrotizing cellulitis
- *Vibrio vulnificus* infection
- Necrotizing fasciitis
- Toxic shock syndrome
- Clostridial cholecystitis (emphysematous cholecystitis)
- Other problems to be considered
- Other causes of necrotizing myositis (Group A streptococci, polymicrobial aerobic-anaerobic flora and nonclostridial anaerobes)
- Cutaneous anthrax
- Acute gout
- Familial mediterranean fever
- Septic arthritis
- Pyoderma gangrenosa
- Carcinoma erysipeloids
- Pyomyositis
- Water-borne skin infections (*Vibrio vulnificus, Aeromonas hydrophila, Mycobacterium marinum,* etc.)
- Other causes of soft tissue gas (e.g. pneumomediastinum, pneumothorax, fractured larynx, fractured trachea, etc.).

Laboratory Studies

- Gram stain and culture of bullae fluid, *Clostridia* species are known to be large, Gram-positive rods (box-car appearance)
- The presence of Gram-positive or gram variable rods with few white blood cells is indicative of clostridial etiology
- Complete blood count may reveal anemia, thrombocytopenia and evidence of intravascular hemolysis on smear
- *Electrolyte level:* Hyperkalemia can result from cell breakdown. Hypocalcemia may result from subcutaneous fat necrosis
- *Renal panel:* Kidney dysfunction may occur secondary to hypotension, hemoglobinuria, and myoglobinuria or direct toxin effect
- *Coagulation panel:* Coagulopathy and thrombocytopenia can also result
- *Liver function tests:* Hyperbilirubinemia and liver dysfunction may result from release of toxins
- *Arterial blood gas determination:* Gas gangrene can cause metabolic acidosis, with significant lactic acidosis secondary to tissue death and ischemia

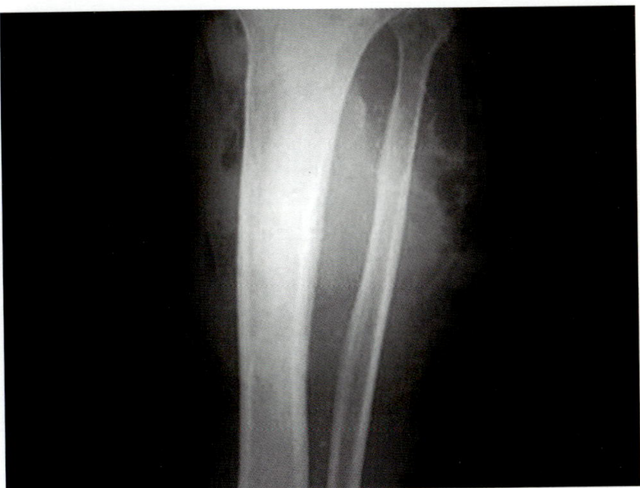

Fig. 8: X-ray of extremity taken, with gas gangrene.

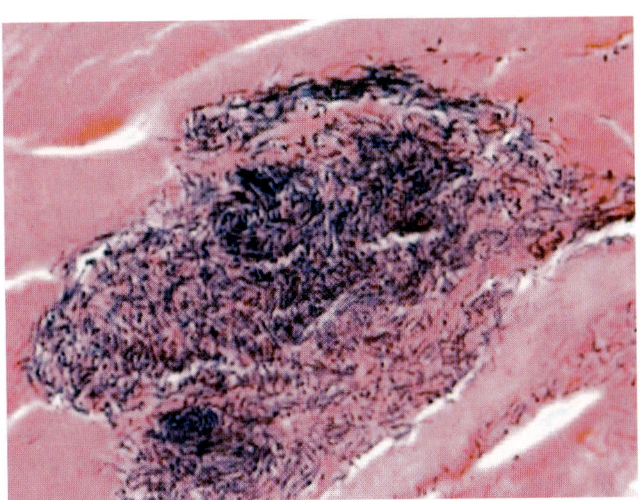

Fig. 9: Destructive changes as seen in histological findings in gas gangrene.

- *Myoglobin level:* Myoglobinemia and myoglobinuria can result from cellular breakdown
- *Blood cultures:* This may help narrow antibiotic coverage.

Imaging Studies (Fig. 8)

- Gas in the soft tissues is neither sensitive nor specific for gas gangrene. Many different bacteria, trauma, and visceral perforation can cause soft tissue gas. Plain radiographs or ultrasonography can be used to look for the presence of gas.
- Computed tomography or magnetic resonance imaging can help to evaluate the depth of soft tissue inflammation.

Other Tests

- Once *Clostridia* are isolated from culture, identification of the lecithinase function of alpha toxin may be elicited by inoculating blood agar with the isolated bacteria. A double area of hemolysis will develop around the colonies, demonstrating the presence of lecithinase. Inoculation of the colonies with antitoxin will halt the hemolysis.
- Rapid detection of alpha toxin or sialidases (i.e. neuraminidases) in infected tissues through enzyme linked immunosorbent assay (ELISA).
- Although, not widely available for clinical practice, *in vitro* amplification of the alpha-toxin or DNA by polymerase chain reaction (PCR) has been used to isolate clostridial species.

Procedures

- Tissue biopsy with culture and Gram stain is the criterion standard in helping to make the diagnosis of gas gangrene.
- Surgical exploration confirms the diagnosis of myonecrosis. Affected muscle appears pale and shows no contractile function, when incised or electrically stimulated.
- Under local anesthesia, bedside biopsy with immediate frozen section can be performed, to provide early and accurate diagnosis of gas gangrene.
- Patients with gas gangrene frequently develop massive hemolysis, shock, acute respiratory distress syndrome (ARDS), and renal failure, which often requires invasive procedures (e.g. right-sided heart catheterization, mechanical ventilation, hemodialysis, etc.).

Histologic Findings (Fig. 9)

Histopathologic findings in gas gangrene consist of widespread myonecrosis, destruction of other connective tissues, and a paucity of neutrophils in the infected area. Leukocyte aggregates are found in the border regions.

TREATMENT

The combination of aggressive surgical debridement and effective antibiotic therapy is the determining factor for successful treatment of gas gangrene.

Prehospital Care

- Oxygenation;
- Intravenous (IV) fluids.

Emergency Department Care

- Gas gangrene is a true emergency and concurrent evaluation, treatment, and coordination of care should be carried out
- *Airway and breathing:* Oxygen and airway management as necessitated
- *Circulation:* Good vascular access and liberal use of IV fluids is indicated
- Administer tetanus toxoid, if indicated
- Administer antibiotics
- Correct electrolyte abnormalities
- Check compartment pressures, if severe pain and evidence of compartment syndrome are present with minimal cutaneous evidence of infection.

Antibiotics

- Historically, penicillin G in dosages of 10–24 million unit/day was the drug of choice. Currently, a combination of penicillin and clindamycin is widely used.
- Recent studies show that protein synthesis inhibitors (e.g. clindamycin, chloramphenicol, rifampin, tetracycline, etc.) may be more effective because they inhibit the synthesis of clostridial exotoxins and lessen the local and systemic toxic effects of these proteins.
- A combination of clindamycin and metronidazole is a good choice for patients allergic to penicillin.

- Although, approved for treating complicated skin and soft-tissue infections, latest antibiotics such as daptomycin, linezolid, and tigecycline have not been studied in patients with gas gangrene, therefore, they should not be used as primary antibiotics for treating this condition.
- *Adjuvant therapy:* Recombinant human activated protein C has been used as an adjuvant therapy for patients with severe sepsis, but aside from the serious bleeding that may be associated, repeated surgical debridement in patients with gas gangrene requires frequent interruption of the continuous infusion of this product. Therefore, is not widely used.

Surgical Care

- Fasciotomy, for compartment syndrome may be necessary and should not be delayed in patients with involvement of extremities.
- Perform debridement, as needed to remove all necrotic tissue.
- Exposure of all the affected muscle groups, by long incisions or in the subcutaneous infections, multiple subcutaneous drainage, and slough extraction by incisions into the subcutaneous tissue may be done.
- Amputation of the extremity may be necessary and life-saving.
- Abdominal involvement requires excision of the body wall musculature.
- Uterine gas gangrene following septic abortion, usually necessitates hysterectomy.

Hyperbaric Oxygen (HBO)

- Use is controversial.
- Can be used to supplement surgical debridement and antibiotics.
- Particularly helpful in areas, where complete surgical resection of necrotic tissue is difficult, such as the paraspinal muscles or abdominal wall (Fig. 10).
- Potential benefits include improved neutrophil-mediated killing of bacteria, direct bactericidal effect on anaerobes, improved activity of some antibiotics and enhanced wound healing.

Deterrence/Prevention

Avoid suturing wounds, due to a crush injury or open fractures with devitalized muscle and soil contamination.

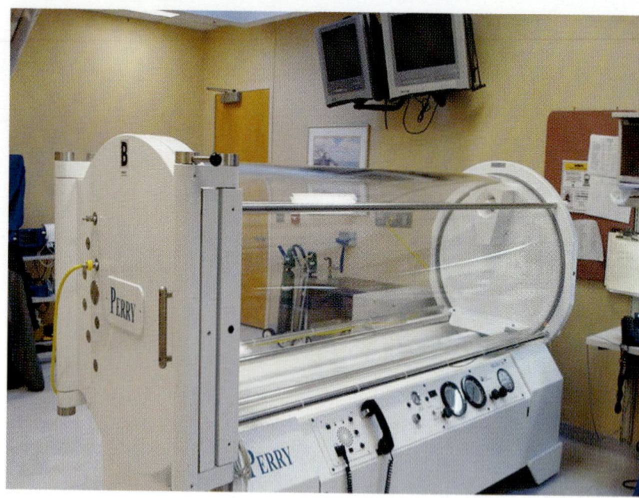

Fig. 10: Hyperbaric oxygen, set up.

PROGNOSIS

- Failure to provide an early diagnosis and inadequate surgical intervention are the two most common mistakes in the management of gas gangrene. These are the factors which eventually dictate the outcome.
  The prognosis of gas gangrene is better, if the incubation period is shorter than 30 hours, if the patient has limb involvement and if he or she does not have concomitant serious medical conditions or complications, [e.g. shock, disseminated intravascular coagulation (DIC), ARDS, renal failure, etc.].
- Spontaneous gas gangrene frequently carries a worse prognosis than other forms of gas gangrene.

COMPLICATIONS

- Massive hemolysis, which may require repeated blood transfusion
- Disseminated intravascular coagulation, which may cause severe bleeding and may complicate aggressive surgical debridement
- Acute renal failure
- Acute respiratory distress syndrome
- Shock
- The most important factors in the successful treatment of gas gangrene are early diagnosis and prompt treatment.

CHAPTER

21

Head Injury

OBJECTIVES

- Anatomical Considerations
- Injuries to Brain
- Intracranial Hematomas
- Fractures of Skull
- Evaluation of Head Injury Patient
- Management of Head Injury
- Complications of Head Injury

INTRODUCTION

Head injuries account for the maximum number of trauma deaths, about 9 deaths per 100,000 population every year. Out of all cases, half die before arrival, half are below 31 years of age, and half are in drunken state, or after assault. A head injury can occur due to road traffic accidents, falls, assaults, sports accidents, industrial accidents or birth trauma. Majority does not need surgery, but a general surgeon must be aware of the need for special investigations and the indications of urgent operation.

ANATOMICAL CONSIDERATIONS

Brain is well encased in the cranial cavity, covered by three layers of meninges. The outermost dura is closely adherent to the bony skull while the arachnoid membrane lies just underneath the intervening space being the subdural space. The brain itself is lined closely by pia mater, and the space between arachnoid and pia mater is called the subarachnoid space containing the cerebrospinal fluid (CSF). The meningeal layers form *Falx cerebri* in between frontal lobes and *Tentorium cerebelli* in between the cerebrum and cerebellum around the brain stem. Fractures of the skull can cause accumulation of blood in the extradural, subdural, or subarachnoid spaces, while the brain itself may suffer various types of injuries due to various mechanisms (Fig. 1).

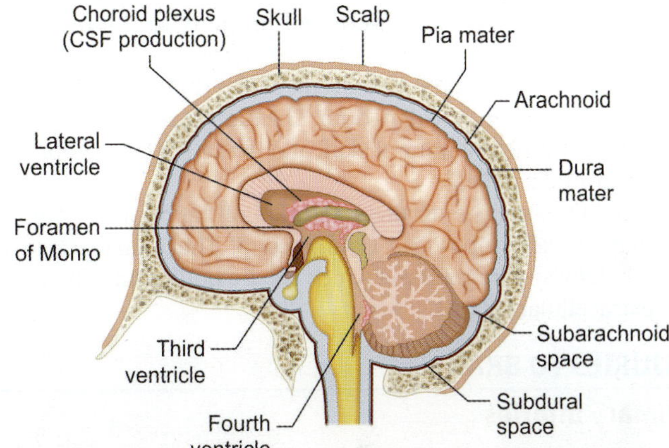

Fig. 1: Cross section of head showing underlying brain, meninges, and skull.

Classification of Head Injuries

- *Depending on the communication to exterior:*
  - *Closed*—where scalp is intact.
  - *Open*—where the wound communicates with cranial cavity (Figs. 2 and 3).
- *Depending on the extent of injury:*
  - *Focal*—localized injury.
  - *Diffuse*—widespread injury in the brain tissue.
- *Depending on the severity:*
  - *Minor*—brief/no loss of consciousness; no fracture.
  - *Major*—loss of consciousness usually associated with fracture.
- *Location of injury:*
  - *Scalp injury*—bruises/lacerations.
  - *Skull injury*—fractures of skull involving vault/base.

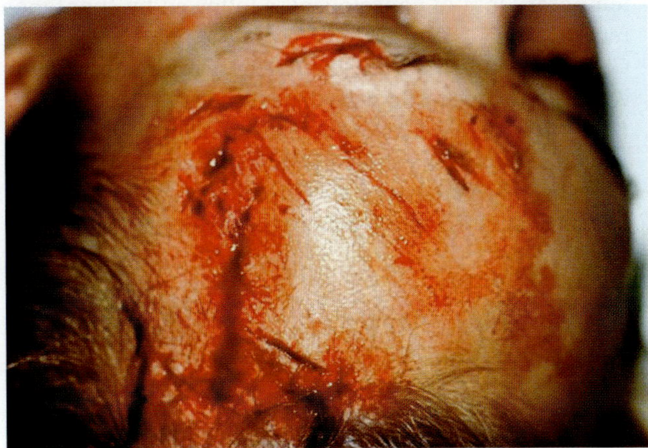

Fig. 2: Closed head injury.

  - *Intracranial hematomas*—extradural, subdural, subarachnoid, intracerebral, and intraventricular hematomas.
  - *Brain injuries*—concussion, contusion, laceration, and diffuse axonal injury (DAI).

Factors Affecting Head Injury

- Brain is protected well in bony shell and cushioned by CSF. Because of its soft consistency and slight mobility,

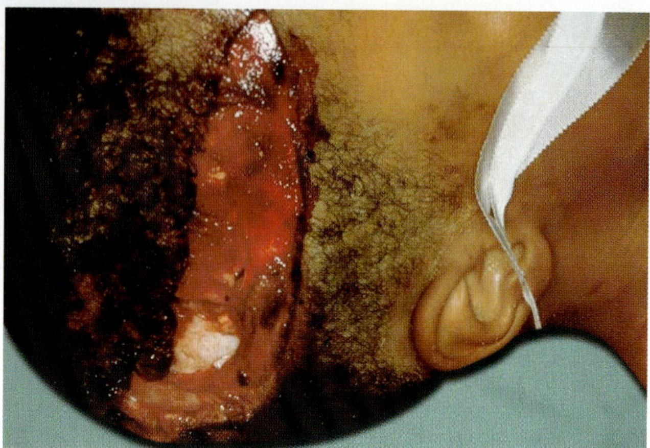

Fig. 3: Open head injury.

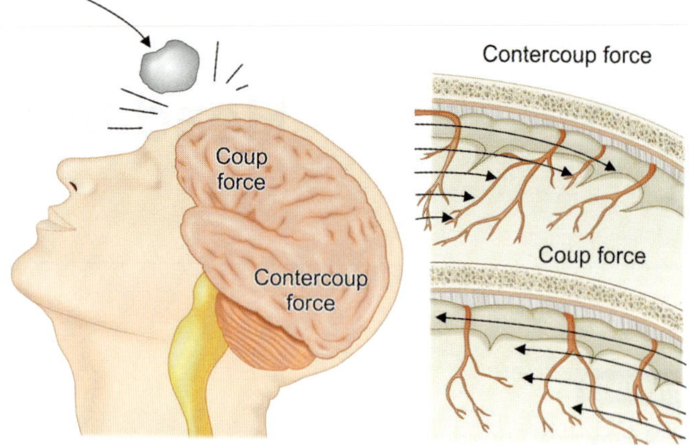

Fig. 4: Coup and countercoup injuries.

it is vulnerable to injury due to sudden acceleration and deceleration forces imparted because of direct and indirect trauma. The morbidity further increases in old age with atrophic brain having increased mobility in the increased space.

- The intracranial cerebral movement can rupture cerebral vein especially where it enters dura. The damage is marked due to irregular inner contour of skull and the tough falx cerebri and tentorium cerebelli.
- The injury can be on the same side of the blow—"Coup" or diametrically opposite—"Countercoup." The brain reacts to the insult by swelling/edema which can be both intracellular and extracellular (Fig. 4).

INJURIES TO BRAIN

Primary Injuries

- *Concussion:* Brief physiological paralysis without organic damage. There is transient brain distortion producing temporary loss of consciousness followed by spontaneous recovery.
- *Contusion:* Bruising with small hemorrhages and swelling of brain tissue causing damage to nerve cells and axons.
- *Laceration:* Cerebral tear with effusion of blood in CSF.
- *Diffuse axonal injury:* Rotational forces causing disruption of axons in brain stem and corpus callosum with widespread petechial hemorrhages leading to persistent coma.

Secondary Factors

Intracranial Factors

- *Edema*—intracellular/extracellular due to underlying tissue injury.
- *Necrosis*—combined with swelling/ischemia of the tissue.
- *Hematoma*—pressure due to associated intracranial hematomas.
- *Vascular*—further ischemia due to increased intracranial tension.
- *Coning*—herniation of uncus on the side of supratentorial mass, causing pressure on the ipsilateral 3rd cranial nerve and midbrain.
- *Coup and countercoup*—craniocerebral damage due to injury on same side (coup) and diametrically opposite side (countercoup).

Extracranial Factors

- *Respiration*—respiratory failure causing brain edema and congestion.
- *Blood pressure*—hypotension causing decreased cardiac output and irreversible brain damage. Head injury *per se* never causes hypotension in adults, hence look for other factors if hypotension is evident.
- *Fluids*—hypotonic fluids like 5% glucose avoided as they increase brain edema.
- *Infection*—open injuries more prone to develop meningitis.
- *Hypoxia*—due to increased intracranial pressure and decreased cerebral blood flow further aggravates the damage.

INTRACRANIAL HEMATOMAS

They account for one-third of deaths occurring in head injury and are also common causes of significant morbidity.

Extradural Hematoma

Occurs due to direct trauma causing fracture of temporal/parietal bone, causing tear in anterior/posterior branch of middle meningeal artery/vein. The blood passes upward in the parietal region, downward in middle cranial fossa, and outward under temporalis muscle.

Clinical presentation is characterized by a *classic "triphasic" response*—initial trauma causes immediate *loss of consciousness* due to distortion of brain stem and reticular formation which is followed by *state of alertness ("lucid interval")*. The accumulating blood keeps on collecting causing pressure and *second episode of unconsciousness* which may rapidly prove fatal (Fig. 5).

- The patient is *confused and irritable* with restlessness and headache due to the stripping of dura from skull as he slowly lapses into unconsciousness.
- There is *ipsilateral dilatation of pupil ("Hutchinson's pupil")* due to inward displacement of temporal lobe against oculomotor nerve above the edge of tentorium and *contralateral hemiparesis* due to pressure on the crossed pyramidal tracts (Fig. 6).
- Further increase in intracranial tension due to the expanding hematoma causes further displacement of brain to opposite side causing *contralateral papillary dilatation and ipsilateral hemiparesis.*
- Further progression of the condition causes transtentorial herniation leading to *bilateral fixed dilated pupils and decerebrate rigidity.*

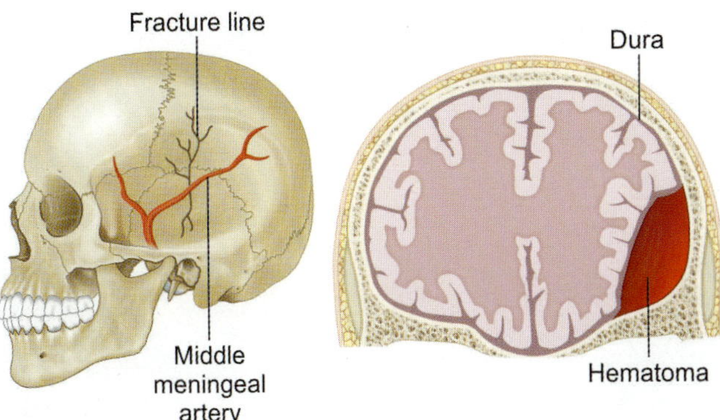

Fig. 5: Extradural hematoma.

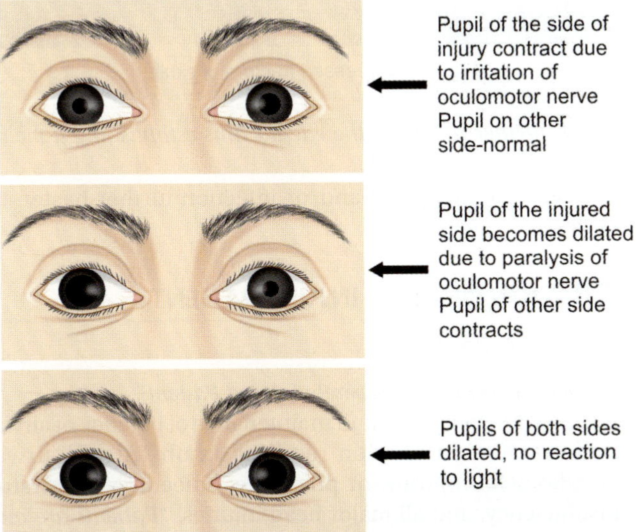

Fig. 6: Hutchinson's pupil.

Extradural hematoma is a life-threatening emergency and needs immediate surgical intervention. *Beware of a drowsy irritable patient with a swelling in temporal region. He could be harboring a potentially lethal extradural hematoma underneath!*

Subdural Hematoma (Acute)

Subdural hematoma occurs due to rupture of large cortical veins at junction of their fixed part with dural sinuses, causing extensive hematoma and severe brain damage (Fig. 7).

Clinical Presentation

- Always associated with initial and persistent unconsciousness *(No lucid interval)* and faster deterioration.
- Hematoma may be coup/countercoup, extending below frontal and temporal lobes.
- Pupillary dilation, same as in extradural hematoma although march of paralysis, may not be typically progressive from face to limbs.
- *Chronic subdural hematoma*—due to small tear in cortical vein with extravasation of blood giving rise to space occupying lesion or coma several days after the injury.

Other Intracranial Hematomas

They can be subarachnoid, intracerebral, or intraventricular hematomas. They are rare but are always associated with cortical

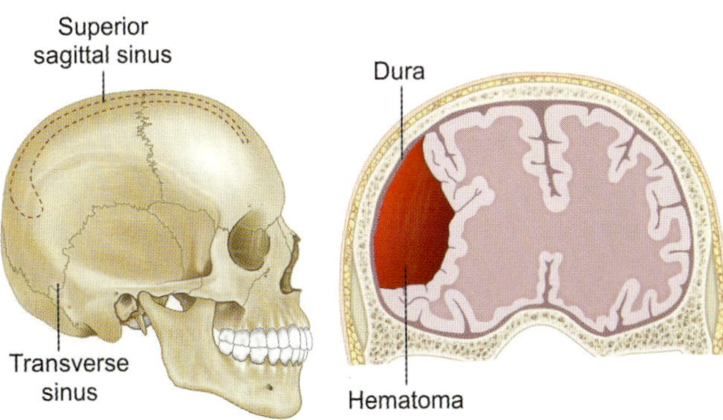

Fig. 7: Subdural hematoma.

laceration/necrosis and widespread brain injury with worse prognosis.

FRACTURES OF SKULL

They may be simple (closed) or compound (open), linear or depressed, and comminuted or noncomminuted (Fig. 8).

- *Fractures of vault:* They may not be of special significance except when they cross line of vessels, signifying underlying hematoma.
- *Fractures of base:* May need special radiological views for diagnosis.
  - *Anterior cranial fossa fractures*—indicated by bruising within orbital margins, hematoma of eyelids and conjunctiva, periorbital ecchymosis ("Raccoon eyes"), involvement of 1st to 6th cranial nerves, CSF rhinorrhea, due to involvement of frontal or paranasal sinuses, or bleeding through nose (Fig. 9).
  - *Middle cranial fossa fractures*—indicated by bruising over mastoid region ("Battle's sign"), involvement of 7th or 8th cranial nerve, CSF otorrhea, or bleeding through the ear (Fig. 10).
  - *Posterior cranial fossa fractures*—usually associated with respiratory depression proceeding to loss of consciousness, bruising over occipital region, involvement of 9th, 10th, or 11th cranial nerve, or bleeding through the throat.
- *Depressed fractures*: Usually significant if outer table of fractured fragment lies below the inner table as the surrounding skull appears as double density in X-rays. Complications can occur such as dural tear, an underlying hematoma, pressure on cerebral cortex, epilepsy (early/late), cosmetic deformity ("Pond's fracture") in infants due to forceps applied during delivery, and pressure on dural sinuses causing increased intracranial tension. They are confused with large scalp hematoma, which feels soft in center (Fig. 11).

Cause of Death in Head Injury

- Extensive injury to vital areas indicated by unconsciousness right from beginning, bilateral fixed dilated pupils, flaccidity in all four limbs or autonomic disturbances (loss of bladder and/or bowel control).
- Associated injuries to chest, abdomen, spine, or limbs.
- Improper management of secondary factors, e.g. hypoxia, infection, and fluid balance. *Injury to brain causes edema and increased intracranial tension which leads to decreased cerebral blood flow, hypoxia, infarction, and necrosis of brain tissue*

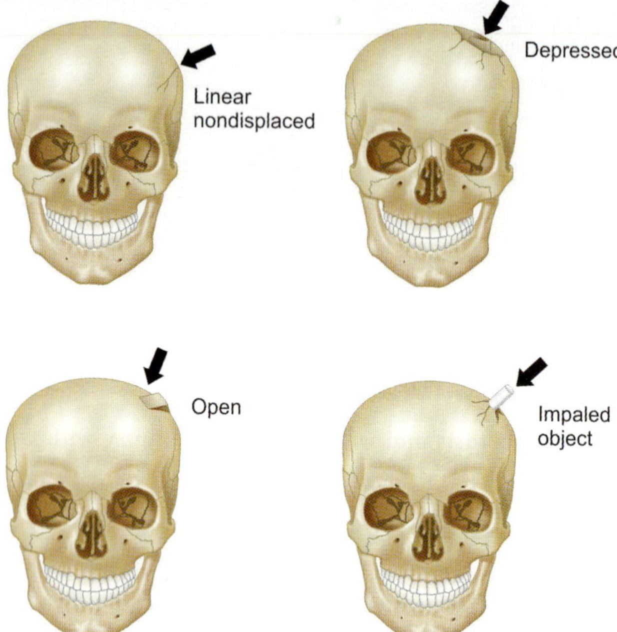

Fig. 8: Fractures of skull.

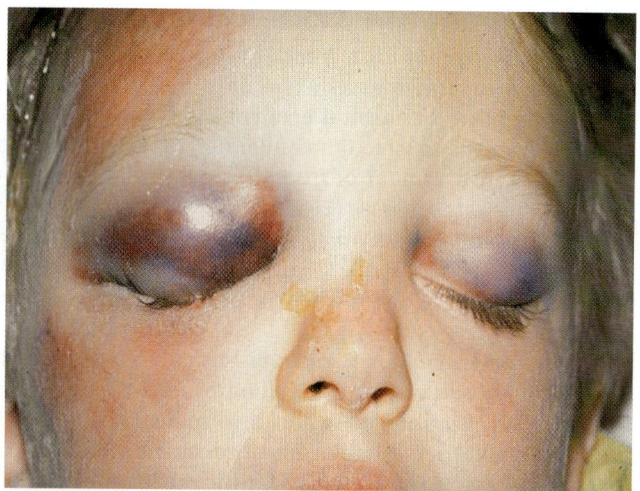

Fig. 9: "Raccoon eyes" in anterior cranial fossa fractures.

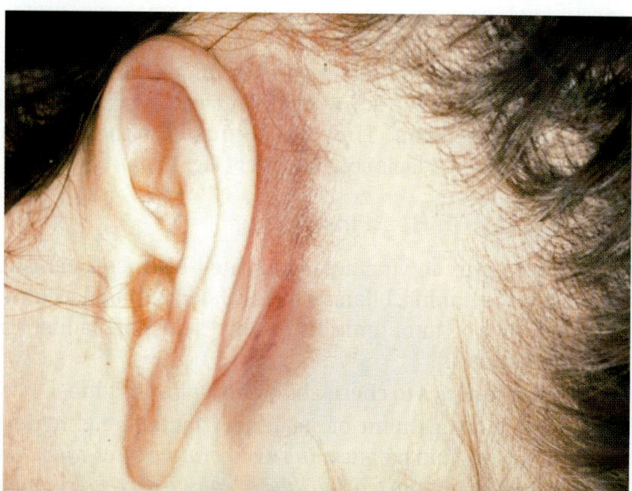

Fig. 10: "Battle's sign" in middle cranial fossa fractures.

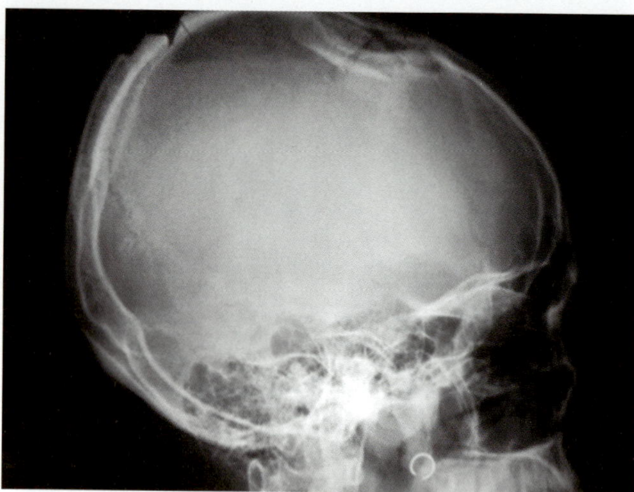

Fig. 11: Depressed fracture of skull.

which further increases the edema thus establishing a vicious cycle.

- Increased temperature and/or infection further hasten the cycle.

EVALUATION OF HEAD INJURY PATIENT

General Examination

"Protocol for Reception of Severely Injured Patient"

- *A (Airway)*—clearance and maintenance of patency of airway. Endotracheal intubation required in obstructed airway, maxillofacial injuries, or pharyngeal bleeding, respiratory insufficiency, and all major head injuries. *"Patients are more likely to die of airway obstruction than any other cause."*
- *B (Breathing)*—care of breathing/oxygen/intermittent positive pressure respiration (IPPR) instituted if required.
- *C (Circulation)*—establishment of intravenous line and infusion of intravenous fluids/blood as required. *"A picture of surgical shock should not be ascribed to head injury and cause of internal bleeding is always to be looked for."*
- *D (Deformity)*—splintage of fractures/care of external wounds.
- *E (Examination and further evaluation): Examine—*
  - Vital signs—temperature/pulse/respiration/blood pressure;
  - Scalp/skull/face/ear/nose/throat;
  - Cervical spine injury/neck stiffness;
  - Thorax/abdomen/spine/pelvis/extremities.

Neurological Examination

- *Level of consciousness:* Determined by "*Glasgow Coma Scale" (GCS)*. This is now the most widely accepted scale for head injury and the grade of injury is classified as minor, moderate, or severe head injury. *Note that the minimum score in GCS is 3 and a score between 3 and 8 constitutes a severe head injury (Table 1 and Fig. 12).*
- *Head*: Look for wounds, fractures, periorbital, or retromastoid bruising, and temporal hematoma. A *"Red eye"*, usually bilateral, occurs due to fracture of anterior cranial fossa and is characterized by hematoma confined to orbital margins, subconjunctival hemorrhage, and mild exophthalmos. It needs to be distinguished from a *"Black eye"*, usually unilateral, and

TABLE 1: Glasgow Coma Scale (mild 12–15; moderate 9–12; severe 3–8).

Eye opening		*Verbal response*		*Motor response*	
	Points		*Points*		*Points*
Spontaneous	4	Oriented Confused	5	Obeys commands	6
To voice	3	Inappropriate words	4	Localizes pain	5
To pain	2	Incomprehensible	3	Withdraws	4
		sounds	2	Abnormal flexion	3*
None	1	Silent	1	Abnormal extension	2**
				No movement	1

*Decorticate posturing to pain
** Decerebrate posturing to pain

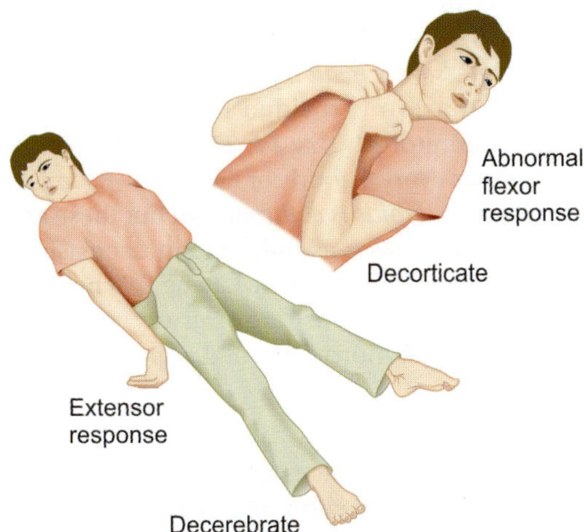

Fig. 12: Decorticate and decerebrate posturing.

occurring due to direct trauma, characterized by grazing of surrounding skin, conjunctival hemorrhage and absence of exophthalmos.

- *Face:* Look for fractures, CSF rhinorrhea, CSF otorrhea, and bleeding through ear/nose/throat.
- *Neck:* Carefully look for any cervical fractures. *"In comatose patients, it should be assumed that cervical spine is unstable and to be immobilized by sandbags on either sides/cervical collar till X-ray rules out cervical fractures."*
- *Eyes:*
  - *Pupils:* Failure of pupil to react to both direct and consensual light indicates *3rd cranial nerve lesion*, ipsilateral dilated pupil is seen in *extradural hematoma*, while bilateral fixed dilated pupils are indicative of *increased intracranial tension* with tentorial herniation.
  - *Eye movements:* Conjugate deviation indicates damage to same side visual field/failure to elicit oculocephalic reflex ("Doll's eye movements,"—i.e. movement of eyes to opposite side of head movement) in comatose patient indicates severe brain stem damage.
- *Neurological deficit in limbs:* Asymmetrical weakness/hemiparesis/hemiplegia in the limb contralateral to the lesion.
- *Other neurological signs*:
  - *Increased intracranial pressure: Hypertension, bradycardia, Cheyne-Stokes respiration (periodic breathing), and papilledema.*
  - *Other localizing signs: Jacksonian epilepsy, dysphagia/aphasia, homonymous hemianopia on opposite side of the lesion, absence of corneal reflex on both sides due to 5th cranial nerve lesion, and facial palsy.*

Special Evaluation and Care

Investigations

- *X-ray*: X-ray (skull–AP, lateral/cervical spine–AP, lateral/chest PA/paranasal sinuses if indicated). Look for site/type of fracture in X-ray skull and shift of calcified pineal to one side.

  Indications for skull X-rays—History of amnesia or level of consciousness (LOC), any neurological symptoms or signs, discharge of blood, or CSF from nose/ear, bruising or swelling over scalp, alcohol intoxication, and medicolegal cases.
- *Computed tomography (CT) scan: This is now the gold standard in management of all head injury cases and has now replaced carotid angiography which used to be done in the past.*
  - *Indications for CT scan*—deteriorating/prolonged/fluctuating level of unconsciousness, localizing signs, GCS 7 or less, penetrating head injury, and late indications (CSF fistula, infection, hydrocephalus, chronic subdural hematoma). *Biconvex hyperdense shadow is seen in extradural hematoma while irregular concavo-convex shadow indicates subdural hematoma (Figs. 13 and 14).*
- *Other investigations*: Electroencephalography, intracranial pressure monitoring, and carotid angiography are rarely done in selected cases.

Observation of Head Injury Cases

- *Continuous monitoring of clinical state* is done in all head injury cases:
  - *Vital signs*—temperature, pulse, blood pressure, and respiration
  - *Neurological status*—GCS, pupils, limb movements, and other deficits.

  Great majority of cases recover but a small number pass into progressive deeper coma due to cerebral edema or intracranial hemorrhage indicated by developments of signs of increased intracranial pressure.
- *Features of cerebral compression (increased intracranial pressure)—deteriorating LOC, dilatation of pupil and loss of light reflex, increasing blood pressure, decreasing pulse rate, Cheyne-Stokes respiration, and localizing signs—(Jacksonian fits/limb weakness or paralysis/other neurological deficits).*
- *It is very important to recognize these signs of cerebral compression and in all such cases CT scan must be done to distinguish between the cases of diffuse cerebral edema, or a space occupying lesion such as intracranial hematoma as surgical intervention is a must in the latter.*

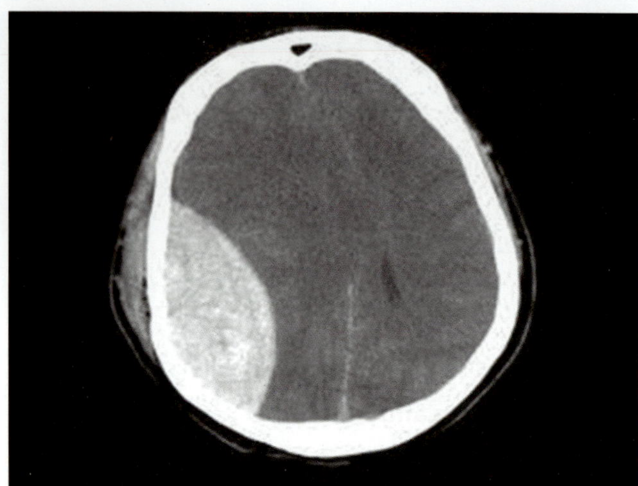

Fig. 13: Computed tomography (CT) scan showing "biconvex" shadow of extradural hematoma.

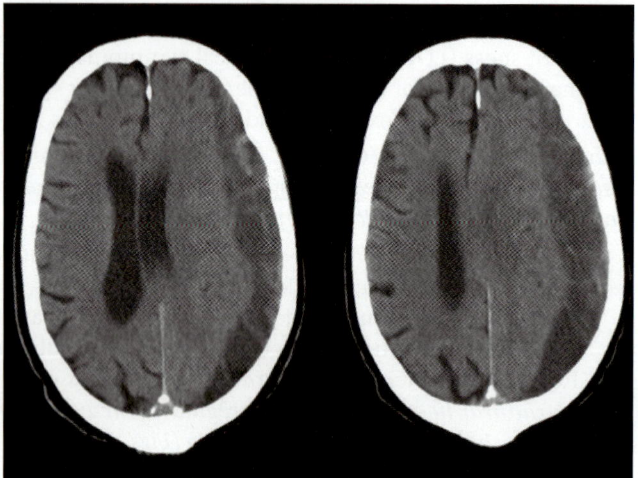

Fig. 14: Computed tomography (CT) scan showing "concavo-convex" irregular shadow of subdural hematoma.

MANAGEMENT OF HEAD INJURY

All patients with *minor head injuries (GCS 9 or above)* and without skull fractures may be allowed to go home after initial evaluation and treatment, provided relatives are warned to bring back if headache/drowsiness/vomiting/visual disturbances develop.

- *Indications for admission*:
  - Confusion/decreased LOC
  - Skull fracture
  - Any neurological signs/headache/vomiting
  - Difficulty in assessment, e.g. alcoholics/epileptics
  - Associated other medical condition
  - Social factors (lack of relatives)
  - All medicolegal cases.

All patients are observed carefully after admission and if they develop any symptoms/signs of increased ICT or localizing signs, they are subjected to immediate CT scan. *All patients with fracture skull are admitted regardless of GCS and have an elective CT scan done for a review.*

All *major head injury* cases are admitted in intensive care unit (ICU), intubated, and IPPR instituted. A CT Scan is done in all cases for further assessment. *All cases who develop localizing signs may have immediately to be shifted to operation theater if CT scan is not available.*

Patients with *polytrauma and unstable vital signs* with GCS 8 or below are stabilized first, as hypovolemia and hypoxia themselves result in decreased LOC.

Nonsurgical Therapy

- *Close monitoring of the patient*: Vital signs, neurological status, and input/output chart.
- *Intravenous fluids*: Maintenance fluids as required; avoid 5% dextrose as it will increase cerebral edema.
- *Tetanus prophylaxis/antibiotics.*
- *H2 receptor blockers*: To prevent *"Cushing's ulcers",* i.e. stomach ulcers developing in head injury patients.
- *In all cases of open head injuries/seizures*: *Anticonvulsants—phenytoin* 300 mg tds IV/orally.
- *In all moderate/severe head injury cases*: To prevent increased intracranial tension (provided intracranial hematoma is excluded), mannitol—1 g/kg IV; 250 mL of 20% mannitol IV over 20 minutes every 8 hourly or Lasix—40–80 mg IV 8 hourly.
- *Steroids*: *Role of steroids is controversial* but these are useful in severe head injury cases as they help in decreasing the brain edema. Dexamethasone is given 4–8 mg IV 8 hourly.
- *Care of unconscious patient*: Care of airway/eye/skin/bladder/bowel/mouth/limbs/nutrition—oral or parenteral.

Surgical Management

About 10% of head injury patients need surgical intervention. The importance of prompt detection and evacuation of intracranial mass lesion before it produces secondary damage is very important. *An urgent CT scan is very useful for this, but if it is not available or there is an unacceptable delay in arranging it, exploratory burr hole can be considered as a primary diagnostic procedure in patients with clinical suspicion of traumatic transtentorial herniation.*

Exploratory Burr Hole Operation

- *Indications for exploratory burr hole operation*:
  - All patients with traumatic tentorial herniation with stable vital signs.
  - Patients with progressive neurological symptoms/signs indicative of mass lesion causing cerebral compression.
- *Technique of operation*:
  - *Site of burr hole*: Initial *burr hole* is made in temporal region 3 cm above and midway between orbit and external auditory meatus on the side indicated by findings in the x-ray and CT scan. If CT scan is not available, it is done on *same side of dilated pupil/obvious external evidence of trauma (contusion/raccoon eye/battle's sign/skull fracture) or the side contralateral to any progressive motor deficit, e.g. hemiparesis/hemiplegia.*
  - If significant hematoma is found (>75 mm thick), a standard *craniotomy* is done by making further burr holes and raising the skull flap to evacuate the hematoma, ligating or clipping the bleeding vessel, arrest of all hemorrhage, clearing of all the dead necrotic tissue and clots, and hitching of dura before closing the wound.
  - In case of negative findings after the temporal burr hole, a frontal or a parietal burr hole, or even a contralateral burr hole (countercoup injury) may have to be performed to clinch the diagnosis and management of the intracranial lesion (Fig. 15).

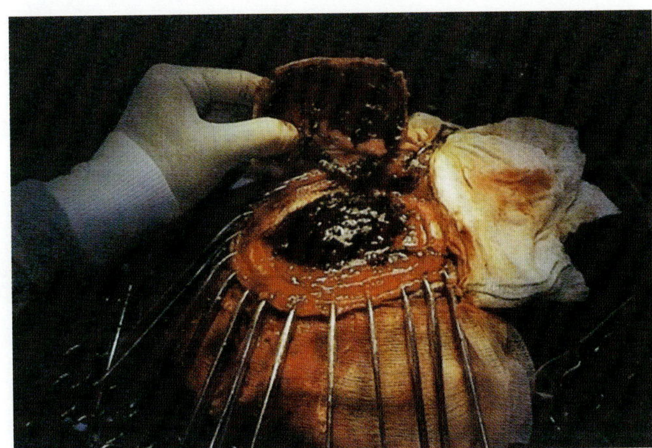

Fig. 15: Craniotomy in a case of head injury.

Treatment of Specific Conditions

Depressed Skull Fractures

The most common indication for surgery in depressed fractures is for cosmetic deformity. Surgery is also indicated in suspicion of dural tear, underlying intracranial hematoma, or depressed fragment occluding a dural venous sinus. In all cases elevation of the fracture fragment done with taking utmost care of underlying dural sinus. A compound fracture will require removal of all contaminated tissues and contused brain tissue, evacuation of hematoma, control of hemorrhage with repair of underlying dura, and restoration of bony defect by reconstructive surgery.

Penetrating Injuries

Most of the intracranial bullet injuries are usually fatal. In rare cases which survive, debridement of scalp wound, evacuation of hematoma, and pulped brain done with appropriate dural closure and overlying defect.

Traumatic Cerebrospinal Fluid Leakage

Traumatic otorrhea usually closes spontaneously but will require repair of leak if persists for more than 2 weeks. Traumatic rhinorrhea associated with fracture of underlying bones requires reduction of fracture and repair of tear.

COMPLICATIONS OF HEAD INJURY

- *Early complications*: Brain stem injury, posterior fossa compression, CSF rhinorrhea/otorrhea, aerocele, meningitis, pituitary failure.
- *Late complications*: Chronic subdural hematoma, post-traumatic epilepsy (early/late), post-traumatic headache, and psychiatric disorders.

Out of all severe head injury cases, the mortality is 50% while 10% have severe disability throughout life. The remaining 40% cases have good recovery with moderate disability.

A general surgeon's acumen lies in identifying the cases which need emergency surgery, at times even without CT scan and need of the referral of the patient to specialized neurological center.

CHAPTER

22 Chest Trauma

OBJECTIVES

- Thoracic Wall Injuries
- Subcutaneous Emphysema
- Pulmonary Contusion
- Pulmonary Laceration
- Pneumothorax
- Hemothorax
- Other Injuries

INTRODUCTION

Trauma is a leading cause of morbidity and mortality all over the world. About 25% of all trauma deaths are contributed by thoracic injuries. Frequently, thoracic trauma is accompanied by multiorgan damage which adds to the morbidity. Early diagnosis and management are the key to reduce morbidity and mortality. The management is essentially multidisciplinary, beginning right at the accident site, continuing through transport and into the hospital.

Thoracic injuries can be classified on the basis of the anatomical region involved as:

- Thoracic wall
- Lung
- Mediastinum
- Diaphragm.

On the basis of mode of injury, they can further be classified as:

- Blunt or nonpenetrating
- Penetrating.

THORACIC WALL INJURIES

Thoracic wall injuries account for 50% of all chest traumas. An intact thoracic wall includes the ribs, the sternum, and the intervening muscles. An injury to any one of these components disturbs the normal physiology of breathing by affecting adequate chest expansion. The most common form of chest wall injury is rib fracture. The others include sternal fracture, costochondral separation, flail chest, and traumatic asphyxia.

Rib Fracture

One or more ribs may be fractured due to either blunt or penetrating injury. They are more common in adults due to inelasticity of the chest wall as compared to children who are resistant due to compliant chest wall. Older people are more susceptible to rib fractures due to osteoporotic changes consistent with age.

The susceptibility to rib fracture increases with age. The importance of this injury is not the fracture itself but rather the associated potential complications, particularly pneumothorax, hemothorax, pulmonary contusions, and post-traumatic pneumonia. Rib fractures in children signify serious trauma to the thorax and have a high incidence of underlying injury.

The fourth through ninth ribs are most commonly involved. Ribs 1–3 are relatively protected while ribs 10–12 are free-floating anteriorly. Ribs fracture usually posteriorly, near the posterior angle as it is the weakest point.

Simple rib fractures *per se* do not cause much morbidity, but the main symptoms are due to underlying organ damage, notably, lungs, liver, and spleen. Trauma to the lungs may result in pneumothorax, hemothorax, pulmonary contusion, and pneumonia. Lower rib fractures should be viewed with high suspicion of hepatic and splenic injuries. Patients with right-sided rib fractures are almost three times more likely to have a hepatic injury, and patients with left-sided rib fractures are almost four times more likely to have a splenic injury. Fractures of ribs 1–3 may indicate severe intrathoracic injury. The presence of two or more rib fractures at any level is associated with a higher incidence of internal injuries. Elderly patients with multiple rib fractures have a greater incidence of pneumonia and a higher mortality compared with patients younger than age 65 years.

Clinical Features

The patient presents with symptoms of pain at the concerned site and rapid breathing due to pain or underlying lung contusion. Clinically, diagnosis may be suspected on the basis of bony tenderness, crepitus, overlying ecchymosis, and overlying muscle spasm. Diagnosis can also be made by demonstrating mobility at the fracture site by barrel compression test (bimanual compression of the thoracic cage remote from the site of injury).

Diagnosis

Diagnosis can be made clinically with proper examination. Chest radiograph is the most common investigation ordered in emergency department. But single rib fractures are easily missed on chest radiograph. CT scan of the thorax is highly sensitive for the diagnosis. However, CT scan is not routinely needed unless other intrathoracic pathologies or other accompanied injuries need to be ruled out. X-ray studies are often ordered, even though 50% of single-rib fractures are not seen on the initial X-ray film. A CT scan should be considered based on the mechanism of injury, physical examination, hemodynamic and respiratory parameters, abnormal findings on chest X-ray examination (especially widened mediastinum), or clinical evidence of multiple rib fractures, especially of the lower ribs (which may herald a splenic or hepatic injury).

Management

Basic management includes adequate analgesia and maintenance of pulmonary function. Oral analgesics are sufficient for young and fit people with no other comorbidities. They should be encouraged to perform deep breathing exercises preferably incentive spirometry 30–40 minutes after having analgesic.

Patients with three or more rib fractures should be admitted in indoor patient department and closely watched for development of complications like pneumothorax, hemothorax, and pneumonia. Analgesia can be provided either intravenously or with local nerve block using lignocaine or bupivacaine. Such intercostal nerve blocks are achieved by administration of 1–2% lidocaine or 0.25% bupivacaine along the inferior rib margin several centimeters posterior to the site of the fracture. One rib above and one rib below the fractured rib should also be blocked for optimal analgesia. Thoracic epidural analgesia is also an effective choice.

Strapping or chest binders should be avoided because even though they reduce pain, they also reduce pulmonary excursion by the splinting action hence reducing the reserve.

Elderly patients should particularly be monitored for development of atelectasis and pneumonia.

Prognosis

Rib fractures with no accompanying injuries usually heal uneventfully in 3–4 weeks. Higher the number of ribs involved, higher the morbidity and mortality associated with it. Associated comorbidities like old age, chronic obstructive pulmonary disease (COPD), and multiple organ injuries are associated with a longer hospital stay.

Sternal Fracture

Sternal fractures and displacements are caused by blunt trauma to anterior chest wall due to restraints like seatbelts and steering wheel in motor vehicle accidents. Risk factors for sternal fracture from blunt trauma include types of vehicular passenger restraint systems and patient age. Restrained passengers are more likely than unrestrained passengers to sustain sternal fracture. In fact, the rate of occurrence of sternal fractures has increased threefold since the use of across-the-shoulder seat belts became widespread. The location of the sternal fracture varies depending on the position of the belt, patient size, the magnitude of the impact, and the vector of the forces.

They may be associated with blunt trauma to intrathoracic organs like myocardial contusion or lung contusion. Aortic rupture is extremely rare, but hematomas due to avulsion of minor vessels are common. Rib fractures may be associated with sternal injuries. Sternal fractures are more common in older patients than in younger patients, and they are slightly more common in women than in men. It is believed that the more elastic and pliable chest wall of younger people allow more efficient transmission of kinetic energy to the underlying mediastinum. Although skeletal injury is less likely to occur in younger patients, damage to soft tissue structures underneath is greater. In older patients, the energy of impact is dissipated in the sternum, resulting in fewer intrathoracic injuries but a higher frequency of sternal fractures. Multiple rib fractures and lung contusion are concomitant injuries in more than 10% of diagnosed sternal fractures.

Diagnosis can be made clinically by the presence of crepitus, bony tenderness, ecchymosis, or deformity. Lateral chest radiograph is diagnostic as most sterna fractures are transverse, unlike posteroanterior view in which minor fractures may be missed. It is advisable to order a chest computed tomography (CT) as underlying mediastinal injuries can be ruled out. These fractures can be missed radiographically because a lateral plain chest X-ray film is not usually obtained during the initial trauma evaluation. Furthermore, plain films are sometimes inconclusive. Even if the sternal fracture is diagnosed by plain radiographs, the extent of the injury is often underappreciated. The advent of helical CT, especially with three-dimensional images of the skeletal system, has resulted in markedly improved diagnosis of sternal fractures. Emerging literature suggests that ultrasound (US) may be more sensitive than plain radiography.

Treatment includes providing adequate analgesia. Majority of the patients with undisplaced fractures can be discharged home on oral analgesics with conservative management. But patients with displaced fractures or bony fragments impinging on skin and those with respiratory compromise should undergo operative fixation.

Costochondral Separation

This form of injury is also caused by blunt trauma to anterior chest wall. It may be associated with rib fracture. Bilateral costochondral joint separation can sometimes result in flail chest, but it is very rare. Chest radiograph is usually normal but there is a snapping sensation with deep respiration. Management is conservative, but healing takes longer due to poor vascularity at the cartilage.

Flail Chest

Flail chest is a fairly rare form of chest injury that is most often accompanied by a significant underlying pulmonary parenchymal injury and can be a life-threatening thoracic injury. Cause is usually high velocity blunt trauma to the chest. Flail chest occurs when three or more adjacent ribs are fractured at two or more sites allowing a freely moving segment of the chest wall to move in paradoxical motion. It can also occur with costochondral separation or vertical sternal fracture in combination with rib fractures. Because of its common association with pulmonary contusion, it is one of the most serious chest wall injuries.

Flail chest results in derangement of respiratory physiology. Paradoxical movement of the flail segment is the hallmark feature. The flail segment moves in with inspiration and out with expiration. This reduces the respiratory reserve. Accompanying pulmonary contusion and atelectasis due to splinting due to pain also result in decreased pulmonary function. This may result in hypoxemia and decreased cardiac output.

Clinical Features

Patient comes to emergency department in respiratory distress. There is pain, tenderness, and crepitus at the concerned site. The paradoxical movement can be appreciated with proper examination. Endotracheal intubation and positive-pressure ventilation will internally splint the chest wall, making the flail segment difficult to detect on physical examination.

Diagnosis: Diagnosis is made on physical examination. Endotracheal intubation may make the diagnosis difficult due to internal splinting by positive-pressure ventilation.

Patient may have associated tension pneumothorax or hemopneumothorax.

Multiple rib fractures are readily identified on chest radiograph. However, for major chest trauma CT thorax is the preferred option as it also identifies underlying lung contusion.

Management

Out-of-hospital or emergency department (ED) stabilization of the flail segment by positioning the person with the injured side down or placing a sandbag on the affected segments has been abandoned. These interventions actually inhibit expansion of the chest and increase atelectasis of the injured lung.

Oxygen should be administered, cardiac and oximetry monitors applied if available, and the patient observed for signs of an associated injury such as tension pneumothorax. A 12-lead electrocardiogram (ECG) and cardiac enzymes should be obtained, with consideration given to obtaining an echocardiogram for significant dysrhythmias, high-grade blocks, or hemodynamic instability unexplained by other causes such as hemorrhage.

The cornerstones of management include adequate analgesia, oxygenation, chest physiotherapy, selective intubation, and close observation for respiratory compromise. Associated pulmonary injuries add to the morbidity caused by flail chest. Respiratory decompensation is the primary indication for endotracheal intubation and mechanical ventilation for patients with flail chest. Obvious problems, such as hemopneumothorax or severe pain, should be corrected before intubation and ventilation are presumed necessary. In fact, in the awake and cooperative patient, noninvasive continuous positive airway pressure (CPAP) by mask may obviate the need for intubation. In general, the most conservative methods for maintaining adequate oxygenation and preventing complications should be used.

In a cooperative patient, noninvasive ventilation by continuous positive airway pressure is better tolerated and associated with least complications. Analgesia can be provided by intercostal nerve block or high epidural or patient controlled analgesia. Patients treated with intercostal nerve blocks or high segmental epidural analgesia, oxygen, intensive chest physiotherapy, careful fluid management, and CPAP, with intubation reserved for patients in whom this therapy fails, have shorter hospital courses, fewer complications, and lower mortality rates.

Recovery is faster with internal fixation of fractured segments. Endotracheal intubation should be avoided as far as possible as it increases the chances of pneumonia. Internal fixation has better cosmetic and functional results, and it is cost-effective. Indications for open fixation for flail chest include patients who are unable to be weaned from the ventilator secondary to the mechanics of flail chest, persistent pain, severe chest wall instability, and a progressive decline in pulmonary functions.

SUBCUTANEOUS EMPHYSEMA

Subcutaneous emphysema in the presence of chest wall trauma usually indicates a more serious thoracic injury. Although the presence of air in the tissues is a benign condition, in the context of chest trauma it usually represents serious injury to any air-containing structure within the thorax. Air enters the tissues either extrapleurally or intrapleurally. Extrapleural tears in the tracheobronchial tree allow air to leak into the mediastinum and soft tissues of the anterior neck, producing a pneumomediastinum, which rarely may progress to a tension pneumomediastinum. This most often occurs in patients who are undergoing positive-pressure ventilation and have a pneumopericardium visible on chest X-ray examination. They may also have Hamman's crunch, which is a crackling sound with each heartbeat, heard on cardiac auscultation. Intrapleural lesions, however, usually produce a pneumothorax by allowing air to escape the lung through the visceral pleura into the pleural space and then through the parietal pleura into the thoracic wall.

An esophageal tear resulting from Boerhaaves syndrome or penetrating injury may also produce a pneumomediastinum manifested by subcutaneous emphysema over the supraclavicular area and anterior neck. An additional cause of subcutaneous emphysema, which may or may not be indicative of intrathoracic injury, is found immediately adjacent to a penetrating wound of the thorax. A small amount of air may be introduced into the adjacent subcutaneous tissues from the outside at the time of penetration.

Although subcutaneous emphysema is a benign condition, massive accumulations can be uncomfortable to the patient. The underlying cause, such as pneumothorax, ruptured bronchus, or ruptured esophagus, is treated appropriately. Benign pneumomediastinum secondary to a Valsalva maneuver is treated with observation and high-flow oxygen to facilitate the reabsorption of nitrogen from tissues because the volume of nitrogen causes the discomfort.

PULMONARY CONTUSION

Pulmonary contusion is reported to be present in 30–75% of patients with significant blunt chest trauma, most often from motor vehicle crash (MVCs) with rapid deceleration. Pulmonary contusion can also be caused by high-velocity missile wounds and the high-energy shock waves of an explosion in air or water. Pulmonary contusion is the most common significant chest injury in children.

Pulmonary contusion is a direct bruise of the lung parenchyma followed by alveolar edema and hemorrhage but without an accompanying pulmonary laceration.

Clinical Features

The clinical manifestations include dyspnea, tachypnea, cyanosis, tachycardia, hypotension, and chest wall bruising. There are no specific signs for pulmonary contusion, but hemoptysis may be seen sometime during the patient's course, and moist rales or absent breath sounds may be heard on auscultation. Palpation of the chest wall commonly reveals fractured ribs. If flail chest is discovered, pulmonary contusion is commonly present.

Diagnosis

Typical radiographic findings begin to appear within minutes of injury and range from patchy, irregular, and alveolar infiltrate to frank consolidation. Usually, these changes are present on the initial examination, and they are almost always present within 6 hours. The rapidity of changes on chest X-ray visualization usually correlates with the severity of the contusion. Pulmonary contusion should be differentiated from acute respiratory distress syndrome (ARDS), with which it is often confused because the radiographic appearance of the two conditions may be similar. The contusion usually manifests within minutes of the initial injury, is usually localized to a segment or a lobe, is often apparent on the initial chest study, and tends to last 48–72 hours. ARDS is diffuse, and its development is usually delayed, with onset typically between 24 and 72 hours after injury.

The increased frequency of CT scans for blunt trauma patients has resulted in a corresponding increase in the diagnosis of pulmonary contusion. CT scans have been shown to detect twice as many pulmonary contusions as plain radiographs. Some authors suggest that pulmonary contusions visible only on CT scan and not on plain radiographs may not be clinically significant.

Chest CT scan is particularly valuable to identify a pulmonary contusion in the acute phase after injury because plain chest X-ray films have a low sensitivity. Arterial blood gases may be helpful in making the diagnosis of pulmonary contusion because most patients are hypoxemic at the time of admission. A low partial pressure of oxygen (PO_2) alone may be reason to suspect pulmonary contusion. A widening alveolar-arterial oxygen difference indicates a decreasing pulmonary diffusion capacity of the patient's contused lung, and it is one of the earliest and most accurate means of assessing the current status, progress, and prognosis.

Management

Treatment for pulmonary contusion is primarily supportive. When only one lung has been severely contused and has caused significant hypoxemia, consideration should be given to intubating and ventilating each lung separately with a dual-lumen endotracheal tube and two ventilators. This allows for the difference in compliance between the injured and the normal lung and prevents hyperexpansion of one lung and gradual collapse of the other. As with flail chest, however, intubation and mechanical ventilation should be avoided if possible because they are associated with an increase in morbidity, including pneumonia, sepsis, pneumothorax, hypercoagulability, and longer hospitalization. The need for mechanical ventilation increases significantly when the area of pulmonary contusion exceeds 20% of total lung volume.

Certain patients may benefit from a trial of noninvasive positive-pressure ventilation with bilevel positive airway pressure (BPAP) or CPAP to avoid intubation and mechanical ventilation. Certain procedures may ameliorate the pulmonary contusion, including the restriction of intravenous fluids to maintain intravascular volume within strict limits and aggressive supportive care consisting of vigorous tracheobronchial toilet, suctioning, and pain relief. These maneuvers may preclude the need for ventilator support and allow a more selective approach to flail chest and pulmonary contusion.

PULMONARY LACERATION

The lungs are most often lacerated from penetrating injury, but they may also be injured by the inward projection of a fractured rib or avulsion of a pleural adhesion. These injuries are usually minor and rarely life-threatening, and they can usually be treated with continuous oxygen therapy, observation, or tube thoracostomy. Severe lacerations are present in only 3% of patients with thoracic trauma, and they are usually associated with hemopneumothorax, multiple displaced rib fractures, and hemoptysis. Often, these life-threatening lacerations require thoracotomy with resection or tractotomy to control bleeding.

PNEUMOTHORAX

Pneumothorax, which is the accumulation of air in the pleural space, is a common complication of chest trauma. It is reported to be present in 15–50% of patients who sustain significant chest trauma, and it is invariably present in those with transpleural penetrating injuries.

Depending on whether there is a communication with the atmosphere, pneumothorax is divided into three types:

1. Simple
2. Communicating
3. Tension.

A pneumothorax is considered simple when there is no communication with the atmosphere or any shift of the mediastinum or hemidiaphragm resulting from the accumulation of air. It can be graded according to the degree of collapse as visualized on the chest radiograph. A small pneumothorax occupies 15% or less of the pleural cavity, a moderate one 15–60%, and a large pneumothorax more than 60%. Traumatic pneumothorax is most often caused by a fractured rib that is driven inward, lacerating the pleura. It may also occur without a fracture when the impact is delivered at full inspiration with the glottis closed, leading to a tremendous increase in intra-alveolar pressure and the subsequent rupture of the alveoli. A penetrating injury, such as a gunshot or stab wound, may also produce a simple pneumothorax if there is no free communication with the atmosphere.

A communicating pneumothorax is associated with a defect in the chest wall and most commonly occurs in combat injuries. In the civilian sector, this injury is typically secondary to shotgun wounds. Air can sometimes be heard flowing sonorously in and out of the defect, prompting the term "sucking chest wound." The loss of chest wall integrity causes the involved lung to paradoxically collapse on inspiration and expand slightly on expiration, forcing air in and out of the wound. This results in a large functional dead space for the normal lung and, together with the loss of ventilation of the involved lung, produces a severe ventilatory disturbance.

The progressive accumulation of air under pressure within the pleural cavity, with shift of the mediastinum to the opposite hemithorax and compression of the contralateral lung and great vessels, is the constellations of findings in tension pneumothorax. It occurs when the injury acts like a one-way valve, and prevents free bilateral communication with the atmosphere, and leads to a progressive increase of intrapleural pressure. Air enters on inspiration but cannot exit with expiration. The resulting shift of mediastinal contents compresses the vena cava and distorts the cavoatrial junction, leading to decreased diastolic filling of the heart and subsequent decreased cardiac output. These changes result in the rapid onset of hypoxia, acidosis, and shock.

Clinical Features

Shortness of breath and chest pain is the most common presenting complaints of pneumothorax. The patient's appearance is highly variable, ranging from acutely ill with cyanosis and tachypnea to misleadingly healthy. The signs and symptoms are not always correlated with the degree of pneumothorax. The physical examination may reveal decreased or absent breath sounds and hyper-resonance over the involved side as well as subcutaneous emphysema, but small pneumothoraces may not be detectable on physical examination.

Patients with tension pneumothorax become acutely ill within minutes and develop severe cardiovascular and respiratory distress. They are dyspneic, agitated, restless, cyanotic, tachycardic, and hypotensive, and display decreasing mental activity. The cardinal signs of tension pneumothorax are tachycardia, jugular venous distention (JVD), and absent breath sounds on the ipsilateral side. However, JVD may not reliably be present with massive blood loss. Hypotension will not occur as early as hypoxia and may represent a preterminal event.

Diagnostic Strategies

Because intrapleural air tends to collect at the apex of the lung, the initial chest radiograph should be an upright full inspiratory film if the patient's condition permits. An upright film will often reveal small pleural effusions that are not visible on supine films, and it also allows better visualization of the mediastinum. Although the chest radiograph has traditionally been the preferred initial study for diagnosing a simple pneumothorax, emerging literature suggests that a simple pneumothorax can be identified during the initial US examination of the trauma patient as part of the extended focused assessment with sonography in trauma (E-FAST) examination.

If a pneumothorax is suspected but not visualized on the initial inspiratory film, an expiratory film should be obtained because it makes the pneumothorax more apparent by reducing the lung volume. Notably, as many as one-third of initial chest X-ray films will not detect a pneumothorax in trauma patients. Although it is not recommended as a primary method of diagnosing pneumothorax, CT is very sensitive in finding small pneumothoraces even in supine patients.

Management

Simple Pneumothorax

Treatment of a simple pneumothorax depends on its cause and size. Most advocate treating a traumatic pneumothorax with a chest tube to correct any respiratory compromise; treatment with a chest tube is generally thought to be safer than observation in these patients. Small pneumothoraces (i.e. <15%), whether spontaneous or traumatic, have been treated with hospitalization and careful observation if the patient is otherwise healthy and symptom-free, if the patient does not need anesthesia or positive-pressure ventilation, and the pneumothorax is not increasing in size.

Isolated apical pneumothoraces of less than 25% may be observed in patients with stab wounds. This conservative method seldom has application in multisystem trauma, and a chest tube should be inserted immediately on any signs of deterioration. Some suggest that because it is small and lacks symptoms, occult traumatic pneumothorax found only on CT scan can be managed with observation and does not need treatment. Studies indicate that these injuries can be handled as small but initially detectable pneumothoraces, with observation in hemodynamically stable patients without symptoms. The data regarding the frequency with which patients with occult pneumothorax on mechanical ventilation will require tube thoracostomy are conflicting. However, an occult pneumothorax may be observed in a stable patient even if he or she is placed on positive-pressure ventilation.

Any moderate to large pneumothorax should be treated with a chest tube. The preferred site for insertion is the fourth or fifth intercostal space at the midaxillary line. If the tube is positioned posteriorly and directed toward the apex, it can effectively remove both air and fluid. This lateral placement of the tube is preferred not only because it is more efficient but also because it does not produce an easily visible cosmetic defect, as does the anterior site at the second interspace at the midclavicular line.

Care is taken to be certain the vent holes along the side of the tube are all inside the chest cavity. A radiopaque line along the side of the tube with interruptions at these drainage holes helps greatly in radiographically interpreting tube position. The tube should be attached to a water seal drainage system that allows re-expansion of the pneumothorax. If there is significant air leak or a large hemothorax, the tube may be connected to a source of constant vacuum at 20–30 cm H_2O for more rapid re-expansion.

Tube thoracostomy does have some potentially serious complications, including the formation of a hemothorax, pulmonary edema, bronchopleural fistula, pleural leaks, empyema, subcutaneous emphysema, infection, intercostal artery laceration, contralateral pneumothorax, and parenchymal injury. To reduce the incidence of empyema and pneumonitis, current recommendations include the administration of empirical antibiotics with all tube thoracostomy placements. Pneumothoraces that have been present for more than 3 days should be re-expanded gradually without suction to avoid re-expansion pulmonary edema.

Communicating Pneumothorax

For a patient with a communicating pneumothorax in the out-of-hospital setting, the defect should be covered immediately, which helps convert the condition to a closed pneumothorax and eliminates the major physiologic abnormality. An occlusive dressing of petrolatum gauze can be applied, but care should be taken because this can convert the injury to a tension pneumothorax, especially in patients who are intubated and undergoing positive-pressure ventilation. The wound should never be packed because the negative-pressure during inspiration can suck the dressing into the chest cavity. These considerations are not as important once the patient is in the ED, where endotracheal intubation and tube thoracostomy can be performed. Positive-pressure ventilation can then be started without the fear of producing a tension pneumothorax, and the patient can be prepared for definitive surgical repair.

Tension Pneumothorax

When the diagnosis of tension pneumothorax is suspected clinically, the pressure should be relieved immediately with needle thoracostomy, which is performed by inserting a large-bore (14-gauge or larger) catheter, at least 5 cm in length, through the second or third interspace anteriorly or the fourth or fifth interspace laterally on the involved side. Recent studies have suggested that some catheters may not be of sufficient length to penetrate the pleural space and that the lateral approach may be preferred. This method can be easily performed in the field or ED, allowing vital signs to improve during transport or preparation for a tube thoracostomy.

The intubated patient in the ED who is receiving positive-pressure ventilation and external cardiac compressions is at particular risk for developing tension pneumothorax. Fractured ribs from cardiopulmonary resuscitation (CPR) can penetrate lung parenchyma and cause pneumothorax. Positive-pressure ventilation then increases intrapleural pressure and produces a tension pneumothorax. The earliest sign of this complication is an increase in resistance to ventilation. If the patient has vital signs, the blood pressure will fall and the central venous pressure (CVP) will rise. Misplacement of an endotracheal tube does not result in tension pneumothorax but, rather, asymmetry of breath sounds. If tension pneumothorax is suggested, the clinician should proceed with empirical emergent therapy.

HEMOTHORAX

Hemothorax is the collection of blood in pleural cavity. It is commonly associated with pneumothorax (25% of cases) as well as extrathoracic injuries (73% of cases).

Hemorrhage from injured lung parenchyma is the most common cause of hemothorax, but this tends to be self-limited unless there is a major laceration. Specific vessels are less often the source of hemorrhage, with intercostal and internal mammary arteries causing hemothorax more often than hilar or great vessels. Bleeding from the intercostal arteries may be brisk, however, because they branch directly from the aorta.

Close monitoring of the initial and ongoing rate of blood loss is performed. Immediate drainage of more than 1,500 mL of blood from the pleural cavity is usually considered an indication for urgent thoracotomy. Perhaps even more predictive of the need for thoracotomy is a continued output of at least 200 mL/hour for 3 hours.

Clinical Features

Depending on the rate and quantity of hemorrhage, varying degrees of hypovolemic shock will be manifested. Tactile fremitus is decreased, and breath sounds are diminished or absent.

Diagnostic Strategies

The upright chest radiograph remains the primary diagnostic study in the acute evaluation of hemothorax. A hemothorax is noted as meniscus of fluid blunting the costophrenic angle and tracking up the pleural margins of the chest wall when viewed on the upright chest X-ray film. Blunting of the costophrenic angles on upright chest radiograph requires at least 200–300 mL of fluid. The supine view chest film is less accurate, and it may be more difficult to make the diagnosis with the patient in this position. Unfortunately, this is often the only film available because of the patient's unstable condition. In the supine patient, blood layers posteriorly, creating a diffuse haziness that can be rather subtle, depending on the volume of the hemothorax. With a massive hemothorax, the large volume of blood can create a tension hemothorax, with signs and symptoms of both obstructive and hemorrhagic shock.

As is the case with pneumothoraces, US has much greater sensitivity than chest radiography in the detection of a small hemothorax, but CT scanning has the highest sensitivity.

Management

Treatment of hemothorax consists of restoring the circulating blood volume, controlling the airway as necessary, and evacuating the accumulated blood. Tube thoracostomy allows constant monitoring of the blood loss, and serial chest radiographs help monitor lung re-expansion. A large-bore tube should be inserted in the fifth interspace at the anterior axillary line and connected to underwater seal drainage and suction (20–30 mL H_2O).

Close monitoring of the initial and ongoing rate of blood loss is performed. Immediate drainage of more than 1,500 mL of blood from the pleural cavity is usually considered an indication for urgent thoracotomy. Perhaps even more predictive of the need for thoracotomy is a continued output of at least 200 mL/hour for 3 hours.

Although small hemothoraces may be observed in stable patients, a moderate hemothorax or any hemothorax in an unstable or symptomatic patient requires tube thoracostomy. Severe or persistent hemorrhage requires thoracostomy or open thoracotomy. Studies are required to better delineate the size of a hemothorax detected on CT scan that requires tube thoracostomy drainage.

Autotransfusion has been successfully used in tube thoracostomy. Recent simplification and commercial availability of the equipment have made autotransfusion feasible in most EDs. Autotransfusion also eliminates the risk of incompatibility reactions and transmission of certain diseases such as hepatitis C. Because the majority of blood loss occurs immediately after tube thoracostomy placement, autotransfusion apparatus should be immediately available in the ED.

Video-assisted thoracic surgery (VATS) is particularly useful for evaluation and evacuation of retained hemothorax, control of bleeding from intercostal vessels, and diagnosis and repair of diaphragmatic injuries.

OTHER INJURIES

Other mediastinal structures can also be injured in thoracic trauma patients, namely, tracheobronchial tree, esophagus, aorta and major vessels, heart and diaphragm.

Depending on the structure injured, patient will present with different clinical features. Tracheobronchial tree injury may present with air-leak or subcutaneous emphysema. Esophageal injury may present with chest pain and food particles in chest tube. Injury to heart and major vessels is usually fatal and may present with cardiac tamponade or hemothorax. Diaphragmatic injuries may go unnoticed or may present with herniation of abdominal organs into thoracic cavity.

Diagnosis is made clinically and with CT thorax and abdomen.

Management includes initial stabilization followed by surgical correction of presenting organ injury.

CHAPTER

23 Abdominal Trauma

OBJECTIVES

- Pathophysiology
- Evaluation of Abdominal Trauma
- Investigations
- Management of Abdominal Injuries
- Laparotomy for Abdominal Injuries

INTRODUCTION

Abdominal trauma is the third leading cause of traumatic death after head and thoracic injuries in polytrauma cases and almost 27–55% of cases have history of alcoholic intoxication. Surgical intervention is needed in 25% cases of all abdominal injuries. *As Hippocrates knew, gut can be ruptured even if there is no visible external mark on abdominal wall.* A patient can die bleeding into his peritoneal cavity, especially from his ruptured liver, or spleen, or may succumb to peritonitis developing after a perforated bowel.

Abdominal cavity is the largest hollow space in body, lined by peritoneum and separated from the thoracic cavity by diaphragm. It contains various hollow organs of the digestive tract, gallbladder, and urinary bladder, as well as solid organs such as liver, spleen, pancreas, and kidneys. Any of these organs can be injured by different types of injuries especially due to a blunt or penetrating trauma or rarely, could be iatrogenic (Figs. 1A and B).

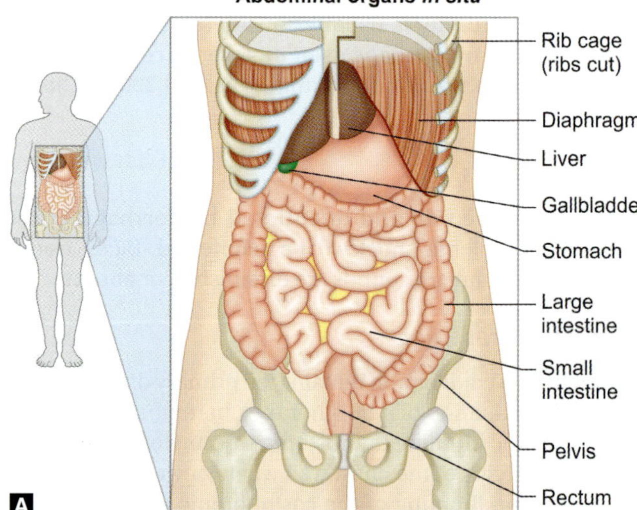

Figs. 1A and B: Abdominal organs.

Blunt Abdominal Injuries

Majority of the blunt injuries, i.e. 75%, are caused by road traffic accidents and common in elderly people. Compression forces from seatbelts or steering wheel can cause rupture of hollow organs and capsule of solid organs. Deceleration forces can tear organs from the peritoneum or blood vessel. Solid organs are more commonly involved than hollow organs in blunt injuries. Spleen is involved in 49% of all blunt injuries while liver is injured in 5% of cases. *They may be commonly associated with head injury, thoracic injury, and fractures of limb bones which should never be overlooked.*

Blunt abdominal injuries are notoriously difficult to diagnose accurately in initial stages due to variety of reasons. There may be no clearcut history available especially in children. Other more obvious injuries may distract the attention from abdomen which itself may be deceptively normal for first few hours after the injury. The patient may be drunk or unconscious from associated head injury. Even rupture of gut may not be associated with any external visible mark. Some injuries may not reveal themselves for many days, e.g. subcapsular hematoma of spleen, or a retroperitoneal injury of duodenum or pancreas. Thus, one has to be extra vigilant in all such cases.

A careful and repeated assessment of the patient is essential even if there is a slightest possibility of a patient having abdominal injury and such patients are always admitted for further observation and management.

Penetrating Abdominal Injuries (Fig. 2)

They are caused by penetrating sharp objects like knives, bullets, or animal horns. Stab wounds are three times more common than gunshot wounds. It is the depth of wound that matters

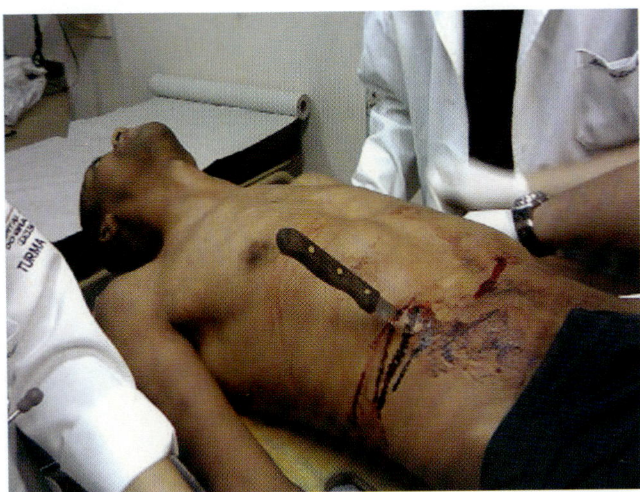

Fig. 2: Stab injury abdomen.

than its length. More severe injuries are often multiple and may penetrate patient's thorax and abdomen. Stab wounds often involve only the organs which they penetrate but bullet wounds may change the direction and involve multiple organs causing unpredictable damage. Liver, bowel, and diaphragm are more commonly involved. Midline wounds are more dangerous than flank wounds.

Wounds can enter the abdomen through chest/back/buttocks, or thigh. Always rule out hemothorax or hemopneumothorax in case of all thoracoabdominal injuries.

Iatrogenic Injuries

A small proportion of abdominal injuries can be iatrogenic occurring during some surgical procedures such as endoscopy, laparoscopy, percutaneous transhepatic cholangiograhy, liver biopsy, or peritoneal dialysis.

PATHOPHYSIOLOGY

Abdominal trauma can cause damage to the abdominal viscera in varieties of ways leading to increased morbidity and mortality.

- *Hemorrhage:* Severe hemorrhage could occur either intraperitoneally or extraperitoneally, leading to hemorrhagic shock evident clinically.
- *Disruption:* A hollow or solid organ may be disrupted leading to peritonitis presenting early or late. Small bowel is ruptured by compression forces or avulsed by shearing forces.
- *Infection:* Can be superimposed over initial chemical peritonitis, causing abscess or septicemia later.
- *Neurological deficit:* May accompany spinal/nerve root injuries.
- *Concurrent injuries:* Always rule out accompanying head injuries, thoracic injuries, diaphragmatic injuries, spinal injuries, and pelvic injuries in suspected abdominal trauma.

EVALUATION OF ABDOMINAL TRAUMA

Patient's History

A detailed history is essential of the abdominal injury cases. Exact mechanism of injury and point of impact is ascertained.

If blunt injury, type of road traffic accident or height of fall is noted. Whether the patient was wearing seatbelt and what was the vehicular damage is inquired. Almost all patients with blunt trauma will have persistent pain and/or vomiting. Severity and radiation of pain is important as shoulder tip pain will indicate liver or spleen injury because of irritation of diaphragm by blood (Kehr's sign). Any leaking gut or internal hemorrhage will be accompanied by concomittent abdominal pain.

In case of penetrating injury, ascertain the type of weapon, direction, and distance of impact, and amount of blood loss at the scene of accident.

Admit and observe the patient if you think that he might have abdominal injury as almost half of the patients will have it!

Examination of the Patient

- *Mental status*: Patient may be drowsy or unconscious if there is accompanying head injury, shock, or alcohol consumption.
- *Signs of shock*: May be evident by rapid thready pulse or hypotension as in case of internal hemorrhage. *If he has lost more blood than accounted for by known injuries or if he fails to improve after initial rapid resuscitation, it is a good indicator of internal bleeding!*
- *Breathing*: Shallow, irregular, grunting respiration may be indicative of underlying abdominal injury.
- *Inspect abdomen*: Note abdominal contour, movement of abdominal wall with respiration, and external wounds/bruises. Observe for ecchymosis in flanks ("Grey Turner's sign"), or around umbilicus ("Cullen's sign"), indicative of retroperitoneal bleeding. Bruising just below umbilical region in region of seatbelt may indicate intraabdominal injury ("Seatbelt sign") (Figs. 3 to 5).
- *Tenderness*: It is less marked in hemoperitoneum than in septic peritonitis but may be confused with muscle bruising. Pain on coughing and on percussion is more reliable. Note also intercostal tenderness (rib fractures) and back tenderness (retroperitoneal collection/pancreatic or kidney injuries).
- *Guarding and rigidity*: Guarding progressing to rigidity is a reliable sign of peritonitis, evident in cases of bowel injuries and perforation.
- *Dullness in flanks/shifting dullness*: Indicate intraperitoneal collection of blood or fluid.
- *Auscultation*: A "silent abdomen", i.e. absence of peristaltic sounds, or one which becomes silent later is a reliable sign of peritonitis.
- *Other examination*: Look for fractured ribs on left side indicative of splenic and right indicative of liver injuries. Examine head, thorax, spine, pelvis, and limbs to rule out any other concomittent injury. Be alert to rule out kidney injury in fracture of posterior rib or urethral/bladder injury in case of pelvic fractures.
- *Per rectum/Per vaginal (PR/PV) examination*: Fullness or tenderness in rectovesical (RV) pouch may indicate hemoperitoneum.

Special Methods of Examination

- *Insertion of nasogastric tube (NGT) and urinary catheter*: If blood is aspirated from stomach, it may indicate stomach injury while blood in urine may indicate bladder/kidney injury.
- *Abdominal girth*: It is important to measure the abdominal girth after putting NGT and keep a serial record of it by measuring it at the same place. Any increase in girth (2–3 cm is significant) will indicate paralytic ileus following hemoperitoneum or peritonitis.

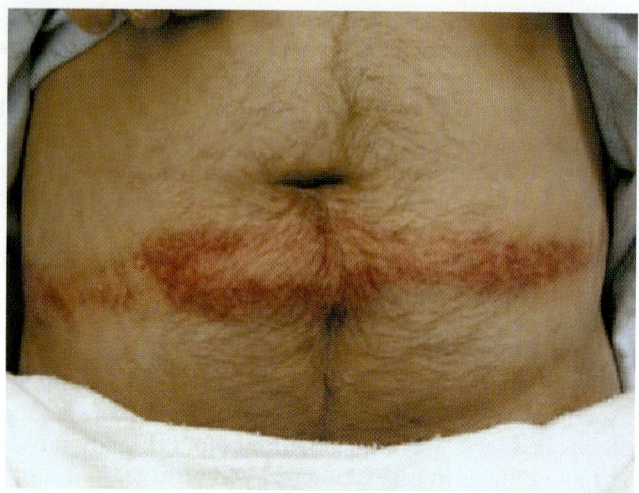

Fig. 3: Seatbelt sign.

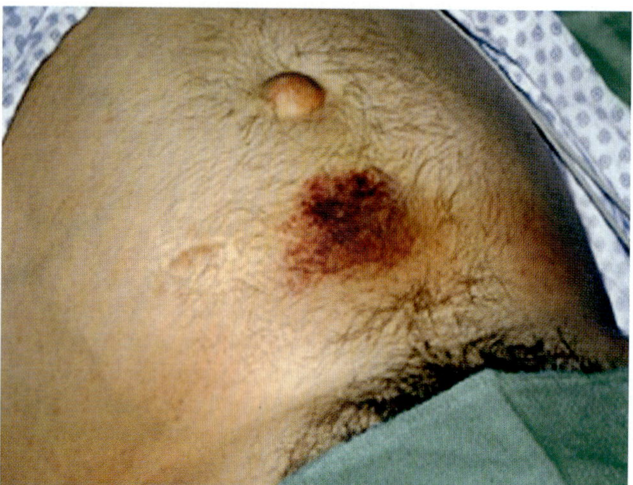

Fig. 4: Cullen's sign.

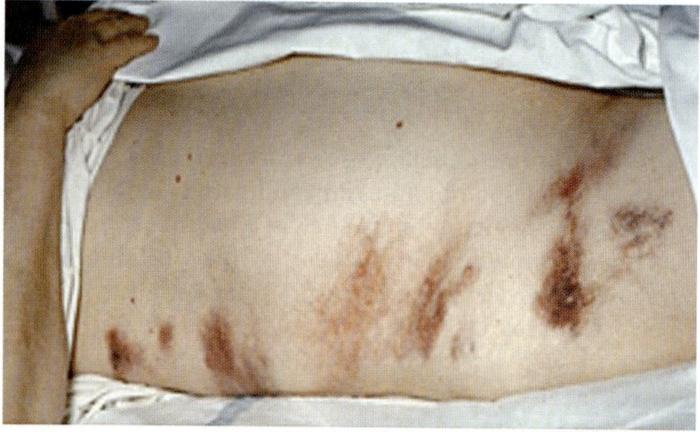

Fig. 5: Grey Turner's sign.

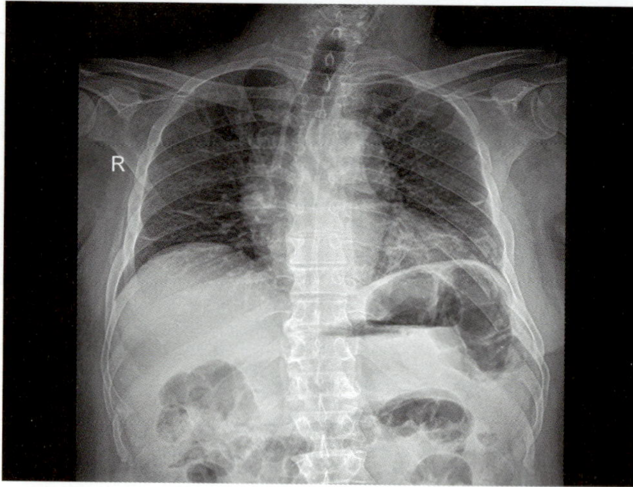

Fig. 6: Fractures of left lower ribs in splenic injury.

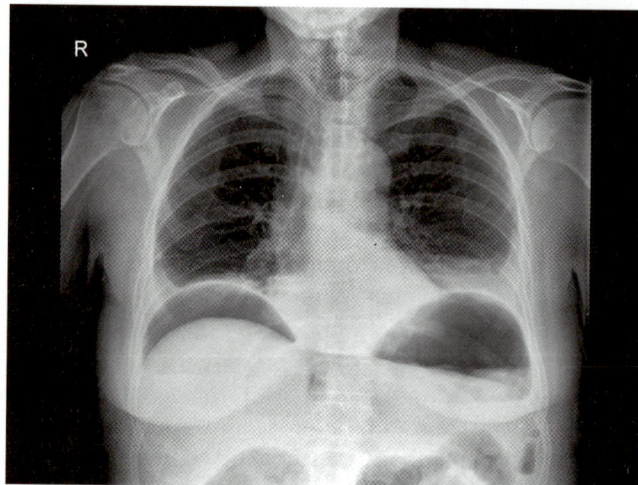

Fig. 7: Gas under diaphragm in case of bowel perforation.

INVESTIGATIONS

An unstable patient may have to be taken to operation theater directly!

- *Baseline investigations*: Complete hemogram, blood sugar, blood urea nitrogen (BUN) and serum creatinine, blood grouping and cross matching, bleeding and clotting time, serum amylase, serum electrolytes, blood gases, and urine examination are sent urgently.

  Leukocytosis of 15,000 or more is common in hemoperitoneum. A rupture of hollow organ does not raise the count so high. A low hemoglobin (Hb)/packed cell volume (PCV) may not be reliable as the patient will not become anemic until there is time for his blood to dilute.
- *X-rays*: X-rays of erect chest/abdomen may reveal gas under diaphragm in case of bowel perforation. Other relevant X-rays are also obtained of skull, spine, and limbs if indicated. Always take two X-rays—AP and lateral in case of bullet injuries to determine exact location of it and consider the possibility of the structures it may have traversed (Figs. 6 and 7).

  Signs of intra-abdominal injury on abdominal X-rays are:
  - Fractures of lower ribs indicating splenic/liver injuries
  - Gas under diaphragm indicating bowel rupture
  - Herniated viscera in pleural space
  - *"Ground glass appearance"* between intestinal loops suggestive of hemoperitoneum
  - Presence of bullets/foreign bodies in abdominal cavity
  - Obliteration of psoas shadow
  - Signs of "splenic injury" are—elevation of left hemi-diaphragm/opacity in left hypochondrium/indentation of stomach/displacement of stomach and splenic flexture medially

- *Diagnostic paracentesis*: Aspiration by a needle is performed in all four quadrants of abdomen ("4 Quadrant Tap"). Aspiration of 1–2 mL of blood (which is usually unclotted as it is defibrinated) is significant and indicates hemoperitoneum.
  A negative result does not rule out abdominal injury. If the aspiration is negative, it is repeated in a few hours. One may also occasionally aspirate urine (ruptured bladder), bile (perforated gut/peptic ulcer), feces, or pus (peritonitis).
- *Diagnostic peritoneal lavage (DPL)*: It is useful in doubtful cases especially in unconscious patients or multiple injuries with suspected abdominal injury. It is the mainstay of diagnosis in blunt injuries and has got 97% accuracy. A peritoneal dialysis catheter is put after putting a trocar and cannula and 500 mL of saline is infused in peritoneal cavity. The patient is put in supine position tilting him side-to-side for some time and infusion bottle lowered in position.
  A significant result suggesting abdominal injury is indicated by RBCs more than 10,000/cm, WBCs more than 500/cm, a bloody tap more than 20 mL or serum amylase more than 175 units, or presence of bile/bacteria/feces/food in the returning fluid, although a negative result does not exclude it.
- *Culdocentesis*: It is also a very useful method of diagnosing intraperitoneal bleeding in female patients.

Other Tests

- Contrast studies—gastrografin (bowel leaks)/intravenous pyelography (genitourinary injuries)/cystogram (bladder injury).
- *Abdominal ultrasonography (USG)*—very important in diagnosing liver/spleen/organ injuries, internal bleeding, presence of fluid/gas/fluid/foreign bodies in abdominal and genitourinary injuries (Fig. 8).
- *FAST (Focused Assessment with Sonography for Trauma)*—very useful investigation gaining importance in doubtful cases of internal bleed by focusing ultrasound beam in particular areas. Generally perihepatic, perisplenic, pericardial, and pelvic areas are specially examined. It takes 4–5 minutes and is 94% accurate in diagnosis.
- *Computed tomography (CT) scan and magnetic resonance imaging (MRI)*—are now frequently being used for more accurate diagnosis of site and extent of injury, genitourinary injuries, and detection of retroperitoneal hematomas.
- *Arteriograms*—done in selected cases of solid organ injury, renal arterial injury, and for therapeutic embolization.

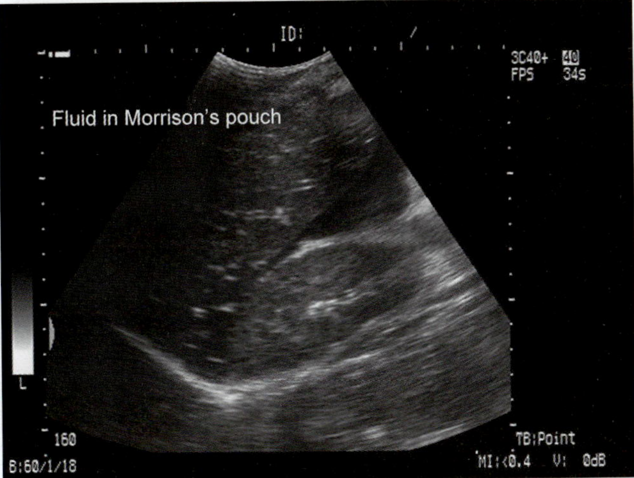

Fig. 8: Abdominal ultrasonography (USG) showing collection of fluid in Morrison's pouch.

MANAGEMENT OF ABDOMINAL INJURIES

- *Resuscitation and evaluation*:
  - A, B, C, D, E of resuscitation (maintenance of Airway, control of Breathing, restoration of Circulation, Care of Deformities and Evaluation of neurological status) instituted promptly.
  - Penetrating object not removed immediately and extruded viscera covered with sterile sheets.
- *On admission*:
  - Intravenous (IV) line/central venous pressure (CVP) inserted immediately, baseline investigations sent, and adequate amount of R.L./plasma/blood infused for control of shock.
  - Administration of oxygen.
  - Insertion of NGT for aspiration and indwelling urinary catheter for hourly monitoring of urine output done.
  - Injection tetanus toxoid (TT)/antibiotics/analgesics/H2 receptor inhibitors and other medications as indicated.
- *Blunt abdominal injuries*:
  - Continuous monitoring of patient—level of consciousness, pulse, blood pressure, respiration, input-output, oxygen saturation, abdominal girth every ½ hourly.
  - *"Don't wait too long for laparotomy, as the difference between best and worst surgery is much less than early and late surgery"!* Increasing pain, development of shock, and signs of peritonitis indicate the need for surgical intervention.
  - *If in doubt-"OPERATE"!* Few patients survive if peritonitis has been developing for 16 hours but most live if you operate within the first 6 hours. Occasional negative laparotomy is better than waiting for obvious signs of intra-abdominal injury.
- *Penetrating abdominal injuries*:
  - *Operate on all bullet wounds.*
  - *In case of stab wounds,* explore them in operation theater excising down up to peritoneum. If peritoneum is intact, close the wound by primary/delayed primary suture. If peritoneum is opened, laparotomy is done through standard incision. If plug of omentum is protruding through the wound, enlarge and explore the wound to rule out any injured viscera underneath.
  - Do not try to explore the abdomen by extending the wound as you may face anatomical difficulty. Always make a separate laparotomy incision.

LAPAROTOMY FOR ABDOMINAL INJURIES

- *Indications for laparotomy*: Laparotomy is indicated in abdominal injuries in following circumstances:
  - Signs of severe intraperitoneal bleeding (tachycardia, hypotension, restlessness, increasing pallor)
  - Signs of peritonitis (increasing tenderness, rebound tenderness, guarding, rigidity of abdominal wall)
  - Herniation of viscera through diaphragm, abdominal wall, and tag of omentum protruding through the wound

- Hematemesis, blood in gastric aspirate, or rectal bleeding
- Positive findings on gastric lavage, paracentesis, DPL, and increasing abdominal girth
- All bullet wounds, penetrating wounds, penetrating anal or vaginal injuries, and thoraco-abdominal wounds.

- Principles of laparotomy—perform the laparotomy as soon as adequate resuscitation is done within few hours of admission. If bleeding exceeds your efforts at replacements, operate urgently to control it (Figs. 9 and 10).
  - Adequate preoperative resuscitation, work up and perioperative broad-spectrum antibiotics, and appropriate anesthesia is given.
  - Standard midline or paramedian incision is taken for exploration.
  - Look for blood (splenic, hepatic, or mesenteric injuries), bile [hepatic/common bile duct (CBD)/duodenal injuries], and intestinal contents (perforated gut with peritonitis).
  - Adequate suction is done to remove as much of blood, pus, or intestinal contents as possible. Bleeding vessels secured and bleeding arrested.
  - Exploration of abdominal viscera is done preferably in following order—diaphragm, stomach, spleen, liver, large gut, small gut, rectum, bladder, pancreas, kidney, and gynecological organs.
  - Opening of lesser sac can be done from anterior part of transverse colon to detect pancreatic injuries/Kocherization of duodenum can be done by incising peritoneum on its lateral aspect to visualize retroperitoneal region for kidney and ureteric injuries. In case of large retroperitoneal hematoma in flank due to kidney injuries, do not open it.
  - Meticulous search is done for gunshot injuries and organs injured.
  - Treatment of the injury done which may require splenectomy, suturing of liver lacerations, closure of intestinal perforations, resection anastomosis of injured segment of intestine/colon, diverting colostomy/ileostomy, suturing of mesenteric laceration, and other operative procedures as required for the injury.
  - Suction is done to remove as much blood, pus, and intestinal contents as possible and good peritoneal wash given with saline.
  - All bleeding points secured and drain kept in abdominal cavity.
  - After closing peritoneum, thorough irrigation of abdominal wall done and single layer closure is done/tension sutures employed in closing.

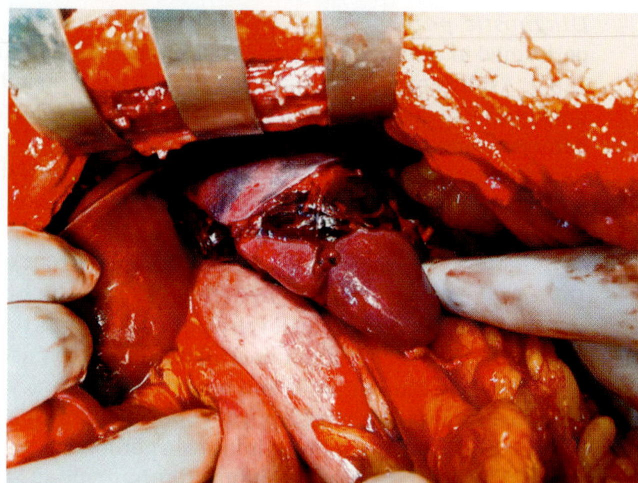

Fig. 9: Rupture of spleen.

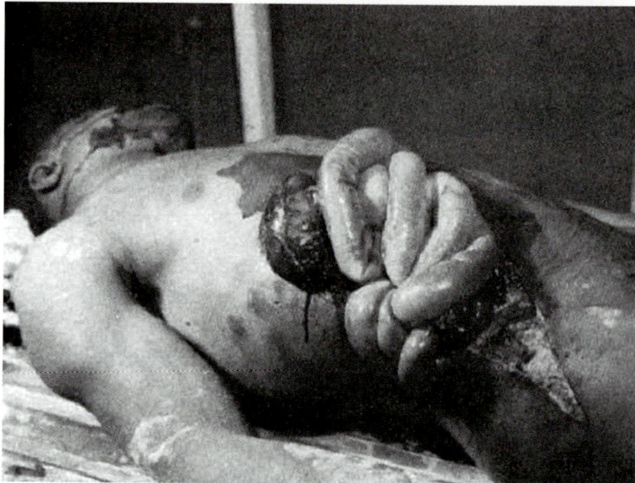

Fig. 10: Evisceration of gut.

  - Appropriate postoperative management including suitable antibiotics, care of wound, correction of anemia, and nutritional deficiencies done along with careful monitoring of the patient.

Thus, abdomen is a *"Black box,"* i.e. it is very difficult to know exact nature of the abdominal injury at initial evaluation. *A watchful eye and high index of suspicion with timely operative intervention is essential for appropriate management of the same.* The key to saving lives in abdominal trauma is *not* to make an accurate diagnosis but the need to recognize that there is an abdominal injury.

CHAPTER

24 Polytrauma and Management of Polytrauma Patient

OBJECTIVES

- Polytrauma Definition
- Management of Polytrauma
- Damage Control Surgery
- Nutrition of Polytrauma Patient

POLYTRAUMA DEFINITION

An injury to one or more body regions, or organs of which one or their combinations is life-threatening.

Injury to more body regions following which, during treatment, we have to make compromises.

Accidental death is the most common cause of death in people below 50 years of age. The death distribution in polytrauma patient is divided into three parts:

1. *Trimodal death distribution*:
   - *Immediate*: Seconds to minutes following injury.
   - *Causes*: Brain, cervical spine, and large vessel injury.
2. *1-2 hours following injury*:
   - *Causes*: Epidural hematomas and bleedings.
3. *Several days following injury*: Due to multiple organ failure (M.O.F.) and sepsis.

Golden Hour Concept

Prompt and proper supervised treatment in the first 1 or 2 hours will decrease the mortality by almost 40% as shown in the graph in Figure 1.

MANAGEMENT OF POLYTRAUMA

Needs of trauma patient:

- To treat life-threatening injuries to maximize the likelihood of survival.
- To treat potentially disabling injuries to maximize return to independence.
- To minimize pain and suffering.

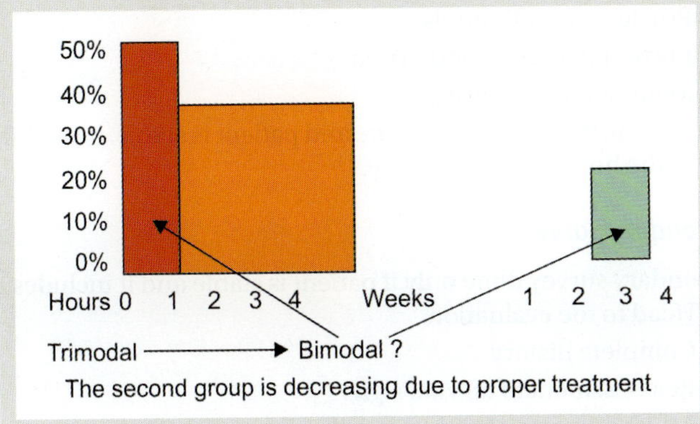

Fig. 1: Trimodal death distribution.

Management of polytrauma patient has been divided into three stages:

1. *Pre-hospitalization care:*
   - Maintain airway/breathing.
   - Control of external bleeding and shock.
   - Immobilization with padded, prepared, splint spinal brace and board.
   - Drug therapy injectable analgesics, intravenous infusion, and continuous oxygenation.
   - While transferring to closest trauma center.
2. *Hospital care*: The same as 1, but proper equipment/staff (trauma surgeon).
3. *Posthospital recovery*: Physiotherapy and prevention of late complications like sepsis.

Pre-hospitalization Care

The most important part in pre-hospitalization is triage.

Triage

Definition: It refers to the evaluation and categorization of sick or wounded when there are insufficient resources for medical care of everyone at once.

In mass casualty situations, triage is used to decide who is most urgently in need of transportation to hospital for care and whose injuries are less severe and can wait for medical care.

Advanced triage system involves a color coding system using red, yellow, green, white, and black tags to different patients depending upon severity.

- *Red tags*: (Immediate) Used to label those who cannot survive without immediate treatment but who have a chance of survival.
- *Yellow tags*: (Observation) Used for those who require observation (and possible later re-triage). Their condition is stable for the moment and, they are not in immediate danger of death. These victims will still need hospital care and would be treated immediately under normal circumstances.
- *Green tags*: (Wait) Reserved for the walking "wounded" who will need medical care at some point after more critical injuries are treated.

- *White tags*: (Dismiss) Given to those with minor injuries for whom a doctor's care is not required.
- *Black tags*: Used for the deceased and for those injuries are so extensive that they will not be able to survive given the care that is available.
- To define which patients have critical injuries, certain scoring system is used in triage as:
  - Abbreviated injury severity score (ISS):
    - Mild
    - Medium
    - Severe
    - Very severe
    - Critical
    - Not survivable.
  - Injury Severity Score (ISS)

The body is divided into six regions (Table 1):

1. Head and neck
2. Face
3. Chest
4. Abdomen
5. Extremities (pelvis)
6. Skin.

The three most severely injured body regions are identified and their injuries are classified as per the abbreviated injury severity score (ISS).

Then the square of each value is taken and then added to get the final injury severity score.

Problems of ISS:

- In one body region only one injury is considered as severe.
- Sometimes severity can be defined after surgery, only the 2nd most severe in one region can be worse than the most severe in another region.
- Physiology data not taken into consideration.
- Every region with the same importance?

Pre-hospitalization Treatment

Guidelines for pre-hospitalization have been given by advanced trauma life support (ATLS) which include:

- *Primary survey*:
  - Airway
  - Breathing
  - Control of external bleeding
  - Disability
  - Environment.
- *Secondary survey*.

TABLE 1: Injury Severity Score.

Example		*Value*	*Value²*
Head, Neck	Brain contusion	3	9
Face	None	0	
Chest	Unstable chest	4	16
Abdomen	Severe liver rupture	2 5	25
Extremities	Fracture of the femur	3	
Skin	Bruises	1	
	Sum		**50**

Severe: More than 20

Airway Management

First step is to determine the consciousness of the patient using either Glasgow Coma Scale or AVPU (alert, verbal stimuli, painful stimuli, unresponsive) method. If patient is unconscious, the first step is to prevent the avoidable causes of hypoxia like tongue fall, secretions in pharynx, and vomit. In this case airway is managed by head-tilt and chin-lift method or by jaw-thrust method in patients with suspected cervical spine injury.

In conscious patient, airway problem should be suspected if there is paradoxical breathing, cyanosis, patient using accessory muscles of respiration, and tracheal deviation.

Breathing

Unconscious patients: After airway management, next step in unconscious patient is to assess the breathing. Normal respiratory rate is 12–30 breaths per minute in adult. If patient is breathing below this rate, patient should be started on cardiopulmonary resuscitation (CPR), and if patient is breathing normally, he should be shifted immediately to higher center.

In conscious patient, next step is to check for life-threatening conditions like hemothorax and tension pneumothorax.

Circulation

Next step is to prevent external or internal bleeding and maintain the circulation. Visible external bleed should be stopped immediately by compression method. Patient's blood pressure should be checked and it should be maintained to the optimum using crystalloids. If there are long bone fractures, they should be immobilized immediately to prevent further loss. If there are suspected internal bleeds, fast ultrasonography (USG) abdomen and pelvis should be done.

Disability

The most common causes which lead to disability in polytrauma patients include spinal cord injury and vertebral fracture, brain contusion, brain hypoxia, subdural hemorrhage (SDH) < extradural hemorrhage (EDH).

To prevent the disability, patient's neurological level should be checked repeatedly using Glasgow Coma Scale or AVPU scale.

Environment

This last step in primary survey involves:

- Undress patient completely
- Maintain body temperature to normal
- Provide warm IV fluids
- Prevent patient hypothermia
- Maintain patient privacy
- Once primary survey is done and patient is stable, he is shifted to the hospital immediately.

Secondary Survey

Secondary survey done only if patient is stable and it includes:

- Head to toe evaluation
- Complete history
- Reassessment of all vital signs
- All body parts should be fully examined. Necessary X-ray should be taken.

Hospital Care of Polytrauma Patient

It is a multidisciplinary approach and needs a team work which includes general surgeon, orthopedician, intensive care specialist, and good nursing team nutritionist.

Once polytrauma patient has arrived at hospital, his ABCs are again evaluated and maintained, patient is further evaluated with fast USG abdomen and pelvis, chest X-ray, cervical spine, and PBH X-rays to rule out any serious injuries.

Patient is then evaluated by all specialties to determine if there is any serious injuries which can lead to death or which will deteriorate the physiology of patient and if multiple such injuries are present, they are prioritized and dealt with according to priority.

DAMAGE CONTROL SURGERY

Definition

It is a form of surgery typically done by trauma surgeon on severely injured patient which puts more emphasis on prevention of triad of death rather than restoring normal anatomy.

Trauma Triad of Death

- Hypothermia
- Acidosis
- Coagulopathy.

Hypothermia—main causes are:
- Heat loss by evaporation and conduction
- Inability to produce heat.

Acidosis:
- Massive transfusion
- Vasopressor
- Diminished cardiac function.

Coagulopathy causes are:
- Consumption dilution
- Acidosis
- Hypothermia.

Concept of Damage Control Surgery

Earlier polytrauma patients used to undergo definitive management as early as possible to restore the anatomy to its normal, but it has shown excess mortality because of postoperative complication. 30–40% deaths in polytrauma patients result in uncontrolled hemorrhage.

Damage control surgery is meant to be utilized as a measure that saves lives. While this life-saving method has resulted in a significant decrease in the morbidity and mortality of critically ill patients, complications can result and do exist. This procedure is generally indicated when a person sustains a severe injury that impairs the ability to maintain homeostasis due to severe hemorrhage leading to metabolic acidosis, hypothermia, and increased coagulopathy. The approach would provide a limited surgical intervention in order to control both hemorrhage and contamination. This will subsequently allow for clinicians to focus on reversing the physiologic insult prior to completing a definitive repair. While the temptation to perform a definitive operation exists, surgeons should avoid this practice because of the deleterious effects on patients which results in them succumbing to the physiologic effects of the injury, despite the anatomical correction.

Damage Control Surgery Stages

Initial management:
- Resuscitation to reverse the physiology to normal
- Definitive reconstruction.

Principle of initial management:
- Abdomen should not be opened for a long time as it causes hypothermia due to evaporation
- Concomitant opening of thorax should be avoided as it aggravates hypothermia
- All measures to be taken to prevent lethal triad of death formation
- All bleeding surfaces like liver should be packed with laparotomy pads
- Pancreatic and kidney injuries should not be touched if they are not bleeding
- Small enteric injuries should be stapled
- Clamps may be left on unrepaired vascular injuries or vessels can be ligated
- Vessels which cannot be ligated without loss of life or limb should be treated with temporary indwelling shunts
- No drain should be put
- Abdomen closed with sharp towels rather than suture as it will close abdomen in 30–60 seconds and do not bleed
- Closure of just skin allows to accommodate excess fluid without increasing pressure a lot
- Towels used to cover skin should be covered with mob and adhesive dressing applied to prevent fluid from escaping on patients bed
- Long bone fractures should be properly immobilized either in splints or by external fixator.

Resuscitation: The aim of resuscitation is to bring the physiology to normal and aim is to prevent hypothermia, acidosis, and coagulopathy.

Definitive reconstruction: It is usually planned once patient's physiology is maintained. Surgeries are planned according to priority. More serious or life-threatening injuries should be operated first.

NUTRITION OF POLYTRAUMA PATIENT

This is the most important part in the management of polytrauma patient.

The metabolic changes taking place in polytrauma patients are divided into two phases—(1) Ebb phase and (2) flow phase. Ebb phase occurs in first few hours and is characterized by hypothermia, decreased oxygen consumption aimed toward reducing energy depletion. The flow phase is characterized by increased catabolic state which includes increased body temperature, increased oxygen consumption, negative nitrogen balance, increased cortisol level, hyperglycemia, insulin intolerance, gluconeogenesis, and proteolysis. Proteolysis and glycolysis are increased in order to provide substrate for hepatic neoglucogenesis and the hepatic synthesis of acute phase reactant.

The state of hypercatabolism after severe injury can lead to severe complications associated with post-traumatic hyperglycemia, hypoproteinemia, lactate acidosis, and immunosuppression. Thus, the presence and significance of these metabolic alterations must be recognized and appreciated in severely injured patients. An optimal therapeutic regimen should include the concept of a "metabolic control" in addition to the initial measures of resuscitation by hemorrhage control, and securing airways and oxygenation. The post-traumatic catabolic state requires an adjusted energetic balance with early protein substitution and hypercaloric nutrition. The specialized nutritional support for severely injured patients includes the administration of "immune nutrient cocktails" which have been shown to improve the survival of septic patients during the intensive care period. The concept of "immunonutrition" has been established in recent years and exemplified by the enteral supplementation of glutamine, one of the most promising new nutritional concepts for severely injured patients in recent years. Glutamine is an essential amino acid which exerts metabolic benefits beyond its nutritional value by mediating immunological effects, such as induction of neutrophil phagocytic activity and oxidative burst and cellular protection from ischemia/reper. Glutamine was also shown to protect neutrophils from undergoing apoptosis *in vivo*. In addition, glutamine is a precursor to the reducing agent glutathione and thus, contributes to antioxidant effects and cellular protection against reperfusion injury. Furthermore, glutamine has been shown to restore cellular energy reserves to normal levels after hemorrhagic shock and to attenuate the extent of shock induced cellular apoptosis.

In addition to glutamine, Ω-3 fatty acids have become an important nutritional supplementation for severely injured patients in recent years. These long-chain polyunsaturated fatty acids derived from fish oil were shown to exert potent anti-inflammatory properties in trauma patients, such as attenuation of arachidonic acid-derived metabolites like prostaglandin PGE2 and leukotriene LTB4, inhibition of leukocyte activation, activation and chemotaxis, and attenuation of pro-inflammatory gene expression.

As far as possible polytrauma patient should be started on enteral nutrition supplemented with glutamine and polyunsaturated fatty acids at a rate calculated by Weir equation or Harris Benedict's equation.

Posthospital Care

It includes physiotherapy to maintain mobility and prevent deformity and contractures.

CHAPTER 25

Soft Tissue Coverage in Orthopedics

OBJECTIVES

- Historical Aspects
- Skin Grafting
- Graft Survival and Healing
- Graft Application
- Flap Cover

INTRODUCTION

The incidence of polytrauma in our country is increasing every year due to increase in the incidence of motor vehicle accidents and poor traffic discipline. Management of such cases, especially open fractures of extremities, has been a major challenge to the team of trauma surgeons involved in the management (Fig. 1).

The need for primary thorough debridement, adequate fracture fixation, followed by suitable soft tissue coverage in reducing the morbidity cannot be overemphasized (Fig. 2). This warrants a collective approach to the problem by specialists in orthopedics and plastic surgery. But in an unfortunate situation where a plastic surgeon is not available, an orthopedic surgeon possessing the theoretical knowledge of the local vascular anatomy may have to harvest a local flap to cover the exposed bone or metal in fracture tibia. This approach to the common problem will lessen the burden of referring all the cases to the tertiary care centers.

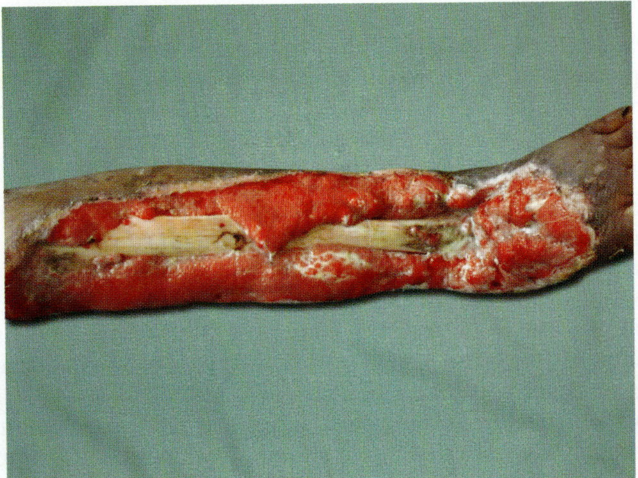

Fig. 1: Extensive soft tissue defect of lower extremity with exposed tibia.

HISTORICAL ASPECTS

- Sushruta "the father of surgery" in 600 BC gave the first detailed description of plastic surgical procedures, as mentioned in the "Sushruta Samhita". Amputation of nose used to be a punishment during that period and Sushruta described a skin flap raised from cheek for reconstruction of such noses.[1]
- Branca family from Sicily described delayed pedicle flap in year 1400.
- Pare described vascular anatomy of skin in year 1500.
- Skin grafting was described in the 19th century, by Reverdin who used pinch graft in 1869.[2] Subsequently, Ollier and Thiersch used split-thickness grafts in 1872 and 1886, respectively[3] and Wolfe described use of the full-thickness graft in 1875.[4]
- Sir Harold Gillies, father of modern plastic surgery, described staged pedicle flaps in 1900. He was actively involved in managing war casualties during first and second World Wars.
- Tansini in 1917 described latissimus dorsi myocutaneous flap for breast reconstruction.
- Zeiss developed commercial operating microscope in 1951 which ultimately helped in microvascular surgery.
- McGregor and Jackson described groin flap in 1972.[5]
- Fasciocutaneous flaps (containing deep fascia and skin) were described in the 1980s.
- Microvascular free flaps were described in 1975.

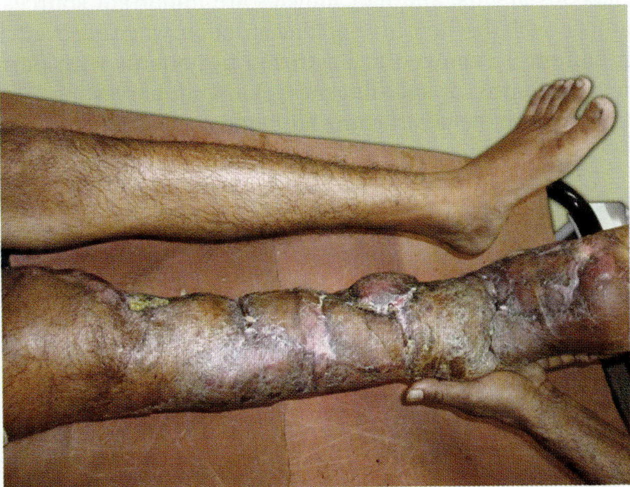

Fig. 2: Complete coverage obtained by multistage local flaps and split-thickness skin graft.

SKIN GRAFTING

Skin grafting is the transplantation of skin from one part of body to another location in the same/other individual. Skin graft is the most commonly used tissue for soft tissue coverage.

It can be used for reconstruction after the surgical removal of skin malignancies to cover chronic nonhealing ulcers or to replace tissue lost in full-thickness burns.

Anatomical Aspects

The skin consists of two layers—the outer layer or epidermis and the thicker inner layer or dermis. The epidermis constitutes about 5% of the skin, and the remaining 95% is dermis.

Structure of Skin

The skin varies in thickness depending on the anatomical location, gender, and age of the individual. Skin is found to be thickest on the palms and soles of the feet, while it happens to be thinnest on the eyelids. Male skin is characteristically thicker as compared to female skin. Children have relatively thin skin, but around puberty, the skin progressively thickens. This thickening continues until the fourth or fifth decade of life, when the skin begins to thin, primarily due to loss of dermal elastic fibers, epithelial appendages, and ground substance.

Epidermis: The epidermis or the outer skin layer is a stratified squamous epithelium consisting primarily of keratinocytes. The epidermis has no blood vessels; hence, it receives nutrition by diffusion from the underlying dermis through the basement membrane, which separates the two layers.

Dermis: The dermis is also composed of two layers, the superficial papillary dermis and the deeper reticular dermis. The papillary dermis is thinner, consisting of loose connective tissue that contains capillaries, elastic fibers, reticular fibers, and some collagen. The reticular dermis consists of a thicker layer of dense connective tissue containing larger blood vessels, closely interlaced elastic fibers, and coarse, branching collagen fibers arranged in layers parallel to the surface. The reticular layer also contains fibroblasts, mast cells, nerve endings, lymphatics, and some epidermal appendages (Fig. 3).

Epithelial cell sources: Epidermal appendages like sweat glands, sebaceous glands, and hair follicles are important sources of epithelial cells that help in re-epithelialization, when the overlying epithelium is removed or destroyed in patients with partial thickness, burns, or split-thickness skin graft harvesting. These intradermal epithelial structures are found deep within the dermis.

GRAFT SURVIVAL AND HEALING

The success of a skin graft, or its "take," depends on nutrient uptake and vascular ingrowth from the recipient bed, which occurs in three phases. The first phase takes place during the first 24–48 hours. The graft is initially bound to the recipient site through formation of a fibrin layer and undergoes diffusion of nutrients by capillary action from the recipient bed by a process called plasmatic imbibition (Fig. 4). The second phase involves the process of inosculation, in which the donor and recipient end capillaries are aligned and establish a vascular network.

Revascularization of the graft is accomplished through those capillaries as well as by ingrowth of new vessels through neovascularization in the third and final phase, which is generally complete within 4–7 days. Reinnervation of skin grafts begins approximately 2–4 weeks after grafting and occurs by ingrowth of nerve fibers from the recipient bed and surrounding tissue.

Operative Technique

Wound Preparation

For obvious reasons, a well-vascularized recipient bed is of utmost importance for survival of the skin graft. Skin grafts rarely take up when placed on bare bone, cartilage, or tendon without the presence of periosteum, perichondrium, or paratenon.

Recipient Bed Preparation

Meticulous hemostasis of the recipient bed is a key in preventing hematoma formation between the graft and wound bed. Hemostasis is typically achieved through use of epinephrine and saline-soaked gauze, particularly in freshly excised burns, in combination with precise electrocoagulation. Infection also compromises graft survival; therefore, careful preparation of the recipient bed is necessary. A recipient bed that contains a bacteria concentration greater than 10^5 organisms per gram of tissue will not allow a skin graft to be taken up.

Donor Site Selection

Donor site selection is based on multiple factors, including skin color, texture, dermal thickness, vascularity, and anticipated donor site morbidity.

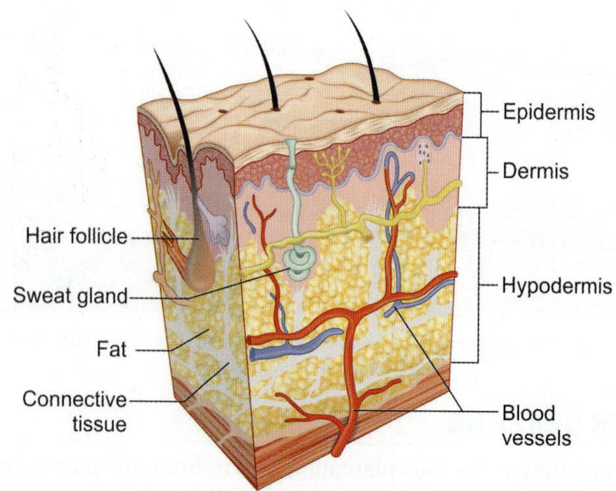

Fig. 3: Structure of skin.

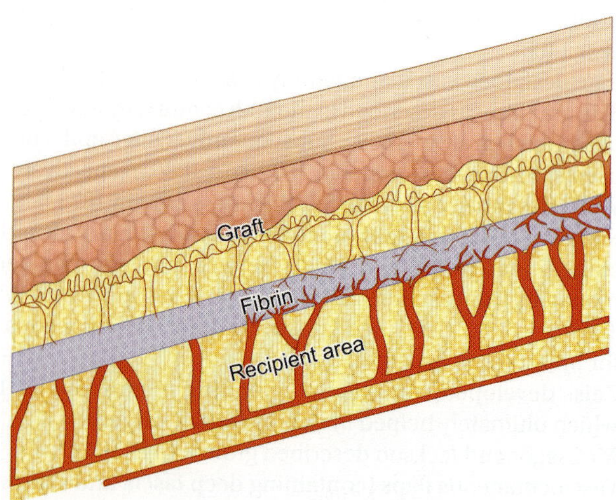

Fig. 4: "Take up" of split skin graft.

Full-thickness grafts are generally taken from the supraclavicular area, pre- or post-auricular areas (Fig. 5). Full thickness skin from these sites provides a suitable color match for defects of the face. The full-thickness skin graft is excised with a scalpel at the subdermal level. The residual adipose tissue should be subsequently removed with sharp curved scissors prior to placement of the graft on the recipient bed. Donor site defects resulting from full-thickness grafts are generally closed primarily or covered some times, with a split-thickness graft if the defect area is large.

Split-thickness skin grafts are commonly harvested from the thigh, buttocks, and abdominal wall.[6] The method of harvesting the split-thickness skin graft depends primarily on the size and thickness needed for coverage of the defect. Powered electric dermatomes or handheld Humby's dermatomes are most commonly used to harvest split-thickness skin grafts.

GRAFT APPLICATION

One of the more common and faster methods of affixing a graft to the recipient site is with surgical staples, particularly to large recipient areas. In children or in sensitive areas of adults, anchoring the graft into place using absorbable sutures may be more advantageous.

Donor Site Care

The split-thickness skin graft donor site epidermis regenerates by secondary epithelialization from the wound edges and from migration of epithelial cells originating in the shafts of hair follicles as well as sweat and sebaceous glands remaining in the dermis.

FLAP COVER

Flap is a piece of tissue partly detached from surrounding tissue and transferred to another area. It maintains its vascularity and is not dependent on its survival from vascularity from recipient area.

Anatomical Parts of a Flap

The proximal part of flap still attached to donor area is known as base, whereas pivot point is referred to the point around which flaps rotate and is a fixed point.

Distal segment of the flap is inserted into the defect and pedicle is the part of flap which carries its vascularity.

Composition of Flaps

- *Skin flap:* Consists of skin and superficial fascia only
- *Fascial flap:* Flap raised from deep fascia only
- *Fasciocutaneous:* Skin and deep fascia
- *Muscle flap:* Muscle detached from one end and transferred to recipient area
- *Myocutaneous:* Muscle and fasciocutaneous
- *Osteomyocutaneous:* Bone, attached muscle, and overlying skin transferred
- *Free flap:* When a flap is transferred along its vessels and nerve and vascular and nerve attachment is carried out at recipient site by microvascular technique using very fine suture material.

Methods of Transfer

- *Advancement flap:* Wherein skin from adjacent area is advanced without rotation.
- *Transposition flap:* It is transposed to adjoining defect and rotates at pivot point. Donor area is split skin grafted.
- *Rotation:* A larger flap is raised in a semicircle and rotated into defect and donor area is generally directly closed (Fig. 6).
- *Direct:* Flap directly transferred to the defect area
- *Indirect (tubed-now obsolete):* Tubed flap were used extensively during first and second world wars.
- *Free flaps:* Flap is raised along with its arterial supply, venous drainage, and vascular anastomosis has to be carried out at recipient site for its survival.

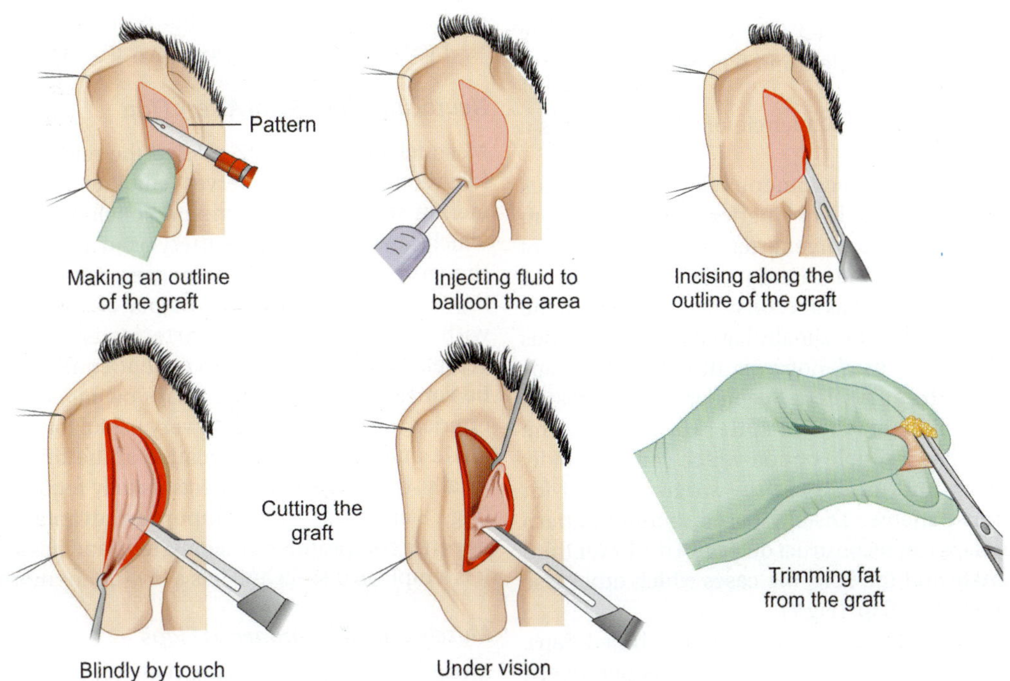

Fig. 5: Full-thickness skin graft harvest.

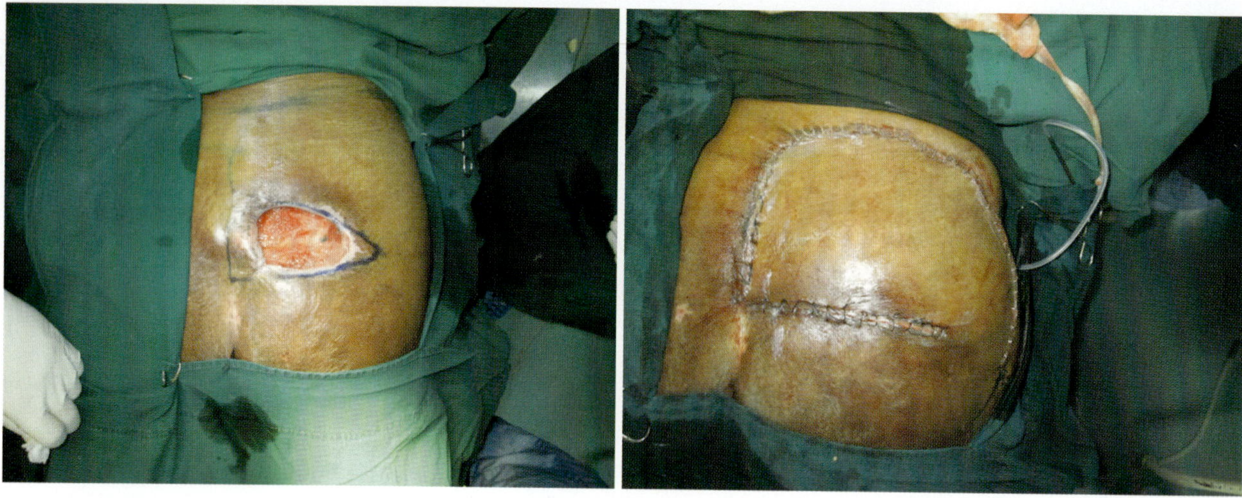

Fig. 6: Rotation flap.

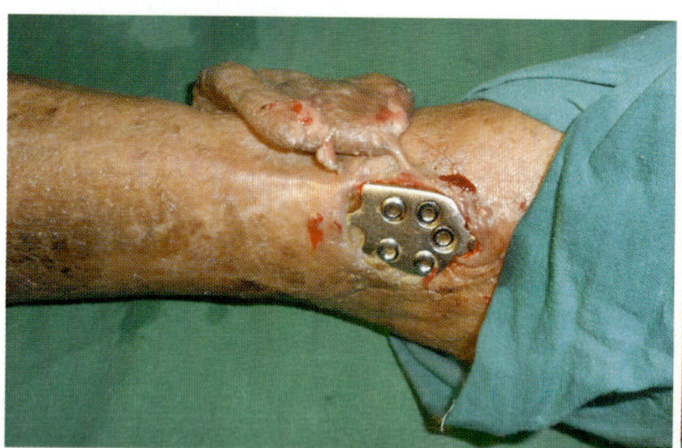

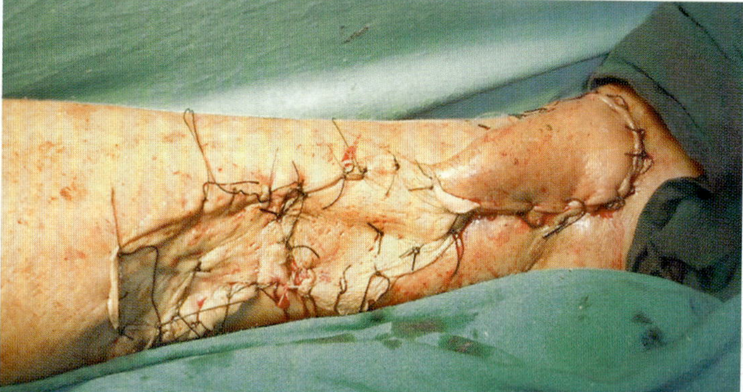

Fig. 7: Exposed implant and a failed flap: cover achieved by distally based fasciocutaneous flap.

Planning for the Flap

- *Triangulation of the defect:* Applicable in all transposition and rotation flaps.
- *Transposition flap:* It is designed as a square immediately adjacent to the triangulated defect and flap moves laterally to close the defect.
- *Rotation flap:* It is raised in a semicircle of which defect is a segment.
- *Fasciocutaneous flaps:* Fasciocutaneous flaps carry plexus of vessels on the deep fascia, fed by perforating vessels from underneath muscle or deeper larger arteries. The inclusion of the deep fascia during elevation of random skin flaps enhances the viability of large local flaps as a reconstructive option in the lower leg.[7] In the extremities, proximally based fasciocutaneous flaps are most frequently used, however, distally based flaps can also be raised with equal safety. Secondary defect created after raising these flaps has to be split skin grafted. The fasciocutaneous flap is a simple option which can be rapidly elevated and inset, and minimizes the surgical insult for many multitrauma patients.[7] Distally-based random pattern fasciocutaneous flaps can reconstruct defects of the lower third of the leg, the ankle and the heel, the cases which otherwise would have required free flap[8] (Fig 7).
- *Perforator-based flaps:* More recently, perforator-based flaps, rather than random pattern flaps, are used. Preoperatively, identification of the perforator vascular basis of such flaps must be carried out. Perforators from post-tibial vessels on medial side and perforators from peroneal vessels on lateral side are generally used. Site of emergence of perforators should be assessed by handheld Doppler and while raising these flaps perforators must be safeguarded to ensure survival of flaps.[9]

Neurocutaneous Sural Artery Flap

Masquelet et al. in 1992 studied the role of the vascular axis that follows the superficial nerves (sural nerve and saphenous nerves, etc.) in supplying the skin and concluded that the vascular axis, which can be either a true artery or an interlacing network, ensures the vascularization of the nerves, gives off several cutaneous branches in the suprafascial course of the nerve, and anastomoses with the septocutaneous arteries issuing from a deep main vessel. The superficial nerves that course the leg can therefore be considered as vascular relays owing to their neurocutaneous arteries.[10] Sural artery flap is very useful for reconstruction around ankle and heel defects because of the limited tissues available locally, otherwise such defects usually require free flap coverage[11] (Figs. 8 and 9). The most important advantage of this flap is that it does not compromise a major artery, and has a wide arc of rotation. It is simple to dissect and has a low-donor morbidity.[12,13]

Muscle and Myocutaneous Flaps

Muscle and myocutaneous flaps which have a neurovascular bundle either at proximal or distal ends can be used as flaps.

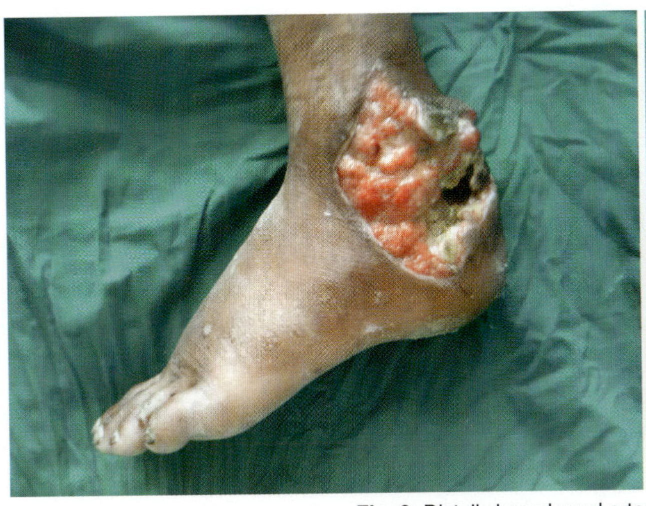
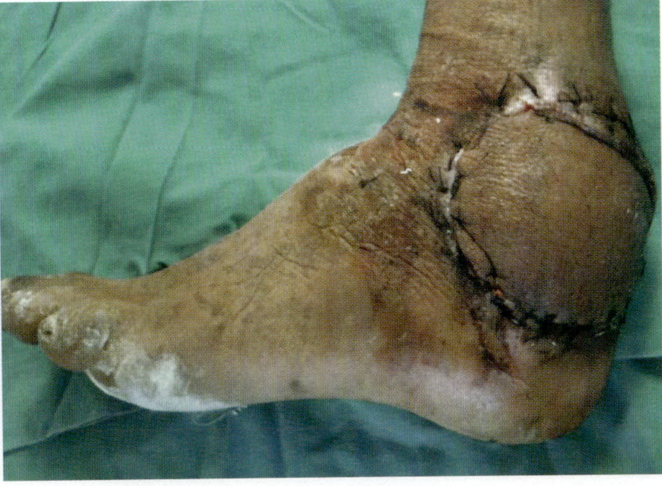

Fig. 8: Distally based sural artery flap for soft tissue defect over ankle region.

Neurovascular bundles act as pivot point around which these flaps are moved for transfer. These flaps are simple to raise, found reliable, fill the cavities, bring in more vascularity, and leave a minimum disability from loss of function of that particular muscle. Gastrocnemius muscle is frequently used for defects over knee and upper third of tibia. One head of gastrocnemius is used since each head has got separate neurovascular bundle proximally (Figs. 10 and 11) and there is hardly any postoperative disability. If there is bony gap in long bone, patient may require bone grafting as well. It has been observed that patients who undergo bone grafting after complete re-epithelialization of the wound, regardless of the method of closure, have a lower rate of infection.[12]

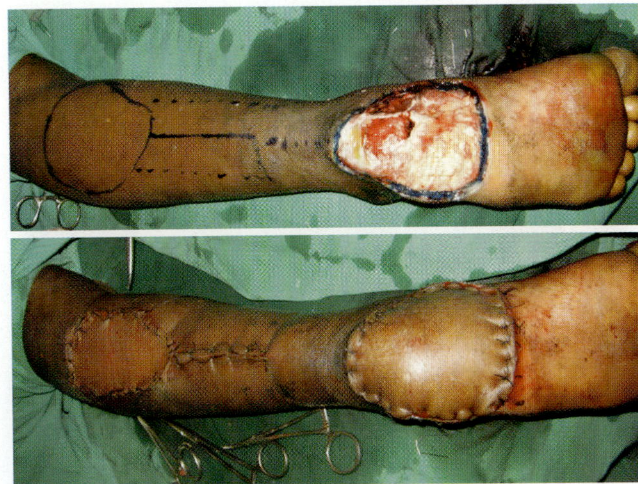

Fig. 9: Distally based sural artery flap for soft tissue defect over heel region.

Free Flaps

To plan a free flap, anatomical knowledge of the local vascular anatomy is essential to get an idea as to which particular vessel will be used for anastomosis at recipient site. If the flap is required post-trauma, the effect of trauma on local vasculature must be carefully assessed. There are definite indications for free flaps in type III tibial fractures, where radical removal of dead bone, stable external fixation, and transfer of vascularized bone may salvage the majority of type III B and C tibial fracture with function superior to that after amputation.[14]

Soft Tissue Cover in Hands

- Cross finger flap
- Radial artery forearm flap
- Groin flap
- Posterior interosseous artery flap.

Cross-finger Flap

Cross-finger flap was first described by Gurdin and Pangman by using the dorsal skin and subcutaneous tissue from an adjacent finger for volar defect coverage.[15] A rectangular flap is raised from three sides of the dorsal surface of middle phalanx of the adjacent finger. Flap is raised through the subcutaneous tissue and down to epitenon. The flap is swung to cover the defect and donor area is split skin grafted. Flap is generally divided after 2–3 weeks.

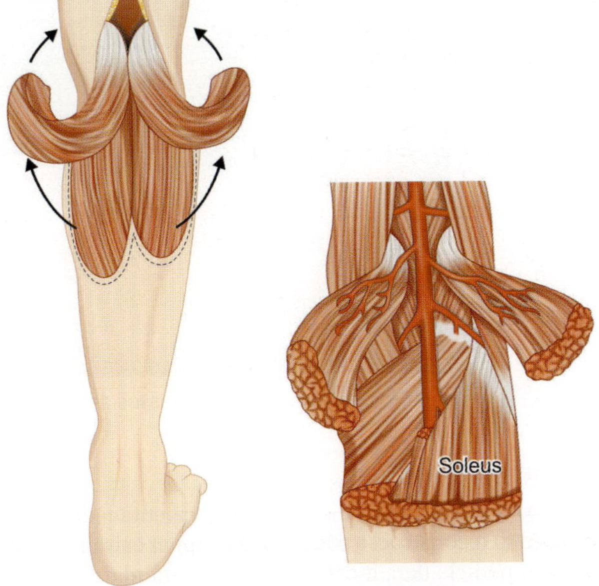

Fig. 10: Gastrocnemius muscle flap.

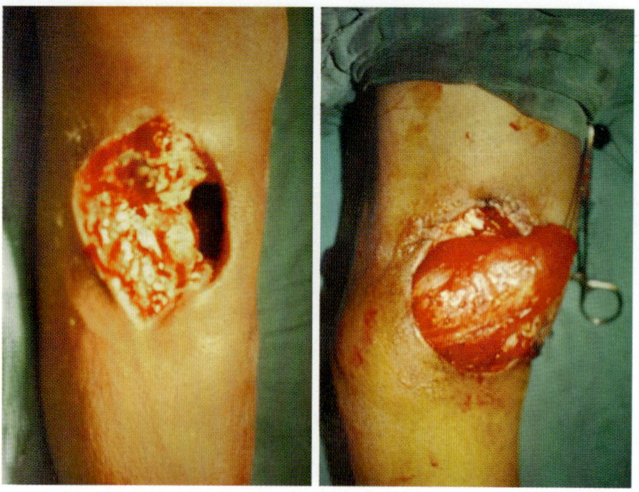

Fig. 11: Soft tissue defect and comminuted fracture upper end tibia: cover by gastrocnemius flap.

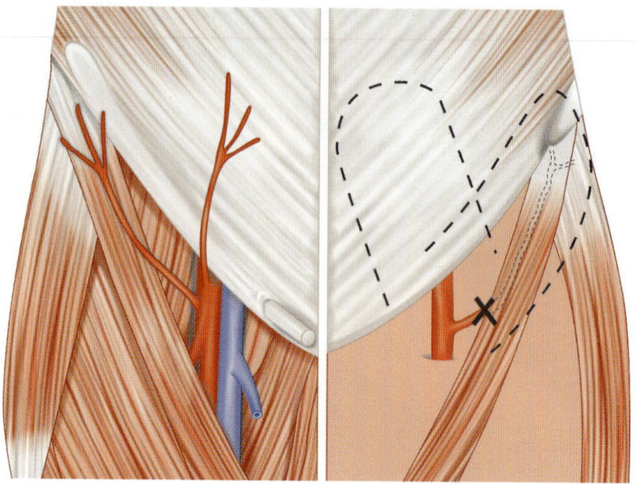

Fig. 12: Groin flap and its anatomy.

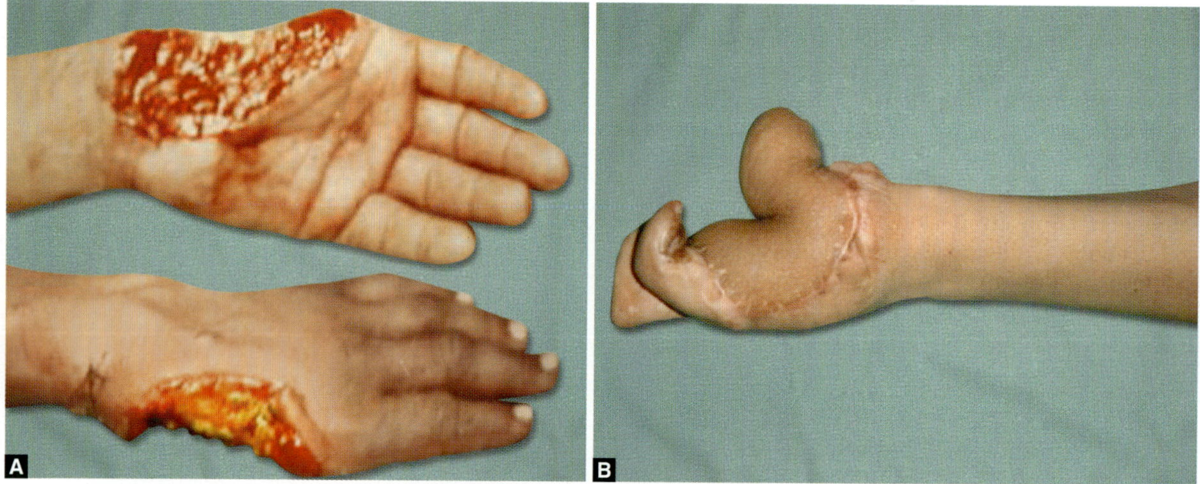

Figs. 13A and B: Amputation of thumb with large soft tissue defect; (B) Groin flap cover provided.

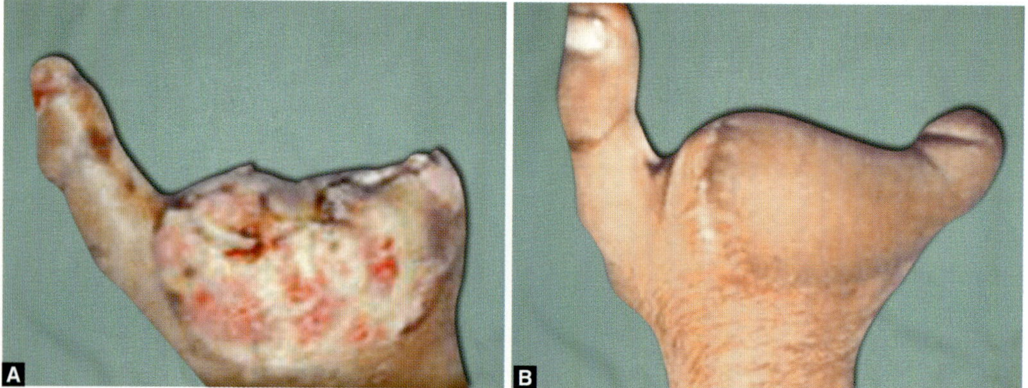

Figs. 14A and B: (A) Soft tissue defect hand with amputation all fingers; (B) Groin flap cover provided.

Radial Artery Forearm Flap

Radial artery forearm flap is a versatile fasciocutaneous flap that can be used to reconstruct a wide range of upper extremity defects. If used as a pedicle flap, it can be used in a standard or reversed fashion to provide coverage of the forearm, elbow, wrist, hand, and thumb defects. If used as a free flap, it is more versatile and can be raised in various shapes and sizes. This flap is based on the radial artery and its accompanying venae comitantes, which drain the flap. For distally based pedicle flap, it is raised on volar aspect of forearm, the vessels are identified proximally, and ligated. Flap is then turned over and raw area is covered over the hand. Since a major vessel is sacrificed, it is essential that continuity and dominance of ulnar artery is ensured by preoperative Allen's test, before undertaking this flap.

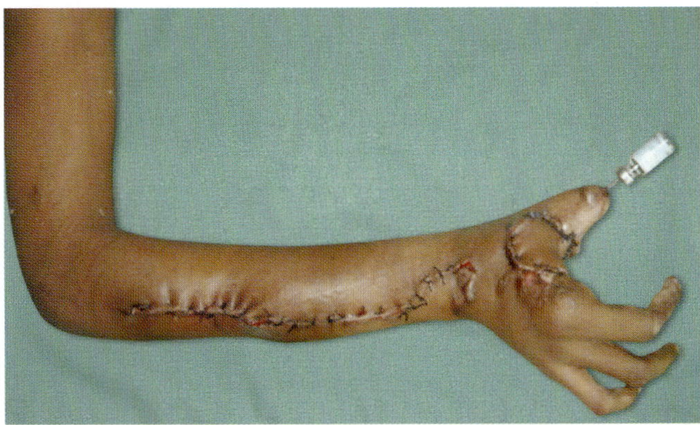
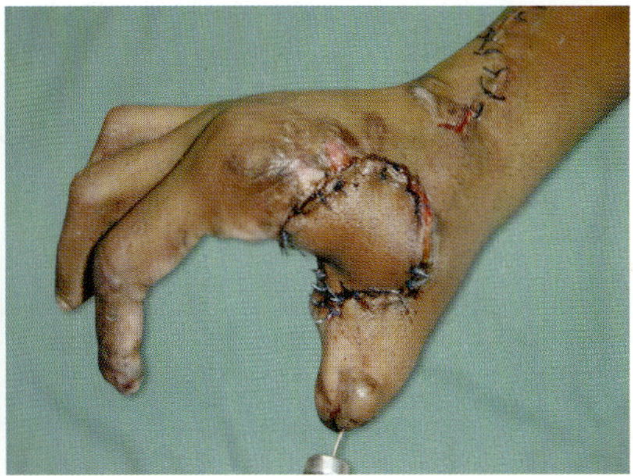

Fig. 15: Posterior interosseous artery flap.

Groin Flap

Groin flap is based on superficial circumflex iliac branch of femoral artery and arises 2–3 cm below the inguinal ligament and runs laterally parallel to the inguinal ligament (Fig. 12). At the level of medial border of sartorius it gives away a deep branch and gradually becomes superficial. Groin flap is thus raised parallel to the inguinal ligament keeping vascular pedicle in center of the flap. Usual width is about 10 cm and length of flap can be beyond the anterior superior iliac spine in 1:1 ratio. This flap is very handy for soft tissue cover over dorsum of hand. The pedicle is divided 3 weeks later and final inset is then carried out (Figs. 13 and 14).

Posterior Interosseous Artery Flap

The posterior interosseous artery based flap is another flap which can be used for soft tissue coverage over dorsum of hand and 1st web space. Advantage of this flap is that no major vessel is sacrificed and it offers thin pliable skin from extensor surface of proximal forearm (Fig. 15).

REFERENCES

1. Hauben DJ, Baruchin A, Mahler A. On the history of the free skin graft. Ann Plast Surg. 1982;9(3):242-5.
2. Davis JS. The story of plastic surgery. Ann Surg. 1994;113:641.
3. Smahel J. The healing of skin grafts. Clin Plast Surg. 1977;4(3):409-24.
4. Hexsel CL, Loosemore M, Goldberg LH, et al. Postauricular skin: an excellent donor site for split-thickness skin grafts for the head, neck, and upper chest. Dermatol Surg. 2015;41(1):48-52.
5. McGregor IA, Jackson IT. The Groin Flap. Br J Plast Surg. 1972;25:3-16.
6. White N, Hettiaratchy S, Papini RP. The choice of split-thickness skin graft donor site: patients' and surgeons' preferences. Plast Reconstr Surg. 2003;112(3):933-4.
7. Hallock GG. Local fasciocutaneous flaps for cutaneous coverage of lower extremity wounds. J Trauma. 1989;29(9): 1240-4.
8. Lagvankar SP. Distally-based random fasciocutaneous flaps for multi-staged reconstruction of defects in the lower third of the leg, ankle and heel. Br J Plast Surg. 1990;43(5):541-5.
9. Kamath BJ, Joshua TV, Pramod S. Perforator based flap coverage from the anterior and lateral compartment of the leg for medium sized traumatic pretibial soft tissue defects—a simple solution for a complex problem. J Plast Reconstr Aesthet Surg. 2006;59(5):515-20.
10. Masquelet AC, Romana MC, Wolf G. Skin island flaps supplied by the vascular axis of the sensitive superficial nerves: anatomic study and clinical experience in the leg. Plast Reconstr Surg. 1992;89(6):1115-21.
11. Schannen AP, Truchan L, Goshima K, et al. Sural versus perforator flaps for distal medial leg wounds. Orthopedics. 2015;38(12):e1059-64.
12. Fischer MD, Gustilo RB, Varecka TF. The timing of flap coverage, bone-grafting, and intramedullary nailing in patients who have a fracture of the tibial shaft with extensive soft-tissue injury. J Bone Joint Surg Am. 1991;73(9):1316-22.
13. Ogün TC, Arazi M, Kutlu A. An easy and versatile method of coverage for distal tibial soft tissue defects. J Trauma. 2001;50(1):53-9.
14. Reigstad A, Hetland KR, Bye K, et al. Free tissue transfer for type III tibial fractures. Microsurgery in 19 cases. Acta Orthop Scand. 1992;63(5):477-81.
15. Gurdin M, Pangman WJ. The repair of surface defects of fingers by trans-digital flaps. Plast Reconstr Surg (1946). 1950;5(4):368-71.

CHAPTER

26 Amputation Surgery

OBJECTIVES

- Historical Review
- Nomenclature
- Types/Classification of Amputation
- Causes of Amputation
- Indications for Amputation
- Ideal Stump
- Preoperative Stage
- Amputations in Special Circumstances
- Prevention of Amputation in Ischemic Limbs
- Some Useful Tips
- Amputation Surgery
- Amputation in Lower Extremity
- Amputation in Upper Extremity
- Complications of Amputation Surgery

INTRODUCTION

Amputation should not be considered as cutting of a limb, rather it is a reconstructive procedure to create a new organ for locomotion. Amputation also includes congenital absence of a limb or part of limb. In olden days, amputation was carried out to save the life, whereas in recent times it is to improve the quality of life.

HISTORICAL REVIEW

Sushruta (600 BCE), ancient Indian surgeon, should be considered as the Father of present day Amputation Surgery.[1] Other known names are Ambroise Pare (1575), Francois Chopart (1791), Sir James Syme (1843), Nikolai Ivanovich Pirogoff (1854), HB Boyd (1939), Jacques Lisfranc de St. Martin (1830), Rocco Gritti (1857), and William Stokes (1870).[2,3] In recent times, Ernest Burgess (1960) is known for long posterior flap technique, Robinson (1981) and Jain (2005) for designing and improving the skew flap technique for below-knee amputation.[4-9]

NOMENCLATURE

Old nomenclature is related to the joint, whereas the new nomenclature is related to the bone or major bone through which the amputation is performed Table 1.

TABLE 1: A comparison in nomenclature.

New nomenclature	*Old nomenclature*
Hip disarticulation	Through hip
Transfemoral	Above knee
Knee disarticulation	Through knee
Transtibial	Below knee
Shoulder disarticulation	Through shoulder
Transhumeral	Above elbow
Elbow disarticulation	Through elbow
Transradial	Below elbow
Wrist disarticulation	Through wrist

TYPES/CLASSIFICATION OF AMPUTATION

- *Guillotine amputation*: Performed as an emergency, as a lifesaving procedure, where all the tissues including bone are divided at the same level (Fig. 1A).
- *Flap amputation*: Skin and deep fascial flaps are planned and all the remaining tissues are divided at the same level and result in a conical stump. It is performed where patient's general condition is poor and a non-limb wearer (Fig. 1B).
- *Myoplastic*: Muscle flaps of opposing groups are sutured over the end of bone, which result in a bulky terminal end of the stump.
- *Osteoplastic (Myodesis)*: The muscle flaps are sutured to the terminal end of the bone resulting in a conical stump (Fig. 1C).
- *Osteomyoplastic*: It is a combination of myoplastic and osteoplastic techniques where deeper muscles are sutured to bone-end and superficial muscles sutured with each other at the end of bone (Fig. 1D).

CAUSES OF AMPUTATION

- *Trauma*: In developing countries, 70% of amputations are due to trauma, mostly as a result of road traffic accidents (Fig. 2A).[10]
- *Vascular*: In developed countries, 80% of amputations are due to poor circulation, resulting from gradually increasing ischemia due to atherosclerosis.[11,12] In younger population, thromboangiitis obliterans (TAO) resulting into chronic ischemia leads to intermittent claudications, rest pain, nonhealing ulcer, and later on gangrene (Fig. 2B). In diabetics, due to vasculopathy, neuropathy, and callus attitude, almost 5% patients lose their limbs.
- *Infection*: Gas gangrene, a life-threatening infection, is managed by amputation (Fig. 2C). Madura mycosis, a fungal infection, and long-standing chronic osteomyelitis also lead to amputation.
- *Neoplastic*: Malignancy, in most of the cases, is managed by amputation (Fig. 2D).
- *Congenital limb deficiency*: For the sake of convenience, the congenital limb deficiency is grouped under amputation. The exact cause of intrauterine limb deficiency is not clear, however

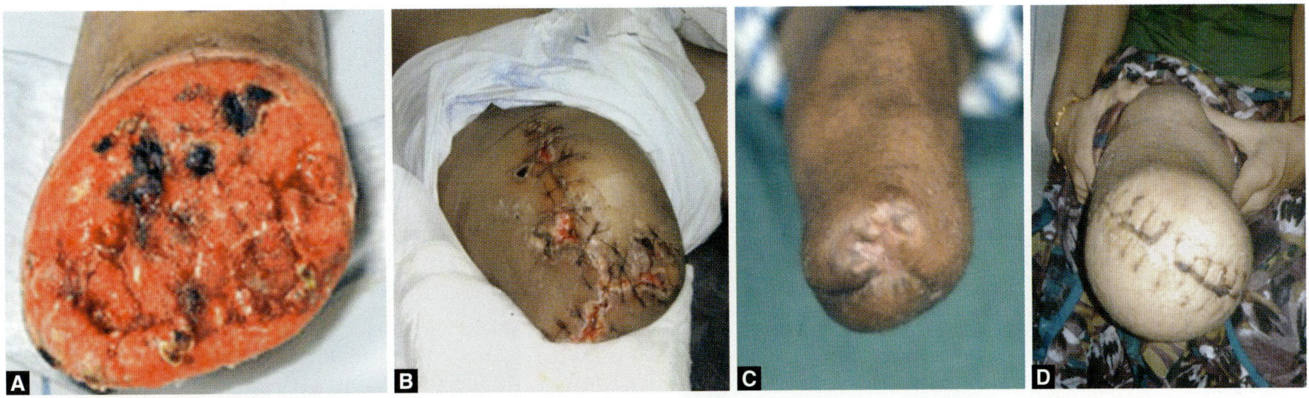

Figs. 1A to D: Amputations. (A) Guillotine; (B) Flap; (C) Osteoplastic; (D) Osteomyoplastic.

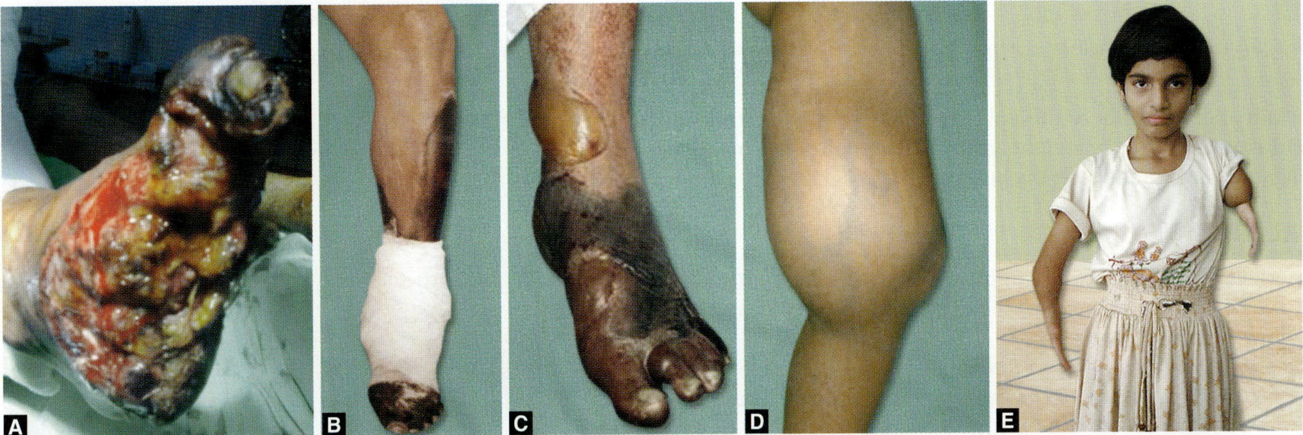

Figs. 2A to E: Causes of amputations. (A) Trauma; (B) Ischemia; (C) Infection (gas gangrene); (D) Neoplasm; (E) Congenital.

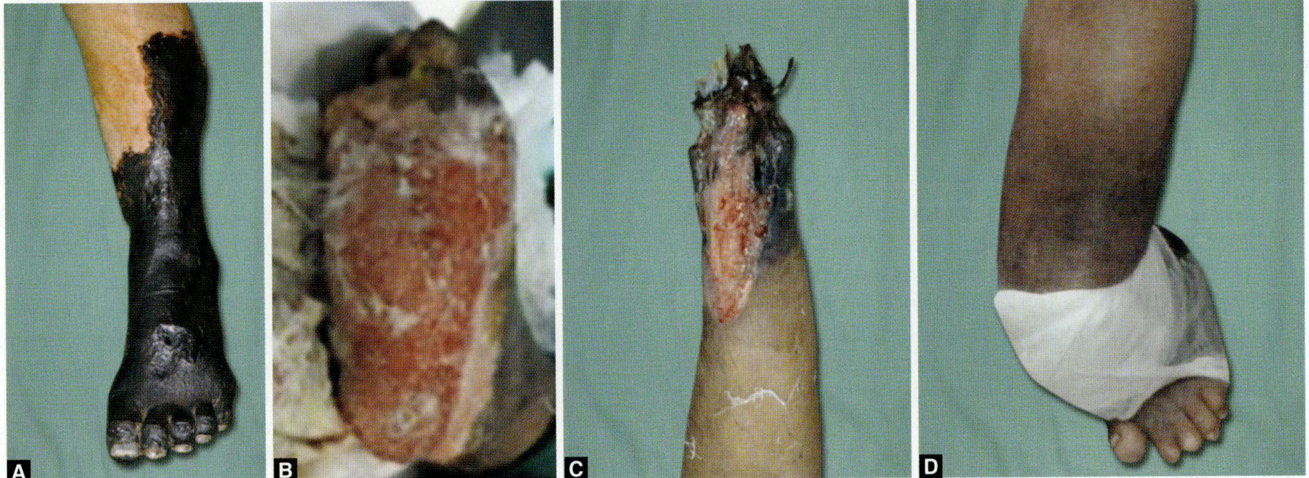

Figs. 3A to D: Indications of amputations. (A) Gangrene; (B) Loss of sole skin; (C) Crush injury; (D) Disorganized ankle and foot.

the most common cause is amniotic band syndrome. The fibrous bands in the amniotic fluid strangulate the growing limb, leading to the restricted blood supply and growth of the limb. Other causes are teratogenic drugs like thalidomide, radiations, intrauterine infections, and trauma during the early stage of pregnancy. The most common congenital limb deficiency is transradial (below elbow) on the left side (Fig. 2E).[13]

- *Legal punishment*: This has also been listed as a cause of amputation that is practiced as a punishment in a number of countries.

INDICATIONS FOR AMPUTATION

Amputation is performed when all the efforts to preserve the limb have failed. One should keep in mind that too much unwarranted effort to save the limb can be life-threatening.

Amputation is indicated when the limb is dead, deadly, or dead loss (debilitating). Gangrene (Fig. 3A), unmanageable claudications, rest pain, loss of the sole skin (Fig. 3B), crush injury (Fig. 3C), if the foot is unsalvageable/potentially life-threatening, and disorganized foot and ankle (Fig. 3D) due to any reason,

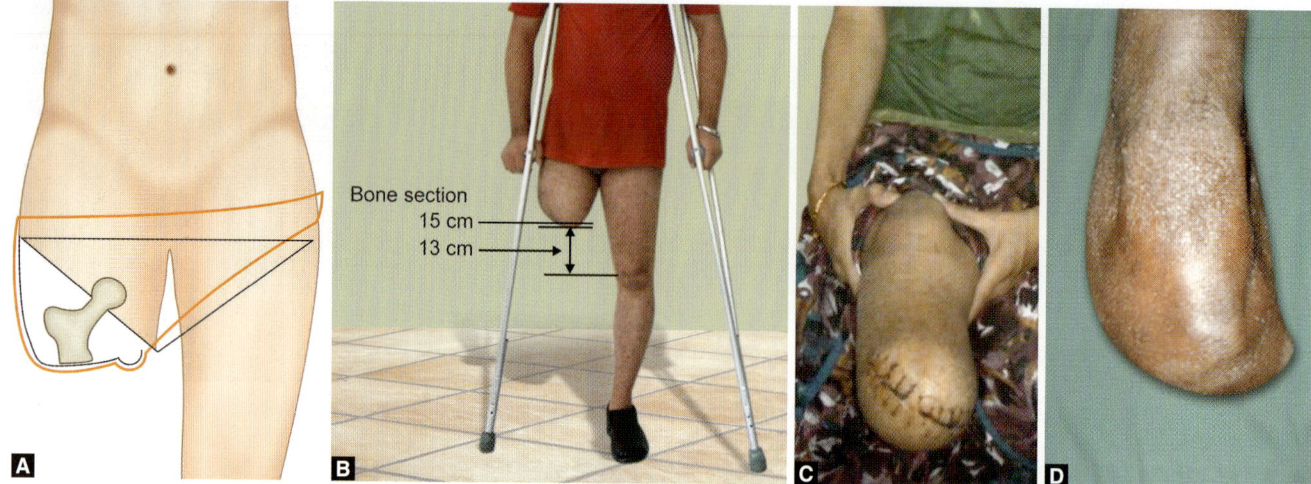

Figs. 4A to D: Ideal length of stump in lower limb. (A) Hip disarticulation; (B) Transfemoral; (C) Transtibial amputation; (D) Transtibial short stump.

especially diabetes, where the ankle is totally destroyed and the patient is unable to take weight and walk even after the orthotic management, amputation is the best option.

IDEAL STUMP

For perfect prosthetic fitting, an ideal stump is needed, though some type of prosthesis can be fitted to any stump. Ideal stump has the following components:

- *Length of the stump—lower limb*:
  - *Hip disarticulation (Through hip amputation)*: There will be a tendency for the prosthesis to migrate upward due to inclined weight-bearing surface while standing with the prosthesis. Head, neck, and greater trochanter of femur should be preserved to provide a horizontal weight-bearing surface (Fig. 4A).
  - *Transfemoral amputation (Above-knee amputation)*: Terminal end of the stump must have a clearance of 10–12 cm (4–5 inch) from opposite knee center, so that after fitting the knee mechanism in the prosthesis, both the knee joints remain at the same level (Fig. 4B). Thus, the bone section should be 14–15 cm (5–6 inch) above the opposite side knee center so that after muscular padding the desired clearance is achieved. A shorter stump, 5 cm from the crotch area, is also acceptable.
  - *Transtibial amputation (Below-knee amputation)*: Ideal length for transtibial amputation in nonischemic limb is 18–20 cm (7–8 inch) to have better pressure distribution, longer lever arm, and better control of prosthesis (Fig. 4C). In ischemic limbs, the idea length should be 12–14 cm (5 inch) to achieve good healing.

  Length of tibia ranges from 35 cm to 40 cm depending upon the height of the individual. Therefore in nonischemic limb, half of the tibia (18–20 cm), and in ischemic limb, one-third of the tibia (12–14 cm) should be preserved.

  Minimum length of the stump should be 8 cm from the joint line; however, 5 cm from the joint line is also acceptable that preserves proprioceptive sensation. Fibular tip, in such a short stump, will deviate outward and cause persistent problem with the prosthetic fitting, and should be completely excised (Fig. 4D).
- *Length of the stump—upper limb*:
  - *Shoulder disarticulation (Through-shoulder amputation)*: Head and some portion of humerus should be preserved providing a horizontal surface for the prosthesis (Fig. 5A).

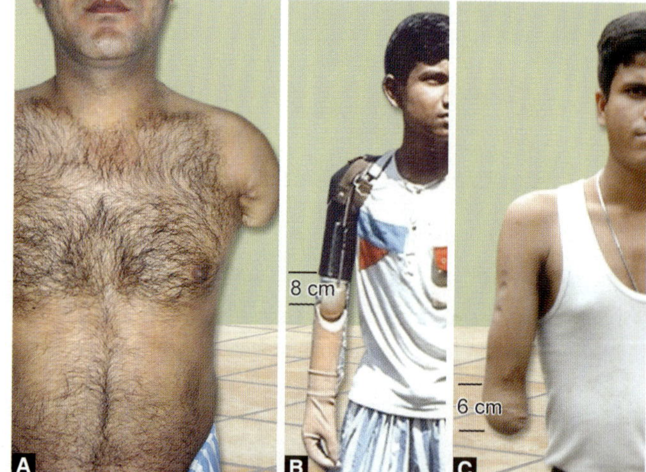

Figs. 5A to C: Ideal length of stump in upper limb. (A) Shoulder disarticulation; (B) Transhumeral; (C) Transradial amputation.

  - *Transhumeral amputation (Above-elbow amputation)*: There should be a clearance of 8 cm from opposite elbow to fit elbow mechanism, so that after fitting the elbow mechanism, both the joints remain at the same level (Fig. 5B).
  - *Transradial amputation (Below-elbow amputation)*: Length for transradial stump should be 6 cm below the elbow crease (Fig. 5C), so that while flexing the elbow the prosthesis will remain in its proper place. There should be a clearance of 6 cm from the wrist joint to fit the wrist mechanism. If the stump is longer than this, the prosthesis will become longer than the other normal side.

  Through-elbow and through-wrist amputation should be avoided, because of poor prosthetic fitting.
- *Scar*: Scar can be placed anywhere provided it is supple and nontender. In transfemoral and knee disarticulation amputees, posterior scar is not preferred since the scar may get compressed between terminal end of the bone and wall of the prosthetic socket during heel strike. In transtibial amputation, the anterior scar should be avoided since it may get crushed between the tibial tip and socket wall. Terminal scar is ideal even for upper limb amputees as well.
- *Joint movements*: All the residual joints should have full and free range of movements. 50% of amputees develop flexion

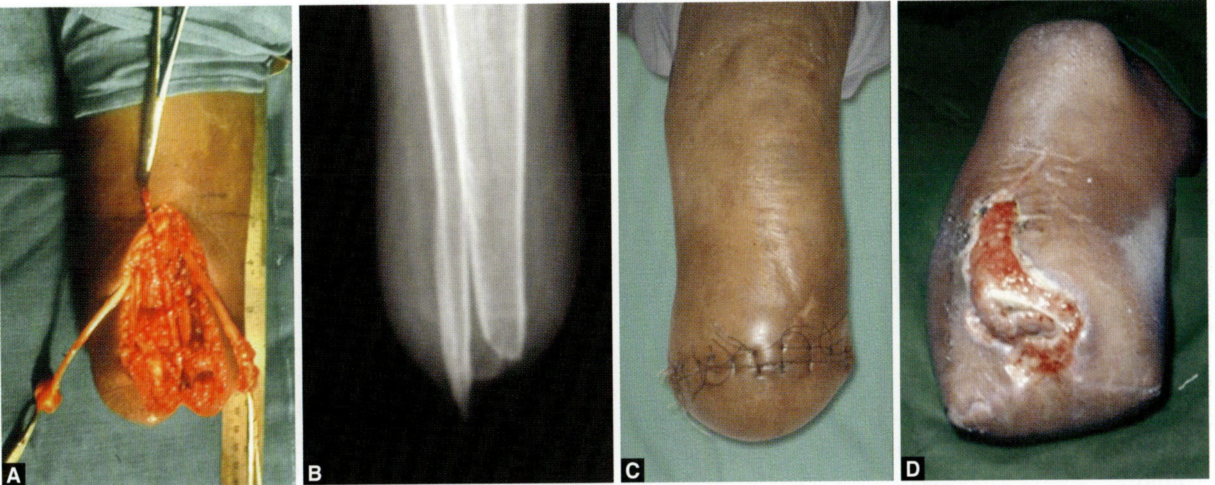

Figs. 6A to D: (A) Terminal scar; (B) Neuroma; (C) Spur formation; (D) Tibial tip.

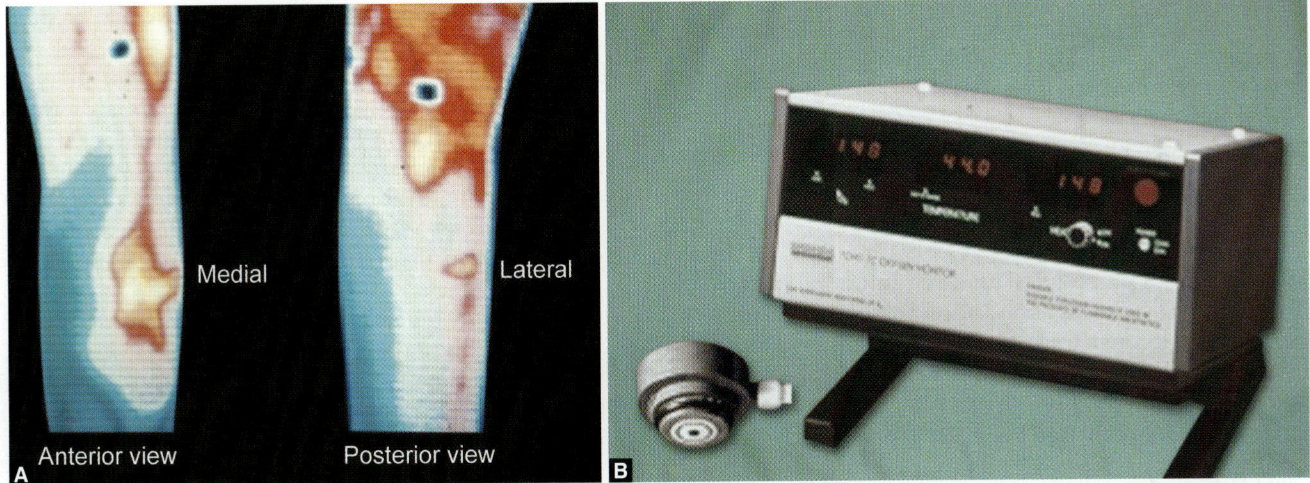

Figs. 7A and B: (A) Thermograph and (B) Clark's electrode and Radiometer's transcutaneous oxygen monitor.

deformity due to keeping a pillow under the stump, especially in ischemic limbs where the muscles undergo fibrosis. No pillow should be used under the stump.

- *Neuroma*: Neuroma formation is a normal physiological process, which under the skin becomes painful while using the prosthesis. To avoid this situation, nerve is pulled, ligated as proximal as possible, and divided just distal to the ligature, allowing the nerve to retract surrounded by the muscles (Fig. 6A).
- *Spur formation*: Spur is formed due to the ossification of the periosteal tags at the terminal end of the bone (Fig. 6B). It can be prevented if the bony side of the periosteum, which is osteogenic and forms the spurs, is buried inside toward the bone.
- *Terminal end of the stump*: Terminal end of the stump should be well-padded with the muscles to provide cushion at the end of the bone (Fig. 6C). The tip of the tibia must be smoothened, otherwise it will pierce through the skin at the end of the stump as shown in Figure 6D.

PREOPERATIVE STAGE

At this stage, counseling and meeting with other amputees plays an important role. Patient should learn walking with crutches and transferring from bed to chair and *vice versa*.

Clinical examination and preoperative investigations are aimed to determine the state of circulation and nutritional state of the tissues.

Clinical Examination

Poor peripheral pulsations, cold skin, loss of hairs, thinning of subcutaneous tissues, bluish discoloration, and blackening indicate poor nutritional state of the limb.

Doppler's Study

Doppler's reading of 75 mm Hg or more supports wound healing. Ischemic index is the ratio of Doppler's reading at the proposed level of amputation and the infraclavicular region. Ischemic index of more than 0.5 supports wound healing. In a state of shock the Doppler's reading would be unreliable.

Thermography

Thermography is the image of the temperature of the limb taken by a thermographic camera where red color indicates good blood flow and bluish-green as poor circulation (Fig. 7A). Thermography results have shown that anteromedial and posterolateral aspect below the knee joint has better blood supply. Based on these observations, skew flap technique of transtibial amputation has been developed.[6,7]

Transcutaneous Partial Pressure of Oxygen Estimations

It is based on the principle that the oxygen carried by the red blood cells (RBCs) comes out through the capillary pores, utilized by the tissues, and under special circumstances it comes out of the skin and can be measured in mm Hg. This indicates the availability of oxygen and healing potential at the recorded area (Fig. 7B). The reading more than 40 mm Hg indicates adequate healing potential. The ratio of transcutaneous partial pressure of oxygen ($TcPO_2$) value at the proposed site of incision with and at control site (infraclavicular region or forehead), if more than 0.5 indicates good healing potential.[14]

Angiography

Angiography visualizes any occlusion in main vessels and may help managing the occlusion with angioplasty or bypass surgery to save the limb.

X-ray

X-ray of the affected limb is done as a routine to assess bony pathology like osteomyelitis or malignancy to decide the level of amputation.

Other routine investigations to assess the fitness for anesthesia are carried out.

Clinical photographs are also recommended for medicolegal purposes.

Preoperative Preparations

Second opinion for amputation and well-informed consent in presence of a witness should always be recorded. Shaving the limb and preoperative through warm water bath with special attention to the limb and perineal area helps in controlling the infection. Preoperative antibiotic, one dose in the evening, and another dose before sending the patient to OT is preferable.

General Principles

Amputation should be performed under pneumatic tourniquet. Tissues holding forceps that damages the tissues should be avoided; using fingers is the best option. Stripping of deep fascia from the skin and periosteum from the bone should be minimal. Major nerves should be gently pulled, ligated as proximal as possible and divided distal to the ligature, so that the nerve-end remains buried in the muscle mass. Main blood vessels should be doubly ligated. A wide bored suction drain under the muscles must be used, which is removed after 48–72 hours or when the drain becomes serous in nature. Operative wound should be closed in layers. Crepe bandaging is done to prevent bleeding keeping the distal pressure more than the proximal. Patient should be covered with proper antibiotics and analgesics.

Pillow under the stump or below the knee joint should never be used. Hyperbaric oxygen should be considered in case of critical ischemia and low molecular weight dextran one unit per day, infused within 2–3 hours for 5 days is found to be advantageous. After removal of drain, the next dressing should be done after 5 days, and repeated after 5 days if everything goes alright. In case of any collection, it should be drained from the side by removing a suture and irrigated with a solution of saline, hydrogen peroxide, and providone iodine in the ratio of 8:1:1. Suture should be removed on 14th day or so and remaining sutures after 48 hours if wound healing is satisfactory.

Physiotherapy

Immediate postoperative physiotherapy should never be done since it encourages capillary oozing. It also increases the oxygen demand, which cannot be met in ischemic limb leading to necrosis of the tissues. However, from 5th day onward gentle movements of the stump should be started. After the wound healing stump shrinker, which is an elastic stump socks with gradient pressure, is recommended.

AMPUTATIONS IN SPECIAL CIRCUMSTANCES

- *Amputation in congenital limb deficiencies:* Surgical intervention, if necessary to fit lower limb prosthesis, should be done at the age, say 18 months, when the child is expected to stand and walk. In case of upper limb, surgery, if required to fit a prosthesis, should be done at the school-going age say 4–5 years.
- *Amputation in children:* Amputation must be avoided or delayed as much as possible unless it is essentially required for prosthesis fitting, and disarticulation should be preferred to preserve the growth plate.
- *Amputation in elderly:* Age is no criteria for denying the amputation in elderly. Elderly patients do fairly well on a wheelchair, even if they are unfit for the prosthesis.
- *Amputation in ischemic limb:* It should be done at the time and at the level where the operative wound is most likely to heal.
- *Amputation in mangled extremity:* In case of massive disruption of tissues where delay threatens life, emergency amputation is indicated.[15,16]
- *Mangled Extremity Severity Score (MESS) is based on:* (1) Injury mechanism (low to very high speed) 1–4, (2) state of shock 1–3, (3) ischemic state 1–4, and (4) age group 1–4. If the mangled extremity severity score is more than 7 in cases of trauma, emergency amputation is indicated.

PREVENTION OF AMPUTATION IN ISCHEMIC LIMBS

Sometimes, amputation can be delayed or prevented by diabetic control, stopping smoking, deep breathing exercises, and hourly oxygen inhalation 5–10 minutes, 3–5 L/min, and hyperbaric oxygen.[17] Omentopexy where omentum along with intact blood supply is brought to calf area through the subcutaneous route and attached to calf muscle. It also helps in cases of ischemic claudications.18 Angioplasty and bypass surgeries have been successfully tried to prevent the amputation and must be tried wherever possible to save the limb.

SOME USEFUL TIPS

- Open wound should be closed as early as possible.
- In case of any collection in the stump, it should be removed by removing one or two sutures from the sides and not from the anterior aspect.
- Split skin graft is not good for stump unless required to preserve the knee joint (Fig. 8A). Stump should not be donor site for skin graft, which affects prosthetic fitting (Fig. 8B).
- Knee joint should be preserved by all possible means even if healing is delayed.
- In case of bilateral amputees, length of the both stumps should be the same as far as possible.

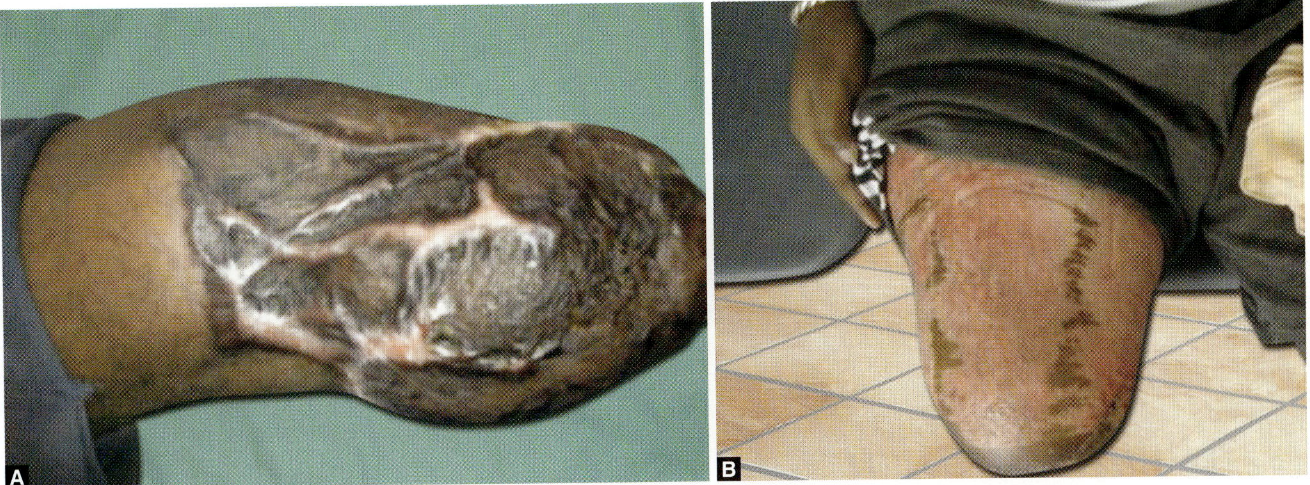

Figs. 8A and B: (A) Skin grafted BK stump and (B) Stump as donor for skin graft.

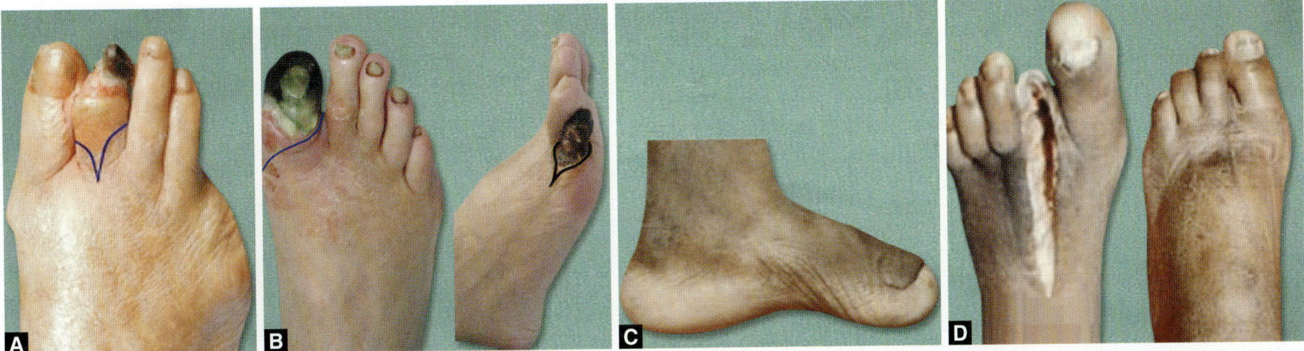

Figs. 9A to D: (A) Amputation of toe; (B) Amputation of great and 5th toes; (C) Tarsometatarsal amputation; (D) Ray amputation.

- In case of malignancy, aim should be to eliminate the disease, even at the cost of stump length.
- Blood transfusion, if patient requires, should be done at the end of the operation.

AMPUTATION SURGERY

Amputation surgery can either be an emergency or planned. Emergency amputation is indicated in severe trauma, irreparable vascular injury, wet gangrene, and severe life-threatening infections like gas gangrene. Amputation should be planned when one can wait to decide the level of amputation. In cases with threatened gangrene, one should wait for the line of demarcation to develop to differentiate between living and dead tissues.

AMPUTATION IN LOWER EXTREMITY

Forefoot Amputation

Amputation of Toes

Under suitable anesthesia, anteroposterior or mediolateral elliptical incision is made as shown in Figure 9A. In case of great toe and 5th toe racket shaped incision is made (Fig. 9B). Preservation of single toe, except great toe, should be avoided. Proximal portion of the base of phalanges should be preserved if possible, when all the toes are to be amputated (Fig. 9C). Ray amputation involves amputation of single toe along with distal metatarsal, which helps maintaining function as well as cosmetic appearance (Fig. 9D).

Transmetatarsal Amputations

The amputation is done through the metatarsals. One should make all efforts to preserve the foot length and sole skin, which is brought dorsally so that terminal portion of residual foot is covered with normal sole skin. Terminal inferior end of metatarsals should be rounded off.

Midfoot Amputation

Tarsometatarsal Amputation (Lisfranc's Amputation)

The amputation is performed at the tarsometatarsal junction (Fig. 10A). Principle of the amputation is the same as that of transmetatarsal amputation. The base of second metatarsal should be preserved to provide smooth distal surface (Fig. 10B). Invariably, the residual foot goes into equinovarus deformity due to strong plantar flexors (tendo Achilles) and weak dorsiflexors, and unopposed action of tibialis anterior and posterior. To overcome the varus deformity, base of fifth metatarsal is saved and peroneus longus is attached to it. Tibialis anterior is transferred to head of the talus in addition to weakening the temporal arteritis (TA) to prevent equinus deformity (Fig. 10C).

Chopart's Amputation

It is amputation of the foot through the midtarsal joint, retaining calcaneum and talus. Residual foot goes into equinovarus deformity, due to similar reasons as in Lisfranc's amputation.

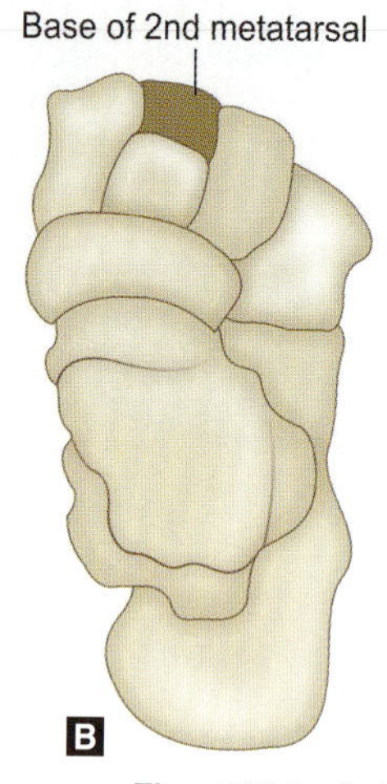

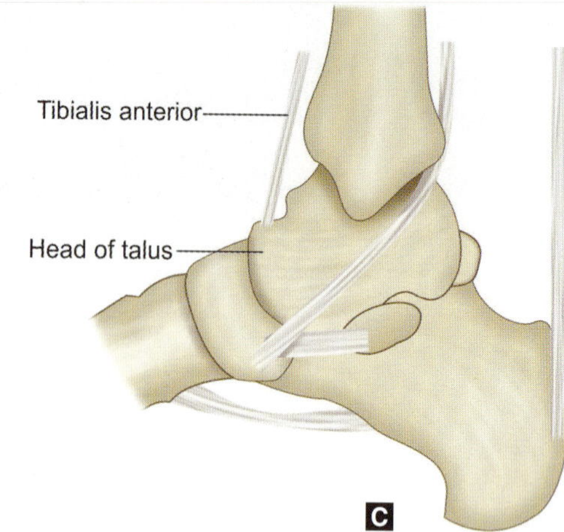

Figs. 10A to C: Lisfranc's amputation.

Procedure: The flaps are marked keeping the planter flap longer, incision is made, and deepened without separating the layers. The interosseous ligaments connecting calcaneum, cuboid and talus, navicular bones are divided to separate the distal foot. To prevent the equinovarus deformity, tendo-Achilles tendon is partially divided and tibialis anterior and extensor tendons are transferred to head of the talus.

Modified Chopart's Amputation

It includes talocalcaneal arthrodesis with anterior shifting of calcaneum to prevent the equinus deformity. Tibiotalocalcaneal arthrodesis (Pantalar arthrodesis) with anterior shifting of calcaneum is also recommended (Figs. 11A and B).

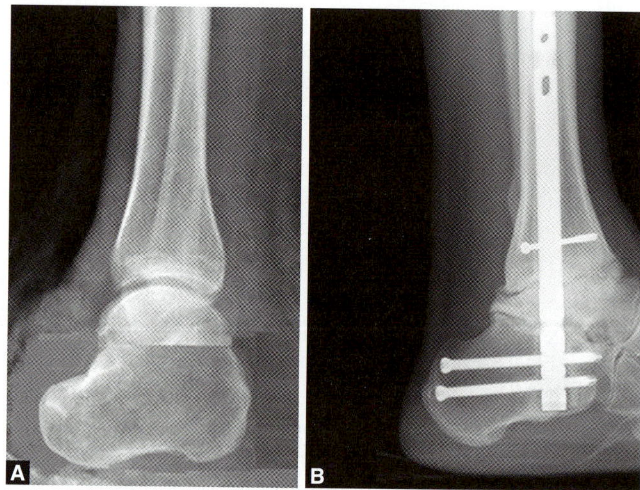

Figs. 11A and B: (A) Talocalcaneal arthrodesis and (B) Tibiotalocalcaneal arthrodesis.

Hindfoot Amputation

Boyd's Amputation (Talectomy and Calcaneotibial Arthrodesis)

Boyd's amputation is at the level of ankle where talus is removed and calcaneum with its heel pad is preserved and fused with tibia.

- Procedure—it is similar to that of Chopart's amputation. Tibia and fibula are divided horizontally just above the articular surface. Talus is removed, foot is dislocated posteriorly, and Achilles tendon is divided since it has no role to play. Superior surface of the calcaneum is roughened and shifted anteriorly and fixed with tibia with two screws (Fig. 12A). It allows weight-bearing through the sole skin that maintains its position.

Pirogoff's (Pirigov's) Amputation (Talectomy and Vertical Osteotomy of Calcaneum)

Pirogoff's amputation is similar to the Boyd's amputation, with a difference that the calcaneum is divided vertically at the middle, rotated and fixed to the tibia and fibula with the help of screws (Fig. 12B). This amputation provides a very narrow area for weight-bearing and therefore has not become popular.

In both, Boyd and Pirogoff amputations, the tibiocalcaneal bony fusion gives good stability. The skin flap does not show necrosis since it is not separated from calcaneum; limb length discrepancy is also minimal that makes it easier for the patient to walk without prosthesis indoors. However, both these procedures have not gained popularity.

Syme's Amputation

Syme's amputation is where the tibial section is done just above the articular surface and heel flap is retained. This gives fairly good results where patient can move around short distances without any prosthesis though with a limp due to limb length discrepancy. On most of the occasions, heel flap migrates posteriorly due to its poor adhesion with tibia and pull by calf muscles.[19]

Marking of flaps: A line is drawn from the tips of the lateral malleolus to medial malleolus over the anterior surface of the ankle through the shortest route. From the tips of malleoli a vertical line is drawn to meet at the planter surface (Figs. 13A and B).

Procedure: Under tourniquet, incision is made on the anterior aspect and deepened to divide deep fascia and tendons, to expose the ankle joint. Vertical incisions are made from both the malleoli to meet at the planter aspect. Incision is deepened up to the calcaneum, with care to avoid any injury to the posterior tibial artery. The foot is now dislocated posteriorly, medial and lateral collateral ligaments are divided, visualizing the posterior aspect of calcaneum. The Achilles tendon is released from the calcaneum by keeping the knife very close to the bone. Foot is further dislocated and calcaneum is now

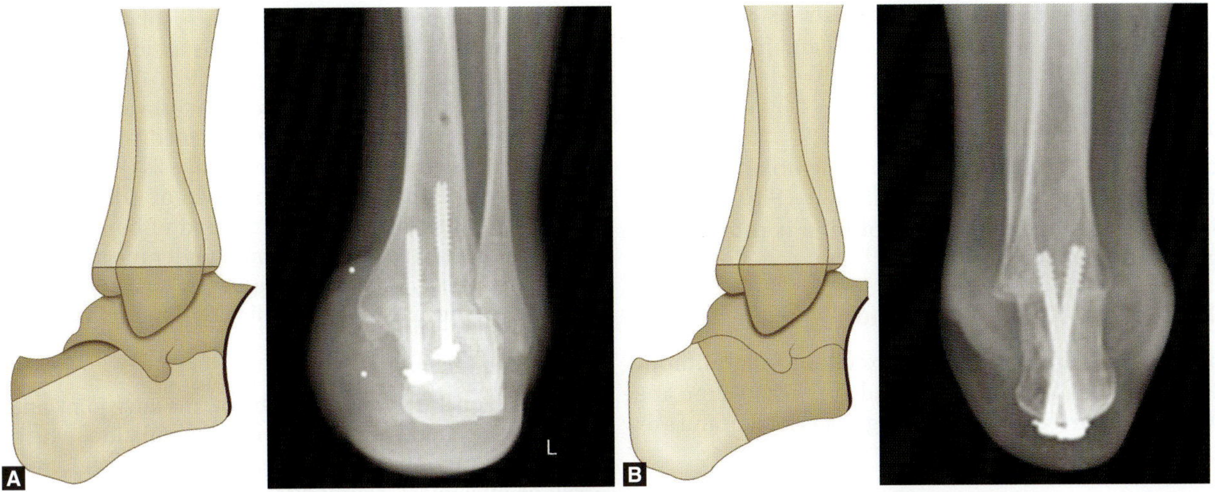

Figs. 12A and B: (A) Boyd's amputation and (B) Pirogoff's amputation.

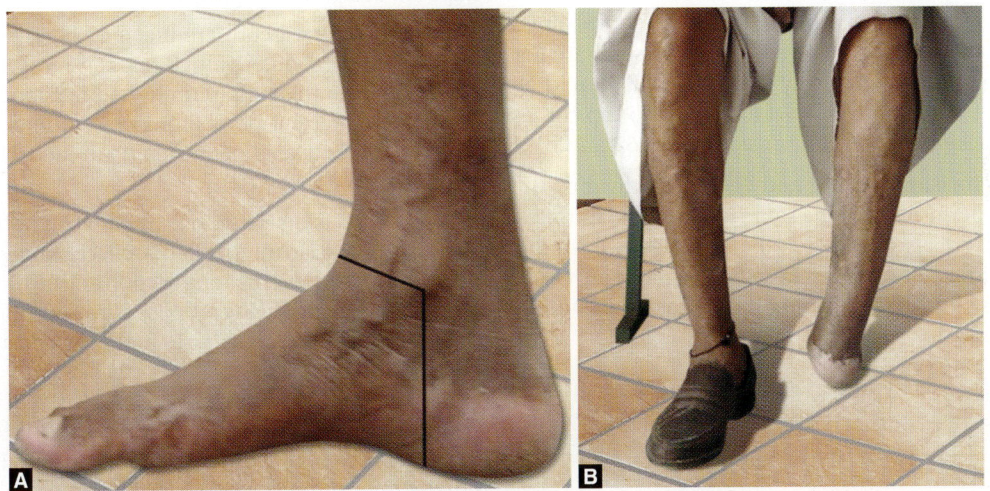

Figs. 13A and B: Syme's amputation: (A) Marking of flaps and (B) Syme's stump.

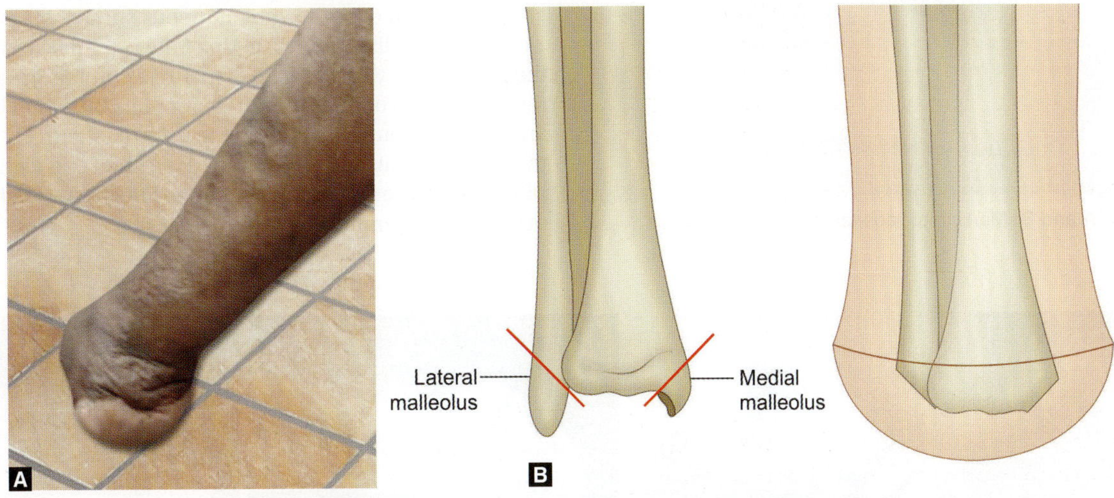

Figs. 14A and B: (A) Migrating heel flap and (B) Modified Syme's amputation.

separated from its periosteum with sharp dissection keeping it close to the bone, thus separating foot from the ankle. Tibia and fibula are divided horizontally just above its articular surface. Periosteum of the plantar flap is sutured with periosteum of tibia on the anterior aspect, which is an important step to prevent posterior migration of plantar flap (Fig. 14A). Achilles tenodesis also helps preventing the heel flap migration posteriorly.[19] The wound now is closed in layers with a drainage tube coming out from the sides. Dog ears, if any, should not be disturbed, since this may damage the blood supply to the plantar flap.

Dressing is done with elastic adhesive straps compressing plantar flap against the lower cut end of tibia and fibula to assist its adhesion.

Modified Syme's Amputation

The articular surface of tibia is retained, while tibial and fibular malleoli are removed by dividing obliquely (Fig. 14B). The cartilaginous weight-bearing surface of tibia is proven to be advantageous in many cases.

Transtibial (Below-Knee) Amputation

Transtibial amputation provides an excellent rehabilitation; therefore all possible efforts must be made to preserve the knee joint. Commonly used techniques are long posterior flap and skew flap techniques.[5-9]

Long Posterior Flap Technique

Marking of flaps: At the proposed level of bone sections, two points are marked on lateral and medial aspects. These points are joined to form the anterior flap. From these two points, a semicircular posterior flap is marked in such a way that its length should be equal to half of the circumference so that the tip of the flap comes up to the anterior incision without any tension (Figs. 15A and B).[4,5]

Procedure: Anterior incision is made and deepened, dividing the deep fascia and the periosteum at the same level. All the muscles, except calf muscles, are also divided at the same level. Posterior incision is made dividing the deep fascia without separating it from the underlying muscles. After reflecting the periosteum, tibia is divided at the proposed level. Fibula is isolated and divided 1–1.5 cm proximal to tibial section. The distal tibia is pulled distally to expose the posterior muscle mass (Fig. 16A), which is divided keeping the knife close to the bone to form a myofascial flap (Fig. 16B). Tibial tip is beveled and smoothened; otherwise it will pierce through the skin while using the prosthesis (Figs. 16C and D).

Posterior flap, which is comprised of calf muscles and skin, is brought anteriorly covering the end of bones, and sutured in layers, after placing a suction drain under the muscle flap. Stump is dressed with crepe bandage. A few surgeons advocate rigid dressing to prevent edema and flexion contracture.

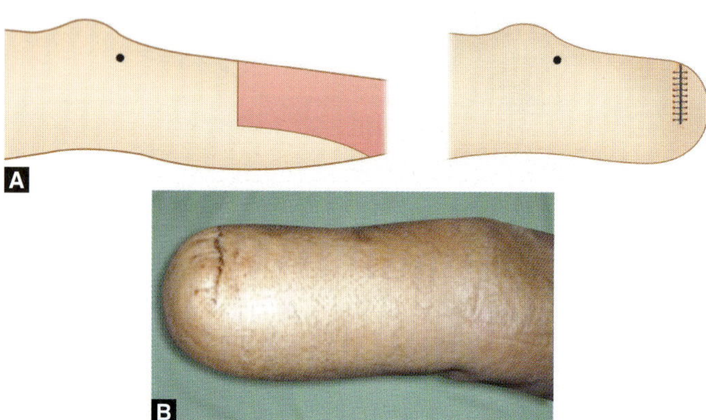

Figs. 15A and B: Marking of flaps and transtibial stump.

Skew Flap Technique

It is based on the principle that below the knee joint, anteromedial and posterolateral areas have better circulation, which has been proved by thermography, transcutaneous oxygen monitoring as well as by clinical examination (Figs. 17A and B).[7-10,20] Based on these observations, equal anteromedial and posterolateral skin flaps are designed, keeping the long muscle flap.

Marking of flaps: Circumferential marking is made at the proposed level of bone section. A point is marked 2.5–3 cm lateral to the tibial crest and from this point another equidistant point is marked on the posterolateral aspect. From these points, equal semicircular flaps are marked keeping the length of each flap, one-fourth of the circumference (Fig. 17C).

Procedure: Incision is made as planned on both the sides up to the level of deep fascia. Anterior flap is reflected along with the deep fascia till the proposed level of bone section and all the muscles except calf muscles are divided at the proposed level of bone section. Thereafter, the procedure remains same as in the long posterior flap technique (Fig. 17D).

Modified Skew Flap Technique (Jain's Modification)

In due course of time, the posterior muscles fall back, due to the pull by the calf muscles, leaving the tip of tibia just covered with skin and deep fascia without any muscular padding (Fig. 18A). This remains a constant source of problem during prosthetic fitting.

Periosteum over the subcutaneous surface of tibia is stripped 1 cm from the distal end. The tip of the calf muscle is sutured with the periosteum with the help of mattress sutures, in such a way that the beveled tip of the calf muscle remains buried in between tibia and its periosteum as if it has been inserted there (Fig. 18B).[9,10] This procedure results in a well-padded terminal end of the stump. The same procedure is also applied for the long posterior flap technique of transtibial amputation (Fig. 18C).

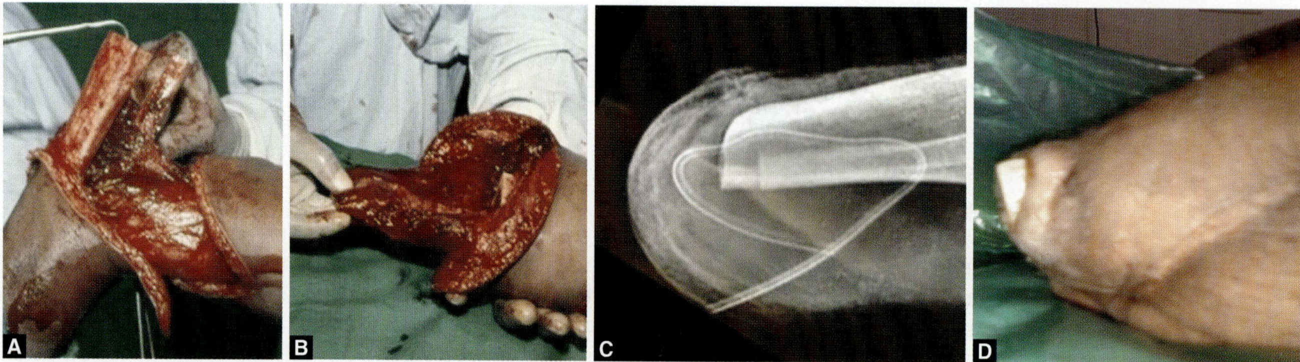

Figs. 16A to D: (A) Exposed calf muscles; (B) Long posterior flap; (C) Beveled smoothened tibia; and (D) Sharp tibial tip piercing through the skin.

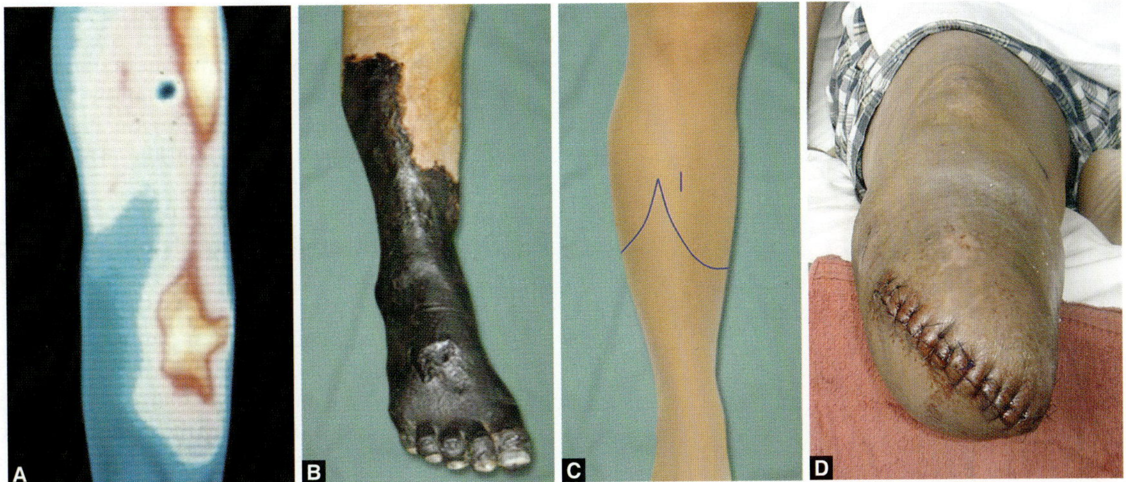

Figs. 17A to D: (A) Thermography anterior view; (B) Anteromedial viable skin; (C) Marking of skew flaps; (D) Postoperative picture—after flap placement.

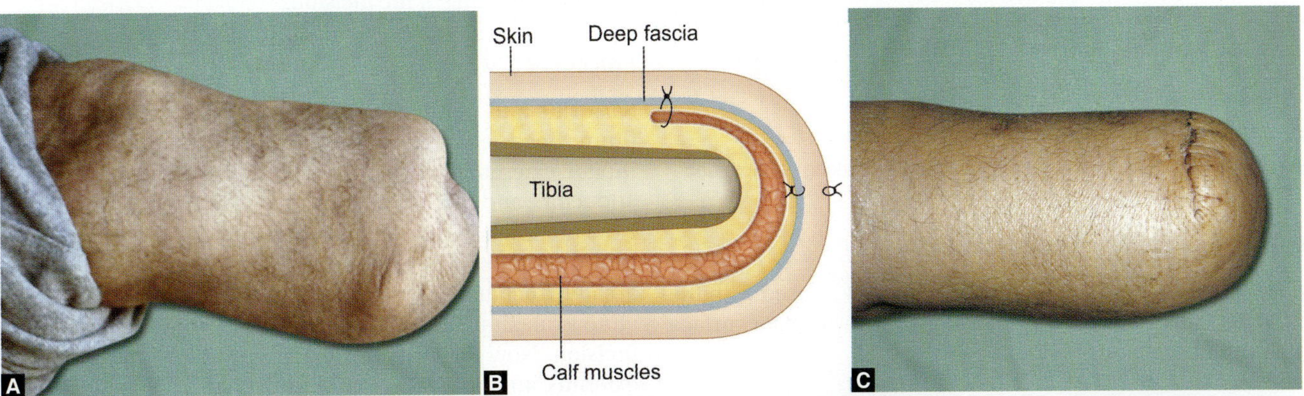

Figs. 18A to C: Modified skew flap technique and stump.

Other Variations of Transtibial Amputation

Bone-Bridging (Ertl Procedure)

The Ertl procedure is bone bridging between the distal ends of tibia and fibula achieved by a fibular osteotomy rotated and fixed to the tibia (Fig. 19).[21,22] This procedure has not gained popularity.

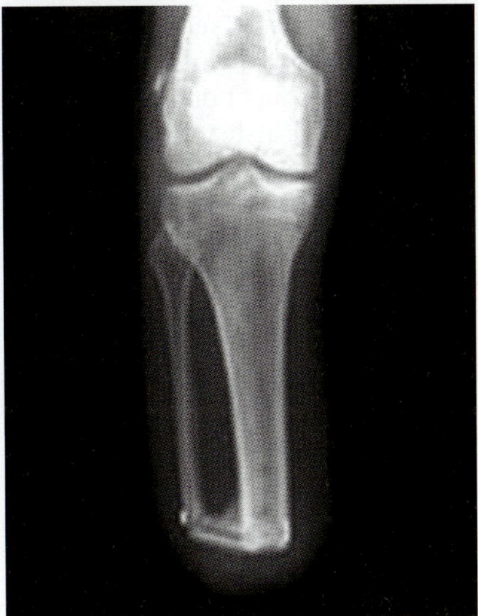

Fig. 19: Ertl bone bridging procedure.

Knee Disarticulation

Knee disarticulation has many advantages like—(1) Large weight-bearing surfaces; (2) Prosthesis can be self suspending due to its broad terminal end; (3) Muscle balance remains undisturbed; (4) Knee disarticulation is helpful in healthy sexual life; (5) In children and young adults with congenital tibial deficiency, knee disarticulation allows femur to grow to its full extent; and (6) May have some proprioceptive sensations due to preserved articular surface.[23] Knee disarticulation may have poor cosmetic appearance while sitting.

Marking of flaps: A circumferential marking is made 8 cm below the knee joint line as shown in Figure 20A.

Procedure: Under tourniquet, incision is made over the circumferential marking and deepened. Patellar tendon is detached from its insertion, joint is exposed by dividing the capsule and the cruciate ligaments are divided at their tibial attachments. Tibia is dislocated posteriorly, collateral ligaments and hamstrings are divided, and then posterior joint capsule is carefully divided. Popliteal vessels are doubly ligated, tibial and peroneal nerves are isolated, pulled gently, ligated as proximal as possible and divided. The patellar tendon and the hamstring tendons are stitched to the cruciate ligaments in such a way that the patella must remain above the condylar level. Wound is closed by converting the circularly divided skin into anteroposterior or lateral flaps. Author prefers equal mediolateral flaps (Fig. 20B), so that the suture line passes through intercondylar groove, avoiding weight-bearing on the scar.

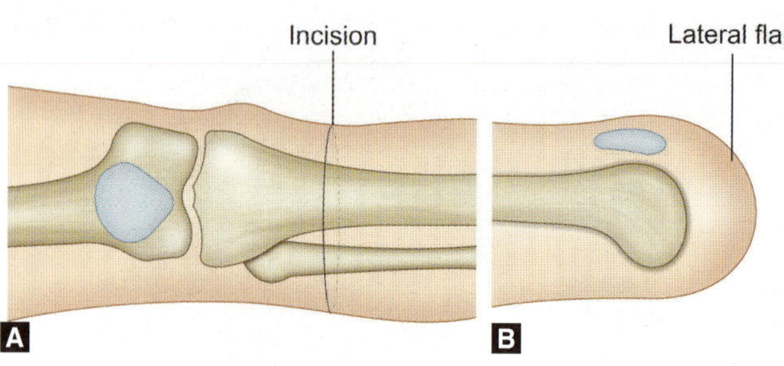

Figs. 20A and B: Knee disarticulation flap marking. (A) Circumferential and (B) Lateral flaps.

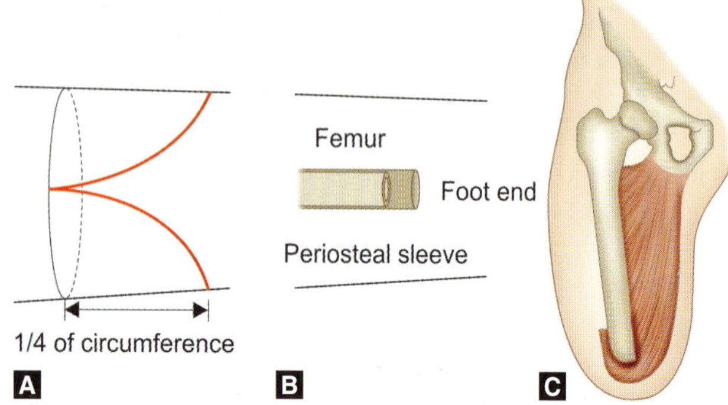

Figs. 21A to C: (A) Transfemoral amputation; (B) Marking of flaps; and (C) periosteal sleeve.

Other Variations of Knee Disarticulation

Gritti stokes procedure: In this procedure, patella is fused with the terminal portion of distal femur after shaving the articular surface of patella and distal end of femur.

Transfemoral (Above-Knee) Amputation

Most of the patients who require transfemoral amputation have traumatic severe soft tissue, vascular, neurologic, and bone injuries. Initially, through debridement followed by closure after 4–5 days, the infection is brought under control. Fractures of the femur should be stabilized instead of amputating through the fracture site, to preserve the appropriate length. In case of tumor, its eradication it more important than the length.

Marking of Flaps

A circumferential marking is made at the proposed level of bone section, which is divided in two equal anterior and posterior halves. Semicircular flaps are now marked from these points keeping the length of each flap one-fourth of the circumference of thigh (Fig. 21A).

Procedure

After applying the pneumatic tourniquet, incision is made on both the sides dividing the deep fascia. Muscles are then incised to expose the femur. Periosteum is now divided circumferentially 3 cm distal to the proposed level of bone section, which is stripped proximally as a periosteal tube (Fig. 21B). Bone is now divided at the proposed level, separating the limb. Periosteal tube is closed over the cut end of the femur, in such a way that the bony side of periosteum is buried inside. Blood vessels and nerves are managed and wound is closed in layers after putting a drain. Stump is dressed and crepe bandage is applied.

Gottschalk's Procedure

The stump has tendency to go into abduction due to unopposed action of the hip abductors. This situation can be overcome by preserving the adductor magnus, bringing it across the cut end of the femur and suturing it on terminal lateral aspect, keeping stump in slight adduction (Fig. 21C).[24]

Hip Disarticulation (Through Hip Amputation)

Marking of Flaps

Incision is marked beginning at a point just below the anterior superior iliac spine, almost parallel with the inguinal ligament to a point on the medial aspect of the thigh 5 cm distal to crotch area, then continue the incision around the posterior aspect of the thigh about 5 cm distal to the ischial tuberosity reaching to the lateral aspect of the thigh about 8 cm distal to the base of the greater trochanter. From this point the incision is brought proximally to join the beginning of the incision.

Procedure

Sartorius and rectus femoris muscles are detached from their ilium; pectineus is divided 1 cm from the pubis. The thigh is rotated externally, the iliopsoas tendon is divided at its insertion, adductors, and gracilis muscles are divided 1 cm from their origins. Now the thigh is rotated internally, and the gluteus medius and minimus muscles are detached from their insertions on the greater trochanter. The fascia lata and the distal portion of the gluteus maximus muscle are now divided in the line of the skin incision. Now piriformis, gemelli, obturator internus, obturator externus, and quadratus femoris are divided from their insertions on the femur and hamstring muscles are released from the ischial tuberosity. Capsule and the ligamentum teres are divided to complete the disarticulation. Gluteal muscle flap is brought anteriorly, and sutured with the pectineus and adductor muscles.[25] Wound is closed in layers after putting a drain.

Hemipelvectomy

Anterior Flap Hemipelvectomy

Hemipelvectomy is indicated for lesions of the buttock, posterior proximal thigh, and tumors around the proximal thigh and hip that cannot be adequately treated by limb-saving procedures. Pelvis is excised with careful dissection, without damaging the bladder, urethra, and rectum. The disarticulation at sacroiliac junction is not required. The larger posterior defect is covered by the quadriceps and the skin from the anterior aspect of the thigh.

AMPUTATION IN UPPER EXTREMITY

Amputation through the Fingers and Hand

During initial surgery one should preserve the fingers as much as possible, especially the thumb, since its loss results in almost 50% loss of function in extremity.

Amputation of Fingers

In case of index finger, the metacarpal should be obliquely divided to have a better cosmetic appearance (Fig. 22A). However, in case of manual workers the head of the metacarpal should be

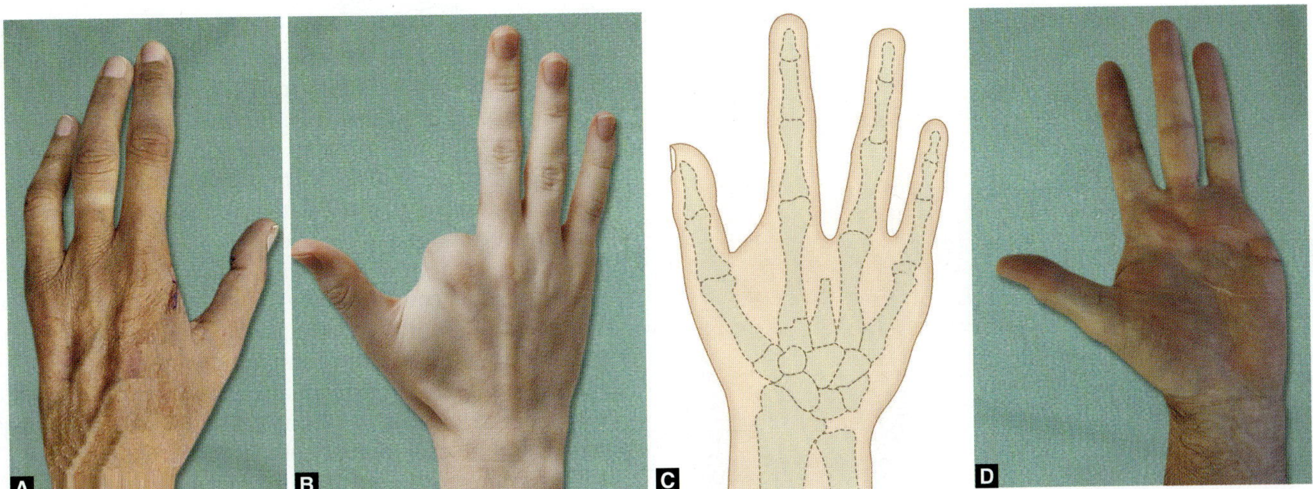

Figs. 22A to D: Amputation of fingers.

preserved (Fig. 22B). In case of amputation of middle or ring fingers the metacarpal should be excised from its base, to have a good cosmetic appearance (Fig. 22C). While amputating the little finger the metacarpal should be excised oblique to achieve good cosmetic appearance (Fig. 22D). The length should be preserved as much as possible in case of multiple fingers amputation.

Amputation of Thumb

Thumb is the most important part of hand, and should be preserved by all possible means. In case of loss of thumb pollicization of the index finger is a good option.

Transmetacarpal Amputation

Amputation through the metacarpals, where all the metacarpals are involved, results into almost useless stump. If thumb is preserved, it would be a good functional partial hand; therefore, one must preserve the thumb by all possible means.

Wrist Disarticulation

Wrist disarticulation is only suitable for cosmetic hand. A circular incision is made 3 cm distal to the proposed level, deepened, and all the tissues are divided. All the carpal bones are removed and wound is closed in layers after managing dog ears.

Transradial Amputation

The length of the stump ranges 8 cm from olecranon to 5 cm proximal from the wrist joint. A circular incision is made 4 cm distal to the proposed level of bone section, deepened up to the bones. Periosteum is divided at the same level around both the bones and reflected up to proposed level of bone section as a periosteal tube. Bones are divided and the periosteal tube along with muscles and tendons sutured the end of the bones. Dog ears are managed by dividing the skin and deep fascia by 2 cm on either excising the corners. Deep fascia and skin are closed in layers.

Elbow Disarticulation

In an elbow disarticulation, the entire radius and ulna are separated at the level of the elbow. A circular incision is made 5 cm distal to the epicondyles exposing the muscles. All the muscles are detached from their incretion at radius and ulna.

The triceps tendon is brought forward over the trochlea and sutured with brachialis muscle. The biceps tendon is also sutured with brachialis muscle as distal as possible. Suturing muscles at the end of the bone may result in a sling-like effect, reducing the effectiveness of the muscles. A myodesis by suturing the muscles with the bone through drill holes at the distal humerus is advisable. It results in a long stump with bulky terminal end, and does not provide sufficient space for fitting the wrist mechanism of the prosthesis. The wrist disarticulation prosthesis is poor functionally and cosmetically.

Transhumeral Amputation

The stump should have a clearance of 8 cm from the elbow joint to fit the elbow mechanism in the prosthesis, therefore the bone section should be 10 cm above the elbow joint and this is marked on the skin. A circumferential marking is made 3 cm below this marking. An incision is made and deepened; all the tissues including the periosteum are divided. Periosteum is reflected a few mm proximal to the proposed bone section. Humerus is divided, periosteal tube, and all the muscles are allowed to fall back over the terminal end of the bone. Periosteal tube is closed and opposing muscles are sutured in layers, deep fascia and skin is closed in layers after managing the dog ears.

Through Shoulder Amputation

It is advisable to preserve the head of humerus (Fig. 23A). Anteriorly the incision is made from coracoid process, along anterior border of the deltoid muscle up to its insertion. Posterior incision is made along posterior deltoid border to posterior axillary fold; both the proximal ends are connected by an incision through the axilla. Deltoid muscle is reflected from its insertion along with the skin flap, pectoralis tendon is divided at its insertion and reflected medially to expose neurovascular bundle. Teres major and latissimus dorsi are divided at bicipital groove. Biceps, coracobrachialis, and triceps are divided 2–3 cm distal to the proposed bone section through its neck. Triceps, biceps, and coracobrachialis are sutured over the end of humerus, wound is closed in layers.

Shoulder Disarticulation

Deltoid muscle is reflected superiorly to expose shoulder joint capsule, teres major, and latissimus dorsi are divided at their insertions. After internally rotating the arm, posterior rotator

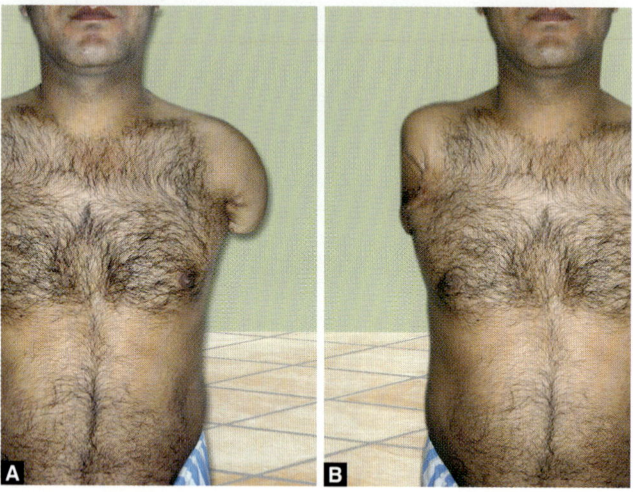

Figs. 23A and B: Through shoulder amputation.

muscles along with posterior capsule are divided. Subscapularis and anterior joint capsule are divided after externally rotating the arm, which is separated by dividing triceps at its insertion on infraglenoid tubercle and inferior capsule. Acromion process is trim to produce smoothly rounded contour. Deltoid is sutured to inferior glenoid region to fill the hollow. Wound is closed in layers (Fig. 23B).

COMPLICATIONS OF AMPUTATION SURGERY

Early Complications

Hematoma

Slipping of ligature from a major vessel and poor drainage are the common causes for hematoma inside the stump. Adequate drainage and compression dressings prevent hematoma formation. In case of increasing hematoma exploration, managing the bleeders is the best option.

Infection

In spite of all the measures, the infection can still take place. This can be managed by antibiotic coverage and draining the collection by removing one or two sutures from the side and irrigating the wound with diluted povidone-iodine and hydrogen peroxide.

Disruption of the Suture Line

It may either be due to hematoma or sutures cutting through. This can be prevented by drainage and compression dressing.

Wound Necrosis

Poor nutrition is the usual cause of necrosis at the margins. Small area of necrosis can be managed by dressing and skin grafting, otherwise shortening the bone and closure without tension is a good option.

Late Complications

- Contracture at the proximal joint usually takes place by keeping a pillow under the stump, gradual stretching is helpful. In ischemic limb sometimes the contracture is unavoidable due to the fibrosis in the muscles.
- Spur formation at the end of the bone takes place due to ossification of the periosteal tags excising is the best option. Spur formation can be prevented by closing the periosteum carefully, keeping the bony side of periosteum buried inside.
- Neuroma formation is a normal physiological process and becomes painful when it is compressed while using the prosthesis. It is managed by exploring it, gently pulling it, ligating the nerve as proximal as possible and dividing it distal to the ligature, so that the cut-end of the nerve retracts and remains surrounded by muscles.
- Phantom sensations are when an amputee experiences sensations that come from the limb that has been amputated. The term phantom does not mean that the symptoms are imaginary. In most of the amputees, within 1 year they feel that the amputated limb gradually shortens and then gradually disappears. However, in 10% of cases the phantom limb pain remains troublesome, especially in those amputees who had suffered from preoperative pain for long duration.[26]

It is difficult to treat established phantom pain, however some may benefit by various measures such as ice, heat, massage, compression socks, local nerve block, sympathetic block, epidural block, ultrasound, and transcutaneous electric nerve stimulation (TENS). Prolonged prosthetic use may also be helpful. Various medications such as—(1) Nonsteroidal anti-inflammatory drugs; (2) Anticonvulsants; (3) Antidepressants; (4) Opioids; and (5) Corticosteroids may be helpful.

Mirror visual feedback is a new concept for phantom limb pain invented by Vilayanur S Ramachandran.[27,28] A mirror is used to create a reflection of the normal limb as amputated limb. The amputee is asked to exercise the amputated limb looking at the image of the normal limb. It has been found to relieve pain from a phantom limb.

- *Surgery*: In some cases, excision of neuroma or neurectomy may be considered to relieve phantom limb pain, though it may not be successful.

REFERENCES

1. Loukas M, Lanteri A, Ferrauiola J, et al. Anatomy in ancient India: A focus on the Susruta Samhita. J Anat. 2010;217(6):646-50.
2. Paré A. A Surgeon in the field. In: Ross JB, McLauglin MM (Eds). The Portable Renaissance Reader. New York, Viking Penguin; 1981. pp.58-63.
3. Boyd HB. Amputation of the foot with calcaneotibial arthrodesis. J Bone Joint Surg Am. 1939;21(4):997-1000.
4. Burgess EM. The below-knee amputation. ICIB. 1969;8(4):1-22.
5. Burgess EM, Romano RL, Zettl JH, et al. Amputations of the leg for peripheral vascular insufficiency. J Bone Joint Surg Am. 1971;53(5):874-90.
6. Robinson KP, Hoile R, Coddington T. Skew flap myoplastic below knee amputation: a preliminary report. Br J Surg. 1982;69(9):554-7.
7. Robinson KP. Skew-flap below-knee amputation. Ann R Coll Surg Engl. 1991;73(3):155-7.
8. Jain SK. Below knee amputation: an improved technique. Medical Journal Armed Forces India. 1993;49(2):113-6.
9. Jain SK. Skew flap technique in trans-tibial amputation. Prosthet Orthot Int. 2005;29(3):283-90.
10. Sabzi Sarvestani A, Taheri Azam A. Amputation: A ten-year survey. Trauma Mon. 2013;18(3):126-9.
11. Marks LJ, Michael JW. Science, medicine, and the future: Artificial limbs. BMJ. 2001;323(7315):732-5.
12. Bisseriex H, Rogez D, Thomas M, et al. Amputation in low-income countries: particularities in epidemiological features and management practices. Med Trop (Mars). 2011;71(6):565-71.
13. Jain SK. A study of 200 cases of congenital limb deficiencies. Prosthet Orthot Int. 1994;18(3):174-9.

14. Mustapha NM, Redhead RG, Jain SK, et al. Transcutaneous partial oxygen pressure assessment of the ischemic lower limb. Surg Gynecol Obstet. 1983;156(5):582-4.
15. Patel MB, Richter KM, Shafi S. Mangled extremity: Amputation versus salvage. Curr Trauma Rep. 2015;1(1):45-9.
16. Niinikoski JH. Clinical hyperbaric oxygen therapy, wound perfusion, and transcutaneous oximetry. World J Surg. 2004;28(3):307-11.
17. Talwar S, Choudhary SK. Omentopexy for limb salvage in Buerger's disease: indications, technique and results. J Postgrad Med. 2001;47(2):137-42.
18. Aboyans V, Ho E, Denenberg JO, et al. The association between elevated ankle systolic pressures and peripheral occlusive arterial disease in diabetic and nondiabetic subjects. J Vasc Surg. 2008;48(5):1197-203.
19. Smith DG, Sangeorzan BJ, Hansen ST Jr, et al. Achilles tendon tenodesis to prevent heel pad migration in the Syme's amputation. Foot Ankle Int. 1994;15(1):14-7.
20. Helfet DL, Howey T, Sanders R, et al. Limb salvage versus amputation. Preliminary results of the Mangled Extremity Severity Score. Clin Orthop Real Res. 1990;(256):80-6.
21. von Ertl J. About amputation stumps. Chirurgie. 1949;20:212-8.
22. Pinzur MS, Pinto MA, Saltzman M, et al. Health-related quality of life in patients with transtibial amputation reconstruction with bone bridging of the distal tibia and fibula. Foot Ankle Int. 2006;27(11):907-12.
23. Batch JW, Spittler AW, McFaddin JG. Advantages of the knee disarticulation over amputations through the thigh. J Bone Joint Surg Am. 1954;36-A(5):921-30.
24. Gottschalk F. Transfemoral amputation: In: Bowker JH, Micheal JW (Eds). Atlas of Limb Prosthetics: Surgical, Prosthetic, and Rehabilitation Principles. St Louis, MO: Mosby Year Book; 1992. pp. 479-86.
25. Sugarbaker PH, Chretien PB. A surgical technique for hip disarticulation. Surgery. 1981;90(3):546-53.
26. Jensen TS, Kreb B, Nielsen J, et al. Phantom limb, phantom pain and stump pain in amputees during the first 6 months following limb amputation. Pain. 1983;17(3):243-56.
27. Ramachandran VS, Rogers-Ramachandran D, Cobb S. Touching the phantom limb. Nature. 1995;377(6549):489-90.
28. Ramachandran VS, Rogers-Ramachandran D. Synaesthesia in phantom limbs induced with mirrors. Proc Biol Sci. 1996;263(1369):377-86.

SECTION

3

Regional Orthopedics

- Hand and Wrist
- Elbow
- Shoulder
- Hip Joint
- Knee
- Foot and Ankle
- Spine

CHAPTER

27

Hand and Wrist

OBJECTIVES

- Anatomy of Wrist
- Examination of Wrist Joint
- Congenital Deformities of Hand
- Madelung Deformity
- Hand Infections
- Injuries of the Hand
- Ganglionic Cysts of the Wrist
- Distal Radioulnar Joint
- Distal Radius Fractures
- Complications and Management of Distal Radius Fractures
- External Fixation of Distal Radius Fractures
- Plating of Distal Radius Fractures
- Carpal Bone Fractures
- Scaphoid Fractures
- Scaphocapitate Fracture Syndrome
- Dorsal Intercalated Segment Instability
- Volar Intercalated Segment Instability
- Gamekeeper's Thumb
- Boxer's Fracture
- Bennett's Fracture
- Rolando's Fracture
- Wrist Arthrodesis
- Wrist Arthroplasty

ANATOMY OF WRIST

Anatomy

Wrist joint comprises of the distal end of radius and articular disk overlying the distal end of ulna and the scaphoid, lunate and the triquetrum.

It is an ellipsoid variety of synovial joint, where the joint line is obtained by joining the styloid process of the radius and ulna. X-ray of wrist joint is shown in Figure 1.

Surface Landmarks

Important surface landmarks of this joint include:

- Radial styloid process
- Lister's tubercle

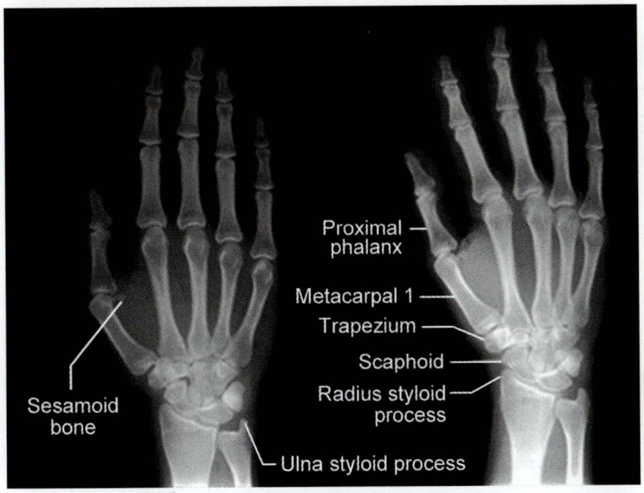

Proximal phalanx
Metacarpal 1
Trapezium
Scaphoid
Radius styloid process
Sesamoid bone
Ulna styloid process

Fig. 1: X-ray showing wrist joint.

- Head of ulna
- Anatomical snuffbox
- Lunate fossa
- Thenar and hypothenar eminences
- Distal wrist flexion crease.

Lister's tubercle: It is dorsal prominence over the distal aspect of the radius, which redirects the extensor pollicis longus (EPL).

Lunate fossa: It is a palpable depression found in the line with the third metacarpal. The lunate bone lies directly below this depression.

Anatomical snuffbox: It is formed ulnarly, by the third dorsal compartment (EPL), radially by the first dorsal compartment [abductor pollicis longus (APL) and extensor pollicis brevis (EPB) and proximally by the extensor retinaculum.

Osteology and Joint Anatomy

The skeletal components (Fig. 2) of wrist joint include:

- Distal radius and ulna
- Carpal bones
- Proximal ends of the five metacarpal bones
- The carpal bones are arranged into proximal and distal rows. The midcarpal joint is the articulation between these rows.
- The proximal row is formed by scaphoid, lunate, triquetrum, and pisiform and has no muscular attachments.
- The distal row is formed by trapezium, trapezoid, capitate, and hamate.
- The articulation of distal radius is composed of two fossae:
  1. Ovoid-shaped lunate fossa
  2. Triangular-shaped scaphoid fossa, which articulates with the lunate and scaphoid bones, respectively (Fig. 3).

Distal Radioulnar Joint

- On the ulnar aspect of the distal radius, sigmoid notch articulates with the distal ulna to form distal radioulnar joint (DRUJ).
- It is a pivot joint, which permits pronation and supination of the wrist joint.
- Other movements at wrist joint are flexion and extension, radial deviation, and ulnar deviation.

Triangular Fibrocartilage Complex

- Triangular fibrocartilage complex (TFCC) (Fig. 4) consists of following structures:
  - Ulnolunate ligament
  - Ulnotriquetral ligament
  - Ulnar collateral ligament
  - Sheath of the extensor carpi ulnaris (ECU)
  - Dorsal radioulnar ligament
  - Palmar radioulnar ligament.
- The DRUJ is primarily stabilized by TFCC. Additional stability is imparted by joint capsule, interosseous membrane, pronator quadratus, and ECU.
- Between the head of the ulna and the carpus, there is a fibrocartilaginous plate, which is a fan-shaped structure spreading from ulnar styloid process to the rim of the radial sigmoid notch.
- The peripheral attachment of the TFCC has a good vascular supply and can heal after surgery.
- The central area of the triangular plate is avascular and tears do not heal.
- The articular surface of the distal radius is typically tilted with:
  - 22° of radial inclination (RI)
  - 12 mm of radial length (RL)
  - 11° of radial tilt (RT)
- These are the various angles to assess in distal radial fractures (Figs. 5A to D).

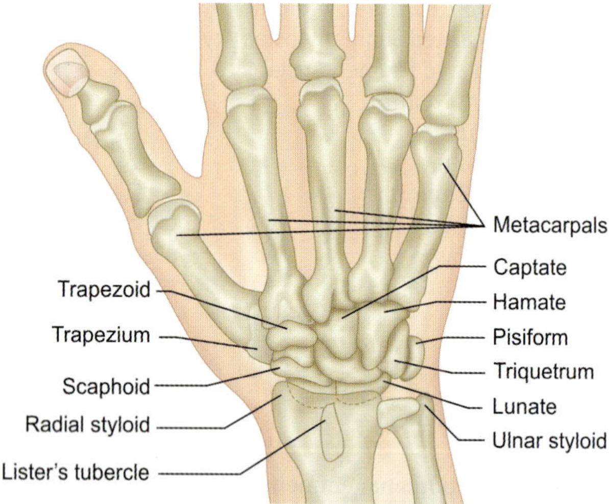

Fig. 2: Skeletal components of the wrist joint.

Ligament Anatomy

Wrist joint ligaments are divided into following subcomponents:

- Extrinsic and intrinsic.
- Palmar and dorsal.
- Extrinsic ligaments span the radiocarpal and midcarpal joints, whereas the intrinsic ligaments connect the carpal bones.
- The extrinsic palmar radiocarpal ligaments originating from the distal radius and travel toward the scaphoid, lunate, and capitate (Fig. 6).
- The radial most extrinsic ligament, the radioscaphocapitate (RSC) ligament originates from the radial styloid, travels across

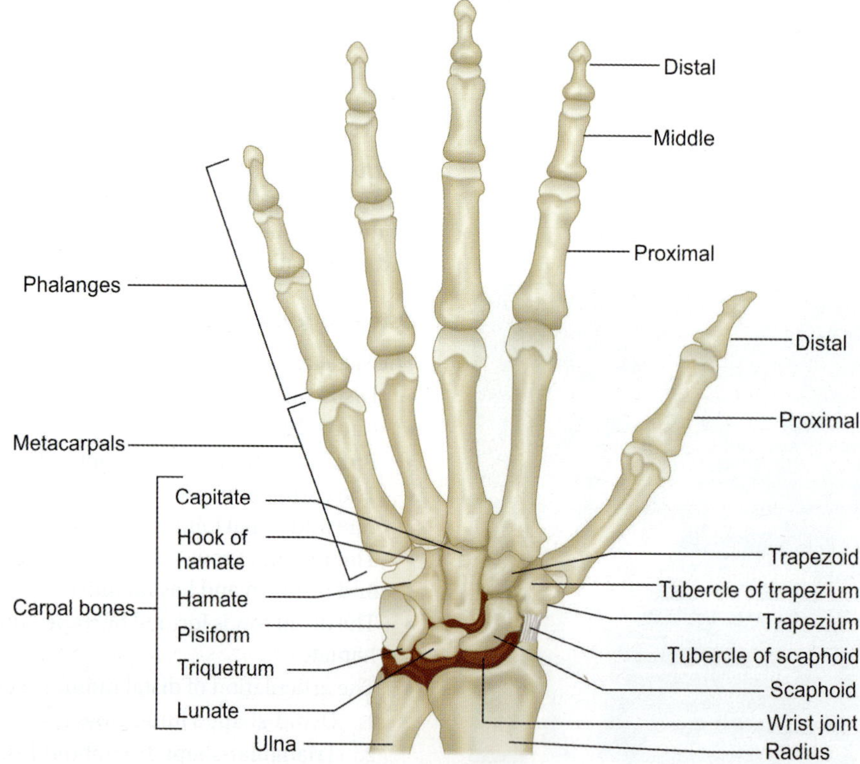

Fig. 3: Lunate fossa and scaphoid fossa.

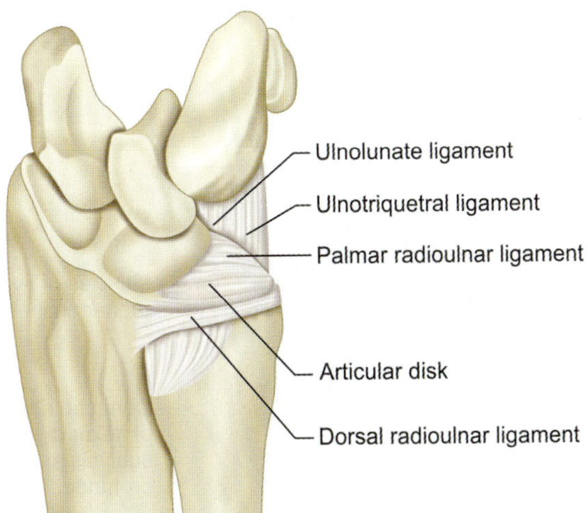

Fig. 4: Triangular fibrocartilage complex.

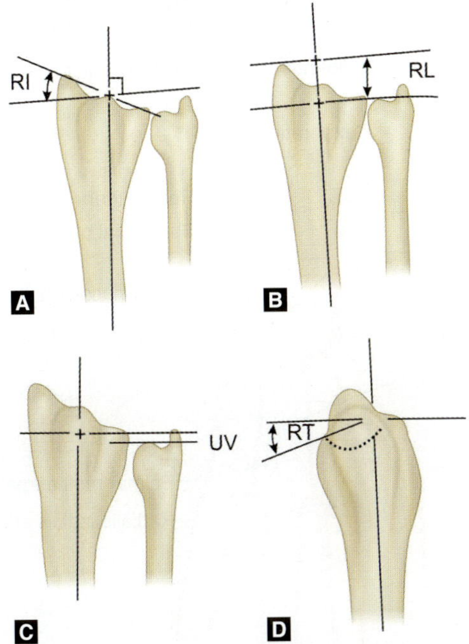

Figs. 5A to D: Various angles for assessing distal radius fractures.

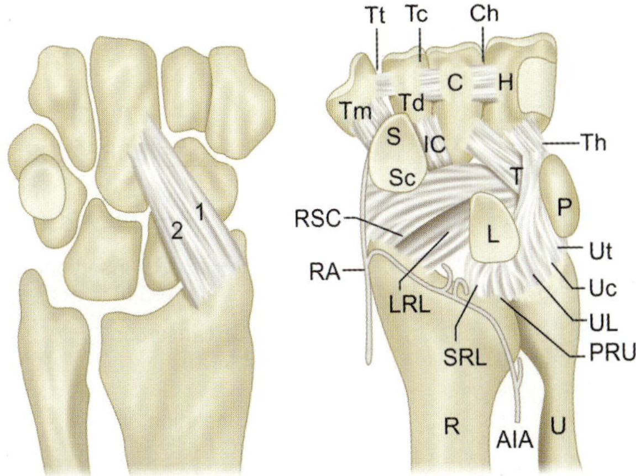

Fig. 6: Wrist from palmar perspective—Bones. (C: capitate; H: hamate; L: lunate; P: pisiform; R: radius; S: scaphoid; Td: trapezoid; Tm: trapezium; U: ulna; Arteries: AIA: anterior interosseous artery; RA: radial artery. Ligaments: Ch: capitohamate; LRL: long radiolunate; PRU: palmar radioulnar; RSC: radioscaphocapitate; Sc: scaphocapitate; SRL: short radiolunate; Tc: triquetrocapitate; Th: triquetrohamate; Tt: trapezio-trapezoid; Uc: ulnocapitate; Ul: ulnolunate; Ut: ulnotriquetral; T: triquetrum; IC: intercarpal)

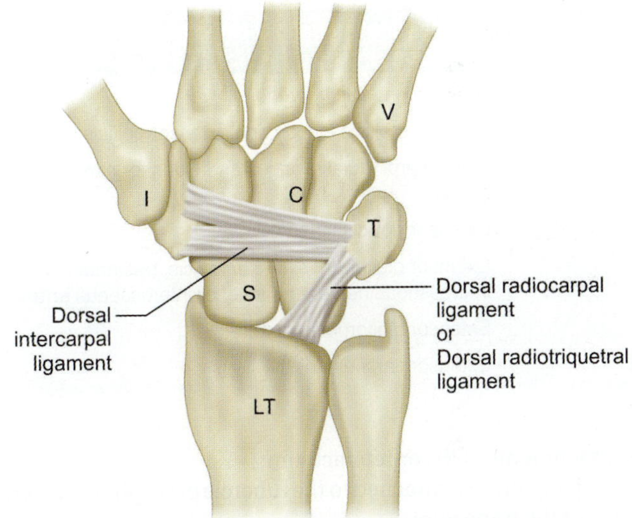

Fig. 7: Ligaments of the dorsal aspect of the wrist joint. (T: triquetral; S: scaphoid; C: capitate; I: first metacarpal; V: fifth metacarpal; LT: lunotriquetral)

the wrist and distal pole of the scaphoid, crosses the capitate and coalesces with the ulnocapitate ligament.
- Dorsally, the dorsal radiotriquetral (radiocarpal) (Fig. 7) ligament and the dorsal intercarpal ligament help to stabilize the wrist.
- The former helps stabilize the lunotriquetral joint, preventing volar intercalated segment instability.
- The latter is an important stabilizer of the proximal pole of the scaphoid.

Collateral ligaments:
- *Radial collateral ligament*: It extends from the tip of the styloid process of radius to the lateral side of scaphoid bone.
- *Ulnar collateral ligament:* It extends from the tip of the styloid process of ulna to triquetral and pisiform bone.

Retinaculum Anatomy

Two retinacula are present in the wrist joint:
1. Extensor retinaculum
2. Flexor retinaculum

Extensor retinaculum:
- Deep fascia on the back of the wrist is thickened to form it, which holds the extensor tendons in place.
- It is an oblique band, which is 2 cm broad directed downwards and medially.
- *Attachments of extensor retinaculum:*
  - *Laterally:* To the lower part of the anterior border of radius
  - *Medially:* To the styloid process of ulna, triquetrum, and pisiform bone.
- *Compartments of extensor retinaculum (Fig. 8):* There are six osteofascial compartments formed over the back of the wrist. Structures passing through each compartment from lateral to medial side are given in Table 1.

Flexor retinaculum:
- This is a strong fibrous band, which bridges the anterior concavity of the carpus and converts it into a tunnel, i.e. the carpal flexor tunnel

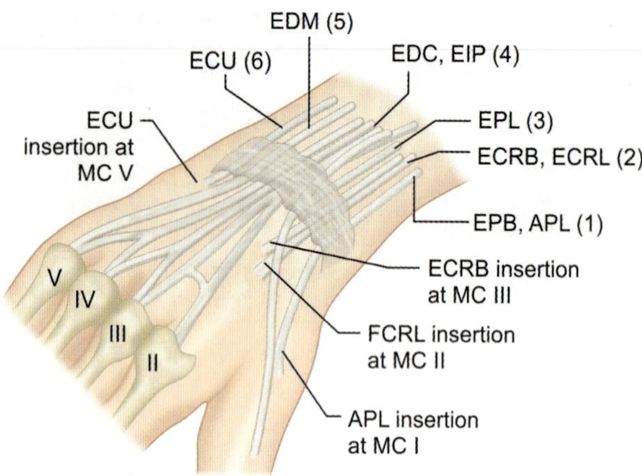

Fig. 8: Compartments of extensor retinaculum and structures passing through it. (APL: abductor pollicis longus; EPB: extensor pollicis brevis; FCRL: flexor carpi radialis longus; ECRB: extensor carpi radialis brevis; EPL: extensor pollicis longus; ED: extensor digitorum; EI: extensor indicis; EDM: extensor digitorum minimi; ECU: extensor carpi ulnaris)

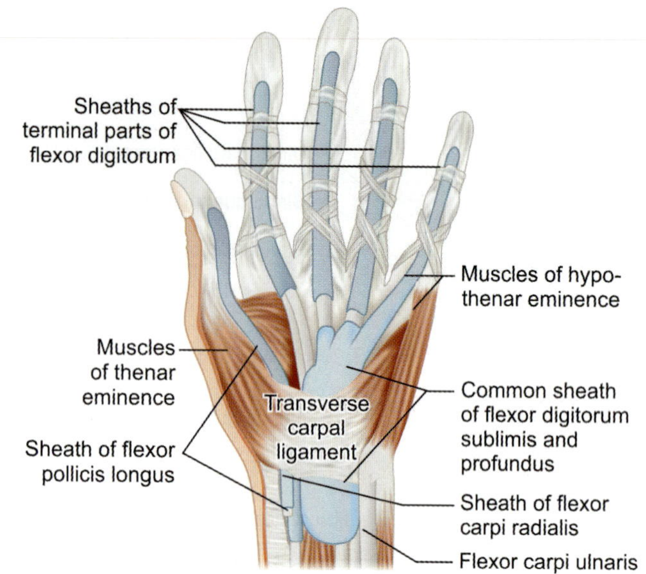

Fig. 9: Boundaries of flexor retinaculum.

TABLE 1: Structures passing through six osteofascial compartments in lateral to medial fashion.

Compartment	*Structures passing through it*
I	Abductor pollicis longus and extensor pollicis brevis
II	Flexor carpi radialis longus and extensor carpi radialis brevis
III	Extensor pollicis longus
IV	Extensor digitorum, extensor indicis, posterior interosseous nerve, and anterior interosseous artery
V	Extensor digitorum minimi
VI	Extensor carpi ulnaris

- Attachments of flexor retinaculum:
  - Laterally, it is attached to the tubercle of scaphoid and crest of the trapezium
  - Medially, it is attached to pisiform bone and the hook of the hamate.
- *Structures passing through flexor retinaculum:* These can be superficial or deep-seated structures:
  - *Structures passing superficial to flexor retinaculum*: Tendon of palmaris longus, palmar cutaneous branch of median nerve, and palmar cutaneous branch of ulnar nerve and ulnar vessels
  - *Structures passing deep to flexor retinaculum*: Median nerve, tendons of flexor digitorum superficialis (FDS), tendon of flexor digitorum profundus (*FDP)*, tendon of flexor pollicis longus, ulnar bursa, and radial bursa.
- *Guyon's canal:* Lies ulnar to the carpal canal and contains ulnar nerve and ulnar artery
- *Boundaries of flexor retinaculum (Fig. 9)*
  - *Floor:* Transverse carpal ligament (between pisiform and hook of the hamate)
  - *Roof:* Volar carpal ligament and palmaris brevis
  - *Radially:* Hook of hamate and the digital flexor tendons
  - *Ulnarly:* Pisiform, flexor carpi ulnaris, and abductor digiti minimi.

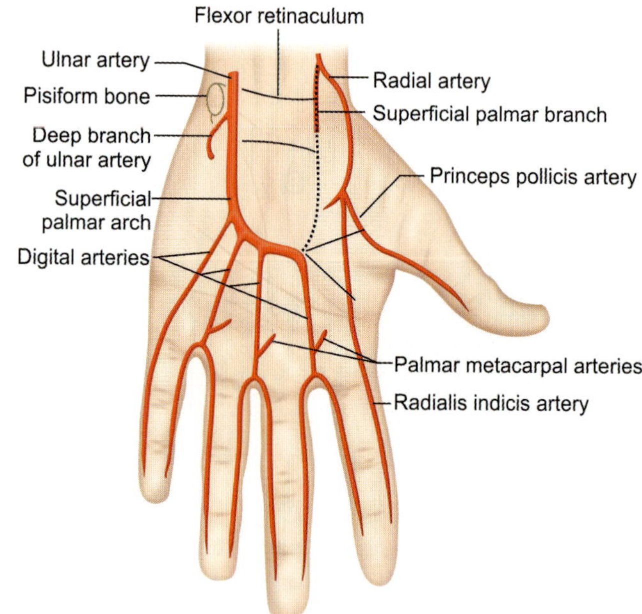

Fig. 10: Superficial palmar arch—formation and branches.

Vascular Anatomy

Blood supply to the hand is by radial and the ulnar arteries, which form two interconnected vascular arches. These are:

1. Superficial palmar arch
2. Deep palmar arch.

Superficial palmar arch:

- *Formation:* It is formed as the direct continuation of ulnar artery beyond the flexor retinaculum (Fig. 10). On the lateral side, the arch is completed by one of the following branches of the radial artery:
  - Superficial palmar branches
  - Radialis indices
  - Princeps pollicis.
- *Relations of the superficial palmar arch:* It lies deep to palmaris brevis and palmar aponeurosis (Fig. 10).

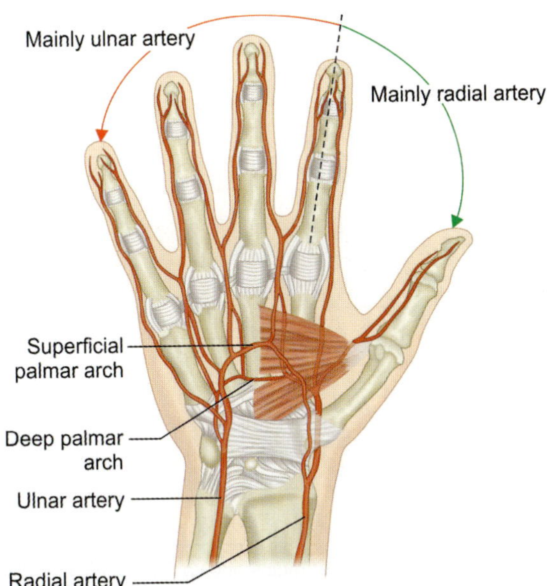

Fig. 11: Deep palmar arch: formation and its branches.

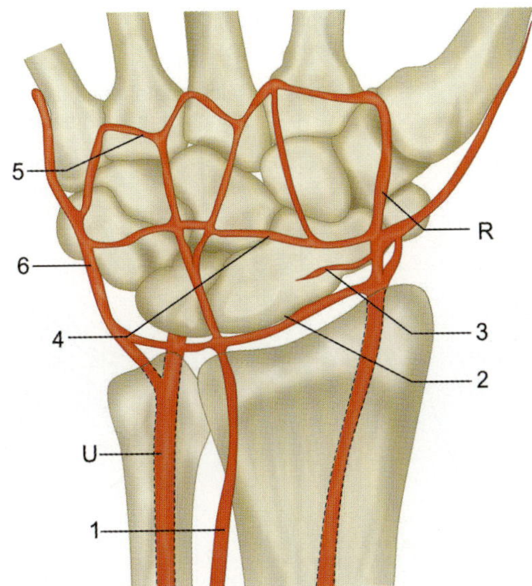

Fig. 12: Vascular supply of wrist joint. (R: radial artery; U: ulnar artery; 1: Dorsal branch of anterior interosseous artery; 2: dorsal radiocarpal arch; 3: branch to dorsal ridge of scaphoid; 4: dorsal intercarpal arch; 5: basal metacarpal arch; 6: medial branch of ulnar artery)

- Medial three and half fingers are supplied by ulnar artery and lateral one and a half fingers are supplied by radial artery.

Deep palmar arch:

- This arterial arch provides second channel connecting the radial and ulnar arteries in the palm. It is situated deep to the long flexor tendon.
- *Formation*: Formation is done by the terminal part of radial artery and is completed medially by the deep palmar branch of the ulnar artery (Fig. 11).
- *Branches of deep palmar arch:* It gives off three palmar metacarpal arteries, which run distally in the second, third, and fourth spaces. Dorsally, the arch gives off three perforating arteries. Recurrent branches arise from concavity of the arch and supply carpal bones (Fig. 11).

Vascular supply of wrist joint: Vascular supply of wrist joint is shown in Figure 12.

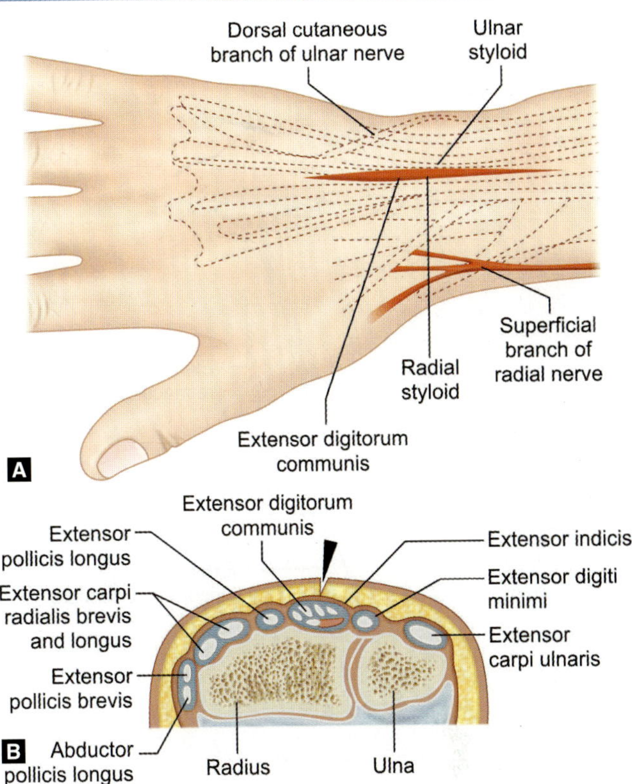

Figs. 13A and B: Surgical approach to wrist in dorsal fashion.

Surgical Approaches to Wrist

- Dorsal approach to the wrist
- Volar approach to the wrist
- Volar approach to scaphoid
- Dorsolateral approach to scaphoid.

Dorsal Approach to the Wrist

Dorsal approach to wrist is shown in Figures 13A and B.

- *Indications*
  - Synovectomy
  - Repair of extensor tendons in case of rheumatoid arthritis
  - Dorsal stabilization of wrist
  - Wrist fusion
  - Excision of lower end of radius for benign and malignant tumor
  - Open reduction and internal fixation for certain distal radial and carpal fractures and dislocation
  - Proximal row carpalectomy.
- *Position*
  - Patient supine
  - Arm on arm table
  - Forearm in supination.
- *Landmarks*
  - Radial styloid process
  - Ulnar styloid process
  - Lister's tubercle.
- *Incision*
  - Take an 8 cm longitudinal incision on dorsal aspect of wrist, crossing midway between radial styloid and ulnar styloid.
  - Incision begins 3 cm proximal to wrist joint and ends 5 cm distal to it.
- *Internervous plane:* There is no true internervous plane.

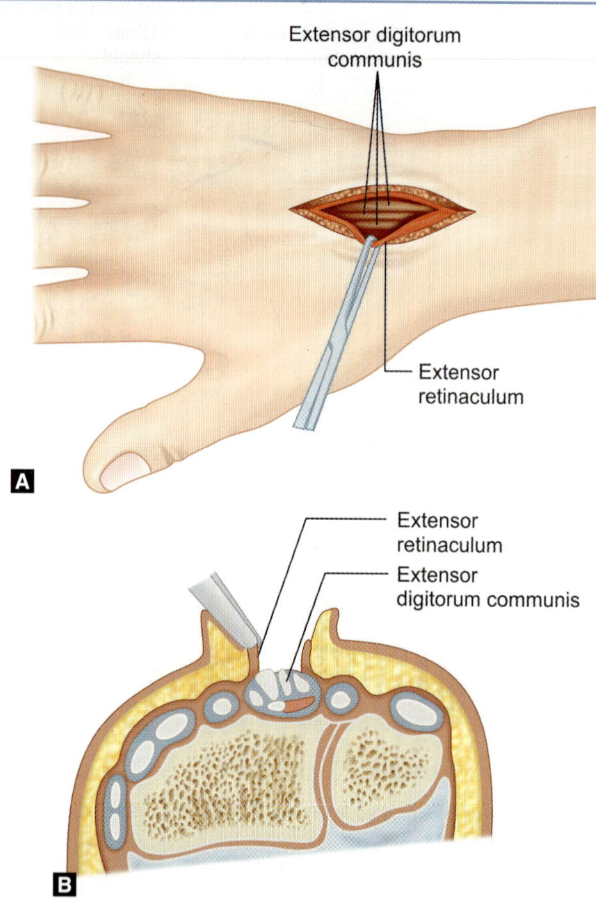

Figs. 14A and B: Incision of extensor retinaculum.

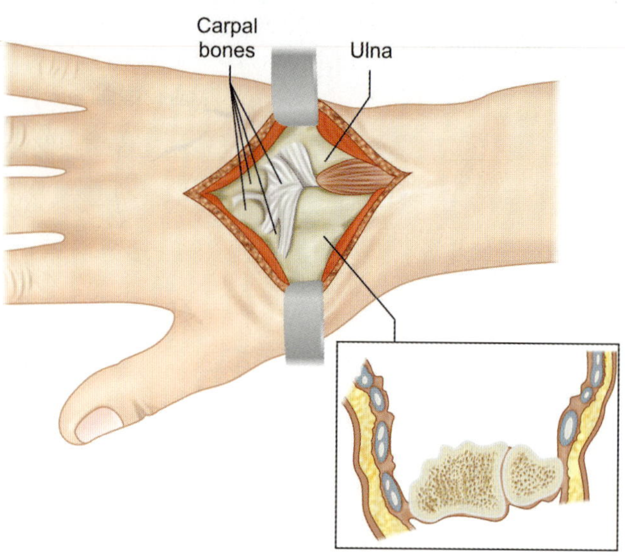

Fig. 15: Exposure of distal end of radius and carpal bones after dissection is made below the capsule.

- *Superficial and deep surgical dissection:* It involves following steps:
  - Incise the skin, subcutaneous tissue and fat to expose the extensor retinaculum.
  - Extensor retinaculum is visualized and incised between third and fourth dorsal compartment (Figs. 14A and B).
  - Extensor pollicis longus is retracted radially and fourth compartment is retracted laterally.
  - Subperiosteal dissection is continued to expose distal radius and carpal capsule.
  - A longitudinal incision is taken over the joint capsule on dorsal aspect of radius and carpus.
  - Dissect below the capsule toward radial side of the radius to expose entire distal end of radius and carpal bones (Fig. 15).
- *Dangers*
  - The superficial radial nerve emerges just above the wrist joint before traveling to the dorsum of the hand. Cutting a cutaneous nerve may result in a painful neuroma.
  - Radial artery crosses the wrist joint on its lateral aspect and is at high-risk of injury.

Volar Approach to the Wrist

- *Indications:*
  - Decompression of median nerve
  - Synovectomy
  - Excision of tumors within the carpal tunnel
  - Repair of lacerated tendon and nerves within carpal tunnel
  - Open reduction and internal fixation of some fractures of distal radius and carpal bones.

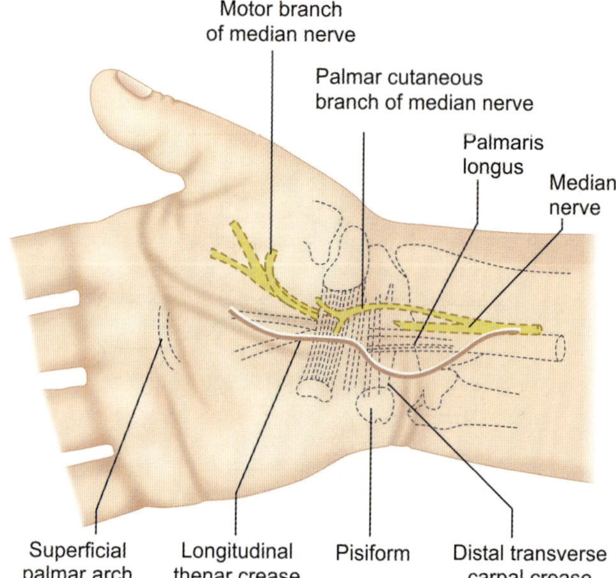

Fig. 16: Landmarks of volar approach to wrist.

- *Position of the patient:*
  - Place the patient in supine position
  - Rest the hand in supinated position on arm board.
- *Landmarks (Fig. 16):*
  - Thenar crease
  - Transverse skin crease of wrist joint
  - Tendon of the palmaris longus muscle.
- *Incision:*
  - Begin the incision just to the ulnar side of the thenar crease
  - Curve the incision toward ulnar side of forearm, so that flexion crease not crossed transversely
  - Incision made on ulnar side of the palmaris longus tendon to protect the palmar cutaneous branch of the median nerve.
- *Internervous plane:* There is no intervenous plane.
- *Superficial and deep surgical dissection.*
  - Incise the skin and subcutaneous tissue.

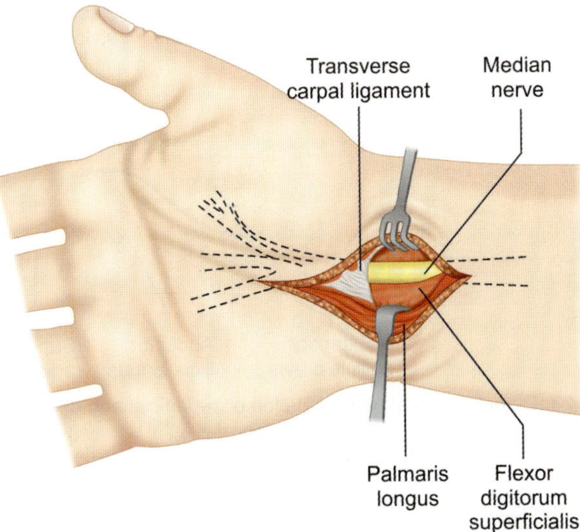

Fig. 17: Median nerve between tendon of palmaris longus muscle and flexor carpi radialis muscle.

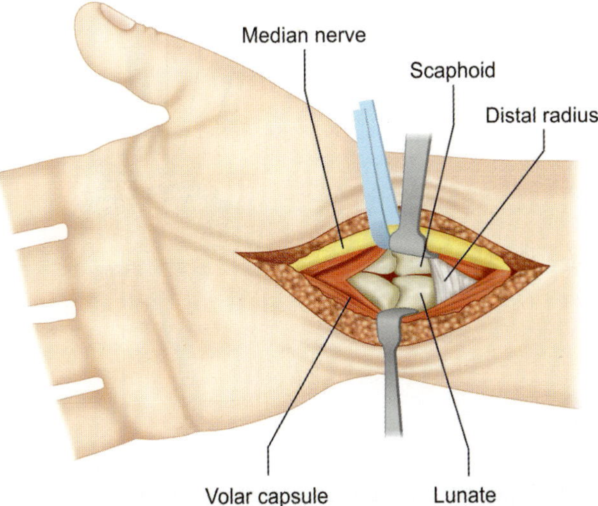

Fig. 19: Volar approach to scaphoid. It is also known as "Russe" approach.

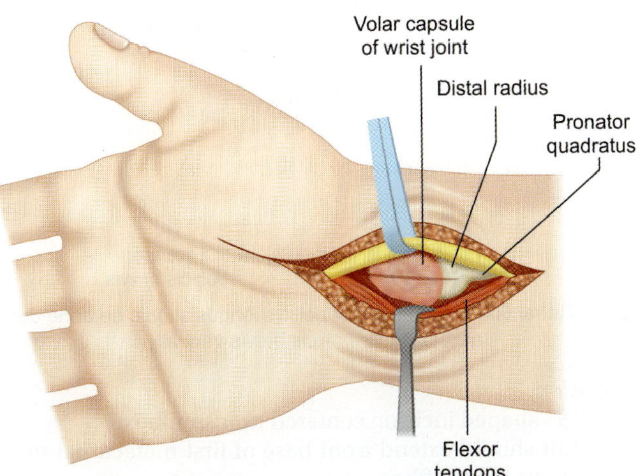

Fig. 18: Exposure of volar aspect of carpus and distal radioulnar joint is done after longitudinal incision.

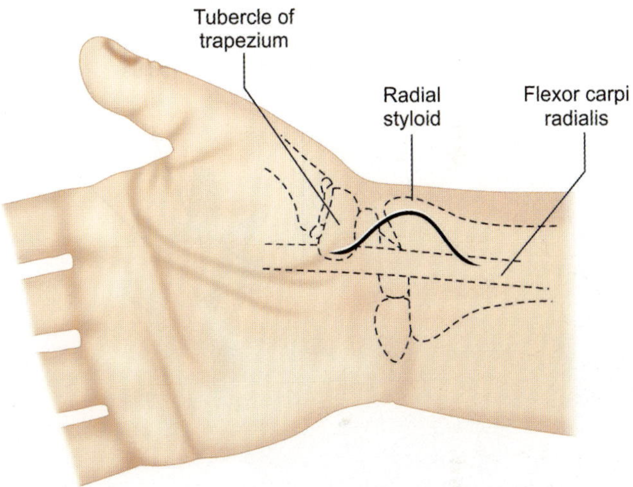

Fig. 20: Landmarks of volar approach to scaphoid.

- Identify superficial palmar fascia and tendon of palmaris longus.
  - Superficial palmar fascia incised.
  - Retract the palmaris tendon to the ulnar side.
  - Identify median nerve between tendon of palmaris longus muscle and flexor carpi radialis (FCR) muscle (Fig. 17).
  - Flexor retinaculum identified and cut along the length of the retinaculum.
- Median nerve retracted radially.
  - Later base of the carpal tunnel is incised longitudinally to expose the volar aspect of the carpus and DRUJ (Fig. 18).

Volar Approach to the Scaphoid

It is also known as "Russe" approach (Fig. 19).

- *Indications:*
  - Bone grafting for nonunion of scaphoid
  - Excision of proximal one-third of scaphoid
  - Excision of radial styloid.
- *Procedure:* Open reduction and internal fixation (screw fixation) for fracture of scaphoid.
- *Position:* Supinate the forearm.
- *Landmarks (Fig. 20):* Tuberosity of the scaphoid (palpate it just distal to the skin crease of wrist joint) at level of tubercle of trapezium. FCR tendon (FCR muscle crosses the scaphoid before inserting into the base of second and third metacarpal).
- *Incision:* Vertical or curvilinear incision 2–3 cm long. Base the incision on the scaphoid tuberosity and extend it proximally between tendon of flexi carpi radialis muscle and radial artery. Incision should cross the wrist crease at 45° angle.
- *Internervous plane:* No internervous plane because the only muscle mobilized is FCR, which is supplied by median nerve.
- *Superficial and deep surgical dissection (Fig. 21):*
  - Incise skin, subcutaneous tissue, and deep fascia
  - Identify the radial artery on the radial aspect
  - Retract the radial artery and subcutaneous tissue radially
  - Identify the tendon of FCR muscle, trace it distally and free it from flexor retinaculum after incising it
  - Retract it medially, to expose the wrist joint
  - Incise the capsule of the wrist joint longitudinally over the scaphoid (Fig. 22)

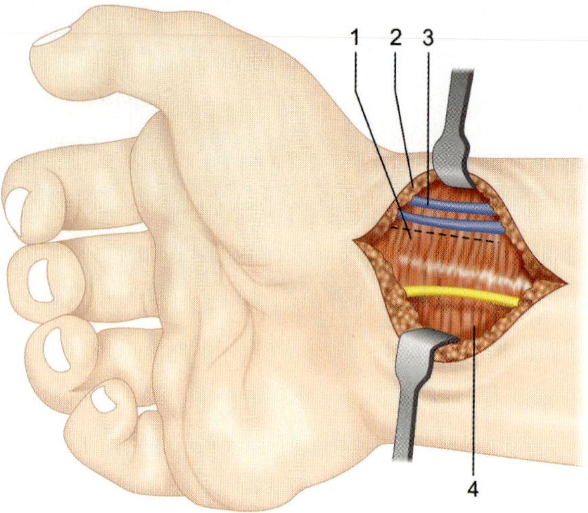

Fig. 21: Superficial and deep surgical dissection of the volar approach. (1: palmar cutaneous branch of median N; 2: fascia over flexor carpi radialis; 3: radial artery and venae comitantes; 4: palmaris longus)

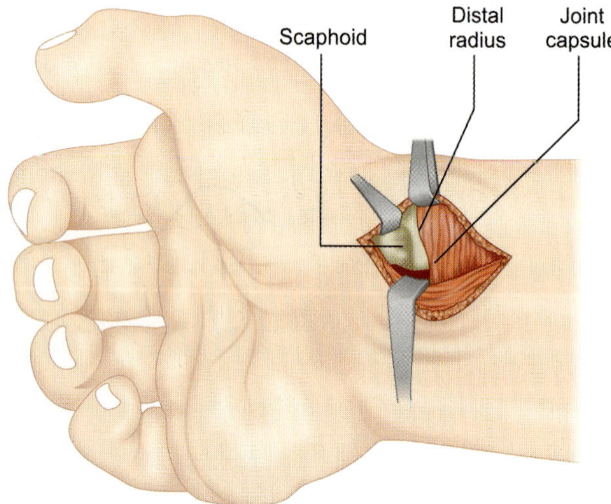

Fig. 22: Capsule of wrist joint is incised longitudinally over the scaphoid.

- Place the wrist in marked dorsiflexion to get a better view of the joint.
- *Dangers*
  - Radial artery lies laterally and is prone to be incised.
  - Care should be taken to prevent palmar cutaneous branch of median nerve (in superficial dissection).
- *Advantages*
  - It avoids damaging the dorsal blood supply to the bone's proximal half.
  - Avoids damage to superficial branch of radial nerve.

Dorsolateral Approach to the Scaphoid

- *Indications*:
  - Bone grafting for nonunion scaphoid
  - Excision of proximal fragment of scaphoid
  - Excision of radial styloid
  - Open reduction and internal fixation of fracture of scaphoid.
- *Position:* Pronate the forearm.
- *Landmarks*
  - Radial styloid process
  - Anatomical snuffbox.

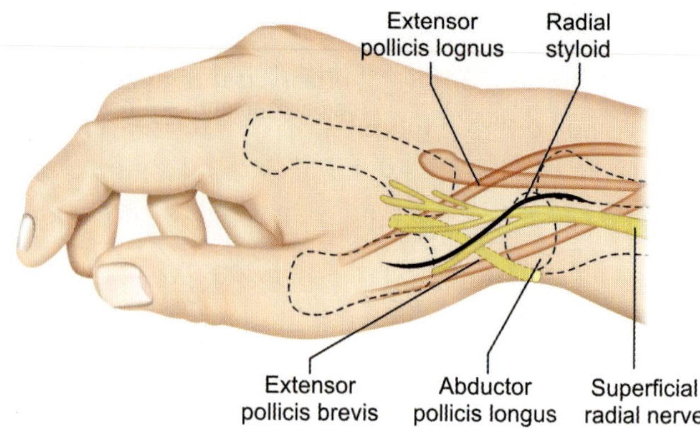

Fig. 23: Diagrammatical representation of superficial and deep surgical dissection.

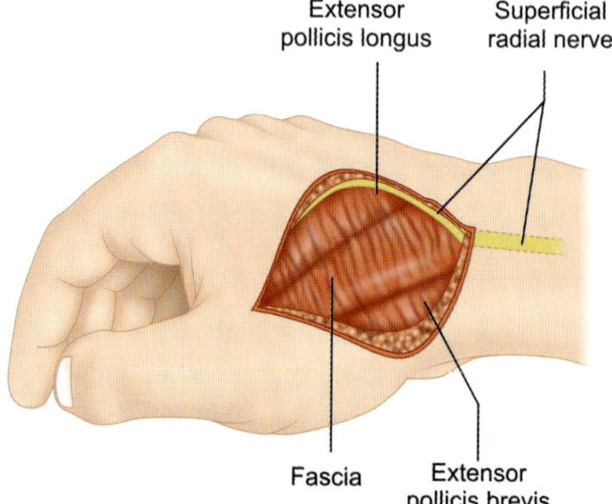

Fig. 24: Retraction of the extensor pollicis longus should be done dorsally and extensor pollicis brevis ventrally.

- *Incision*
  - "S"-shaped incision centered over snuffbox.
  - Cut should extend from base of first metacarpal to 3 cm above the snuffbox.
- *Internervous plane*: No true internervous plane.
- *Superficial and deep surgical dissection (Fig. 23):*
  - Cut skin and subcutaneous tissue
  - Identify tendon of EPL (dorsally) and EPB (ventrally)
  - Open fascia between the two tendons
  - Retract the EPL dorsally and EPB ventrally (Fig. 24)
  - Identify radial artery lying on the bone and retract it radially
  - Incise capsule of the wrist joint longitudinally
  - Expose the articulation between distal end radius and proximal end of scaphoid
  - Place the wrist in ulnar deviation to expose the joint completely (Figs. 25A to C).
- *Dangers:*
  - Superficial radial nerve is at risk during exposure (because it lies directly over the tendon of EPL muscle and can get cut during mobilization of extensor pollicis tendon)
  - Incising the nerve may produce:
    - Neuroma
    - Hypoesthesia (area on dorsal aspect of hand).

EXAMINATION OF WRIST JOINT

Introduction

Wrist joint as shown in Figure 26 is a synovial joint of ellipsoid variety. It is formed by inferior surface of lower end of radius,

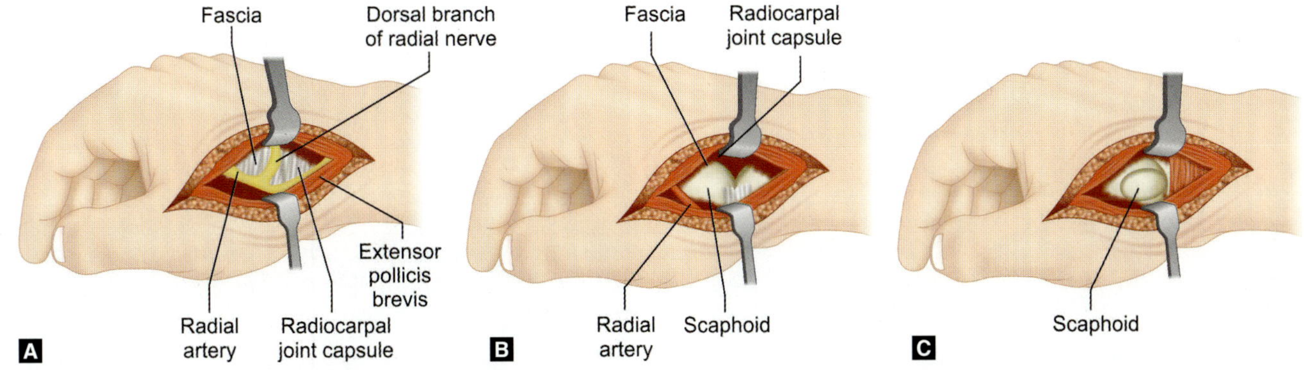

Figs. 25A to C: Radial artery should be identified and retracted radially. After longitudinal incision of wrist joint capsule, articulation between distal end radius and proximal end of scaphoid should be exposed.

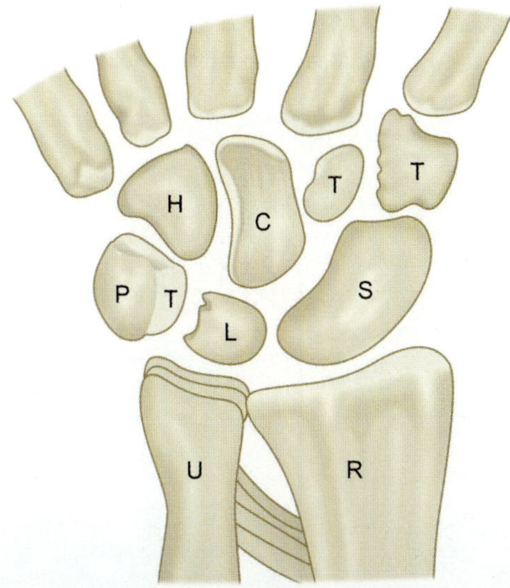

Fig. 26: Wrist joint. (S: scaphoid; L: lunate; T: triquetrum; P: pisiform; T: trapezium; T: trapezoid; C: capitate; H: hamate; R: radius; U: ulna)

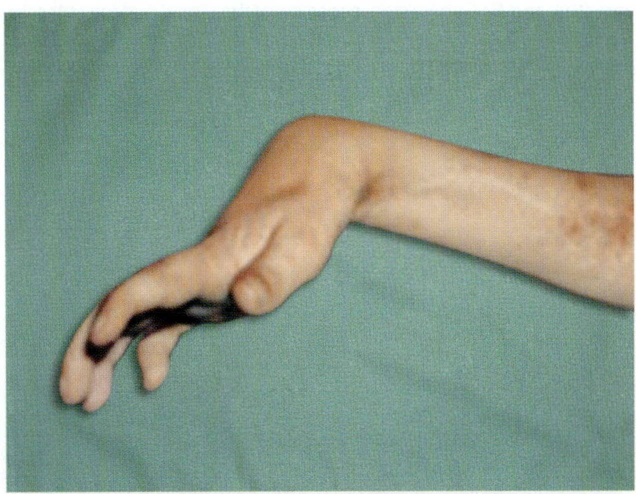

Fig. 28: Volkmann's ischemic contracture.

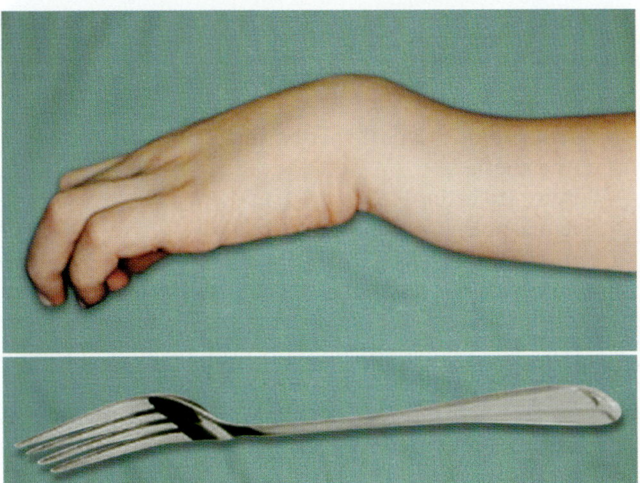

Fig. 27: Dinner fork deformity in Colles' fracture.

articular disk of inferior radioulnar joint, scaphoid, lunate, and triquetral bone.

History

Patient with any wrist pathology usually presents with a history of:
- Swelling, trauma
- Deformity
- Restricted movements, etc.

Attitude

- Dinner fork deformity, e.g. Colles' fracture (Fig. 27)
- Flexion contracture of wrist and finger, e.g. Volkmann's ischemic contracture (VIC) (Fig. 28).

Inspection

- *Dorsal surface localized:*
  - Ganglion
  - Rheumatoid nodule
  - Tumor.
- *Generalized (Figs. 29A and B)*
  - Traumatic
  - *Skin condition:* Any scar, sinuses, venous prominence, contracture, etc.
- *Palmar surface (Fig. 30):*
  - Swelling
  - Muscle wasting, e.g. RA, TB
  - Anterior tilting, e.g. Smith fracture
  - Posterior tilting, e.g. Colles' fracture.

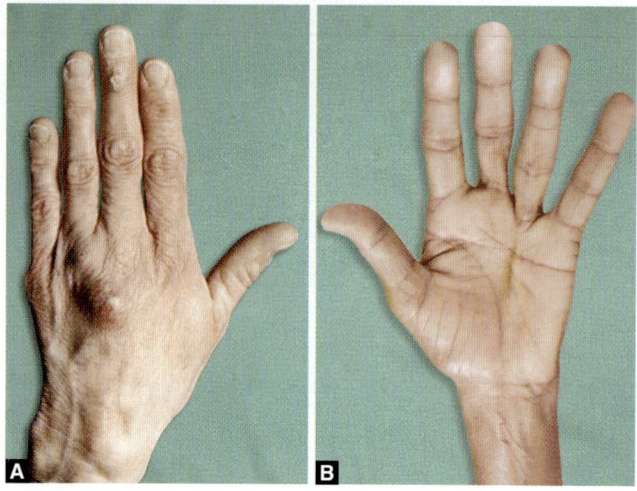

Figs. 29A and B: Generalized inspection of the dorsal surface of the wrist.

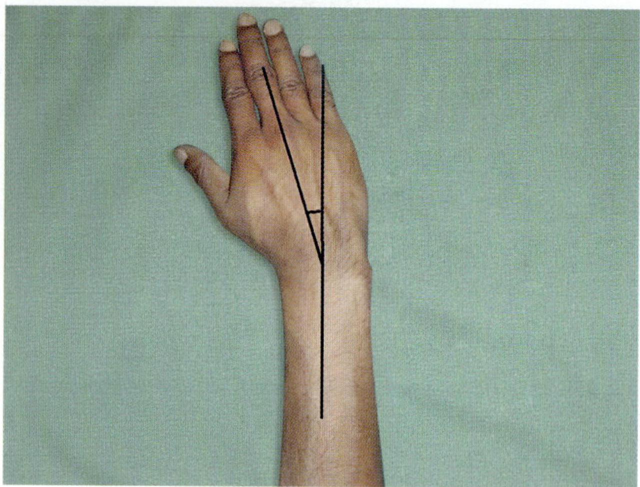

Fig. 32: Measuring radial deviation.

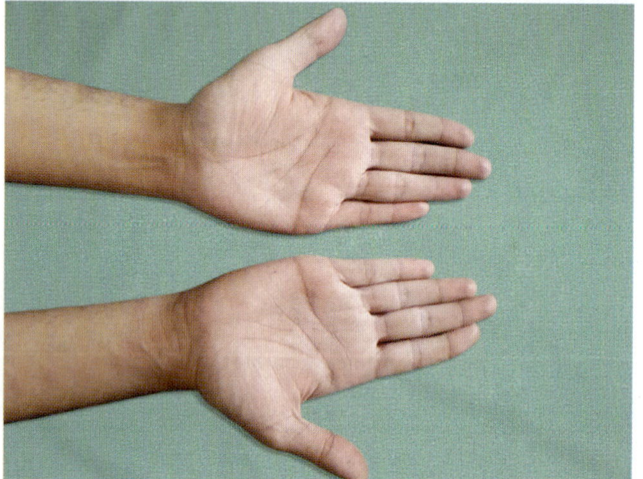

Fig. 30: Inspecting palmar surface of the wrist and hands for any pathological signs.

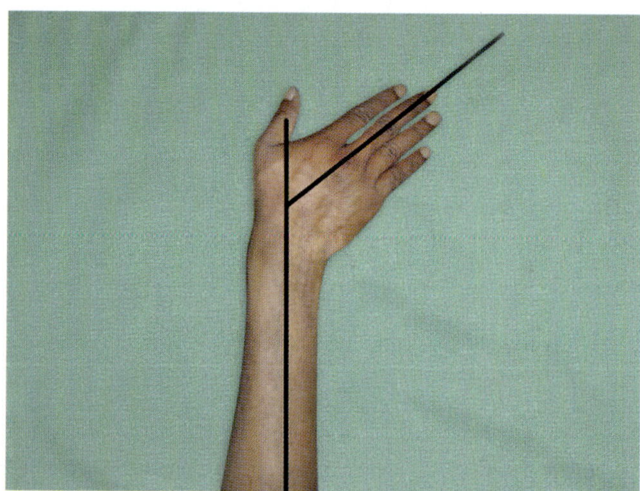

Fig. 33: Measuring ulnar deviation.

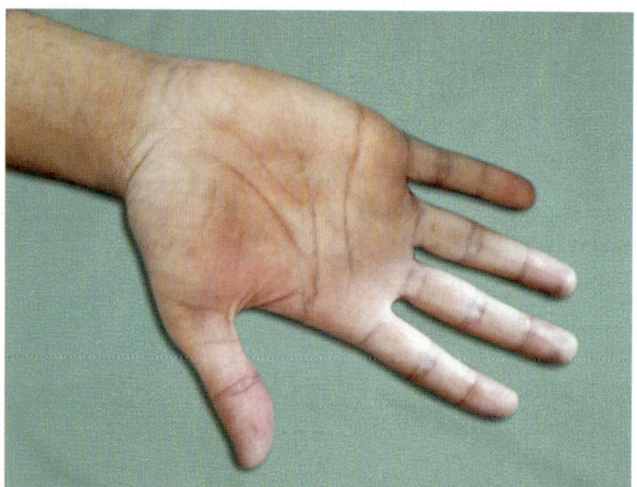

Fig. 31: Hypothenar eminence.

- *Radial surface:* Swelling in anatomical snuffbox.
- *Ulnar surface:* Hypothenar eminence (Fig. 31).
- *Deformity:*
  - Radial deviation (Fig. 32), e.g. in Colles' fracture
  - Ulnar deviation (Fig. 33), e.g. rheumatoid arthritis.

Palpation

- *Superficial*
  - *Temperature:* Hypo/hyperthermia
  - Anesthesia
  - Bony projection
  - Radial pulse.
- *Deep*
  - *Palpate ulnar and radial styloid process:* Normally, radial styloid process is 1 cm distal to the ulnar styloid process (Fig. 34). Tenderness presents over anatomical snuffbox, indicates scaphoid fracture.
  - *De Quervain's disease (Fig. 35):* Tenderness presents over sheath of abductor pollicis longus and extensor pollicis brevis:
    - *Step sign:* In case of any injury to the wrist joint, note for step sign (Figs. 36A to C), pass down your index finger on outer aspect of forearm over radial shaft. In case of outer shift of lower fragment (Fig. 36A), finger will step over the hard underlying structure and can be seen on dorsal aspect also (lateral step-up). In Colles' fracture (posterior stepping up) (Fig. 36B) and reverse in Smith's (posterior stepping down) (Fig. 36C).

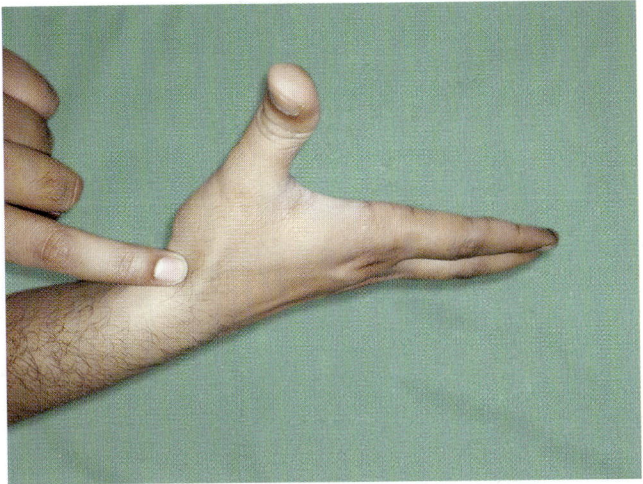

Fig. 34: Tenderness present over anatomical snuffbox: scaphoid fracture.

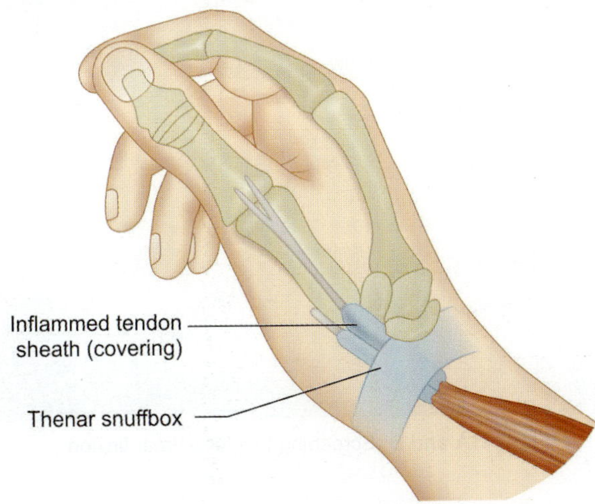

Fig. 35: De Quervain's disease.

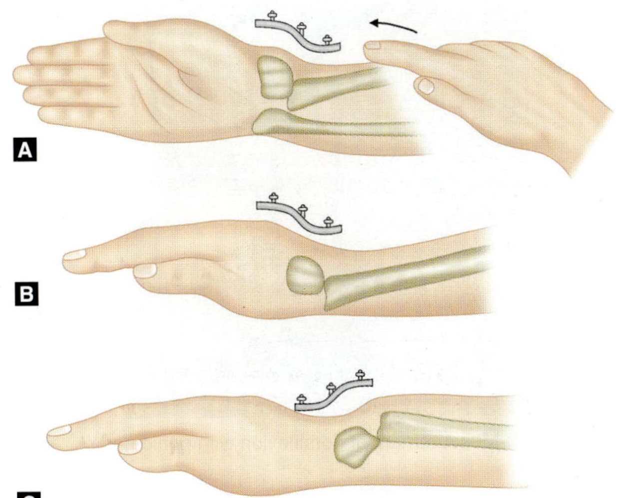

Figs. 36A to C: Step sign—(A) Lateral step-up; (B) Posterior step-up; and (C) Posterior step-down.

- *Styloid process of radius and ulna (Fig. 37):* Patient forearm is pronated. Wrist is in neutral position. Support the palm in one hand.

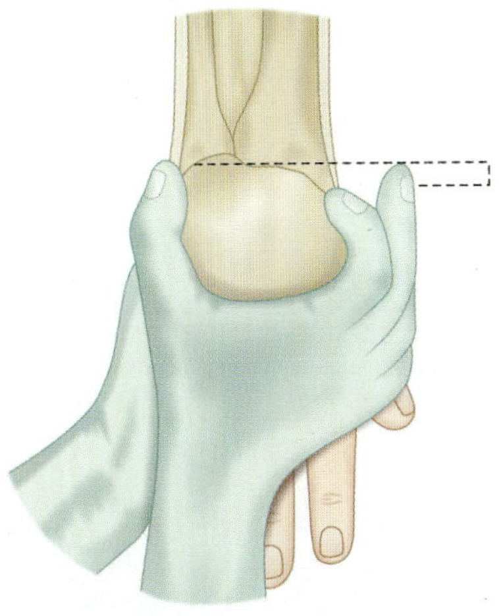

Fig. 37: Styloid process of radius and ulna.

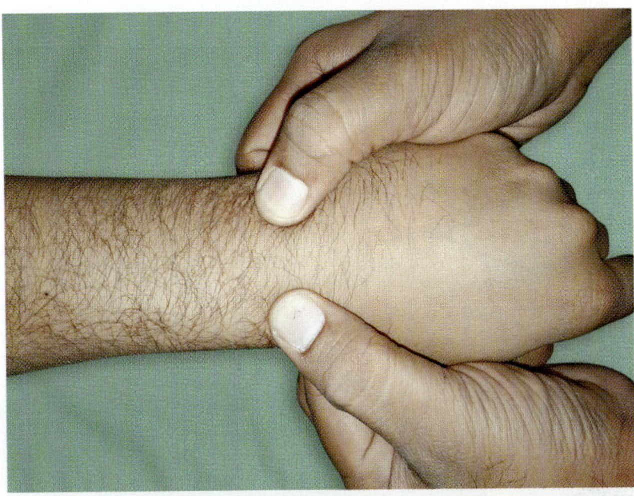

Fig. 38: Palpation of joint line (wrist).

- Put thumb and index fingertip of opposite hand on two sides of wrist from dorsal aspect. Gently squeeze within and at the same time shift your fingertip proximally styloid process will be felt.

- *Palpation of joint line (Fig. 38):*
  - *Crepitus radioulnar joint (Figs. 39A and B):* Place index finger and thumb over joint, then, supinate and pronate the wrist. Crepitus comes when joint is disorganized.
  - *Crepitus radiocarpal joint:* Encircle the wrist with the hand and ask the patient to dorsiflex, palmarflex, radial deviate, and ulnar deviate the wrist (Figs. 40A and B). Osteoarthritis of wrist is uncommon but occurs after scaphoid and distal radius fracture and Kienbock's disease.

Range of Motion

Palmar Flexion

- *Normal range*: 75°
- *Screening test:* Ask the patient to put the backs of the hands in contact and then to bring forearm into horizontal position (Figs. 41A and B).

Dorsiflexion

- Measured with goniometer (Fig. 42)
- Normal range: 75°

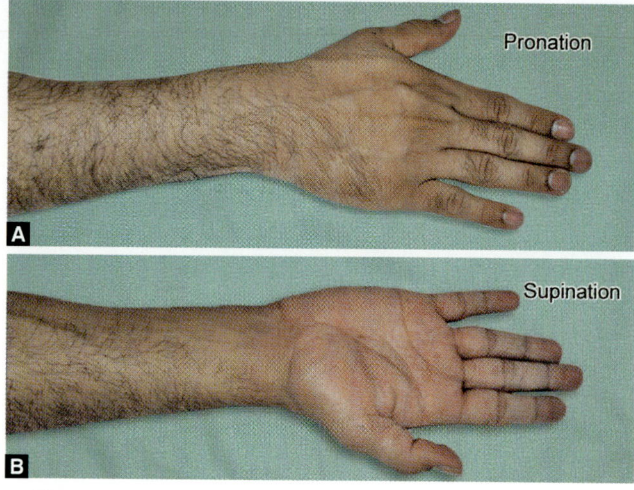

Figs. 39A and B: Pronation and supination movement of wrist.

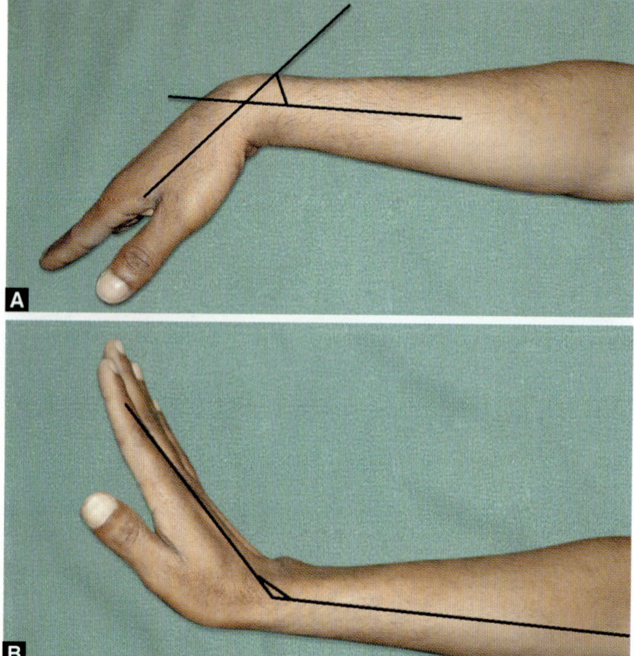

Figs. 40A and B: Dorsiflexion, palmar flexion of wrist.

- Restricted in:
  - Ankylosis of joint secondary to infection
  - Reduced Colles' fracture.

Joint Hypermobility (Fig. 43)

Try to bring the thumb into contact with forearm and measure gap. Average separation is 4.5 cm at 17.5 years. It increases with age due to loss of elasticity of ligament.

Radial Deviation (Fig. 44)

It is an angle formed between forearm and middle metacarpal. Normal range is 20°.

Ulnar Deviation (Fig. 45)

- *Normal range:* 35°
- It is measured with goniometer.

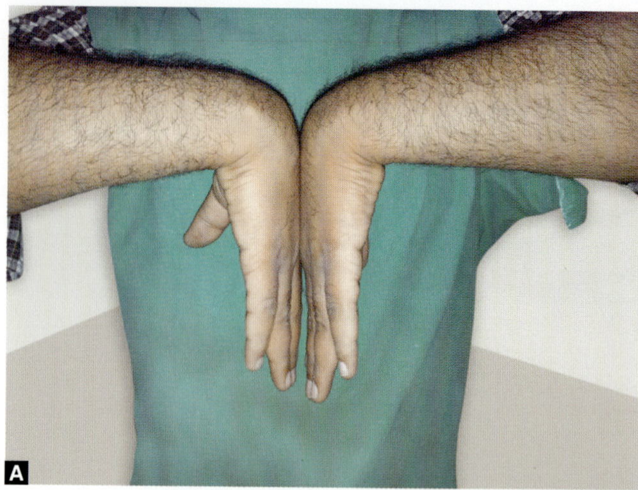

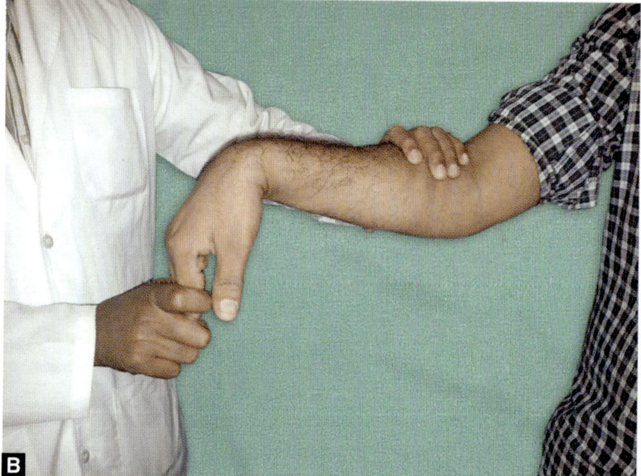

Figs. 41A and B: Screening test for palmar flexion.

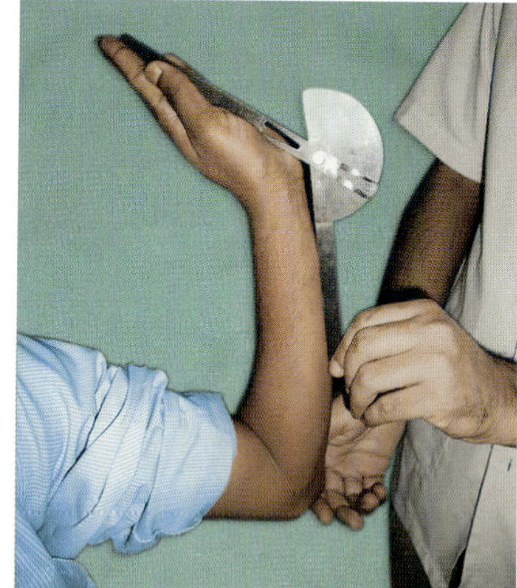

Fig. 42: Measurement of dorsiflexion with goniometer.

Supination

- *Normal range:* 90°
- It is defined by the degree to which radius can rotate over ulna
- *Tests*: Tell the patient to hold the pencil in each hand, then move both forearm simultaneously into supination (Fig. 46). Normally, pencils are parallel to floor.

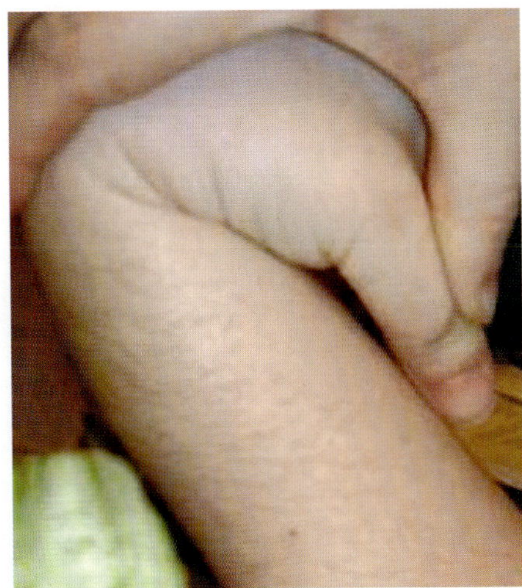

Fig. 43: Depiction of joint hypermobility.

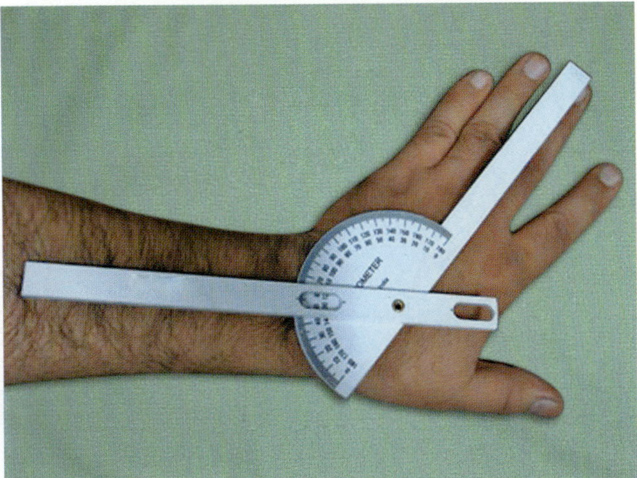

Fig. 44: Radial deviation.

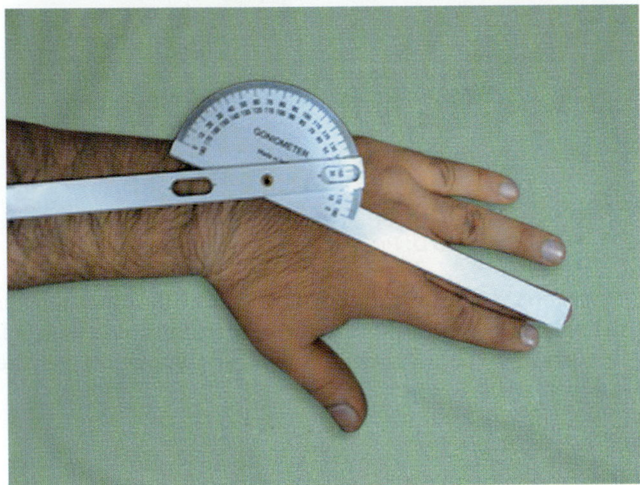

Fig. 45: Measurement of ulnar deviation.

Pronation

Ask the patient to flex elbow to 90° at his waist fist holding the pencil. Ask the patient to rotate his fist from fully supinated position until his palm faces downward. Normally, palm faces downwards and pencil parallel to floor (Fig. 46). Any dissimilarity implies restricted range of motion (ROM).

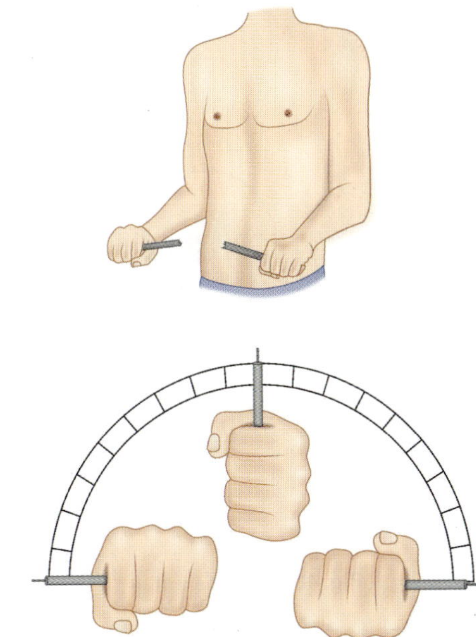

Fig. 46: The elbow range of motion in supination and pronation.

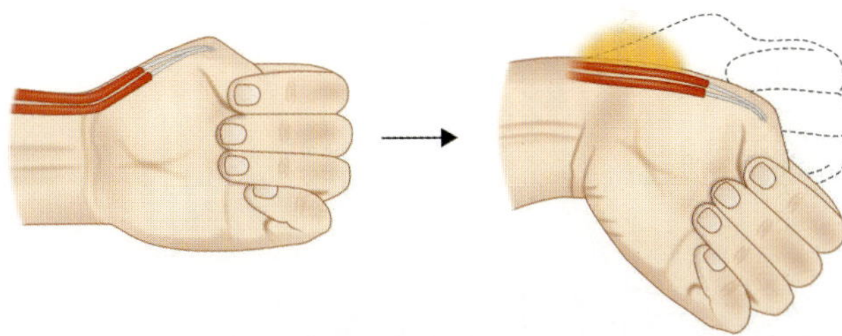

Fig. 47: Finkelstein's test.

Special Tests

Finkelstein's Test (Fig. 47)

- Ask the patient to flex the thumb and close the finger over it
- Now, move the hand in ulnar deviation in De Quervain's disease, and excruciating pain accompanies this maneuver. It is used for carpal instabilities.

Watson's Test (Fig. 48)

Press the thumb against tubercle of scaphoid. With the other hand palmarflex and radially deviate the patient wrist. A click sound should be felt. The scaphoid subluxates over distal radius and reduction occurs, if pressure of thumb is slacked. Accompanying pain is confirmatory. It is for scapholunate instability.

Ballottement Test (Fig. 49)

Triquetral and lunate are grasped with thumb and index finger. An attempt is made to displace them relative to each other, first in dorsal then in volar direction note any associated pain and crepitus. It is for lunotriquetral instability.

Midcarpal Instability (Fig. 50)

With one hand steady the forearm and with other hand grasp the patient's hand. Push the carpus against radius and gently swing the wrist from position of full ulnar deviation to full radial deviation. The test is positive, if this normal smooth movement is irregular.

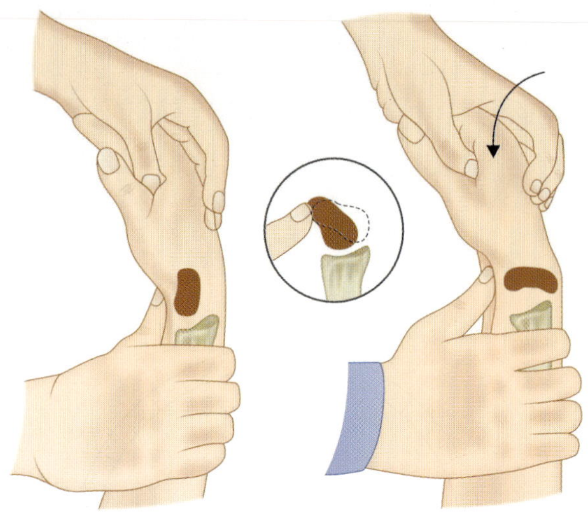

Fig. 48: Watson's test.

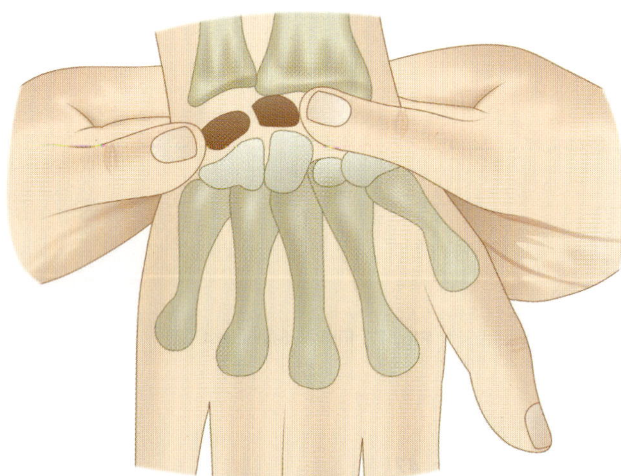

Fig. 49: Ballottement test.

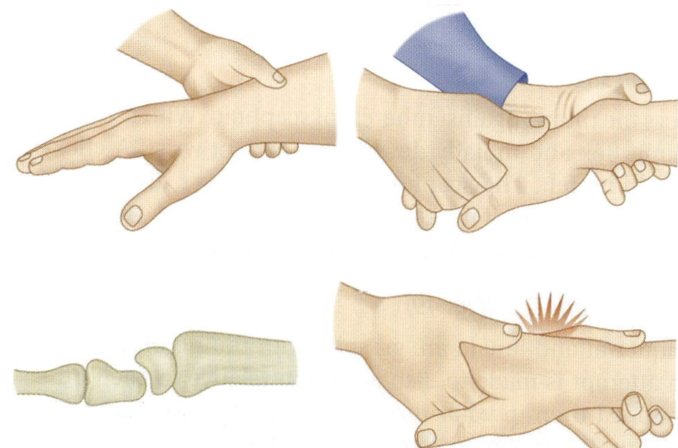

Fig. 50: Test for midcarpal instability.

Test for DRUJ Laxity (Fig. 51)

- It is to test weakness of wrist. Clicking sensation is present, if ulnar nerve involvement is present.

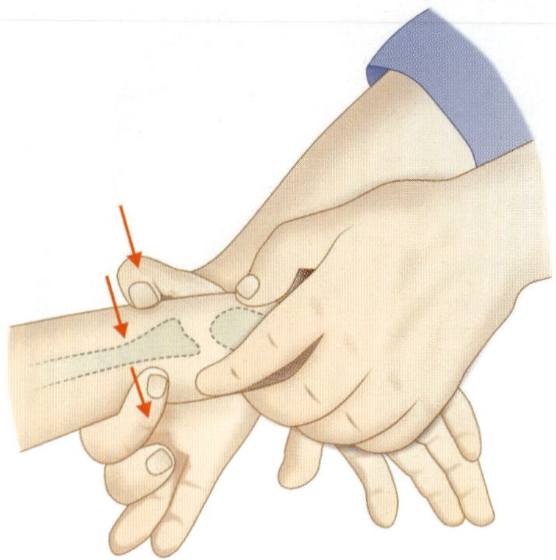

Fig. 51: Test for distal radioulnar joint laxity.

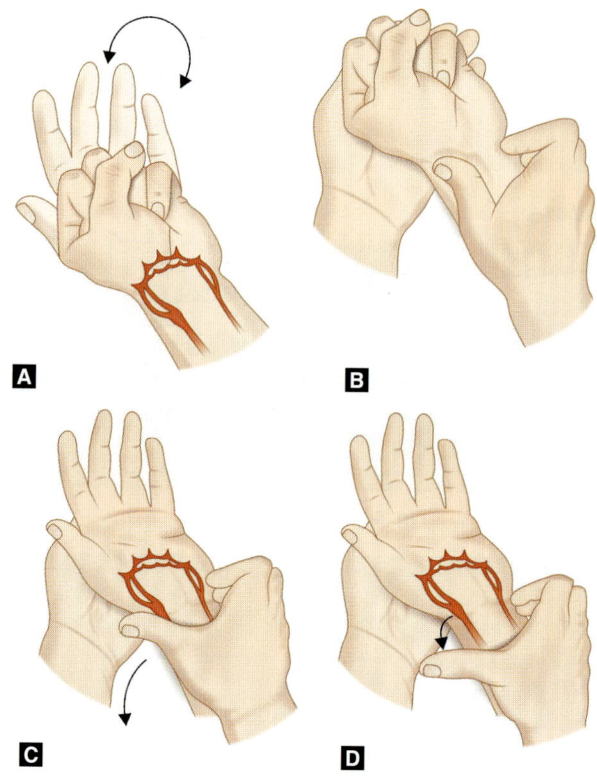

Figs. 52A to D: Procedure to perform Allen's test.

- *Procedure*: Steady the carpus with one hand, the other hand use to hold distal ulna and attempt to move in dorsal and then volar direction. Note, if any click sensation and complain of pain then compare other side.

Allen Test (Figs. 52A to D)

- It determines patency of radial and ulnar arteries.
- *Procedure*:
  - To perform this test, open and close the fist several times. Squeeze the fist tightly so that venous blood comes out of palm. Place your thumb over radial artery, index and middle finger over ulnar artery. Press them against underlying bone to occlude them.
  - Instruct the patient to open his palm. It should be pale. Release one of the artery at wrist, while maintaining

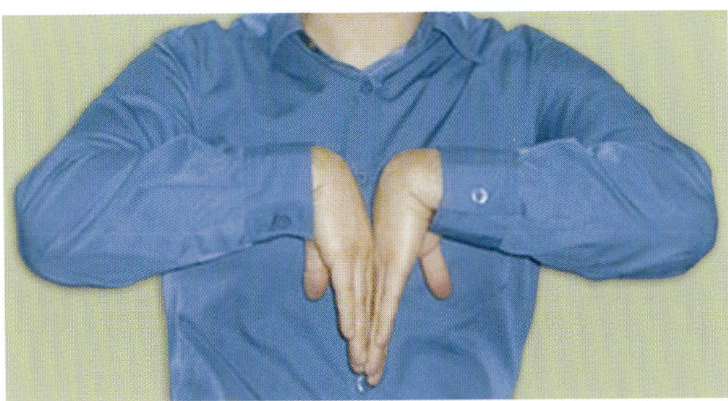

Fig. 53: Phalen test.

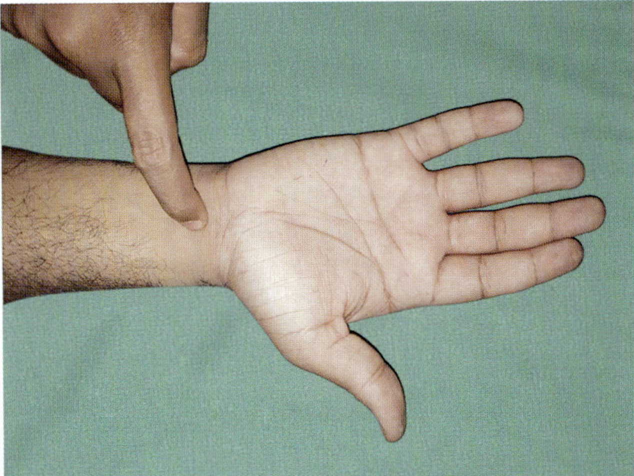

Fig. 54: Tinel's sign.

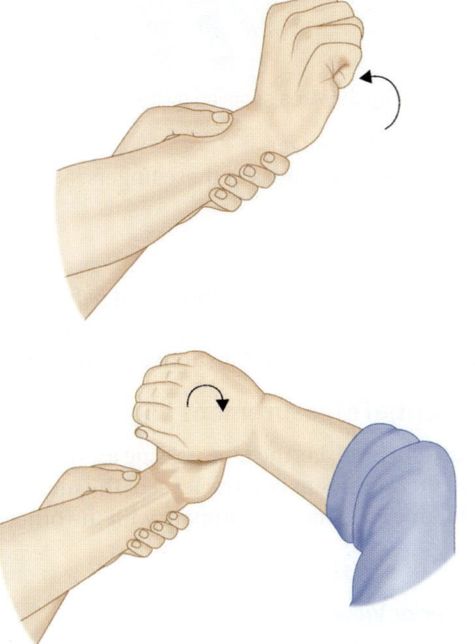

Fig. 55: Extension of wrist.

pressure over other. Normally, hand flushes immediately. If flushed slowly then released artery is partially or completely occluded, so other artery should be tested. Similarly, other hand should be checked for comparison.

Phalen Test (Fig. 53)

Ask the patient to hold both wrists in fully flexed position for 1–2 minutes. The appearance or exacerbation of paresthesia in median nerve distribution is suggestive of carpal tunnel syndrome.

Tinel's Sign (Fig. 54)

Test is positive, if gentle finger percussion over median nerve produces paresthesia in its distribution.

Finsterer's Sign

- Percuss at the head of third metacarpal bone with the arm pronated
- If produces pain then it suggests Kienbock's disease of lunate.

Maisonneuve's Sign

- Arm is pronated with elbow flexed
- The hand and wrist are actively dorsiflexed
- If marked hyperextension of wrist is seen then the test is positive
- It is seen in old malunited Colles'.

Carpal Lift Test

- The finger to be examined is lifted against resistance, while the other fingers are fixed
- If pain is elicited, the test is positive
- It is the earliest sign of carpal bone, even before X-ray.

Neurological Examination

Muscle Power

- Wrist extensor (C6)
- Wrist flexor (C7)
- Supination (C5 and C6)
- Pronation (C6, C8, and T1).

Sensory Examination

- Reflex
  - *Wrist extensors (C6) (Fig. 55):* Primary extensor and their nerve supply:
    - *Extensor carpi radialis longus:* Radial nerve (C6 and C7)
    - *Extensor carpi radialis brevis*: Radial nerve (C6 and C7)
    - *Extensor carpi ulnaris:* Radial nerve (C7).
  - *Wrist flexion (Fig. 56) (C7):* Primary flexors are:
    - *Flexor carpi radialis:* Median nerve (C7)
    - *Flexor carpi ulnaris:* Ulnar nerve (C8).
- *Pronation*
  - Primary pronator are:
    - *Pronator teres:* Median nerve (C6)
    - *Pronator quadratus:* Anterior interosseous branch of the median nerve (C8 and T1).
  - Secondary pronator is FCR.
- *Supination*
  - Primary supinator are—biceps, e.g. musculocutaneous nerve (C5 and C6) and supinator, e.g. radial nerve (C6)
  - Secondary supinator is brachioradialis.

Other Joints Examinations (Fig. 57)

- While examining wrist joint, attention must also be paid to:
  - Cervical spine
  - Shoulder
  - Elbow.

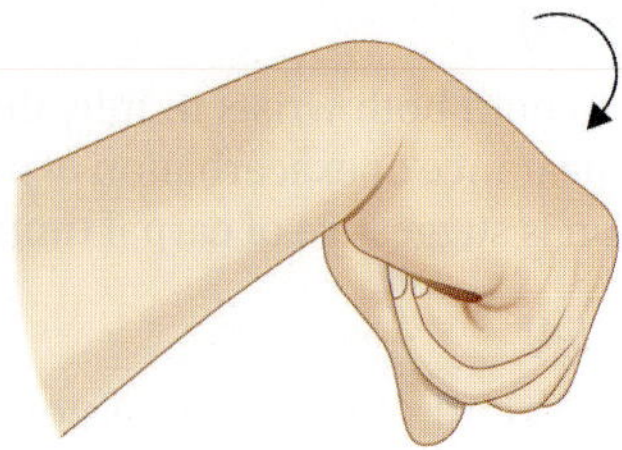

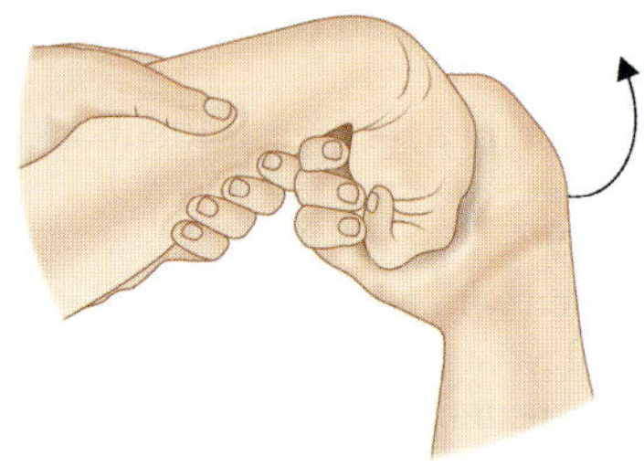

Fig. 56: Muscle test for wrist flexion.

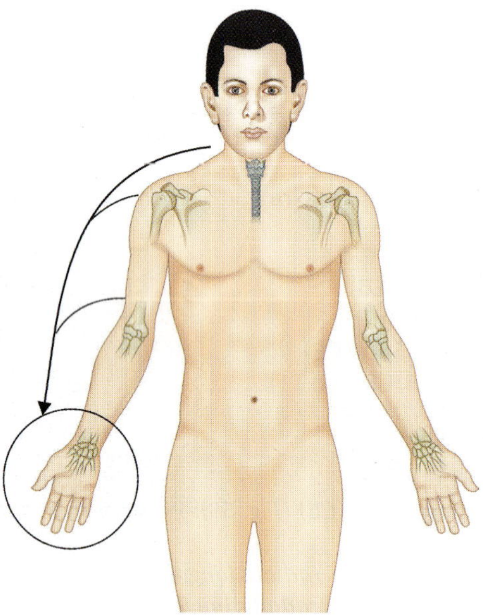

Fig. 57: Other joints, e.g. cervical spine, shoulder, and elbow that need to be examined along with the wrist joint.

- *Evaluate causes of wrist pain:*
  - Herniated cervical disk
  - Osteoarthritis.

Sensation

Radial Nerve

It supplies the dorsum of hand on the (Fig. 58):

- Radial side of third metacarpal
- Dorsal surface of thumb
- Index finger
- Middle finger
- Web space between thumb and index finger (Fig. 58).

Median Nerve

It supplies hand on the (Fig. 59):

- Radial portion of palm
- Palmar surface of thumb

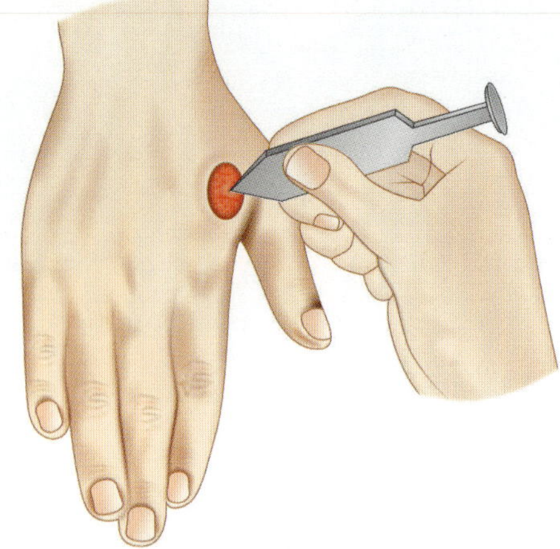

Fig. 58: Web space between thumb and index finger is supplied by the radial nerve.

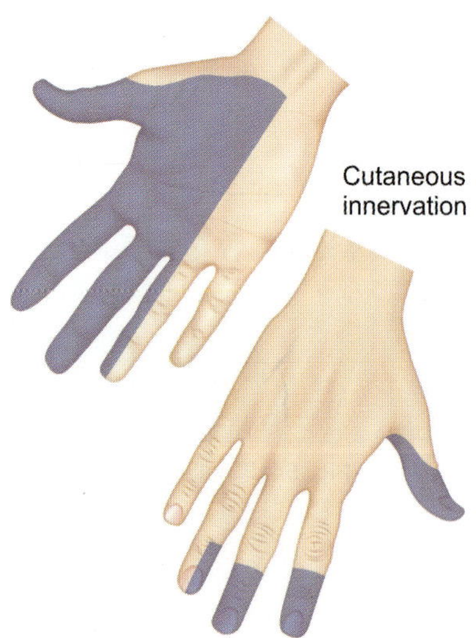

Fig. 59: Area supplied by median nerve.

- Index and middle finger
- It also supplies phalanges of these fingers.

Ulnar Nerve

It supplies hand on the (Fig. 60):

- Ulnar surface of hand (both dorsal and palmar surface)
- Ring and little finger
- Its purest area is on the volar surface of tip of little finger.

Circumferential Measurement (Fig. 61)

- Done at joint level, i.e. the tape passing around both styloid tips
- Second measurement is at the level of the mid forearm
- Look for any wasting and compare with the other side.

Radiology of Wrist

Anteroposterior View

- In anteroposterior view, identify carpal bones and note their shape, density, and position
- There are eight carpal bones (Fig. 62) in two rows. They are as follows:
  1. Pisiform
  2. Triquetrum
  3. Lunate

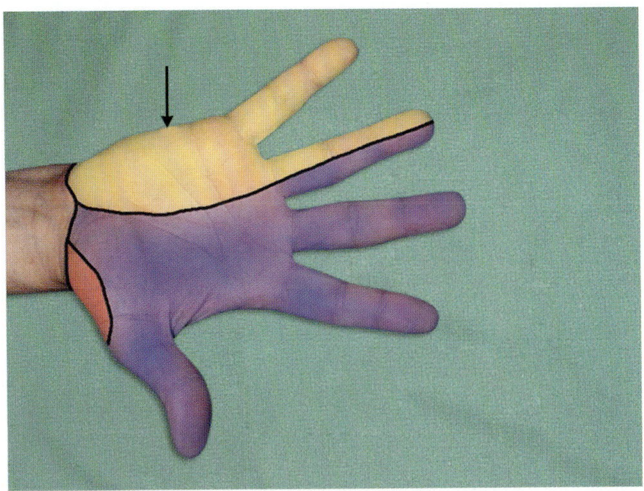

Fig. 60: Area supplied by ulnar nerve.

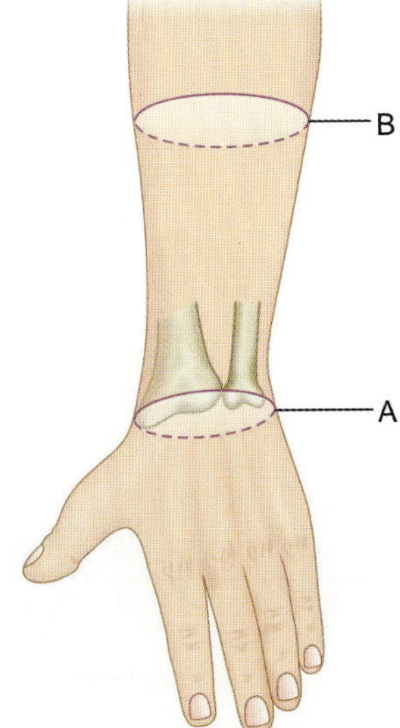

Fig. 61: Circumferential measurement. (A: joint level; B: level of mid forearm)

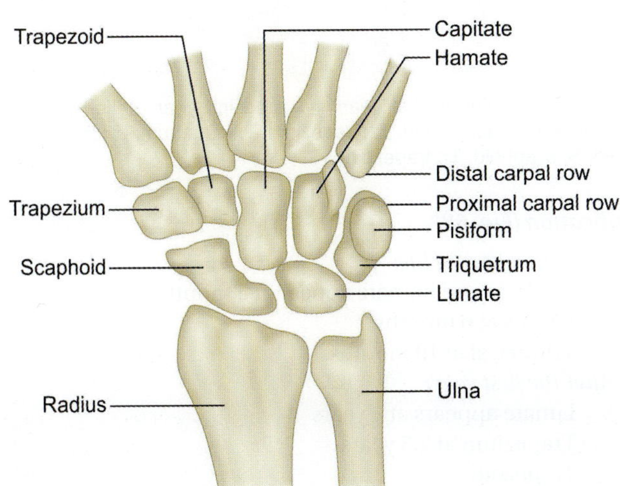

Fig. 62: Anteroposterior view of wrist, note the gap between the carpals.

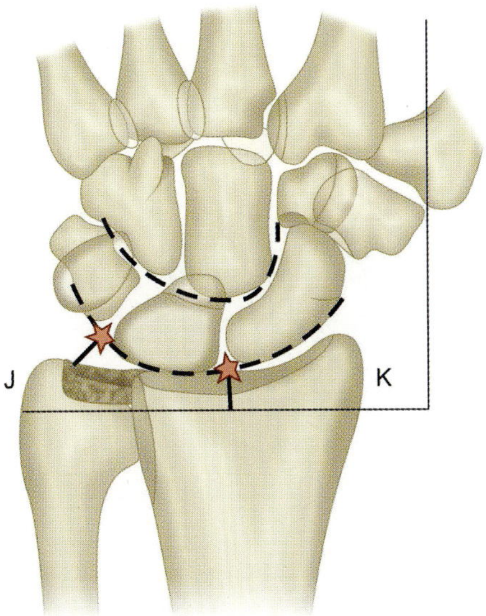

Fig. 63: Distal end of ulna stops short of the radius to make room for triangular fibrocartilage. (J: ulna styloid, K: radial styloid).

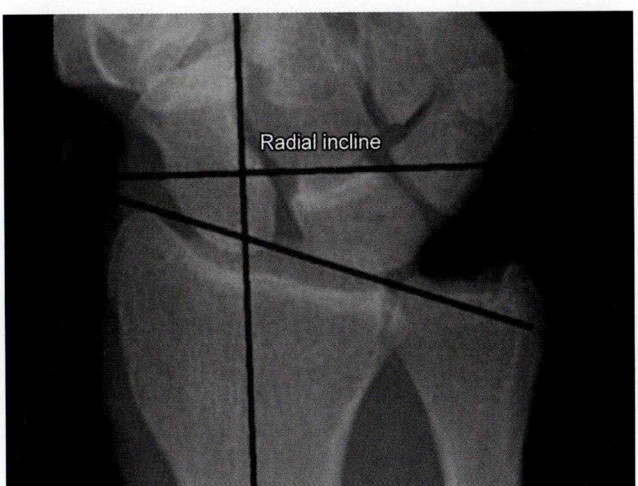

Fig. 64: Radial inclination.

4. Scaphoid
5. Trapezium
6. Trapezoid
7. Capitate
8. Hamate

- Note smooth curve between proximal and distal rows of carpus. The distal end of ulna stops short of the radius, to make room for triangular fibrocartilage (Fig. 63)
- If there is widening of gap between scapholunate and lunotriquetral, obtain additional view in full radial and ulnar deviation and compare with other side.

Radial Inclination (Fig. 64)

- It is an angle between distal articular surface of radius and radial shaft
- It is decreased after Colles' fracture
- Normal range is 19–25°.

Assessment of Carpal Height and Drift (Fig. 65)

A line drawn through middle metacarpal (M), carpus (C), and its distance from radial styloid (RS), ulnar axis (U) expresses these ratios as:

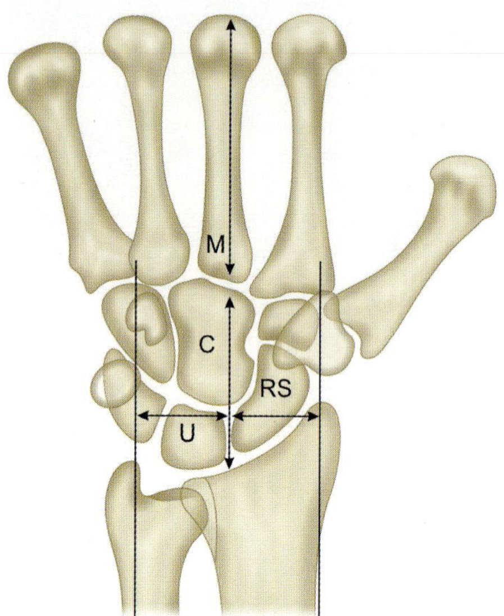

Fig. 65: Assessment of carpal height and drift. (M: middle metacarpal; C: capitate; RS: radial styloid; U: ulnar axis; C: triquetral).

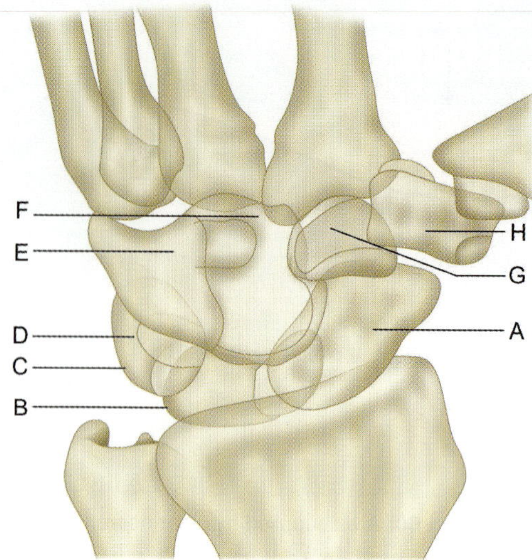

Fig. 67: Wrist shown in oblique view. (A: tubercle of scaphoid; B: crest of lunate; C: triquetral; D: pisiform; E: hamate; F: capitate; G: trapezoid; H: trapezium)

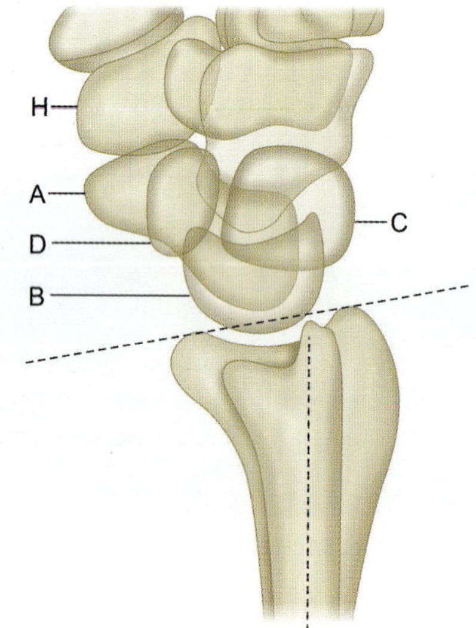

Fig. 66: Structures seen on lateral radiograph. (H: trapezium; A: tubercle and body of scaphoid; D: pisiform one; B: crest of lunate; C: triquetral)

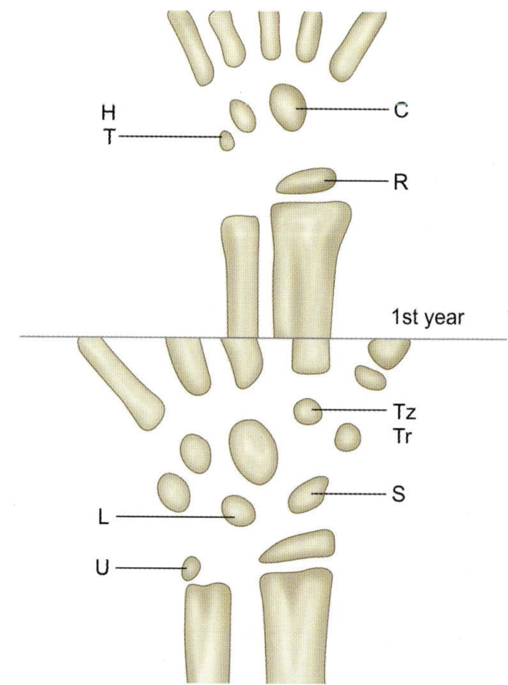

Fig. 68: Ossification in first year and after first year of life. (H: hamate; C: capitate; R: radial styloid; Tz: trapezium; T: triquetrum; L: lunate; U: ulnar styloid; S: scaphoid; Tr: trapezoid)

- *Carpal height ratio*: C/M (Normal—0.51-0.57)
- *Chamy measurement*: U/M (Normal—0.25-0.31)
- *McMurtry's index*: U/M (Normal—0.27-0.33).

Lateral Radiograph

- Structures seen on lateral radiograph (Fig. 66) are as follows:
  - Trapezium
  - Tubercle and body of scaphoid
  - Pisiform bone
  - Crest of lunate
  - Triquetral.
- The plane of wrist joint normally tilted at 5° anteriorly.

Oblique View (Fig. 67)

This is taken, when hairline fracture of carpus is suspected.

Ossification (Fig. 68)

- *In the first year of life:*
  - Capitate and hamate appear at 2 months
  - Radius at 6 months
  - Triquetral at 10 months.
- *After the first year:*
  - Lunate appears at 2 years
  - Trapezium at 2.5 years
  - Trapezoid
  - Scaphoid at 3 years
  - Distal ulna at 4.5 years.

CONGENITAL DEFORMITIES OF HAND

Introduction

A congenital disorder involves defects or damage to a developing fetus. It may be the result of:

- Genetic abnormalities
- The intrauterine environment
- Errors of morphogenesis
- Chromosomal abnormality.

Classification

Swanson, Barsky, and Entin Classification

- Failure of formation (arrest of development)
- Failure of differentiation (or separation)
- Duplication
- Overgrowth
- Undergrowth
- Congenital constriction band syndrome
- Generalized skeletal abnormalities.

Incidence and prevalence: 11 per 10,000 population.

Most common anomalies:

- Syndactyly
- Polydactyly
- Camptodactyly
- Clinodactyly
- Congenital amputations
- Radial clubhand.

Embryology

- The arm arises as a small bud of tissue on the lateral body wall beginning on 26th day of gestation, preceding leg bud formation by only 24 hours
- "Proximal-to-Distal" growth and development fashion
- Growth occurs under apical ectodermal ridge, which produces fibroblast growth factor
- By day 31 of gestation, hand paddle is present
- Programmed cellular death and fissuring of hand paddle are completed by day 36, with central rays forming first, followed by preaxial and postaxial digits
- This is followed by development of:
  - Chondral elements
  - Endochondral ossification
  - Joint, muscle, and vascular development
  - The entire process is completed by 8 weeks of gestation.

Failure of Formation or Arrest of Development (Fig. 69)

The upper limb can fail to develop either:

- Transversely
- Longitudinally.

Transverse Deficiencies

- These include deformities in which there is complete absence of parts distal to some point on the upper extremity, producing amputation-like stumps
- Further classification is by naming the level at which the remaining stump terminates
- About 98% are unilateral and the most common level is upper one-third of forearm.

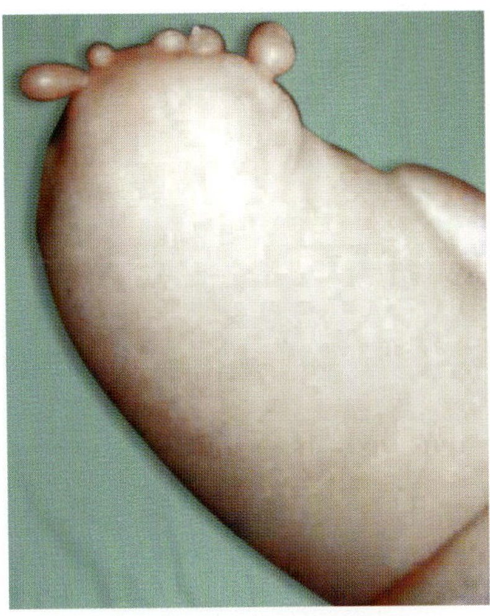

Fig. 69: Failure of formation.

Causes

- Failure of apical ectodermal ridge, possibly secondary to infarct
- Use of misoprostol, to induce abortion
- Usually, slightly bulbous, well-padded stump is present, while in more distal deficiencies, rudimentary vestigial digital "nubbins" are present
- Hypoplasia of more proximal muscles helps differentiate these deficiencies from deficiencies associated with congenital bands
- Usually, forearm is 7 cm at birth and no more than 10 cm in adults.

Management

- *Prosthetic management:* It is useful for patients who do not require surgery:
  - *Timing:* At the time of crawling and certainly at the time of independent ambulation. The fitting of upper limb prosthesis should complement and enhance the normal developmental milestones.
  - Choice of prosthesis depends on following:
    - Level of amputation
    - Age
    - Mental capacity of child
    - Socioeconomic conditions.
- *Surgical management:* Krukenberg reconstruction and Nathan and Trung modification (Figs. 70 to 72):
  - It consists of separation of radius and ulna to allow a sensate, "chop-stick" like forearm
  - Best in bilateral below-elbow amputation
  - Prosthesis can still be used for cosmesis
  - Surgical prerequisites are:
    - Stump length of 8 cm from insertion of biceps
    - Normal forearm musculature
    - Patient and family should be willing to undergo this disfiguring operation, to improve function.

Procedure of Krukenberg reconstruction (Figs. 70 to 72): Skin closure on flexor surface of forearm elliptical area indicates location of any needed split-skin grafts.

Metacarpal lengthening:

- It is usually reserved for transverse deficiencies at level of metacarpophalangeal (MCP) joints in a child with at least one remaining digit

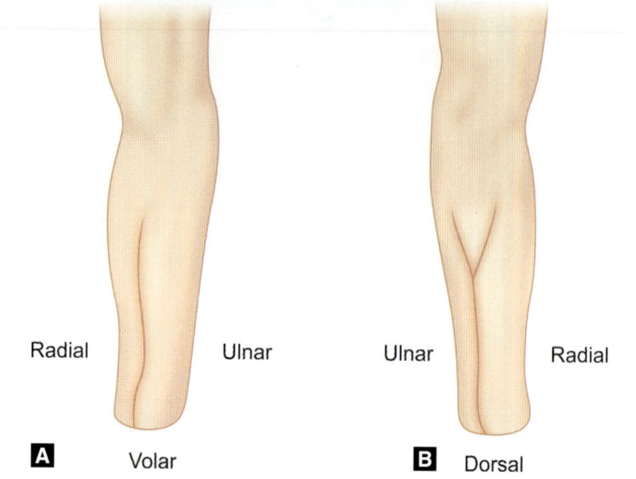

Figs. 70A and B: Incisions on flexor or volar and dorsal surfaces of forearm.

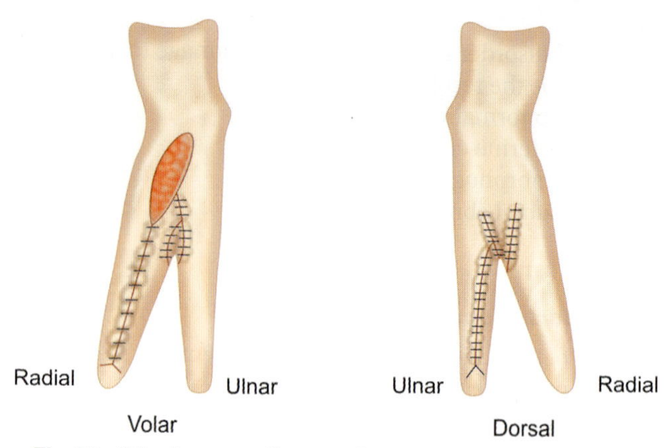

Fig. 72: Skin closure on flexor surface of forearm elliptical area.

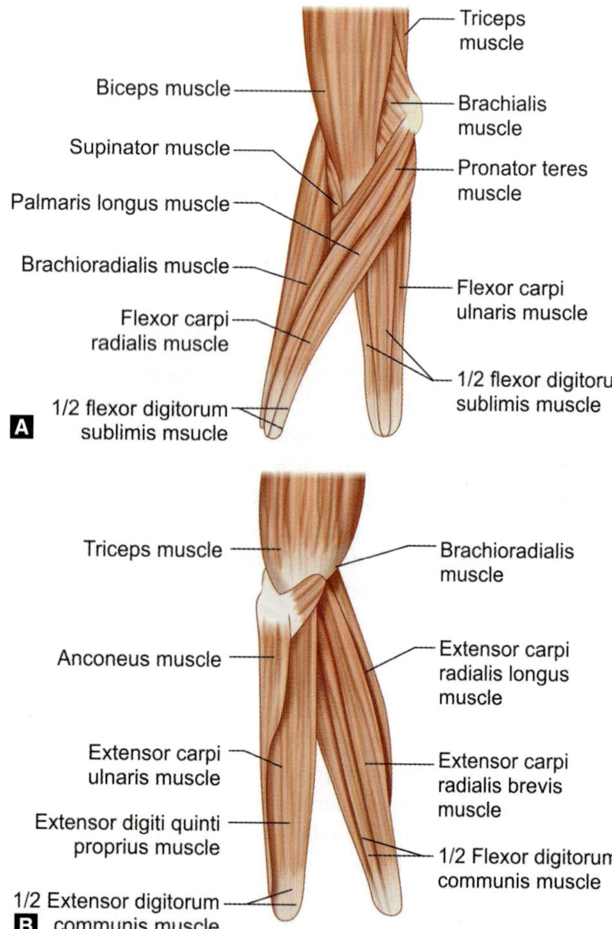

Figs. 71A and B: Forearm muscles have been separated into two groups.

- *Ideal age:* 5–11 years
- Matev (1967) described osteotomy of digital ray with gradual distraction and subsequent bone grafting for a deficient thumb
- An ideal of 4–5 cm of length can be gained, but improved function and cosmesis may not be achieved.

Longitudinal Deficiencies (Figs. 73A to C)

These include all failure-of-formation anomalies that are not transverse deficiencies. These are:

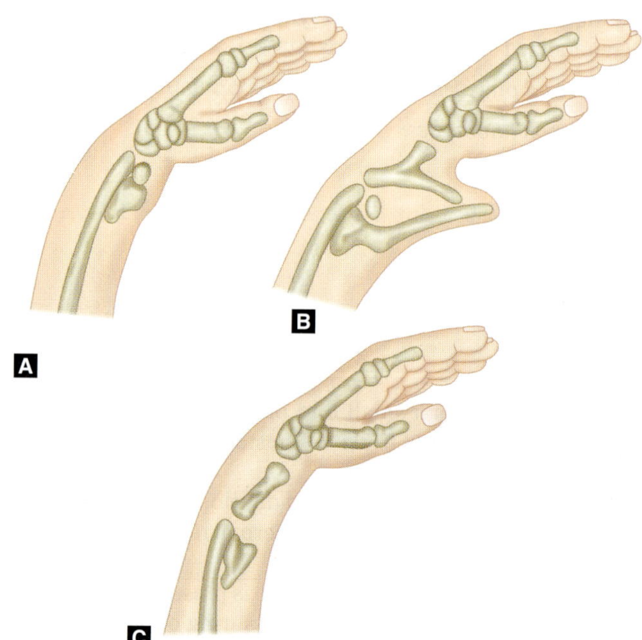

Figs. 73A to C: Different types of longitudinal deficiencies.

- Phocomelia
- Radial ray dysplasia
- Ulnar ray dysplasia
- Central dysplasia.

Phocomelia

Phocomelia is a Greek word, meaning "Seal Limb" or "Flipper". There are three anatomical patterns:

1. *Type 1:* Complete phocomelia with absence of all limb bones proximal to hand
2. *Type 2:* Absence or extreme hypoplasia of proximal limb bones with forearm and hand attached to trunk
3. *Type 3:* Hand attached directly to humerus.

Treatment

- Usually conservative
- Surgery indicated only for shoulder instability, limb shortening, or inadequate thumb opposition
- Prosthesis may help to certain extent.

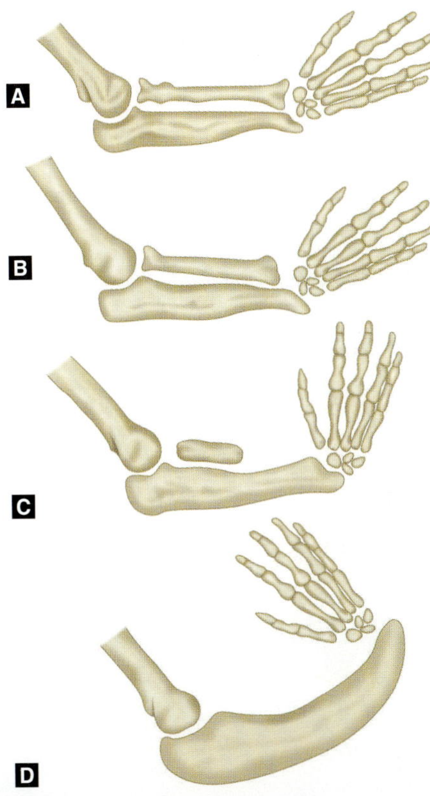

Figs. 74A to D: Different types of radial dysplasia. (A) Type 1. Short distal radius; (B) Type 2. Hypoplastic radius; (C) Type 3. Partial absence of radius; and (D) Type 4. Total absence of radius.

TABLE 2: Manske's modified classification of radial longitudinal deficiency.

Type	*Thumb*	*Carpus*	*Distal radius*	*Proximal radius*
N	Hypoplastic or absent	Normal	Normal	Normal
0	Hypoplastic or absent	Absence, hypoplasia, or coalition	Normal	Normal, radioulnar synostosis, or congenital dislocation of radial head
1	Hypoplastic or absent	Absence, hypoplasia or coalition	> 2 mm shorter than ulna	Normal, radioulnar synostosis, or congenital dislocation of radial head
2	Hypoplastic or absent	Absence, hypoplasia or coalition	Hypoplasia	Hypoplasia
3	Hypoplastic or absent	Absence, hypoplasia or coalition	Physis absent	Variable hypoplasia
4	Hypoplastic or absent	Absence, hypoplasia or coalition	Absent	Absent

Radial Club Hand

Radial Deficiencies

- Include all malformations with longitudinal failure of formation of parts along the preaxial or radial border of upper extremity.
- *Radial club hand:* Deficient or absent thenar muscles, shortened, unstable and absent thumb, shortened, and absent radius
- Thalidomide may play a role in its occurrence.

Heikel's classification of radial dysplasia (Figs. 74A to D)

- *Type 1:* Short distal radius
- *Type 2:* Hypoplastic radius
- *Type 3:* Partial absence of radius
- *Type 4:* Total absence of radius

Manske's modified classification of radial longitudinal deficiency: It is listed in Table 2.

Management

- *Nonsurgical management:* Immediately after birth, early casting and splinting are done. A light, molded plastic short-arm splint is applied along radial side of forearm and removed only for bathing, until infant begins to use his hands and then it is worn only at night. There is no satisfactory conservative treatment for associated significant thumb deformities.
- *Surgical management*: Ideal age—3–6 months. Pollicization, if indicated, follows at 9–12 months.

Specific Contraindications

- Severe associated anomalies, not compatible with life
- Inadequate elbow flexion
- Mild deformity with adequate radial support
- Older patients, who are well adjusted.

Procedures to be considered

- Centralization of the hand
- Centralization of the hand and tendon transfers
- Pollicization for reconstruction of thumb with radial club hand
- Opponensplasty
- Triceps transfer to restore elbow flexion.

Centralization arthroplasty (transverse ulnar approach, by Manske, McCarroll, and Swanson): The procedure is illustrated in Figures 75 to 78.

Centralization arthroplasty (transverse ulnar approach by Watson, Beebe, and Cruz): The procedure is demonstrated in Figures 79A to G.

Centralization of hand by Bayne and Klug (Figs. 80A to C).

Pollicization for reconstruction of thumb with radial club hand by Buck-Grumco (Figs. 81 to 83).

Opponensplasty

- *Operative procedure:* Modified Goldner and Riordan procedure.
- *Findings:* Complete absence of first dorsal compartment, i.e. EPB and APL and hypoplastic EPL.
- *Plan*: Rerouting of ring finger FDS tendon and then attaching it to EPL and base of proximal phalanx of thumb through transosseous tunnel (Fig. 84).
  The procedure is demonstrated in Figures 85 to 89.

Splinting

It should be done, while taking care of following things:

- Thumb in abduction
- Metacarpophalangeal joint in extension

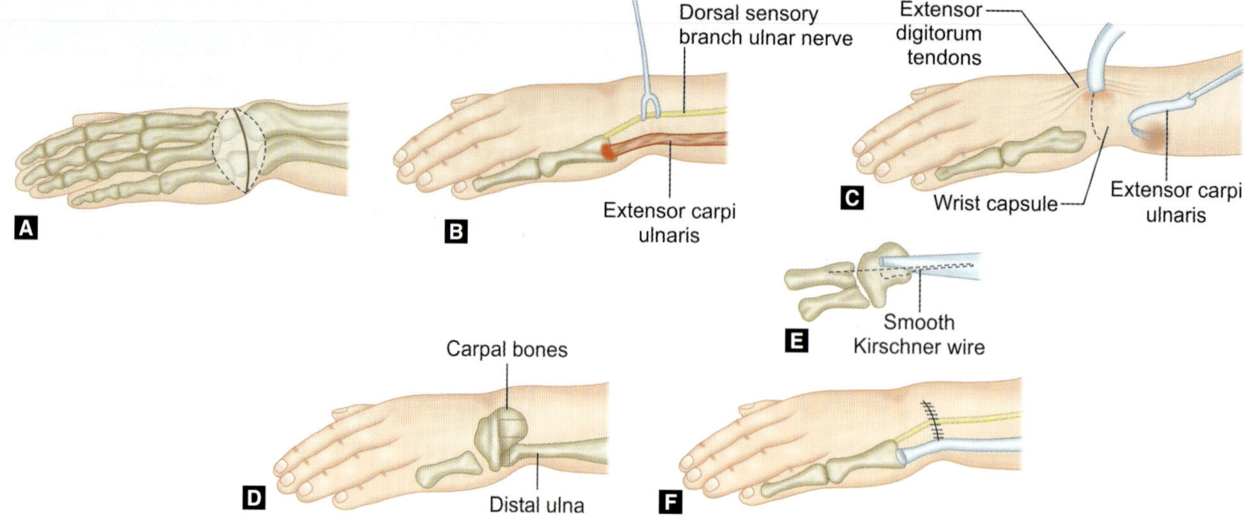

Figs. 75A to F: Different steps of centralization arthroplasty.

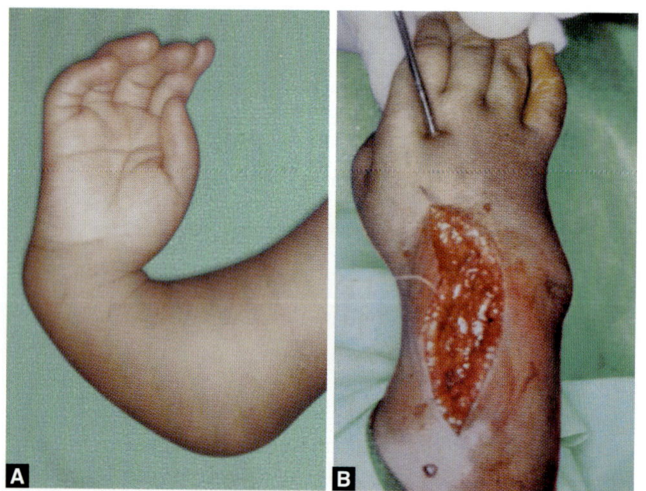

Figs. 76A and B: Centralization arthroplasty, transverse ulnar approach by Manske, McCarroll, and Swanson.

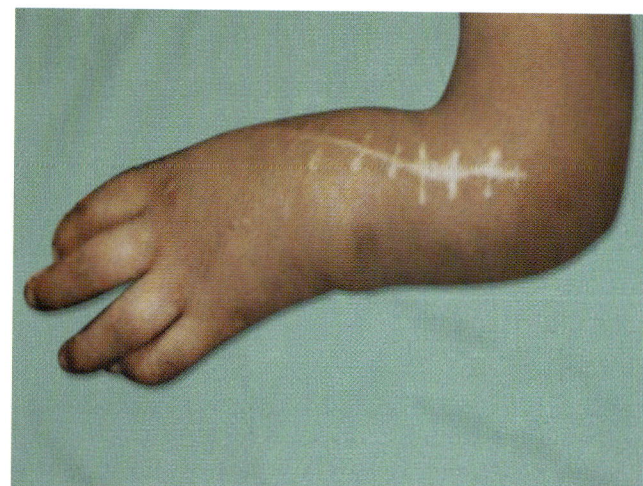

Fig. 78: Centralization arthroplasty performed, by transverse ulnar approach.

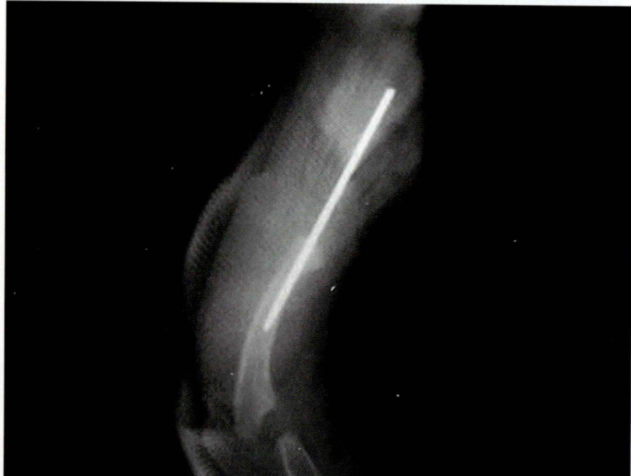

Fig. 77: X-ray taken after performing centralization arthroplasty.

- Distal phalanges (DP) in extension
- Wrist in extension.

Cleft Hand

Central Deficiencies

- Also known as "ectrodactyly", "crab claw", or "lobster claw" (Fig. 90)
- Cleft deficiencies of the hand include malformations, in which there is a longitudinal failure of formation of the second, third, or fourth ray
- It also includes a one-digit (fifth-ray) hand
- Two main patterns of occurrences are:
  1. Typical pattern of central deficiency, with central V-shaped cleft (Fig. 91).
  2. Atypical pattern of central deficiency with U-shaped defect, involving index, and long and ring fingers (Fig. 92).

Flatt's Classification of Central Deficiencies (Figs. 93A to C)

Treatment:

- No definitive treatment
- Operative treatment must be Tailor-made

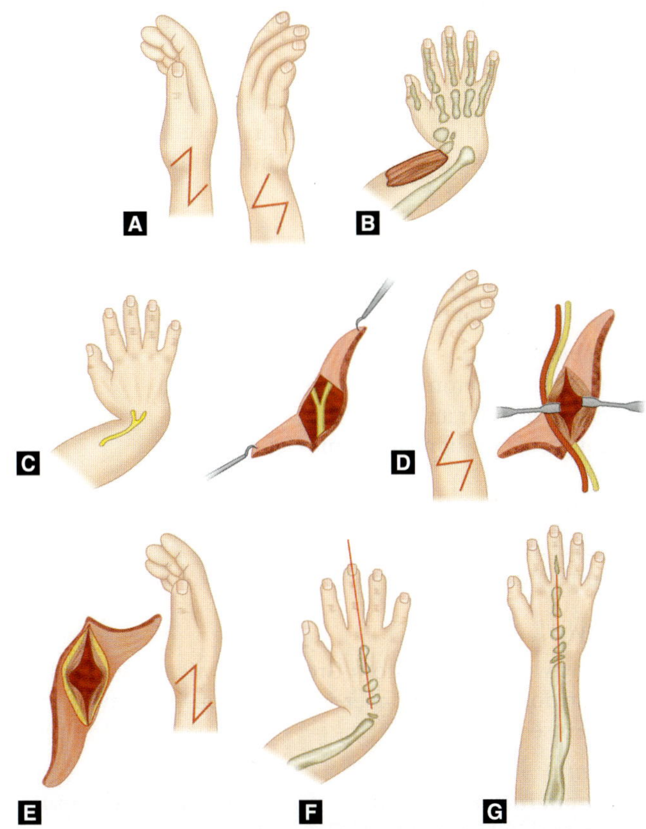

Figs. 79A to G: Different steps of centralization arthroplasty (transverse ulnar approach by Watson, Bebee, and Cruz).

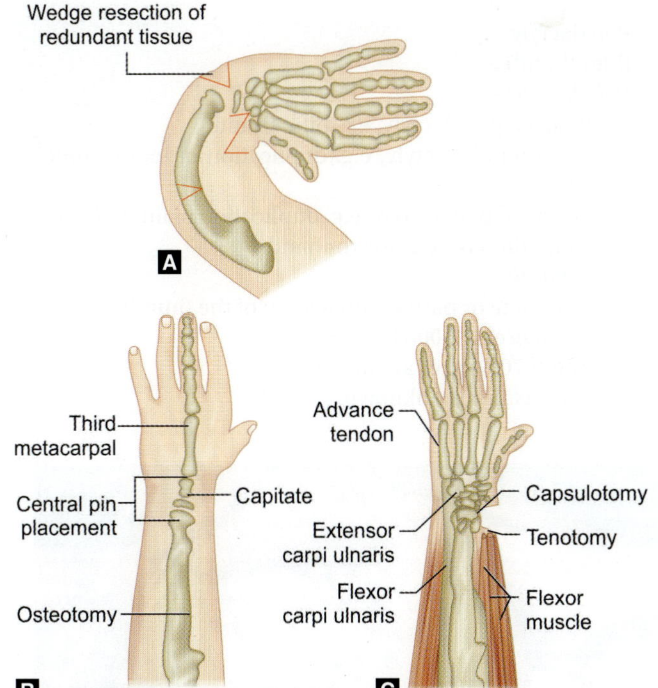

Figs. 80A to C: Different steps of carrying out centralization of hand procedure as given by Bayne and Klug.

- Surgical reconstruction includes:
  - Closure of cleft
  - Release of syndactyly

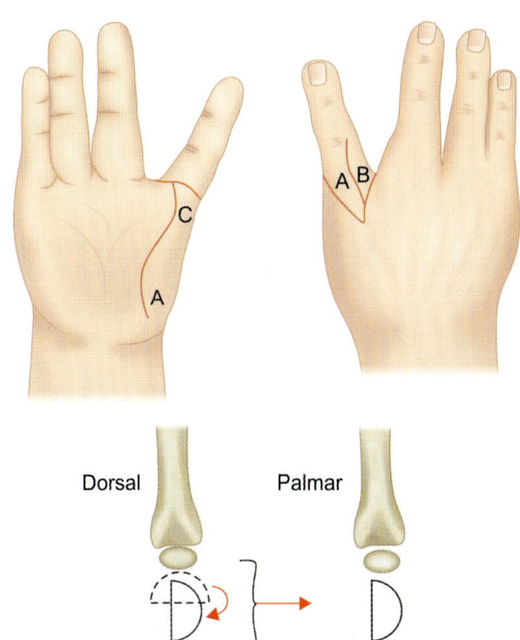

Fig. 81: Pollicization of index finger. (A: palmar skin incision; B: dorsal skin incision; C: rotation of metacarpal head into flexon to prevent postoperative hyperextension)

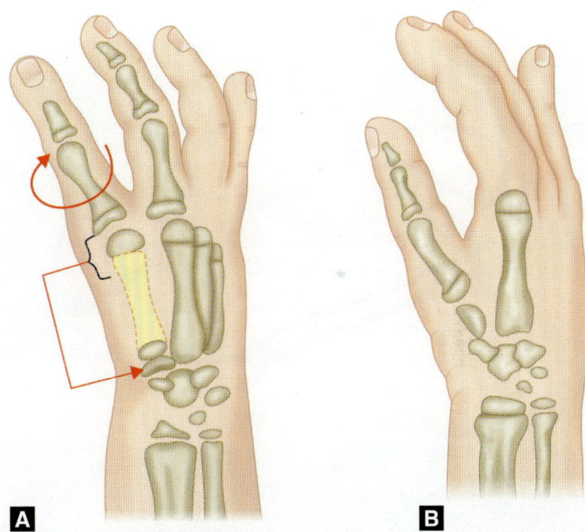

Figs. 82A and B: (A) Index finger rotated about 160° along long axis; (B) final positioning in about 40° of palmar abduction with metacarpal head secured to metacarpal base or carpus.

  - Correction of thumb adduction contracture
  - Removal of deforming bony elements
  - Correction of delta phalanx.
- In atypical pattern, deepening of palm for grasp, tendon transfers, etc. are required.

Ulnar Club Hand

- Ulnar deficiencies are malformations, in which there is longitudinal failure of formation along the postaxial border of the upper extremity.
- Other terms used are:
  - Dysmelia
  - Paraxial ulnar hemimelia
  - Congenital absence of ulna.

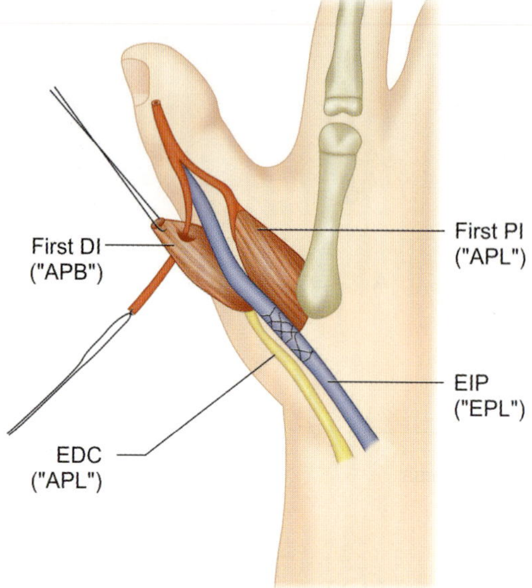

Fig. 83: Reattachment of tendons to provide control of new thumb. First palmar interosseous (PI) functions as adductor pollicis (AP); First dorsal interosseous (DI) as abductor pollicis brevis (APB); Extensor digitorum communis (EDC) as abductor pollicis longus (APL); and extensor indicis proprius (EIP) as extensor pollicis longus (EPL).

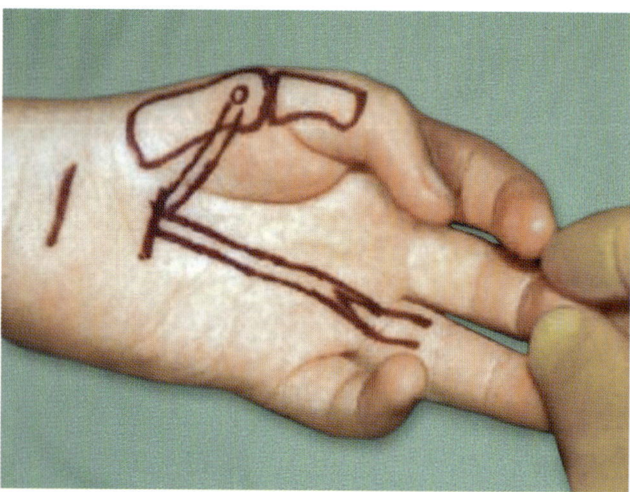

Fig. 84: Planning of the opponensplasty procedure (as seen by markings on hand).

Swanson's Classification of Ulnar Deficiency (Figs. 94A to D)

Treatment:
- *Nonoperative:* Serial corrective casting and splinting, followed by surgery if indicated, for more than 6 months of age
- *Operative:* Indications for surgical intervention are:
  - Syndactyly
  - Radial bowing
  - Presence of ulnar anlage
  - Dislocation of radial head
  - Internal rotation deformity of humerus.

Surgical procedures:
- Rotational osteotomy of first metacarpal
- Excision of ulnar anlage
- Creation of one-bone forearm (Figs. 95A to C).

Failure of Differentiation

- Syndactyly
- Alpert syndrome.

Syndactyly

Syndactyly word derived from Greek "syn" meaning together or plus "dàktydos" meaning finger, is a condition where two or more digits are fused together.

Treatment:
- *Intraoperative or Whitey's technique:* The procedure is illustrated in Figures 96A to C.
- *Postoperative follow-up:* This has been shown in Figures 97A to C.

Duplication

- Polydactyly
- Bifid thumb
- *Polydactyly:*
  - Preaxial polydactyly, e.g. bifid thumb
  - Central polydactyly, e.g. duplication of index, middle, or ring finger
  - Postaxial polydactyly, e.g. duplication of little finger
  - Ulnar dimelia, e.g. mirror hand.
- *Bifid thumb:*
  - Complete or partial duplication of the thumb
  - *Incidence:* 1/3,000 live births
  - About 70% cases are unilateral
  - Exact cause is unknown.

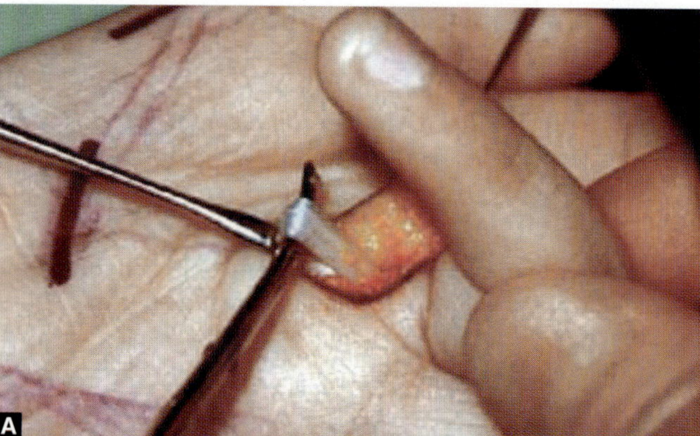

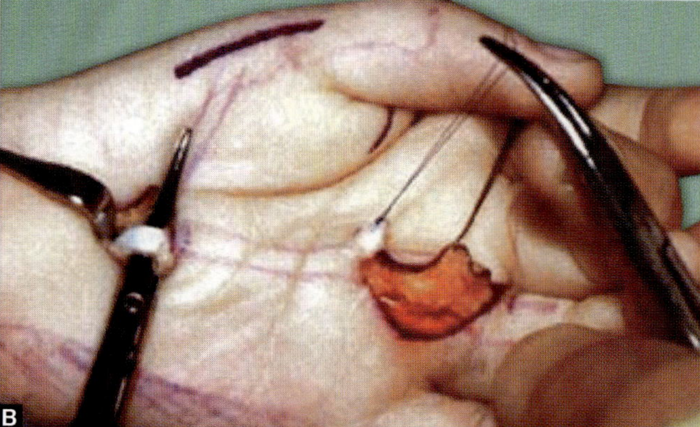

Figs. 85A and B: The two slips of flexor digitorum superficialis detached from ring finger.

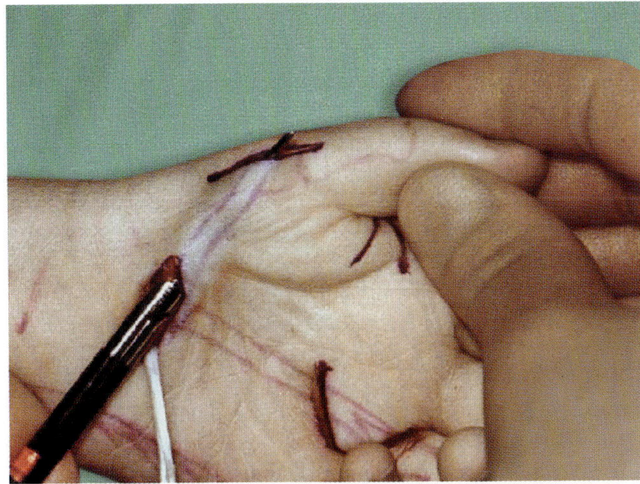

Fig. 86: Flexor digitorum superficialis tendon passed through flexor carpi ulnaris (FCU) pulley.

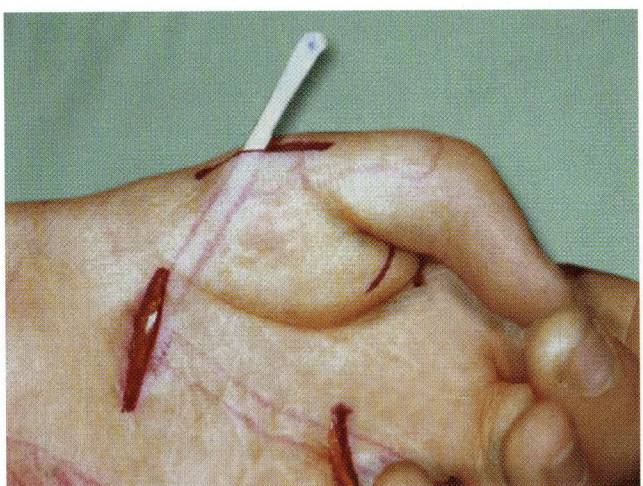

Fig. 87: Flexor digitorum superficialis tendon then passed through subcutaneous tunnel towards the MP joint.

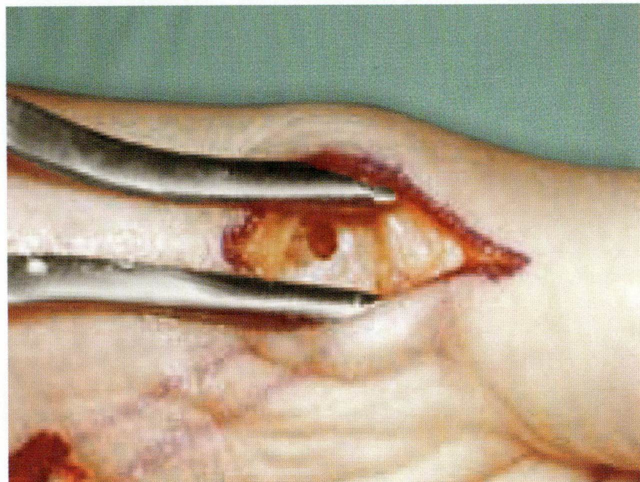

Fig. 88: A transverse hole drilled into the proximal phalanx and one slip of flexor digitorum superficialis attached to it.

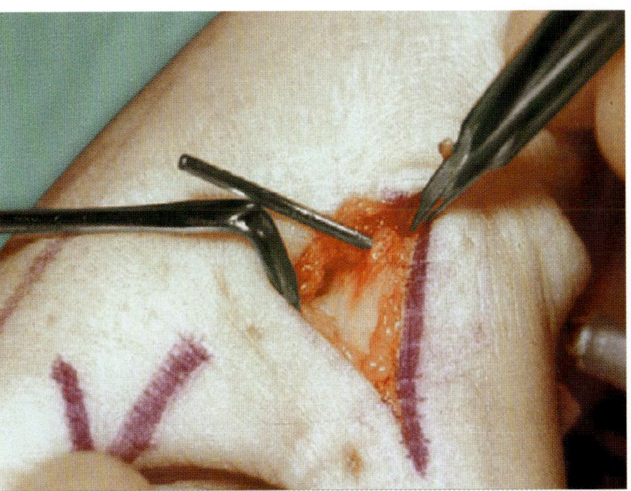

Fig. 89: The second slip attached to the EPL tendon.

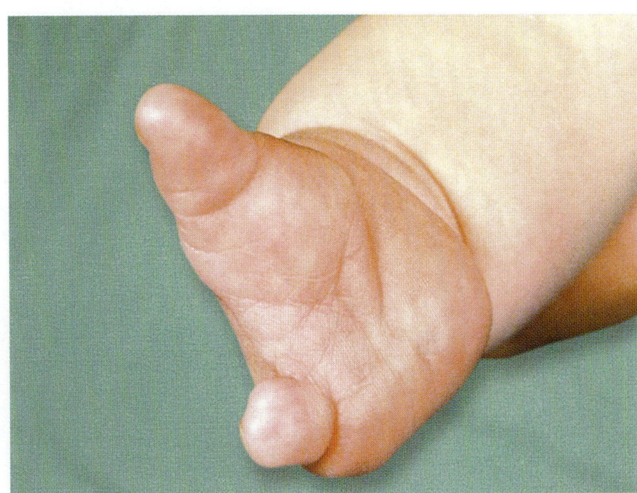

Fig. 90: Cleft hand.

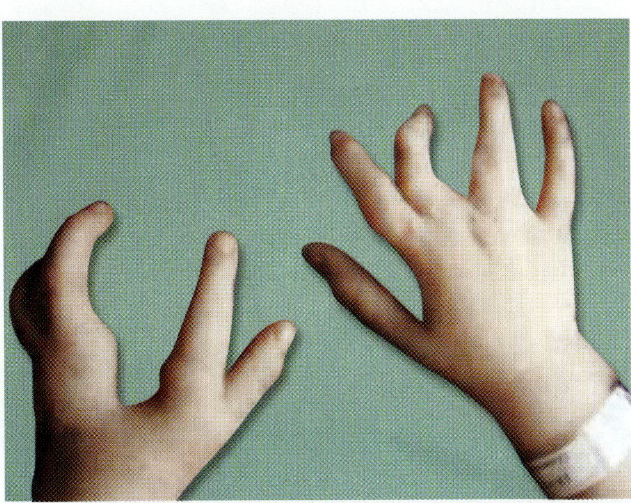

Fig. 91: Typical pattern of central deficiency with central V-shaped cleft.

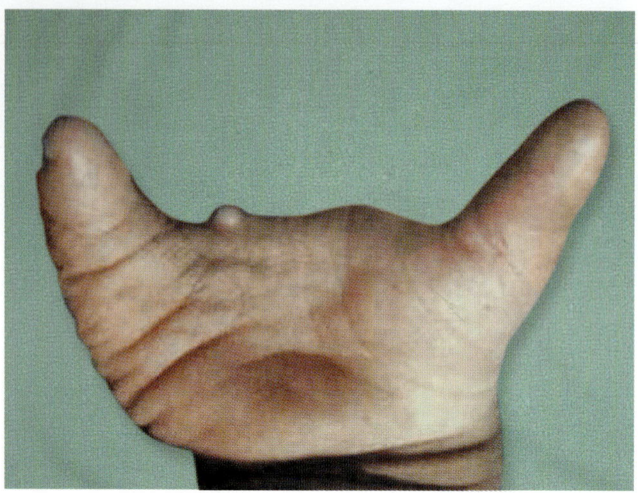

Fig. 92: Atypical pattern of central deficiency with U-shaped defect, involving index, and long and ring fingers.

Wessel Classification (Fig. 98)

Treatment:

- Surgical correction almost always warranted for better function and cosmesis
- Surgery generally, done greater than 18 months of age, but not beyond 5 years
- Types 1 and 2 are treated by "combination procedure"
- More proximal duplication requires excision of the more hypoplastic thumb
- Usually, the ulnar side thumb is preserved.

Bilhaut-Cloquet "combination procedure" (Figs. 99A and B).

Triphalangeal Thumb

- It has three phalanges instead of normal two (Fig. 100)
- These are of two types:
    1. *Wedge-shaped extraossicle:* Angular deformity
    2. *Normal-sized extraossicle*: "Five-finger hand".
- Also classified as "opposable and nonopposable".

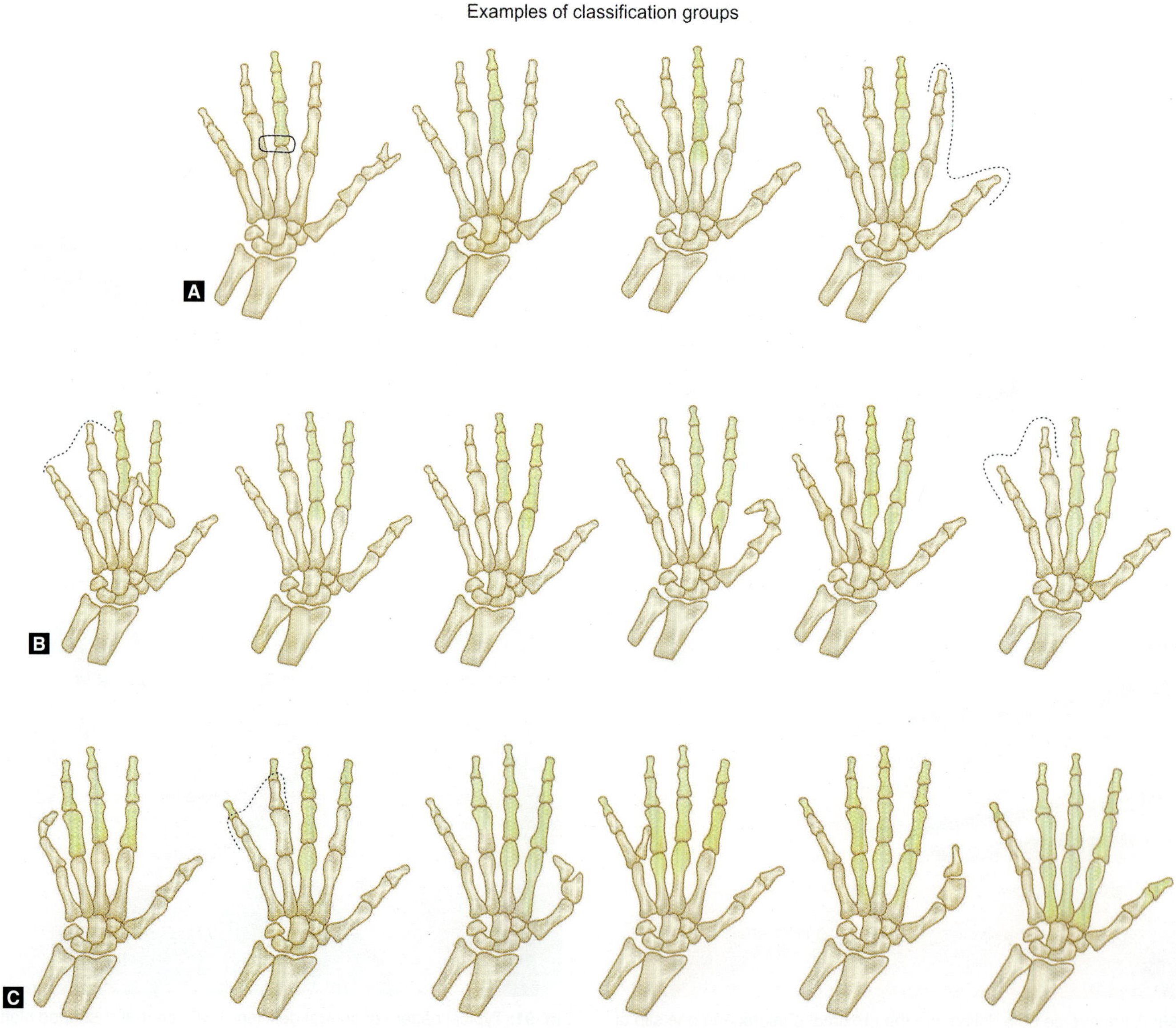

Examples of classification groups

A

B

C

Figs. 93A to C: Flatt's classification of central deficiencies.

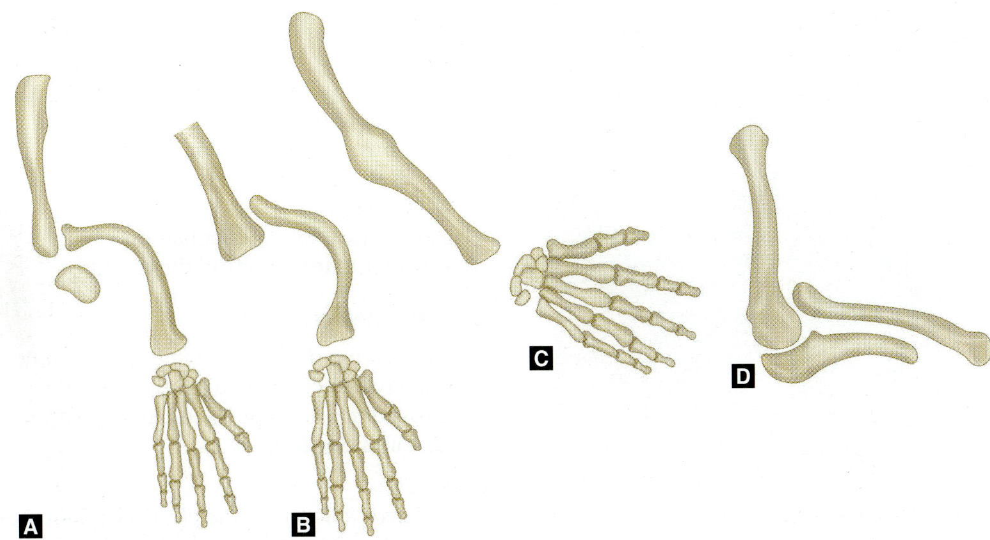

Figs. 94A to D: Swanson's classification of ulnar deficiency—(A) Hypoplasia or partial defect of ulna; (B) Total defect of ulna; (C) Partial or total defect of ulna, with humeroradial synostosis; (D) Total or partial defect of ulna, with congenital amputation at wrist.

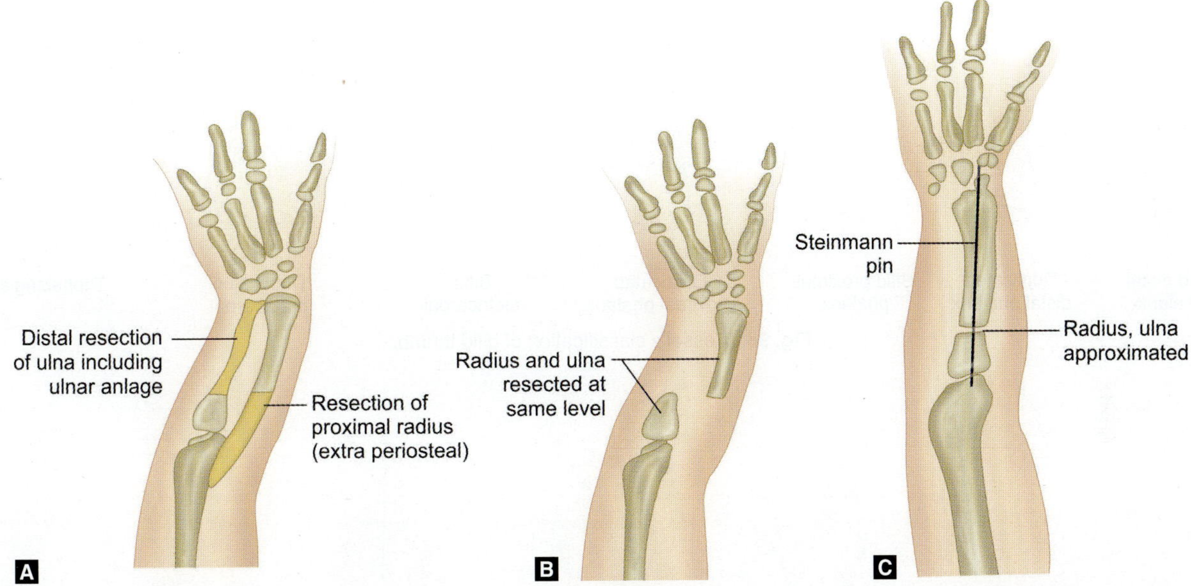

Figs. 95A to C: Different steps of surgical correction of ulnar club hand: Creation of one-bone forearm—(A) resection of distal ulnar anlage and proximal radius (shaded areas); (B) Alignment of distal radius and proximal ulna; (C) Kirschner wire extending into carpals used to stabilize radial and ulnar segments.

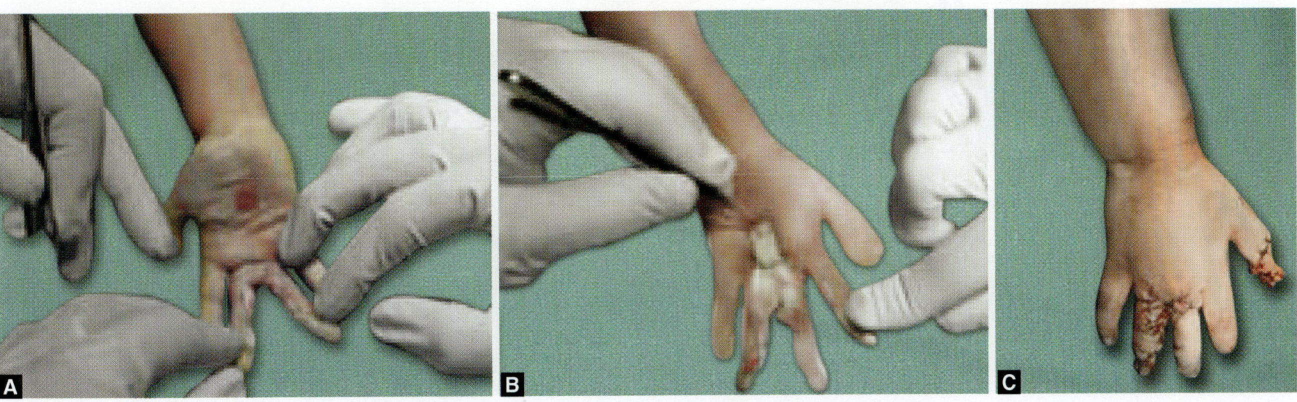

Figs. 96A to C: Whitey's technique of correction of syndactyly.

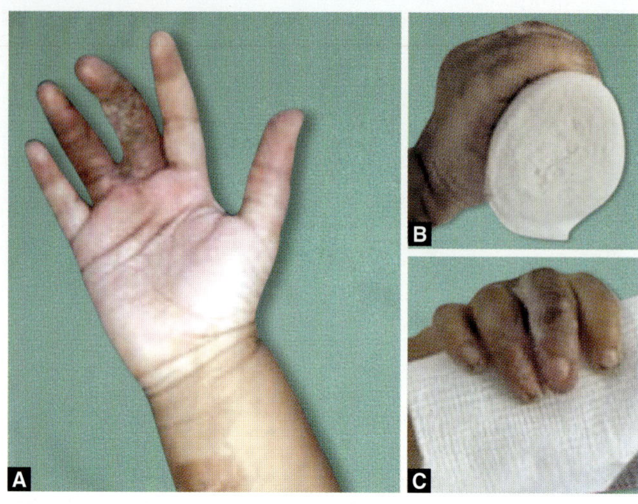
Figs. 97A to C: Postoperative follow-up after correcting syndactyly.

Treatment

- *Nonoperative treatment:* It is not very useful
- *Operative treatment (Figs. 101A to D):* Goals of an operative treatment are:
  - Correction of angular deformity
  - Restoration of normal length
  - Correction of web contracture
  - Improvement of opposition
  - Adequate stability of the thumb.

Central Polydactyly

- Duplication of index, middle, or ring finger
- Usually associated with complex syndactyly
- *Most common:* Type 2, concealed within syndactyly between long and ring fingers.

Treatment:

- *Isolated central polydactyly:* Excision of most hypoplastic digit

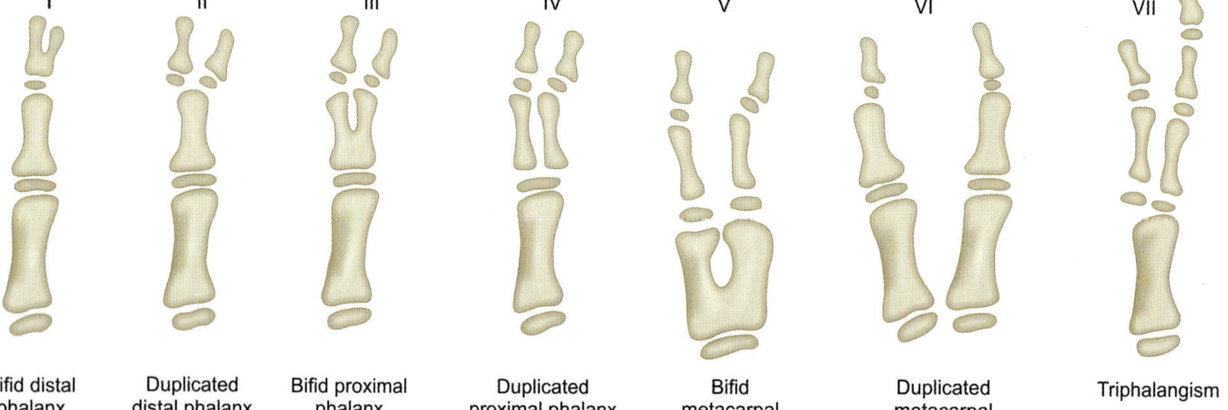

Fig. 98: Wessel's classification of bifid thumb.

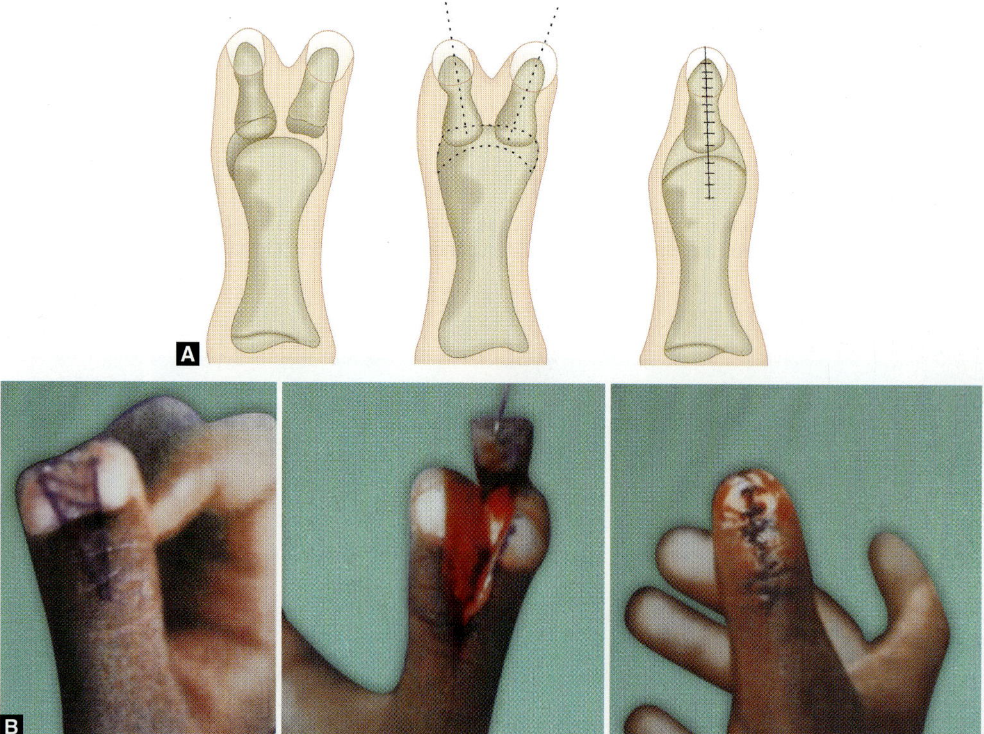
Figs. 99A and B: Bilhaut–Cloquet "combination procedure".

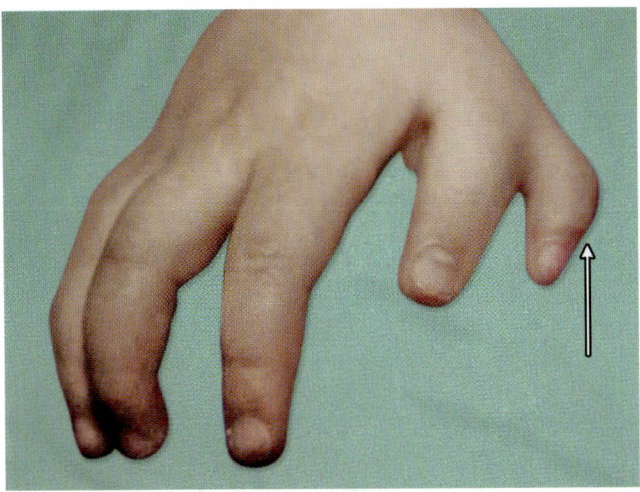

Fig. 100: A triphalangeal thumb.

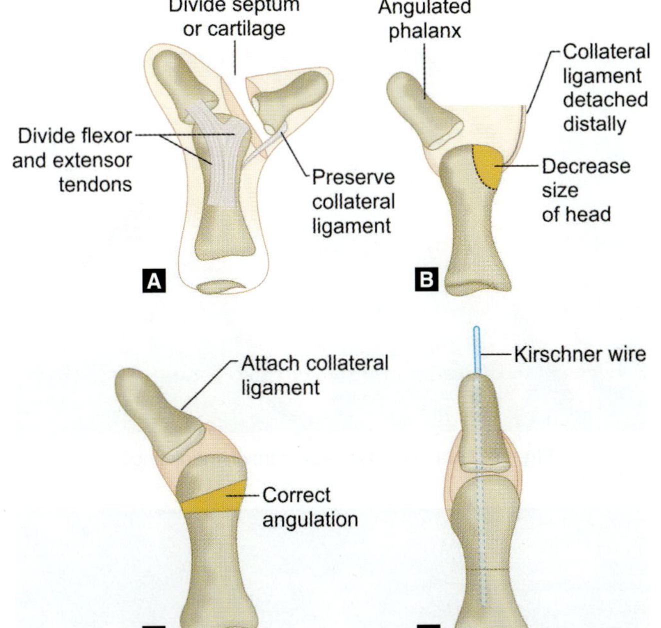

Figs. 101A to D: Operative procedure for correcting triphalangeal thumb.

- *Central polysyndactyly:*
  - Reconstruction with excision of extra digit or
  - Creation of three-fingered hand
  - To be done at 6 months of age, to prevent further angular deformity
  - Amputation of functionless digits may be performed later.

Postaxial Polydactyly

Duplication of Little Finger

- Most common in black population (1 per 300 live births)
- Stelling and Turek classification:
  - *Type 1:* Duplication of soft parts only
  - *Type 2:* Partial duplication of digits, including osseous structures
  - *Type 3:* Complete duplication of the ray, including the metacarpal.
- It can be due to autosomal dominant inheritance, although the perfect cause is not known.

Treatment

Treatment procedures for different types of polydactyly are:

- *Type 1:* Use of ligatures at base not recommended due to reports of fatal hemorrhage
- *Type 2:* Excision of extra digit at 1 year of age
- *Type 3:* No definitive treatment.

Ulnar Dimelia

- Also called "mirror hand"
- Very rare, only a few cases reported worldwide
- Radial and ulnar clusters of fingers in the same hand that are nearly mirror images of each other
- It is considered a duplication phenomenon of ulnar half of the forearm, wrist, and hand, but there is complete substitution of the radial components as well
- Usually associated with some degree of hypoplasia of arm and scapula.

Clinical Features

- Deformity is usually unilateral, with multiple fingers dangling from the palm
- Six to eight, well-formed fingers in same plane
- Postaxial digits more normal than preaxial
- Thumb is absent
- Syndactyly may be present
- Digits may be flexed, absence of extensors
- Hand is radially deviated
- Wrist and elbow are thick
- Elbow motion is decreased
- Arm is shortened
- Ulna and ulnar carpal bones are completely duplicated
- Distal ulnar epiphysis is broadened
- At the elbow, each of the duplicated ulna articulate with humerus separately
- No capitellum on distal humerus.

Treatment

- Parents encouraged to maintain passive ROM in fingers, wrist, elbow, and shoulders by gentle stretching exercises, until child reaches 2 years of age
- Child should be carefully observed during play, to see which radial digit may function best as the opposable thumb
- Surgery should be done early, to prevent psychological trauma to parents and child
- The reconstruction of hand as described by Entin et al. is shown in Figures 102A to C.

Overgrowth: Macrodactyly

- A rare congenital anomaly, in which there is enlargement of the finger
- Incidence (0.9%)
- Index finger most commonly involved (Fig. 103)
- *Barsky classification:* They are of two types:
  1. *Static enlargement:* Enlargement of the digit without further growth with growth of the child
  2. *Progressive enlargement:* Continuous growth of the digit with the growth of the child.

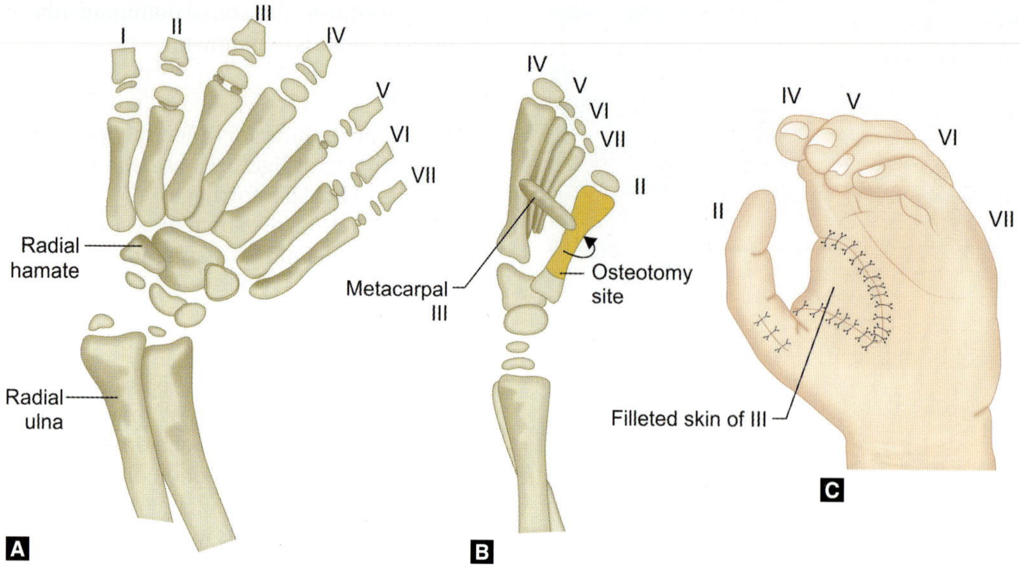

Figs. 102A to C: Hand reconstruction (by Entin et al.).

- Usually unilateral, involves greater than two fingers
- With advancing age, the enlarged digits begin to lose function
- The phalanges are always involved and metacarpals may be involved
- If thumb is involved, usually an abduction and hyperextension deformity results.

Treatment

Nonsurgical methods are unsatisfactory

Operative procedure:

- Indications for surgery are:
  - Excessive enlargement
  - Angulation
  - Carpal tunnel syndrome
  - Causalgia.
- Procedure is called "debulking"
- Most common complication is recurrence.

Undergrowth: Hypoplastic Thumb (Fig. 104)

- Short thumb
- Adducted thumb
- Abducted thumb
- Floating thumb (pouce flottant)
- Absent thumb
- Clasped thumb
- Hypoplastic hands and digits
- Hypoplastic thumb
- Some degree of deficiency in its anatomical parts, e.g. osseous, musculotendinous, or ectodermal.

Short Thumb

If normal thumb extends to the level of proximal interphalangeal (PIP) joint of the index finger, if it is shorter than this, it is considered a "short thumb".

Treatment

- Surgical correction is rarely indicated
- If prehension is significantly limited, deepening of web space is carried out

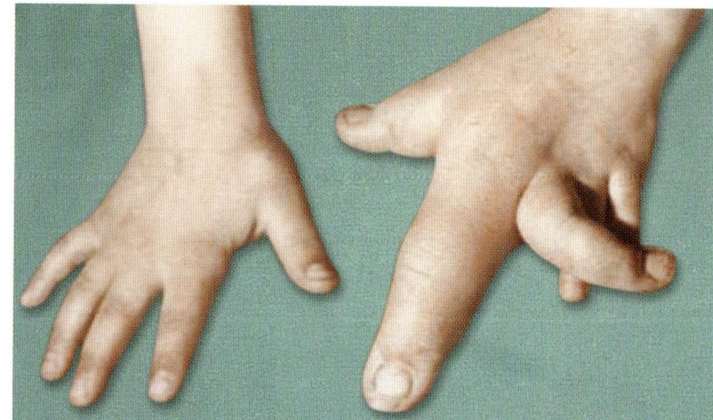

Fig. 103: Macrodactyly—overgrown index finger.

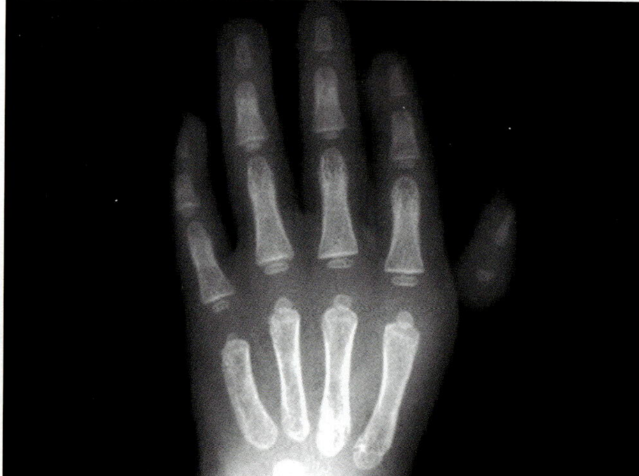

Fig. 104: X-ray showing hypoplastic thumb.

- This creates relative lengthening of the thumb in relation to other digits.

Adducted Thumb

- Absence or deficiency of thenar muscles, resulting in deficient opposition

- Flexor pollicis longus (FPL) often absent
- Radial collateral ligament of thumb's MCP joint may be deficient
- Deformity is transmitted as autosomal dominant trait
- It is usually unilateral.

Treatment

Goals of the treatment are:
- Reconstruction of adducted thumb
- Correction of adduction contractures.

Procedure

Huber, Littler, and Cooley procedure: Ring finger's flexor superficialis tendon opponensplasty and abductor digiti quinti opponensplasty.

Abducted Thumb

- Described by Tupper in 1969
- Also called "pollex abductus"
- Results from abnormal insertion of FPL into an otherwise normal EPL muscle
- This results in marked abduction of proximal phalanx of thumb
- Extremely rare, only few cases are reported.

Treatment

- Many treatments have been proposed
- Release of bifurcated tendon insertion and reattachment to metacarpal neck
- Release of tendon, distally withdrawal at wrist reattachment to distal phalanx
- Also required release of radial collateral ligament and reefing of ulnar collateral ligament of MCP joint.

Floating Thumb: Pouce Flottant (Fig. 105)

- Small and slender thumb that seems to dangle from radial border of hand
- There are two phalanges, a fingernail and no MCP joint and first metacarpal.

Treatment

- Amputation, followed by pollicization of index finger
- In bilateral cases, pollicization of one side should be performed early.

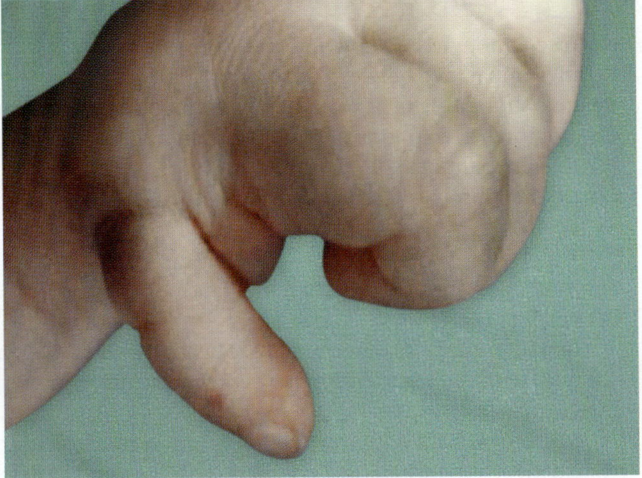

Fig. 105: A floating thumb.

Absent Thumb

- It is most severe manifestation of hypoplastic thumb
- Associated with radial ray deficiencies, ring D chromosomal abnormalities, trisomy 18 syndrome, etc.

Treatment

Choice between two procedures:
- Pollicization of index finger
- Recession of index finger (Figs. 106A to C)
- Done at 6–12 months of age, to allow some growth of hand before surgery.

Congenital Clasped Thumb

- Thumb is positioned in adduction and extreme flexion at MCP joint
- Weckesser, Reed, and Heiple classification:
  - *Group 1:* Deficient extension only
  - *Group 2:* Flexion contracture with deficient extension
  - *Group 3:* Hypoplasia of thumb, including tendon and muscle deficiencies
  - *Group 4:* Other deformities.

Treatment

- *Nonoperative:* Early splinting in extension and abduction
- *Operative:* Useful donor tendons for inadequate EPL muscle are:
  - Palmaris longus
  - Brachioradialis
  - Extensor carpi radialis longus
  - Extensor indicis proprius
  - Flexor superficialis
  - Significant web space reconstruction may also be required.

Congenital Ring Syndrome (Figs. 107A and B)

- Occurs when deep cutaneous creases encircle a limb, as if a string was tightly tied around it
- Other common terms are streeter bands, annular grooves, and intrauterine amputations.

Patterson Classification

- *Type 1:* Simple ring, usually transverse or oblique around a digit
- *Type 2:* Deeper ring with abnormality of part distally, usually lymphedema

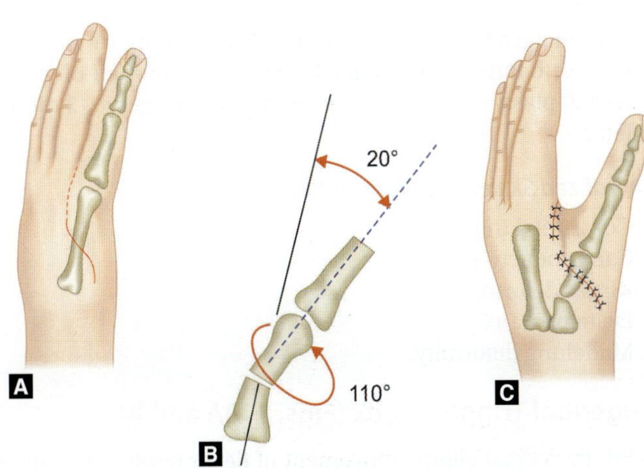

Figs. 106A to C: Recession of index finger.

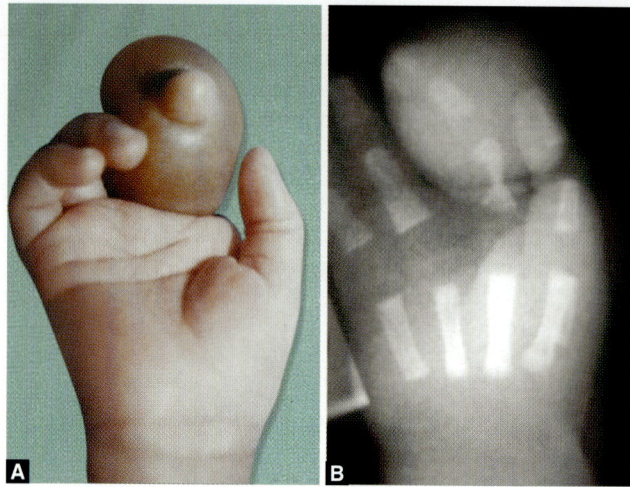

Figs. 107A and B: (A) Congenital ring syndrome; (B) X-ray image of the ring syndrome.

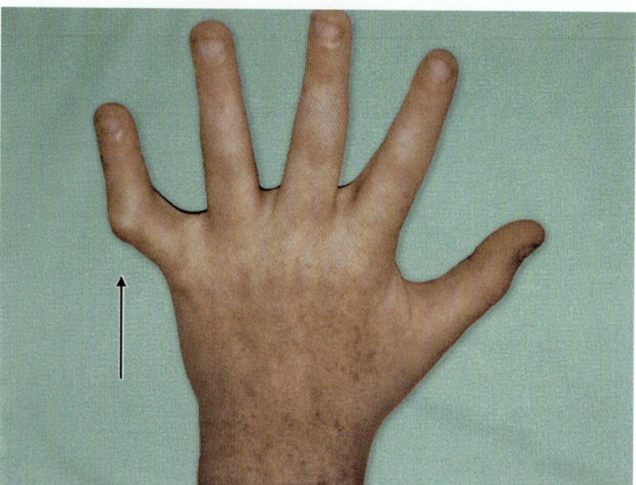

Fig. 109: Camptodactyly, with flexed proximal interphalangeal joint of little finger.

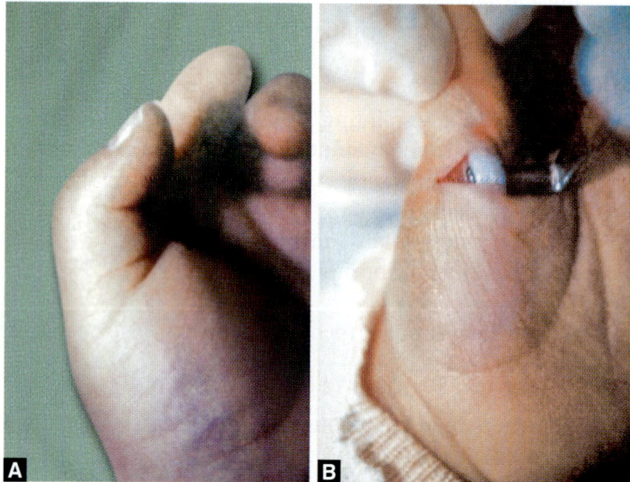

Figs. 108A and B: (A) Trigger thumb and (B) A1 pulley.

- *Type 3:* Fenestrated syndactyly or lateral fusion of adjacent digits at their distal ends, with proximal fenestrations between intervening skin and soft tissue
- *Type 4:* Intrauterine amputation (guillotine amputation).

Treatment

- Superficial bands do not require any treatment
- Deeper bands require staged excision of one-half of groove, with Z-plasty closure, followed by another surgery 2–3 months later.

Generalized Skeletal Abnormalities

- Congenital trigger digits
- Camptodactyly
- Kirner deformity
- Delta phalanx
- Madelung deformity.

Congenital Trigger Digits (Figs. 108A and B)

- When normal gliding movement of flexor tendon is impeded within digital flexor sheath
- In contrast to adult condition (stenosing tenovaginitis), it shows persistent flexion deformity rather than "triggering"
- Sheath is narrowed and thickened, with occasional ganglion cyst.

Treatment

- Conservative treatment is tried first
- Surgery not delayed for more than 3 years
- Surgery at first year of age, if multiple digits involved
- Surgical release of first annular pulley is done
- May also be done percutaneously.

Camptodactyly

- Flexion deformity of PIP joint that usually involves only little finger (Fig. 109)
- Should be distinguished from clinodactyly, in which finger is bent radially or ulnarly.

Classification

- *Type 1:* Occurs in infancy and affects both sexes equally. More common (80%)
- *Type 2:* Occurs during adolescence and affects girls. Less common (20%).

Causes

Exact cause although not known, it may be due to:

- Relative imbalance between flexors and extensors
- Relative shortening in flexor superficialis muscle tendon group
- Contractures of collateral ligaments or volar plate
- Insufficient palmar skin
- Congenital fibrous substrata in subcutaneous tissues.

Treatment

- For mild deformity, no treatment is advised
- In age less than 4 years:
  - In patients, where deformity disappears with wrist flexion, release of sublimis tendon may correct the deformity
- In age greater than 4 years:
  - Release of flexor digitorum sublimis muscle and transfer to extensor apparatus is done as given by Millesi and Lankford (Figs. 110A and B).

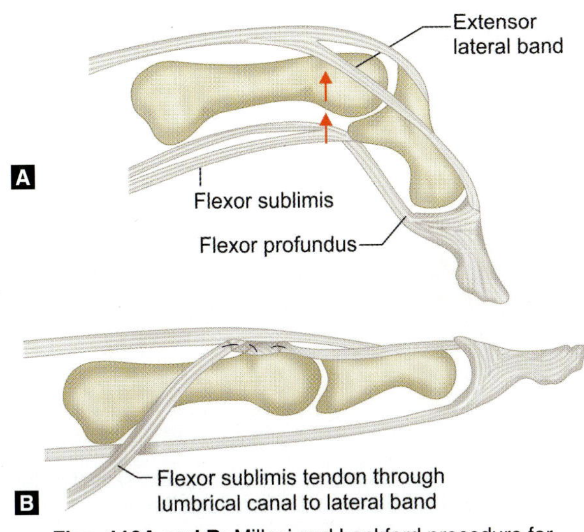

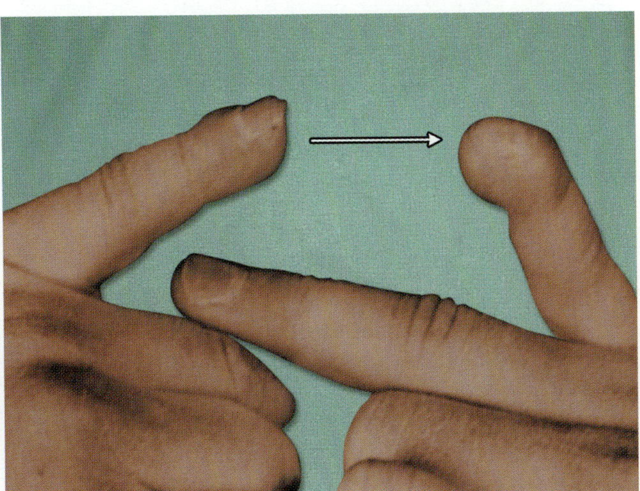

Figs. 110A and B: Millesi and Lankford procedure for correcting camptodactyly.

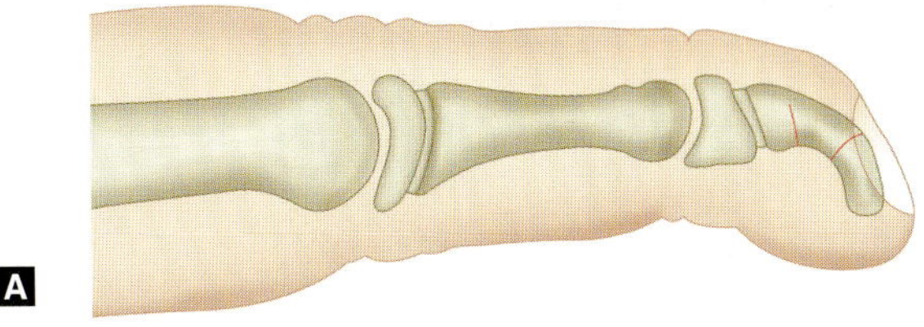

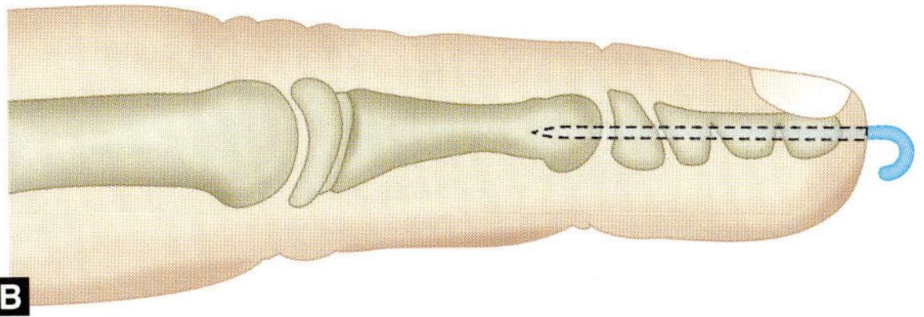

Figs. 112A and B: Correction of Kirner deformity by osteotomy.

Fig. 111: Kirner deformity.

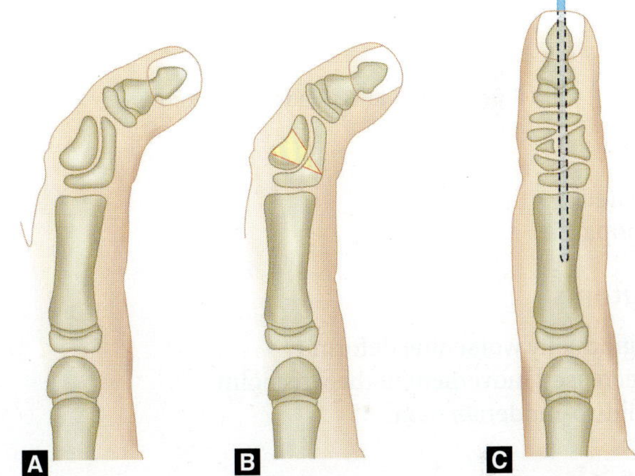

Figs. 113A to C: Reverse wedge osteotomy, for correcting delta phalanx.

Kirner Deformity (Kirner, 1927)

- Palmar and radial curving of distal phalanx of little finger (Fig. 111)
- Appears when child 8–10 years old and appears as a beaked little fingertip, with increased convexity of finger nail
- Fingertip curves radially and toward the palm
- Usually bilateral and symmetrical
- Usually not painful, though progressive
- *X-ray:* Broadened epiphysis, irregularities of metaphysis and typical curvature of distal phalanx.

Treatment

- Mild deformities warrant a conservative treatment
- Severe deformities in skeletally mature patients require one or more osteotomies of terminal phalanx (Carstam and Eiken) (Figs. 112A and B)
- No effective treatment for correction of nail deformity.

Delta Phalanx

- Abnormal, trapezoidal phalanx that appears triangular on radiographs
- It derives its name from a Greek letter "delta"
- Abnormal epiphysis is "J" or "C"-shaped and brackets on one side of phalanx
- Delta phalanx causes an angular deformity of digit in frontal plane
- Most common site is proximal phalanx of ring finger.

Treatment

Reverse wedge osteotomy (Carstam and Theander): This is shown in the Figures 113A to C.

MADELUNG DEFORMITY

Introduction

Abnormality of palmar ulnar part of distal radial physis, in which progressive ulnar and volar tilt develops at distal radial articular surface with dorsal subluxation of distal ulna. It was described by Malgaigne in 1855 and by Madelung in 1878 (Figs. 114A and B).

Vender and Watson Classification

- Post-traumatic
- Dysplastic

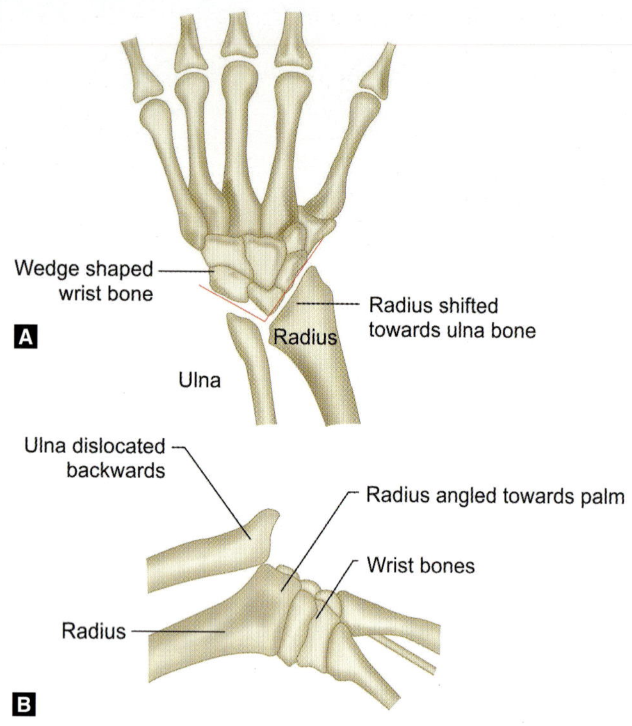

Figs. 114A and B: Madelung deformity.

- Genetic
- Idiopathic.

Symptoms

- A gradually worsening deformity
- Decreased movement in the wrist joint
- Mild-to-moderate pain.

Diagnosis

Confirmed by X-rays of the wrist joint. X-rays findings are:
- Curvature and angulation of the radius
- Shifting of the ulna towards the back of the wrist
- Small bones of the wrist joint are pressed together and appear wedge like.

Treatment

- Initially treated conservatively
- Surgery indicated due to severe pain from ulnocarpal impingement of carpus.

Choice of Surgery

- *Closing wedge osteotomy with Darrach excision of distal ulnar head, by Ranawat, DeFiore, and Straub (Fig. 115):* Dorsal-based and radial-based closing wedge osteotomy of radius is performed in conjunction with Darrach excision. Correct alignment is obtained and plate along with screws is used for fixation.
- *Dome osteotomy and excision of Vicker's ligament, by Carter and Ezaki (Figs. 116A to C):* Ligament of Vicker's is excised, biplanar dome osteotomy is made in metaphysic, and distal fragment is rotated at osteotomy site and secured with Steinmann pins.

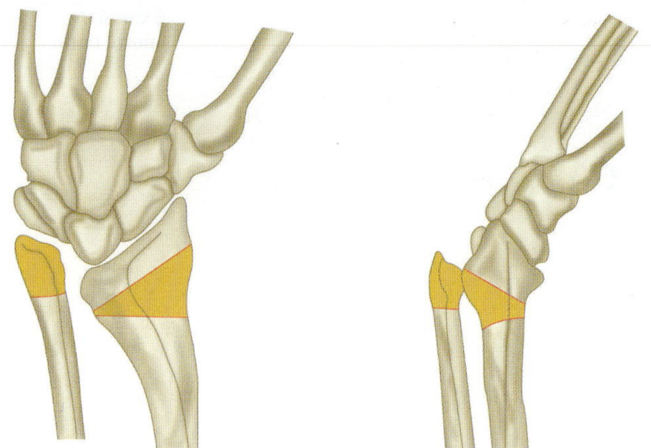
Fig. 115: Closing wedge osteotomy with Darrach excision of distal ulnar head, by Ranawat, DeFiore, and Straub.

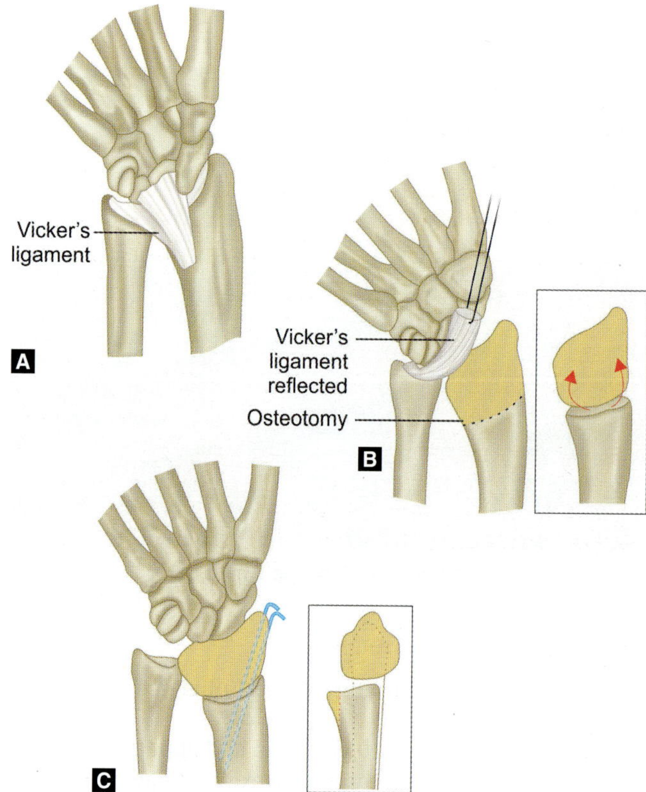

Figs. 116A to C: Dome osteotomy and excision of Vickers ligament, by Carter and Ezaki.

HAND INFECTIONS

Introduction

Hand infections occur commonly due to following reasons:
- It is frequently injured
- It is infrequently infected
- It has abundant blood supply.

Potential Problems

- *Confined spaces*
  - Joints
  - Tendon sheaths
  - Compartments and bursae.

- *Local factors*
  - Soft tissue damage
  - Amount or virulence of organism
  - Type or amount of foreign material.
- *Systemic factors*
  - Malnutrition
  - Alcoholism
  - Diabetes mellitus
  - Steroids
  - Immunosuppression.

Anatomy

The spaces of hand are of practical significance because they may become infected and in consequence become distended with pus. The important spaces are:

- The superficial pulp spaces of the finger
- The synovial tendon sheaths of the second, third, and fourth finger
- The ulnar bursa
- The radial bursa
- The midpalmar space
- The thenar space.

Superficial Pulp Space

- The pulp space of the fingers is a closed fascial compartment situated in front of the terminal phalanx of each finger.
- Each space is subdivided into numerous smaller compartments by fibrous septa (Fig. 117).
- Accumulation of inflammatory exudate within these compartments causes the pressure in the pulp space to rise quickly.
- In children, pressure on the blood vessels could result in necrosis of diaphysis.
- The close relationship of the proximal end of the pulp space to the digital synovial sheath accounts for the involvement of the sheath in the infectious process, when the pulp-space infection has been neglected.

Synovial Tendon Sheath

- The common synovial sheath for the flexor tendons is a synovial sheath in the carpal tunnel
- It contains tendons of the FDS and the *FDP*, but not the flexor pollicis longus
- The sheath, which surrounds the flexor digitorum, extends downward about halfway along the metacarpal bones, where it ends in blind diverticula around the tendons to the index, middle, and ring fingers. It is prolonged on the tendons to the little finger and usually communicates with the mucus sheath of these tendons
- Untreated infection of the synovial sheaths can impair hand function
- Infection of the synovial sheaths of the thumb or little finger may spread readily into the palm and even into the forearm (space of parona) (Fig. 118).

Ulnar and Radial Bursae

- The common and pollicial sheaths are frequently referred to in clinical writing as the ulnar and radial bursae, respectively
- These two sheaths project proximally, a short distance above the flexor retinaculum and they usually communicate with each other in the carpal tunnel
- Hence, infection of the synovial sheaths of the thumb or little finger may spread readily into the palm and even into the forearm.

Ulnar Bursa

- Common flexor synovial sheath (ulnar bursa)
- The long flexor tendons of the fingers (FDS and profundus) are enclosed in a common synovial sheath, while passing deep to the flexor retinaculum
- The sheath has a parietal layer, lining the walls of the carpal tunnel and a visceral layer closely applied to the tendons
- From the arrangement of the sheath, it appears that the synovial sac has been invaginated by the tendons from its lateral side
- In hands, the tendons of the FDS and profundus muscle invaginate a common synovial sheath from the lateral side
- Medial part, common sheath extends distally on the tendons of little finger
- Lateral part, it stops on the middle of palm
- Distal ends of index, middle, and ring finger acquire digital synovial sheaths.

Radial Bursa

- The synovial sheath of the tendon of FPL forms the radial bursa.
- This sheath is usually separate, but may communicate with the common sheath behind the retinaculum.
- Superiorly, it is coextensive with the common sheath and inferiorly, it extends up to the distal phalanx of the thumb.

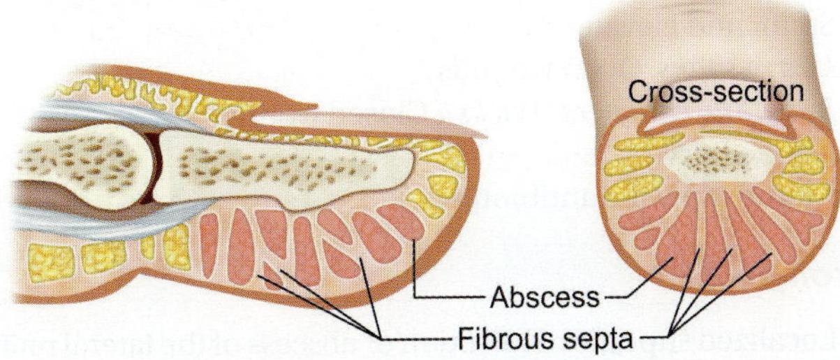

Fig. 117: Superficial pulp space and subdivided smaller compartments divided by fibrous septa.

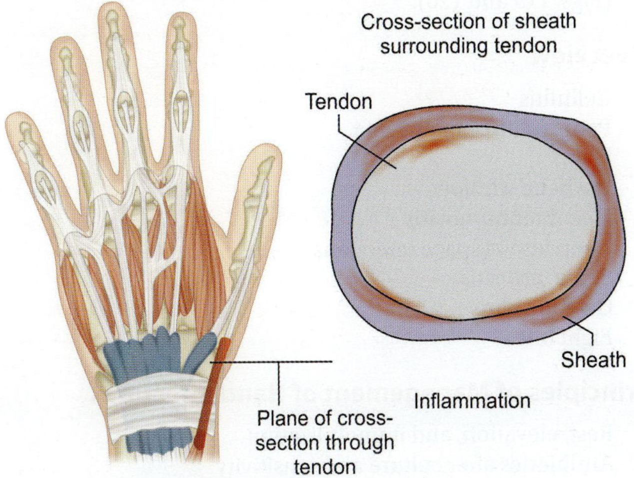

Fig. 118: Routes through which infection of synovial sheath of thumb will spread.

- Flexor pollicis longus tendon has its own synovial sheath that passes into the thumb, which allows the long tendons to move smoothly.
- Synovial sheath of the FPL (radial bursa) communicates with the ulnar bursa, at the level of wrist in about 50% of subjects.

Midpalmar Space (Mid-Central Palmar Space)

- Contains three to five flexor tendons, two to four lumbricals, superficial palmar arch, and three to five digital vessels and nerves.
- Communicates through the subcutaneous tissues at webs and extends dorsally to common flexor sheaths.
- *Location:* The midpalmar space lies posterior to the long flexor tendons to the middle, ring, and little fingers. It lies in front of the interossei and the third, fourth, and fifth metacarpal bone.
- *Boundaries:*
  - *Anterior:* Flexor tendons of medial three fingers are surrounded by synovial sheaths (ulnar bursa)
  - *Posterior:* Third, fourth, and fifth metacarpal bones with its interossei muscles
  - *Medially:* Hypothenar muscles
  - *Laterally:* Septum separating it from thenar space
  - *Distally:* Communicate with web spaces
  - *Proximally:* Communicate with parona space.

Thenar Space (Lateral Central Palmar Space)

- It contains, tendons of flexor pollicis longus, FDS and profundus to index finger, palmar digital nerves, and vessels to thumb and radial side of index finger.
- Communicates through web of thumb and under flexor retinaculum.
- *Location:* The thenar space lies posterior to the long flexor tendons of the index finger and in front of the adductor pollicis muscle.
- *Boundaries*
  - *Radial:* Thenar eminence, radial bursa
  - *Ulnar:* Middle metacarpal, ulnar bursa
  - *Superficial:* Carpal tunnel
  - *Deep:* Adductor pollicis.
- The thenar space lies just superficial to the adductor pollicis muscle, forming a plane connecting the deep aspects of the radial bursa and the ulnar bursa. Abscess or space occupying lesions may spread transversely through the thenar space, deep in the palm between the thumb and the carpal tunnel (Figs. 119 and 120).

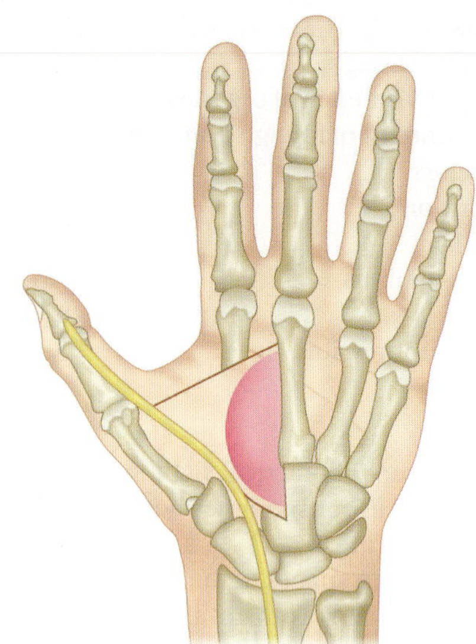

Fig. 119: The thenar space lying just superficial to the adductor pollicis muscle, forming a plane connecting the deep aspects of the radial bursa and the ulnar bursa.

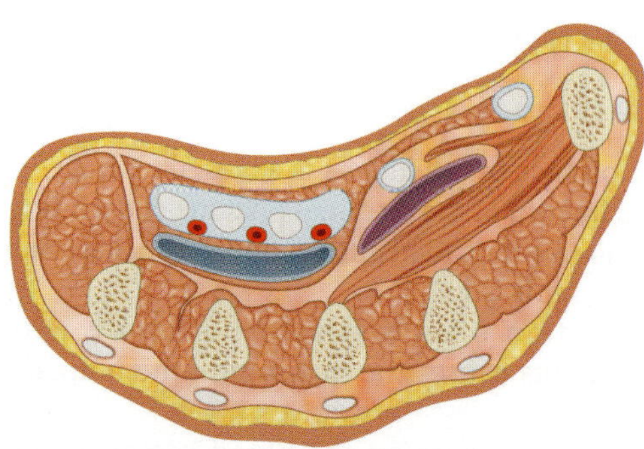

Fig. 120: The thenar space is shown in purple in the figure. In the cross section, the midpalmar space is blue, the radial bursa is light blue, and the ulnar bursa is red.

Overview

- Cellulitis
- Paronychia or eponychia
- Felon
- Herpetic whitlow
- Flexor tenosynovitis
- Deep fascial space infections
- Septic arthritis
- Osteomyelitis
- Fight bites.

Principles of Management of Hand Infections

- Rest, elevation, and immobilization
- Antibiotics after culture and sensitivity
- Incision and drainage
- Tetanus prophylaxis.

Cellulitis of the Hand

- Involves only the skin, erythema, edema, and pain of localized area (Fig. 121).
- One must rule out that deeper structures are not involved. Beware of the dorsal hand cellulitis:
  - Full painless ROM of digits, hand, and wrist
  - No tenderness on palpation of deeper structures.

Causative Organisms

- *Streptococcus pyogenes*
- Occasionally, *Staphylococcus aureus.*

Treatment

- Splint and elevate
- *Warm soaks:* Open wounds
- *Irrigating catheters (Wicks):* Closed wounds
- Gentle ROM
- Culture-specific antibiotics.

Paronychia

- Localized superficial infection or abscess of the lateral nail fold
- Most common infection in the hand
- Caused by frequent trauma to area

- Swelling and tenderness of the soft tissue next to the nail fold (Fig. 122)
- May have associated cellulitis
- If extends to overlying proximal nail, it is called eponychia.

Causative Organisms

- *Staphylococcus aureus*: Thumb sucking and nail biting, and is an anaerobes
- Chronic infection by *Candida*.

Treatment

- *Early cellulitis:* Warm soaks, elevation, and antibiotics
- *Late or fluctuant cellulites:* Treatment includes:
  - Marsupialization
  - Partial nail removal (Figs. 123A and B).
- Mostly resolve in 5–10 days.

Complication

Osteomyelitis of distal phalanx.

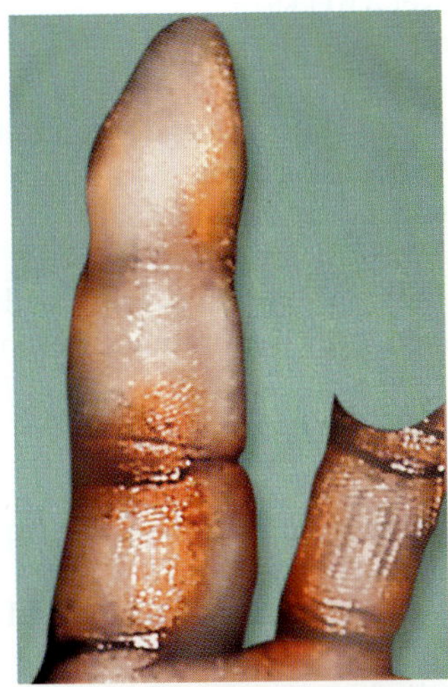

Fig. 121: Cellulitis of hand.

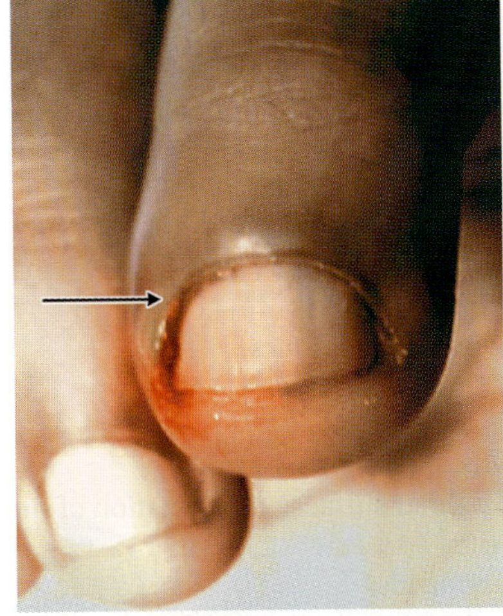

Fig. 122: Swelling and tenderness of the soft tissue next to the nail fold in paronychia.

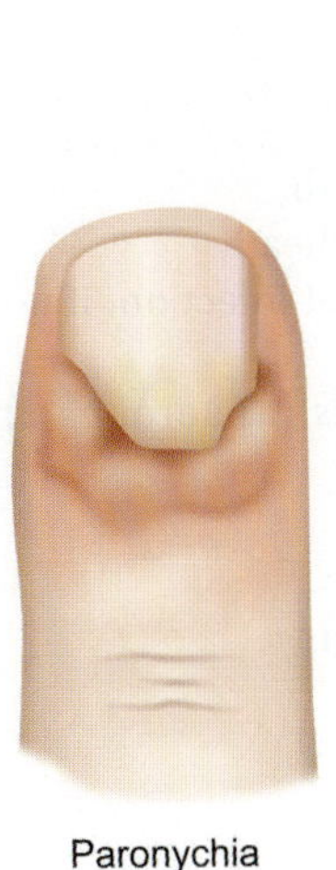

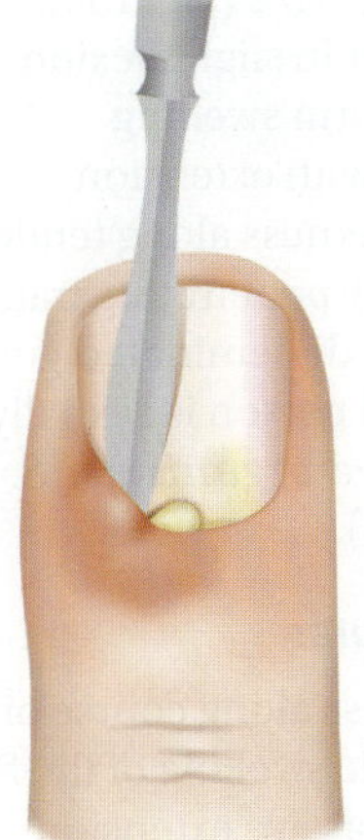

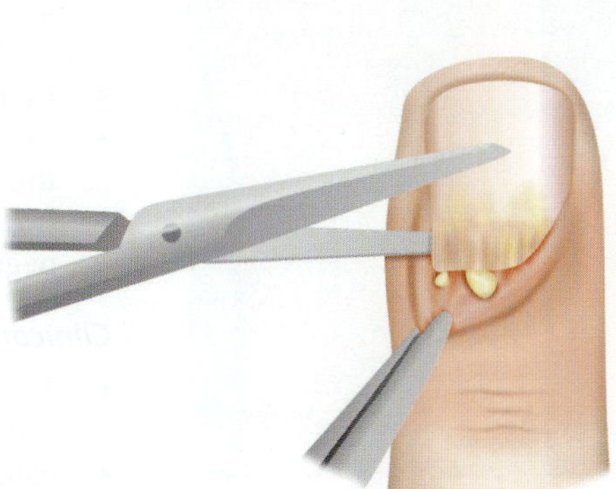

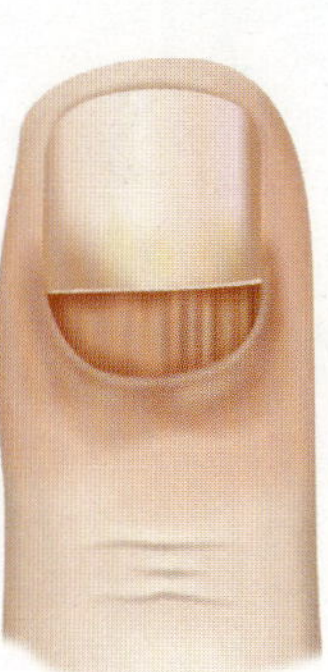

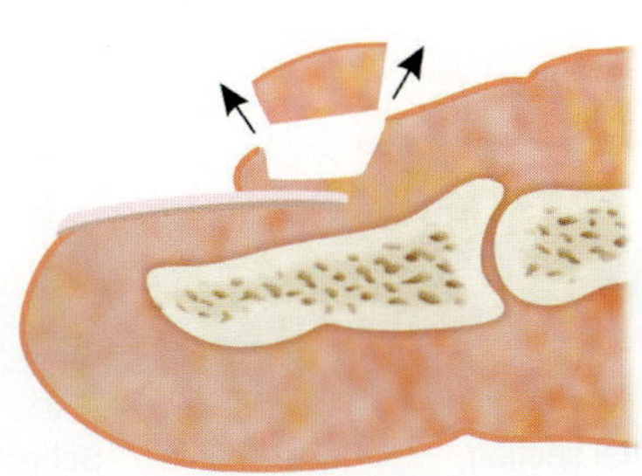

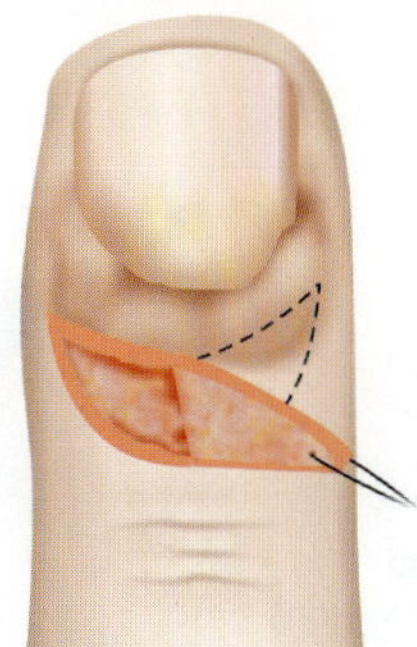

Figs. 123A and B: Partial nail removal procedure.

Felon

Infection of the pulp of the distal finger or thumb (Fig. 124).

- *Septa:*
  - Facilitate infection
  - Inhibit drainage, but acts as a barrier protecting the joint space and tendon sheath and limits proximal spread
- Caused by penetrating trauma and secondary infection
- Causative organism: *S. aureus*
- Area of cellulitis and inflammation rapidly progresses to severe throbbing, pain, redness, swelling, and tense feeling of distal finger.

Treatment

- Early and complete incision through septa (Fig. 125)
- Most drained by single lateral incision with blunt dissection, also volar approach (Fig. 126)
- Send cultures
- Irrigate, dress, elevate, etc.
- Reevaluate in 24–48 hours
- Culture specific IV antibiotics.

Complications

- Osteomyelitis
- Necrosis of palmar surface and formation of sinus tract
- Septic arthritis
- Flexor tenosynovitis.

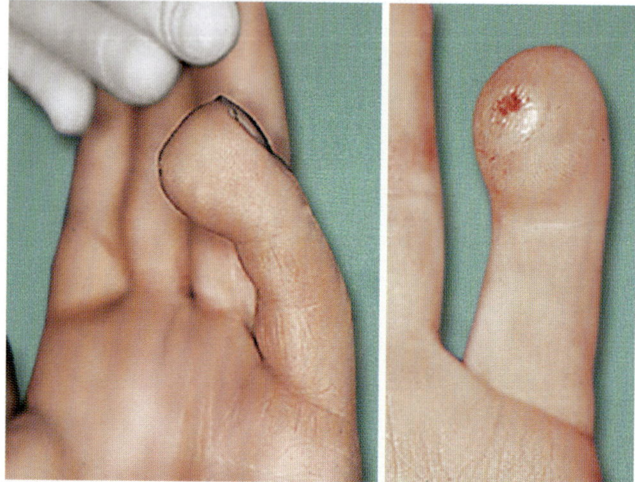

Fig. 124: Felon, with infection of the pulp of the distal finger or thumb.

Herpetic Whitlow

- Herpes simplex virus (HSV) infection of distal finger
- Most common viral infection of the hand
- Caused by direct inoculation through broken skin:
  - Kids with herpetic gingivostomatitis
  - Adults more likely HSV 2
  - Healthcare workers.
- Single finger involved
- Pain, pruritis, and swelling
- Vesicles (Fig. 127)
- Coalescence over 2 weeks
- Ulcer formation
- Hemorrhagic base
- May look like a felon, but drainage is contraindicated
- Careful history should be taken
- Tender distal finger, but soft pulp space
- Resolves spontaneously in 3–4 weeks
- Prevent oral inoculation by covering with a dry dressing. Acyclovir is given, only if immunocompromised or frequent infections.

Flexor Tenosynovitis

- This is a surgical emergency and should act quickly to preserve function of digit and hand
- Usually involves flexor tendon sheaths and radial and ulnar bursae (Fig. 128)
- Infection spreads along course of flexor tendon sheaths, which may spread to midpalmar, thenar, and lumbrical compartments (Fig. 129)
- *Kanavel's signs* (Fig. 130):
  - Finger in slight flexion
  - Fusiform swelling
  - Pain with extension
  - Tenderness along tendon sheath.
- Caused by penetrating trauma to sheath
- Consider disseminated gonococcal infection, if no trauma is there and person is sexually active
- *Causative organisms: S. aureus* (anaerobes and Gram-negatives).

Clinical Features

- Tenderness along course of tendon
- Symmetric swelling of the finger
- Pain on passive extension
- Flexed posture of finger.

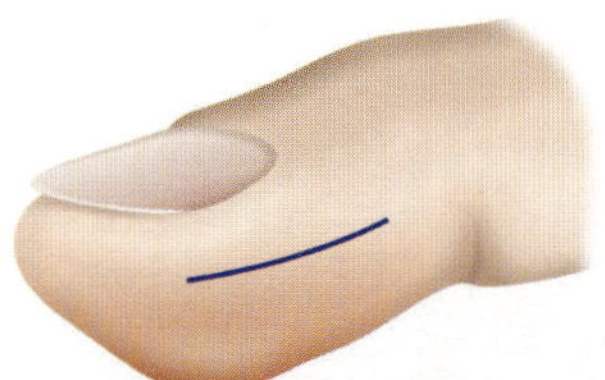

Felon
(Showing incision)

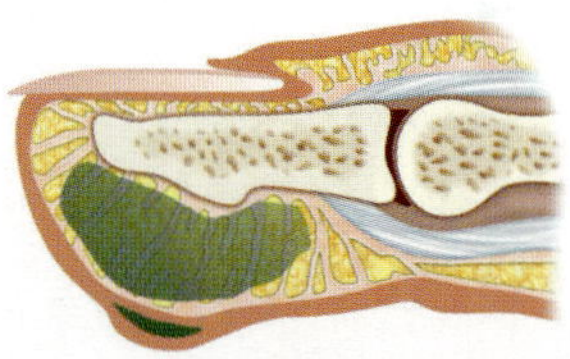

Sagittal section
showing pus (green)
between septa

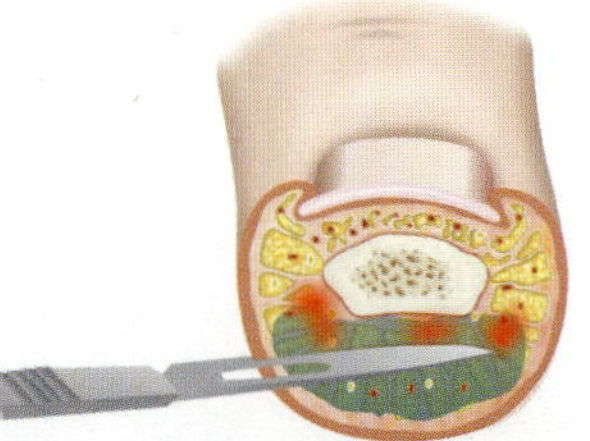

Schematic cross-section
showing how incision
divides septa

Fig. 125: Felon: Pus drained by incision made on the septa.

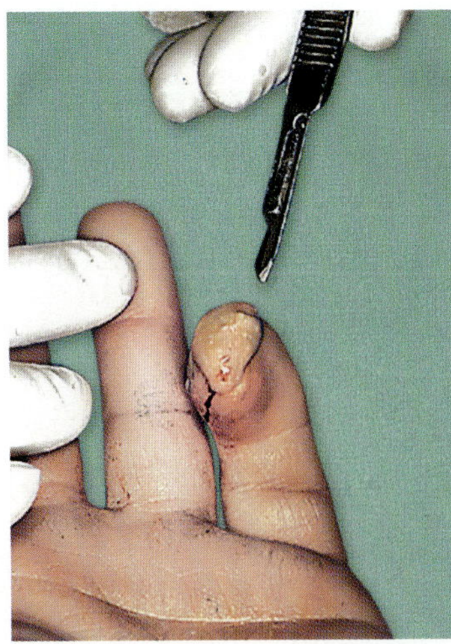

Fig. 126: Pus drainage by single lateral incision with blunt dissection (volar approach).

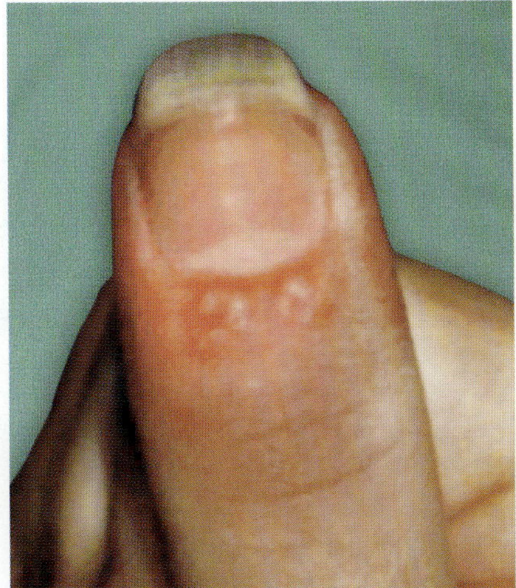

Fig. 127: Vesicles in herpetic whitlow.

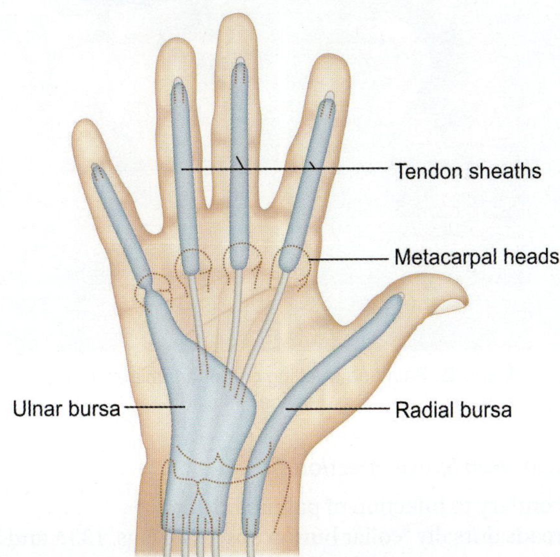

Fig. 128: Flexor tendon sheaths and radial or ulnar bursae, involved most commonly in tenosynovitis. (L: little finger; R: ring finger; M: middle finger; I: index finger; Th: thumb).

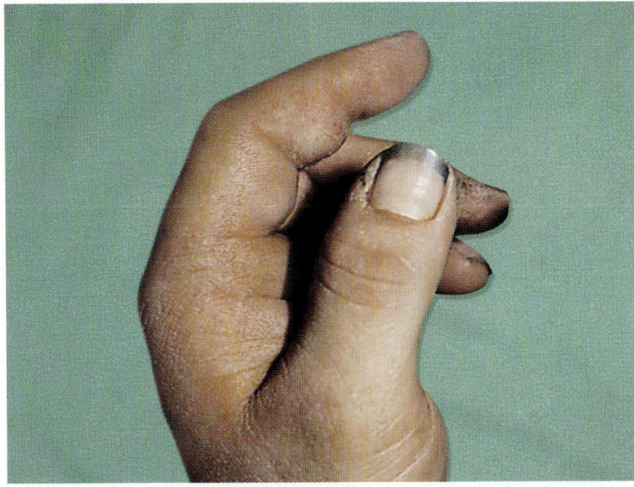

Fig. 129: Infection spread from flexor tendon sheaths to midpalmar, thenar, and lumbrical compartments.

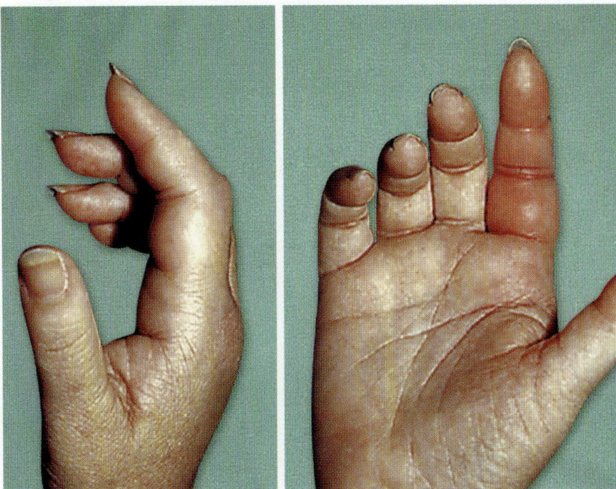

Fig. 130: Kanavel's signs.

Treatment

- Splint and elevate
- Incision and drainage (Fig. 131)
- Irrigation
- Intravenous antibiotics.

Deep Fascial Space Infection

- Palm is relatively fixed, the infection is seen on the dorsal side of the hand
- Four potential spaces, shown in Figures 132A to C
  - Dorsal subaponeurotic space
  - Subfascial web space
  - Thenar space
  - Midpalmar space.

Route of Infection

- Direct penetrating trauma
- Contiguous spread
- Hematogenous spread.

Causative Organisms

- *Staphylococcus aureus, Streptococcus*
- Occasionally coliforms and anaerobes.

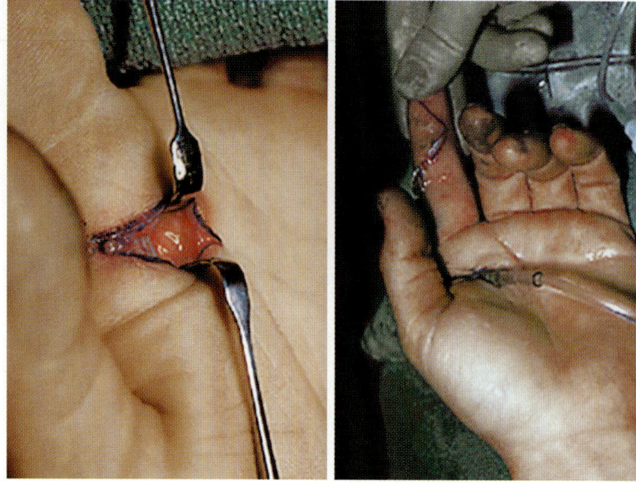

Fig. 131: Incision and drainage of pus in infected tenosynovitis.

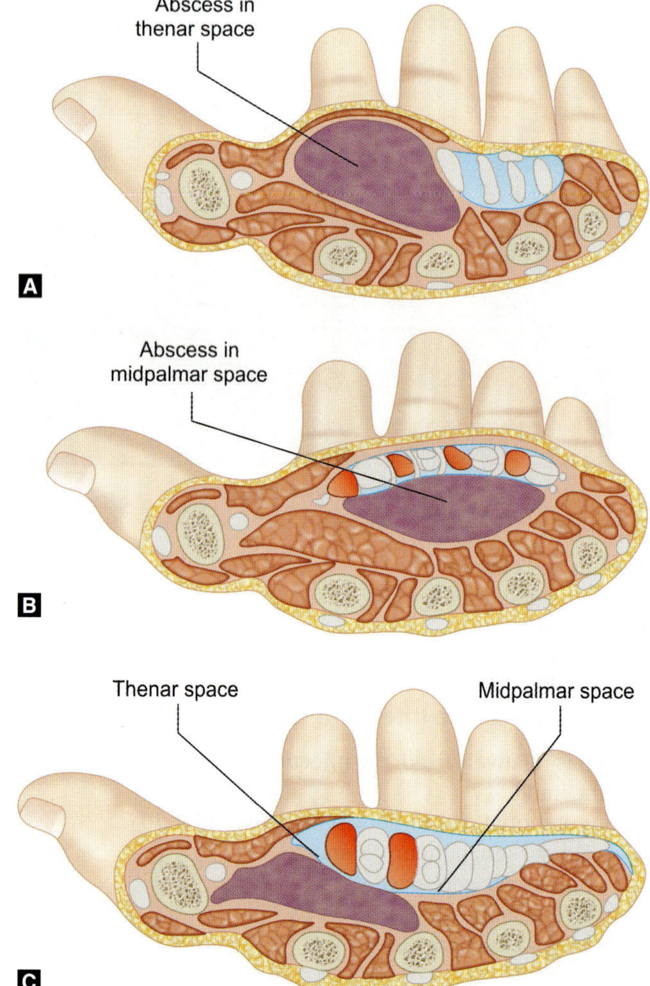

Figs. 132A to C: Four potential deep fascial spaces.

Dorsal Subaponeurotic Abscess

- Swelling and erythema on dorsum of hand
- Pain with passive movement of extensor tendons
- Looks like cellulitis.

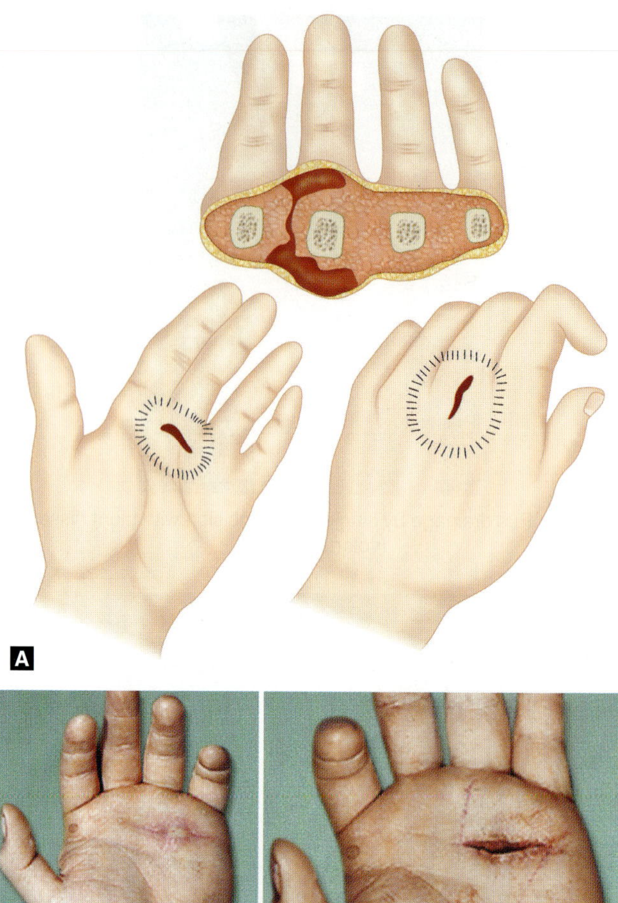

Figs. 133A and B: Collar button abscess.

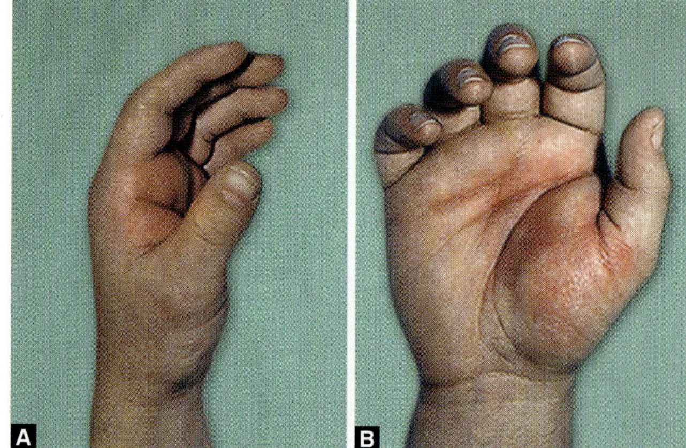

Figs. 134A and B: Pain and swelling of thenar eminence and first web space.

Subfascial Web Space Infection

- Secondary to infection of palmar blisters
- Spreads dorsally "collar button abscess" (Figs. 133A and B).

Thenar Space Infection

- Pain and swelling of thenar eminence and first web space (Figs. 134A and B)

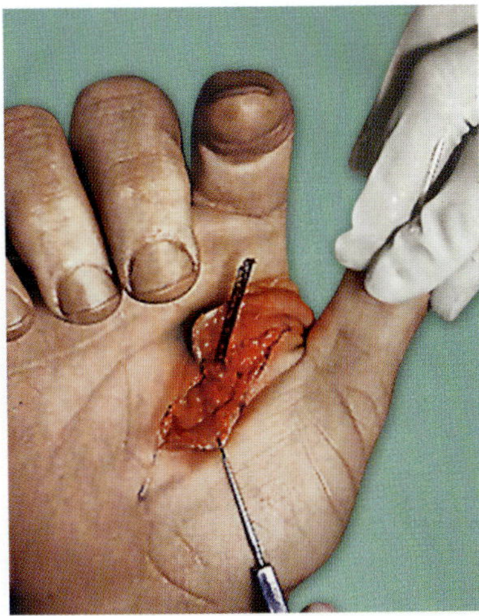

Fig. 135: Incision and drainage.

- Can be from tenosynovitis of second digit with rupture proximally
- Thumb is held, abducted, and flexed.

Midpalmar Infection

- Loss of normal hand concavity
- Tenderness of central palm
- Pain with movement of third and fourth digits
- Can be from tenosynovitis of third, fourth, and fifth digits.

Treatment

- Incision and drainage (Fig. 135)
- Culture sensitivity
- Intravenous antibiotics
- Resting splint.

Septic Arthritis

- Any joint may be involved
- Can spread from direct inoculation, from penetrating trauma or contiguous spread
- *Causative organism*: *S. aureus* (rarely others).

Clinical Features

- Joint is red, swollen, tender, and localized (unlike flexor tenosynovitis)
- May have overlying puncture wound
- Held in position to maximize joint volume
- Very painful passive flexion and axial load
- Diagnosed by arthrocentesis.

Treatment

- Intravenous antibiotics
- Open drainage.

Osteomyelitis

- Most common with open fractures or soft tissue infections
- Fever, redness, swelling, warmth, tenderness, and pseudoparalysis (in kids)
- *Plain film:* Bony destruction or periosteal elevation.

Treatment

- Debridement
- Intravenous antibiotics (long-term).

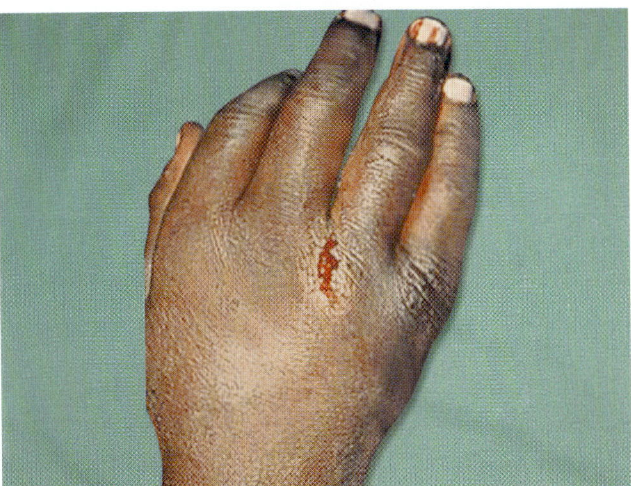

Fig. 136: Puncture wound, with surrounding area of cellulitis.

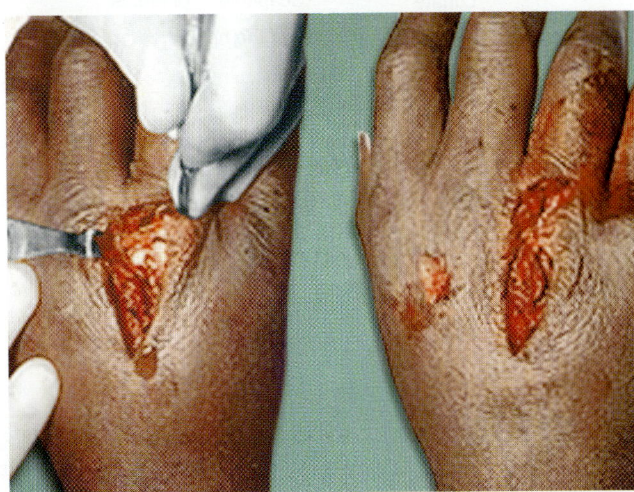

Fig. 137: Clean and irrigate the wound thoroughly.

Fight Bites

During fights, when a person bites the other person's hand, the oral flora of the incisors gets deposited in the deep layers, thus facilitating rapid spread of infection.

Physical Examination

- Puncture wound with area of cellulitis surrounding it (Fig. 136)
- Tendon may be visible inside the wound
- Plain film is indicated, often associated with fractures.

Treatment

- Clean and irrigate the wound thoroughly (Fig. 137)
- Leave it open
- Intravenous antibiotics
- Immobilize the hand
- Elevate the hand.

Summary

- Most common organisms are Gram-positive
- Sleepless night indicates pus under pressure
- Pus should be drained
- The shortest distance to the pus is the best (felon, tendon sheath, and deep space abscess)

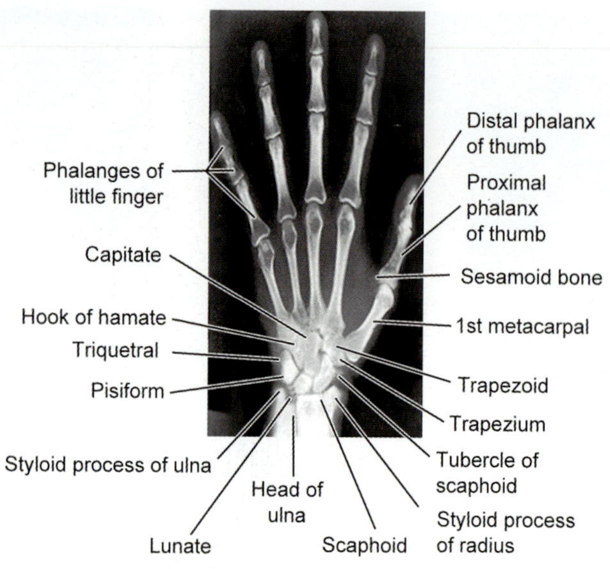

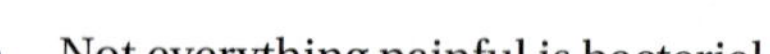

Fig. 138: Anatomy of the hand.

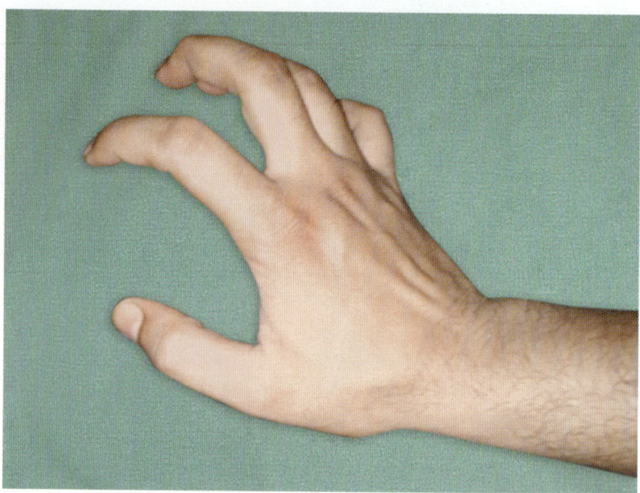

Fig. 139: Extensor tendons pass under the extensor retinaculum and separate it into six compartments.

- Not everything painful is bacterial
- Things that grow slowly and painlessly are either very bad (metastasis) or are associated with tuberculosis
- Even simple infections can be lethal
- Inexpensive antibiotics are usually adequate.

INJURIES OF THE HAND

Anatomy

Bones

Hand consists of 27 bones. Wrist bones are shown in Figure 138.

- Phalangeal bones (14)
- Metacarpal bones (5)
- Carpal bones (8)
  - Carpal bones are made up of two rows of four bones bridged by flexor retinaculum which forms the carpal tunnel
  - Carpal tunnel consists of the median nerve and the nine long flexor of the fingers.

Intrinsic muscles:

- Intrinsic muscles have their origins and insertions within the hand. Consist of the following muscles:
  - Thenar
  - Hypothenar
  - Adductor pollicis
  - Interossei
  - Lumbricals.

Extensor Tendons

- Courses over the dorsal side of the forearm, wrist, and hand.
- Nine extensor tendons pass under the extensor retinaculum and separate it into six compartments (Fig. 139).
- The tendons that are palpated, with thumb abducted and extended, form an anatomical snuffbox.
- Extensor digitorum communis (EDC) is connected by junctura and because of this, a complete tendon laceration proximal to the junction may still result in normal extensor function.

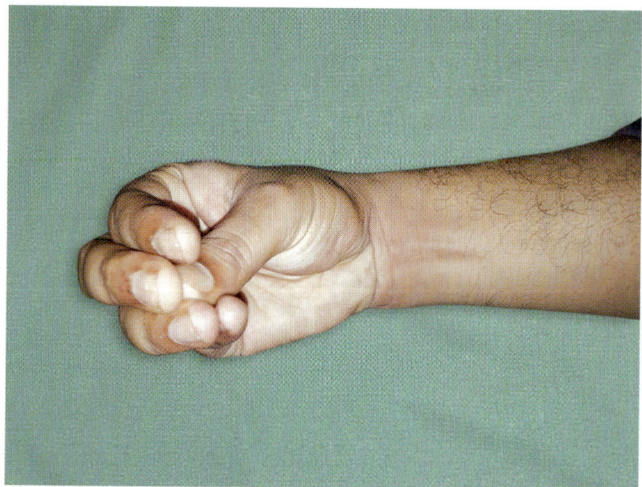

Fig. 140: Flexor carpi radialis, flexor carpi ulnaris, and palmaris longus tendons are visible and are prime flexors of the wrist.

Flexor Tendons

- Courses over the volar side of the forearm, wrist, and hand.
- Unlike the extensor tendons, the flexor tendons are enclosed in synovial sheaths, making them prone to deep space infections.
- Flexor carpi radialis, flexor carpi ulnaris, and palmaris longus primarily flex the wrist (Fig. 140).
- Nine flexor tendons pass through the carpel tunnel:
  - One tendon (FPS) goes to the base of the distal phalanx of the thumb
  - The other four digits have two tendons each (FDS and FDP).

Flexor digitorum superficialis:

- *Origin (two muscle bellies):* Medial epicondyle and radial shaft
- Insert into the middle phalanx of the four fingers (Fig. 141).

Flexor digitorum profundus:

- *Origin:* Ulna and interosseous membrane
- Inserts at the base of the distal phalanx (Fig. 141).

Tendon Sheaths

Anatomy of the synovial sheaths of the fingers and the radial and ulnar bursae is depicted in Figure 142.

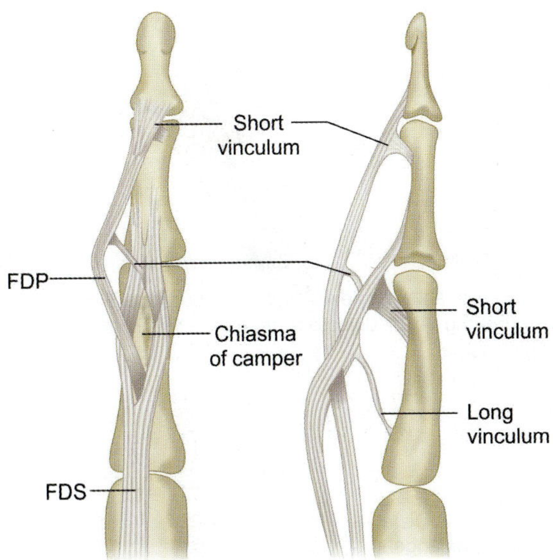

Fig. 141: Insertion of flexor digitorum superficialis (FDS) into the middle phalanx of the four fingers and insertion of flexor digitorum profundus (FDP) at the base of the distal phalanx.

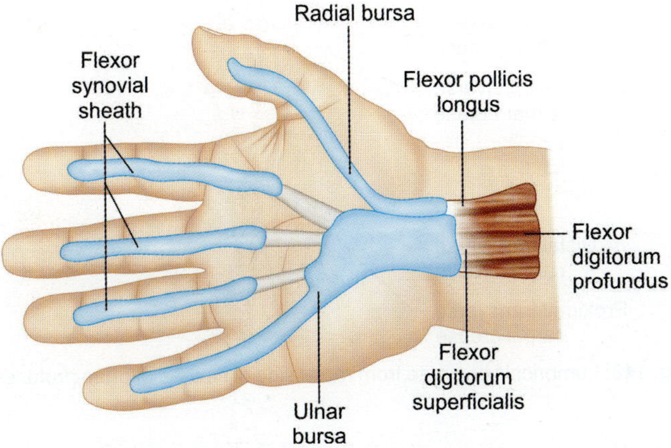

Fig. 142: Anatomy of the synovial sheaths of the fingers and the radial and ulnar bursae.

Zones (by Milford)

- The anatomy of the finger flexor tendons encompasses five zones, each of which is separated from the others by anatomic landmarks (Figs. 143 to 145)
- All the zones must be treated differently in cases of tendon laceration.

Zone I:

- It is the area distal to the insertion of the superficialis tendon
- Although the profundus tendon is still enclosed tightly within a fibro-osseous sheath here, it runs alone
- Therefore, the prognosis for the repair of lacerations in this zone is better than that for zone 2, although not as good as that for zones III, IV, and V.

Zone II:

- Stretches from the distal palmar crease to the middle of the middle phalanx
- In this area, the two tendons for each finger run together in a common fibro-osseous sheath

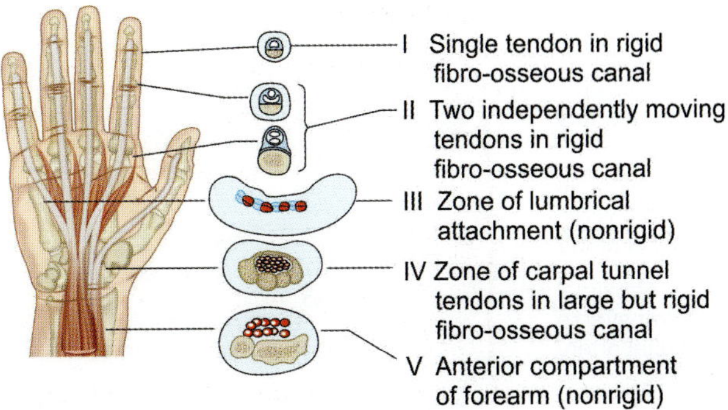

Fig. 143: Anatomy of the finger flexor tendons encompasses five zones.

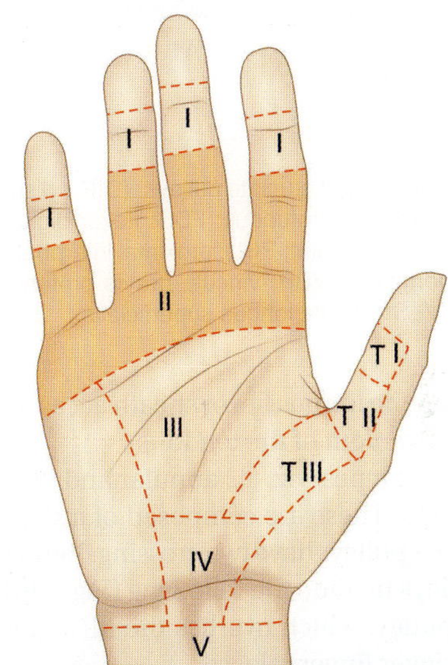

Fig. 144: Five zones of finger flexor tendons.

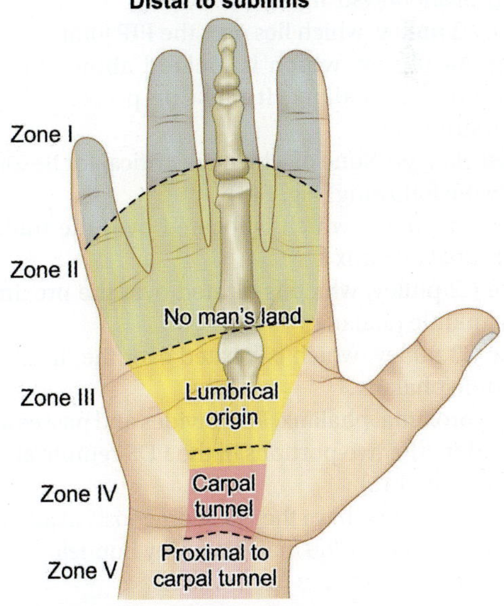

Fig. 145: Zones of the finger flexor tendons. (Zone I: distal to superficialis tendon; Zone II: distal palmar crease to proximal interphalangeal crease; Zone III: palm; Zone IV: within the carpal tunnel; Zone V: forearm proximal to the carpal tunnel)

- The sheaths run from the level of the metacarpal heads (the distal palmar crease) to the DP. They are attached to the underlying bone and prevent the tendons from bowstringing

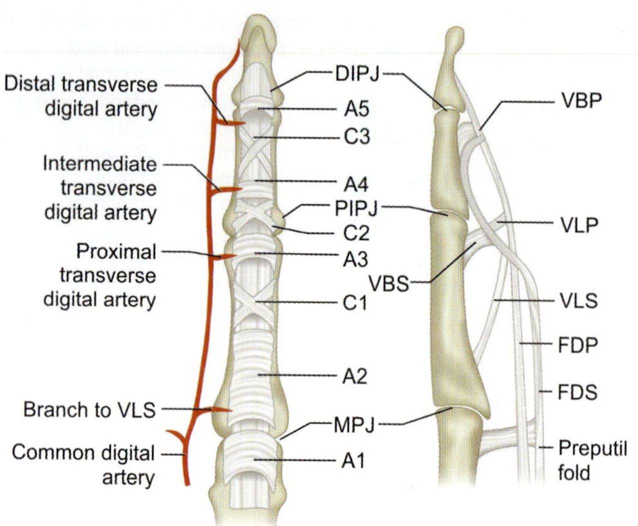

Fig. 146: Annular pulleys and cruciate pulleys. (DIPJ: distal interphalangeal joint; FDP: flexor digitorum profundus; FDS: flexor digitorum superficialis; MPJ: metacarpophalangeal joint; PIPJ: proximal interphalangeal joint; VBS: vincula brevis superficialis; VBP: vincula brevis profundus; VLP: vincula longus profundus; VLS: vincula longus superficialis)

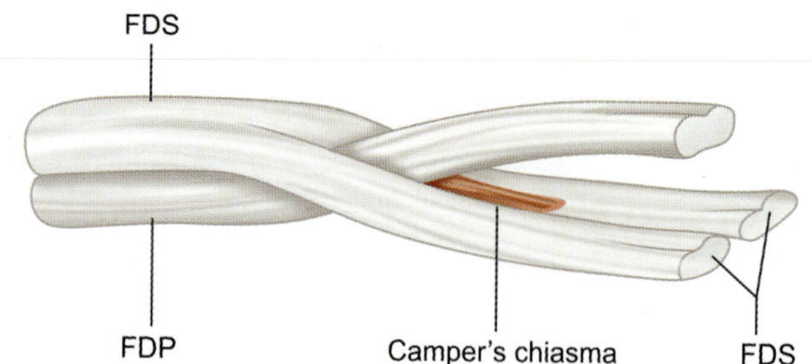

Fig. 147: Diagram showing flexor digitorum superficialis (FDS) divides and passes around the flexor digitorum profundus (FDP) tendon to reunite at "Camper's chiasma".

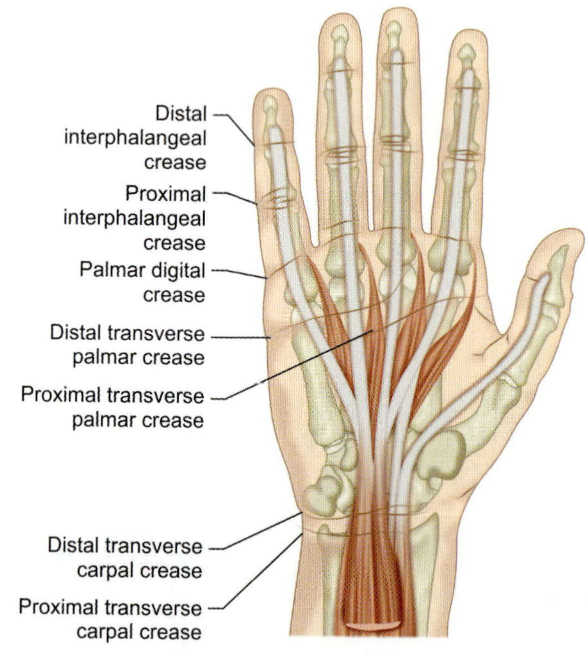

Fig. 148: Lumbricals originate from radial side of flexor digitorum profundus.

- Thickenings in the fibrous flexor sheath act as pulleys, directing the sliding movement of the tendons
- There are of two types, viz. (1) annular and (2) cruciate
- *Annular pulleys*: These are composed of a single fibrous band (ring). Cruciate pulleys have two crossing fibrous strands (cross)
- Annular pulleys include the following (Fig. 146):
  - The A1 pulley, which overlies the MCP joint. It is incised during trigger finger release
  - The A2 pulley, which overlies the proximal end of the proximal phalanx. It must be preserved (if at all possible) to prevent bowstringing
  - The A3 pulley, which lies over the PIP joint
  - The A4 pulley, which is located about the middle of the middle phalanx. It must be preserved to prevent bowstringing.
- *Cruciate pulleys:* None of which are critical for flexor function, include the following (Fig. 146):
  - The C1 pulley, which is located over the middle of the proximal phalanx
  - The C2 pulley, which is located over the proximal end of the middle phalanx
  - The C3 pulley, which is located over the distal end of the middle phalanx.
- Over the proximal phalanx, FDS divides and passes around the FDP tendon, the two portions of the FDS reunite at "Camper's chiasma" (Fig. 147)
- Repairs in this zone have the worst prognosis of all the zones. It has been nicknamed "no man's land" by Bunnell.

Zone III:
- It is the zone of the lumbrical origin
- Lumbricals originate from radial side of FDP (Fig. 148).
- The tendons of the lumbricals pass along the radial sides of the MCP joints, before they insert into the dorsal expansion.
- They pass volar to the axes of the MCP joints. Thus, they act as flexors of those joints, even as they extend the interphalangeal joints.

Zone IV:
- Encompasses the tendons, as they run through the carpal tunnel.
- All the tendons remain in a common synovial sheath throughout the carpal tunnel.

Zone V:
It is in the anterior compartment of the forearm, proximal to the flexor retinaculum and the carpal tunnel.

Blood Supply

- Segmental branches of digital arteries, which enter the tendon through:
  - *Vincula:* Vincula longa and brevia are the main blood supplies to the flexor tendons (Fig. 149)
  - Osseous insertions.
- Synovial fluid diffusion.

Hand Injuries

Etiology

- Needle puncture
- Blade, knife cut, broken glass, or edge of metal
- Burn, road traffic accidents, and explosion
- Boxing and allied sports

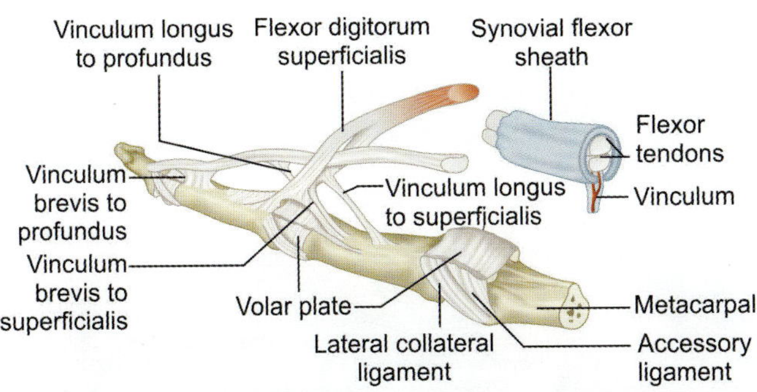

Fig. 149: Vincula longa and brevia are the main blood supplies to the flexor tendons.

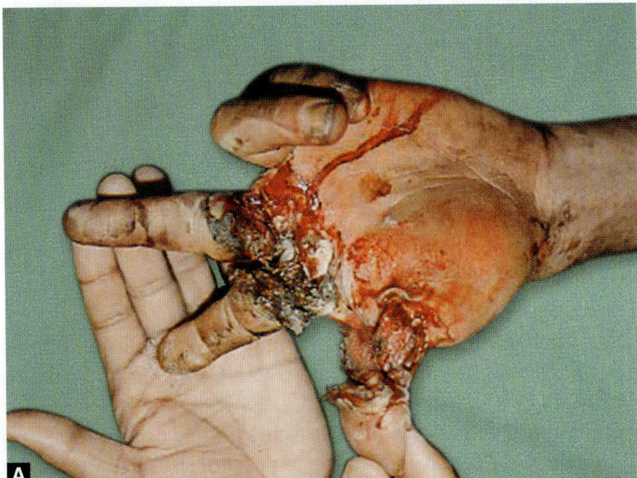

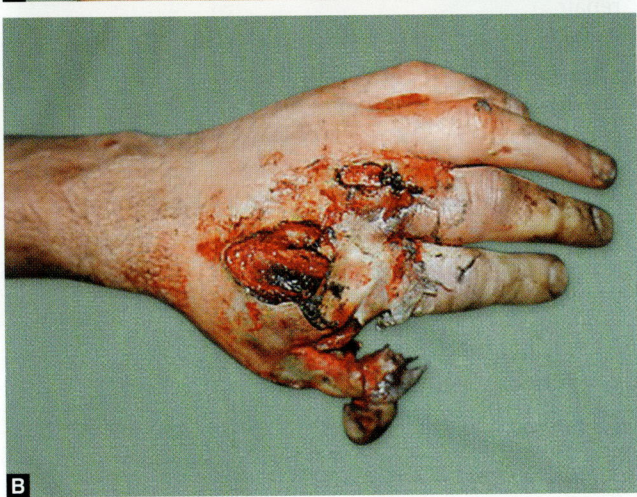

Figs. 150A and B: Untidy wound.

- Machine parts, e.g. fan belt, grinding mechanism, guillotine, hot press machine, like those used in sealing wrappers and those used in plastic manufacturing industries.

Classification

- Tidy wound
- Untidy wound (Figs. 150A and B)
- Injury may involve nerves, tendons, intrinsic hand muscles as well as bones and joints.

Principles of Evaluation

- The position of the hand at the time of injury should be determined.
- Injuries with the digits in flexion may result in retraction of the cut end of the tendon, when the digit is examined in neutral position.

Clinical Examination

One should detail the extent of injury by documenting the following:

- Amount of devascularization
- Status of the skin
- Posture of the fingers
- Presence of deformity
- Active bleeding
- Bilateral grip strength
- The ROM and strength should be tested against resistance.

Radiography

- X-rays should include posteroanterior (PA), lateral, and oblique views
- Rule out dislocations and fractures.

Nerve Testing—Motor

Test for median nerve:

- Have the patient flex the distal phalanx of the thumb against resistance. Test opposition by touching the tip of the thumb to the tip of the little finger. The patient will be unable to oppose against resistance, if median nerve function is lost
- Test thumb abduction by placing the hand palm up and raising the thumb to the perpendicular while palpating the belly of the abductor pollicis muscle to insure, it is contracting.

Test for ulnar nerve:

- Spread the fingers apart against resistance and then push them together against resistance
- Test the hypothenar muscle, extend the fingers and then move the fifth finger away from the others
- Test thumb adduction (ulnar nerve innervates the adductor pollicis muscles), bring the thumb tightly against the side of the index finger. Adductor strength can be further tested by interposing a piece of paper between the thumb and the side of the index finger and then trying to pull the paper away.

Test for radial nerve:

- Extend the fingers and wrist
- With the thumb in the hitchhiking position, test its resistance to further extension.

Nerve Testing—Sensory

- Determined by two-point discrimination
- Normal two-point discrimination is less than 6 mm at the fingertips and is often less than 2 mm. Both injured and noninjured fingers must be compared
- Repeat two-point discrimination testing two to four times on each side of the digit (80% accuracy is considered acceptable)
- A sensory deficit implies a potential digital artery laceration because of the close proximity of the two.

Nerve Injury Management (Table 3)

Tendon testing:

- Full ROM of each tendon against resistance should be assessed and compared with the uninjured side.
- Important to test resistance because up to 90% of a tendon can be lacerated with preservation of ROM without resistance.

TABLE 3: Seddon's classification of nerve injuries, their treatment and prognosis.

Seddon's classification of nerve injury	*Disruption*	*Treatment*	*Prognosis*
I Neuropraxia	Minimal axonal	Conservative	Complete in days or months
II Axonotmesis	Total axonal	Conservative	Complete in months
III Neurotmesis	Axon and endoneurium perineurium	Repair	Moderate reduction of function

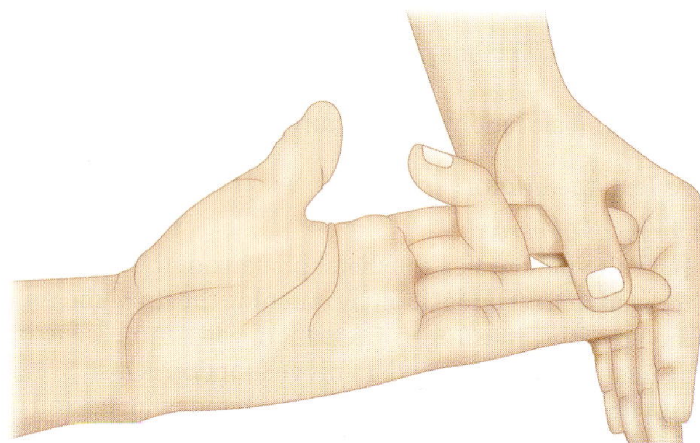

Fig. 151: Testing flexor digitorum superficialis, by flexing the proximal interphalangeal against resistance.

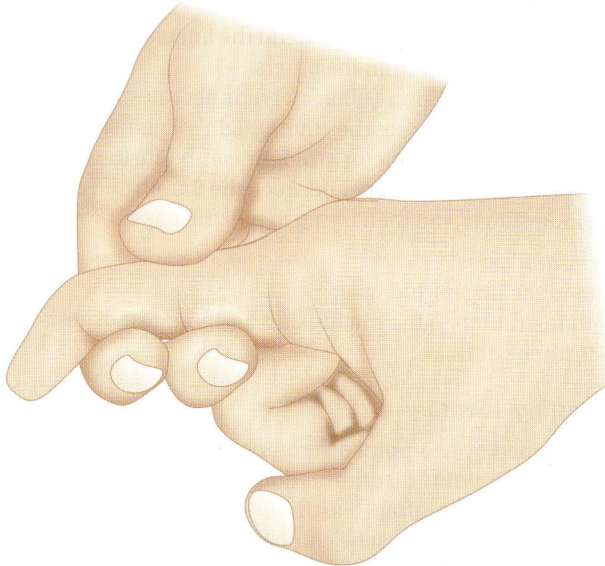

Fig. 152: Flexor digitorum profundus is tested by flexing the distal interphalangeal against resistance.

- Pain along the course of the tendon, during resistance, testing suggests a partial laceration even if the strength appears adequate.

Flexor digitorum superficialis: FDS is tested by flexing the PIP against resistance, while the remaining fingers are held (Fig. 151).

Flexor digitorum profundus: FDP is tested by flexing the distal interphalangeal (DIP) against resistance, while the metacarpal-phalangeal (MP) and PIP are held in extension (Fig. 152).

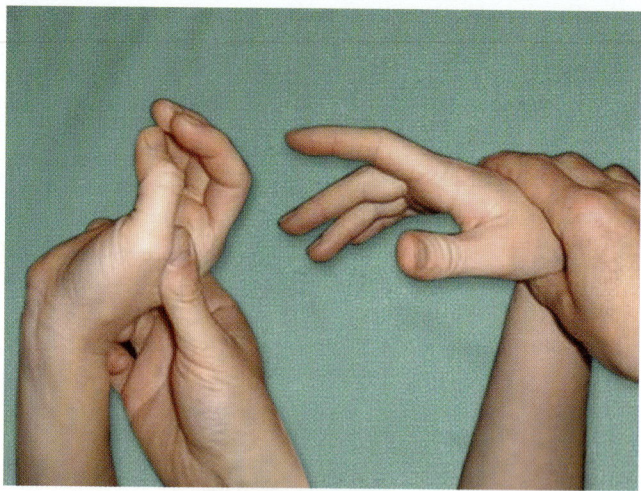

Fig. 153: Tenodesis effect.

Tenodesis effect: Passive extension of the wrist does not produce the normal "tenodesis" flexion of the fingers, if flexors are injured (Fig. 153).

Principles of Treatment of Hand Injury

Tidy wounds:
- Early debridement, irrigation, and primary repair of damaged structures including soft tissue cover. Occasionally, a delayed primary closure is necessitated
- Elevation and early mobilization based on one of the several regimens, e.g. Kleinert traction to prevent stiffness after tendon repair
- Antitetanus and antibiotic cover as well as analgesics.

Untidy wounds:
- Debridement and irrigation
- Secondary repair of damaged soft tissues
- Immobilization by external fixation and elevation
- Antitetanus and culture specific antibiotics cover.

Fractures:
- K-wire fixation or Joshi's external stabilization system (JESS) fixation depending on the type and site of injury
- Immobilization by plaster of Paris (POP) slab or cast.

Flexor Tendon Injuries

Zone 1 Injuries

Jersey Finger (Figs. 154 and 155):
- *Leddy's classification of Jersey finger:*
  - *Type 1:* Retraction into palm
  - *Type 2:* Retraction to PIP level
  - *Type 3:* Bony avulsion (tendon attached)
  - *Type 4:* Bony avulsion (tendon attached not attached to bony fragment).
- Repair within 7–10 days
  - *Types of repair:* These can be classified as follows:
    - *Direct repair:* If laceration is more than 1 cm from FDP insertion
    - *Tendon advancement:* If the laceration is less than 1 cm from insertion (Figs. 156A to D)
    - Previously advocated for zone 1 repairs, as moving the repair site out of the sheath was felt, to decrease adhesion formation.

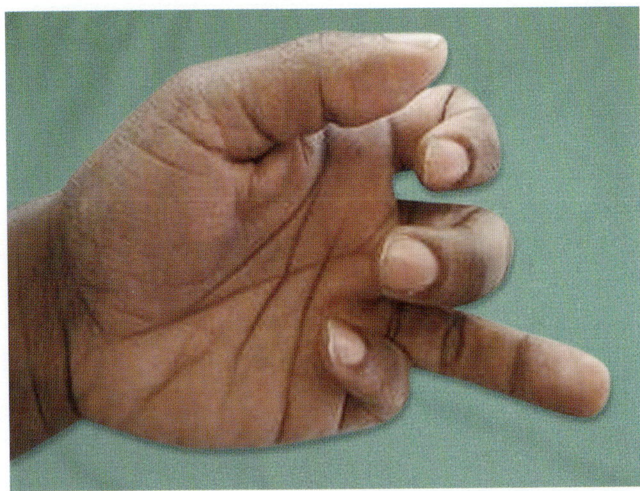

Fig. 154: Jersey finger.

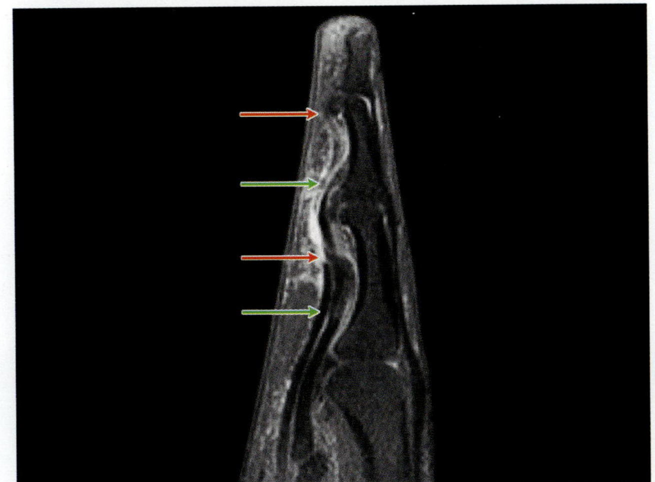

Fig. 155: The sagittal image of the ring finger reveals the gap (red arrows) between the torn ends of the flexor digitorum profundus and also depicts the intact flexor digitorum superficialis tendon (green arrows).

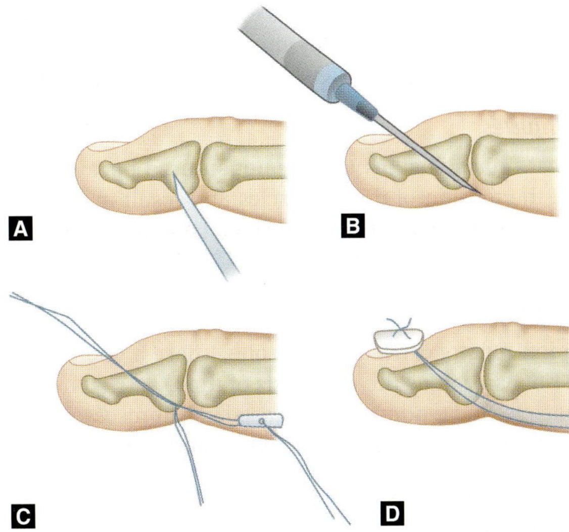

Figs. 156A to D: Tendon advancement.

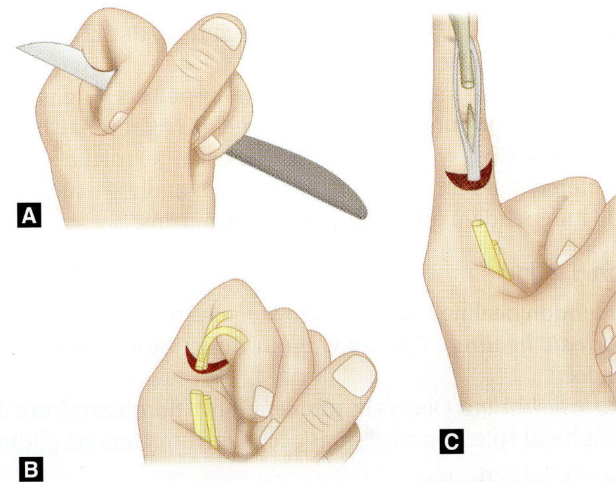

Figs. 157A to C: Injury (lacerated) in this zone causes tendons to retract.

Disadvantages:
- Shortening of flexor system
- Contracture
- Quadriga effect.

Quadriga effect:
- If FDP tendon advanced too distally
- Entire muscle bells get pulled distally
- Tendon excursion of FDP of other digits is limited
- Loss of grip strength.

Zone 2 Injuries

- Deep and superficial flexor gliding inside tendon sheets
- Traditionally, "no man's land", stiffness after repair
- Injury (lacerated) in this zone causes tendons to retract (Figs. 157A to C).

Partial lacerations:
- No repair if 40% of the tendon intact
- Potential complications:
  - Triggering
  - Tendon entrapment.
- Evaluate for the risk of triggering debride, if necessary
- Dorsal block splinting with wrist in 10° of flexion for 6–8 weeks
- It is better not to fix a partial laceration because the dissection necessary to fix it, might cause too much scarring, which might outweigh the benefit.

Complete lacerations:
- Repair of the flexor tendons by multiple strand sutures
- Ultimate strength and repair are proportional to number of strands
- Six and eight strand repairs are strongest, but have got a disadvantage of increased adhesion formation, due to increased tendon handling
- Usually, four-strand repair provides adequate strength.

Injuries to both FDP and FDS:
- Fix FDP and FDS
- As the blood supply to the FDP tendon is jeopardized, the FDS is not also fixed (due to the vinculae anatomy).

Complications:
- Stiffness
- Rerupture

- Tenolysis may be required in an estimated 18–25% of patients
  - No earlier than 3 months after repair
  - If no ROM, improvement for 1–2 months.

Zone 3 Injuries

Lumbrical muscle bellies usually not sutured because this can increase the tension of these muscles and result in a "lumbrical plus" finger (paradoxical PIP extension on attempted active finger flexion).

Zone 4 Injuries

- Tendon repairs carried out in zone 4 have a good prognosis, but not as good as the prognosis of those carried out in zone 5, because the tendons are enclosed in a fibro-osseous tunnel
- The tunnel must be opened for repairs and adhesions may form after surgery.

Zone 5 Injuries

- In this zone 5, distinct tendons run into the hand toward the digits
- Each finger has two tendons, one each from the FDS muscle and the *FDP* muscle
- The thumb has one long flexor, the flexor pollicis longus
- The tendons in zone 5 are not enclosed in a tight canal, but are surrounded by a synovial sheath in the distal part of the forearm
- Tendon repairs carried out in this area generally are successful and independent finger flexion usually returns.

Tendon Healing

Flexor tendon healing can be of following two types:
- *Intrinsic healing* : Occurs without direct blood flow to the tendon
- *Extrinsic healing*: Occurs by proliferation of fibroblasts from the peripheral epitenon adhesions occur and limit tendon gliding.

Phases of tendon healing:
- *Inflammatory (0–5 days):* Strength of the repair is reliant on the strength of the suture itself.
- *Fibroblastic (5–28 days):* Also called as collagen-producing phase.
- Remodeling (28 days–4 months).

Postoperative rehabilitation:
- Evaluate the ROM of the repaired fingers
- Too much motion, indicates rupture of the tendon
- Too little motion, indicates stiffness.

Postoperative protocols:
- *Kleinert:* Active extension, passive flexion by rubber bands (Figs. 158 and 159).
- *Duran:* Controlled passive motion methods
- *Strickland:* Early active ROM.
  - *Kleinert*: Goal is to achieve full active ROM by 10–12 weeks.
  - *Duran Protocol (Figs. 160 and 161)*
    - Dorsal splint in 20° wrist flexion
    - No rubber bands
    - Passive flexion
    - Designed in response to notion that 3–5 mm of tendon gliding is sufficient to prevent restrictive adhesions.
  - *Strickland (1980s–1990s)*
    - Uses a four-strand repair with epitendinous suture
    - Dorsal blocking splint with wrist at 20° of flexion

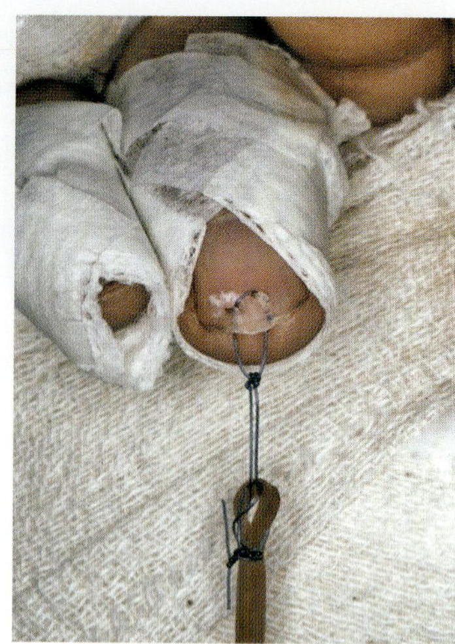

Fig. 158: Active extension, passive flexion by rubber bands.

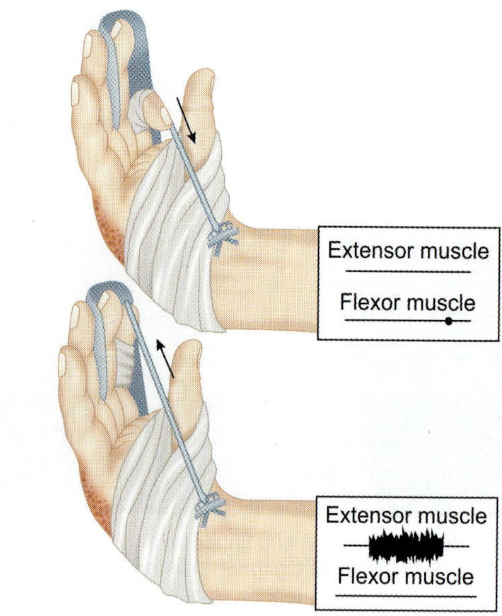

Fig. 159: Mechanism of Kleinert protocol of active extension and passive flexion by rubber bands.

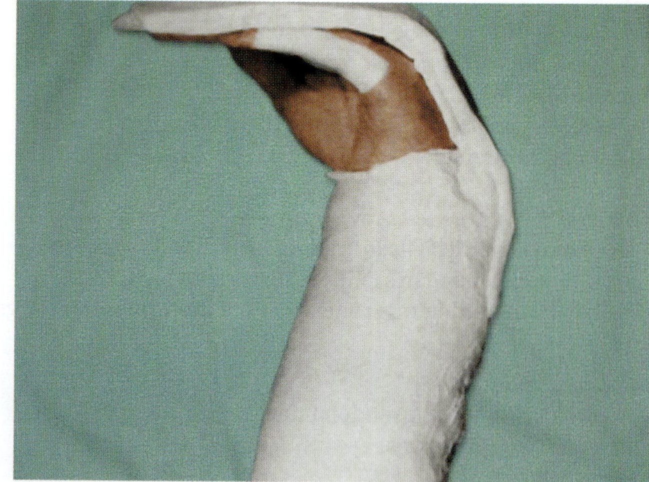

Fig. 160: Dorsal splint in 20° of wrist flexion.

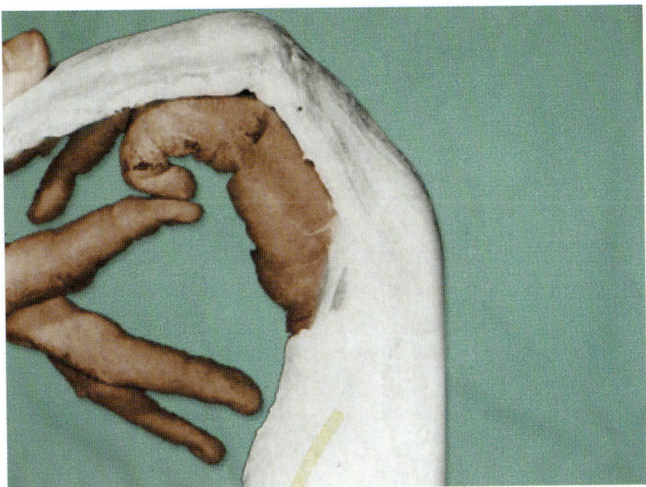

Fig. 161: Passive flexion exercises are performed, to promote tendon gliding and to prevent restrictive adhesions.

- Supervised active ROM starts on postoperative day 3
- Unsupervised active ROM at 4 weeks
- Rarely used, because it requires a pretty extensive "bulky" repair to allow for early active ROM. A lot of surgeons think that too much suture material may be problematic for tendon healing.

In children:
- They are usually not able to reliably participate in rehabilitation programs
- No benefit to early mobilization in patients under 16 years
- Immobilization greater than 4 weeks may lead to poorer outcomes.

Delayed Reconstruction

Single stage tendon grafting:

Indications for single stage tendon gliding are:
- Segmental tendon loss
- Delay in definitive repair (more than 3–6 weeks)
- Patient should be having:
  - Full passive ROM (PROM)
  - Competent pulleys.
- Graft donors are:
  - Palmaris longus
  - Plantaris
  - Long toe extensors
  - Flexor digitorum superficialis
  - Extensor indicis proprius
  - Extensor digiti minimi (EDM).

Two stage reconstruction:

Indications for two stage reconstructions are:
- Extensive soft tissue scarring
  - Crush injuries
  - Associated fractures, nerve injuries, etc.
- Loss of significant portion of pulley system.

Stages of reconstructions:
- *Stage 1*
  - Excision of tendon remnants
  - Hunter rod then placed through pulley system and fixed distally
  - Reconstruct pulleys as needed, if implant bowstrings.

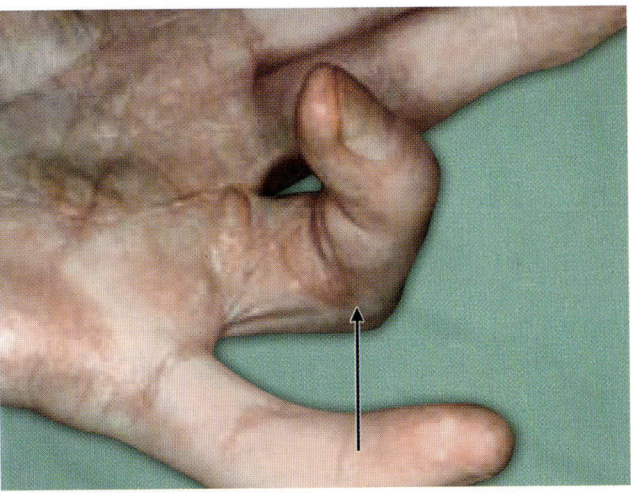

Fig. 162: Joint contracture after reconstruction.

- *Stage 2*
  - Implant removal and tendon graft insertion
  - The FDS transfer from adjacent digit described
  - *Postoperative:* Early controlled motion for 3 weeks, then slow progression to active motion.

Complications:
- Joint contracture (Fig. 162)
- Adhesions
- Rupture
- Bowstringing
- Infection.

Amputation and replantation:
- Care of amputated part needs to be done. The part should be:
  - Washed gently with saline
  - Wrapped in moist saline gauze
  - Tucked into polythene bag (or bread wrapper)
  - Put in a container of a mixture of ice block and water.
- *Absolute contraindications to replantation*:
  - Concomitant life-threatening injury
  - Inhibiting systemic illness
  - Severe crushing
  - Extreme contamination
  - Prolonged ischemia time
  - Multiple levels injuries
  - Previous surgery to the amputated part.

Replantation

Steps followed are illustrated below as:
- Bone shortening and fixation
- Arterial repair
- Venous anastomosis
- Nerve and tendon repair
- Skin closure.

Note: The reader is requested to refer other special books on hand surgery for details of reimplantation.

GANGLIONIC CYSTS OF THE WRIST

Introduction

- It is a type of mucinous filled cyst, which is found adjacent to joint capsule or tendon sheath.

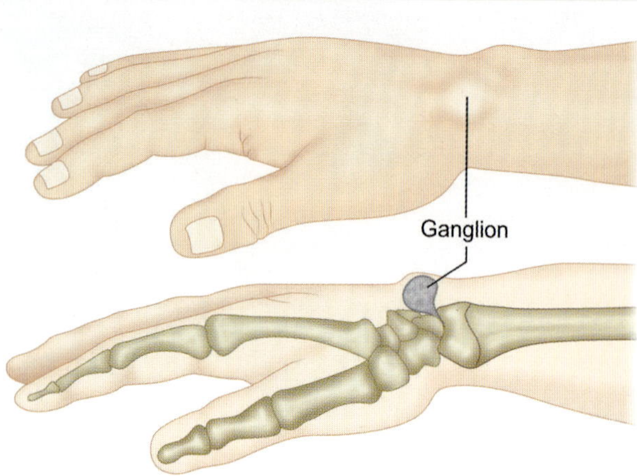

Fig. 163: Ganglion on wrist.

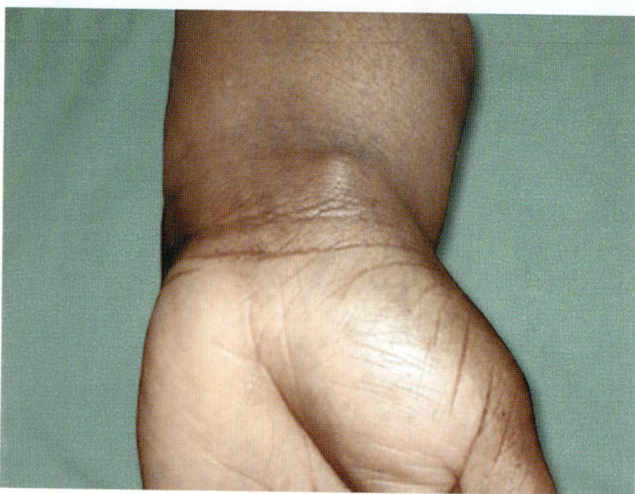

Fig. 164: Volar ganglion.

- It consists of an outer fibrous coat and an inner synovial lining along with a clear, colorless, and gelatinous fluid
- Ganglions usually occurs singly, but may be multilocular
- More common in women.

Age

- Seventy percent occur between the second and fourth decades
- Ganglions occurring at DIP joint (mucus cyst) are associated with osteoarthritis and occur at older ages
- Rarely seen in children.

Location

- Frequent in hand and wrist (Fig. 163), less often in ankle, foot, and knee
- Most common soft tissue mass of hand is ganglion
- *Dorsal ganglion*: 60–70% of all ganglia occur over scapholunate ligament
- *Volar ganglion*: 20% of all ganglia occur at volar wrist (Fig. 164). Most common site is at volar wrist crease between the FCR and APL at the scaphotrapezoid joint.

Differential Diagnosis

- Synovial sarcoma
- Extraskeletal chondrosarcoma
- Avascular necrosis (AVN)
- Venous aneurysm.

Clinical Presentation and Examination

- Dorsal wrist pain, which is made worse with repeated use; a slow growing, localized swelling, with mild aching, and weakness
- Cyst is firm, smooth, rubbery, rounded, slightly fluctuant, and at times tender
- Cysts will transilluminate
- It is usually fixed but may be slightly movable, if it involves tendon sheath
- Mass may become obvious with wrist flexion
- Palpation of cyst with compression may not only increase the extent of the cyst, but also the direction of pedicle.

Occult Ganglia

- Source of similar symptoms occur especially in young gymnasts. Discomfort is usually maximal in extension
- Point tenderness is directly over scapholunate interval
- Attempt to palpate mass over scapholunate ligament with wrist in volar flexion.

Radiographs

- Usually negative
- Arthrography is usually not helpful
- Dorsal ganglions may be found with scapholunate diastasis.

Surgical Treatment

- Aspiration
- Complete excision
- In a few cases, cysts return following needle aspiration or surgical treatment.

DISTAL RADIOULNAR JOINT

Carpal Bones

There are eight carpal bones, arranged in two rows, as shown in Figure 165.

Proximal Row (Lateral to Medial)

- Articulates with inferior surface of lower end of radius and articular disk of inferior radioulnar joint.
  - Scaphoid (S)
  - Lunate (L)
  - Triquetral (Tq)
  - Pisiform (P).

Distal Row (Lateral to Medial)

- Articulates with the base of metacarpals:
  - Trapezium (Tm)
  - Trapezoid (Td)
  - Capitate (C)
  - Hamate (H).

Ligaments

There are 33 ligaments around the wrist. These can further be classified as follows:

Taleisnik and Kelly's Classification

- Extrinsic ligaments
- Intrinsic ligaments.

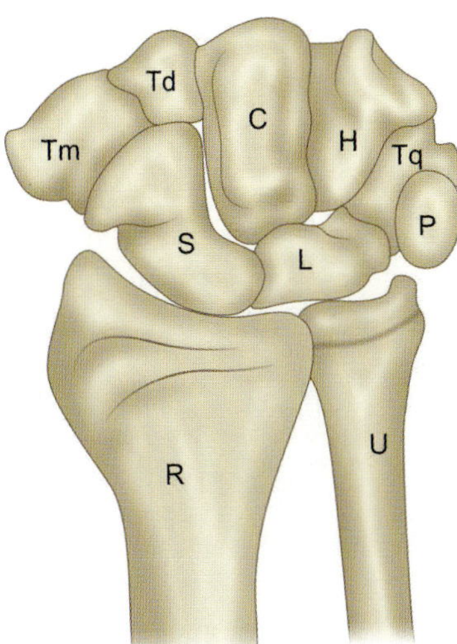

Fig. 165: Radiocarpal joint. (C: capitate; H: hamate; L: lunate; P: pisiform; S: scaphoid; Td: trapezoid; Tm: trapezium; Tq: triquetrum; R: radius; U: ulna)

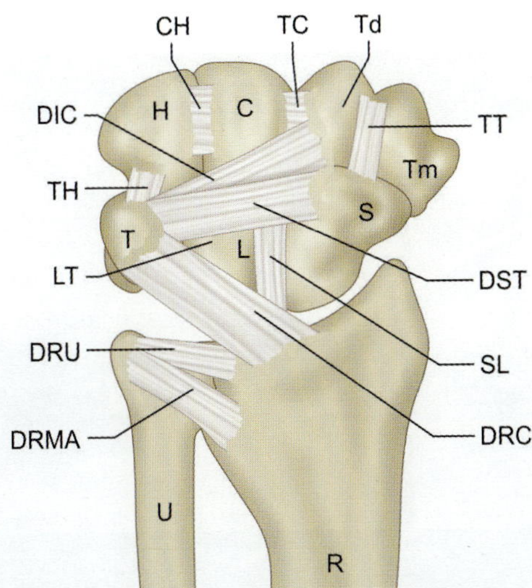

Fig. 166: Wrist from dorsal perspective. (Bones—C: capitate; H: hamate; L: lunate; R: radius; S: scaphoid; T: triquetrum; Td: trapezoid; Tm: trapezium; U: ulna; Ligaments—CH: capitohamate; DIC: dorsal intercarpal; DRC: dorsal radiocarpal; DRMA: dorsal radial metaphyseal; DRU: dorsal radioulnar; LT: lunotriquetral; SL: scapholunate; TC: trapezocapitate; TH: triquetrohamate; TT: trapezio-trapezoid; DST: dorsal scaphotriquetral)

Extrinsic ligaments: These are radiocarpal and carpometacarpal ligaments (Fig. 166). These can further be divided into ligaments on volar and dorsal aspects.

1. Volar ligaments
2. Dorsal ligaments.

1. *Volar ligaments:* Extrinsic ligaments on volar aspects are enumerated below:
   - Radioscaphocapitate
   - Long radiolunate
   - Radioscapholunate (ligament of Testut)
   - Short radiolunate
   - Ulnolunate
   - Ulnotriquetral
   - Ulnocapitate.

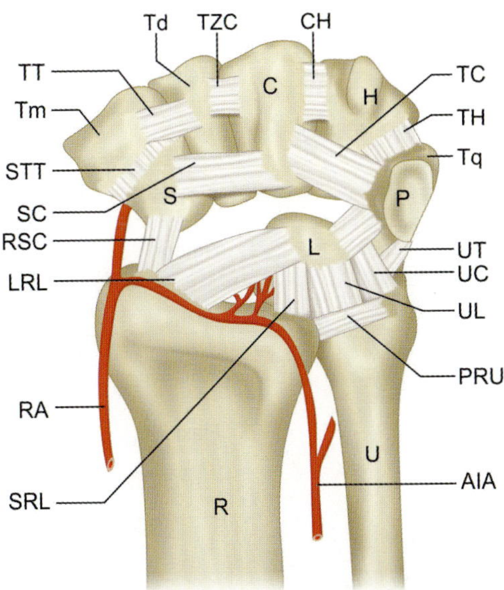

Fig. 167: Wrist from palmar perspective. (Bones—C: capitate; H: hamate; L: lunate; P: pisiform; R: radius; S: scaphoid; Td: trapezoid; Tm: trapezium; Tq: triquetrum; U: ulna, Ligaments—CH: capitohamate; LRL: long radiolunate; PRU: palmar radioulnar ligament; RSC: radioscaphocapitate; SC: scaphocapitate; SRL: short radiolunate; STT: scaphotrapeziotrapezoid; TZC: trapezocapitate; TC: triquetrocapitate; TH: triquetrohamate; TT: trapezio-trapezoid; UC: ulnocapitate; UL: ulnolunate; UT: ulnotriquetral; RA: radial artery; AIA: anterior interosseous artery)

2. *Dorsal ligaments:* These include following ligaments:
   - Dorsal intercarpal
   - Dorsal radiotriquetral.

Intrinsic ligaments (Fig. 167): These are intercarpal ligaments and include following ligaments:

- Scapholunate
- Lunotriquetral
- Scaphotrapeziotrapezoidal
- Scaphocapitate
- Triquetral capitate
- Triquetral hamate
- Capitohamate
- Capitotrapezoidal
- Trapeziotrapezoidal.

Angles

Radiolunate Angle (Fig. 168)

- It is an angle between axis of radius and axis of lunate
- Normal movement can be up to 15° in flexion and up to 20° in extension.

Capitolunate Angle

- It is an angle between axis of capitate and axis of lunate
- There is some abnormality, if movement is more than 15°.

Scapholunate Angle (Fig. 169)

It is an angle between axis of lunate and axis of scaphoid. Normal range 30–70°.

Carpal Height Ratio (Fig. 170)

It is the distance between distal edge of radius and base of third metacarpal divided by the length of third metacarpal. Normal ratio 0.53 ± 0.03.

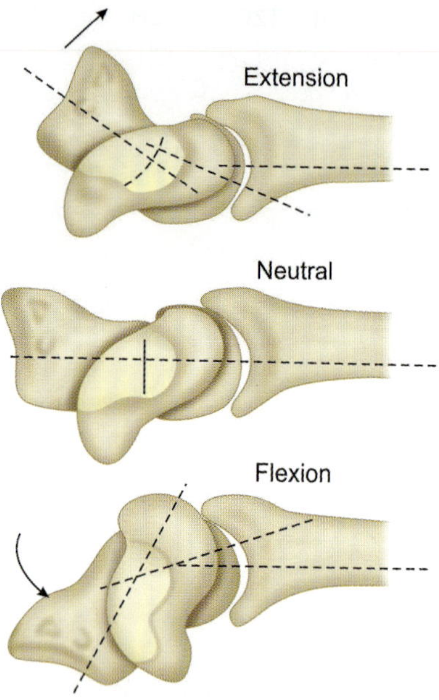

Fig. 168: Radiolunate angle.

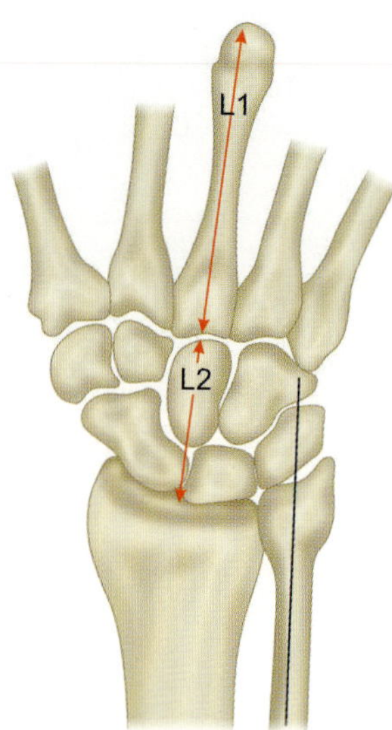

Fig. 170: Carpal height ratio. (L1: length of the third metacarpal; L2: distance between distal edge of radius and base of third metacarpal)

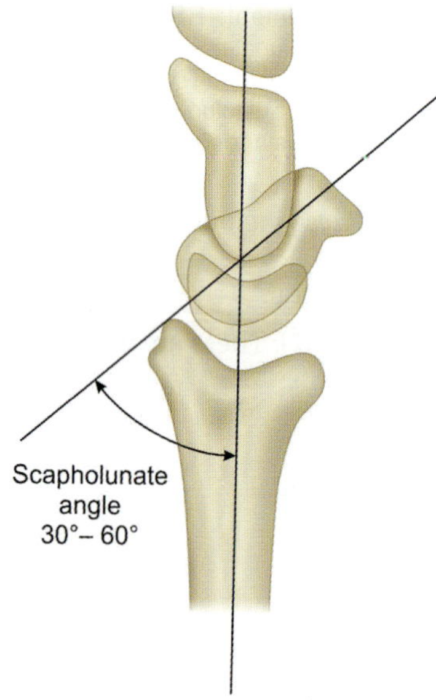

Fig. 169: Scapholunate angle.

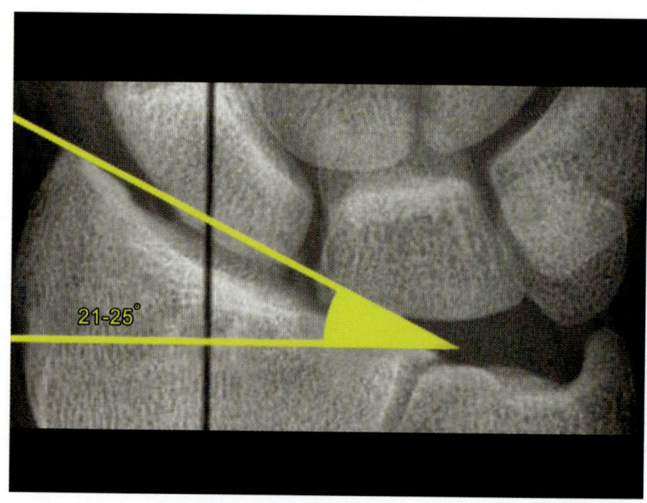

Fig. 171: Radial angulation.

Radial Angulation (Fig. 171)

It is an angle between articular surface of ulna and radius. Normal range 23°.

Palmar Angulation (Fig. 172)

It is an angle between axis of radius and axis of lunate in lateral view. Normal range 11°.

Radial Length

- It is the distance between radial styloid and ulnar styloid.
- Normal length is 12 mm.

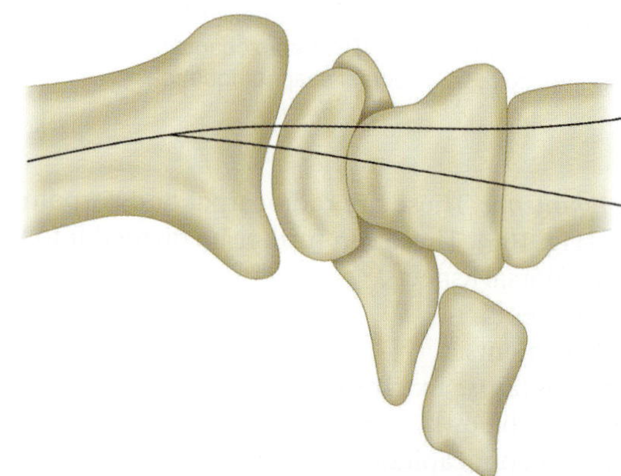

Fig. 172: Palmar angulation.

Anatomy of Distal Radioulnar Joint

Distal radioulnar joint is a pivot type synovial joint, where head of ulna articulates with ulnar notch of radius. It consists of the following features:

- *Articular disk:* Fibrocartilage apex attached to the base of styloid of ulna and base to lower margin of ulnar notch of radius.
- *Capsule:* Upper part is weak and evaginated by synovial membrane, forming recessus sacciformis.
- Triangular fibrocartilage complex of Werner and Palmer.

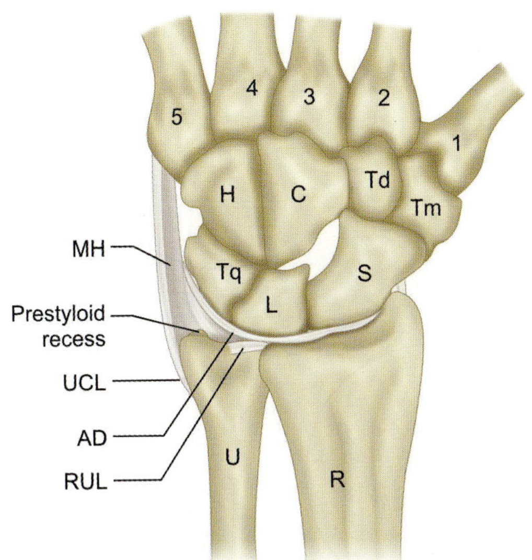

Fig. 173: Components of triangular fibrocartilage complex. (AD: articular disk; MH: meniscus homologue; RUL: dorsal and volar radioulnar ligaments; UCL: ulnar collateral ligament. Other structures shown are metacarpal bones (1, 2, 3, 4, and 5), carpal bones; C: capitate; H: hamate; S: scaphoid; Td: trapezoid; Tq: triquetrum; R: radius; U: ulna; L: lunate; Tm: trapezium)

Triangular Fibrocartilage Complex

Triangular fibrocartilage complex begins on ulnar side of lunate fossa of radius and attaches to ulnar head and base of ulnar styloid (Fig. 173).

It has following components:

- Volar and dorsal radioulnar ligament
- Ulnar collateral ligament
- Meniscal homologue
- Articular disk
- Extensor carpi ulnaris sheath
- Ulnolunate ligament
- Ulnotriquetral ligament.

It consists of following features:

- Stable radioulnar connection
- Stable ulnocarpal connection
- Mechanism for transmitting forces from hand
- Suspensory ligament function for ulnar side of carpus from radius
- Extending dividing surface for proximal row across distal end of forearm bones.

Acute Instability

Subluxation

There can be two reasons for subluxation:

1. *Forcible excess pronation:*
   - Radius engages ulnar prominence
   - Painful and limited supination
   - No deformity.

Treatment:

- Passive manipulation to supination
- Immobilization in above elbow cast for 4–6 weeks.

2. *Forcible excess supination:*
   - Radius engages posterolateral aspect of ulna
   - Slight anterior prominence of ulnar head.

Treatment:

- Reduction, while forearm is pronated
- Immobilization in above elbow cast for 4–6 weeks.

Dislocation

Acute Traumatic

- Complete volar or dorsal displacement of ulna, associated with disruption of volar or dorsal radioulnar capsular ligament.
- Radiocarpal unit displaces, abducted fixed inferior end of ulna.
- Excessive prominence of ulnar head and narrow wrist.

Treatment:

- Reduction by pressure on ulna and above elbow cast for 4–6 weeks.

Associated Instability

- *Galeazzi fracture:*
  - Fracture of lower third radius with dislocation of DRUJ
  - *Treatment:* Open reduction internal fixation (ORIF) with plating
  - If DRUJ not reduced, fixation with K-wire for 6 weeks in supination.
- *Essex lopresti fracture dislocation*:
  - Fracture radial head or neck with disruption of DRUJ with interosseous membrane tear.
  - *Treatment:* ORIF with DRUJ fixation by K-wire for 6 weeks
- Fractures of lower end of radius
- Fractures of lower end of ulna.

Chronic Instabilities

- Malunited fractures of radius and ulna
- Nonunited fractures of radius and ulna
- Undetected dislocations
- Triangular fibrocartilage complex tear
- Madelung deformity
- Post-traumatic arthritis
- Rheumatoid and osteoarthritis
- Subluxation of ulna
- Subluxation of ECU tendon.

Treatment Modalities

- Ulnar hemiresection-interposition arthroplasty (Bowers)
- Ulnar shortening procedures
- Distal radioulnar arthrodesis with distal ulnar pseudoarthrosis (Sauve–Kapandji)
- Procedures to stabilize DRUJ.

Ulnar Hemiresection Interposition Arthroplasty (Bowers) (Figs. 174 and 175)

Indications:

- Unreconstructable fractures of ulnar head
- Ulnocarpal impingement syndrome
- Rheumatoid arthritis
- Chronic painful TFCC tear
- Post-traumatic and osteoarthritis

Ulnar Shortening Procedure Darrach Resection (Figs. 176A and E)

Indications

- Malunited Colles' fracture
- Malunion or nonunion of radius
- Abnormality of growth of distal radius.

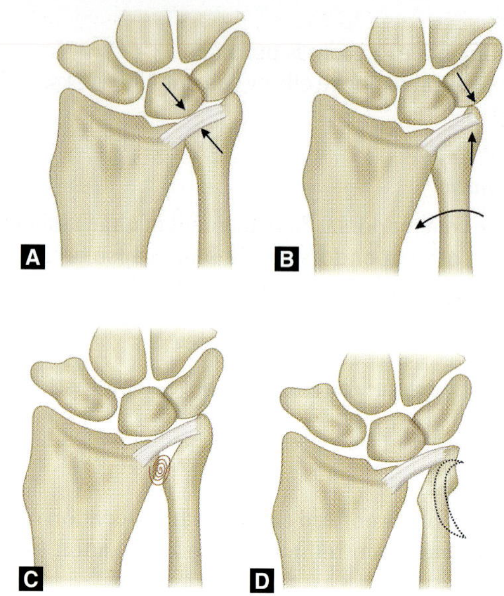

Figs. 174A to D: Steps followed, while performing ulnar hemiresection interposition arthroplasty (Bowers arthroplasty).

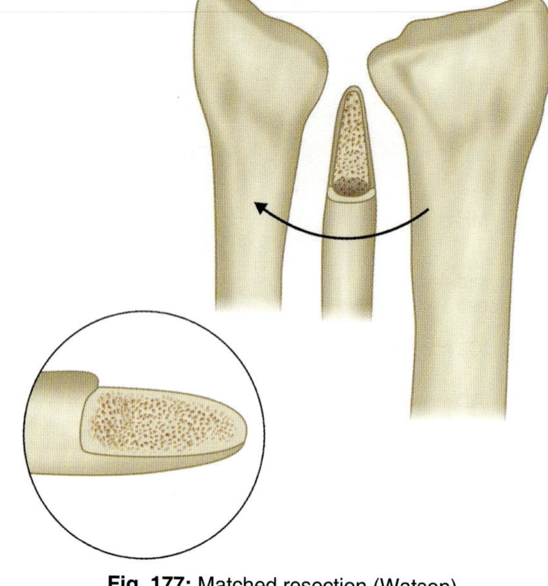

Fig. 177: Matched resection (Watson).

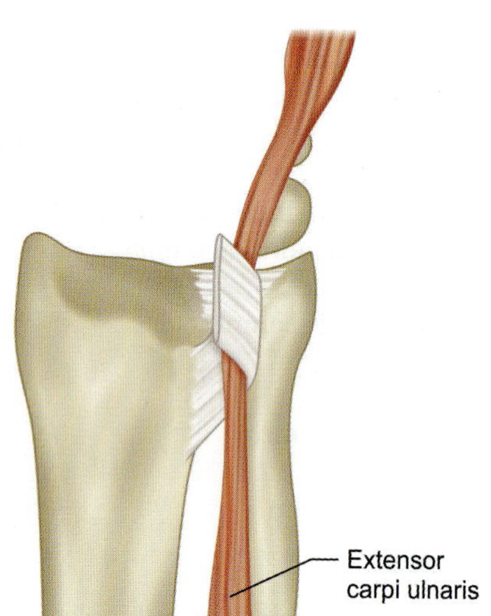

Fig. 175: Ulnar hemiresection interposition arthroplasty (Bowers).

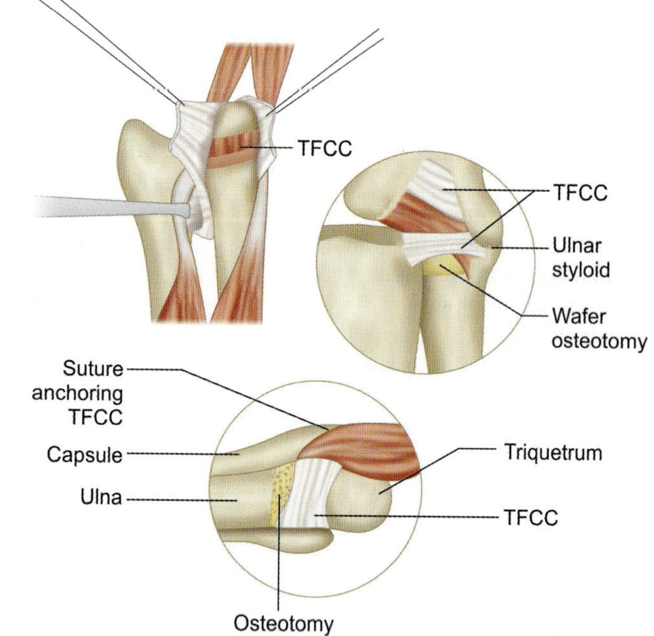

Fig. 178: Wafer resection (Feldon).

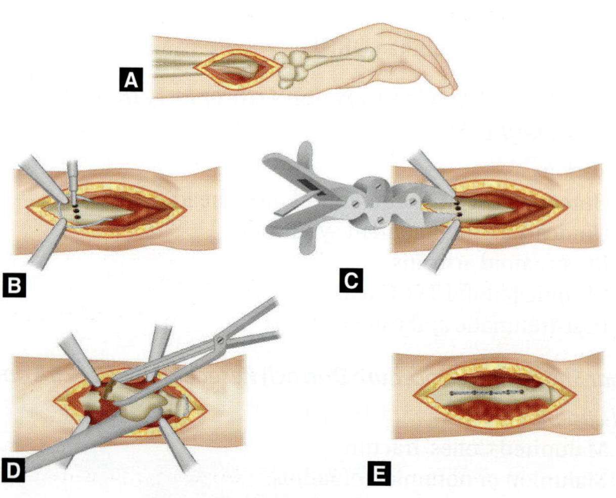

Figs. 176A to E: Darrach resection.

Matched resection (Watson) (Fig. 177):

- *Indications:*
  - Rheumatoid arthritis
  - Trauma.

Wafer resection (Feldon) (Fig. 178):

- *Indications*
  - Triangular fibrocartilage complex tear
  - Ulnar impaction syndrome.

Milch cuff resection (See Figs. 207A to C):

- *Indications*
  - Malunited Colles' fracture
  - Malunion or nonunion of radius
  - Cessation or abnormality of growth of distal radius.

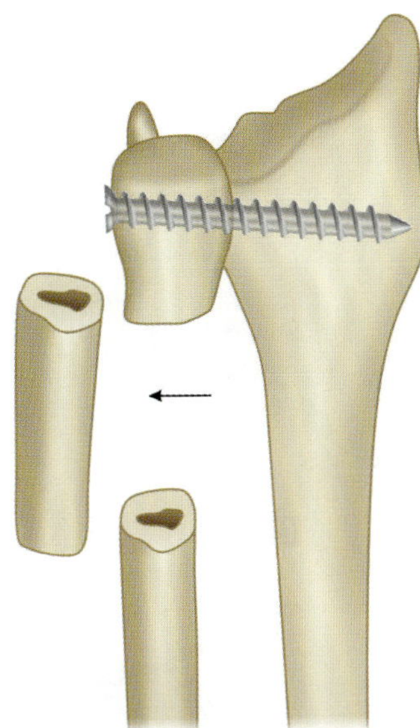

Fig. 179: Distal radioulnar arthrodesis with distal ulnar pseudarthrosis (Sauve-Kapandji).

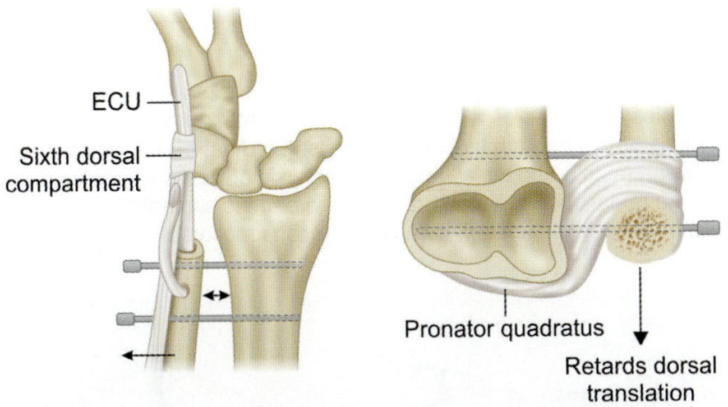

Fig. 180: Tenodesis of extensor carpi ulnaris (ECU) and transfer of pronator quadratus (Kleinman and Greenberg).

Distal radioulnar arthrodesis: Distal radioulnar arthrodesis with distal ulnar pseudarthrosis (Sauve-Kapandji) is shown in Figure 179.

- *Indications*
  - Painful wrist by previous surgery
  - Traumatic arthritis
  - Rheumatoid arthritis.

Procedures for Stabilization

The DRUJ should be stabilized:

- After undetected dislocation
- After surgical procedure to resect distal ulna:
  - Tenodesis of ECU and transfer of pronator quadratus (Kleinman and Greenberg) (Fig. 180)
  - Reconstruction of dorsal ligament of TFCC (Scheker) (Figs. 181A to G).

DISTAL RADIUS FRACTURES

To be effective, a classification system must accurately categorize the fracture type and injury severity to serve as a guideline for treatment and prognosis.

Although many classification systems have attempted to provide a more accurate representation of various distal radius fracture patterns, some have proven more useful than others in guiding treatment and predicting outcome.

Classification

- *Gartland and Werley classification:* This has been illustrated in the Table 4 and shown in Figure 182.
- *Melone's classification:* Intra-articular fractures are classified, as demonstrated in Table 5 and shown in Figure 183.
- McMurtry and Jupiter classification (Table 6).
- Mayo classification (Table 7).
- *Fernandez classification:* This has been illustrated in Table 8 and shown in Figure. 184.
- Lidstrom and Andres classification (Table 9).
- Sarmiento classification (Table 10).
- AO classification (Figs. 185 to 187) (Table 11).
- Frykman's classification (Table 12).

Nonoperative Management

Indications:

- Elderly patients
- Low demand patients
- Fractures with less articular involvement
- Associated comorbid conditions
- Fractures, which can be maintained in acceptable position.

Guidelines for reduction:

- Radial shortening less than 5 mm at DRUJ
- Radial inclination on PA radiographs greater than 15°
- Sagittal tilt on lateral projection between 15° dorsal tilt and 20° volar tilt
- Intra-articular step-off or gap less than 2 mm of radiocarpal joint
- Articular incongruity less than 2 mm of sigmoid notch of distal radius.

Reduction techniques:

Typical dorsally angulated fractures with minimal displacement of volar cortex:

- Adequate analgesia
- Longitudinal traction
- Increase the dorsal angulation (to unlock volar cortex if overlapped)
- Direct pressure on the distal fragment to correct the angulation
- Palpate the volar and dorsal rim (estimation of correction).

Cast application (Fig. 188):

- Mechanical analogy in reducing Colles' fracture (disimpaction reduction, locking the fracture by pronation).
- The squeezing grip is for reduction and for molding the cast into an oval cross-section.
- If the thenar eminence is liberated from the plaster with the object of encouraging movement in the thumb, a pressure sore often results at the proximal part of the aperture. This is inevitable, if the radius collapses toward the ulna.
- By incorporating the whole thumb, as in the scaphoid cast, a pressure sore at the base of the thumb is avoided.
- Showing the ideal shape of the cast for function of the hand. Full opposition of the thumb is imperative.
- X-ray appearance of a Colles' plaster in strong ulnar deviation, as shown in Figure 189.

Follow-up and aftercare:

- Follow-up radiographs to assess for redisplacement and healing

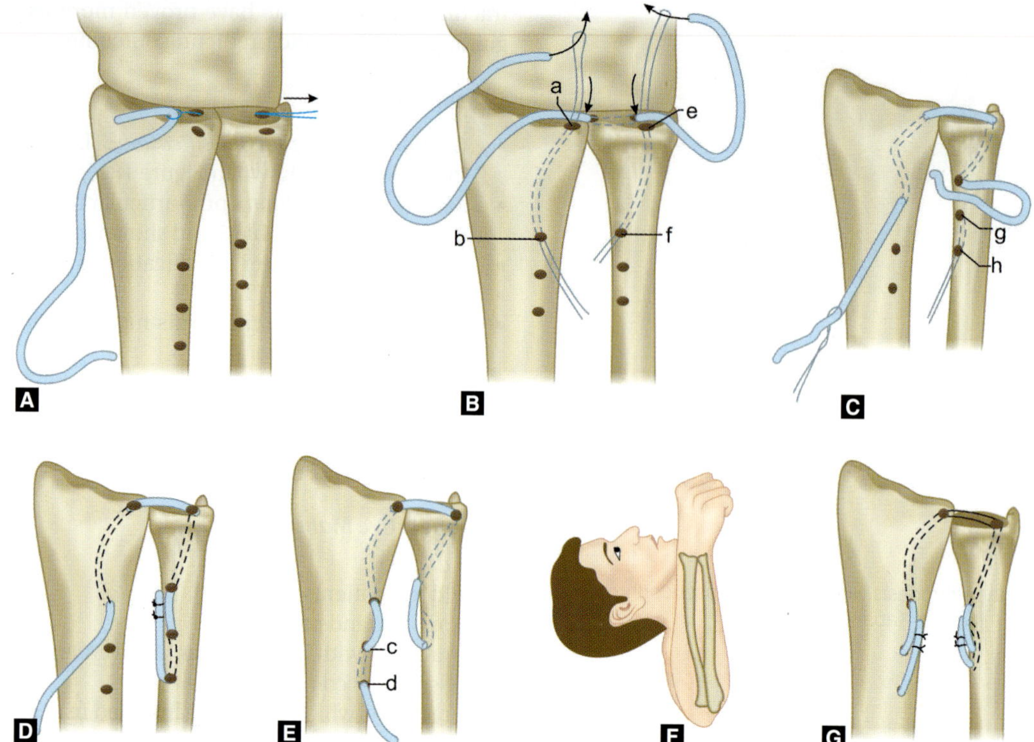

Figs. 181A to G: Schekar technique: (A) Tendon graft is drawn through capsulotomies; (B) Ends of tendon graft inserted into loops of wire emerging from tunnels in ulnar fovea and dorsal lip of sigmoid notch of radius; (C) Tendon graft is drawn through two distal tunnels; (D) Ulnar end of tendon graft is threaded through second tunnel and sutures to itself; (E) Tendon graft is pulled between middle and distal hole in metaphysic of radius to ensure that full tension has been applied between fovea and sigmoid notch; (F) With tension applied to radial end of tendon graft while forearm is supinated, joint stability is tested through full range of motion; (G) On radial side, graft is sutures to itself with forearm is supinated, completing reconstruction of dorsal ligament.

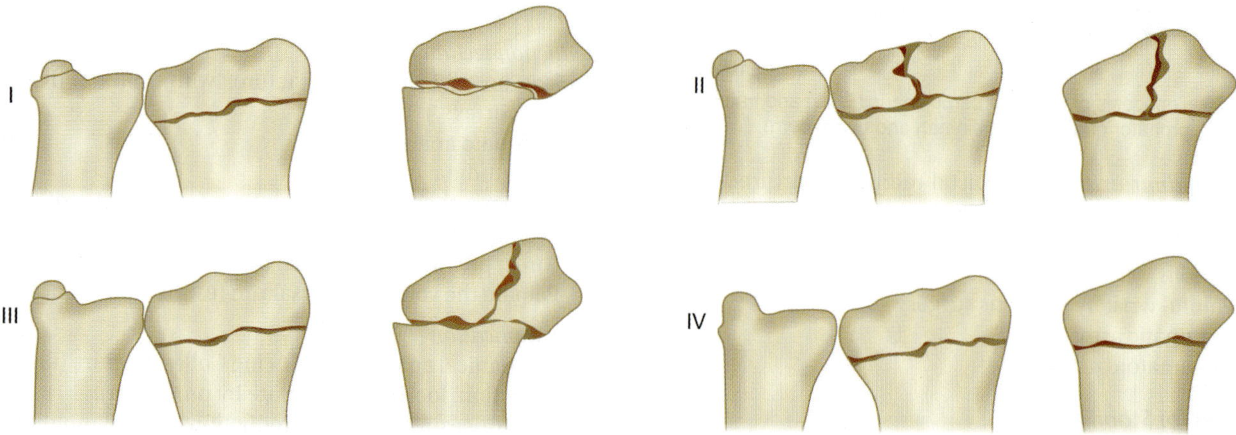

Fig. 182: Gartland and Werley classification for distal radial fractures.

TABLE 4: Gartland and Werley classification of distal radius fractures.

Group 1	Simple Colles' fracture
Group 2	Comminuted Colles' fracture with undisplaced intra-articular fragments
Group 3	Comminuted Colles' fracture with displaced intra-articular fragments

TABLE 5: Melone's intra-articular fractures classification.

Type I	Minimal comminution—stable
Type II	• Comminuted—stable • Displacement of medial complex: – *Posterior:* Die–punch and barton – *Anterior:* Smith
Type III	Displacement of medial complex as a unit + anterior spike
Type IV	Wide separation or rotation of the dorsal fragment and palmar fragment rotation

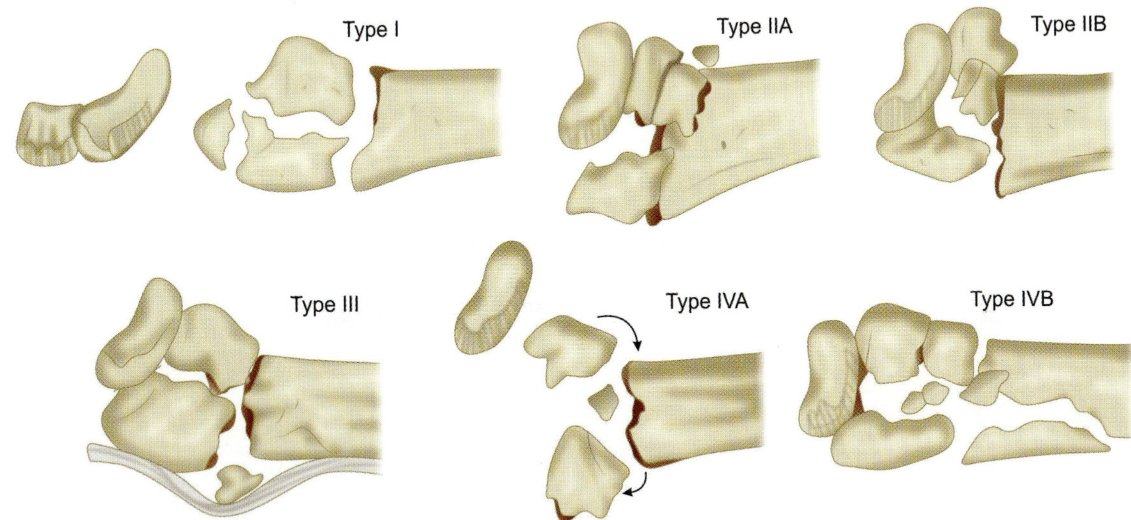

Fig. 183: Melone's classification.

TABLE 6: McMurtry and Jupiter classification.

Group 1 *Two parts:* (The opposite portion of the radiocarpal joint remains intact) • Dorsal barton • Volar barton • Chauffeur • Die–punch
Group 2 *Three parts:* The lunate and scaphoid facets separate from each other and the proximal portion of the radius
Group 3 *Four parts:* Groups 2 + lunate facet fractured in dorsal and volar fragment
Group 4 Five parts or more.

TABLE 7: Mayo classification.

Type 1	Extra-articular radiocarpal
Type 2	Intra-articular radioulnar
Type 3	Intra-articular scaphoid fossa of distal radius
Type 4	Intra-articular, scaphoid fossa, lunate fossa, and sigmoid fossa of the distal radius.

TABLE 8: Fernandez classification.

Type I	Metaphyseal bending fractures
Type II	Shearing fractures
Type III	Compression of the articular surface without the characteristic fragmentation
Type IV	Avulsion fractures or radiocarpal fracture dislocations
Type V	Combined injuries with significant soft tissue involvement due to high energy nature of these fractures

- Loss of reduction most commonly occurs during the second week of cast treatment or later, especially in the elderly osteopenic patient
- This suggests that the timing and number of follow-up visits need to be individualized to both the patient and fracture
- For those fractures that are less stable, immobilization for at least 6 weeks is indicated.

TABLE 9: Lidstrom and Andres classification.

Group 1	Undisplaced
Group 2a	Dorsal angulation, extra-articular
Group 2b	Dorsal angulation, intra-articular but without gross separation of fragments
Group 2c	Dorsal angulation articular plus dorsal displacement, extra-articular
Group 2d	Dorsal angulation plus dorsal displacement, intra-articular but without gross separation of fragments
Group 2e	Dorsal angulation plus dorsal displacement, intra-articular with separation of fragments

TABLE 10: Sarmiento classification.

Group 1	Nondisplaced fractures without radiocarpal joint involvement
Group 2	Displaced fractures without radiocarpal joint involvement
Group 3	Nondisplaced fractures with radiocarpal joint involvement
Group 4	Displaced fractures with radiocarpal joint involvement

TABLE 11: AO classification.

Group 1	Extra-articular
Group 2	Partial articular
Group 3	Complete articular
C1	Simple articular and metaphyseal
C2	Simple articular and complex metaphyseal
C3	Complex articular and complex metaphyseal.

TABLE 12: Frykman's classification.

Type I	Extra-articular
Type II	Extra-articular fracture with ulnar styloid fracture
Type III	Radiocarpal articular involvement
Type IV	Radiocarpal involvement with ulnar styloid fracture
Type V	Radioulnar involvement
Type VI	Radioulnar involvement with ulnar styloid fracture
Type VII	Radiocarpal and radioulnar involvement
Type VIII	Radiocarpal and radioulnar involvement with ulnar styloid fracture

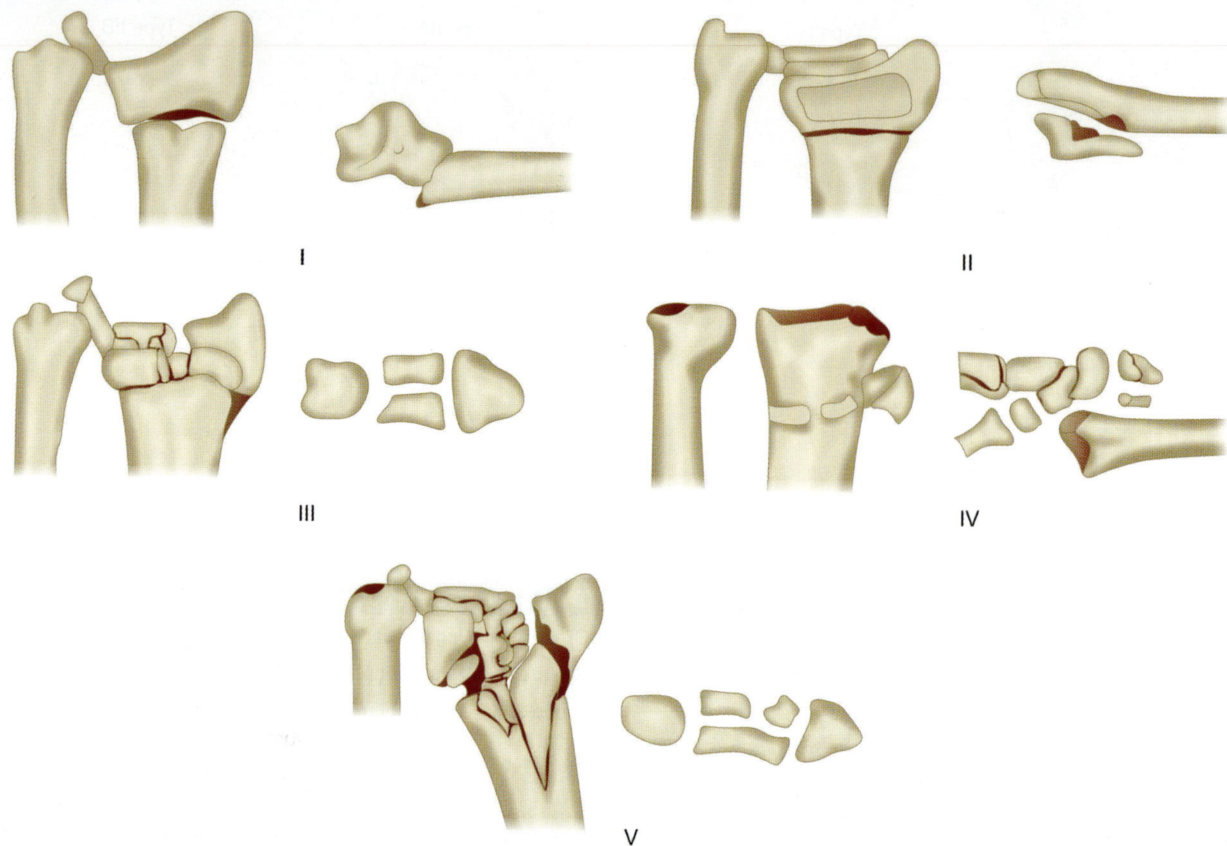

Fig. 184: Fernandez classification.

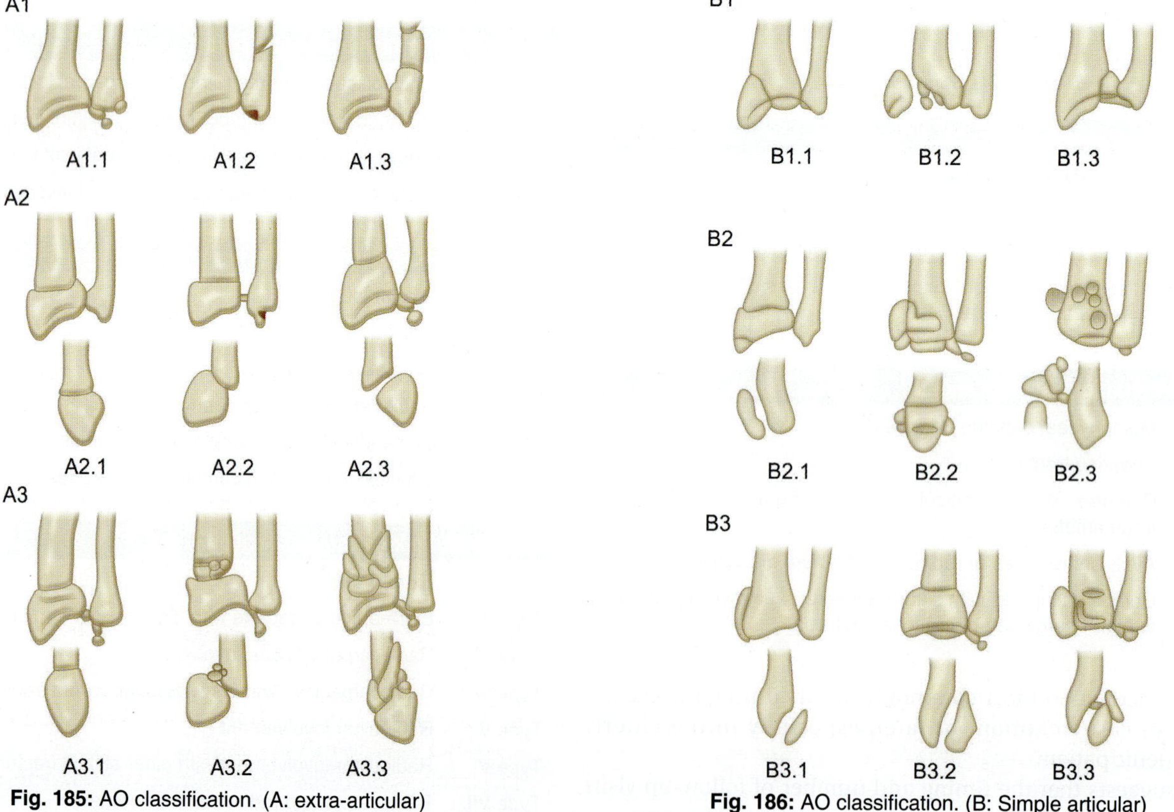

Fig. 185: AO classification. (A: extra-articular)

Fig. 186: AO classification. (B: Simple articular)

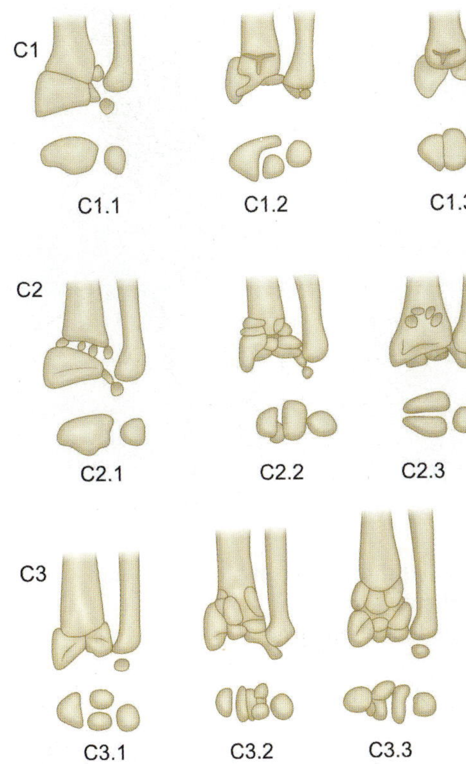

Fig. 187: AO classification. (C: Complex articular)

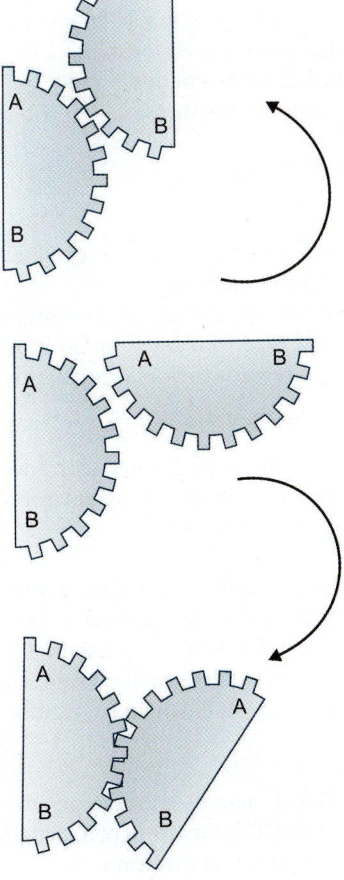

Fig. 188: Cast application.

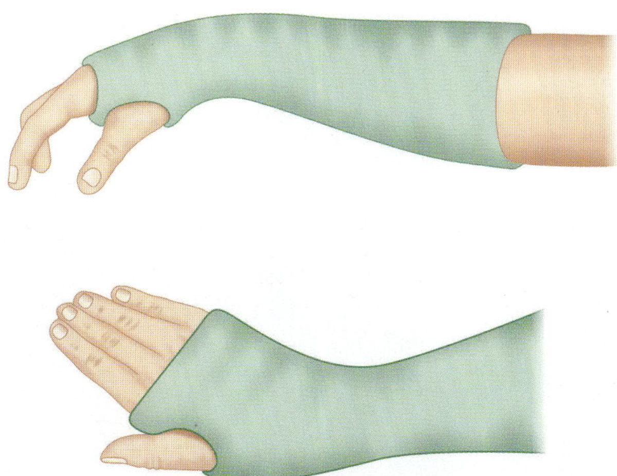

Fig. 189: Colles' plaster in strong ulnar deviation.

Predicting successful nonoperative treatment:

- Careful patient selection
- Initial satisfactory reduction
- Maintenance of reduction throughout the follow-up period to final fracture healing
- At present, we can conclude that radial shortening followed by dorsal comminution is most predictive of instability
- Increasing age significantly increases the risk of both early and late loss of reduction, even with minimal initial displacement
- In recent times, adjunctive modalities such as ultrasound and electrical stimulation have been postulated to quicken healing and subsequently prevent redisplacement.

Complications

- May be associated with the injury itself, its management or failure to restore the anatomy
- Some of the common complications are:
  - Compression neuropathies, which can be acute or delayed
  - Malunion
  - Midcarpal instability
  - Post-traumatic arthritis
  - Residual wrist and hand stiffness
  - Attrition ruptures of the EPL
  - Complex regional pain syndrome (CRPS) Type 1 and 2
  - Ugly deformity of radial deviation is cosmeticologically corrected by resection of lower end of ulna (Figs. 190A and B). This also restores full rotation and abolishes residual pain round the prominent head of the ulna.

Outcomes:

- Preservation of RL is most important for the preservation of function, followed by palmar angulation
- Loss of RL can lead to ulnar impaction or dysfunction of the DRUJ, with limited ROM in pronation and supination, depending on the volar or dorsal subluxation of the ulnar head within the sigmoid notch
- Residual dorsal angulation can precipitate ulnar impaction, midcarpal instability, and altered stress concentrations, which may lead to early arthritis
- Poor outcomes are more common in malunions and include at least one of the following:
  - The DRUJ pain
  - Nerve compression

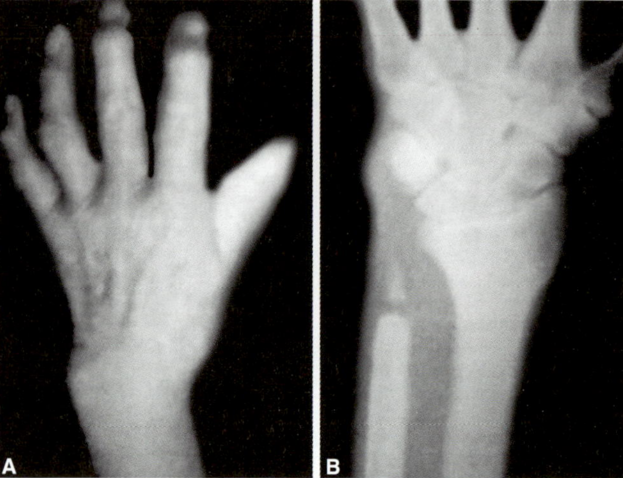

Figs. 190A and B: Ugly deformity of radial deviation corrected by cosmetological resection of lower end of ulna.

- Radial deviation of the wrist
- Osteoarthritis
- Dorsal angulation
- Reduced grip strength
- Prominent ulnar styloid.

Indications for Surgery

- Patient factors
- Fracture pattern
- Fracture stability
- Associated injuries.

Patient Factors

- Lifestyle
- Mental attitude
- Associated medical conditions
- Compliance with treatment
- Chronological age.

Fracture Pattern

- For extra-articular distal radius fractures, adequacy of closed reduction is assessed by reducing the fracture to normal radiographic parameters and maintaining them till the fracture heals.
- For intra-articular fractures, articular congruity must be assessed in addition to the normal radiographic parameters of the distal radius.
- Guidelines for acceptable closed reduction are:
  - Radial inclination greater than or equal to 15° on PA view
  - Radial length less than or equal to 5 mm shortening on PA view
  - Radial tilt less than 15° dorsal or 20° volar tilt on lateral view
  - Articular incongruity less than 2 mm of step-off.

Fracture Stability

- Radiographic signs that should alert the surgeon that the fracture is probably unstable and closed reduction will be insufficient include following:
  - Palmar metaphyseal comminution
  - Initial dorsal tilt greater than 20°
  - Initial displacement (fragment translation) greater than 1 cm
  - Initial radial shortening greater than 5 mm
  - Intra-articular disruption
  - Associated ulna fracture
  - Severe osteoporosis.
- Other factors that influence the stability of distal radius fractures are:
  - Radiocarpal intra-articular involvement
  - Age of the patient.

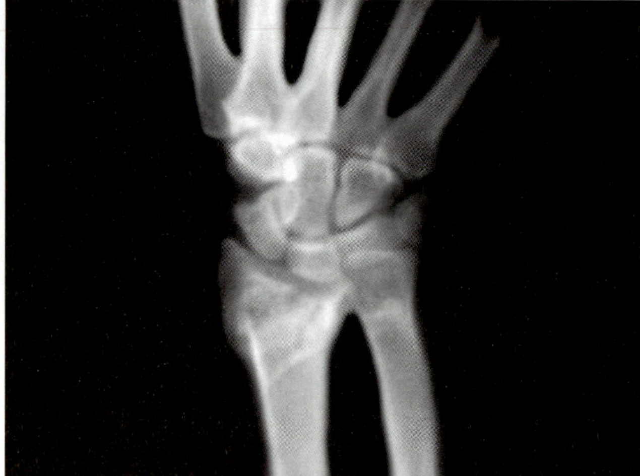

Fig. 191: Distal radial fracture before percutaneous pinning.

Associated Injuries

- Open fractures
- Bilateral distal radius fractures
- Ipsilateral concomitant fractures of upper extremity
- Carpal bone fractures and dislocations
- Acute median nerve dysfunction
- Raised compartment pressures.

Percutaneous Pinning

Indications

- Younger patients who have reduced or reducible fractures with predicted or proven instability
- Fractures without significant shortening, comminution of the volar cortex and that have failed closed reduction or redisplaced with regards to dorsal angulation.

Technique

- Percutaneous pinning is performed with adequate anesthesia, fluoroscopy, and a sterile operating environment. Techniques can be broadly classified into:
  - Extrafocal
  - Intrafocal (passing through the fracture site).
- Irrespective of the preferred method of fixation, the selected technique should achieve fracture stability, minimize injury to nerves, vessels, and tendons as well as avoid injury to the articular surface. This technique is illustrated in Figures 191 to 194.

Complications

Includes those previously described in nonoperative treatment as well as those directly attributed to the use of percutaneous pins such as:

- Tendon tethering, injury, or rupture
- Pin migration

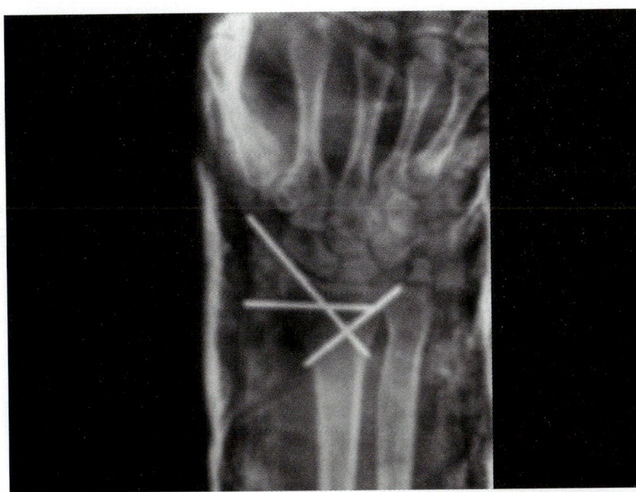

Fig. 192: Distal radial fracture after percutaneous pinning.

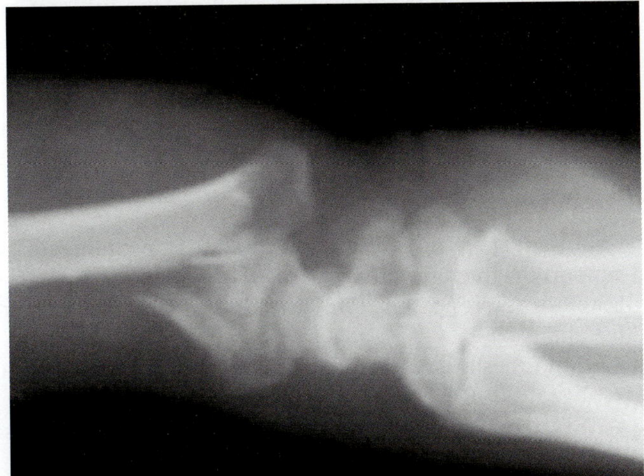

Fig. 193: Distal radial fracture before percutaneous pinning (lateral view).

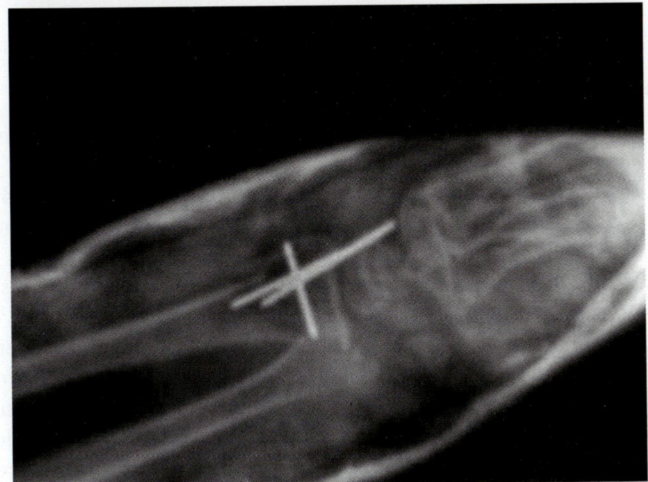

Fig. 194: Distal radial fracture after percutaneous pinning lateral view.

- Nerve injury
- Pin site infection
- Superficial radial nerve irritation and injury.

Summary

- Percutaneous pinning demonstrates good reproducible outcomes with minimal risk in appropriately selected fracture patterns. It is well suited for younger patients who have unstable, but reducible extra or intra-articular distal radial fractures.
- This technique can provide adequate fracture stability and soft tissue and vascular preservation in addition to minimal patient morbidity, which may facilitate a more rapid return to function compared with more invasive methods of treatment.

TABLE 13: Complications and incidences of distal radius fractures.

Complication	*Incidence*
Ligament damage	98%
Arthritis or arthrosis	7–65%
Loss of motion (marked deformity, decreased ROM)	2–31%
Osteomyelitis	4–9%
Malunion	5%
Others like delayed union, nerve compression, neuritis hardware complications tendon rupture, radioulnar disturbance.	0.5–1.2%

COMPLICATIONS AND MANAGEMENT OF DISTAL RADIUS FRACTURES

Introduction

- Fractures occur at the distal end of the radius more commonly than at any other location. They comprise about 10–12% of all fractures. The reported complication rate varies from 6% to 60%.
- McKay and colleagues reviewed the overall incidence of complications after distal radius fracture in their literature and subsequently in their series of 250 consecutive patients treated for distal radius fractures. The results are shown in Table 13.

Immediate Complications

- Nerve injury
- Open injury
- Compartment syndrome
- Skin injury during manipulation
- Missed associated injury.

Nerve Injury

- Incidence of nerve injuries varies from 0 to17%
- The median nerve is the most commonly involved, followed by the radial and the ulnar nerves (Fig. 195)
- The radial nerve's sensory branch is particularly vulnerable to injury during the K-wire fixation, as the nerve exists beneath the dense fascia between the tendons of brachioradialis and extensor carpi radialis longus
- Neuromas in this area are particularly troublesome because they can be irritated by rubbing against shirt cuffs, watches, and bracelets.

Carpal Tunnel Syndrome

- Acute carpal tunnel syndrome is more common in patients, who have more severe and comminuted fractures. It may also occur in those people, who undergo multiple closed reduction attempts

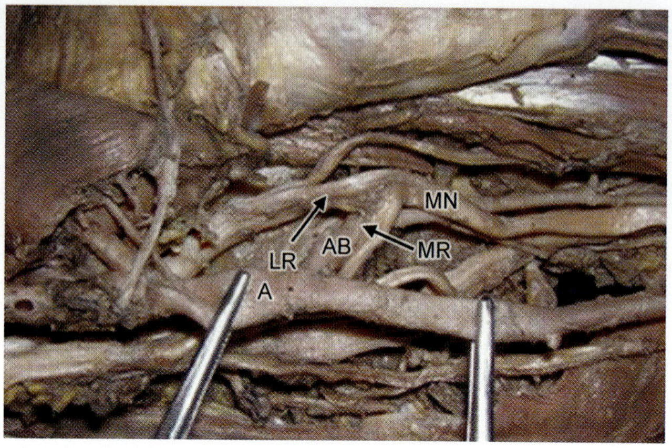

Fig. 195: Dissection showing median nerve and adjoining structures. (A: third part of axillary artery; AB: anomalous branch; MR: medial root of median nerve; LR: lateral root of median nerve; MN: median nerve).

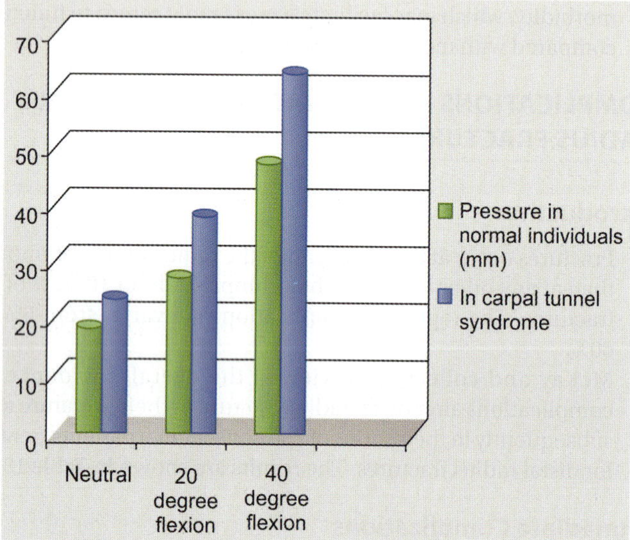

Fig. 196: Carpal tunnel pressure variations, as studied by Gelberman and colleagues.

- Gelberman and colleagues studied the mean carpal tunnel pressures and made the graph shown in Figure 196.

How to avoid?

- Careful examination of the patients to rule out neurological injury
- Splinting and casting to be avoided in extreme wrist flexion
- Encourage patients to keep the hand elevated and actively flex and extend their fingers
- In patients with significant hand and wrist swellings splints or bivalved casts should be used rather than circumferential casts
- If symptoms get worse then surgical intervention must be considered as early release has a better long-term outcome.

Open Injury

- They are infrequent and the largest reported series of open fractures included 18 consecutive patients collected over 8 years
- Type I Gustilo and Anderson injuries were most common with an incidence of 50% followed by Type III with 34% and lastly Type II with 16%. Four patients in this series had nerve and tendon injuries and two had vascular injuries
- They were promptly irrigated and debrided, intravenous antibiotics were given and tetanus status was assessed in emergency. Fracture was stabilized and patients were subjected to multiple operative procedures
- Eight out of 18 patients developed postoperative infections (five soft tissues and three osteomyelitis) and five developed a nonunion.

Early Complications (Less than 6 Weeks)

- Cast issues
- Loss of reduction
- Infection
- Tendon rupture.

Cast Issues

- Depending upon the degree of swelling, the full cast and noncircumferential splint should be applied
- Cast should support the fracture and permit free movement of the fingers and thumb
- Patient should be encouraged to exercise the fingers, to prevent stiffness and reduce the risk of dystrophy.

Loss of Reduction

- Charnley's three-point fixation technique is recommended to support the fracture within the cast
- MacKenney reported following findings in case of early instability:
  - Ten times more common in patients, more than 80 years age
  - Six times more common in fractures with dorsal comminution
  - Five times more common in fractures maintaining 5–10° of dorsal angulation
  - Greater risk of displacement with percutaneous K-wire in older individuals and fractures with dorsal comminution.

Infection

- Compound fractures and fractures treated operative are at risk for infection
- Largest reported series of compound fractures reported 44% infection rate with 62% of infections involving the soft tissues and 38% as osteomyelitis
- A randomized trial reported that burning K-wire percutaneously reduces the risk of infection by half
- Percutaneous K-wires should not be used to supplement internal fixation because this can act as a pathway for superficial infection to spread to the deeper tissues and bone
- Soft tissue infections should be treated with oral antibiotics and those involving the bone; causing osteomyelitis requires surgical intervention.

Tendon Rupture

- It may occur as an early or as a late complication.
- Extensor pollicis longus tendon is the most commonly ruptured tendon (Fig. 197).
- The ruptured tendon usually cannot be repaired and function can be well restored by performing an extensor indicis proprius transfer.

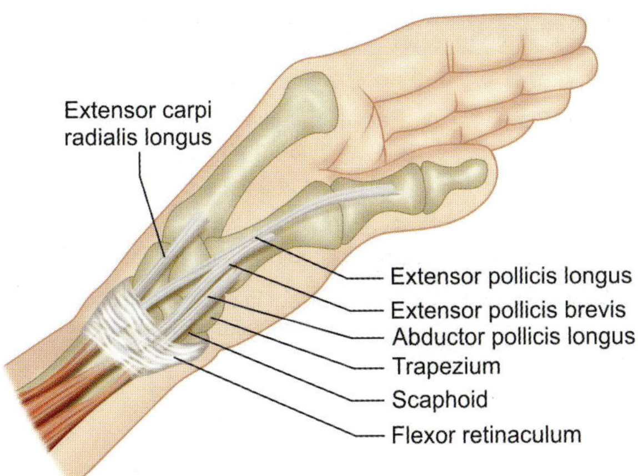

Fig. 197: Different tendons of hand.

Late Complications (More than 6 Weeks)

- Nerve complications and CRPS
- Arthrosis
- Nonunion or delayed union
- Malunion.

Complex Regional Pain Syndrome

- It refers to a pattern of symptoms and signs that are disproportionate to those from the degree of trauma, leading to functional impairment. It was formerly referred to as reflex sympathetic dystrophy (RSD) and symptoms include:
  - Increased pain
  - Swelling, stiffness, discoloration, and hyperhidrosis
  - Osteoporosis.
- The condition was first observed by Mitchell, Morehouse, and Keen in 1867. Mitchell coined the term "Causalgia", a Greek word meaning, "burning pain".
- Other eponyms in the literature are Sudeck's atrophy, shoulder-hand syndrome, and Leriche post-traumatic pain syndrome.
- The CRPS type I now replaces RSD and CRPS type II replaces causalgia.
- Various theories have been proposed including short-circuiting effects at the area of injury, permitting irritation of the sensory afferent fibers by the efferent sympathetic impulses, periarteritis involving the vessels around the injured neural segments and abnormal feedback into the internuncial centers of the spinal cord.
- Lankford stated that the following triad must be present to develop RSD:
  - Persistent painful stimulus
  - Diathesis (inherent sympathetic overactivity or insecure fearful personality)
  - Abnormal sympathetic reflex.

Classification:

- Lankford further classified RSD in order of increasing severity as shown in Table 14.

Clinical features:

- Excruciating burning pain often described as having superimposed throbbing, aching, bursting pressure with a knifelike stabbing, twisting, or crushing component. It usually begins around the first week.

TABLE 14: Lankford classification of reflex sympathetic dystrophy (RSD).

Type	*Cause*
Minor causalgia	Injury to purely sensory nerve, cutaneous branch of median, and radial nerve
Minor traumatic dystrophy	Minor crush injuries, sprains, and fractures
Shoulder-hand syndrome	Proximal injury to neck, chest, shoulder, or visceral lesion like cervical disk, heart attack, stroke, and pancoast tumor
Major traumatic dystrophy	Severe crush injuries or Colles' fracture
Major causalgia	After injury to major mixed nerve (median nerve)

- Clinical picture in early stage is that of pain and vasomotor instability with sympathetic overactivity, edema, redness, increased warmth, hyperhidrosis, and stiffness.
- Intermediate stage starts by around third month and is characterized by pale and dry extremity with increasing stiffness and trophic changes. Patient may be comfortable at rest but pain persists on motion.
- Late stage is seen around the end of first year and is characterized by stiff, cool, atrophic, and osteoporotic extremity.

Investigations:

- Three-phase radionucleotide bone scan can aid in early diagnosis. A diffusely increased uptake in the delayed images was found to be diagnostic of RSD with a sensitivity of 96% and specificity of 98%.
- In severe causalgia, local anesthetic block of the second and third sympathetic ganglia also confirms the diagnosis.

Treatment of CRPS:

- No specific treatment.
- Early sympathetic (Stellate ganglion) block with physical therapy is widely recommended.
- Surgical preganglionic sympathectomy in resistant cases.

Arthrosis

- A review of patients at a mean of 6.7 years after an intra-articular fracture of the distal radius fractures found that 65% had radiographic evidence of post-traumatic arthrosis.
- Fractures with residual radiocarpal incongruity had a higher rate of radiographic arthrosis.
- It is a challenge in young patients and treatment options include activity modification, oral analgesics, splinting, or surgery.
- Surgical options include partial or complete wrist fusions with arthroplasty.

Nonunion or Delayed Union

- Fractures with no radiographic signs of bridging trabeculae across the fracture site at 4 months are categorized as delayed unions and as nonunions after 6 months, although later is uncommon.
- Factors affecting it are open fractures, severe comminution, infection, devascularization of the bone ends, overdistraction of fracture, with inadequate stabilization, diabetes, prolapsed vertebral disk (PVD), peripheral neuropathy, smoking, and alcoholism.

- Diagnosis may be confirmed through mobility of the fracture noted on lateral radiographs of wrists in dorsiflexion and volar flexion. Computed tomography (CT) scan helps to confirm diagnosis and surgical planning.
- Surgical treatment includes wrist arthrodesis or bone grafting stabilization with internal fixation as a single stage procedure or primary distraction lengthening with tenotomy of brachioradialis with secondary stabilization and bone grafting.

Malunion and Its Management

Despite improved treatment since early 1980s, malunion remains to be a common cause of residual disability after distal radius fractures. It can be caused due to failure to achieve or maintain an accurate reduction or by inadequate duration or type of immobilization. It is associated with extra-articular deformities, intra-articular malalignment, distal radioulnar incongruity or instability, or a combination of these features.

Clinical evaluation:

- Pain, stiffness, weakness, and cosmetic deformity are common complaints in patients with distal radial malunion
- Decreased wrist flexion is typical in dorsally tilted malunions and extension is limited with volarly tilted malunions. Loss of RI may cause impaired ulnar deviation. Incongruity at DRUJ leads to decreased pronation and supination with supination more affected
- Grip strength is impaired because of a combination of pain and altered wrist mechanics.

Radiographic evaluation:

- Plain anteroposterior and lateral radiographs of both wrists are in neutral rotation. Uninjured wrist is used as a template for surgical reconstruction, if osteotomy is chosen.
- The CT scan to evaluate potential for conguity of the DRUJ and malunions of ulnar styloid.
- Magnetic resonance imaging (MRI) or arthrography can be used to evaluate the integrity of the TFCC and intercarpal ligaments.
- Radiographic criteria are shown in Table 15.

TABLE 15: Radiographic criteria.

Radiographic criteria	*Acceptable measurement*
Radioulnar length	Radial shortening of <5 mm at distal radioulnar joint compared with contralateral wrist
Radial inclination	Inclination of >15° on posteroanterior film
Radial tilt	Sagittal tilt on lateral projection between 15° dorsal tilt and 20° volar tilt
Articular incongruity	Incongruity of intra-articular fracture < 2 mm at radiocarpal joint

Operative treatment: Procedures used to treat malunions of the distal radius fall into three general categories:

1. Correction of deformity of radius by intra-articular and extra-articular osteotomies.
2. Treatment of pathology of DRUJ by ulnar shortening, hemiresection arthroplasty, Sauve-Kapandji procedure, and Darrach resection of distal ulna.
3. Salvage procedures like partial and total wrist arthrodesis, total wrist arthroplasty, and proximal row carpectomy.
   - *Extra-articular malunion with dorsal angulation (Figs. 198 and 199)*
     - Osteotomy and grafting are the most commonly performed procedure and are indicated in patients younger than 45 years. It can be performed in older patients with good bone quality and high functional demands.
     - Contraindications are active RSD, acceptable function despite deformity, poor soft tissue envelope, severe osteopenia, and advanced radiocarpal or intercarpal arthritis.
     - Wrist is immobilized for 2 weeks in a volar plaster splint and 2 weeks ROM exercises are begun. No lifting work is allowed until osteotomy has healed radiographically.

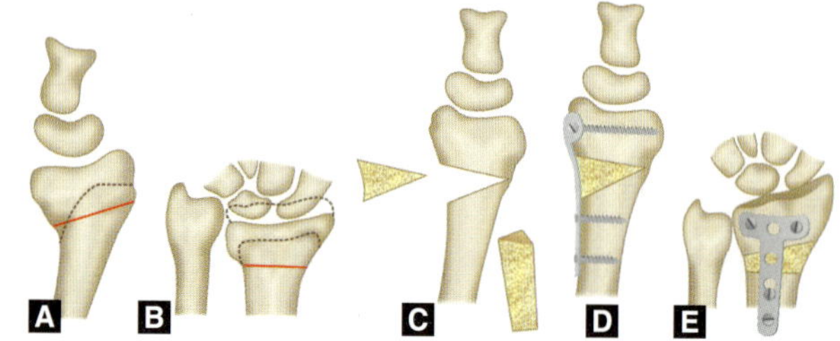

Figs. 198A to E: Fernandez technique of osteotomy and grafting of distal radius—(A and B) site of osteotomy is marked; (C) Osteotomy is opened dorsally and graft is prepared; (D and E) Graft is inserted and plate applied.

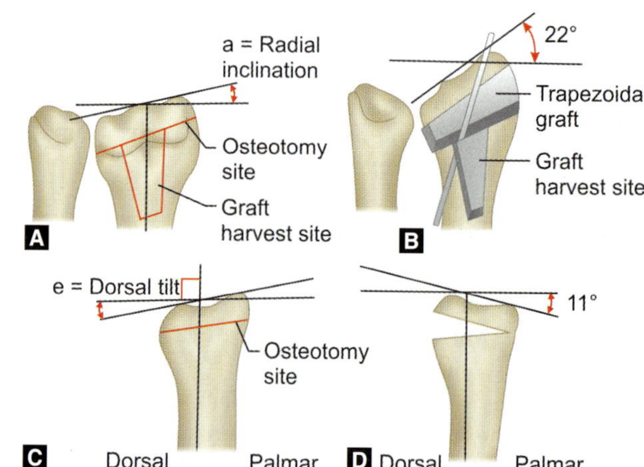

Figs. 199A to D: Trapezoidal osteotomy of distal radius—(A) Preoperative posteroanterior view with decreased radial inclination, osteotomy and trapezoidal graft site are outlined; (B) Postoperative posteroanterior view shows normal radial tilt and single "caging" pin; (C) Abnormal dorsal tilt of radial articular surface reverses all loads across carpals and does not tolerate loading in active patients; (D) Postoperative lateral view shows restorations of 11° of palmar tilt before insertion of graft.

   - *Extra-articular malunion with volar angulation (Figs. 200A to E):*
     - Indications and contraindications are similar to that of dorsal osteotomy and plating
     - Volar open wedge osteotomy with bone grafting and plating is advocated
     - Postoperational volar splint for 2 weeks should be advised. If lengthening of 10 mm or more is necessary, then 6 weeks or below elbow cast is worn. Activities against resistance and manual labor are not permitted until union has been confirmed radiographically.

External fixator:

- Melendez advocated a technique of opening wedge osteotomy, bone grafting, and external fixation for symptomatic extra-articular distal radius malunions

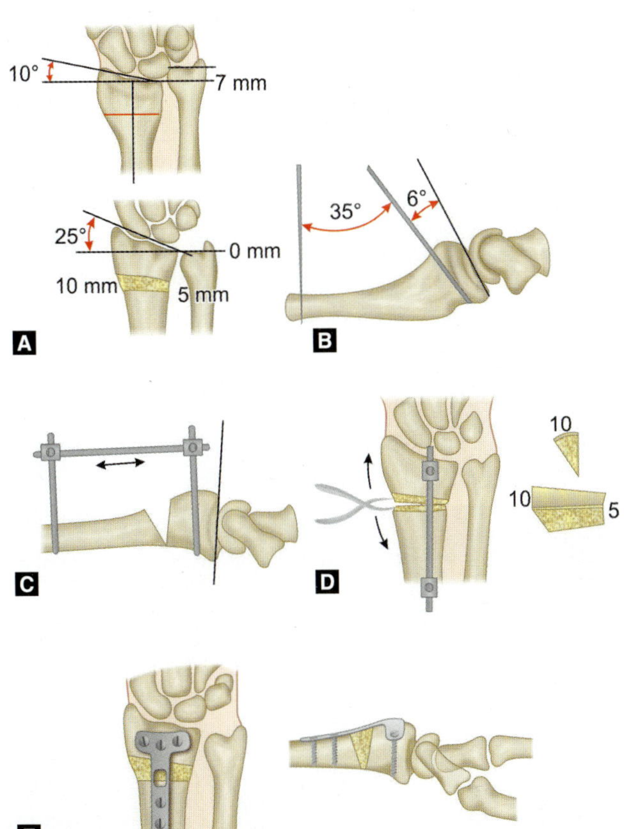

Figs. 200A to E: Volar osteotomy for malunited distal radial fracture—(A) Preoperative planning; (B) K-wire drilled into radial shaft proximal to osteotomy site; (C) Fixator used to maintain corrected alignment; (D) Osteotomy wedged open with lamina; (E) Iliac graft inserted and osteotomy stabilized with T-plate.

- All osteotomies healed at around 7.5 weeks, pain was reduced and mobility was increased, with improved radiographic parameters in all patients
- Postoperative motion was average 88% of that of contralateral wrist
- Contraindications to the technique include osteoporosis, greater than 8 mm radial shortening, intra-articular malunions, and malunions associated with radiocarpal and midcarpal arthritis.

Intra-articular malunions:

- They lead to functional disability and the procedures in this group are divided into:
  - Prevent post-traumatic arthritis (osteotomies).
  - Salvage procedures (carpal arthrodesis, proximal row carpectomy, and wrist arthroplasty).
  - Intra-articular osteotomies are indicated in young, active patients with high functional demands, greater than 2 mm step-off, and no evidence of post-traumatic arthritis. Contraindications are advanced osteoarthritis, massive articular comminution, poor bone quality, low functional demands, RSD, and poor soft tissue coverage.

Triangular Fibrocartilage Complex Abnormalities (See Fig. 4)

It begins on ulnar side of lunate fossa of radius and attaches to ulnar head and base of ulnar styloid.

Box 1: Classification of TFCC abnormalities.

Class 1 Traumatic
- Central perforation
- Ulnar avulsion
  - With distal ulnar fracture
  - Without distal ulnar fracture
- Distal avulsion
- Radial avulsion:
  - With sigmoid notch fracture
  - Without sigmoid notch fracture

Class 2 Degenerative (Ulnocarpal abutment syndrome)
- TFCC wear
- TFCC wear
  - Plus lunate and/or ulnar chondromalacia
- TFCC perforation
  - Plus lunate and/or ulnar chondromalacia
- TFCC perforation
  - Plus lunate and/or ulnar chondromalacia
  - Plus lunotriquetral ligament perforation
- TFCC perforation
  - Plus lunate and/or ulnar chondromalacia
  - Plus lunotriquetral ligament perforation
  - Plus ulnocarpal arthritis

Components:
- Volar and dorsal radioulnar ligament
- Ulnar collateral ligament
- Meniscal homologue
- Articular disk
- Extensor carpi ulnaris sheath
- Ulnolunate ligament
- Lunotriquetral ligament.

Functions:
- Stable radioulnar connection
- Stable ulnocarpal connection
- Mechanism for transmitting forces from hand
- Suspensory ligament function for ulnar side of carpus from radius
- Extending dividing surface for proximal row across distal end of forearm bones.

Classification:

Triangular fibrocartilage complex abnormalities are illustrated in Box 1 and Figures 201 to 203.

Treatment:

Arthroscopic treatment (Figs. 204 and 205): Arthroscopic debridement only in negative ulnar variance and arthroscopic debridement with ulnar head debridement in neutral ulnar variance and with ulnar shortening osteotomy in positive ulnar variance.

Wafer resection (Feldon):
- *Indications*
  - The TFCC tear (Fig. 204)
  - Ulnar impaction syndrome (Fig. 206)

Treatment modalities of DRUJ:
- Ulnar hemiresection interposition arthroplasty (Bowers) (Fig. 206)
- Matched resection (Watson)

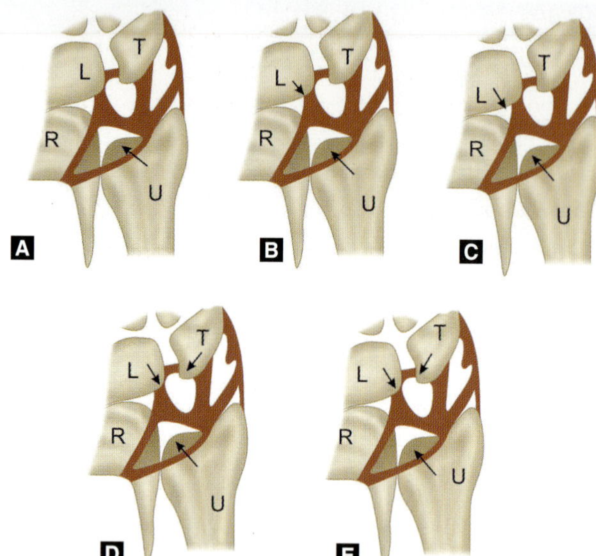

Figs. 201A to E: Diagrammatic representation of degenerative or class 2 abnormalities of the triangular fibrocartilage complex (TFCC)—(A) Class 2A TFCC wear (arrow); (B) Class 2B, TFCC wear with lunate (small arrow) and/or ulnar (long arrow) chondromalacia; (C) Class 2C, TFCC perforation with lunate (small arrow) and/or ulnar (long arrow) chondromalacia; (D) Class 2D, TFCC perforation with lunate (arrow) and/or ulnar (long arrow) chondromalacia and lunotriquetral ligament perforation (small arrows); (E) Class 2E, TFCC perforation with lunate (arrow) and/or ulnar (long arrow) chondromalacia, lunotriquetral ligament perforation (small arrows) and ulnocarpal arthritis. (L: lunate; R: radius; T: triquetrum; U: ulna)

- Milch cuff resection
- Ulnar shortening procedures—Darrach resection
- Distal radioulnar arthrodesis with distal ulnar pseudoarthrosis (Sauve-Kapandji)
- Procedures to stabilize DRUJ.

Ulnar hemiresection interposition arthroplasty (Bowers) indications:
- Unreconstructable fractures of ulnar head
- Ulnocarpal impingement syndrome
- Rheumatoid arthritis
- Chronic painful TFCC tear
- Post-traumatic and osteoarthritis.

Matched resection (Watson) (See Fig. 177): Matched distal ulnar resection. Ulna is resected 5-6 cm and shaped to match contour of radius through full supination and pronation. Distal resected ulna should be at level of radial articular surface. Large cancellous surface adheres to ulnar sling mechanism.
- *Indications:*
  - Rheumatoid arthritis
  - Trauma.

Milch cuff resection (Figs. 207A to C) indications:
- Malunited Colles' fracture
- Malunion or nonunion of radius
- Cessation or abnormality of growth of distal radius.

Ulnar shortening procedures—Darrach resection indications:
- Malunited Colles' fracture
- Malunion or nonunion of radius
- Abnormality of growth of distal radius.

Distal radioulnar arthrodesis with distal ulnar pseudarthrosis (Sauve-Kapandji) (Figs. 208A and B)

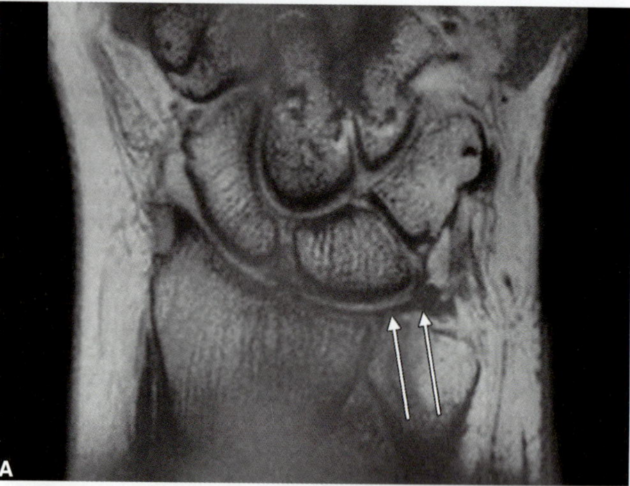

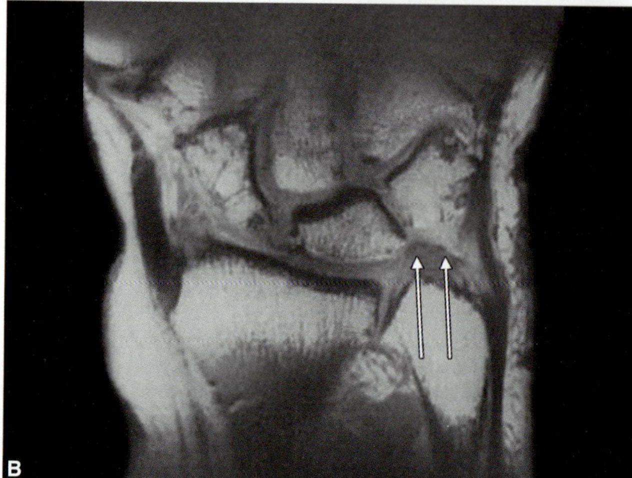

Figs. 202A and B: T1 weighted imaging of the triangular fibrocartilage complex (TFCC), which appears black (arrows)—(A) Normal TFCC: uniform black image extending from the ulnar aspect of the distal radius ulnarward over the ulnar head; (B) Abnormal appearance of the TFCC over the ulnar head as it appears to have lifted from its origin off the radius.

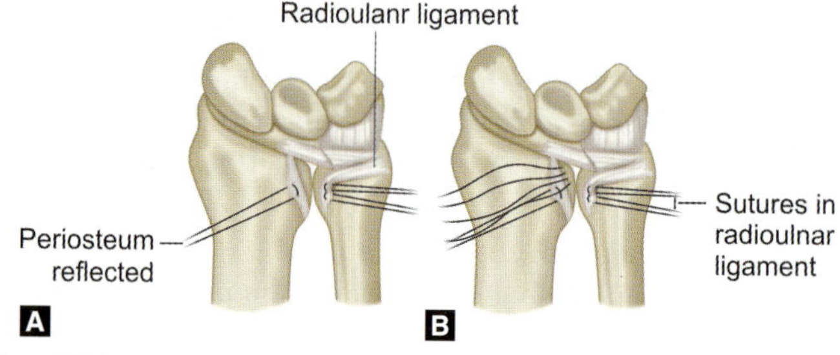

Figs. 203A and B: Open repair of class 1D injuries of triangular fibrocartilage complex (TFCC)—(A) Approach to TFCC, reflection of dorsal radioulnar ligament and periosteum over lunate fossa; and (B) Suture placement into TFCC through holes drills in dorsoulnar aspect of distal radius.

- *Indications:*
  - Painful wrist by previous surgery
  - Traumatic arthritis
  - Rheumatoid arthritis.

Procedures to stabilize DRUJ:
- *Indications:*
  - After undetected dislocation
  - After surgical procedure to resect distal ulna.

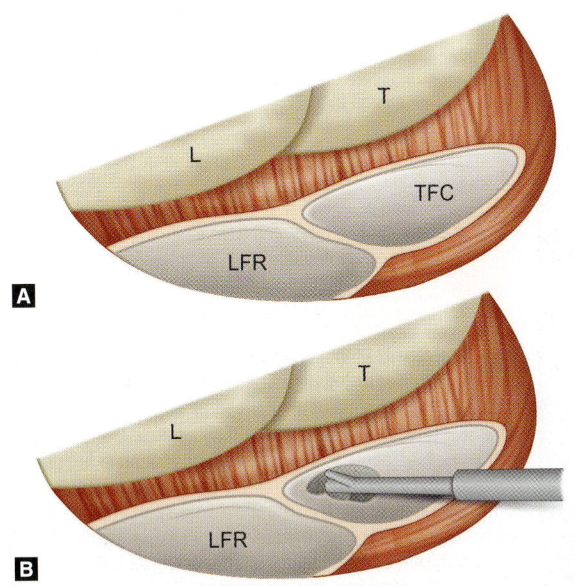

Figs. 204A and B: Arthroscopic debridement of chronic triangular fibrocartilage (TFC) tears. (L: lunate; LFR: lunate facet of radius; T: triquetrum)

- *Methods:*
  - Radioulnar tenodesis (Figs. 209A to H)
  - Reconstruction of dorsal ligament of TFCC (Scheker)
  - Radioulnar tenodesis procedures using ECU, EDC and EDM.
- *Salvage procedures (Figs. 210A to D):*
  - Wrist arthrodesis, partial, and total
  - Total wrist arthroplasty (Fig. 211)
  - Proximal row carpectomy (Figs. 212A and B).

Future trends:

Future trends are as follows (Figs. 213 to 219):

- Computer-assisted surgeries (Figs. 213A to D)
- Bone graft alternates like carbonated hydroxyapatite and calcium phosphate (Figs. 214A to D)
- Volar fixed-angle plate osteosynthesis (Figs. 215 to 217).
  - *Computer-assisted surgeries (Figs. 213 to 216)*
  - Volar fixed angle plates (Fig. 217).

Summary

Symptomatic distal radius malunion algorithms are explained in Flowcharts 1 to 3.

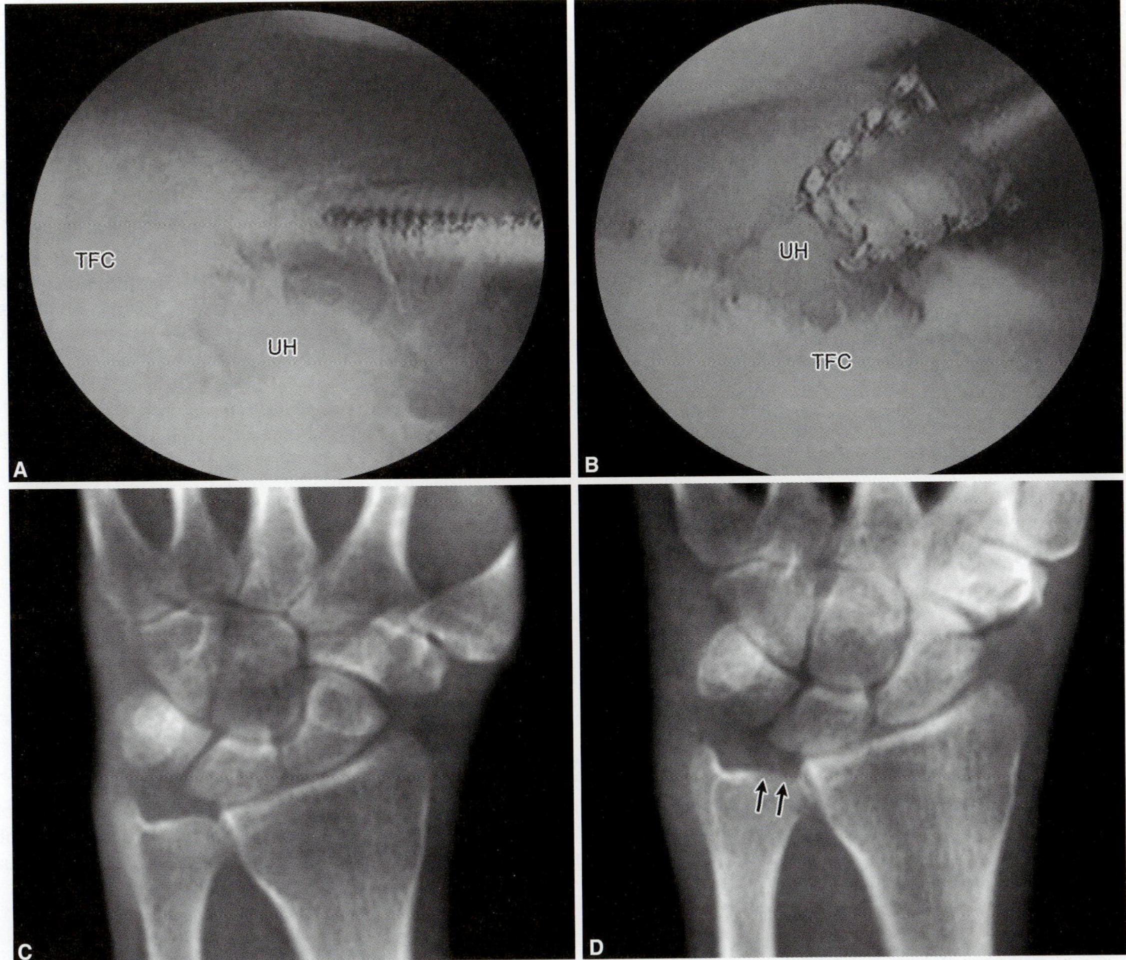

Figs. 205A to D: Arthroscopic Wafer procedure—(A) Arthroscopic view via the radiocarpal portal; (B) Note the better visualization of the ulnar head through the debrided central perforation of the TFCC; (C and D) Preoperative and postoperative radiographs respectively of a patient who underwent an arthroscopic Wafer procedure as a treatment for ulnar impaction syndrome (arrows point to the ulnar head). (TFC: triangular fibrocartilage; TFCC: triangular fibrocartilage complex; UH: ulnar head)

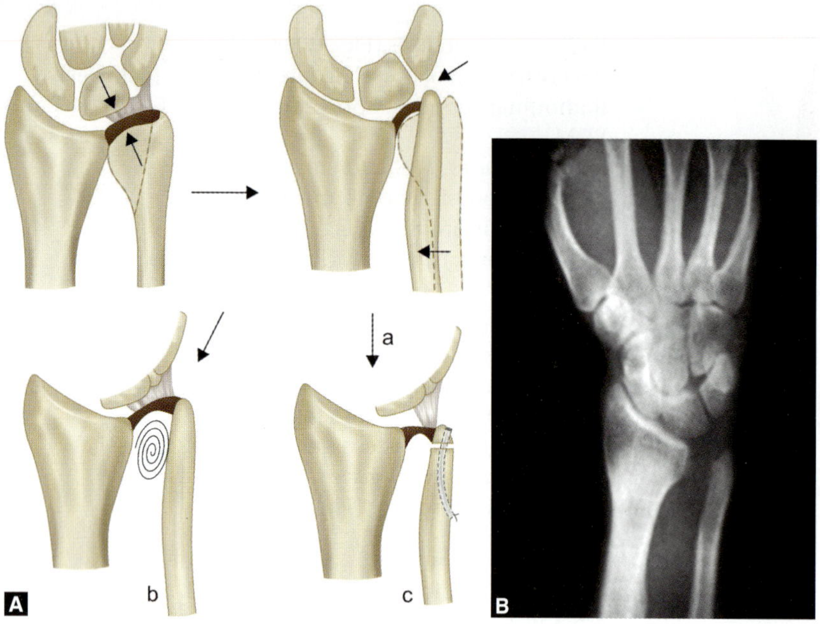

Figs. 206A and B: (A) Hemiresection technique of arthroplasty employed in treatment of the ulnocarpal impingement syndrome. In view "a", the still too-long ulna produces stylocarpal impingement, a condition caused by approximation of the radius and ulna that occurs when the articular dome is removed. To obviate this complication, interposition "b" or shortening "c" is necessary. In every instance in which the hemiresection technique is employed, intraoperative consideration of this possible complication is mandatory; (B) Postoperative radiograph showing the usual case, i.e. no interposition or shortening is necessary.

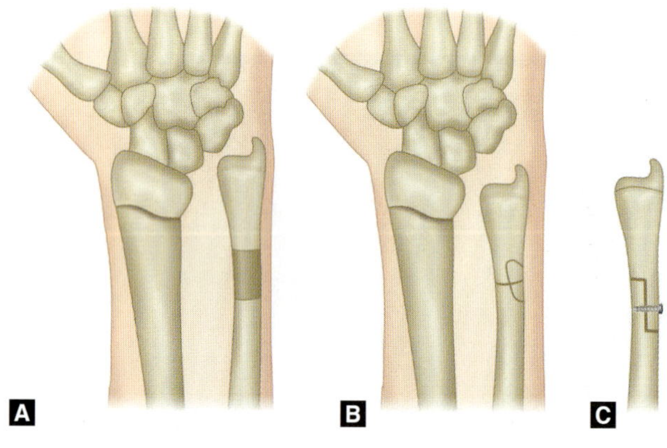

Figs. 207A to C: Milch cuff resection of ulna—(A) Shaded area indicates bone to be resected; (B) Ends of ulna apposed, correcting disproportion in length of radius and ulna; and (C) More stable fixation secured by step-cut procedure and fixation with one screw.

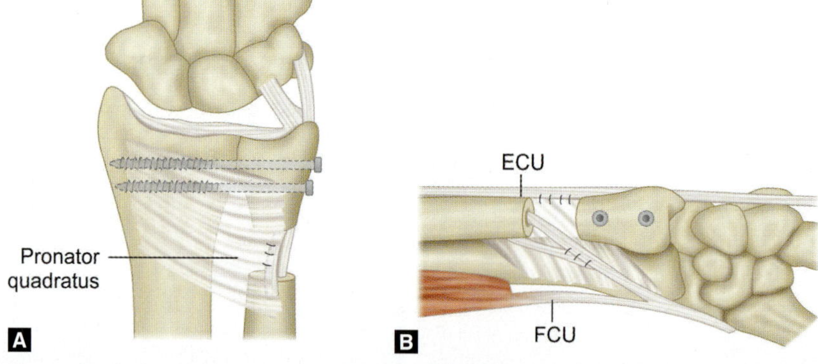

Figs. 208A and B: Distal radioulnar arthrodesis with distal ulnar pseudarthrosis (modified Sauvé-Kapandji procedure)—(A) Posterior view of wrist with two screws fixing ulnar head to sigmoid notch; after resection, gap, which measures 10 mm, is filled with pronator quadratus; (B) Lateral view of wrist showing stabilization of proximal ulnar segment with distally based slip of flexor carpi ulnaris tendon (FCU). Nonunion gap is filled with pronator quadratus, which is sutured to tendon sheath of extensor carpi ulnaris muscle (ECU).

The treatment of distal radius malunions is continually evolving. The advent of new computer technologies, plating systems and bone graft substitutes will likely have a significant impact upon the way distal radius malunions are corrected in the near future. But prevention of malunions through optimal fracture management remains the best option.

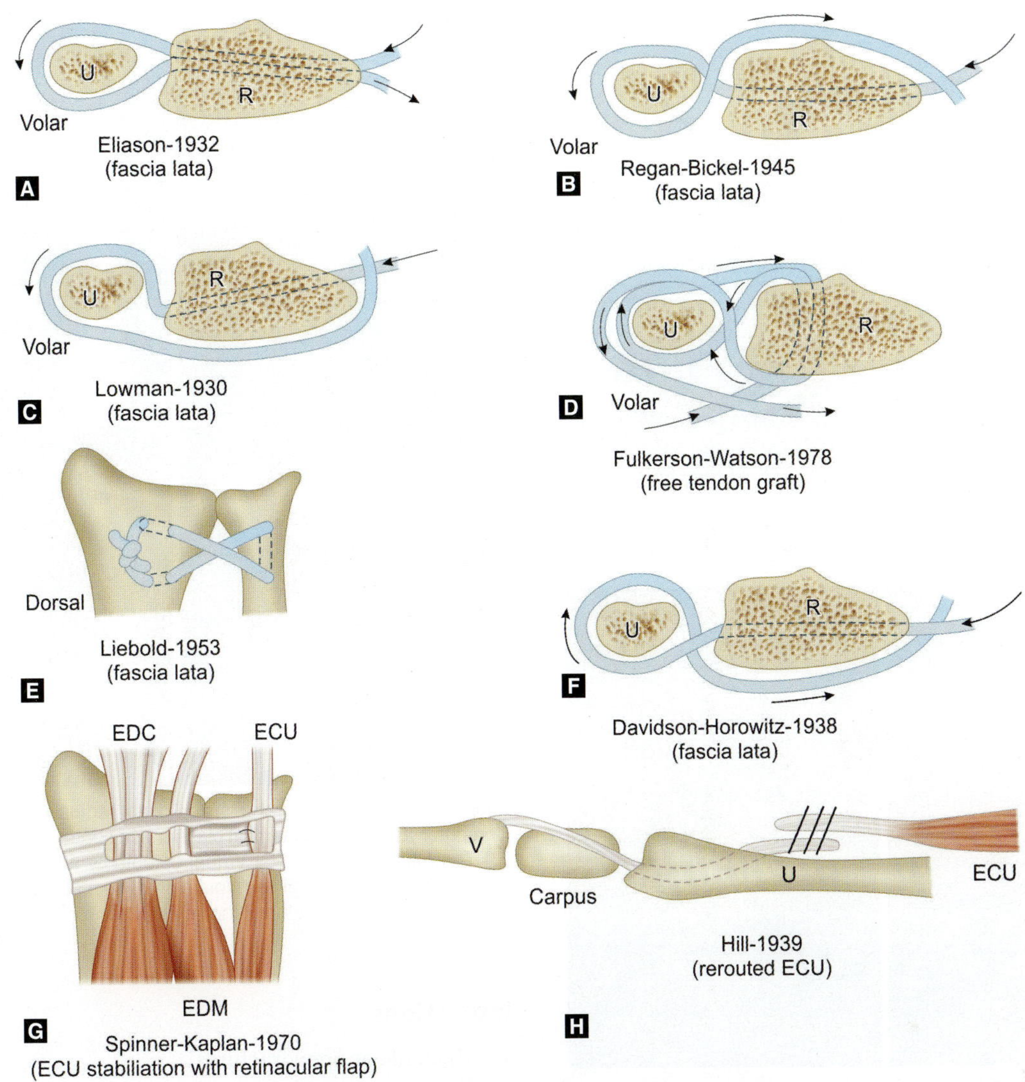

Figs. 209A to H: Different methods of radioulnar tenodesis.
(ECU: extensor carpi ulnaris muscle; EDC: extensor digitorum communis; EDM: extensor digitorum muscle

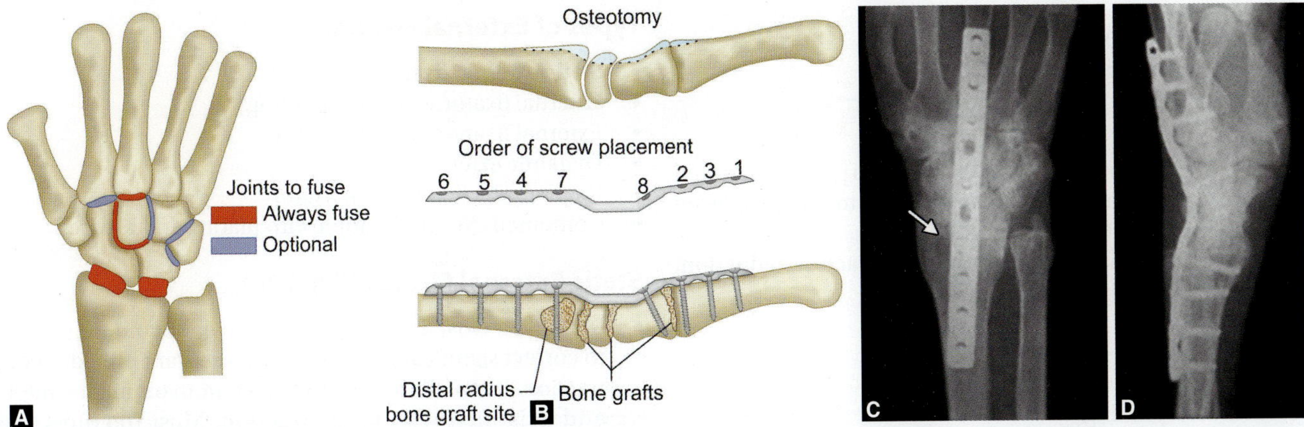

Figs. 210A to D: Wrist fusion with bone grafting and plate fixation—(A) Rigid fusion column through carpus to metacarpal must coincide with the plate placement. All joints spanned directly by plate should be fused if desired; (B) Dorsal cartilage is denuded and plate is applied from distal to proximal, spanning local radial bone graft augmentation; (C) and (D) Placement of 3.5 mm dynamic compression plate, note local distal radial bone graft portal (arrow) and thickness of plate distally.

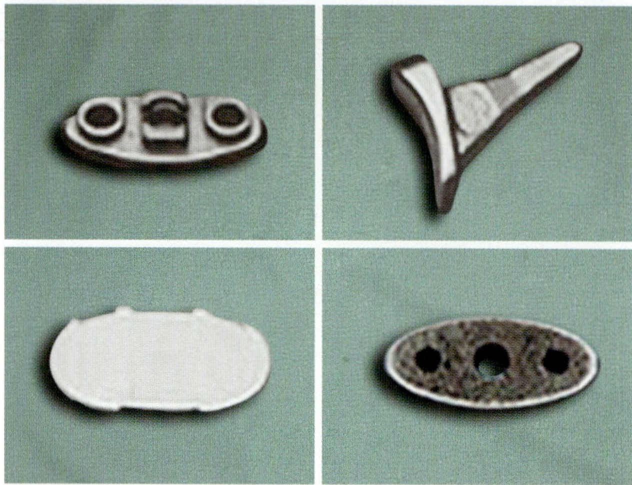

Fig. 211: Different types of Menon prosthesis.

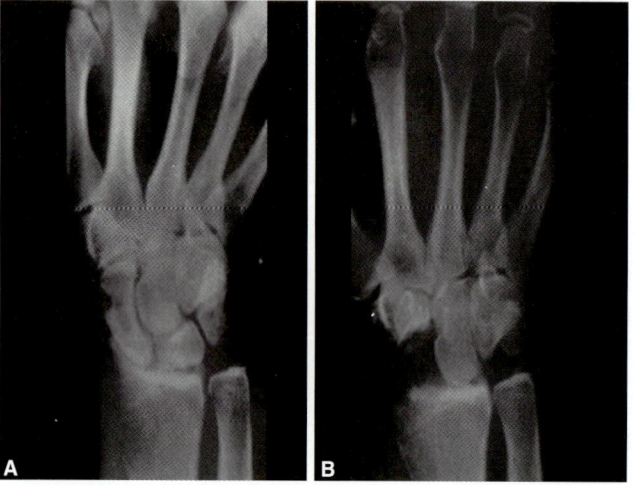

Figs. 212A and B: (A) Degenerative arthritis limited to the radioscaphoid and radiolunate joints; (B) Postoperative radiograph depicting proximal row carpectomy with radial styloidectomy.

EXTERNAL FIXATION OF DISTAL RADIUS FRACTURES

Introduction

They are the most common fractures that occur in patients between ages 15 and 75 years. Many methods are there for treating displaced distal radius fractures (Figs. 219 and 220).

All forms of treatment involve obtaining fracture reduction, which may then be maintained by:

- Casting
- Functional bracing
- External fixation
- Percutaneous pinning
- Internal fixation
- Combination of these methods.

We will be discussing the indications and techniques of fracture treatment with external fixation and when they are required, adjuvant with percutaneous pins.

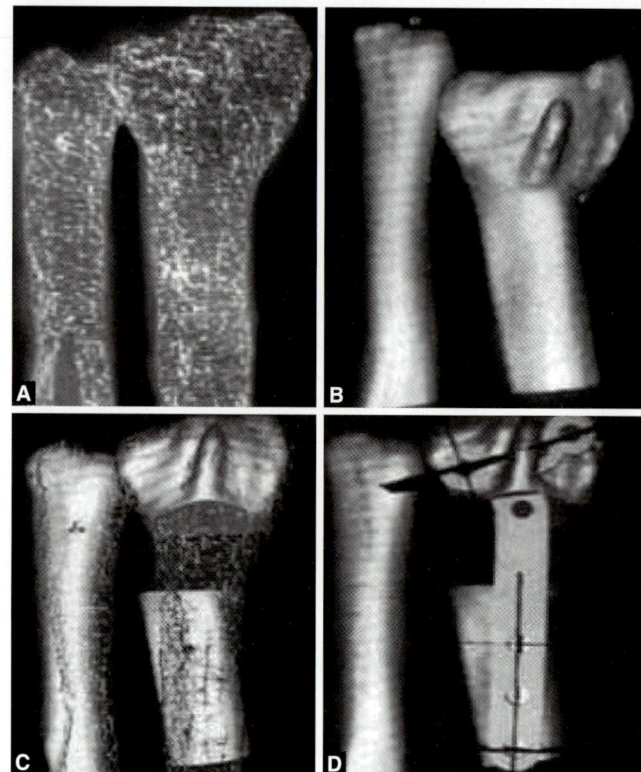

Figs. 213A to D: Computer-assisted distal radius osteotomy planning—(A) Computer-assisted 3-D surgical planner use contralateral wrist as a template; (B) The malunited wrist; (C) Virtual osteotomy and is aligned; and (D) The surgical planner then digitizes a plate onto the realigned radius and saves the coordinates and orientation of the screw holes for intraoperative referencing.

Indications

- Unstable or open fractures
- Fractures occurring in patients with multiple injuries
- Loss of reduction following closed orthopedic treatment
- Bilateral fractures of distal radius
- Acceptable reduction parameters are explained in the Table 16.

Types of External Fixation

- Static external fixator
- External fixator with bone grafting
- External fixation with distractor
- Dynamic external fixator
- Roger Anderson external fixator
- Combined external fixation with plating and K-wires.

Static External Fixator (Fig. 220)

- Initially, a closed reduction maneuver should be performed to correct significant deformity. An assistant provides counter traction at the elbow and the surgeon manipulates the hand and wrist first with inline traction. Most fractures can be reduced with slight volar and ulnar deviation of hand and wrist.
- When the provisional reduction is achieved, the external fixator can be applied. Two pins are inserted into the radial shaft proximal to the zone of injury in the posterolateral aspect of the middle third of radius.

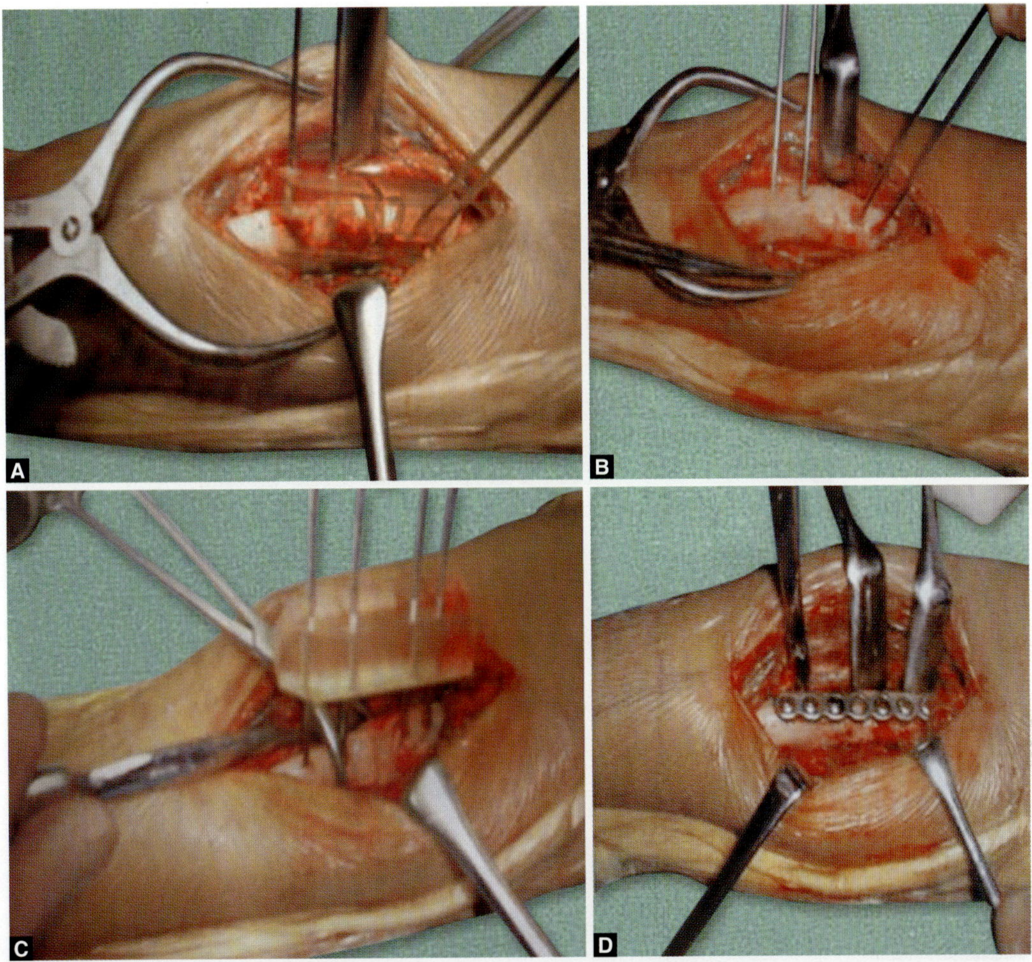

Figs. 214A to D: Bone graft alternates like carbonated hydroxyapatite and calcium phosphate fracture fixed with recon plate.

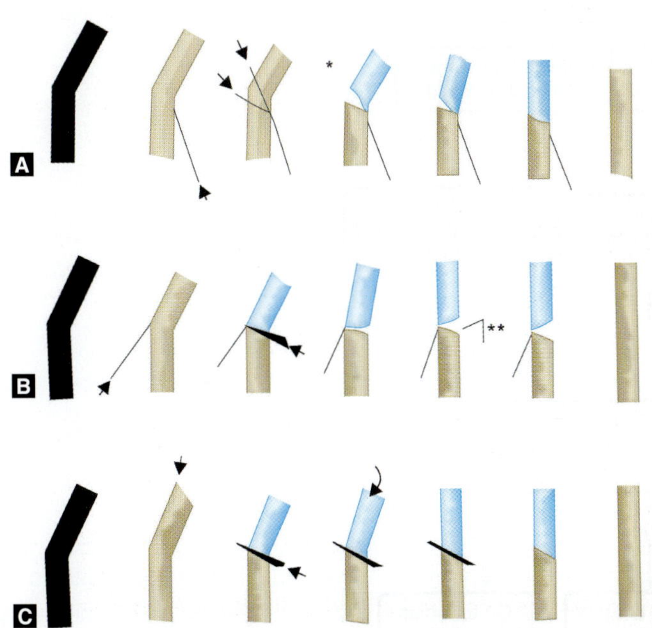

Figs. 215A to C: The bent cylinders represent the deformed bones. Different deformities can show a similar silhouette (the left figures of A, B, and C). The 3-D relationship between the bone and deformity axis (arrowhead of each figure) suggests the most appropriate methods of correction—(A) When the axis runs along the concave side of the deformity, a closing osteotomy after removal of a wedge (asterisk) brings about the rotation of the bone segment around the deformity axis, thereby completing the correction; (B) When the deformity axis is along the convex side, opening wedge osteotomy followed by wedge-shaped bone-grafting (double asterisks are considered appropriate); and (C) If the deformity axis is displaced from the bone, a closing or opening wedge osteotomy with shortening or lengthening is appropriate. The osteotomy planes are indicated by arrows.

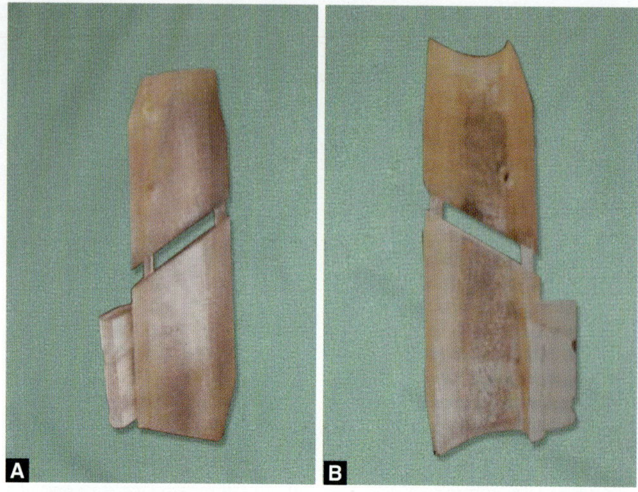

Figs. 216A and B: The osteotomy template was embodied as a real plastic model—(A) The surgeon's side; (B) The template.

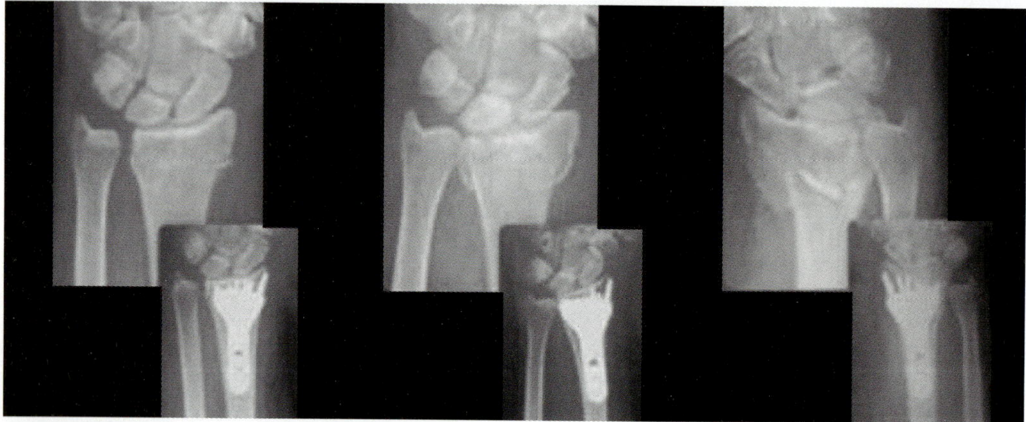

Fig. 217: Different types of volar fixed angle plates applied for correcting distal radial fractures abnormalities.

Flowchart 1: Symptomatic distal radius malunion algorithm number 1.

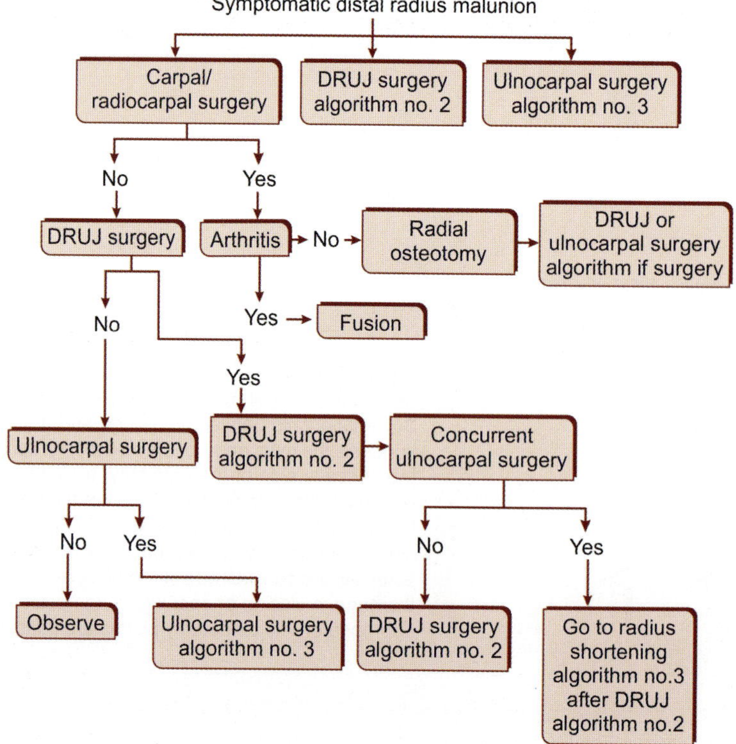

(DRUJ: distal radioulnar joint)

Flowchart 2: Symptomatic distal radius malunion algorithm number 2.

Symptomatic distal radius malunion
- Carpal/radiocarpal surgery algorithm no. 1
- DRUJ surgery
- Ulnocarpal surgery algorithm no. 3

DRUJ surgery
- DRUJ arthritis
- Incongruity → ROM
- Instability

ROM → Painful → (DRUJ arthritis pathway); ROM → Limited → <15° radius malangulation / Instability pathway

- Younger/aggressive → Suave-Kapandji Or Bowers/Watson
- Older/sedentary → Darrach Or Bowers/Watson
- <15° radius malangulation
- Young/active >15° radius malangulation → Corrective osteotomy radius → Persistent instability → Bowers/Watson ± PQ/ECU/FCU stabilization or Darrach
- <15° radius malangulation in young; All older/sedentary

Persistent instability → No → Persistent incongruity → Yes → Bowers/Watson or Suave–Kapandji

Persistent incongruity → No → End

(DRUJ: distal radioulnar joint; ROM: range of motion)

Flowchart 3: Symptomatic distal radius malunion algorithm number 3.

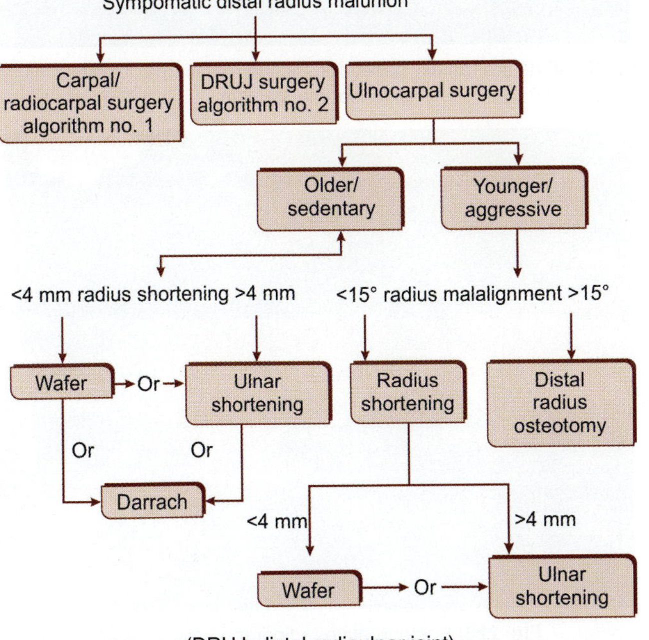

(DRUJ: distal radioulnar joint)

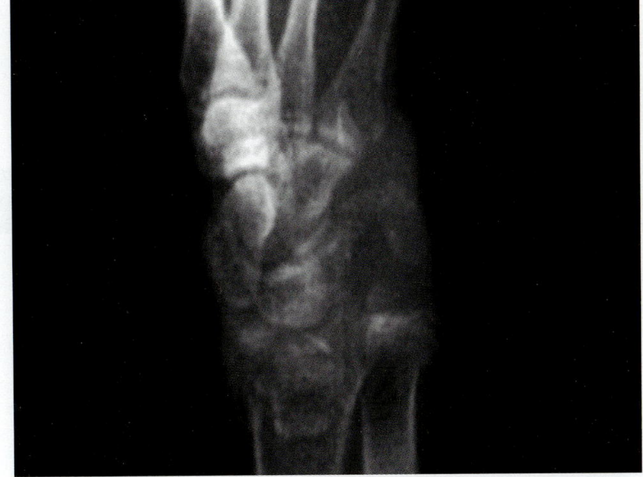

Fig. 218: Preoperative X-ray of wrist (anteroposterior view).

- The distal pins are inserted in the posterolateral aspect of second metacarpal shaft, which is subcutaneous.
- Two pins inserted in each bone, should be in parallel direction, the plane of pins should be varied to construct a quadrangular frame (Fig. 221).
- For the second metacarpal, the pins are radially based to avoid injury to extensor mechanism (Fig. 222).
- The reduction is verified using the image intensifier and once achieved, a second bar is added to frame construct and tightened (Figs. 223 and 224).
- When applying the external fixator, extreme positions of the wrist should be avoided. The goal is to restore radiographic parameters, most importantly the RL.
- The reduction, especially residual intra-articular deformity, must be finely tuned using percutaneous pins or bone grafting (Fig. 225).

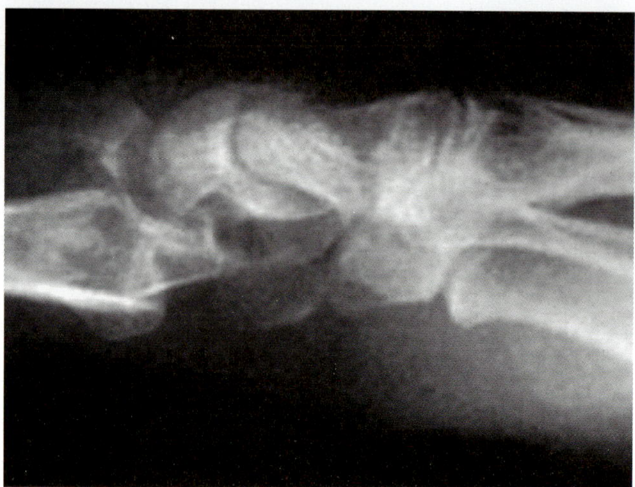

Fig. 219: Preoperative X-ray of wrist lateral view.

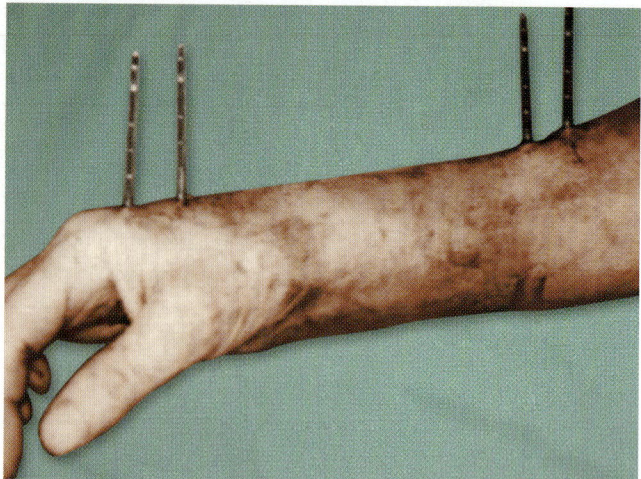

Fig. 221: Two pins are inserted in each bone in parallel direction, the plane of pins are varied to construct a quadrangular frame.

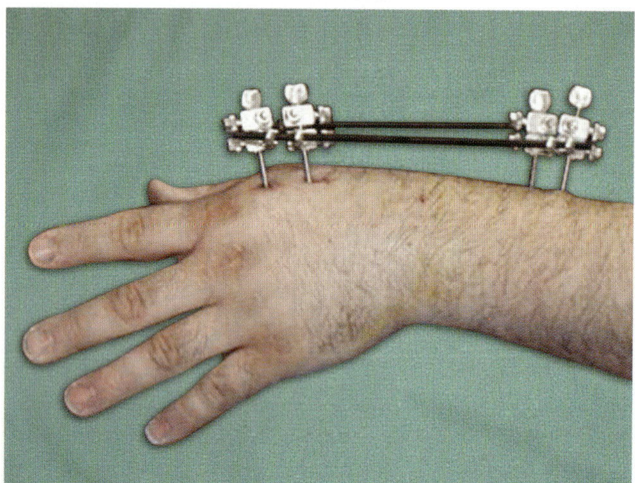

Fig. 220: Static external fixation.

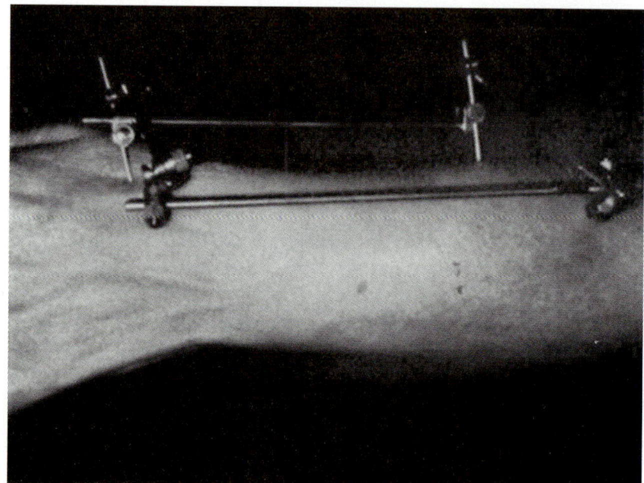

Fig. 222: Pins are radially based for second metacarpal, to avoid injury to extensor mechanism.

TABLE 16: Radiographic parameter for finding acceptable reduction of radial fractures.

Radiographic parameter	*Normal*	*Acceptable*
Radial length	Plus or minus 2 mm comparing level of lunate facet to ulnar head	No more than 2 mm Shortening relative to ulnar head
Radial inclination	20° as measured from lunate facet to radial styloid	No less than 10°
Lateral tilt	11° of volar tilt	Neutral
Intra-articular step or gap	None	Less than 2 mm of either

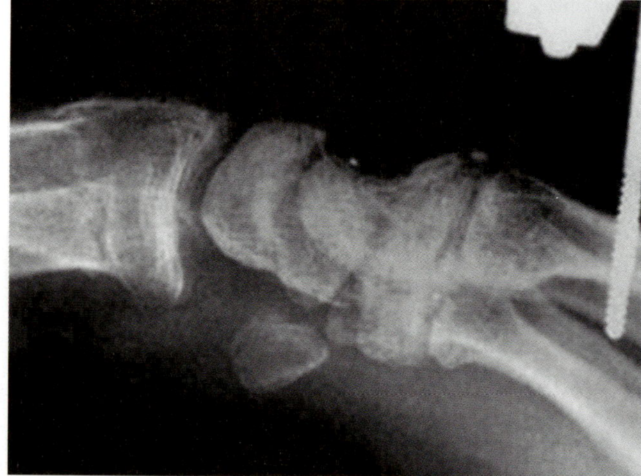

Fig. 223: Postoperative radiograph (lateral view).

Postoperative Care

- Dress the pin sites with the Vaseline-coated gauze and wrap the forearm and wrist in soft bandage
- Keep the sites clean and dry daily
- Patients who have isolated injury can be discharged on the same day from hospital, whereas others stay longer depending on the associated injuries
- Patients are asked to return to clinic within 2 weeks and again 6 weeks postoperatively
- At each visit, plain radiographs are taken, the frame and radiographs are usually removed on 6th week, if the radiographs

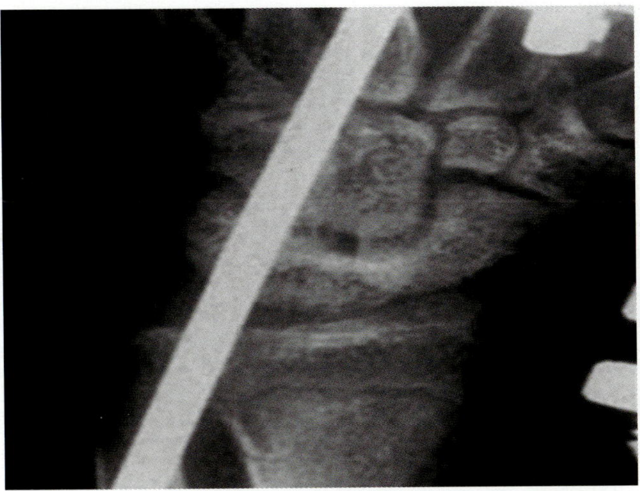

Fig. 224: Postoperative radiograph (anteroposterior view).

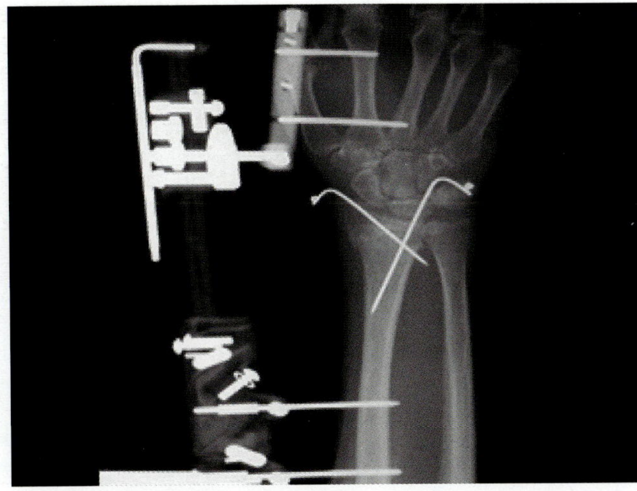

Fig. 225: Reduction using percutaneous pins with external fixator.

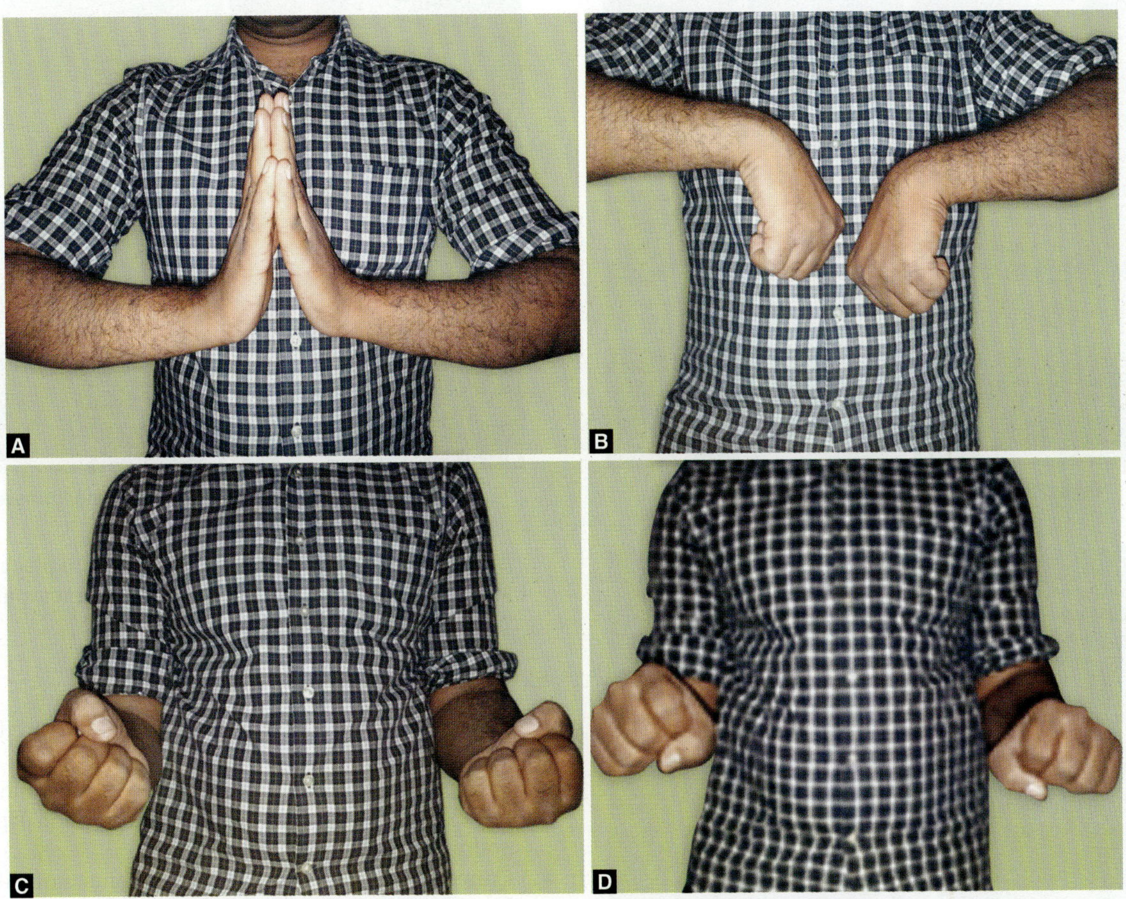

Figs. 226A to D: Wrist exercises initiated after fracture union to increase strength.

show fracture union and a supervised physiotherapy program is initiated to regain the wrist motion and strength (Figs. 226A to D)

- Treating displaced distal radius fractures, including those with an articular component, with external fixation and percutaneous pins yields good results
- Patients experienced improvement in function and pain scores at all points of follow-up
- Grip strength is also superior in those treated with external methods
- Pin tract infections can be treated with an oral antibiotic prescription and local pin care. Fractures are usually healed by 6–8 weeks.

Dynamic External Fixator

- The rationale of this device is a ball joint at proximal part of capitate at the capitolunate joint, since this is the center of rotation of wrist

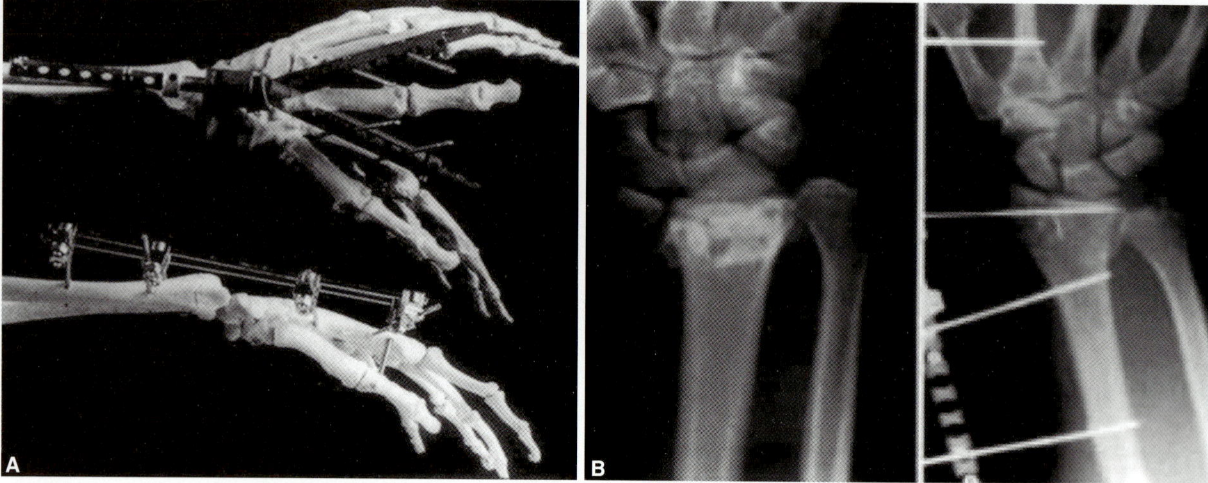

Figs. 227A and B: Proximal pins are placed perpendicularly and distal pins are placed in first and second metacarpal bone.

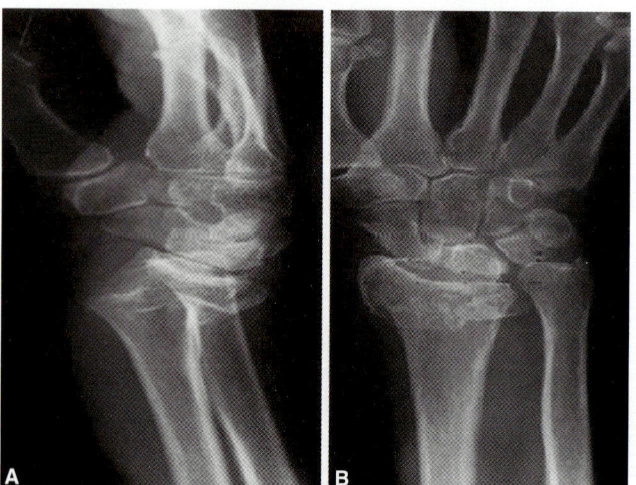

Figs. 228A and B: Preoperative X-rays.

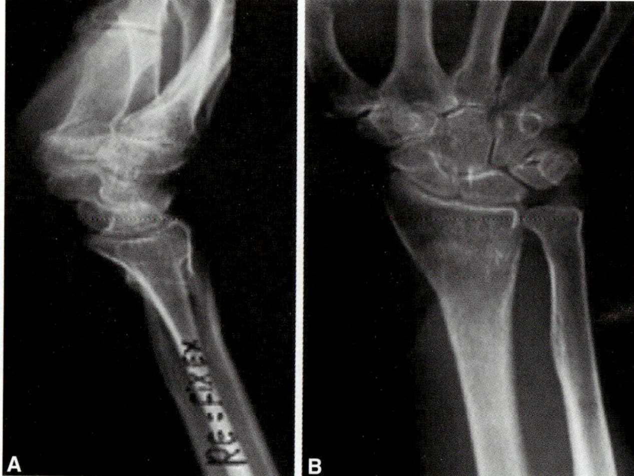

Figs. 230A and B: After external fixator removal.

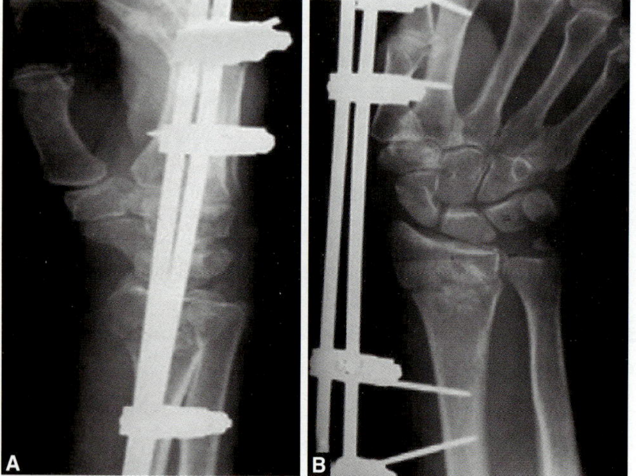

Figs. 229A and B: Postoperative X-rays.

- Advantage of this design is early motion of wrist and hand without any loss of reduction
- The device is placed in radial or coronal plane to permit the movements. Proximal pins are placed in radial bone in perpendicular direction and distal pins are placed in first and second metacarpal bone or second metacarpal bone (Figs. 227A and B).

External Fixation with Bone Graft

- Severely displaced comminuted Colles fracture tends to heal with malunion (Figs. 228A and B).
- Several methods were tried, like plasters, percutaneous K-wires and external fixation. More recently, the option of primary bone grafting has been explored.
- Cancellous bone grafting has both mechanical effects and biological effects, giving intrinsic stability to fracture and speeding the healing process (Figs. 229A and B) and after external fixator removal (Figs. 230A and B).
- We insert a distractor rod instead of a connecting rod in the fixator frame (Figs. 231).
- Principle is distraction could be manually adjusted to aid in the healing process of the fracture union.

Roger Anderson Device (Fig. 232)

It consists of series of pins and rods interconnected with movable clamps, giving a three dimensional configuration to the fixator. The pins are placed at 45° angulation to the shaft (Figs. 233 and 234).

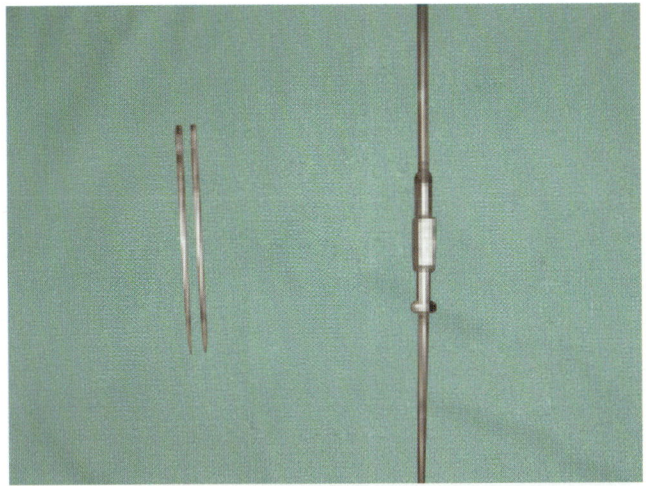

Fig. 231: Schanz screws and distraction rod.

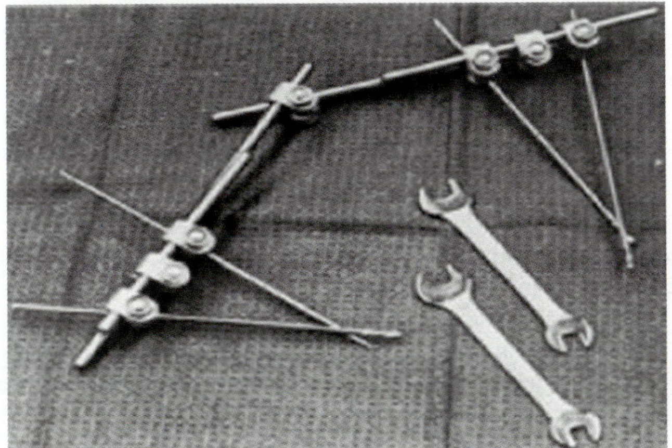

Fig. 232: Roger Anderson devices.

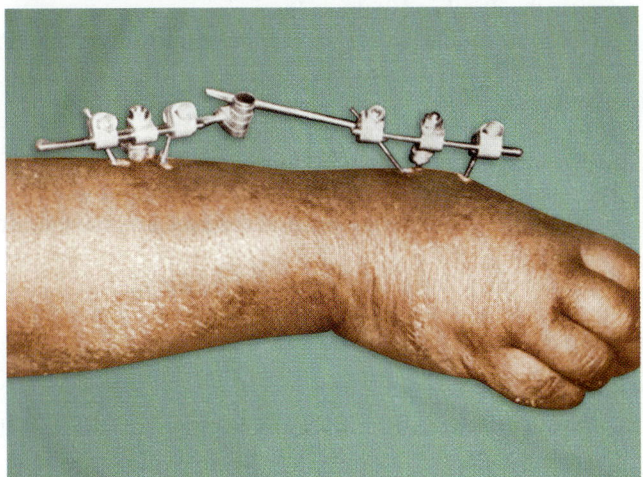

Fig. 233: Roger Anderson devices, applied to externally fixing the fractures fragments.

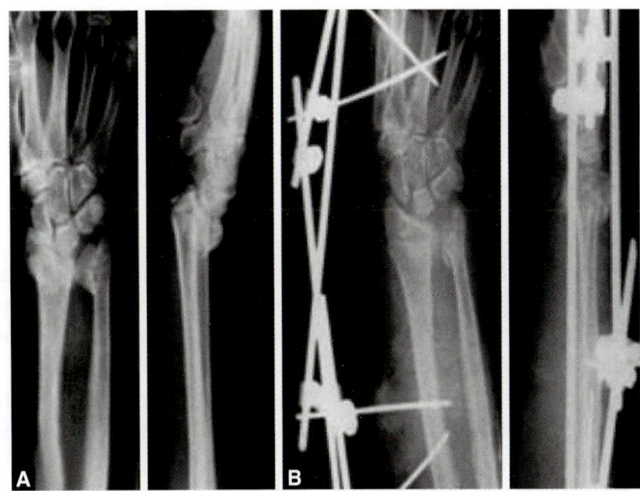

Figs. 234A and B: (A) Preoperative X-ray (anteroposterior and lateral view); (B) X-ray showing Roger Anderson external fixators are applied.

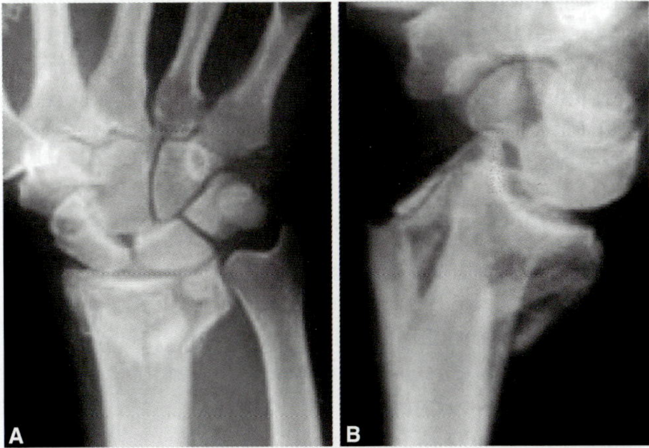

Figs. 235A and B: Preoperative X-rays—(A) Anteroposterior view; (B) Lateral view.

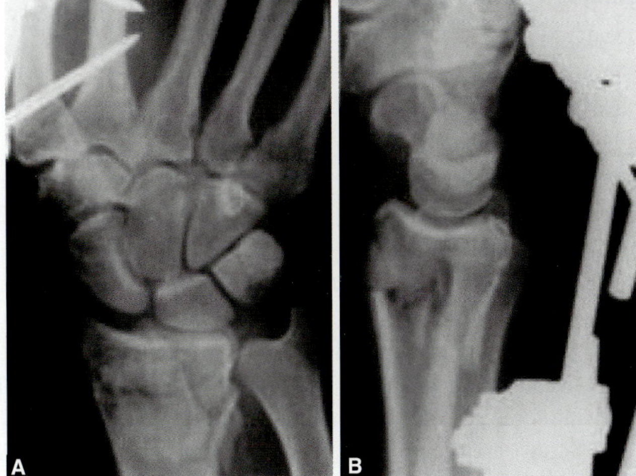

Figs. 236A and B: Postoperative X-ray, with AO fixator applied—(A) Anteroposterior view; (B) Lateral view.

AO External Fixator (Figs. 235 and 236)

Prerequisites

- Severe comminution of fracture
- Extension of fracture to radiocarpal joint
- Dorsal angulation more than 25°
- Articular step off more than 2 mm.

Technique

- 2.5 mm partially threaded AO half pins are used.

- Pins are placed 20–30° off the perpendicular plane, this is done to give convergence to the frame, so that it prevents the loosening of pins.
- Overdrilling of the pins should be avoided, to stripping of threads in far cortex by the smooth shaft of the pins, likewise unicortical placement of pins should also be avoided.

Discussion

- External fixation supplemented with percutaneous pins is an excellent option for treating displaced fractures of the distal radius with reliably good results, showing a low operation rate and a low complication rate.
- The key to success is to restore the anatomic parameters of the distal radius while minimizing insult to the soft tissue envelope.

PLATING OF DISTAL RADIUS FRACTURES

Introduction

No area in fracture management has had a recent explosion of treatment modalities as in distal radius plating. A drift from dorsal to volar plating has occurred. Segment specific fixation has been the new mindset. Other novel approaches for proposed problems include locking plates, nail-plate combinations, and others. Here, some of these approaches are outlined.

Indications for Open Reduction

- Type 2 distal radius fractures (Fernandez classification)
- Type 3 distal radius fractures
- Unstable distal radius fractures
- Partial volar or dorsal (B-type intra-articular fractures)
- Radial styloid fractures
- Lunate fossa split and displaced
- Intra-articular comminuted C2–C3 fractures.

Plating Techniques (See Fig. 263)

- Volar plating
- Dorsal plating
- Combined volar and dorsal plating
- Distraction plate fixation
- Fragment specific fixation.

Volar plating:
- *Surgical approach*
- *AO type C distal radius fracture (Figs. 237 and 238)*
  - Plate is placed
  - A screw is placed in central oval hole (Fig. 239)
  - In each of the distal slot, smooth peg is placed, followed by lag screw to engage the dorsal fragment (Fig. 240)
  - Screws are then placed proximal to holes of the plate (Fig. 241)
  - Brachioradialis and pronator quadratus are sutured
  - Postoperative X-rays after volar plating are shown in Figures 242 to 244.

Postoperative care:
- Patient with stable radioulnar joint are placed in wrist splint
- After 1 week, a fabricated wrist splint is used, during which hand ROMs are started and continued for 6 weeks

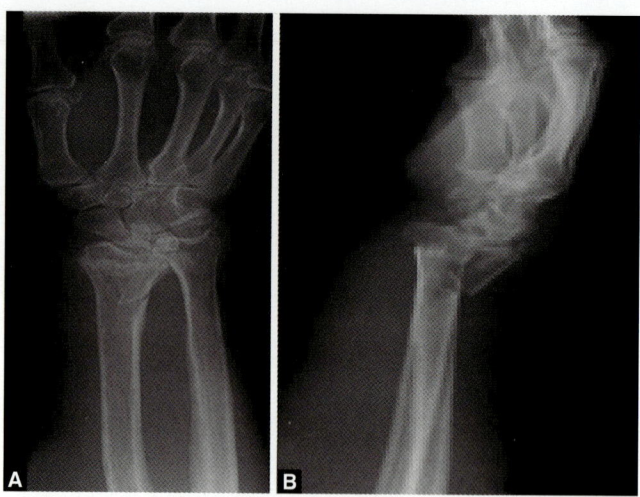

Figs. 237A and B: Preoperative X-ray of AO type C distal radius fracture—(A) Anteroposterior view; (B) Lateral view.

- After 6 weeks, splint is removed and strengthening exercise program is begun
- Unrestricted activities are allowed after 12 weeks
- Patients with DRUJ derangement are placed in supination splint, for 6 weeks, later gentle active pronation and supination exercises are done till another 6 weeks
- After 12 weeks, unrestricted activities are begun.

Dorsal plating: Dorsally displaced distal radial fracture is shown in Figures 245A and B.
- Surgical approach (Fig. 246)
- Incision taken midway of radial and ulnar styloid (Fig. 247)
- Extensor retinaculum incised, extensor communis, and extensor indicis exposed (Fig. 248)
- Fourth compartment muscles are retracted (Fig. 249)
- Dorsal radiocarpal ligament and extensor tendons are elevated
- Extensor tendons in their compartments have been elevated to expose the distal end of the radius.
- Using a low profile plate, stabilization of fracture is done (Fig. 250).

Postoperative care:
- Wrist is immobilized in a volar splint
- Active and passive finger movements are encouraged
- Active and active assisted motions are done after 1 week
- Passive and grip strengthening exercises are started after 6 weeks
- Patients were followed-up with serial radiographs.

Combined Dorsal and Volar Plates Fixation

Indications

- Complex fragmentation of both articular surface and the metaphysis
- AO type C 3.2 fracture
- Percutaneous pinning was attempted, but did not restore the alignment (Fig. 251)
- Note, the inability of K-wires to control the fragments, when there is a metaphyseal comminution (Fig. 252)
- A second procedure of dorsal plate fixation resulted in volar translation of fragments because of absence of volar metaphyseal support (Figs. 253A and B). Application of second volar plate has improved the alignment. The functional result

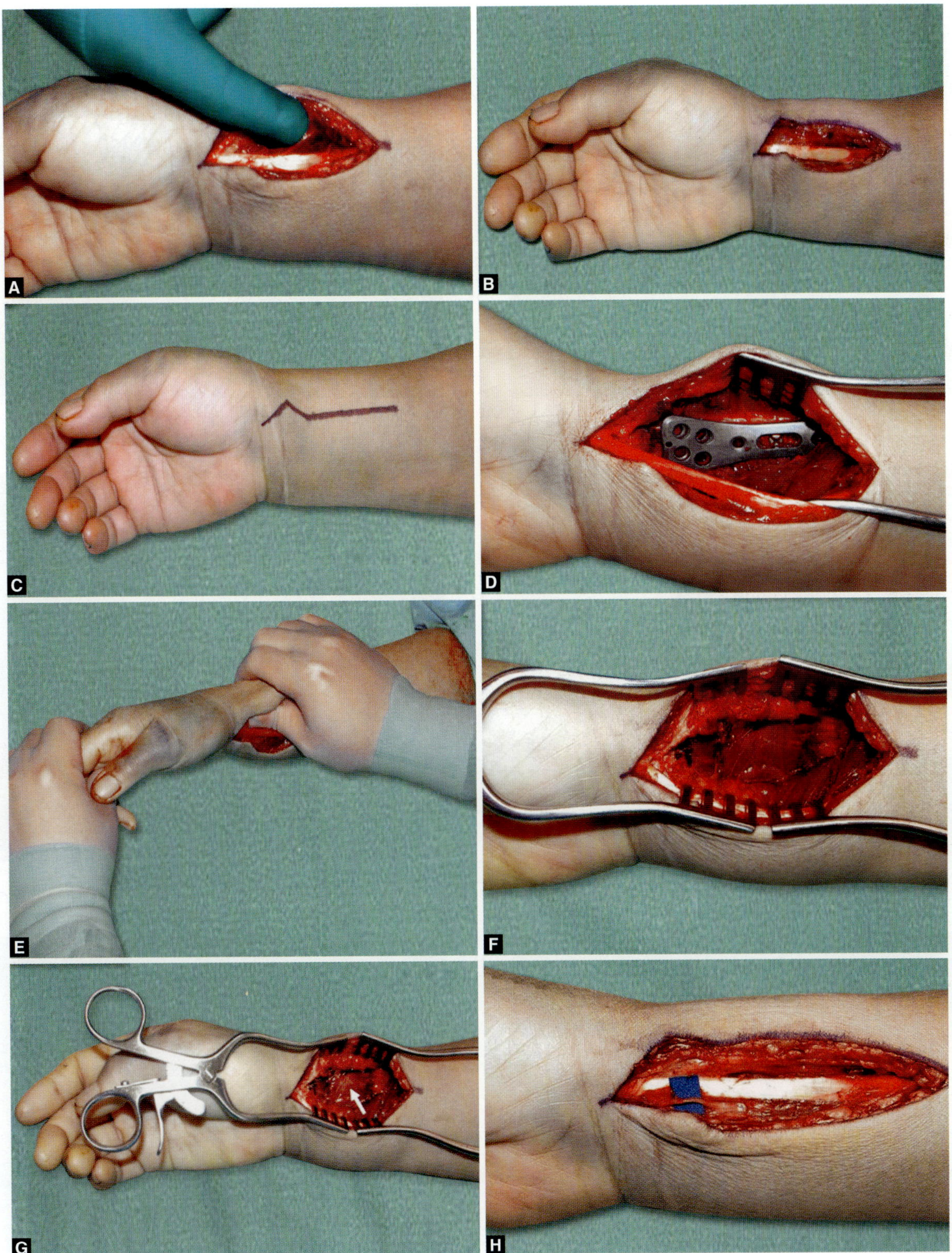

Figs. 238A to H: Surgical approach (AO type C and distal radius fracture).

was rated good according to system of Gartland and Werley. Radiograph after the implant removal, showing healing with reasonable alignment (Fig. 254).

Distraction Plate Fixation

It is indicated in fractures of distal end radius with extensive metaphyseal and diaphyseal comminution (Figs. 255 and 256).

Surgical Technique (Figs. 257 and 258)

- Distal incision is made first over the long finger metacarpal
- Proximal incision is made over dorsal aspect of radial shaft at the anticipated levels of proximal portion of plate
- The level of incision and length of plate are chosen by utilizing fluoroscopy, while holding the plate against the skin to appropriate level of metacarpal and ensuring that at least

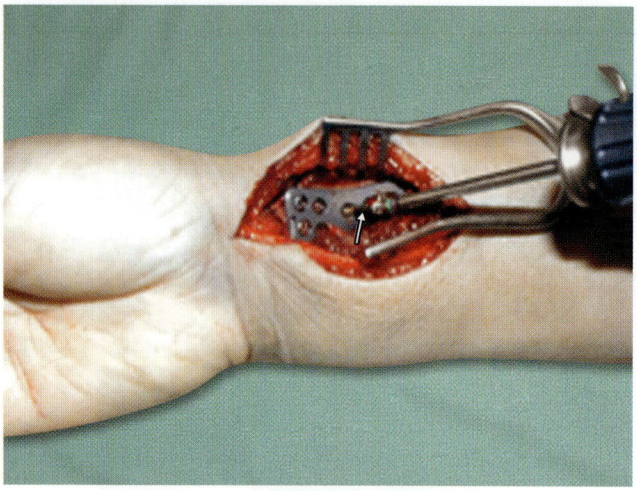

Fig. 239: A screw is placed in central oval hole.

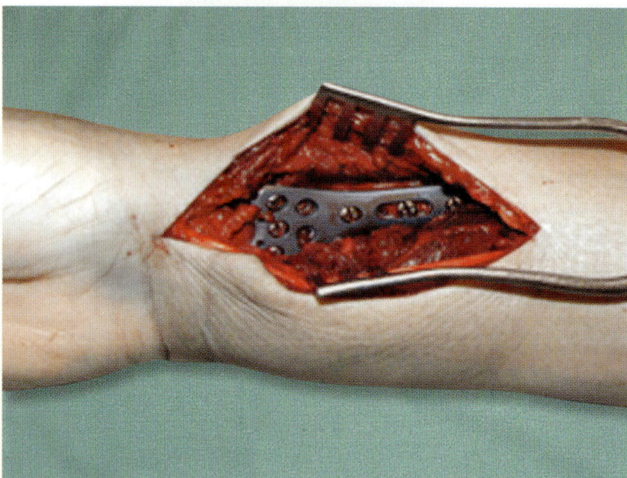

Fig. 240: Placement of smooth peg, followed by lag screw.

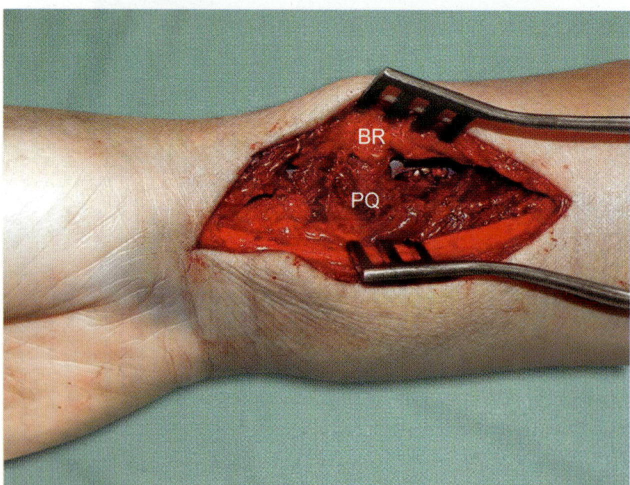

Fig. 241: Placement of screws proximal to holes of the plate. (BR: brachioradialis; PQ: pronator quadratus)

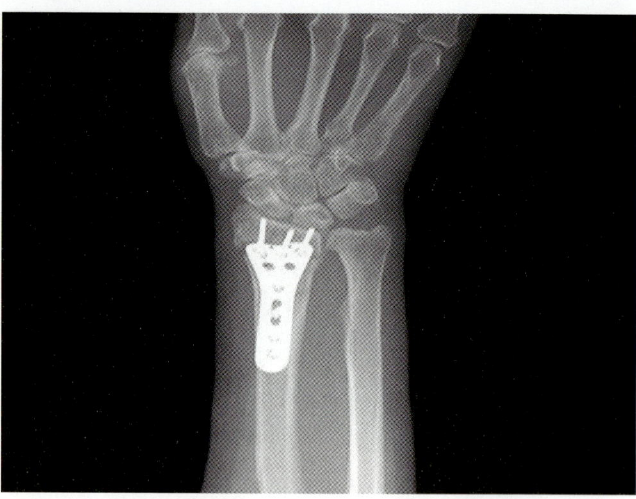

Fig. 242: Posteroanterior view after surgery.

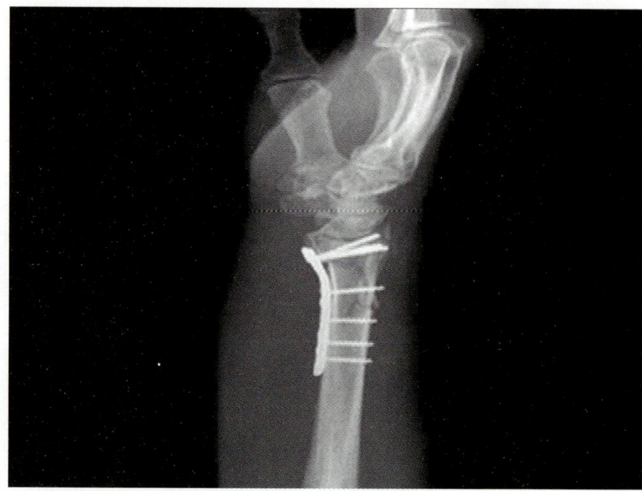

Fig. 243: Lateral view after plating.

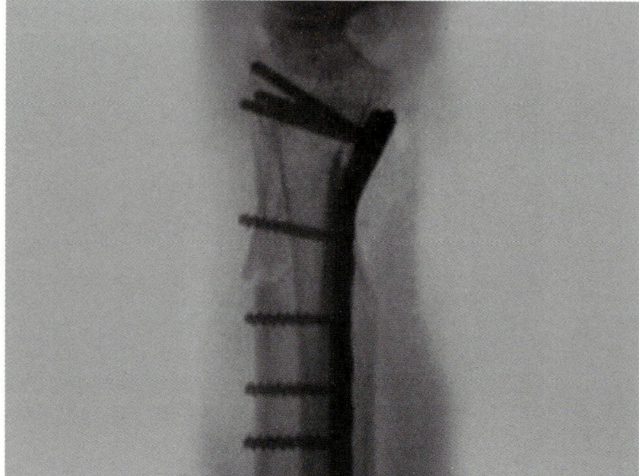

Fig. 244: Lateral view, showing anatomic reduction, protrusion of peg in dorsal cortex less than 1 mm.

four holes of plate are proximal to fracture site (Fig. 257). Intraoperative radiographs taken to check the collect alignment are shown in Figures 259A and B.

- *Postoperative radiographs (Fig. 260):* At 4 months, X- rays show maintenance of RL and palmar tilt with the union of fracture and bridging of bone defect.

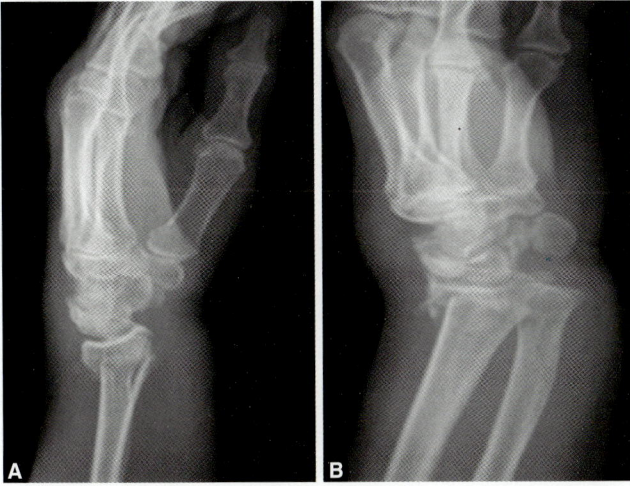

Figs. 245A and B: Dorsally displaced distal radial fractures.

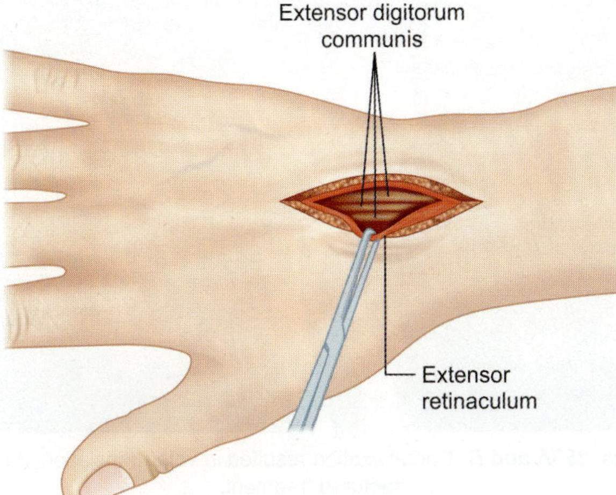

Figs. 246: Surgical approach for dorsal plating.

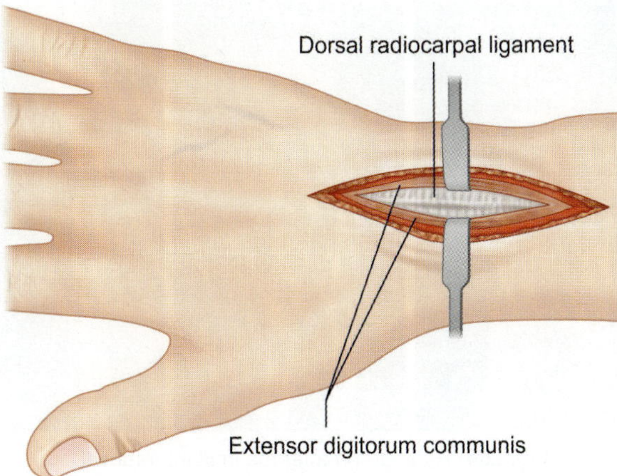

Fig. 247: Site of incision (midway to radial and ulnar styloid).

- Range of motion of operated wrist compared to the normal wrist is shown in Figures 261A to D.
- Dorsal plate (Fig. 262) placements are associated with high rate of complications, like stiffness of joint, tenosynovitis, and tendon rupture (Figs. 263 and 264).

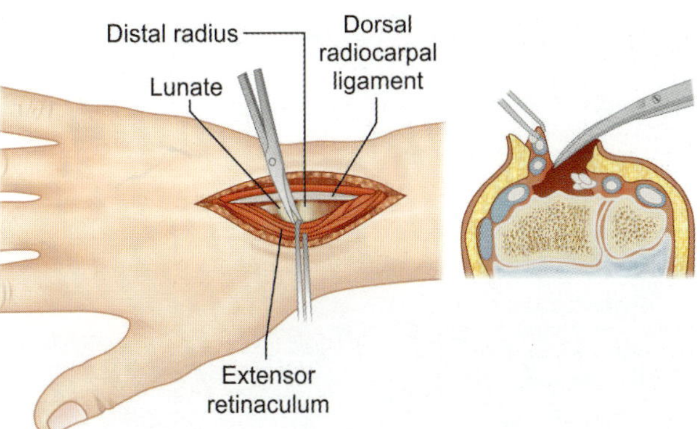

Fig. 248: Extensor communis and extensor indicis are exposed, by making incision through extensor retinaculum.

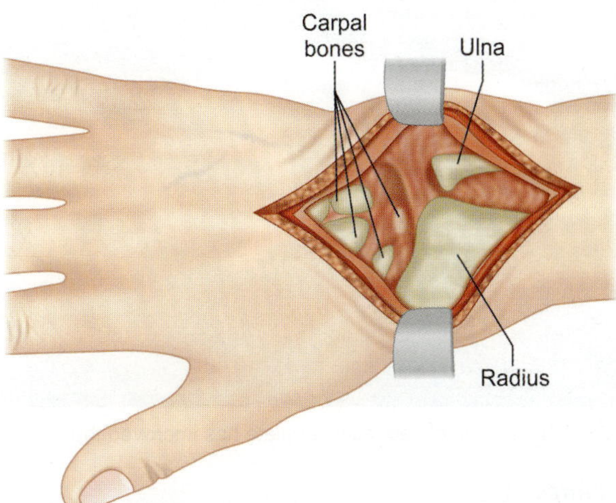

Fig. 249: Muscles of fourth compartment are retracted.

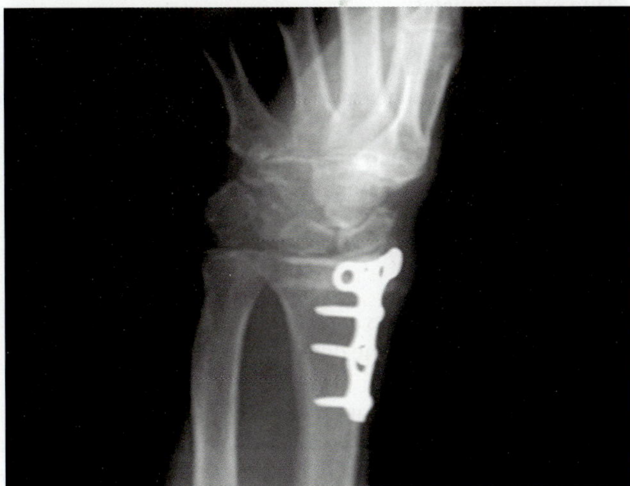

Fig. 250: Postoperative X-ray taken after dorsal plating.

- The effect of attendant scar is difficult to separate from actual location of dorsal plate.
- A volar plate (*See* Fig. 262) placement through FCR approach affords a soft tissue layer between the skin and the plate (*See* Fig. 258).
- With the advent of new fixed angle plates designs, volar fixation has become the standard approach for distal radius fractures with joint congruity.

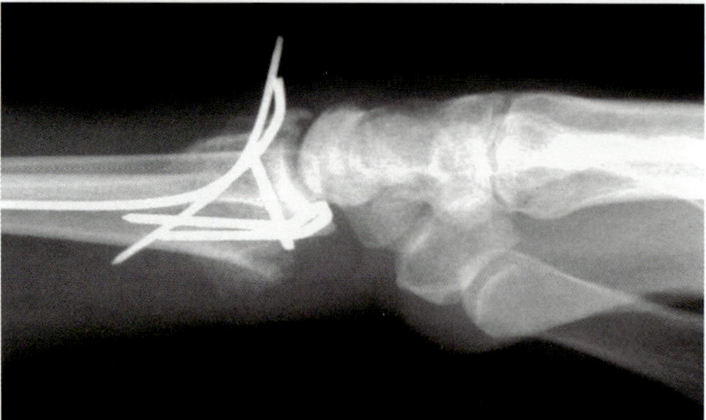

Fig. 251: Failure of percutaneous pinning to restore the alignment.

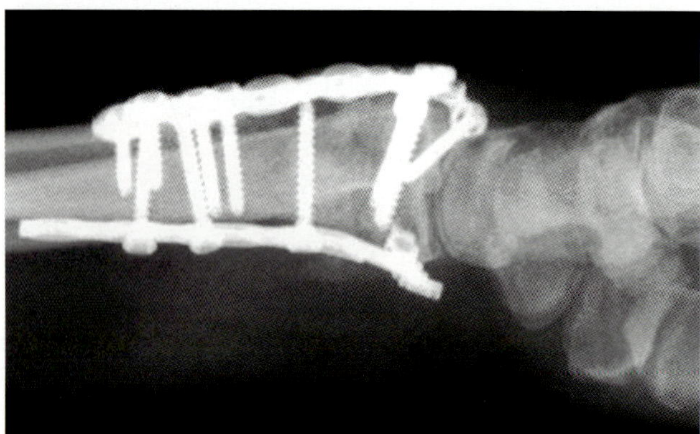

Fig. 252: Application of second volar plate has improved the alignment.

Volar Plates

Volar plates generally fall into four functional categories:

1. Buttress plates with or without distal screws
2. Tine or blade plates
3. Fixed angled locking plates
4. Polyaxial locking plates (Fig. 265).

Different types of volar plates most commonly used are summarized below:

- AOVL: AO 3.5 mm small fragment locking plate
- AOV: AO 3.5 mm small fragment plate
- AOT: AO T-Plate
- DVR: Hand innovations distal single row locking plate
- PI: AO PI plate.

Advantages of locking plates over nonlocking plates (Table 17):

- Produces fixation in bone defects and osteopenic bones
- Early ROM
- Locked plate as an advantage to perform indirect reduction
- Provide an advantage even for comminuted osteoporotic fractures
- Fragment specific fixation
- Designed to independently stabilize each fracture element
- Subchondral support and rigidity can be enhanced
- Increased rigidity provided by implants placed orthogonal planes, taking into consideration complex three-dimensional geometry of the distal radius.

Common fracture types and chosen treatment (Table 18)

Summary

With wide array of options and approaches means that almost all distal radius fractures can be fixed and held in place with open reduction and internal fixation. Whether this procedure is required or can reliably be accomplished with good functional outcome, is open to debate until clinical relevant questions are answered.

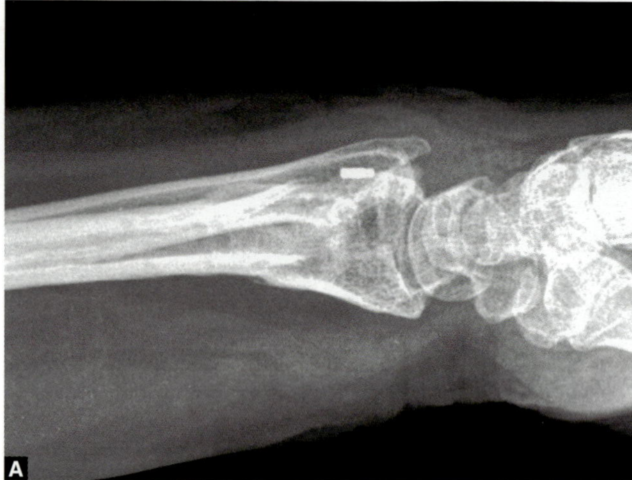

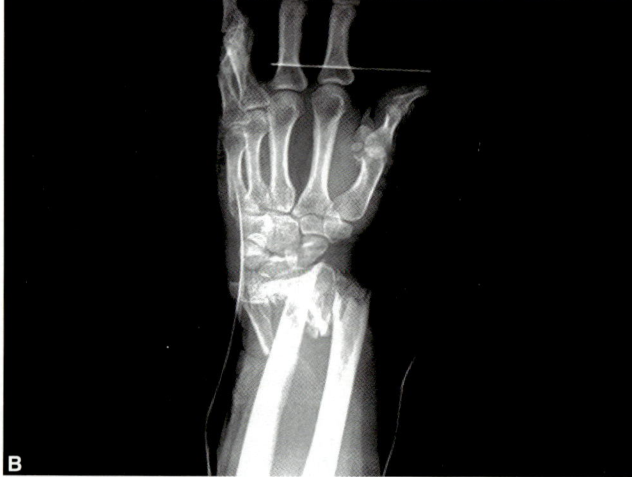

Figs. 253A and B: Dorsal fixation resulted in volar translation of the fractured fragment.

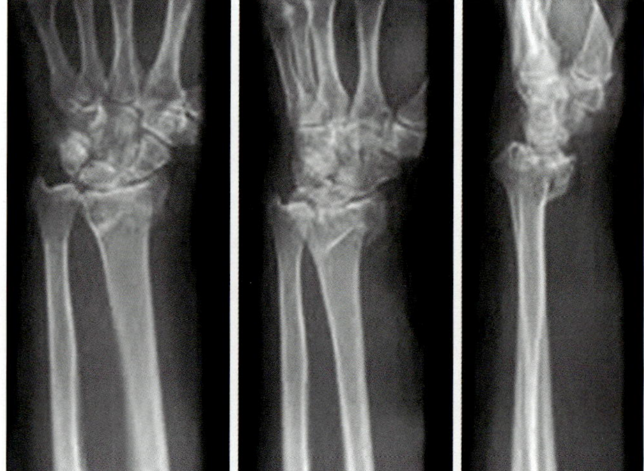

Fig. 254: Radiograph after the implant removal.

CARPAL BONE FRACTURES

Anatomy

Carpal bones and adjoining bones, X-rays are shown in Figures 266 and 267.

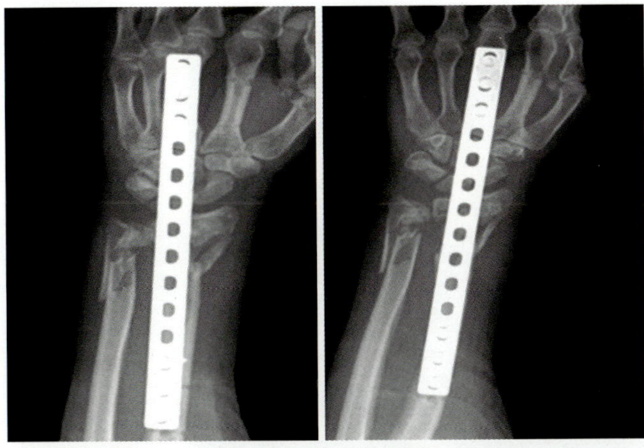

Fig. 255: Distraction plate fixation (anteroposterior view).

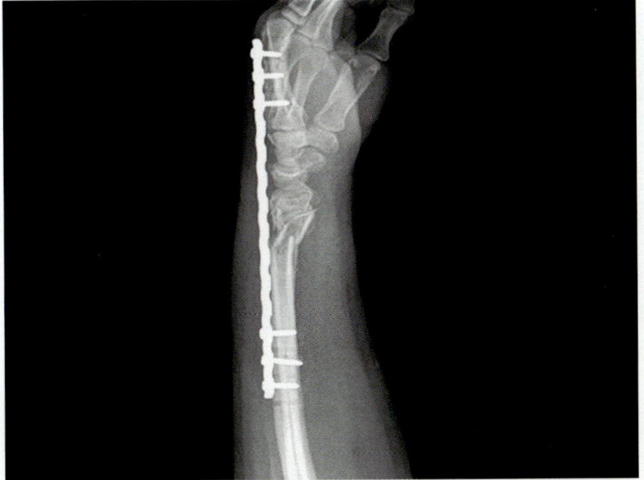

Fig. 256: Distraction plate fixation (an oblique view).

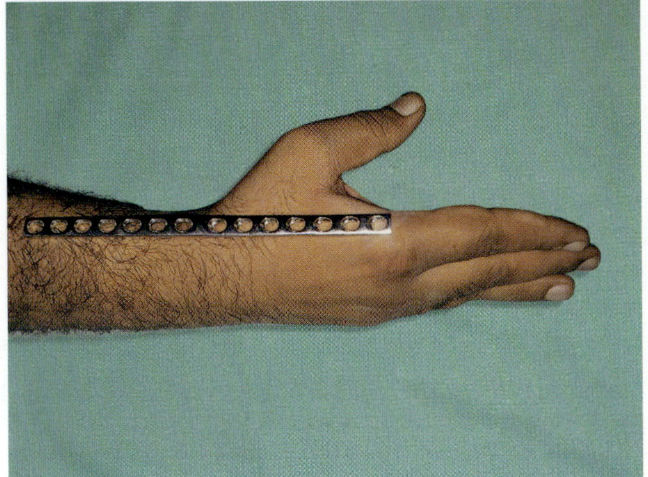

Fig. 257: Measurement taken for the length of the plate.

Lunate Fractures

Introduction

The lunate is the fourth most fractured carpal bone (following the scaphoid, triquetrum, and trapezium) (Fig. 268). They often are not

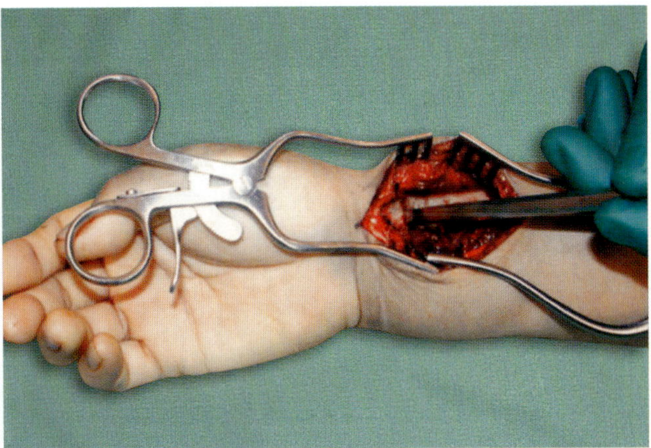

Fig. 258: A volar plate placement through flexor carpi radialis approach is showing elevating pronator quadratus with a periosteal elevator.

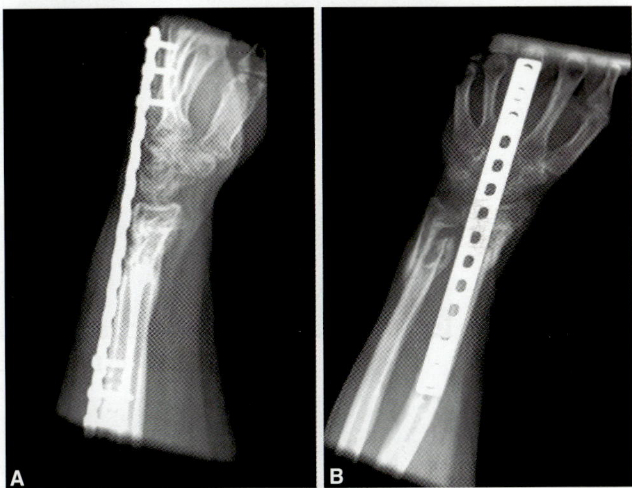

Figs. 259A and B: Intraoperative radiographs.

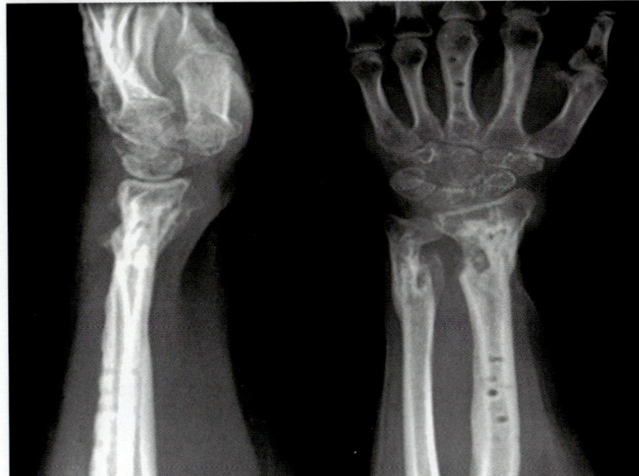

Fig. 260: Postoperative radiographs taken after removal of implant.

diagnosed initially and present delayed as lunate osteonecrosis, which is also known as Kienbock's disease.

Anatomy

- The lunate is shaped like a crescent (Fig. 269)
- *Carpal keystone:* Since it resides within a protected concavity of the distal radius (lunate fossa) and is integral in the flexion or

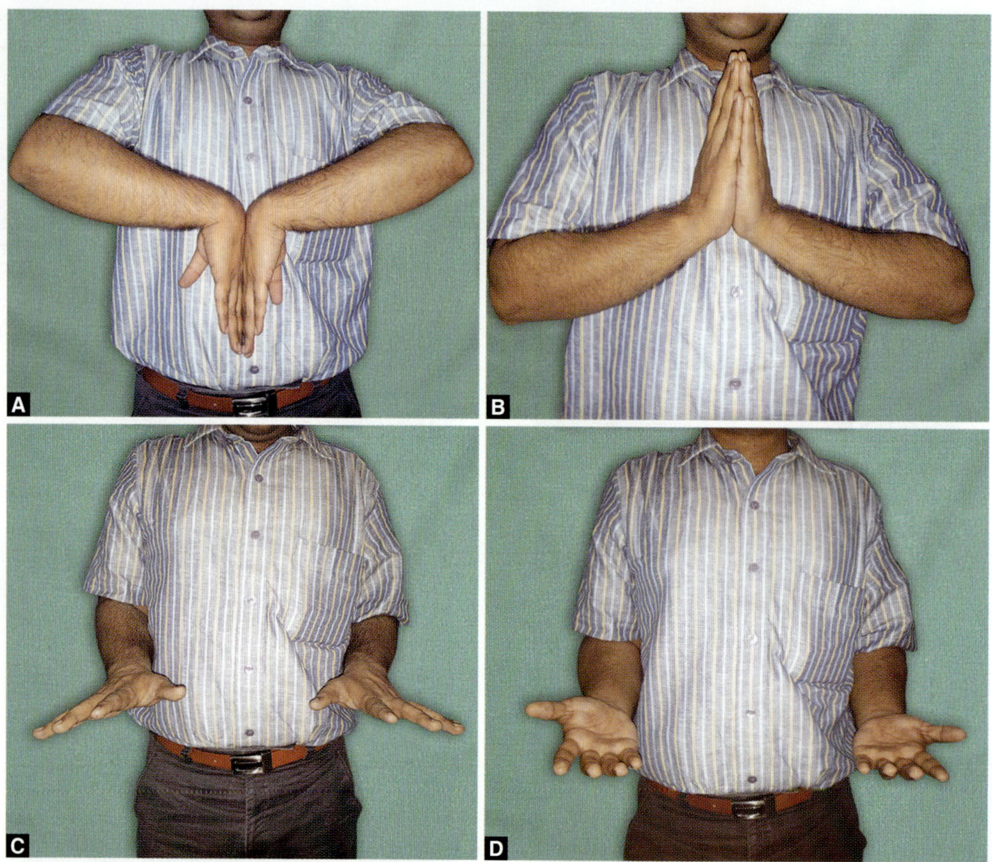

Figs. 261A to D: Range of motion of right wrist after 1 year.

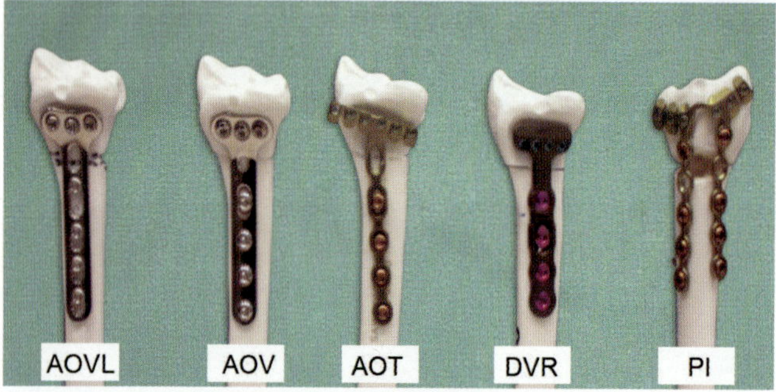

Fig. 262: Different types of volar and dorsal plates.

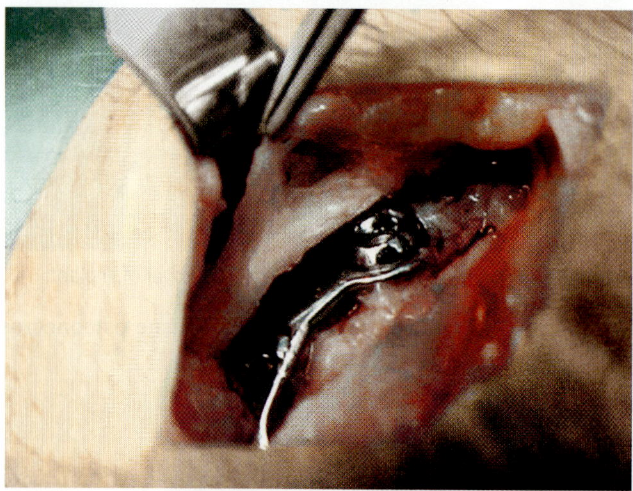

Fig. 263: Extensor tenosynovitis and extensor tendons directly gliding over the dorsal plate.

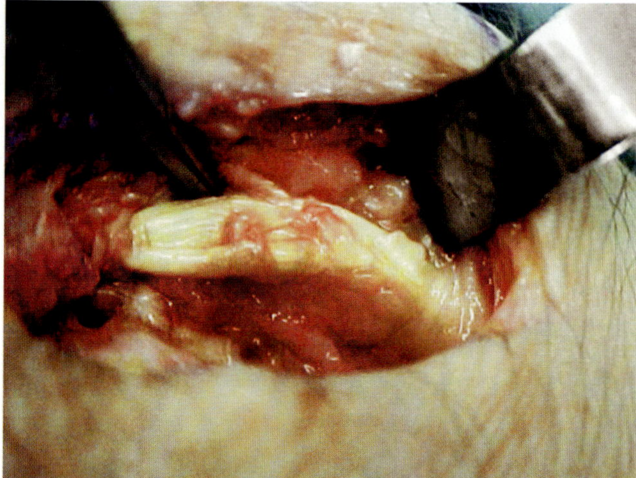

Fig. 264: After implant removal tendons showing visible attritional changes.

extension arc and the radial or ulnar deviation arc, at both the radiocarpal and midcarpal joints.

- The lunate is attached to the scaphoid and triquetrum via interosseous ligaments.
- Distally, it is concave and articulates with the convex head of the capitates and proximally, it articulates with the lunate facet of the distal radius.
- It is supplied by a proximal carpal vascular arcade, volarly, and dorsally. There are three variable intralunate anastomoses.

Mechanism of Injury

The mechanism of injury is typically a fall onto an outstretched hand, with a hyperextended wrist or during a forceful push with an extended wrist.

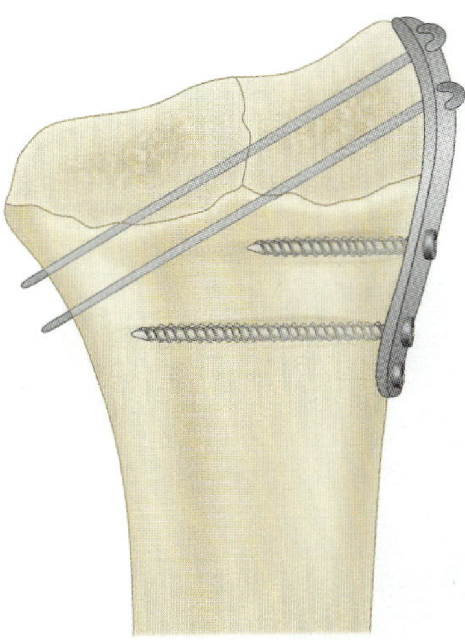

Fig. 265: A polyaxial locking plate.

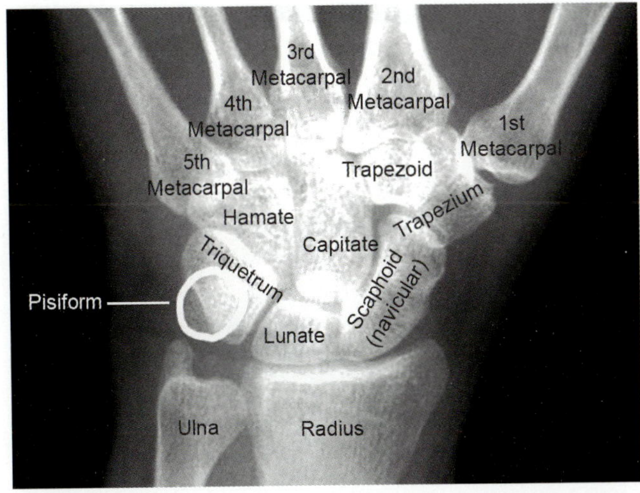

Fig. 266: Identification of carpal bones on X-ray (anteroposterior view).

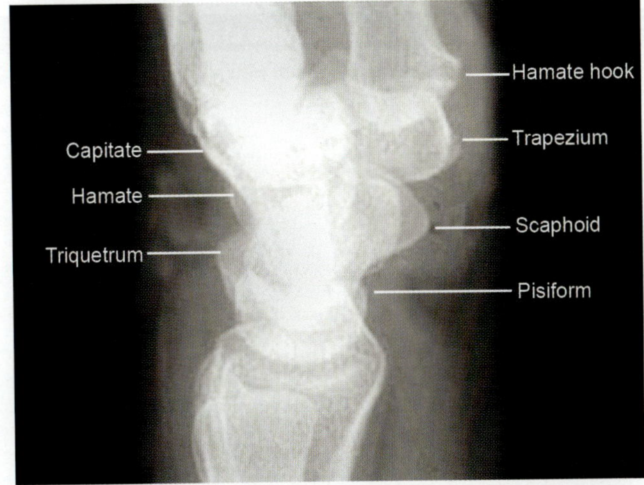

Fig. 267: Identification of carpal bones on X-ray (lateral view).

TABLE 17: Advantages and disadvantages of different locking and nonlocking plates.

Plates	*Advantages*	*Disadvantages*
Buttress plates	Traditional plate design. Can be used with or without distal screw fixation in distal fragment	Since the screws are not locked into plate construct they do not resist angular motion effectively
Blade plates	They offer high strength and stiffness	Having to be placed in a position predetermined to shape and position of times
Fixed angled locking plates	Improved strength and resists angular motion	Fixed trajectory
Polyaxial locking plates	Independent trajectory, matching the distal fixation to variable geometry and surface contour	They tend to be thicker and prominent

TABLE 18: Common fracture types and their chosen treatment.

Fracture type	*Chosen treatment*
Extra-articular and intra-articular	A volar fixed angled locking plate
Partial (B-type) volar	A volar buttress plate
Partial (B-type) dorsal	A volar fixed angled or polyaxial plate
Radial styloid	A volar fixed angled locking plate or fragment specific fixation
Lunate fossa	A volar fixed angled locking plates or polyaxial locking plates. Communition necessitates dorsal reduction then a fragment specific fixation
Lunate fossa split and displaced	A volar locking plate or polyaxial locking displaced plate (complex intra-articular fractures different plate designs and alternate fixation options should be available)
Comminuted (C2–C3)	An extended volar locking plate plus or minus dorsal plates in fragment specific manner
Comminuted (C2) osteoporotic	Extended volar locking plate or distal radius bridge plate
Comminuted with non-reconstructable dorsal rim	Volar plate with dorsal Pi Plate extending over the first carpal row

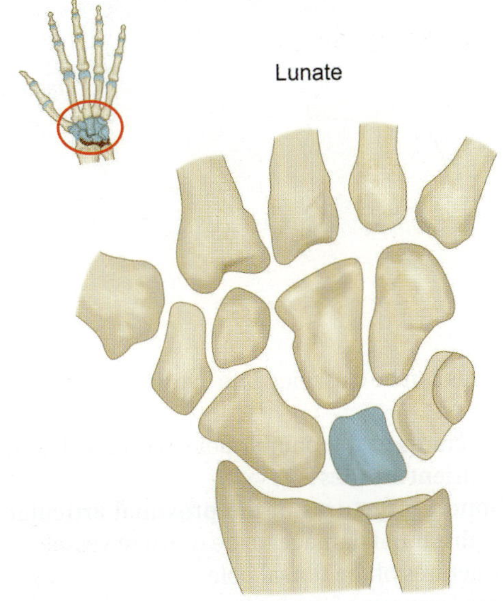

Fig. 268: Carpal bones of wrist with lunate (proximal row).

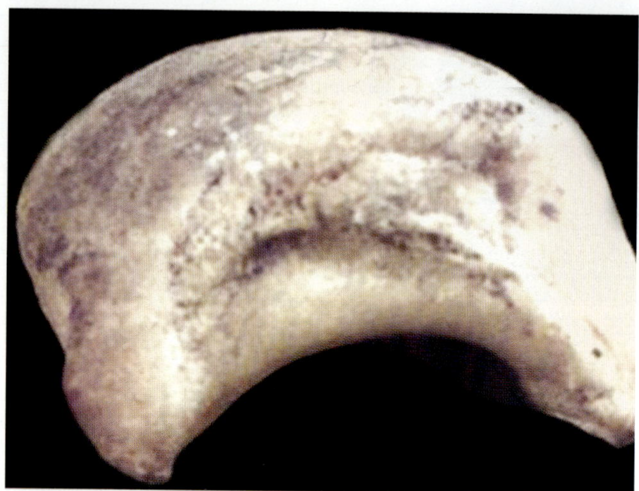

Fig. 269: Lunate is shaped like a crescent.

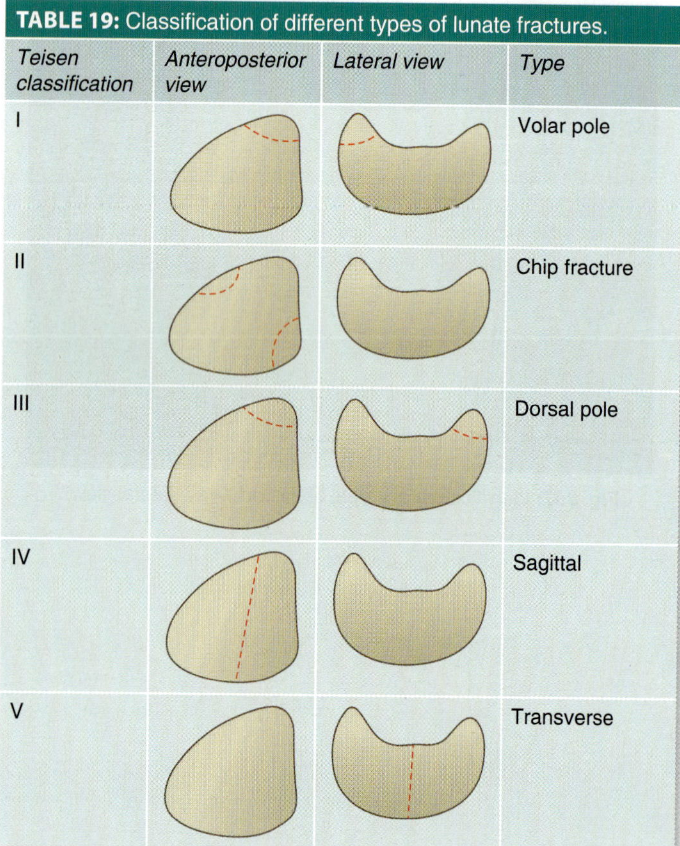

TABLE 19: Classification of different types of lunate fractures.

Teisen classification	*Anteroposterior view*	*Lateral view*	*Type*
I			Volar pole
II			Chip fracture
III			Dorsal pole
IV			Sagittal
V			Transverse

Classification

Lunate fractures can be classified into five groups; this is illustrated in Table 19:

1. Frontal fractures of the palmar pole, with involvement of the palmar nutrient arteries
2. Osteochondral fractures of the proximal articular surface, without substantial damage to the nutrient vessels
3. Frontal fractures of the dorsal pole
4. Transverse fractures of the body
5. Transarticular frontal fractures of the body of the lunate.

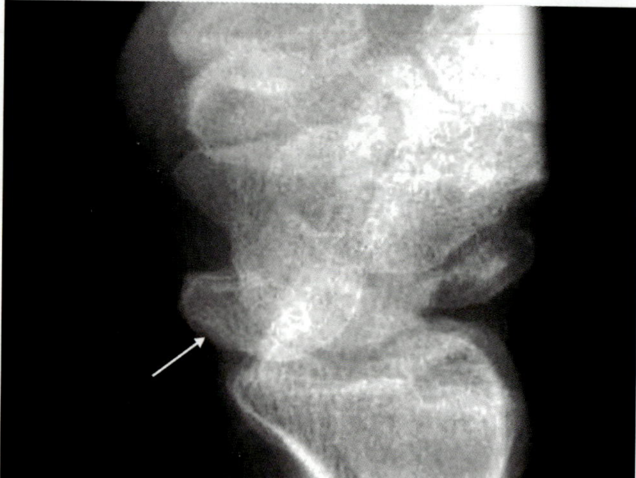

Fig. 270: Radiograph of the wrist, often inadequate to detect a lunate fracture (arrow), due to overlapping radiodensities.

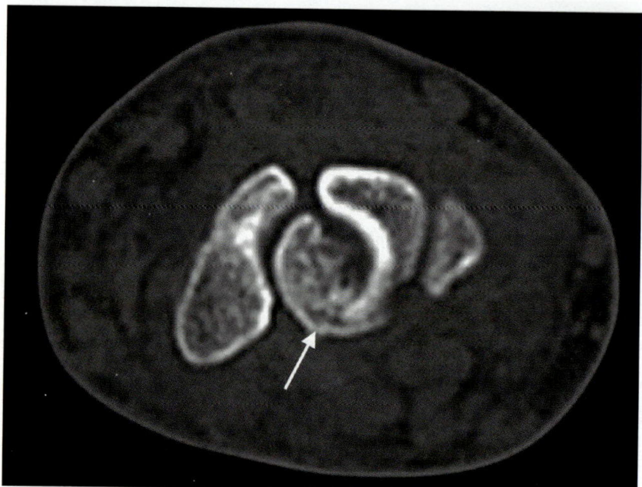

Fig. 271: Magnetic resonance imaging demonstrating healing, vascular injury and signs of osteonecrosis on the fracture site arrow showing a vascular necrosis of lunate.

Presentation

- Patients often present with central dorsal wrist pain, loss of motion at the wrist and diminished grip strength
- Tenderness is demonstrated with direct palpation of the dorsal aspect of the lunate.

Diagnosis

- Standard PA and lateral radiographs of the wrist are often inadequate to detect a lunate fracture because of overlapping radiodensities (Fig. 270)
- Oblique views may be slightly more helpful, however, MRI and CT scans are often needed
- The MRI is also helpful for evaluating healing, vascular injury, and signs of osteonecrosis (Fig. 271).

Treatment

- Nondisplaced fractures can be treated with cast immobilization. Follow-up must proceed at close intervals to monitor healing and possible progression to Kienbock disease
- Displaced or angulated fractures require surgical apposition to allow healing of the vascular supply to the lunate.

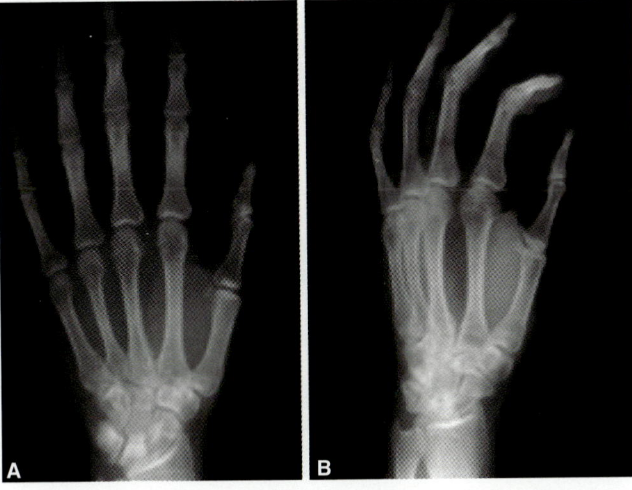

Figs. 272A and B: Radiographs showing Kienbock's disease.

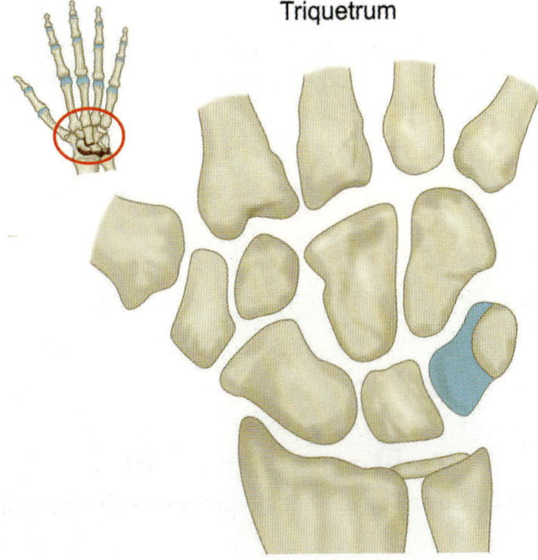

Fig. 273: Triquetrum bone.

Complications

Kienbock's Disease (Figs. 272A and B)

- It is an osteonecrosis of the lunate and can lead to devastating advanced collapse and radiocarpal arthrosis.
- Surgical intervention may be necessary to relieve the severe pain.
- The options for surgical management of Kienbock' disease include:
  - Radial wedge osteotomy
  - Radial shortening
  - Ulnar lengthening
  - Salvage procedures, such as arthrodesis or proximal row carpectomy.

Triquetral Fractures

Introduction

The triquetrum is reported as the second or third most common carpal fracture, representing 3–4% of all carpal bone injuries. It is the second most common carpal fracture in sports (Fig. 273).

Anatomy

- The triquetrum is located just distal to the ulna and the TFCC and proximal to the base of the hamate

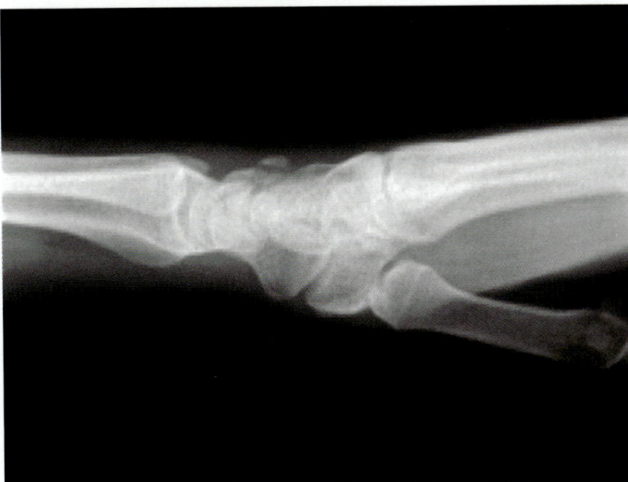

Fig. 274: Chip (dorsal cortical) fractures.

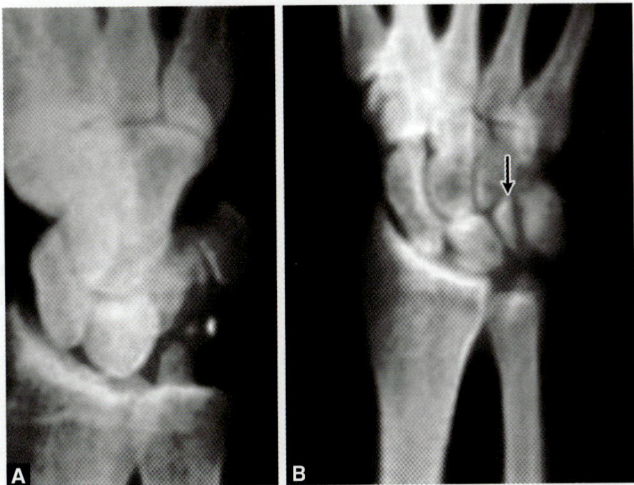

Figs. 275A and B: Arrow shows midbody fracture.

- The triquetrum articulates on its radial side with the lunate, to which it is attached by the lunotriquetral ligament. On the volar (palmar) aspect, there is an articulation with the pisiform.

Mechanism of Injury

- Triquetral fractures typically occur from a hyperextension injury, with the wrist in ulnar deviation. However, injury can also occur with hyperflexion
- The dorsal surface of the triquetrum may be fractured by means of impingement from the ulnar styloid (chisel effect), shear forces, or avulsion from strong ligamentous attachments.

Classification

Triquetral fractures can be divided into two types:

1. *Chip (dorsal cortical) fractures:* A chip fracture typically occurs with a wrist hyperextension (dorsiflexion) and ulnar deviation injury (Fig. 274).
2. *Midbody fracture:* This type of fracture is usually the result of a direct blow or may occur in conjunction with a perilunate dislocation (Figs. 275A and B).

Presentation

- A history of injury and pain on the ulnar aspect of the wrist
- On examination, there will be pain and point tenderness, either dorsally or on the ulnar border of the wrist about 1–2 cm

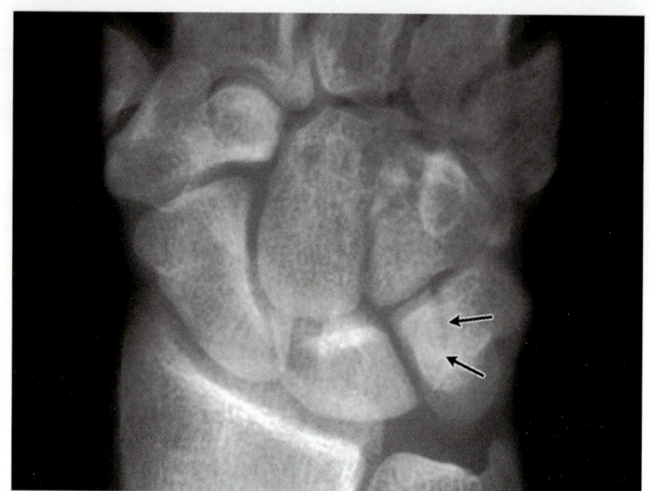

Fig. 276: X-ray anteroposterior view, arrows showing triquetral body fracture.

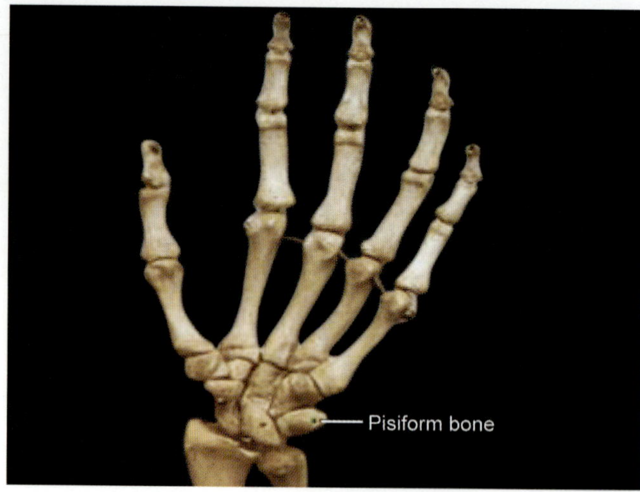

Fig. 277: Location of pisiform bone.

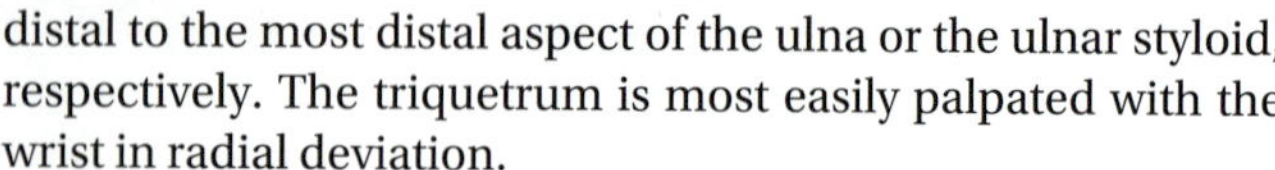

distal to the most distal aspect of the ulna or the ulnar styloid, respectively. The triquetrum is most easily palpated with the wrist in radial deviation.

Diagnosis

- Triquetral body fractures are best visualized on anteroposterior and oblique views (Fig. 276)
- Dorsal chip fractures are best detected on a pronated lateral projection that projects the dorsal triquetrum away from the adjacent carpal bones (Fig. 276)
- The CT scan and/or MRI confirm the diagnosis in suspicion cases.

Treatment

- Immobilization in a cast for a period of 4–6 weeks, usually leads to good long-term functional outcomes for isolated triquetrum fractures
- Fractures in association with perilunate dislocation or those with more than 1 mm of displacement, probably should be considered for surgical treatment to maximize long-term wrist function
- A persistently symptomatic chip fracture may require excision.

Complications

- The deep branch of the ulnar nerve lies in close proximity to the triquetrum and may be compromised in triquetral fractures, with resultant motor impairment
- Pisotriquetral arthritis, secondary to a triquetral malunion can occur. Treatment can be by pisiform excision.

Pisiform Fractures

Introduction

The pisiform is a sesamoid bone in the flexor carpi ulnaris tendon (Fig. 277). It means "pea-shaped". This carpal bone is rare to fracture. Often pisiform fractures are associated with injuries of distal radius, hamate, or triquetrum.

Anatomy

- With the exception of the pisotriquetral ligament and the articular surface with the triquetrum, the pisiform is entirely embedded in the tendon of the flexor carpi ulnaris

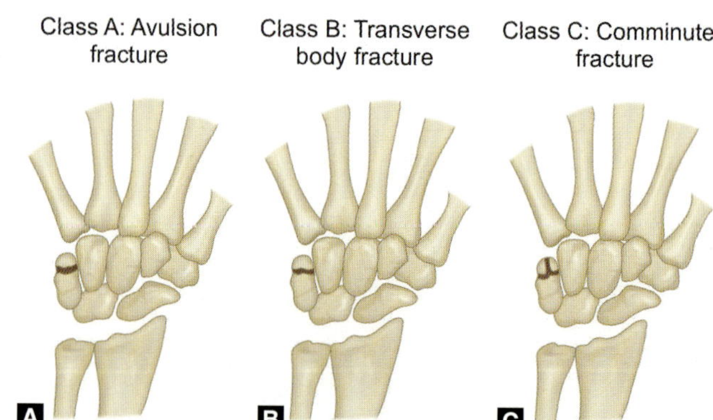

Figs. 278A to C: Classification of different types of pisiform fractures.

- It also serves as the proximal origin of the flexor digiti minimi. The vascular supply to the pisiform is via the ulnar artery with its circumferential foramina on the nonarticular surface.

Mechanism of Injury

The mechanism of injury is usually by a direct blow to the palm, when the wrist is dorsiflexed pulling the pisiform against the triquetrum.

Classification (Figs. 278A to C)

- *Class A:* Avulsion fracture
- *Class B:* Transverse body fracture
- *Class C:* Comminuted fracture.

Presentation

- Pain and swelling at the palmar and ulnar aspects of the wrist
- Tenderness on palpation of the pisiform and over the hypothenar eminence
- Presentation is often delayed, when in isolation and it can be overlooked, when the pisiform fractures are in association with other injuries.

Diagnosis

- Fractures may be missed on AP view. Special views are required to see the pisiform injuries

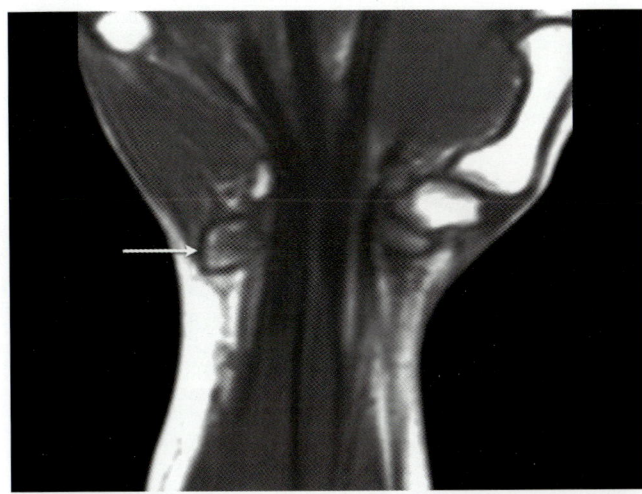

Fig. 279: Computed tomography scan used for making diagnosis, for detecting with arrow showing pisiform bone fracture.

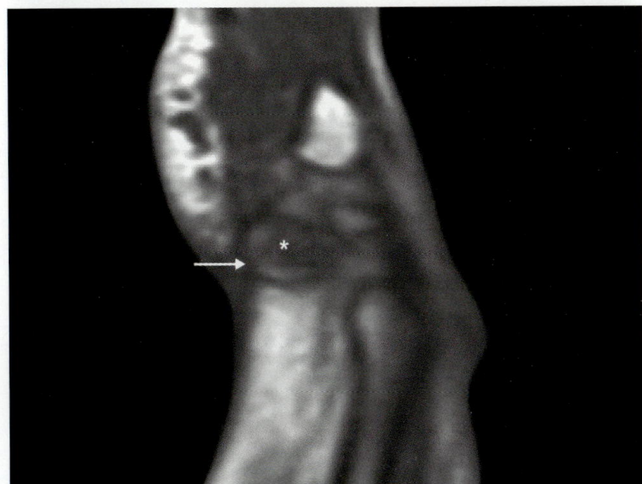

Fig. 280: Computed tomography scan with star (*) showing pisiform and arrow indicates pisciform bone fractures.

- A lateral view of the wrist with the forearm in 20–45° supination and carpal tunnel views are useful
- When in question, a CT may be required to make the diagnosis (Figs. 279 and 280)
- If subluxation of the pisotriquetral joint is suspected, the diagnosis is made when one or more of the following are present: a joint space less than 4 mm in width, loss of parallelism of the joint surfaces greater than 2° proximal or distal over-riding of the pisiform, amounting to more than 15% of the width of the joint surfaces.

Treatment

- Generally, cast immobilization is warranted as a first-line treatment. The cast should be in ulnar deviation with 30° of flexion
- If the fracture progresses to a symptomatic nonunion, the pisiform can be excised.

Complications

- *Nonunions:* In nonunions, bone should be excised. Loss of grip strength occurs after excision, but the difference between hands is not significant.

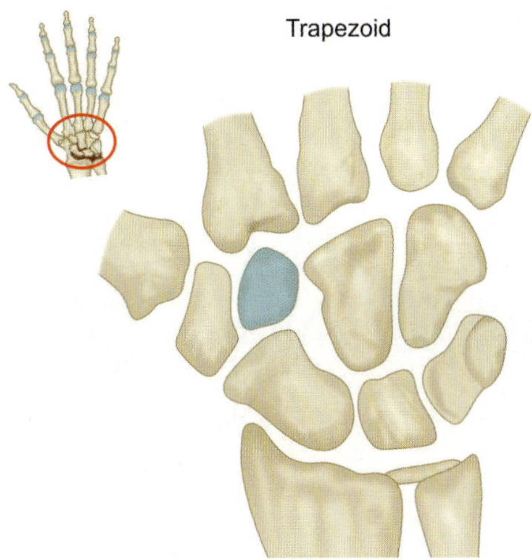

Fig. 281: Trapezium bone (on the radial side of the distal carpal row).

- *Pisotriquetral joint degeneration:* It can also be treated with pisiform excision.

Trapezium Fractures

Introduction

Fractures of the trapezium account for 1–5% of all carpal fractures.

Anatomy

- The trapezium is on the radial side of the distal carpal row (Fig. 281). It articulates distally with the thumb metacarpal and proximally with the scaphoid and the trapezoid
- It forms a double saddle articulation with the base of the thumb metacarpal, allowing motion in two planes, both flexion or extension, and abduction or adduction
- The volar beak ligament from the metacarpal to the trapezium is a key structure in maintaining joint stability and resisting dorsal radial subluxation during key pinch
- A longitudinal ridge is present on the volar surface, which serves as attachment for the transverse carpal ligament.

Mechanism of Injury

- Axial loading of the first metacarpal in the adducted position, typically causes vertical fractures through the articular surface of the trapezium
- Avulsion fractures are caused by capsular and ligamentous attachments that are overloaded in forceful deviation, traction, or rotation
- A direct injury from a blow to the thenar eminence or an avulsion of the transverse carpal ligament will cause a ridge fracture.

Classification

- *Trapezial ridge fractures (Fig. 282):*
  - *Type I*: Basal
  - *Type II*: Apical.
- *Trapezial body fractures:*
  - Vertical
  - Horizontal.
- *Marginal trapeziometacarpal fractures.*

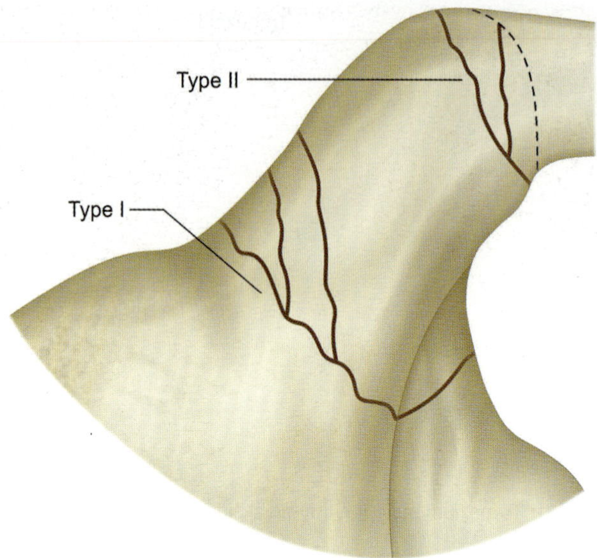

Fig. 282: Trapezial ridge fractures.

Presentation

- Pain and weakness with pinching (making an ok sign or touching the thumb to the tip of the fifth digit)
- Pain with resisted wrist flexion from a dorsiflexed start position may indicate a fracture of the trapezial ridge.

Diagnosis

Special views are required to view the trapezium fractures. These are:

- *Bett's view*: It is obtained with the elbow raised from the cassette, the thumb extended and abducted, the hand somewhat pronated and the hypothenar eminence resting on the plate. The center beam is directed to the scaphotrapeziotrapezoid (STT) joint (Figs. 283A and B).
- *A carpal tunnel view* is mandatory when a fracture of the trapezial ridge is suspected. When there is uncertainty, CT scanning can be diagnostic.

Treatment

- Undisplaced body and marginal trapeziometacarpal fractures can usually be treated with plaster immobilization in a thumb spica cast for 4 weeks, followed by intermittent protective splinting and gradual mobilization
- Displaced body fractures must be exposed surgically open reduction and internal fixation with screws or Kirschner wires
- Type I ridge fractures heal with immobilization, while type II fractures are much likely to heal with immobilization, symptomatic management is therefore advised
- Fractures that remain symptomatic after a period of splinting are treated by surgical excision of the ununited fragment through a palmar approach.

Complications

Progressive degenerative changes of trapeziometacarpal joint are the consequence of intra-articular fractures. With persistent disabling symptoms (aching pain and weakness), trapeziometacarpal arthrodesis or excisional arthroplasty of the trapezium is carried out.

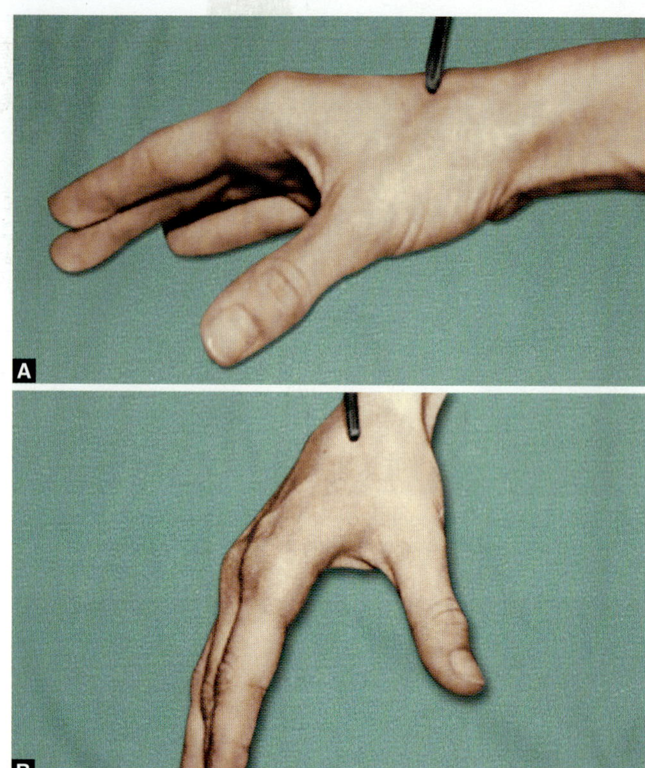

Figs. 283A and B: Bett's view to diagnose trapezium fracture.

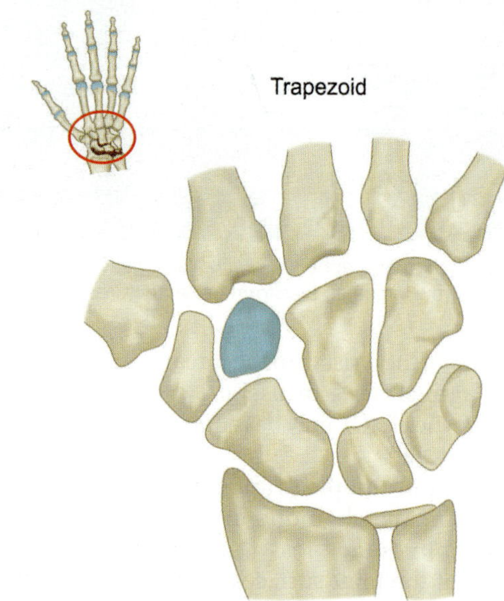

Fig. 284: A wedge-shaped trapezoid bone (distal carpal row).

Trapezoid Fractures

Introduction

Trapezoid fractures are the least common carpal fractures of the wrist, involving less than 1% of all carpal fractures.

Anatomy

The wedge-shaped trapezoid is in the distal carpal row and articulates distally with the index-metacarpal base, radially with the trapezium, ulnarly with the capitate and proximally with the scaphoid (Fig. 284).

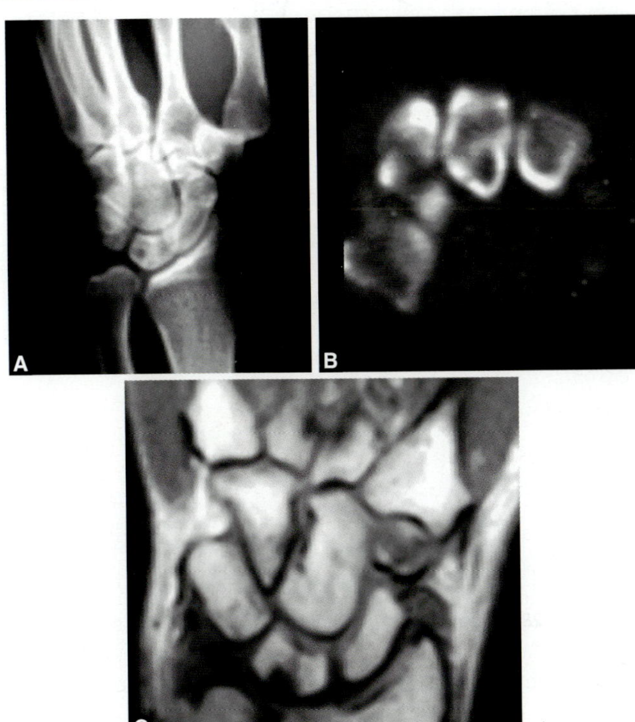

Figs. 285A to C: (A and B) X-rays, showing trapezoid dislocation or fracture; (C) CT scan.

Mechanism of Injury

- Fractures of the trapezoid generally occur with axial loading of the second (index) metacarpal or may rarely occur secondary to direct dorsal trauma
- Wrist hyperflexion with dorsal loading of the index metacarpal and index finger hyperextension with wrist hyperextension, have been suggested as mechanisms and likened to the effect of a nutcracker
- More typically, with a dorsally applied force to the distal aspect of the index metacarpal, a dislocation will occur with the proximal aspect of the metacarpal slipping volar (palmar) to the trapezoid.

Classification

- Vertical fracture
- Osteoligamentary avulsion injury.

Presentation

- Patients will usually have some degree of swelling on the dorsum of the hand and point tenderness dorsally just proximal to the second metacarpal base
- Resisted wrist dorsiflexion may cause pain as the extensor carpi radialis inserts on the proximal aspect of the index metacarpal, which is closely fixed to the trapezoid by firm intercarpal ligamentous attachments.

Diagnosis

- A trapezoid dislocation or fracture dislocation is seen on the anteroposterior X-ray, as a loss of the normal relationship between the second metacarpal base and the trapezoid (Figs. 285A and B).
- The trapezoid may be superimposed over the trapezium or the capitate and the second metacarpal may be proximally displaced.

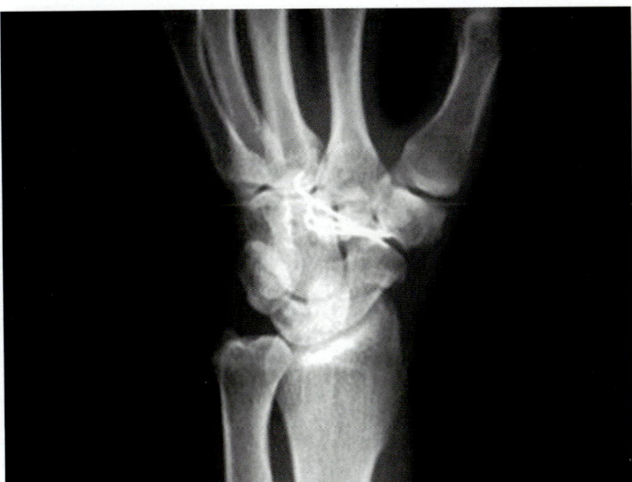

Fig. 286: Large fragment of displaced fracture of trapezoid bone.

- Diagnosis and analysis are best achieved with the CT scans (Fig. 285C).

Treatment

- *Undisplaced fracture:* Cast immobilization
- *Displaced fracture:*
  - *Small fragment:* Closed reduction and casting
  - *Large fragment:* Open reduction and internal fixation (Fig. 286).
- *In chronic injuries:* Open reduction, bone grafting, and carpometacarpal arthrodesis.

Complications

- Malunion
- Delayed union
- Nonunion.

Capitate Fractures

Introduction

The capitate is the largest carpal bone. Injuries to the capitate are often part of complex injuries. Capitate fractures are sometimes seen along with scaphoid waist fractures or distal radius fractures.

Anatomy

The capitate articulates distally with the bases of the third and fourth metacarpals and proximally with the scaphoid and lunate. The trapezoid and the hamate are lateral (radial) and medial, respectively (Fig. 287).

Classification

- Capitate fractures are classified by the anatomic location of the fracture, along with what other concomitant injuries may be present.
- The combination of a capitate fracture and a scaphoid waist fracture is known as scaphocapitate syndrome. The force of injury in this syndrome can propagate leading to perilunate dislocation as well.

Mechanism of Injury

- Direct blow or crushing injuries. These are usually associated with injuries to the metacarpals and other carpal bones.

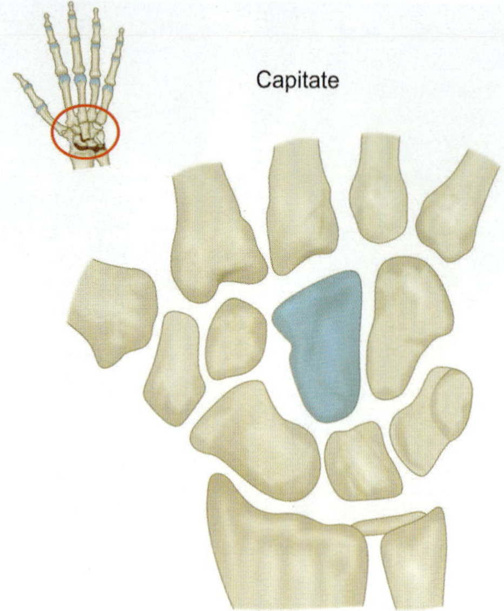

Fig. 287: Capitate bone.

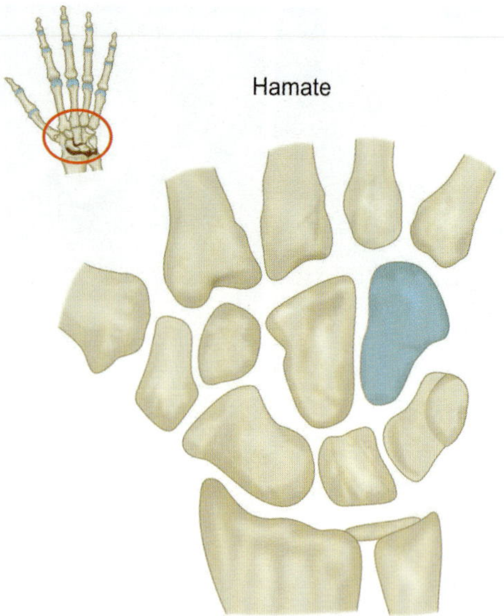

Fig. 289: Hamate bone (distal carpal row on ulnar side).

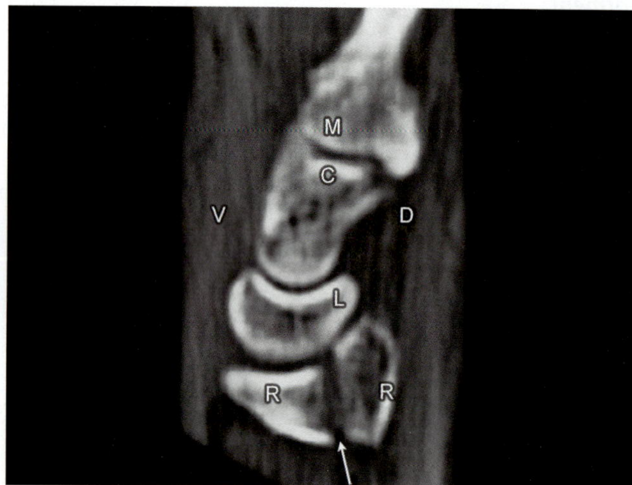

Fig. 288: Standard scaphoid views, lateral views to look for rotation or displacement. (M: metacarpal; C: carpal; L: lunate; R: radius; V: volar; D: dorsal and arrow shows radius fracture)

- A fall with the wrist in dorsiflexion, forcing the capitates onto the dorsal rim of the radius. The dorsal border of the radius will impinge on the capitates and cause a fracture through its waist.
- Scaphocapitate syndrome.

Note: Please refer to scaphocapitate fracture syndrome topic.

Presentation

Patients typically present with wrist pain after an acute injury and a careful examination can pinpoint the area to the capitate.

Diagnosis

- Standard scaphoid views, lateral views to look for rotation or displacement (Fig. 288).
- The CT scan and MRI aid in accurate diagnosis.

Treatment

- *Nondisplaced capitate fractures:* They need to be immobilized in a short arm thumb spica with the wrist in slight dorsiflexion and the thumb immobilized to the interphalangeal joint for 8 weeks.
- *Displaced capitate fractures:* Closed reduction followed by immobilization should be attempted first. If unsuccessful, surgical fixation with a K-wire or a screw, with bone graft, added for significant comminution.

Scaphocapitate Syndrome

- If diagnosed within 3–4 weeks of injury, open reduction is carried out through a dorsal approach with internal fixation for one or both fractures, depending on stability. Cast immobilization is continued until both fractures have healed.
- For fractures diagnosed late, treatment becomes a matter of judgment. If the scaphoid has healed or is healing in a satisfactory position, watchful waiting may be appropriate in as much as some patients will remain symptom free or have tolerable symptoms for many years, despite of capitate head displacement. Patients seen late with significant symptoms and malalignment of both the scaphoid and capitate are probably best treated by a salvage procedure, such as midcarpal arthrodesis.

Complications

- Malunion or AVN
- Post-traumatic arthritis
- Fibrosis after the injury may result in a median nerve neuropathy or a carpal tunnel syndrome.

Hamate Fractures

Introduction

The hamate is the most ulnar carpal bone on the distal row (Fig. 289). Hamate fractures account for 2–4% of the carpal fractures. Hamate fractures mainly occur in two locations, the hook of the hamate or the body.

Anatomy

- The body of the hamate articulates distally with the bases of the fourth and fifth metacarpals, radially with the capitate and proximally with the triquetrum and lunate

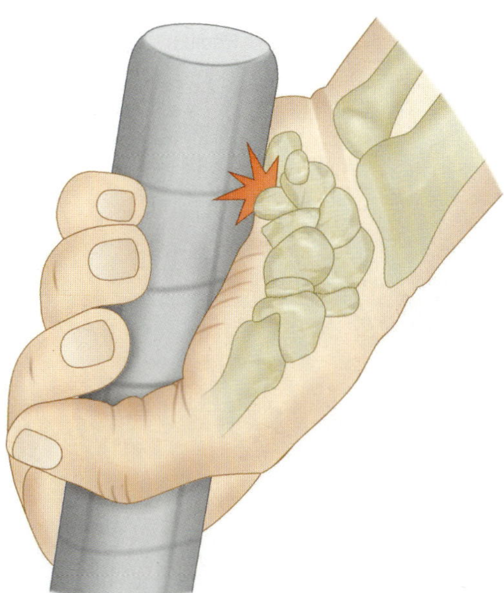

Fig. 290: In sports, fracture of the hook of the hamate results, when a club, racquet or bat is forced into the palm, exerting direct pressure on the hypothenar eminence and thus the hamulus.

- The hook of the hamate (hamulus) is the distal border of Guyon's canal, which contains the ulnar artery and nerve. With injury of the hamate, one should always assure vascular patency and that sensation is intact in the fifth digit and the ulnar border of the fourth
- The hook of the hamate develops from an ossification center separate from the body of the hamate. In some adults, it persists as the os hamulus proprius. This normal variant can present a potential diagnostic pitfall, if misinterpreted as a hamate fracture or nonunion
- Attachments to the hamate include the transverse carpal ligament and flexor carpi ulnaris
- The blood supply to the hamate is variable with 70% having only vascular supply to the body, predisposing hook fractures to nonunion.

Mechanism of Injury

- Fractures of the hook of the hamate are more common
- Fall on the outstretched hand that puts the transverse carpal ligament in tension and causes avulsion of the hook from the body
- In sports, fracture of the hook of the hamate results, when a club, racquet or bat is forced into the palm, exerting direct pressure on the hypothenar eminence and thus the hamulus. This typically occurs on the nondominant hand (Fig. 290)
- Fractures of the hamate body are less common and can be associated with fifth or sometimes fourth metacarpal fractures.

Classification

Fracture of hamate body:

- *Vertical fracture:* These can be on either the ulnar or radial side of the hamulus.
- *Horizontal fracture:* Fracture of the hook (hamulus) of the hamate.

Presentation

- Ulnar sided wrist pain and point tenderness over the hook of the hamate.

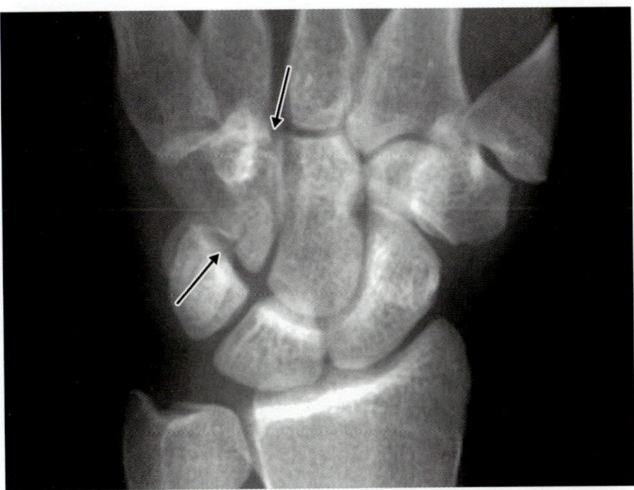

Fig. 291: X-ray showing hamate fractures (arrows).

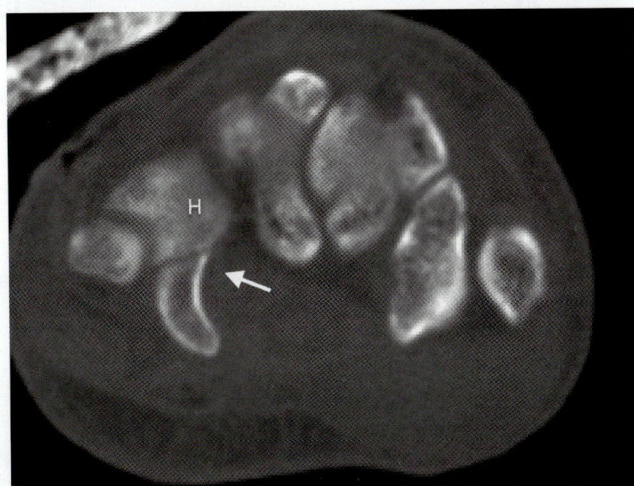

Fig. 292: Computed tomography scanning with the hands in a "praying position" is most diagnostic, in case of a hamate (H) fracture (arrow showing fracture line).

- In acute injuries, pain is present with palpation in hypothenar area.
- Pain also may be present with resisted flexion of the fourth and fifth fingers.

Diagnosis

- Standard radiographs of the wrist (AP and lateral) may be insufficient to make the diagnosis and a carpal tunnel or 45° supination oblique view may be required (Fig. 291)
- A special view (Papilion et al.), involving a lateral radiograph with the thumb maximally opposed (to move it out of the way) and the wrist in ulnar deviation, hand slightly supinated to bring the hook into greatest profile
- The CT scanning with the hands in a praying position is the most sensitive diagnostic study. When in doubt of hook fractures versus os hamulus proprius, an MRI may distinguish the acuity of the injury (Fig. 292).

Treatment

- Acute injuries can be treated closed with cast immobilization
- Hook of the hamate nonunions can be excised with small fragments or fixed with bone graft and screws, when fragments are large enough

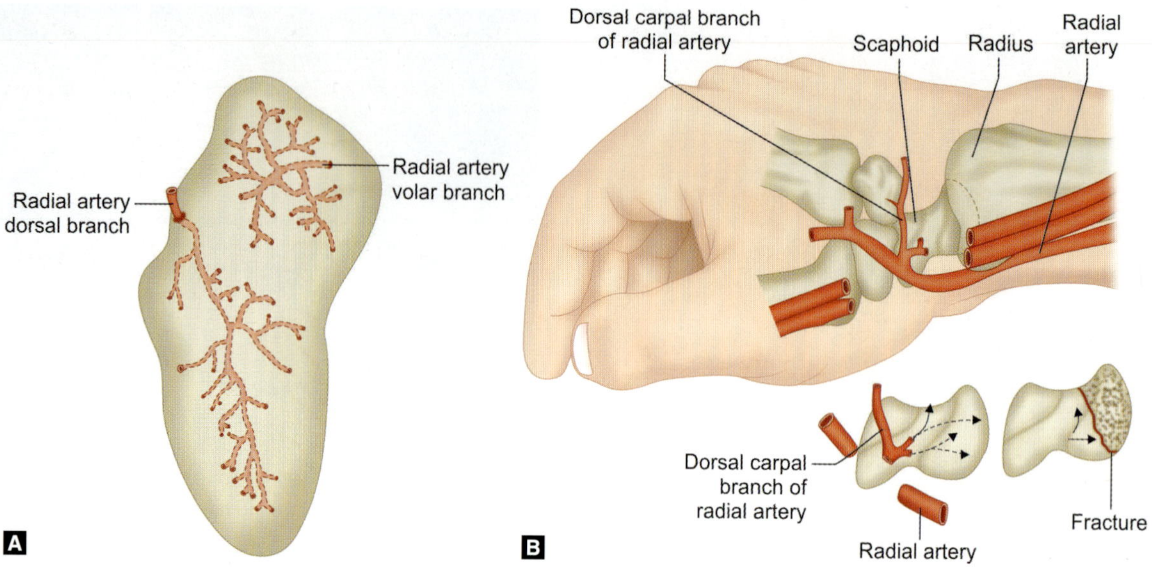

Figs. 293A and B: Blood supply of scaphoid

- Displaced hamate body fractures may either be precutaneously pinned or fixed with an open reduction.

Complications

- Nonunion may occur with vascular disruption
- Ulnar neuropathy may have profound affects
- Flexor tendon rupture over the bony prominence is not an uncommon complication.

SCAPHOID FRACTURES

Anatomy

It is irregularly shaped tubular bone, twisted, and bent into "S"-shaped. More than 80% of its surface is being covered by articular cartilage, which reduces its capacity for periosteal healing and increases chances of nonunion.

It articulates with the distal radius and four of the carpal bones. Scaphoid moves with nearly all carpal motions. Thus, any change in its articular surface will cause severe secondary changes in the carpus.

Blood Supply of Scaphoid

Blood supply of scaphoid bone is shown in Figures 293A and B.

Signs and Symptoms of Scaphoid Fractures

Symptoms:

- Pain in wrist due to fall on outstretched hand
- Usually associated with hyperextension injury and slight radial deviation of the wrist.

Signs:

- Tenderness of anatomical snuffbox and scaphoid tubercle
- Pain with axial compression of thumb
- The ROM is reduced and painful at extremes of motion
- Loss of wrist extension suggests nonunited scaphoid fractures, associated with carpal collapse deformity, and palmar capsular contracture.

Diagnosis

X-rays: Various views of scaphoid, in which X-rays can be taken, are enumerated below and also shown in Figures 294 to 297:

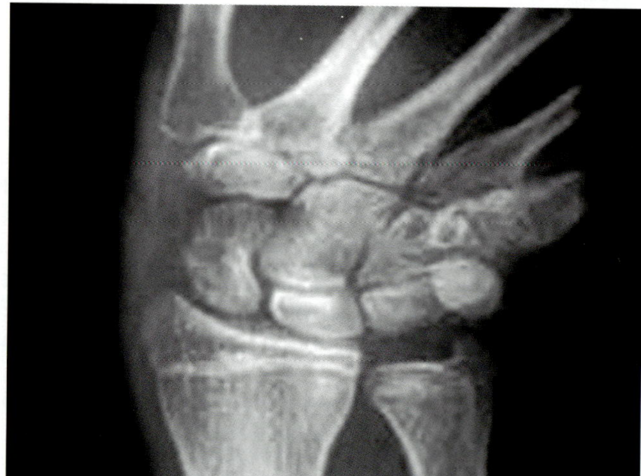

Fig. 294: Normal posteroanterior radiograph of scaphoid (right)

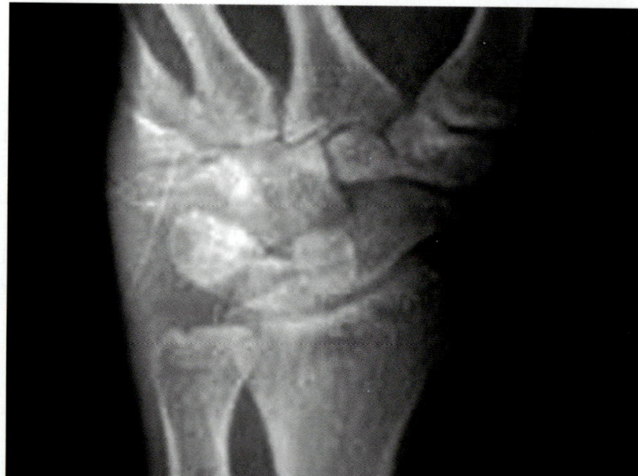

Fig. 295: Normal anterior oblique radiograph of scaphoid (left)

- Posteroanterior ulnar deviation
- Radial oblique ulnar deviation
- True lateral

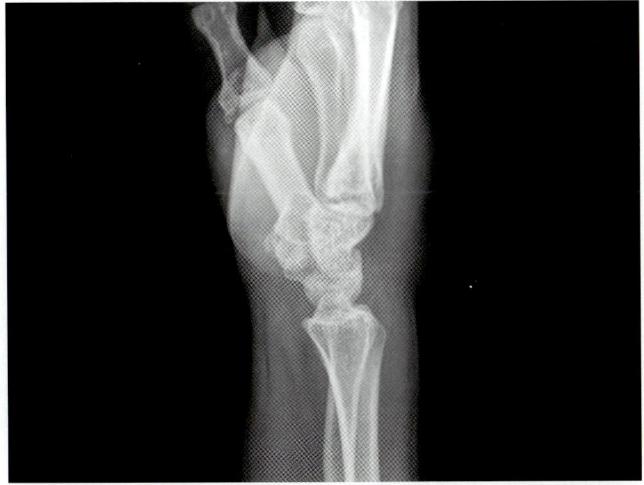

Fig. 296: Normal lateral radiograph of wrist.

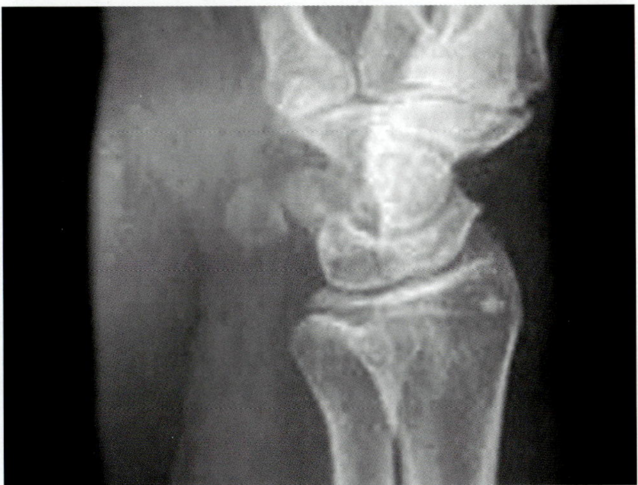

Fig. 297: Normal posterior oblique radiograph of wrist.

- Posterior oblique
- Motion views of scaphoid in flexion extension, along with radial and ulnar deviation will demonstrates fracture displacement.

Reasons of misdiagnosis of scaphoid fracture on X-ray:

- A dark line formed by dorsal lip of radius overlapping the scaphoid.
- Presence of white line formed by proximal end of scaphoid tuberosity.
- Dorsal ridge may appear bent in semisupinated view.

MRI

It is gold standard for diagnosing carpal and wrist injury at an early stage. It is the most effective way of diagnosing scaphoid fractures (Fig. 298).

Classification

Classification of Scaphoid Fractures by Anatomic Location (Fig. 299)

- Proximal pole fracture
- Waist fracture
- Distal body fracture
- Tuberosity fracture.

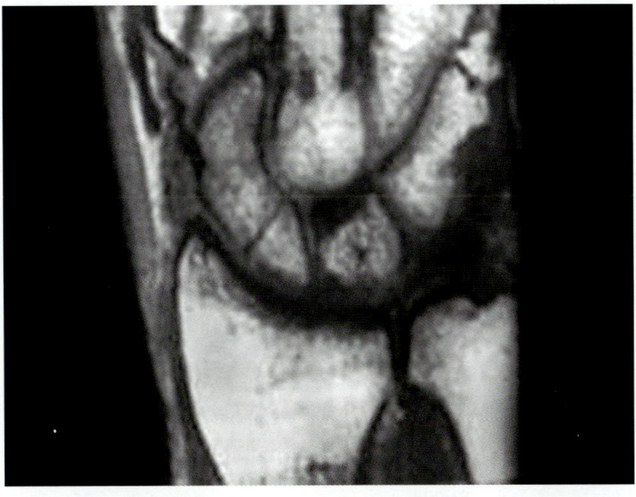

Fig. 298: MRI used for diagnosing scaphoid fracture.

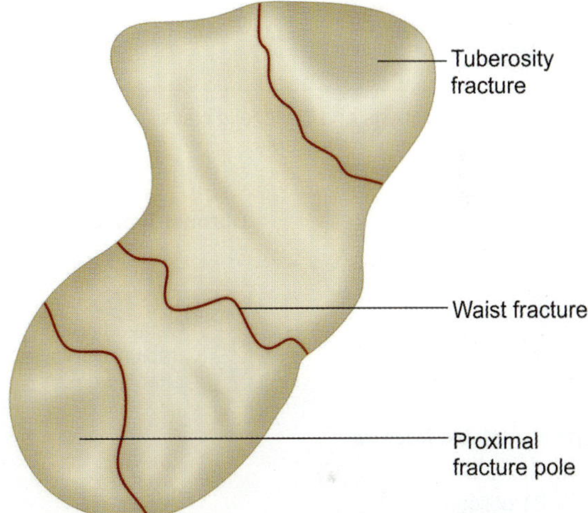

Fig. 299: Classification of scaphoid fractures by anatomic location.

Cooney, Dobyns and Linscheild Classification of Scaphoid Fracture (Fig. 300)

- Undisplaced and stable
- Displaced and unstable

Herbert and Fisherís Classification (Fig. 301)

Type A: Stable acute fractures

- A1: Fracture of tuberosity
- A2: Incomplete fracture through waist

Type B: Unstable acute fractures

- B1: Distal oblique fractures
- B2: Complete fracture of waist
- B3: Proximal pole fracture
- B4: Trans-scaphoid perilunate fracture dislocation
- B5: Comminuted fractures

Type C: Delayed union

Type D: Established nonunion

- D1: Fibrous nonunion
- D2: Pseudarthrosis.

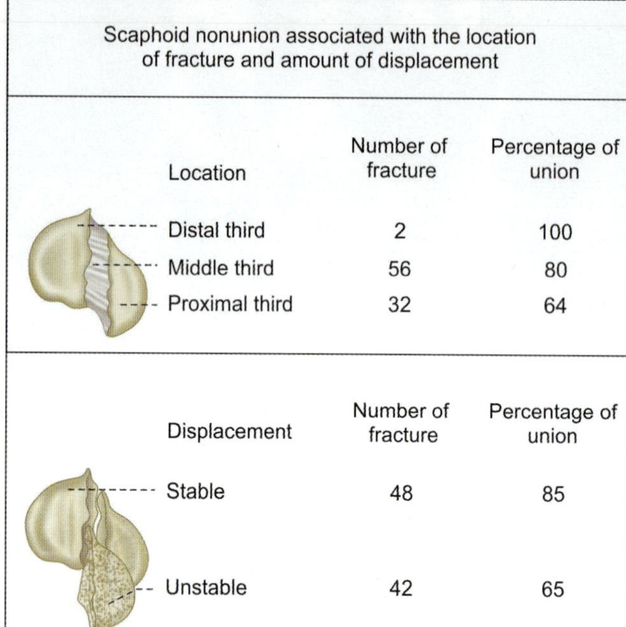

Scaphoid nonunion associated with the location of fracture and amount of displacement

Location	Number of fracture	Percentage of union
Distal third	2	100
Middle third	56	80
Proximal third	32	64

Displacement	Number of fracture	Percentage of union
Stable	48	85
Unstable	42	65

Fig. 300: Cooney, Dobyns and Linscheild classification of scaphoid fractures.

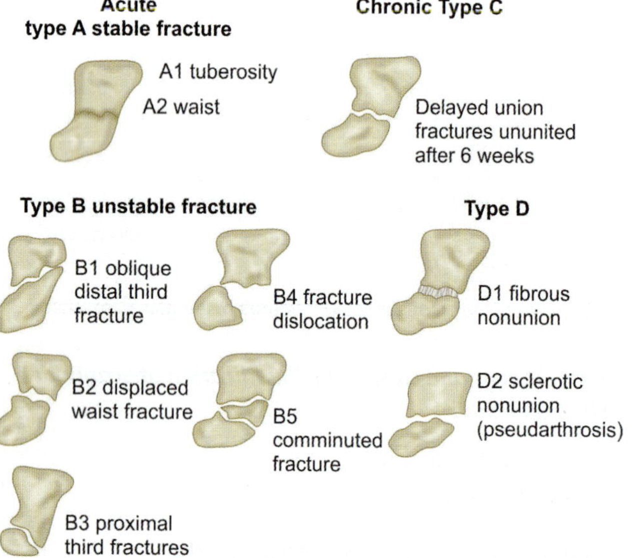

Fig. 301: Herbert and Fisher's classification of scaphoid fracture.

Treatment

- Nondisplaced stable fractures
- Displaced stable fractures.

Treatment for Nondisplaced Stable Scaphoid Fractures

Nonoperative treatment: It is usually recommended. Prognosis is better, if fracture is diagnosed early.

Early diagnosis:

- *Forearm cast or munster type cast (Fig. 302):* It is given from just below the elbow proximally to the base of thumbnail and proximal palmar crease distally. Wrist in slight radial deviation and in neutral flexion. Thumb is maintained in functional position

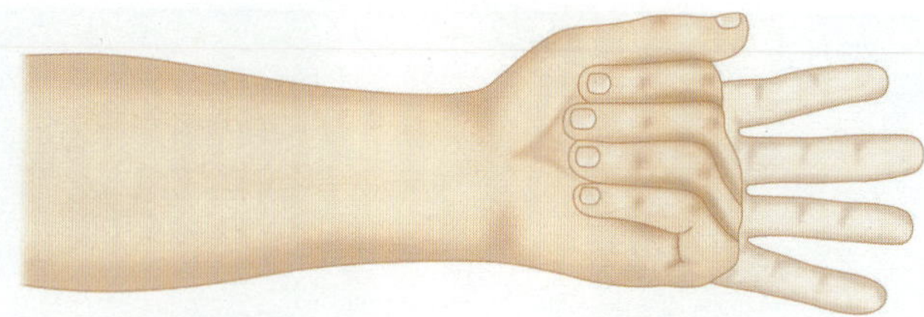

Fig. 302: Forearm cast or munster type cast.

- *Colles' cast:* It may be given for stable nondisplaced fractures
- *Above elbow cast:* Earlier above elbow cast was also given for fracture of scaphoid. The cast is kept for 10–12 weeks. During this time, fracture is observed radiologically for healing. In case of query fracture, cast is applied and X-ray is taken after 2 weeks.

Delayed diagnosis

- *Middle third stable fracture:* It is diagnosed after 1 to 6 months of injury. It is treated with cast immobilization. It usually takes 19 weeks to unite as compared to average of 10 weeks for acute fractures.
- *Proximal third fracture:* Its prognosis is less favorable, but initial long arm thumb spica cast may be justified for 6 weeks.

Operative (Nondisplaced Stable)

Indications:

- Diagnosis is delayed
- Fracture is in proximal third
- Collapse or angulation of the fracture fragment, if found during regular radiological evaluation
- Due to joint stiffness, muscle atrophy and inability to use the hand during and after prolonged immo- bilization, operative treatment may be considered in some patients, e.g. young laborers or athletes.

Operative technique: Percutaneous fixation technique for nondisplaced stable scaphoid fracture. This technique is illustrated in Figures 303A to F.

Treatment for Displaced Stable Scaphoid Fractures

Criteria for fracture to be displaced unstable (Figs. 304A to C)

- Displacement greater than 1 mm in AP or oblique view
- Lunocapitate angulation greater than 15°
- Scapholunate angulation greater than 45° in lateral view
- Lateral intrascaphoid angle greater than 45°
- AP intrascaphoid angle less than 35°.

It is usually treated operatively or and if done with Herbert differential pitch bone screw/AO screw/Acutrak screw, percutaneous fixation of the fracture can also be done.

Advantages of Surgery

- Reduces the time of external fixation
- Provides relatively strong internal fixation
- Produces compression at fracture site
- These screws can be used with bone graft to correct scaphoid angulation.

Exposure of Scaphoid

- *Volar approach (Figs. 305A to D):* Used for scaphoid fracture at or distal to the waist.
- *Dorsal approach (Fig. 306):* Used for proximal pole noncomminuted fractures. Extend skin incision from radial

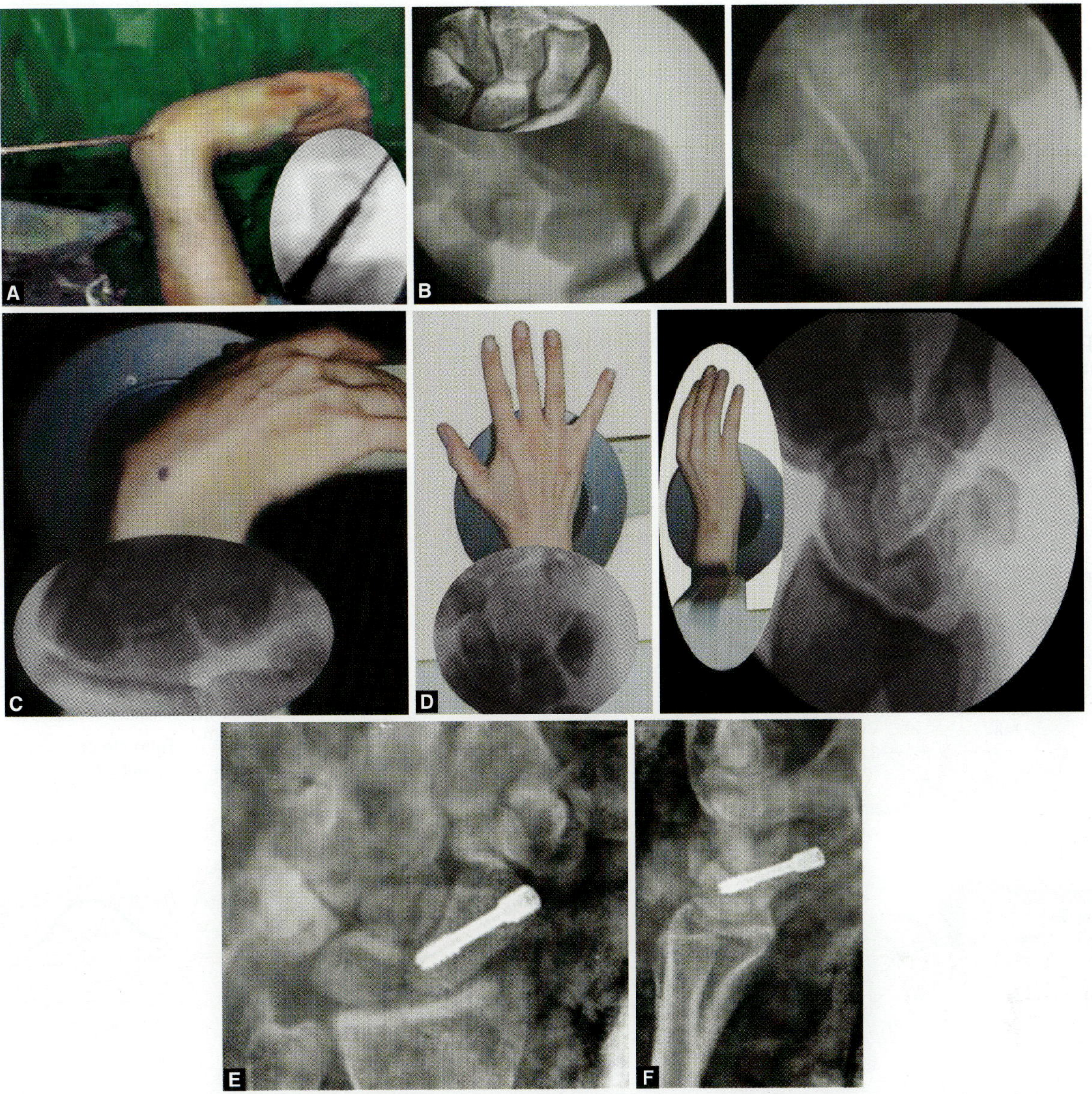

Figs. 303A to F: Techniques for percutaneous fixation.

styloid to ulnar styloid. Make parallel incisions on external retinaculum on each side of external digitorum tendon. Open the dorsal capsule by radially creating base flap and expose fracture.

- *Dorsolateral approach (Figs. 307A to C).*

Scaphoid Nonunion

Nonunion is influenced by:

- Delayed diagnosis
- Gross displacement
- Associated injuries of carpus
- Impaired blood supply.

Radiographic Findings

- Arthritis
- Radioscaphoid narrowing
- Capitolunate narrowing
- Cyst formation
- Pronounced dorsal intercalated segment instability is also called scaphoid nonunion advanced collapse pattern.

Differentiation between Acute Fracture and Nonunion

- Acute fracture is represented by a single line through bone, occasionally with dorsoradial comminution and dorsal angulation.
- Nonunion will show resorption at the fracture site, subchondral sclerosis and displacement on both PA and lateral X-rays.

Stages of Scaphoid Nonunion

Different stages of scaphoid nonunion are shown in Figure 308.

Treatment

Algorithm for treatment of scaphoid nonunion is shown in Flowchart 4.

Following operations can be useful for scaphoid nonunion:

- Radial styloidectomy
- Excision of proximal fragment, distal fragment or entire scaphoid

- Proximal row carpectomy
- Bone grafting
- Vascularized bone grafting
- Partial and total wrist arthrodesis.

Radial Styloidectomy

Image of wrist joint following radial styloidectomy is shown in Figure 309.

Indications

- Arthritic changes in scaphoid fossa. It is indicated with any grafting of scaphoid or excision of its ulnar fragment.
- Older patients with radioscaphoid arthritis and when the proximal fragment not loosen.

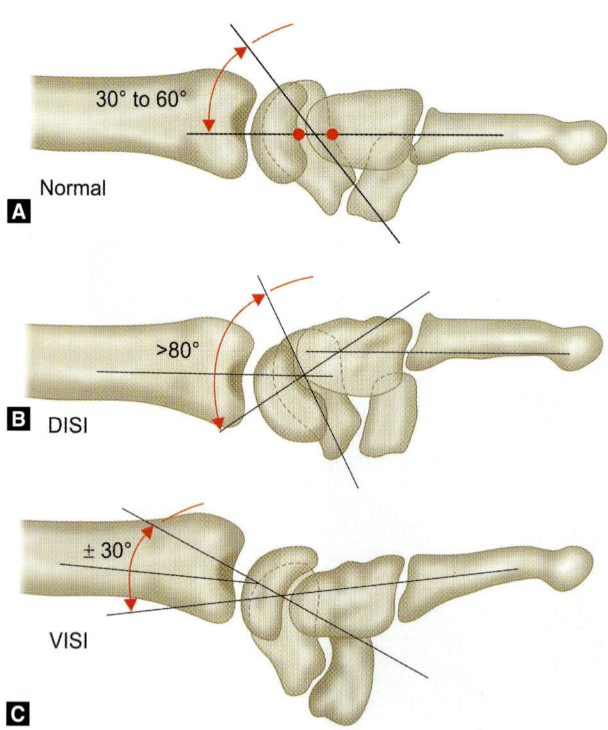

Figs. 304A to C: Criteria for fracture to be displaced unstable.

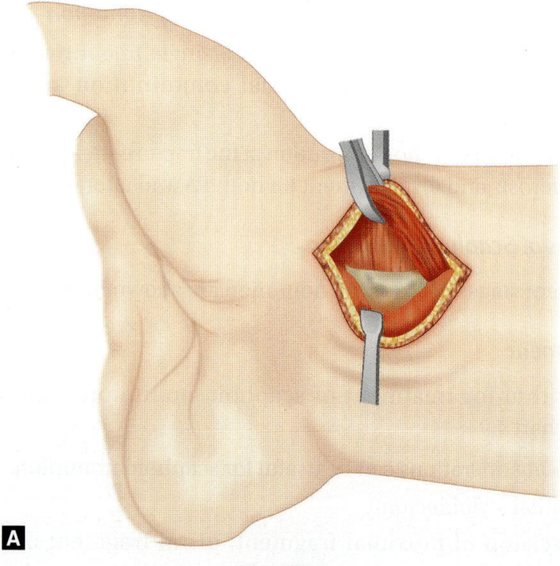

Fig. 305A

Procedure

- Resect enough of the styloid to remove the entire articulation with the scaphoid.

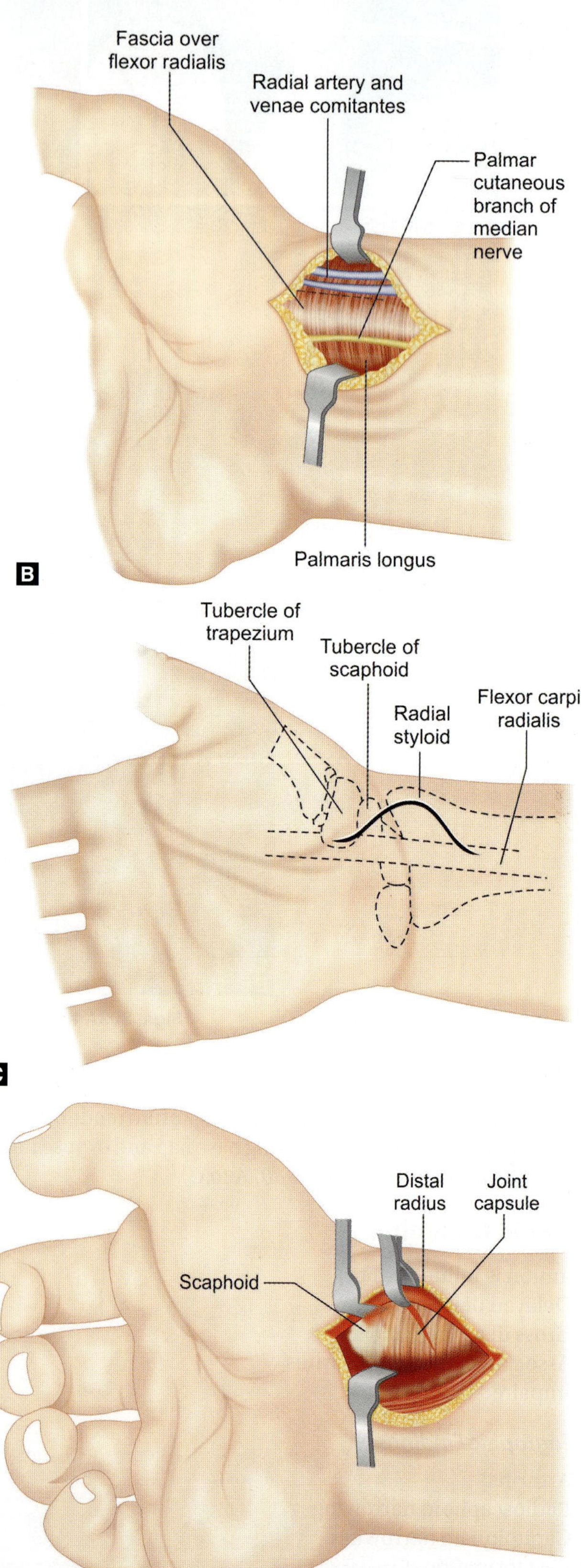

Figs. 305A to D: Exposure of scaphoid—Volar approach.

- Preserve palmar radiocarpal ligaments to avoid ulnar translocation of the carpus.

Excision of Proximal Fragment

Indications

- The fragment is one-fourth or less of the scaphoid
- Above indication and fragment is sclerotic, comminuted or severly displaced
- The fragment is one-fourth or less of the scaphoid and grafting has failed
- Arthritic changes are present in the region of radial styloid.

Excision of the Distal Scaphoid

Indicated in scaphoid nonunions with radioscaphoid arthritis.

Proximal Row Carpectomy

It is reconstructive procedure for post-traumatic degenerative conditions in the wrist, involving the scaphoid and lunate.

Indications

- In patients who have limited requirements for wrist mobility and accept mild persistent pain
- Useful in treating severe open carpal fracture dislocation with significant comminuted fractures of scaphoid and lunate (Figs. 310A and B).

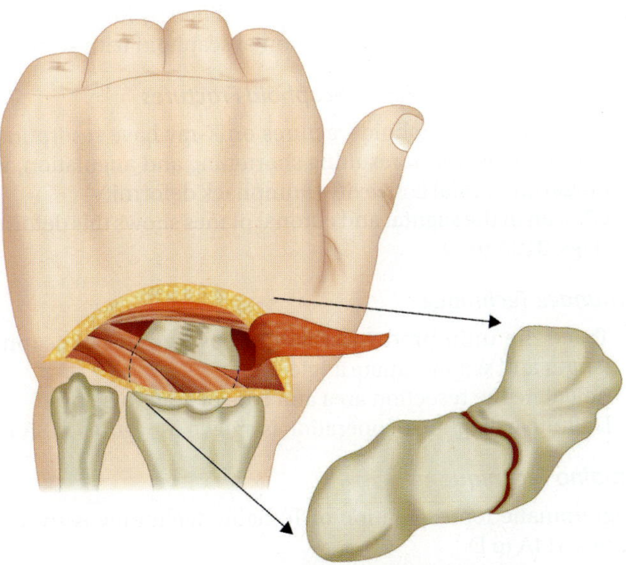

Fig. 306: Dorsal approach to expose scaphoid bone.

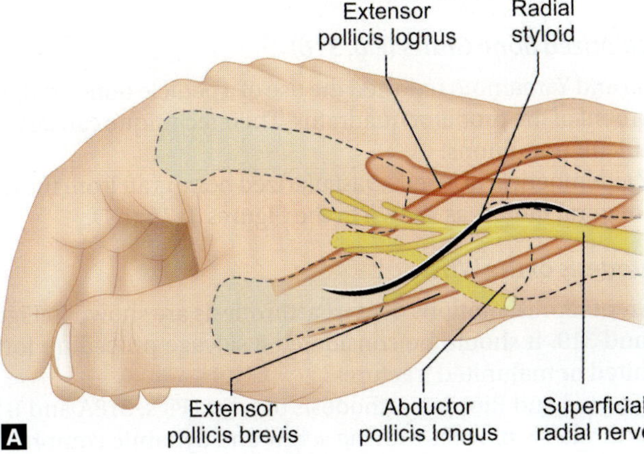

Fig. 307A

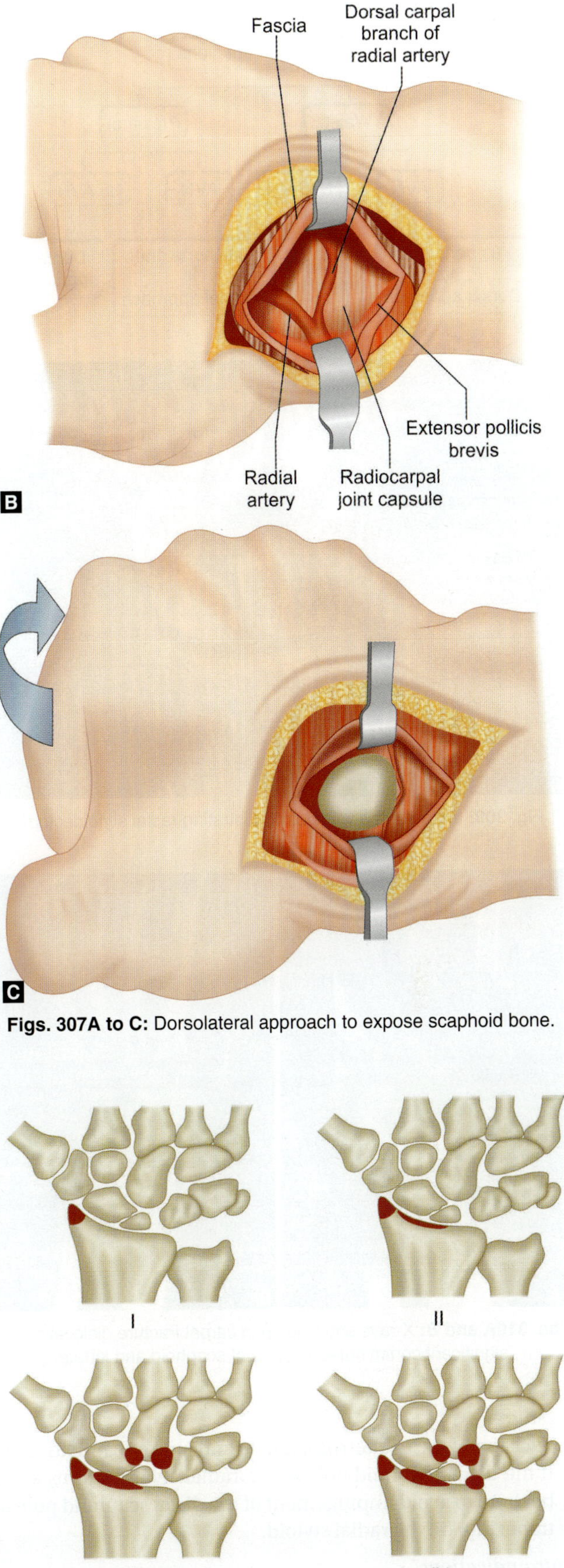

Figs. 307A to C: Dorsolateral approach to expose scaphoid bone.

Fig. 308: Stages of scaphoid nonunion advanced collapse. Stage I: Arthritis at radial styloid; Stage II: Scaphoid fossa arthritis; Stage III: Capitolunate arthritis. Stage IV: Diffuse arthritis of carpus.

Flowchart 4: Algorithm for treatment of scaphoid nonunion.

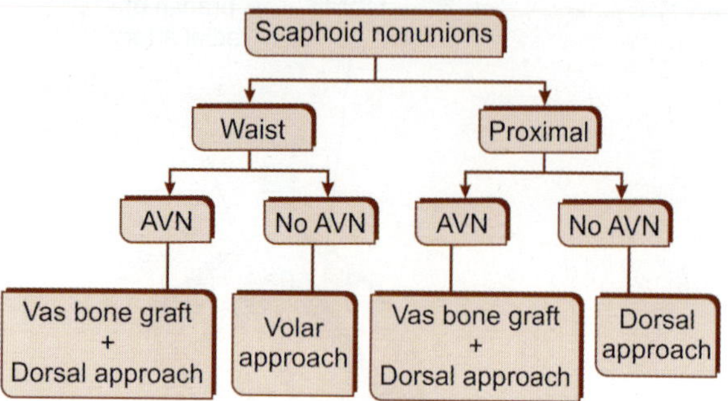

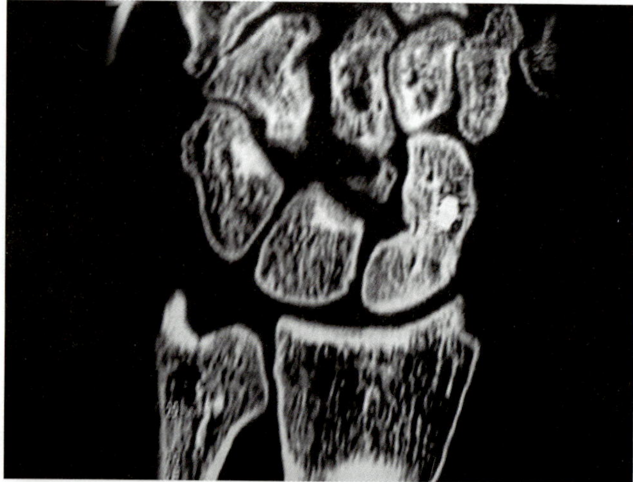

Fig. 309: Image of the wrist joint, illustrating radial styloidectomy.

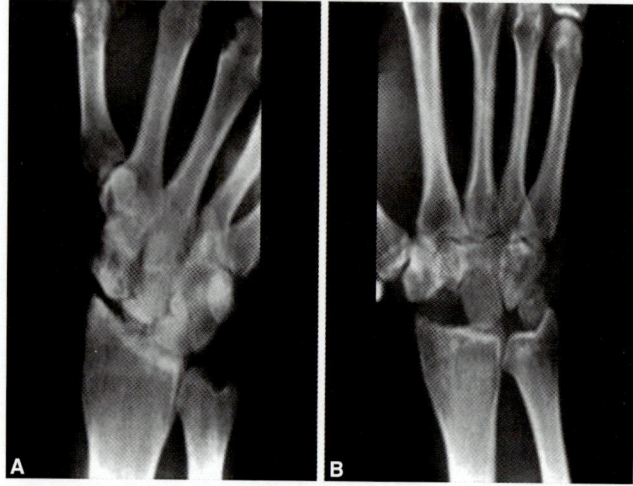

Figs. 310A and B: X-rays showing open carpal fracture dislocation with significant comminuted fracture of scaphoid and lunate.

Procedure

- Excision of the triquetrum, lunate and entire scaphoid is done
- If the distal scaphoid pole is left, radial styloidectomy should be done to avoid impingement of the distal scaphoid pole and trapezium on the radial styloid.

Contraindications

- Severe arthrosis at capitolunate joint
- If mild arthrosis than carpectomy is done with excising proximal pole of capitate and cover that with dorsal capsular flap.

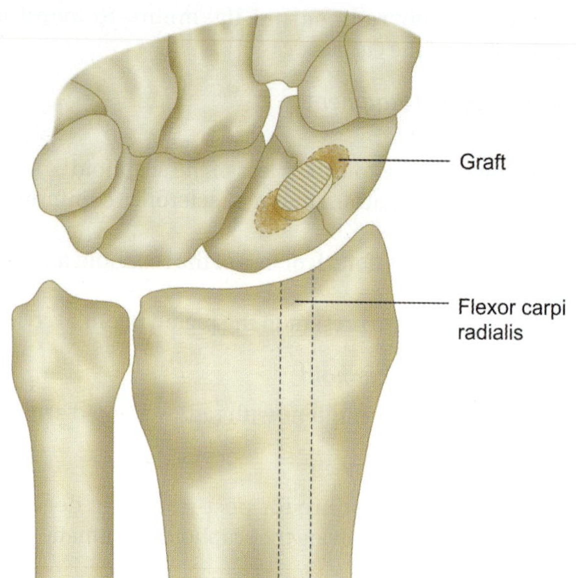

Fig. 311: Grafting operations.

Grafting Operations

- Cancellous bone grafting for scaphoid nonunion that do not have shortening or angulation (Fig. 311)
- It was first describe by Matti and modified by Russe.
- It is done with or without fixation of scaphoid with screw.

Malpositioned Nonunion of Scaphoid Fractures

- Nonunions of scaphoid fractures on X-ray have resorption or comminution, with resulting shortening and angulation, with dorsal and radial convexity (humpback deformity)
- CT scan in the sagittal and coronal planes shows this deformity (Figs. 312A to F).

Fernandez Technique

- Trace the uninjured wrist with measurement of scaphoid length and scapholunate angle
- Calculate the resection area and type of graft to be used
- Definitive diagram of operation is shown in Figures 313A to C.

Tomaino Technique

Diagrammatic representation of Tomaino technique is shown in Figures 314A to D.

Stark Technique: Diagrammatic representation of Stark technique is shown in Figures 315A to C.

Vascularized Bone Grafts (Fig. 316)

Kawai and Yamamoto reported the use of a pedicle bone graft using a segment of the pronator quadratus. Their technique can be useful in difficult nonunions.

Zaidemberg et al. used a vascularized bone graft from the distal dorsolateral radius, as shown in the Figures 317A to D.

Arthrodesis of the Wrist

Different representations of wrist arthrodesis are shown in Figures 318 and 319. It should be considered a salvage procedure for old ununited or malunited fractures.

- Haddad and Riordan arthodesis of wrist (Figs. 318A and B)
- Arthrodesis of wrist with lag screw and dynamic compression plate fixation (Figs. 319A and B).

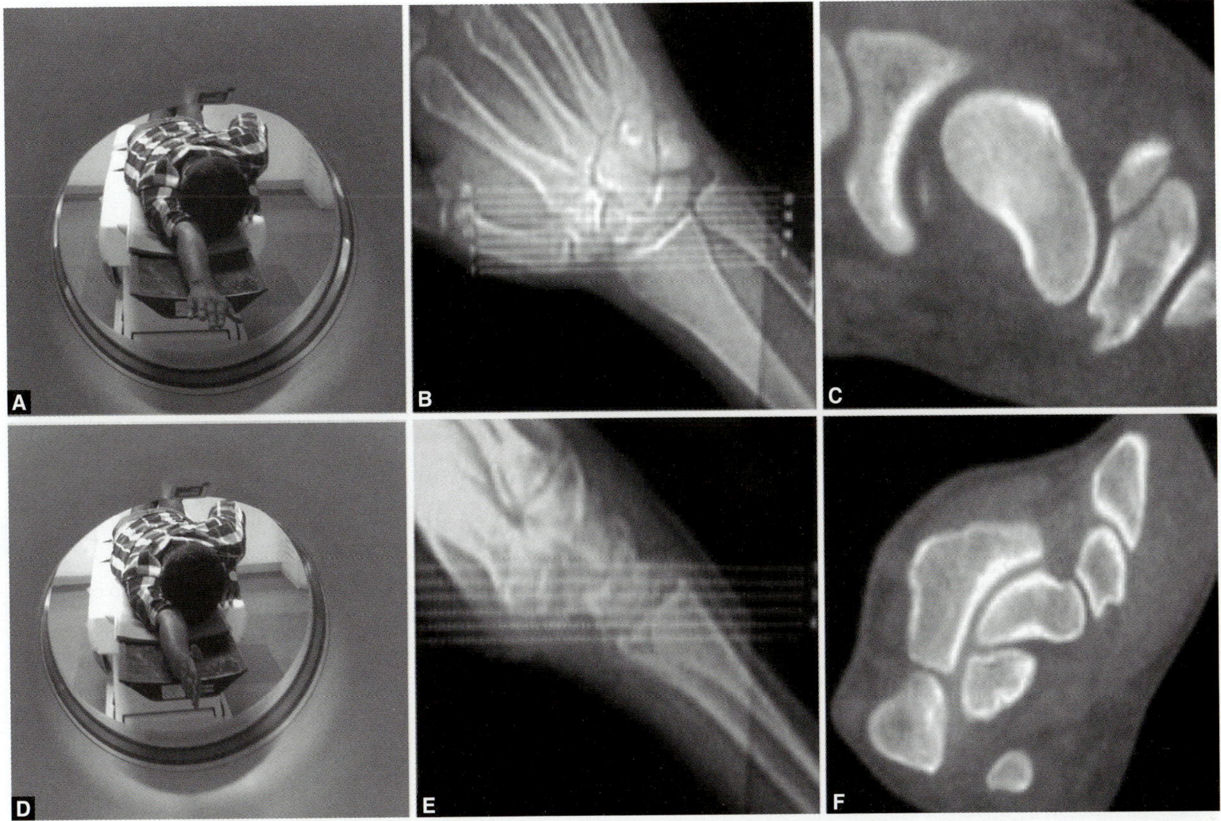

Figs. 312A to F: CT scan in the sagittal and coronal planes showing, humpback deformity.

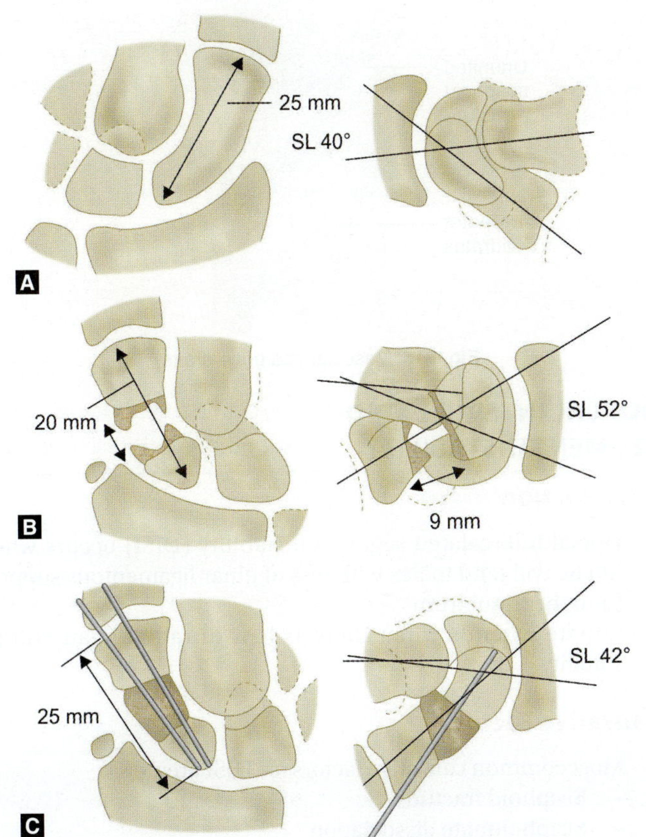

Figs. 313A to C: (A) Tracing of uninjured wrist with measurement of scaphoid length and scapholunate angle; (B) Calculation of resection area and type of graft to be used; (C) Definitive diagram of operation.

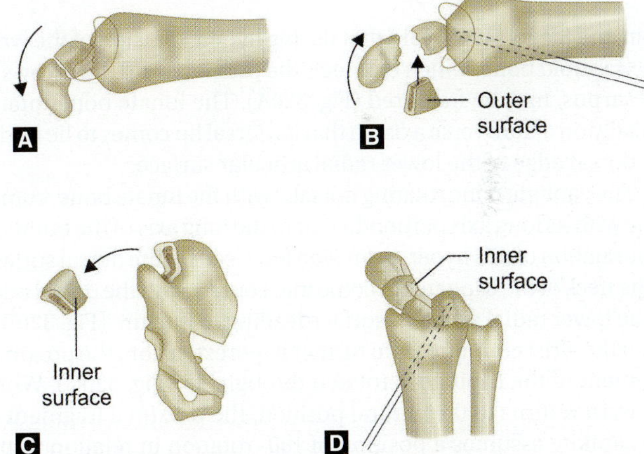

Figs. 314A to D: Tomaino technique—(A) Lunate extension, dorsal intercalated segment instability with scaphoid nonunion; (B) With wrist extension, radiolunate joint is pinned. Scaphoid opens at nonunion site; (C) Tricortical corticocancellous graft is harvested; (D) Graft is placed after that Herbert-Whipple screw is placed and lunate transfixation pin is removed.

Electrical and Ultrasound Stimulation

It has been found to be effective for treatment for scaphoid nonunions. A study shows patients treated with casting alone healed on an average 62 days, whereas patient treated with ultrasound healed in 43 days (Campbell et al.)

Complications following nonunion surgery

- Persistent nonunion
- Hardware malpositioning
- Stiffness
- Pain
- Nerve injury.

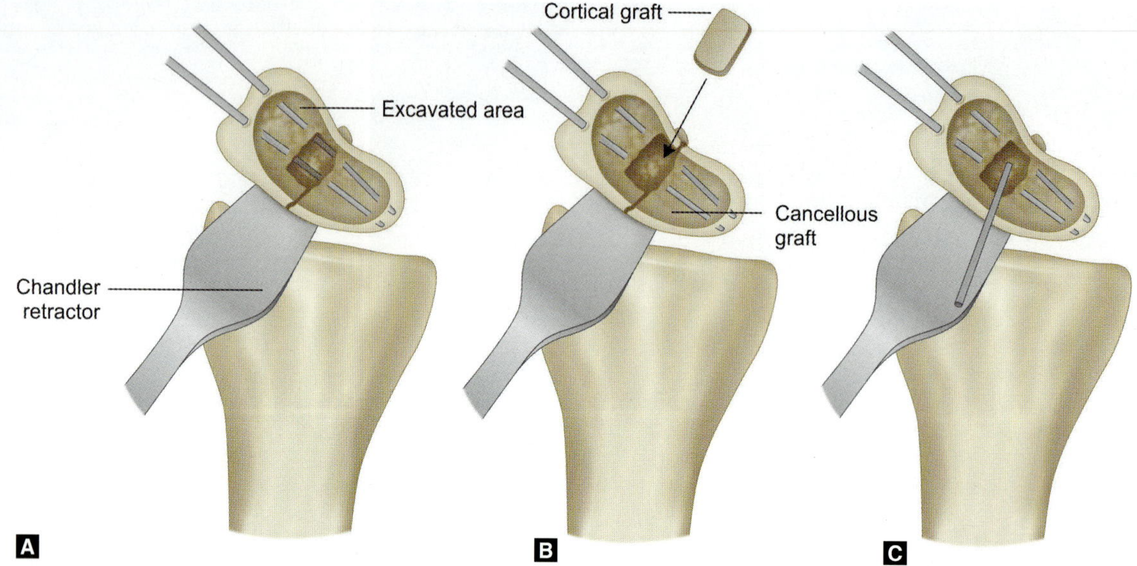

Figs. 315A to C: Stark technique—(A) Excavation of scaphoid and placement of K-wires; (B) Bone graft inserted into cavity; (C) K-wire inserted to stabilize the bone graft.

SCAPHOCAPITATE FRACTURE SYNDROME

Introduction

The scaphocapitate fracture syndrome associated with perilunar dislocation of the carpus is uncommon. There has been some discussion concerning the mechanism of the injury.

Mechanism of Injury

Stein and Siegel (1969) said that during hyperextension of the wrist the scaphoid bone, which connects the proximal and distal rows of the carpus, may be fractured (Fig. 320A). The lunate bone rotates dorsally on a transverse axis, so that its dorsal lip comes to lie under the dorsal edge of the lower radial articular surface.

The capitate bone rotating dorsally with the lunate bone, comes to lie with its long axis perpendicular to the long axis of the radius. A continuation of this hyper- extension force causes the dorsal surface of the neck of the capitates to come into contact with the dorsal edge of the lower radial articular surface leading to fracture (Fig. 320B).

If the wrist continues into further hyperextension, the proximal fragment of the capitate is rotated through 90° (Fig. 320C). When the wrist returns to the neutral position, the proximal fragment of the capitate assumes a position of 180° rotation in relation to the main fragment of the capitate (Fig. 320D).

The axis of this rotation has been discussed by several authors (Fenton 1956, Adler and Shaftan 1962, Stein and Siegel 1969). Stein and Siegel believed that the rotation occurs in the transverse axis. Fenton described two cases of scaphocapitate fracture, not associated with perilunar dislocation, in which the proximal fragment of the capitate had rotated through 180°. He believed that the rotation of the proximal fragment occurred through an axis perpendicular to the palm because the initial displacement of the wrist was one of extension and radial deviation, during which the apex of the radial styloid impinged on the lateral surface of the body of the scaphoid bone, causing it to fracture.

If the force was great enough, the adjacent capitate bone was fractured at the same level as that of the scaphoid bone and a continuation of the force caused the proximal fragment of the capitate to rotate in a perpendicular plane.

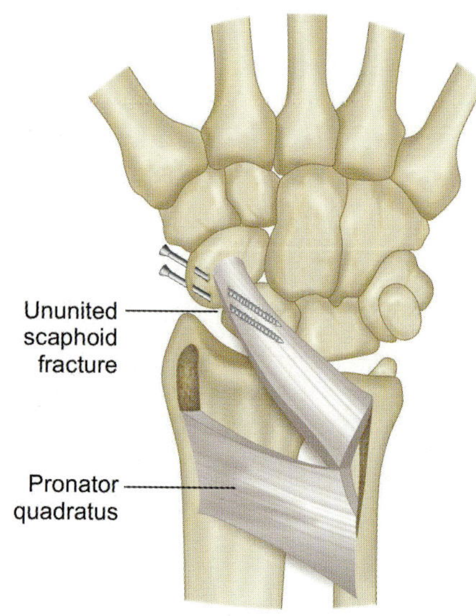

Fig. 316: Vascularized bone grafts.

DORSAL INTERCALATED SEGMENT INSTABILITY

Introduction

- Dorsal intercalated segment instability (DISI) occurs when lunate will tend to flex with loss of ulnar ligamentous support from the triquetrum
- Lunate extends when there is loss of radial ligamentous stability.

Causative Factors

- Most common causative factors for DISI are:
  - Scaphoid fracture
  - Scapholunate dissociation
  - Perilunate dislocation
- End result may be scapholunate advanced collapse (SLAC), refers to a specific pattern of osteoarthritis and subluxation,

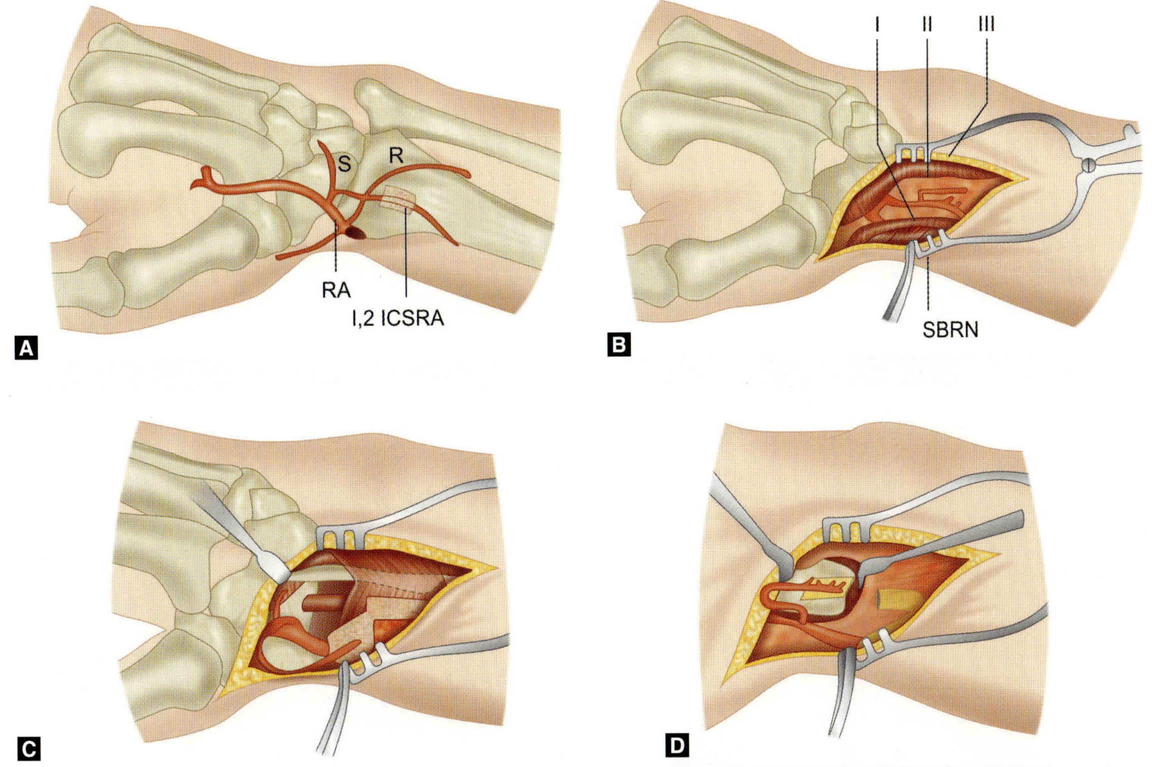

Figs. 317A to D: Vascularized bone graft from the distal dorsolateral radius.

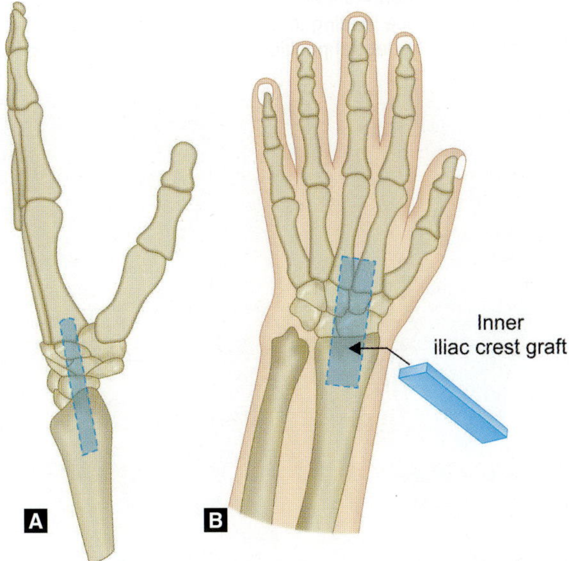

Figs. 318A and B: Haddad and Riordan arthrodesis of wrist—(A) Radial view, showing slot cut in distal radius, carpal bones and second and third metacarpal; (B) Dorsal view, showing shape of the graft and its final position.

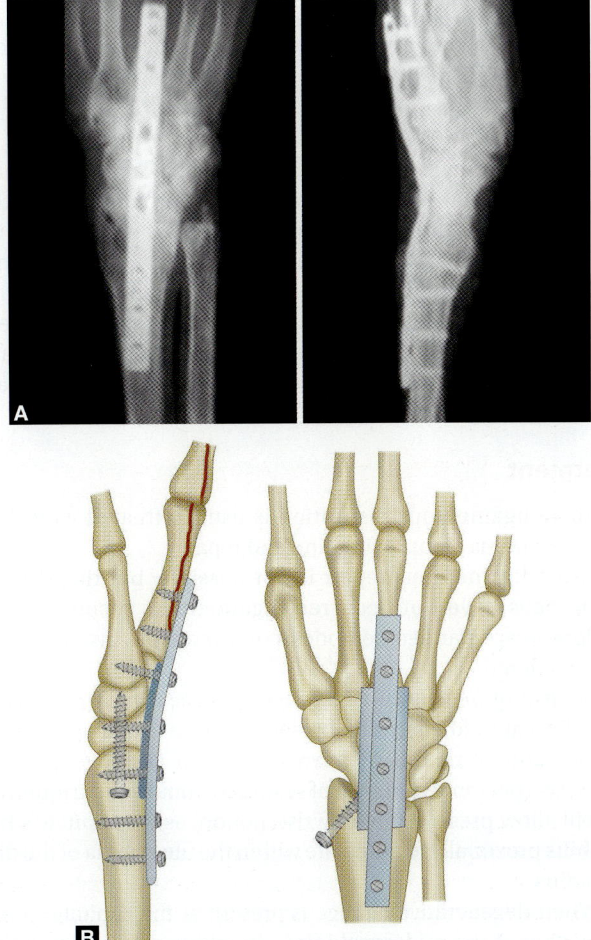

Figs. 319A and B: Arthrodesis of wrist with lag screw and dynamic compression plate fixation.

which results from untreated chronic scapholunate dissociation or from chronic scaphoid nonunion.

Radiographic Analysis

- Radiographic analysis is shown in Figures 321A and B.
- On lateral X-rays, when lunate slips into statically dorsiflexed position greater than 10°, then this condition is defined as DISI. Similarly, when lunate lies palmar to capitate, but faces dorsally, then collapse pattern is also consistent with dorsiflexion instability.

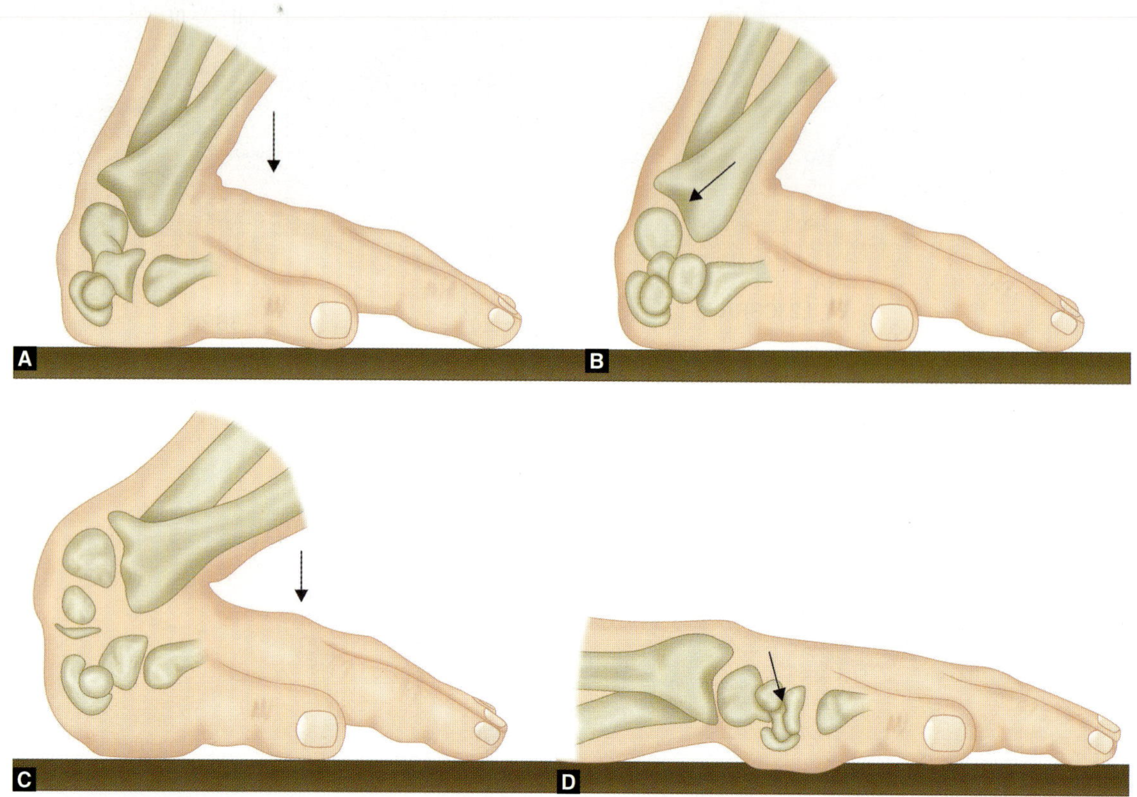

Figs. 320A to D: (A) During hyperextension of the wrist the scaphoid bone may get fractured; (B) If hyperextension force is continued, then dorsal surface of the neck of the capitates to come into contact with the dorsal edge of the lower radial articular surface leading to fracture; (C) If further hyperextension is continued, then the proximal fragment of the capitate is rotated through 90°; (D) As wrist returns to neutral position, the proximal segment of capitate rotates at 180° in relation to the main fragment of capitate.

- DISI deformity is also present, when the scapholunate angle is greater than 60° (signifying scapholunate dissociation. Scapholunate dissociation has been called the "Terry Thomas" sign in which the scapholunate interval is greater than 2 mm).
- Abnormal motion associated with DISI and scapho- lunate dissociation can lead to degeneration and collapse of the medial scaphoid, lateral lunate and radiocarpal joint. This degeneration is termed scapholunate dissociation with advanced collapse (SLAC) of wrist.

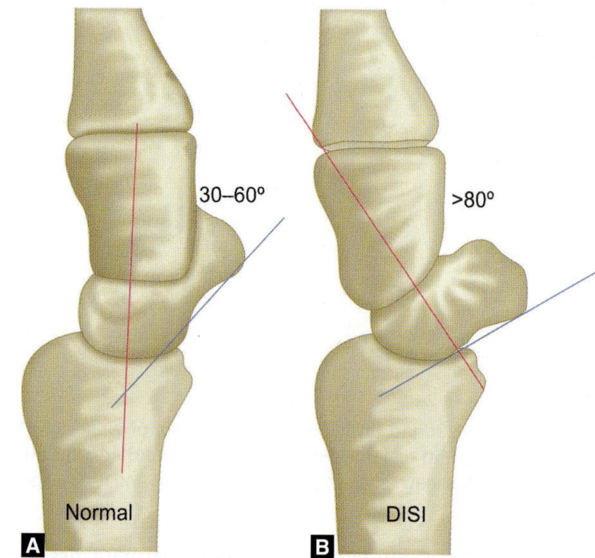

Figs. 321A and B: Radiographic analysis of DISI.

Treatment

- Acute ligamentous disruption is usually treated with direct ligamentous reapproximation and repair
- When ligamentous repair is not possible, but degenerative changes have not occurred, ligamentous reconstruction, dorsal capsular ligamentodesis or intercarpal fusions may be considered
- *In case of degenerative changes (as seen on X-ray):* When radioscaphoid change is present, but the articular surface of the capitate retains its normal articular cartilage, proximal row carpectomy (removal of scaphoid, lunate and triquetrum) will allow preservation of wrist motion, as the capitate's head shifts proximally to articulate within the ulnar fossa of the distal radius
- When degenerative change is present at the capitate's lunate portion of the midcarpal joints, in addition to radioscaphoid change, the scaphoid may be excised and intercarpal fusion of the capitate, lunate, triquetrum and hamate will be accomplished. This selective intercarpal fusion provides motion through the residual radiolunate articulation
- Complete wrist fusion provides reliable pain relief, while permanently sacrificing wrist motion.

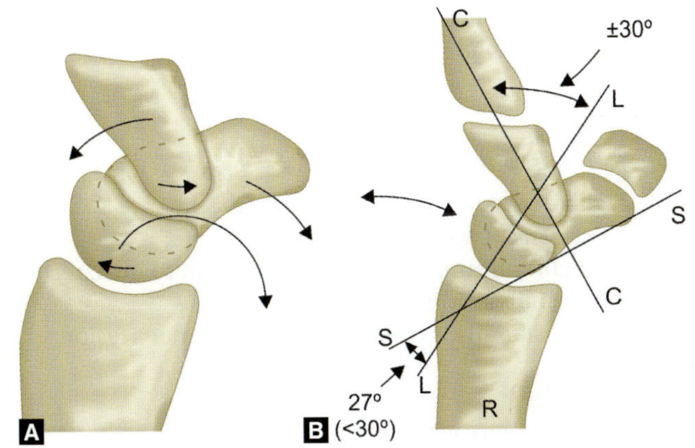

Figs. 322A and B: VISI characterized by scapholunate angle greater than 30°.

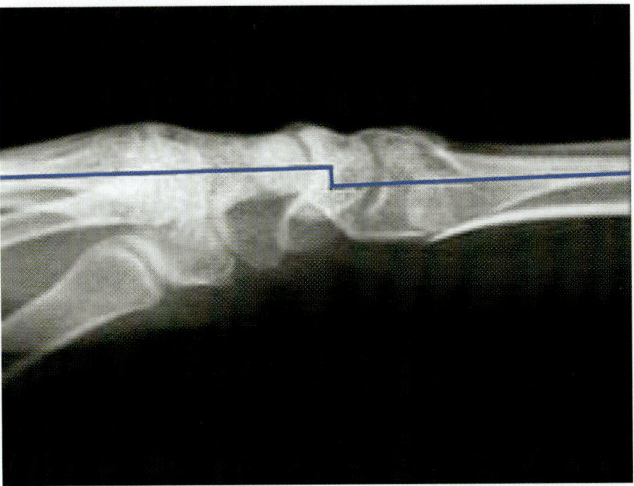

Fig. 323: Lateral view of the wrist in VISI.

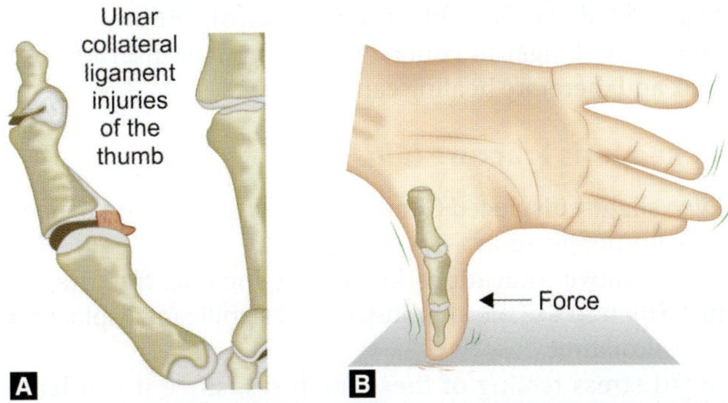

Figs. 324A and B: (A) Injury to the ulnar collateral ligament in Gamekeeper's thumb; (B) Mechanism of injury.

VOLAR INTERCALATED SEGMENT INSTABILITY

Introduction

- Volar inercalated segment instability (VISI) consists of volar flexion of the lunate, relative to the longitudinal axis of the radius and capitate, when the wrist rests in a neutral position
- Lunate will tend to flex, when there is loss of ulnar support from the triquetrum. It may result from disruption of radial carpal ligaments on ulnar side of wrist and is characterized by scapholunate angle less than 30° (Figs. 322A and B)
- Volar flexion instability pattern is usually associated with triquetrolunate dissociation or triquetral-hamate instability
- The dorsal radial triquetral and triquetroscaphoid ligaments have an increased space (increased "V") between them.

Static VISI

- When lunate slips into a statically fixed position greater than 15° of flexion, then it is called static VISI
- *Early treatment:* Closed reduction and casting (with or without K-wires).

Dynamic VISI

- Normal wrist may assume a VISI pattern when relaxed, however this is not considered abnormal unless it is symptomatic
- Etiology may be a laxity in the volar capitotriquetral ligament. These patients may note pain on volar stress testing
- Radiographs may show a widening between the capitate and the triquetrum, when wrist is placed in radial deviation
- *Treatment:* Capitolunate fusion.

Radiographs

- Lateral view of wrist (Fig. 323)
- *Capitolunate angle*
  - Wrist must be placed in a neutral position
  - Normally the distal radius, lunate, capitate and third metacarpal are colinear, however in VISI, there is a zig-zag deformity pattern, so that the lunate is volar flexed in relation to the capitates.

Management

Space of Poirier (it lies at the volar aspect of the proximal capitate, lying between the volar radiocapitate and volar radiotriquetral ligament) is reinforced and is closed, which closes down the space between the triquetrohamate and triquetrocapitate ligaments.

GAMEKEEPER'S THUMB

Introduction

Injury to the ulnar ligament of thumb joint or ulnar collateral ligament is commonly referred to as Gamekeeper's thumb or Skier's thumb (Figs. 324A and B).

It involves injury to ulnar collateral ligament of thumb's MCP joint, causing instability at that joint. Originally it is referred to a chronic injury brought on by chronic stretch of the ulnar collateral ligament, which nearly always separates from the base of first phalanx of the thumb. It frequently becomes lodged between adductor pollicis aponeurosis and its normal position (Stener lesion).

A spectrum of ulnar instability may exist, depending on whether there is an additional injury to the adductor aponeurosis and volar plate.

Stener Lesion

It occurs when torn distal edge of collateral ligament displaces superficially and proximally to the adductor aponeurosis. Proximal margin of aponeurosis slides distal to insertion of ligament.

Creation of Stener lesion requires significant radial deviation of phalanx (up to 60°) along with combined tears of the proper and accessory collateral ligaments, in order for the ligament to

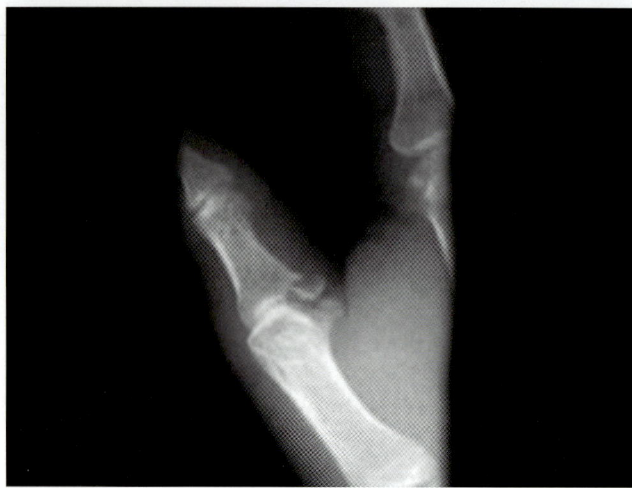

Fig. 325: X-ray showing Gamekeeper's fracture.

be displaced above the adductor aponeurosis. Ruptured end of ligament is no longer in contact with its area of insertion of the phalanx and therefore healing cannot occur.

Gamekeeperís Fracture (Fig. 325)

- Even slightly displaced Gamekeeper's fractures tend to do well with immobilization
- Conservative indications for surgery include, fractures with more than 30% of the joint surface and significant displacement or malrotation
- Avoid stress testing of these fractures, since it can lead to fracture displacement.

Physical Examination

- Examination should begin with normal uninjured thumb
- Note the stability of the uninjured MP joint as well as its ROM
- Look for a supination deformity of the joint (which may be associated with palmar subluxation of the joint) and stability
- This is generally performed in conjunction with X-rays
- Local anesthetic block is required for patient's comfort
- Gamekeeper's fracture is a contraindication to stress testing (but stress testing can proceed with nondis- placed avulsion fractures)
- Stability is documented with stress radiographs.

Palpation

- Determine point of maximum tenderness, noting that generally, the ligament tears distally off the proximal phalanx
- Palpation of torn ligament ends, may identify displaced collateral rupture, i.e. Stener lesion.

Radiographs

- Instability is indicated with radial deviation greater than 40° in extension and deviation greater than 20° in flexion
- Instability in both flexion and extension may indicate tears of both the proper and accessory collateral ligaments (often associated with Stener's lesion)
- More than 3 mm of volar subluxation of the proximal phalanx also indicates gross instability
- Anteroposterior stress radiographs may be obtained of both thumbs for comparison purposes, an injured thumb that shows more than 30° of instability compared with the uninjured side indicates a complete rupture.

Treatment

Nonoperative Treatment

- Treat with a short arm cast with a thumb spica
- Complications of nonoperative treatment are:
  - Main complication is failure of ligament to heal, resulting in instability of joint
  - Gross instability is usually caused by Stener's lesion

Surgical Treatment

Indications for surgery are:

- Gross radiographic instability (which usually represents tears of both the proper and the accessory collateral ligaments)
- Presence of palpable torn ligament ends (Stener's lesion)
- With excessive swelling the Stener's may not be palpable
- Occassionally, significant ligamentous injury may occur without immediate gross instability due to swelling and muscle spasm
- Consider re-examining patients in 5 to 7 days and if motion has not been regained and swelling has not improved consider surgical fixation.

Surgical treatment for injuries of less than 2 to 3 weeks old

- Acute complete rupture of the ulnar collateral ligament should be treated with surgical repair of the ligament. The detached tendinous insertion of the adductor muscle can be advanced and reattached to furnish a dynamic reinforcement
- If the repair is done several months after the injury, a graft can be used to replace the ligament. The graft can be boxlike, with a strip of fascia or palmaris longus tendon passed through the proximal and distal attachments of the ligament or the extensor pollicis brevis tendon, either split or in total, can be threaded through bone and attached by pull-out sutures to reconstruct the ligament.

Chronic Gamekeeper's thumb

- Proximal phalanx tends to volarly subluxate and rotate
- Deformity develops as a result of damage to ulnar collateral ligament and dorsal capsule
- In addition to dorsal joint support provided by capsule, EPB and EPL tendons also contributes to the dorsal stability of MP joint
- When ulnar collateral ligament ruptures, ulnar side of phalanx tends to displace volarly and rotate into supination
- With repeated radial stress, dorsal expansion may attenuate and allow EPL to shift ulnarly, compro- mising its extension effect on the joint
- *Management:* An MP joint with chronic instability and a small flexion arc should be considered for MP joint arthrodesis.

BOXER'S FRACTURE

Introduction

- Metacarpal neck fracture involving little finger (Fig. 326)
- Only collateral ligaments remain attached to the proximal phalanx and therefore metacarpal head is free from any proximal stabilizing influence
- Metacarpal head tilts volarly, causing joint to lie in hyperextension and collateral ligaments become slack.

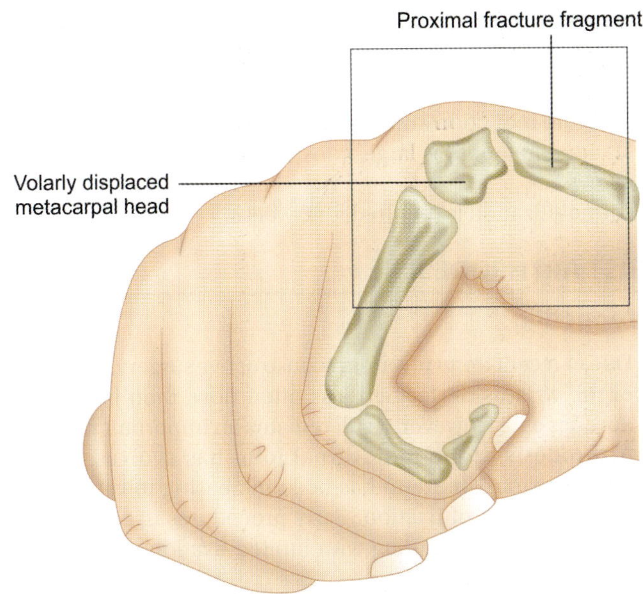

Fig. 326: Boxer fracture—Metacarpal neck fracture of little finger.

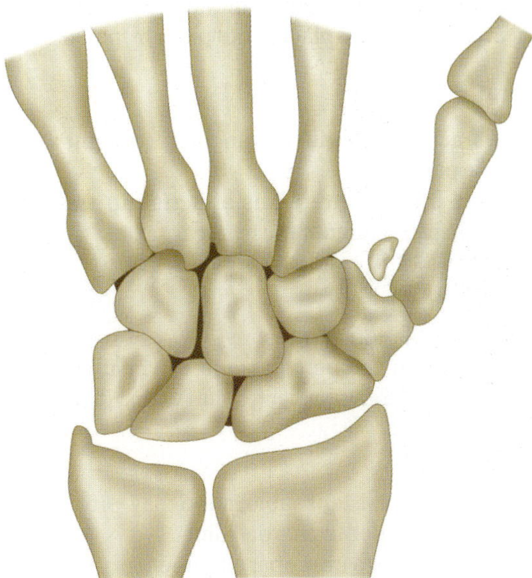

Fig. 327: Palmar beak fragment.

- If joint is allowed to remain in hyperextension, collateral ligaments will shorten, leading to limited MCP flexion
- Little finger CMC articulation allows flexion extension arc of 20° to 30° in addition to a rotatory motion facilitating little finger opposition to thumb
- Ring metacarpal provides 10° to 15° of mobility.

Differential Diagnosis

- *Transverse metacarpal shaft fracture:* This fracture may be amenable to a four holed plate.
- *Fracture of metacarpal head:* It is an infrequent variant of Boxer's fracture. In this injury, impact is received directly on metacarpal head, producing fracture through joint surface. It requires operative fixation.

Radiographs

- True lateral radiograph is necessary with these fractures, in order to measure the angle of displacement of the distal fragment.
- Normal metacarpal neck angle is about 15° and therefore a measured angle on film of 30° is actually 15°.
- When displaced, angulate with dorsal angulation at fracture line and distal metacarpal head displaces towards palmar side.

Treatment

Nonoperative Treatment

- Clawing results from the palmar displacement of the metacarpal head and resulting imbalance of extrinsic tendons
- May have cosmetic deformity, but leads to good function.

Methods of reduction

- As collateral ligaments are the only remaining attachment to metacarpal head, collaterals must be placed in a tightened position to control distal fragment and achieve reduction
- MP joint is flexed at 90° to produce tightening of MP collateral ligaments
- Flexed metacarpal is directed dorsally, which effects reduction of metacarpal head by correction of volar angulation
- *Acceptable reduction:* Following points need to be considered, while accepting the reduced fragment:
  - On lateral view, if angulation greater than 30–40°, a functional deficit (pseudoclawing) may result. Percutaneous pin fixation may be considered then
  - On AP view, little or no angulation should be accepted, since this indicates malrotation of the digit
- *Casting technique:* No matter what casting technique is used, it is essential to "buddy tape" the little and ring fingers (with an intervening of cast padding), in order to control fracture malrotation.

Operative Treatment

Percutaneous K-wire fixation should be done.

BENNETT'S FRACTURE

Introduction

- It is an oblique intra-articular fracture of the base of the first metacarpal with subluxation or dislocation of the metacarpal.
- It was described in 1882 by Dr Edward Bennett. It involves an oblique intra-articular metacarpal fracture (known as the palmar beak fragment), which remains attached to the palmar beak ligament (Fig. 327).

Mechanism of Injury

- Injury results from axial blow, directed against the partially flexed metacarpal (i.e. from fist fights). Fracture starts at ulnar base of thumb metacarpal, as palmar ulnar aspect of thumb is normally stabilized by strong ligaments
- Disruption of the ulnar fragment destabilizes thumb and volar fracture fragment remains attached to CMC, by volar anterior oblique ligament. Anterior oblique ligament anchors volar lip of metacarpal to tubercle of the trapezium, hence small volar lip fragment remains attached to anterior oblique ligament, which is attached to trapezium
- Distal metacarpal fragment (containing most of articular surface) is displaced proximally, radially and dorsally by pull

of APL. It is also rotated in supination by the pull of APL. Metacarpal head is displaced into palm by pull of ADP.

Radiographs

- Oblique fracture line with a triangular fragment at ulnar base of metacarpal
- Triangular fragment remains attached to trapezium with proximal displacement of the metacarpal.

Treatment

- Closed manipulation and casting
- Closed reduction and percutaneous K-wire fixation
- Open reduction and internal fixation with a K-wire or a screw.

Complications

- Malunion with persistent subluxation may progress to painful arthritis of the carpometacarpal joint
- Osteoarthritis, due to improper alignment of the joint surfaces. Treatment by excision of the trapezium in painful arthritis cases.

ROLANDO'S FRACTURE

Introduction

It was described in 1910 by Dr Rolando:

- Involves three part fracture, at base of first metacarpal (Fig. 328)
- In addition to volar lip fracture (as seen with Bennett's fracture), there is also large dorsal fragment, resulting in "Y" or "T" shaped intra-articular fracture
- It is a comminuted intra-articular fracture at the base of thumb metacarpal, even if "Y" or "T" is not present
- It is uncommon, but has a worse prognosis than Bennett's fracture.

Treatment

Nonoperative Treatment

- May be indicated in highly comminuted fracture
- Mold in thumb spica for 3–4 weeks and then begin ROM.

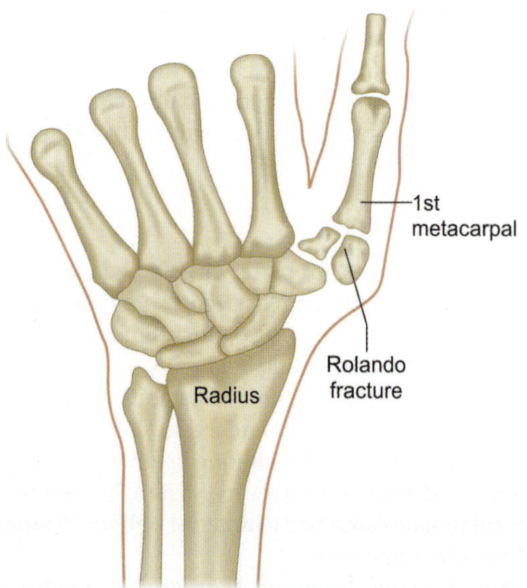

Fig. 328: Rolando fracture.

Surgical Treatment

- Indicated for presence of large volar and dorsal fragments amenable to fixation
- Fracture reduction and K-wire fixation
- If radial fragment is large, consider using 2.0 mm cortical lag screw
- Immobilization is required for 6 weeks.

WRIST ARTHRODESIS

Introduction

- Due to recent trend towards reconstructive surgery, arthrodesis of the wrist is performed less often now, than it was a few decades ago. However, it still remains an important procedure
- Arthrodesis of the radiocarpal joint has evolved over the last 50 years. The trend has been increasing toward stability in the method of fixation. Early procedures used cortical or cancellous bone grafting with limited fixation methods such as pins or screws
- Campbell and Keokarn described an inlay bone grafting technique of wrist fusion in 1964. Haddad and Riordan applied this technique through a lateral (radial) approach. Various fixation methods have been described including screws, multiple staples and multiple Steinmann pins
- In 1970, the AO group described a rigid fixation method, using a dynamic compression plate.

Dynamic Compression Plate

Advantages

- Excellent fusion rates
- Decreased incidence of malposition
- Increased stability allowing early rehabilitation
- Requires less bone grafting than other methods and usually an adequate amount of graft can be harvested from the distal radius.

Indications

- Post-traumatic arthritis
- Neoplastic lesions
- Severely comminuted intra-articular fractures
- Rheumatoid arthritis
- Wrist or hand paralysis
- Spastic hemiplegia
- Failed total joint arthroplasty
- Failed limited arthrodesis.

Contraindications

Includes an open physis of the distal radius. The distal radial physis closes at approximately 17 years of age and care should be taken not to damage it in patients under this age.

Position

- This is usually 10° to 20° of extension (dorsiflexion) with the long axis of the third metacarpal shaft aligned with the long axis of the radial shaft and neutral to 5° of ulnar deviation. Clinically, it is determined by the position that the wrist normally assumes with the fist strongly clenched
- If bilateral wrist fusions are indicated, the position of the wrists should be determined by the needs of the patient. The neutral position for both wrists is thought to provide maximal function.

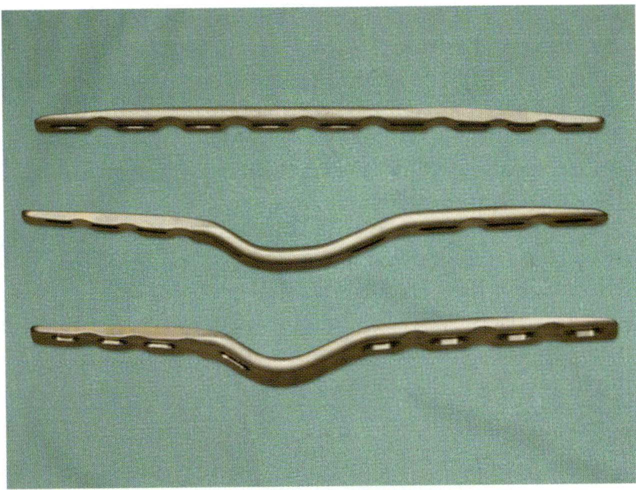

Fig. 329: Different types of AO plates.

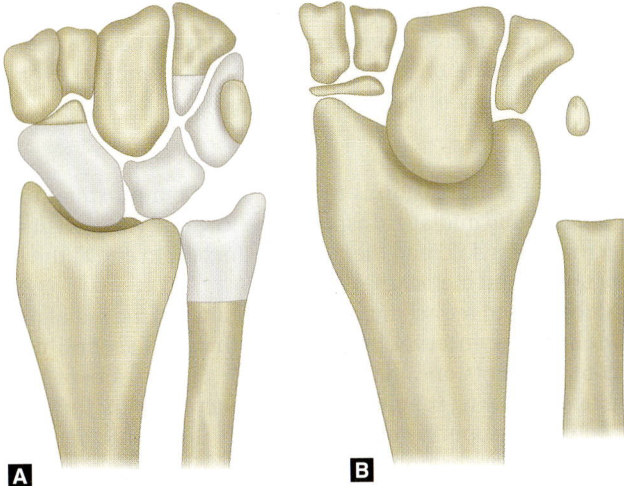

Figs. 330A and B: Fusion with proximal row after carpectomy—(A) Carpectomy (as shown by the shaded portion) performed; (B) Fusion being performed with proximal row.

Techniques

- Of the many techniques that have been described, most include the use of a bone graft. The iliac crest is the most common donor site, but bone graft may be obtained from the distal radius, ulna, tibia or rib
- The distal radius may be exposed through a dorsal, ulnar or radial (lateral) approach. Dorsal approach is the most commonly used approach.

AO Plates (Fig. 329)

- Straight plate use large intercalary graft required
- Long carpal bend in large wrist
- Short carpal bend in short wrist.

Plate Fixation

- Curvilinear skin incision is given, beginning with 2 cm, extending over the distal radioulnar joint and ending over the midshaft of the second and third metacarpals
- Protect the branches of the superficial cutaneous nerve. Make a longitudinal incision between the tendons of the extensor digitorum communis, which are retracted in the ulnar direction and the extensor pollicis longus, which is retracted in the radial direction
- An I-shaped incision is made in the capsule, crossing proximally over the radiocarpal joint and distally over the carpometacarpal joints
- Remove Lister's tubercle and the dorsal cortices of the carpal bones, to allow flat apposition of the precontoured plate
- Denude the radiocarpal and intercarpal joint surfaces of cartilage and fill the gaps with cancellous bone harvested from the excised bone and distal radial metaphysic
- A 3.5 mm cortex lag screw may be placed through the radial styloid in the capitate, to pull the carpus against the radial styloid and help prevent impingement of the distal radioulnar joint
- Secure the appropriate precontoured plate to the dorsal aspect of the third metacarpal. Ensure that the distal end of the plate is centered on the metacarpal.
- Mark the position of the distal hole and remove the plate. Drill a 2.0 mm hole in a dorsal to volar direction, centered in the midline of the metacarpal. Replace the plate, measure, tap and fill the distal hole with a 2.7 mm screw
- Fill the remaining metacarpal holes and compress the radiocarpal and intercarpal joints. This is done using a 3.5 mm screw, placed in compression mode through the second most distal hole in the radius. Fill the remaining holes and close the capsule over a small suction drain.

After Treatment

- A cast is applied from the upper arm to the tips of the fingers and thumb, with the elbow at right angle, the forearm in neutral position and the wrist in 10–15° of extension.
- The fingers and thumb should be slightly flexed. To allow for swelling, the dorsum of the cast is windowed.
- At 3 weeks, a short cast below the elbow, just proximal to the metacarpophalangeal joints, is applied with the wrist in the correct position.
- Support is continued until firm fusion is present, usually at 10 to 12 weeks.

Fusion with Proximal Row (Carpectomy)

- This technique was described by Louis (Figs. 330A and B)
- *Procedure:* Approach the wrist dorsally. Remove approximately 80% of the proximal scaphoid, a portion of the hamate and the entire triquetrum and lunate
- Retain a portion of the scaphoid and hamate to prevent distal carpal row migration. Denude the articular cartilage from the distal radius and proximal capitate. Supporting the fusion site with Kirschner wires or staples and bone graft is not necessary.

After treatment: The wrist is immobilized in a cast or splint for 12 to 16 weeks.

Haddad and Riordan Arthrodesis

- Haddad and Riordan described a technique of arthrodesis of the wrist through a radial or lateral approach (*see* Figs. 318A and B).
- They believed that the formation of scar with the dorsal approach led to more restricted tendon gliding.

- Their technique has several advantages. The distal radioulnar joint is not entered, the extensor tendons to the digits are not disturbed as much and because dorsal thickening is avoided, the appearance of the wrist is not altered.

Technique

- J-shaped skin incision is made, 2.5 to 4 cm proximal to the radial styloid midlateral aspect of the forearm, extend it distally across the styloid and then curve it dorsally to end at the base of the second metacarpal
- Mobilize and retract the superficial branch of the radial nerve. Identify the interval between the first and second dorsal compartments and incise the dorsal carpal ligament in this interval, leaving it attached to the volar aspect of the radius. Mobilize subperiosteally and retract the abductor pollicis longus, extensor pollicis brevis and wrist along with finger extensors
- Divide the extensor carpi radialis longus tendon just proximal to its insertion on the base of the second metacarpal, leaving a stump distally, so that it can be sutured later
- Remove the capsule from the radiocarpal, the intercarpal and the second carpometacarpal joints. Locate the dorsal branch of the radial artery, then ligate and divide it
- Denude the radiocarpal joint of articular cartilage and subchondral bone. Harvest iliac bone graft. With the wrist in 15° of dorsiflexion, cut a slot in the distal end of the radius, the carpal bones and the bases of the second and third metacarpals
- Do not cut through the medial cortex of the radius and enter the distal radioulnar joint. Then place the graft in the prepared bed. If the wrist is unstable, insert another added Kirschner wire obliquely or longitudinally, to engage the base of the second metacarpal and the distal radius
- Cut off the wire under the skin at the palm, to be removed 6 to 8 weeks later. Close the dorsal carpal ligament deep to the abductor pollicis longus and extensor pollicis brevis. Suture the extensor carpi radialis longus tendon and close the wound over a drain.

After Treatment

- Above elbow cast should be applied with elbow at a right angle, the forearm in neutral position and the wrist in 10° to 15° of extension. The fingers and thumb are slightly flexed
- At third-week, below elbow cast is applied just proximal to the metacarpophalangeal joints, with the wrist in the correct position
- Support is continued until firm fusion is present, usually at 10 to 12 weeks.

Watson and Wendor Arthrodesis

Watson and Wendor reported a technique using a radial incision and incorporating iliac bone graft into the fusion site and securing it in place with two removable Kirschner wires.

Technique

- Make a longitudinal incision radially extending 6 cm from the distal radius to the distal second metacarpal. Protect the superficial radial nerve and deep branch of the radial artery. Free and retract the extensor pollicis brevis and abductor pollicis longus in the palmar direction. Retract the extensor pollicis longus and extensor carpi longus with brevis.
- Lift the origin of the first dorsal interosseous from the second metacarpal. Fashion a groove extending 2 cm from distal radius to 1 cm of the second and third metacarpals, by drilling multiple holes and connecting them.
- This trough should include the scaphoid, capitate, lunate and trapezoid. The depth of the groove should be just through the metacarpals and even throughout.
- Place an outer cortical piece of iliac bone graft into the trough with the cancellous side down. Lock the graft into place by bringing the wrist from ulnar deviation to the neutral position. Secure the graft into position, by passing Kirschner wires through the distal radius and graft proximally and the metacarpals and graft distally.

After Treatment

Long arm cast is applied incorporating the thumb, index and long fingers. This is replaced at fourth-week by a short arm splint, which is used for an additional 2 to 4 weeks. The Kirschner wires are removed once the fusion site is solid.

Complications

- Painful hardware
- Tendon adhesions or ruptures
- Early wound infection
- Metacarpophalangeal joint stiffness
- Carpal tunnel syndrome
- Reflex sympathetic dystrophy
- Nonunion
- Persistent pain

WRIST ARTHROPLASTY

- The goal is to provide a mobile, stable and painless wrist with reasonable durability.
- If bilateral bony procedures on the wrist joint are necessary, arthroplasty on at least one side should be considered.
- In some cases, arthroplasty may be indicated initially because eventual collapse of the opposite wrist may require reconstruction.

Total Wrist Arthroplasty

- Total wrist arthroplasty is surgical resection of all or a portion of carpus, removal of the articulating surface of the radius and usually the ulna as well, so that it could be replaced with an articulated implant (Fig. 331).
- The concept of using an articulated non-hinged prosthesis in the wrist was developed by Meuli in Switzerland and by Voltz in Arizona, in early 1970s.

First Designs

Meuli's ball and socket trunnion design (Fig. 332)

- Allows rotation within the articulation in functional mode. Distal cup firmly encompasses the ball and if stress is applied to the hand, with wrist held motionless by soft tissue constraints (capsule or muscle), the resultant forces are transmitted to the stems, as if the prosthesis were constrained
- Two lengths of polyethylene ball insertions are available to adjust tension as necessary.

Voltz's dorsovolar tracking design (Fig. 333)

- It incorporated a flexion-extension arc of motion, but was sloppy fit

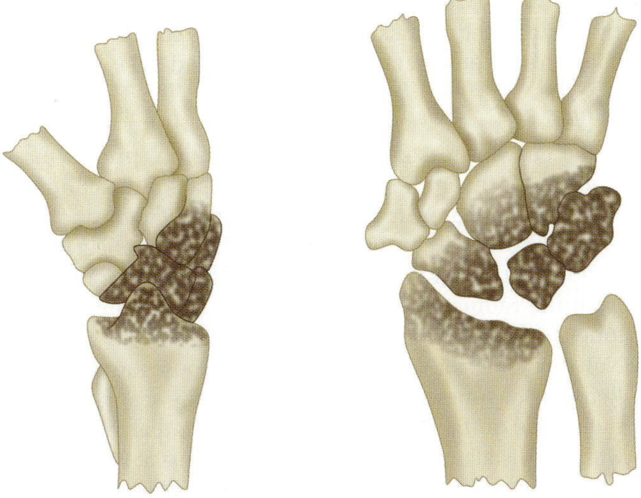

Fig. 331: Total wrist arthroplasty: Surgical resection of all or a portion of carpus (as shown by the shaded portions).

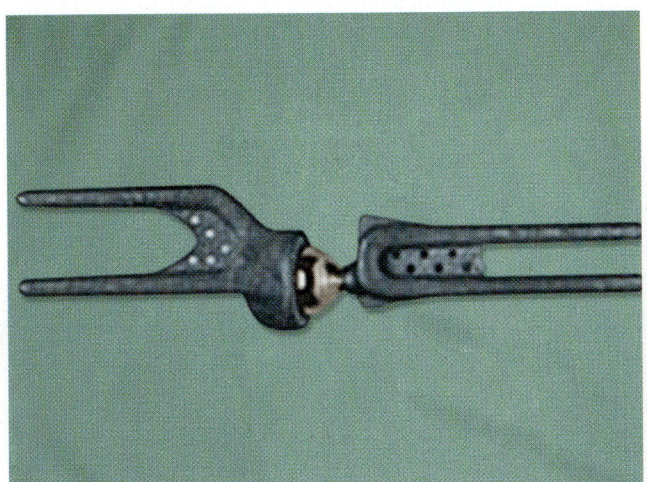

Fig. 332: Ball and socket trunnion design.

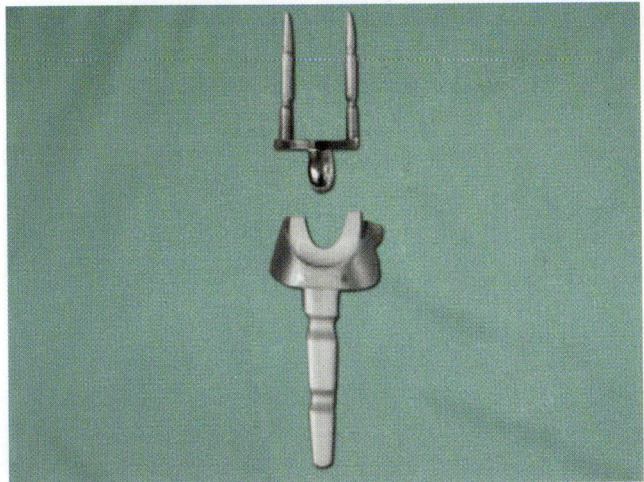

Fig. 333: Dorsovolar tracking design.

- Functionally, it is less constrained than Meuli's design, owing to the loose contact fit between the proximal and distal component

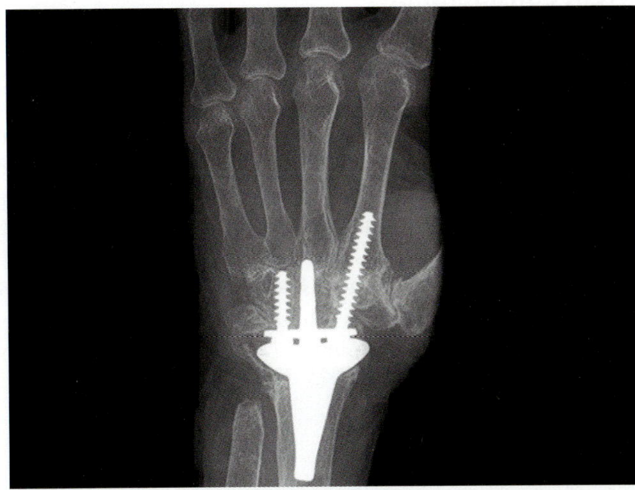

Fig. 334: Ulnar deviation after total wrist arthroplasty.

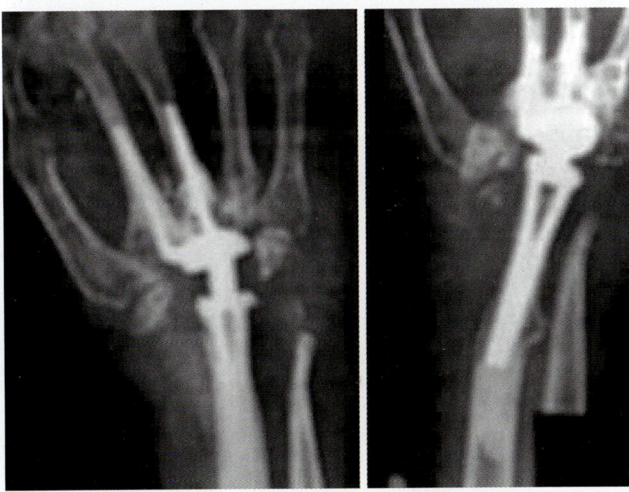

Fig. 335: Stem fixation problem after arthroplasty.

- Both designs utilize two pronged distal components for seating in the modulary canals of the index and long metacarpals.

Problems with Arthroplasty

- *Balancing:* With both the prosthetic designs patients developed ulnar deviation, deformity and contractures (Fig. 334)
- *Infection:* Requires prosthetic removal
- *Dislocation with deformity:* Requires revision surgery
- *Stem fixation problem:* Loosening of the distal component and stress shielding of the proximal component (Fig. 335)
- With the Meuli's design, distal component loosens as it tends to migrate volarly into the carpal canal. This may cause symptoms of the median neuropathy or ruptures of the flexor tendon at the edge of the prosthesis (Fig. 336).

Salvage

Salvage following total wrist arthroplasty done by arthrodesis with bone grafting (Fig. 337).

Current Considerations

As a result of deterioration with the first generation of implants other designs were being developed in an attempt to improve durability, balance and function.

- *Guepar prosthesis by Alnot:* It is backed with polyethylene component proximally and is fixed with screws distally (Fig. 338).
- *Clayton and Ferlic prosthesis:* Clayton and Ferlic developed prosthesis for biologic fixation with proximal ball and distal cup portion.
- *Menon's prosthesis:* It has metal backing at the radial component and screw fixation distally (Fig. 339).

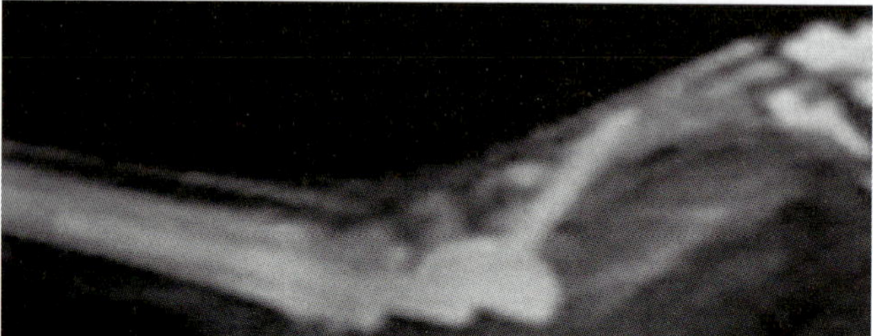

Fig. 336: Meuli's design with distal component loosening and volar migration into carpal canal.

- *Biaxial wrist prosthesis:* The radial component stem is offset radially and the metacarpal component is curved to match the shape of the long metacarpal (Figs. 340 and 341).

Procedure

- Make curved dorsal longitudinal incision, preserving the veins and sensory nerves. Split the dorsal retinaculum over the extensor digitorum tendons and reflect it to the radial side. Detach the dorsal capsule from the radius and reflect it distally as a widely based flap. Detach the radial collateral ligament from the radius and carefully protect the abductor pollicis longus and extensor pollicis brevis tendons
- Now-hyperflex the radiocarpal joint, to expose the distal radius. Remove the lunate, the proximal half of the scaphoid and the radial side of the triquetrum. Resect the radial styloid in line with the distal articular surface of the radius at 90° to the long axis of the radius. Preserve as much cortical bone as possible to provide support. When the joint is dislocated, resect more of the radius as necessary. Align the wrist and prepare the capitate and the base of the third metacarpal to receive the prosthesis
- To ensure proper placement of the reamer in the medullary canal of the third metacarpal, insert a Kirschner wire and check its position by roentgenograms. Then ream with an

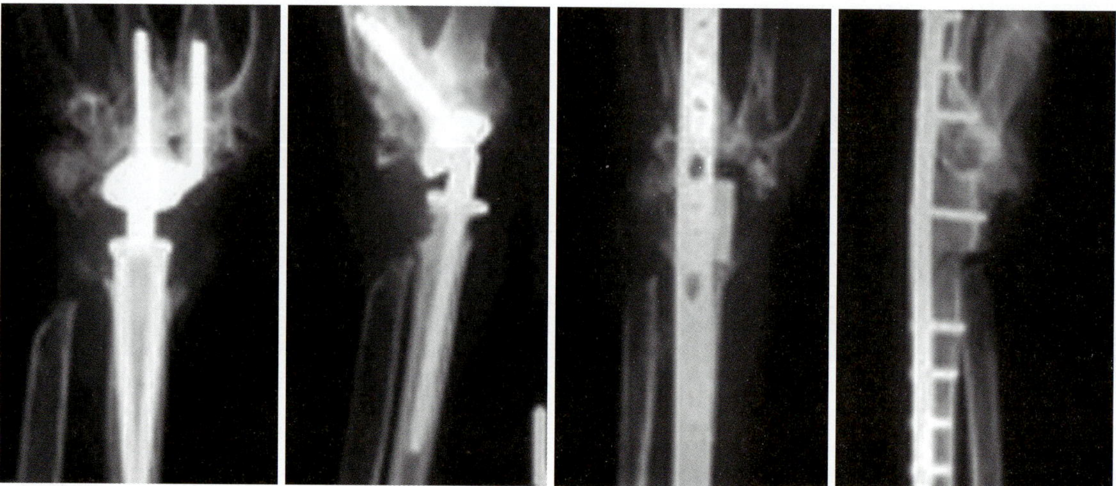

Fig. 337: Salvage after arthroplasty done by arthrodesis with bone grafting.

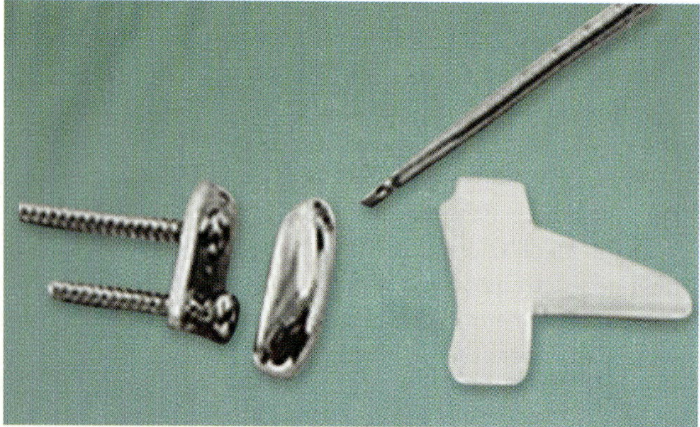

Fig. 338: Guepar prosthesis.

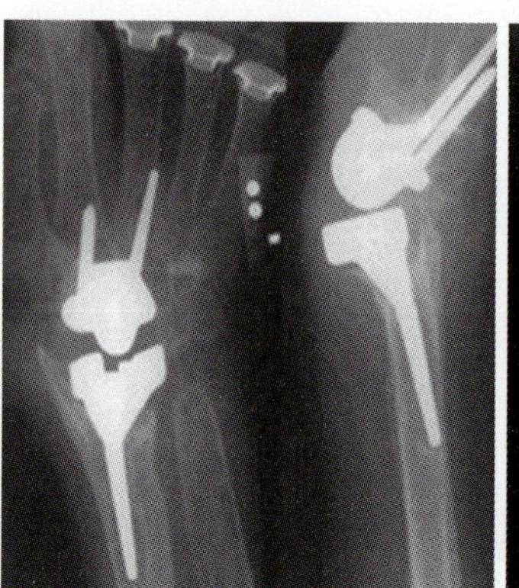

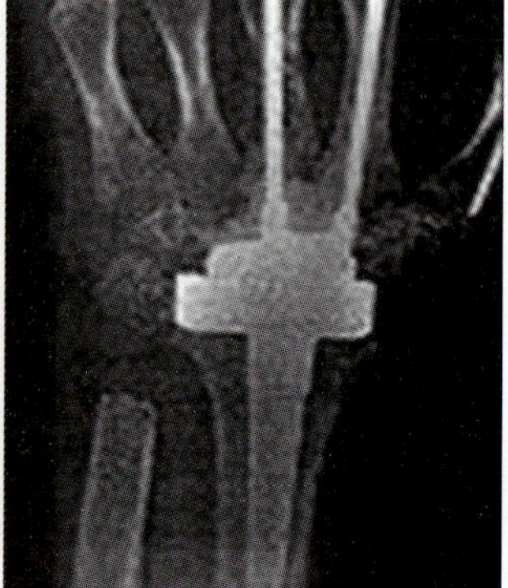

Fig. 339: Clayton and Ferlic prosthesis.

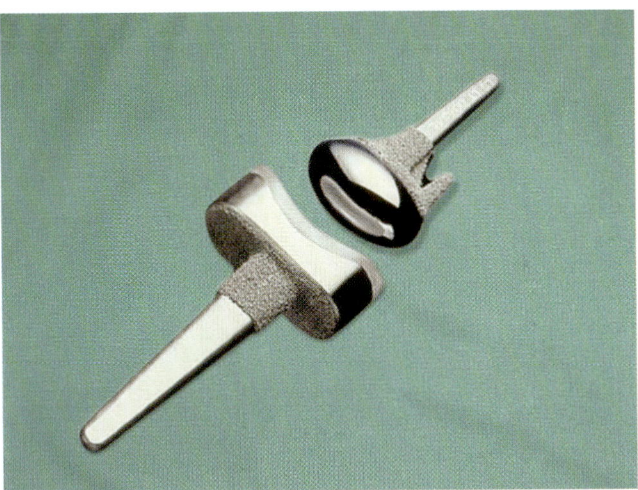

Fig. 340: Biaxial wrist prosthesis.

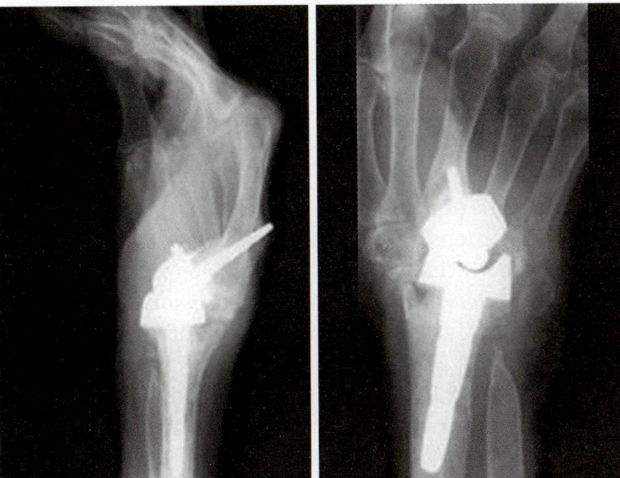

Fig. 341: X-rays of biaxial wrist prosthesis.

awl or if necessary, with a power reamer. Do not perforate the metacarpal shaft. The size of the third metacarpal shaft will determine the size of the prosthesis. Use this shaft for size and then ream the radius to fit the opposite stem of the prosthesis. Smooth the base of the capitate and radius, to eliminate any sharp bony edges that could cause a prosthetic fracture. Use metal sleeve "grommets" as needed. Seat the prosthesis against the radius and capitate, so that there is no tendency for buckling

- Align the hand on the wrist, avoiding ulnar deviation or flexion. See that passive flexion and extension of about 30° each are possible without blockage. Strip the volar capsule, if it is too tight. Next resect the distal ulna. Close the capsule with sutures passed through holes drilled in the dorsal cortex of the distal radius. Reattach the collateral ligament of the radius and realign the dorsal retinaculum under the finger and wrist extensors
- Relocate the extensor carpi ulnaris tendon dorsally, to prevent it from functioning as a wrist flexor. If it has shifted palmar-ward, pass it through a pulley created from a segment of the dorsal retinaculum if necessary. Repair any extensor tendons as indicated and close the wound loosely. Insert a suction drain and apply a bulky dressing and a plaster splint.

After Treatment

- The splint is worn for 5 to 6 weeks
- At third week, limited wrist motion is started and at fourth week active motion is begun.
- A total motion of 60° is considered satisfactory and 95% of patients obtain relief from pain.

Contraindications for Arthroplasty

- Chronic subluxation
- Poor bone
- Prior infection
- Impaired motor or neurologic function
- Use of walker or cane
- Impaired wrist extensor tendons.

CHAPTER

28 Elbow

OBJECTIVES

- Anatomy, Biomechanics, and Examination of the Elbow
- Congenital Anomalies around the Elbow Joint
- Trauma to Elbow Fractures around Elbow
- Myositis Ossificans
- Volkmann's Ischemic Contracture
- Osteochondritis Dissecans of Elbow
- Tennis Elbow and Golfer's Elbow
- Inflammation around Elbow
- Elbow Arthrodesis
- Elbow Arthroplasty
- Tumors around the Elbow

ANATOMY, BIOMECHANICS, AND EXAMINATION OF THE ELBOW

Anatomy

- The elbow joint although a single synovial cavity is made up of three distinct articulations:
  1. *The humeroulnar:* Between the trochlea of the humerus and the trochlear notch of the ulna (a hinge joint).
  2. *The humeroradial*: Between the capitulum and the upper concave surface of the radial head (a ball and socket joint).
  3. *The superior radioulnar*: Between the head of the radius and the radial notch of the ulna, the head being held in place by the tough annular ligament (a pivot joint).
- The capsule of the elbow joint is closely applied around this complex articular arrangement.
- The nonarticular medial and lateral epicondyles are extracapsular.
- The capsule is thin and loose anteriorly and posteriorly to allow flexion and extension, whereas it is strongly thickened on either side to form the medial and lateral collateral ligaments.
- *Two sets of movements take place at the elbow*:
  1. Flexion and extension at the humeroulnar and humeroradial joints (Figs. 1A and B)
  2. Pronation and supination at the proximal radioulnar (in conjunction with associated movements of the distal radioulnar joint) (Figs. 2A and B).

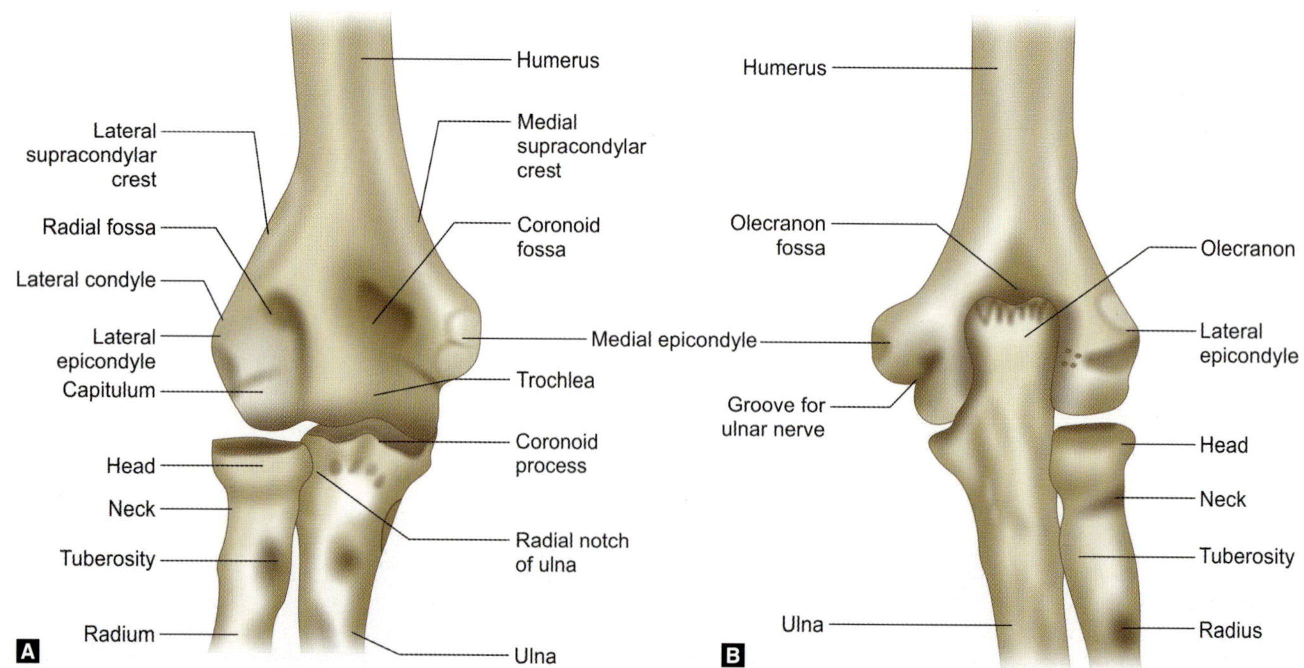

Figs. 1A and B: View of elbow joint in extension: (A) Anterior view; (B) Posterior view.

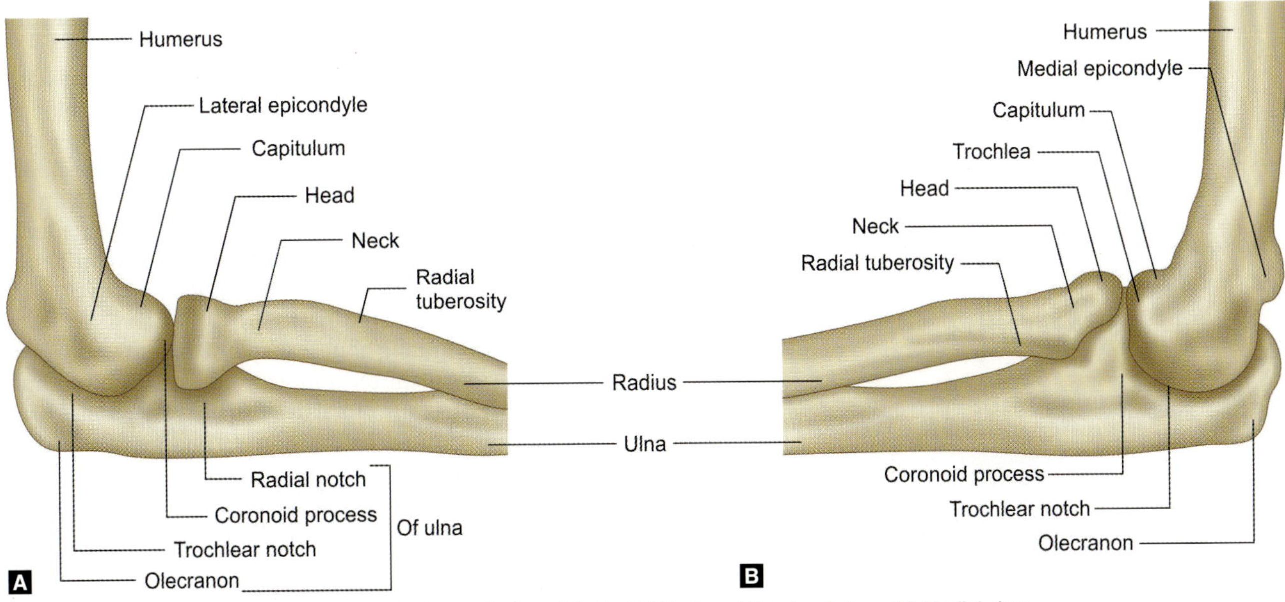

Figs. 2A and B: View of elbow joint in 90° flexion: (A) Lateral view; (B) Medial view.

TABLE 1: Different muscles acting on the elbow.

Flexors	*Extensors*
Biceps	Triceps
Brachialis	Anconeus
Brachioradialis	–
The forearm flexor muscles	–
Pronators	Supinators
Pronator teres	Biceps
Pronator quadratus	Supinator
Flexor carpi ulnaris	• Extensor pollicis longus • Extensor pollicis brevis • Abductor pollicis longus

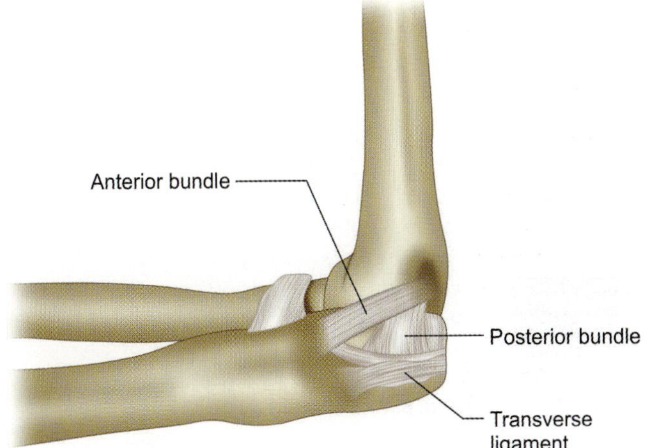

Fig. 3: Medial collateral ligament complex.

Muscles Acting on Elbow

Muscles acting on the elbow are described in Table 1.

Collateral Ligaments of Elbow

Medial collateral ligament complex (Fig. 3):

- The anterior component is the most easily identifiable.
- It is the major portion that inserts along the medial aspect of the coronoid process. It is taut with the elbow in flexion and in extension. The posterior component is taut during flexion.

Lateral ligament complex (Fig. 4):

- The radial collateral ligament arises from the lateral epicondyle and inserts into the annular ligament along with fibers of the capsule.
- The lateral ulnar collateral ligament consists of posterior fibers of the radial collateral ligament, which extend superficial to and across the annular ligament, inserting in a tubercle on the crista supinatoris of the ulna.
- The accessory lateral collateral ligament arises from the lateral epicondyle and inserts into the inferior margin of the annular ligament. It is taut when the elbow is stressed in varus.

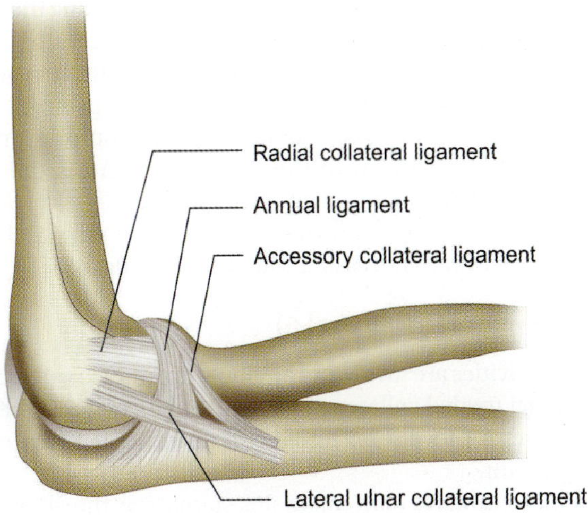

Fig. 4: Lateral ligament complex of elbow.

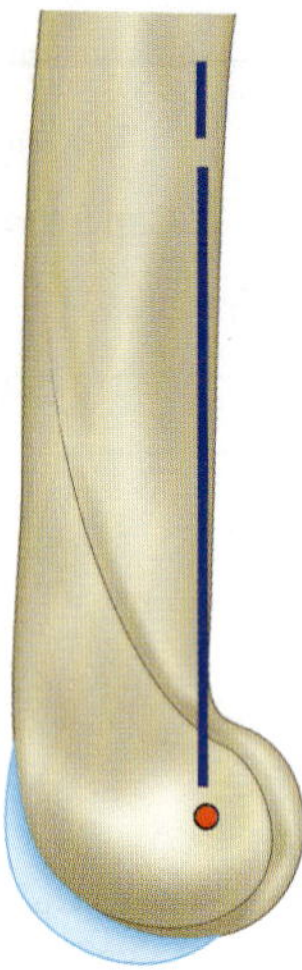

Fig. 5: Instant center of extension and flexion of elbow at the center of trochlea (as viewed from lateral aspect).

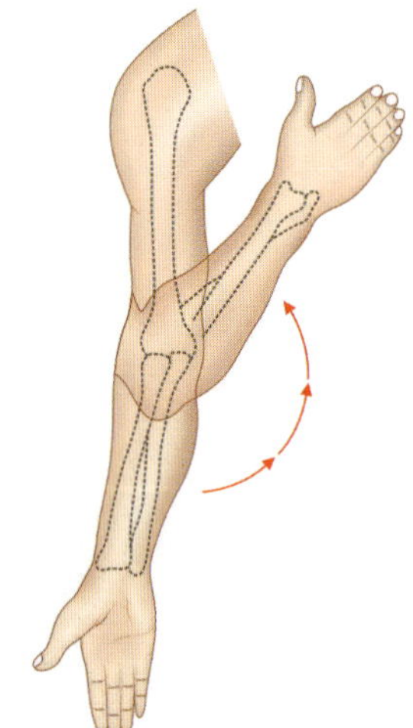

Fig. 6: Axis of elbow rotation.

- The annular ligament arises and inserts on the anterior and posterior margins of the lesser sigmoid notch of the ulna and stabilizes the radial head adjacent to the ulna.
- In extension, the anterior capsule provides approximately 70% of soft-tissue restraint to distraction.
- Valgus stress in extension is divided equally among the medial collateral ligament, capsule, and joint surfaces.
- Varus stress in extension is limited equally by the joint articulation, lateral collateral ligament, and capsule.
- In flexion, the medial collateral ligament complex provides a soft-tissue restraint to the distraction and is the prime stabilizing structure resisting valgus stress.
- The joint articulation provides about 75% of the stability and resistance to varus stressing with the elbow flexed.

Biomechanics (Figs. 5 and 6)

- Most activities are involving the elbow to produce valgus forces.
- An intact medial collateral ligament and intact radial head are essential to prevent posterolateral dislocation of the normal elbow joint.
- The ulnohumeral joint maintains stability as the elbow flexes and extends.
- The radiocapitellar joint resists valgus stress and transmits vertical loading forces of pushing and lifting.
- The elbow is composed of two independent uniaxial joints. One is the humeroulnar joint, which is a hinge joint and the other consists of the humeroradial and proximal radioulnar articulations, a pivot, allowing 2° of freedom in the elbow joint.
- Motion in the elbow involves rotation of the ulna around the humerus, during flexion and extension; and rotation of the radius around the ulna, during supination and pronation.
- *The anatomical restraints of elbow motion include:*
  - The geometry of the joint
  - The surrounding bone, capsule, ligaments, and muscles
  - Impaction of the olecranon process on the olecranon fossa
  - Impaction of the radial head against the radial fossa.
- Rotation is limited by passive resistance of the stretched muscles, ligaments, and impingement of the flexor pollicis longus against the finger flexors.
- The instant center of flexion and extension for the elbow at the center of concentric circles formed by the lateral projection of the capitulum and trochlea of the distal humerus is about 2–3 mm in diameter and is located in the center of the trochlea, when viewed from the lateral aspect (*see* Fig. 5). The axis of rotation of the elbow lies anterior to the humeral midline and on a line drawn along the anterior cortex of the humerus.
- Morrey and Chao found that the carrying angle varied from 11° of valgus with the elbow in full extension to 6° of varus with the elbow in full flexion (*see* Fig. 6).
- The contact surfaces of the elbow change with different elbow positions. In full extension, the contact surfaces are on the inferomedial aspect of the ulna; and in other positions, most of the joint contact occurs along the trochlear notch, which passes from posterolateral to anteromedial.
- Electromyographic studies of elbow muscle activity show that the brachialis is active in most ranges of elbow motion and is the "workhorse" of flexion.
- The joint surfaces slide until the extremes of full flexion and extension are reached and then bony impingement occurs.
- The transverse axis of rotation of the radiohumeral joint coincides with the ulnohumeral axis. The longitudinal axis of the forearm passes through the radial head proximally and the ulnar head distally, and is oblique to the longitudinal axes of the radius and ulna.
- The normal range of motion of the elbow is from 0° (full extension) to approximately 150° (full flexion).
- The forces around the elbow joint forces are greatest in extension. The flexed elbow being able to tolerate higher loads than the extended.
- Elbow joint forces also are found to be greatest in pronation.
- Maximal elbow flexion strength occurs at 90°. One-third to one-half of the maximal lifting force can be generated with the elbow in an extended or a 30°-flexed position.
- A force, three times the body weight, can be developed in the elbow joint during strenuous lifting. Considerable rotatory torque is developed at the distal humerus, when the elbow is flexed to 90° and force is applied to the hand from the side.
- Tensile forces on the medial collateral ligament can approach two times the body weight and compressive forces on the radial head can approach three times the body weight.
- If the radial head is excised, humeroradial force is transmitted to the ulna and the medial collateral ligament tension adds to

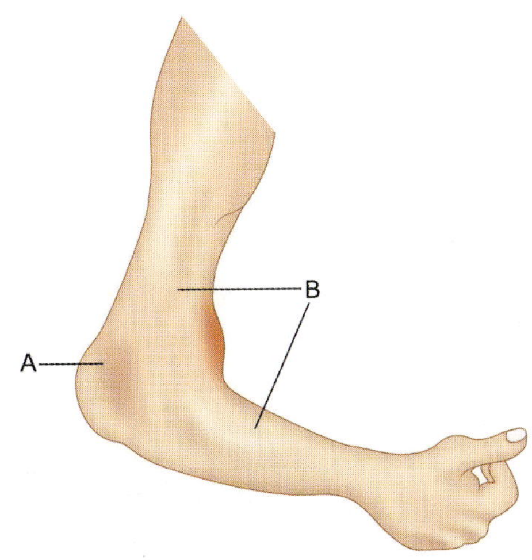

Fig. 7: Earliest sign of effusion, hollows of elbow above olecranon get filled. (A: swelling; B: hollow).

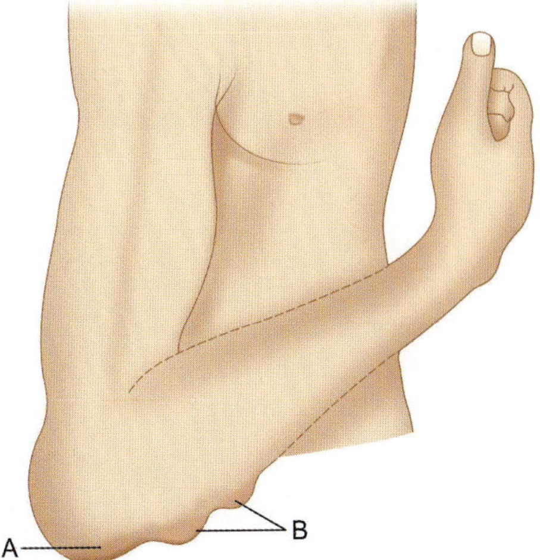

Fig. 9: Inspection done for scars and sinuses. (A: scar; B: sinuses).

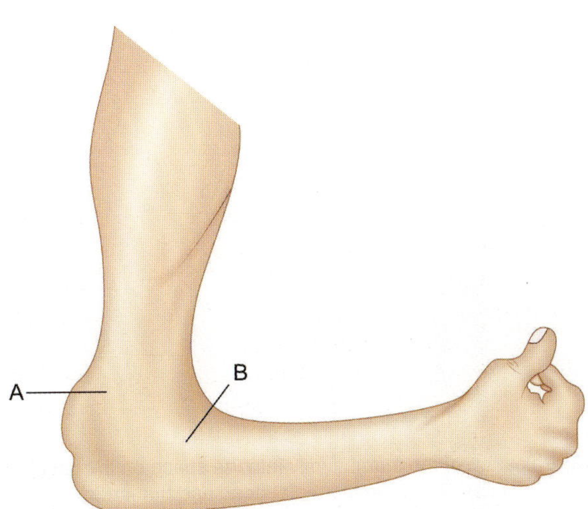

Fig. 8: Inspect for any localized swelling around elbow joint. (A and B: swelling).

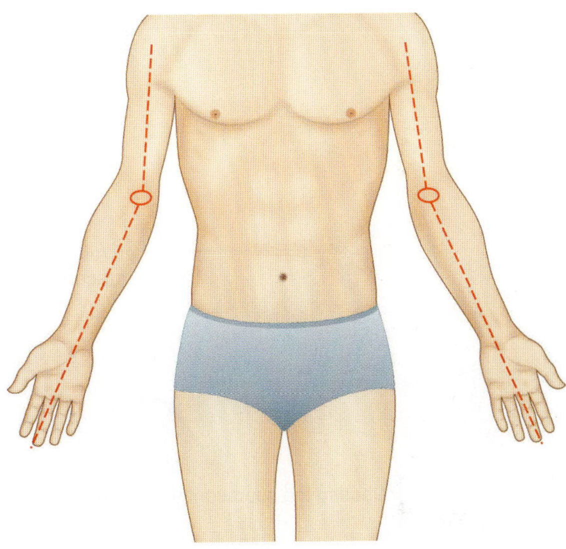

Fig. 10: The carrying angle of the elbow joint (seen as a dotted line joining the axis of rotation of the upper arm and the lower arm at the elbow joint).

the humeroulnar force, which may concentrate the entire load on the lateral edge of the coronoid process. This may apply a force of nine times the body weight to the medial collateral ligament.

Examination

Inspection (Figs. 7 to 10)

- Focus at the attitude of the upper limb and look for:
  - Generalized swelling
  - Muscle wasting.
- Earliest clinical sign of effusion is filling of hollows, which is seen in fixed elbow above the olecranon (Fig. 7).
- Look for any localized swellings around the elbow (Fig. 8), e.g. rheumatoid nodules or olecranon bursitis.
- Look for any scars or sinuses (Fig. 9).
- *The carrying angle (Fig. 10)*: The normal carrying angle is 11° in males and 13° in females. Look for varus (decreased carrying angle) or valgus (increased carrying angle) deformities at the elbow, by extending both the upper limbs fully and comparing them. In cases of fixed flexion deformity of the elbow, the carrying angle cannot be determined and one should not comment on the valgus or varus deformity.

Palpation

- Look for local rise in temperature.
- Look for joint line tenderness.
- Palpate the three prominent bony landmarks, i.e. the medial epicondyles, lateral epicondyles, and the olecranon.
- Sharply localized tenderness at the lateral epicondyle is almost diagnostic of tennis elbow (Fig. 11).
- Sharply localized tenderness at the medial epicondyle is almost diagnostic of golfers' elbow.
- Tenderness over the olecranon is uncommon, except after trauma or infected olecranon bursitis.
- Palpate the supracondylar ridge of humerus (Fig. 12) and look for any thickening, suggestive of old supracondylar fractures.

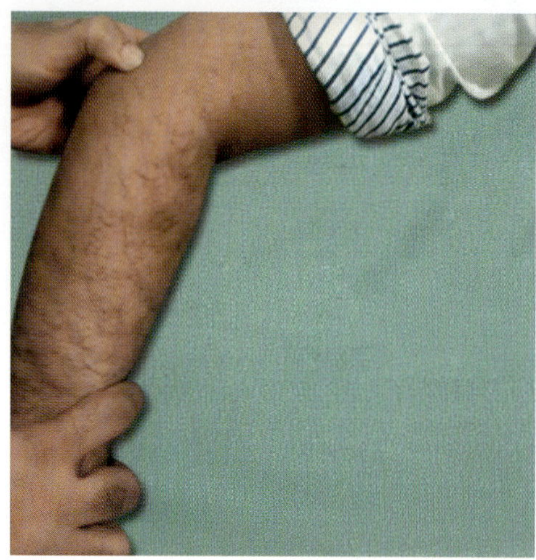

Fig. 11: Eliciting tenderness over lateral epicondyle.

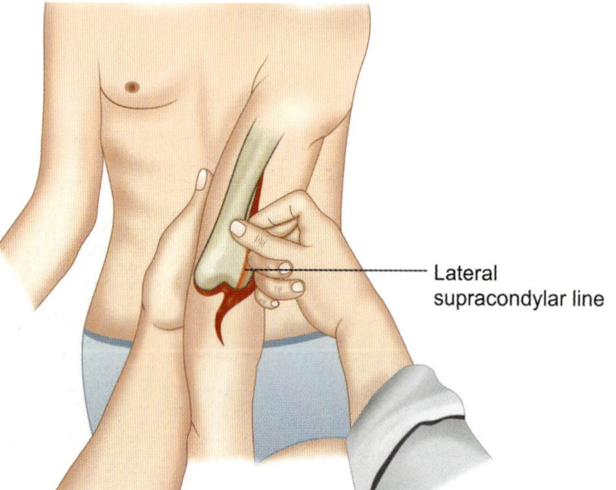

Fig. 12: Palpating the supracondylar ridge.

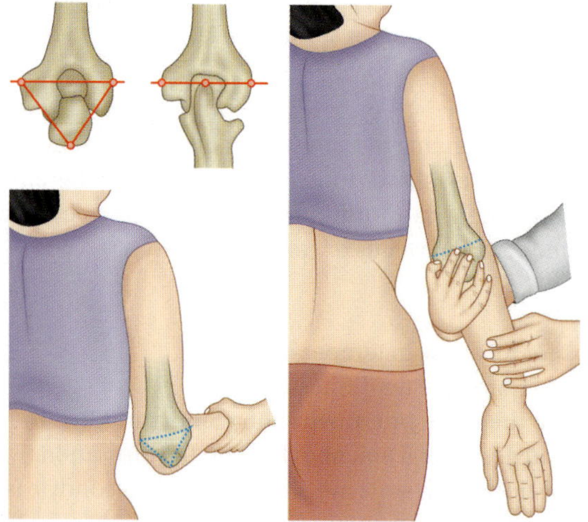

Fig. 13: Isosceles triangle of elbow.

Isosceles triangle of the elbow:

- When the elbow is flexed, the olecranon and the medial and lateral epicondyles form an isosceles triangle, as shown in Figure 13.

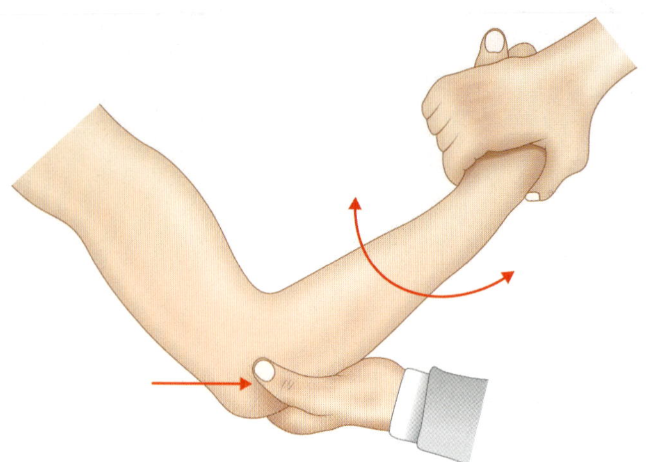

Fig. 14: Pronating and supinating the forearm and palpating its movement under the thumb.

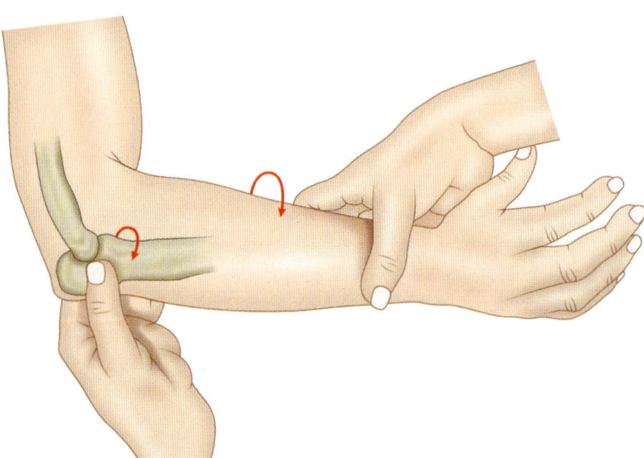

Fig. 15: Palpation of the thumb firmly into the space on the lateral side of elbow between the radial head and humerus.

- These three points come to lie in a straight line, when the elbow is extended.
- Altered distance between the two condyles and olecranon is seen in intercondylar fractures or isolated fracture of medial or lateral condyle.
- Palpate the lateral epicondyle of the humerus and distally the elbow joint, 1 cm more distal to it feels a firm rounded structure under the thumb. This is the radial head.
- Now, pronate and supinate the forearm and feel its movement under the thumb (Fig. 14).
- Palpate the thumb firmly into the space on the lateral side of elbow between the radial head and humerus, any tenderness here is common after injuries to the radial head—osteoarthritis and osteochondritis dissecans (OCD) (Fig. 15).
- For abnormal position of radial head, as occurs in dislocated radial head, one must look for ulnar bow sign, as explained ahead.
- The relationship is disturbed in any pathological condition such as intercondylar fracture of the humerus, elbow dislocation, etc. (Fig. 16).
- Reversal of triangle is seen in posterior dislocation of elbow (Figs. 17A and B).
- There may be an associated Monteggia fracture or dislocation.

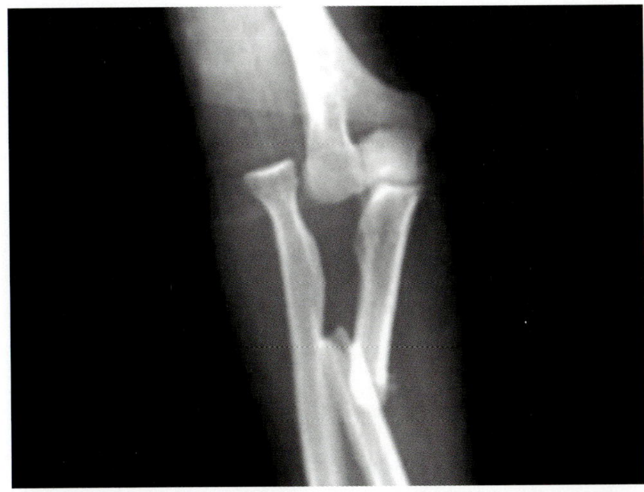

Fig. 16: Disturbed anatomy of the isosceles triangle of elbow in case of fracture forearm.

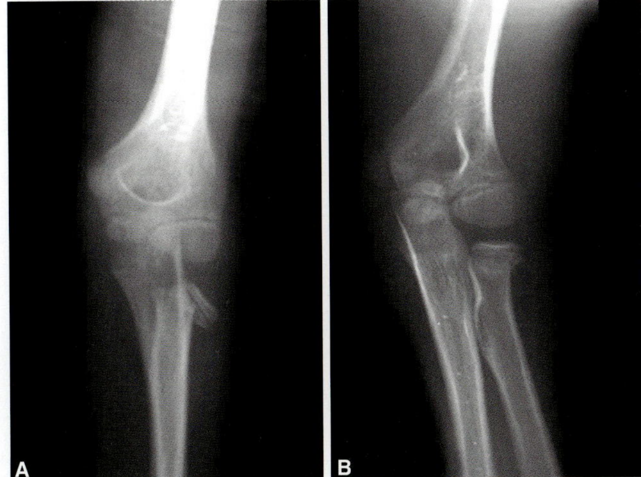

Figs. 17A and B: Disturbed anatomy of the isosceles triangle of elbow in case of elbow dislocation.

Ulnar bow sign:
It is an undetected and isolated radial head dislocation. The shape of ulna indicates persistent plastic deformation of the ulna (Figs. 18 and 19).

- The ulnar bow line is drawn between the distal ulna and olecranon, and it defines the ulnar bow.
- The ulnar bow sign is deviation of more than 1 mm of ulnar border from the reference line.
- Palpate the front of the elbow on both sides of the biceps tendon, while flexing and extending the elbow through 20° (Fig. 20).
- Notice any abnormal masses or thickening of bone (myositis ossificans, loose bodies, or OCD).
- Look for synovial thickening, doughy.

Movements:

- It is defined as the normal range of motion of flexion (Fig. 21). Movement of elbow flexion—135° and extension—0–5°.
- The normal range of motion of pronation and supination is 90° (Fig. 22).
- The range of motion testing should be done passively as well as actively.

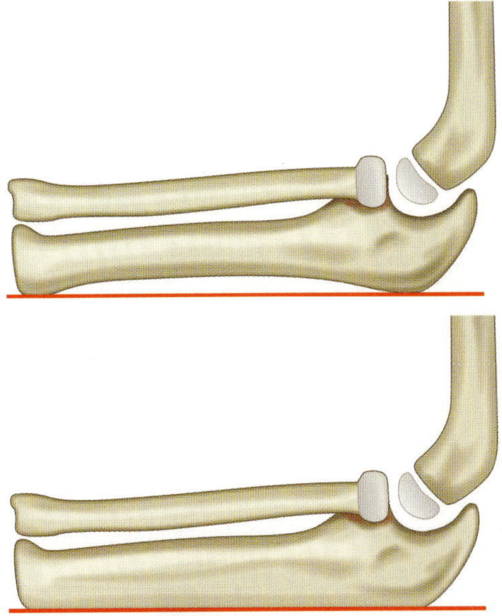

Fig. 18: Ulnar bow sign.

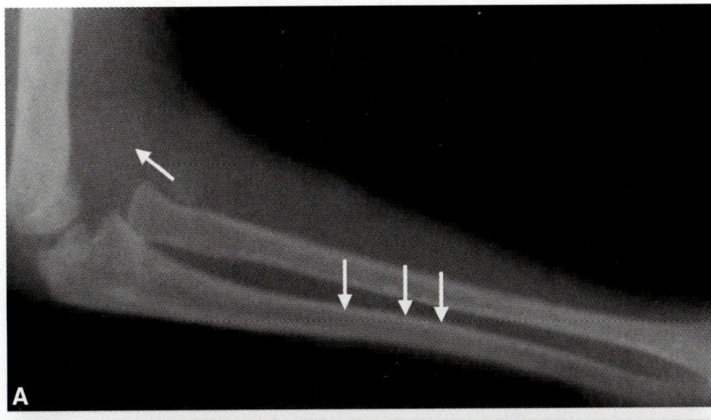

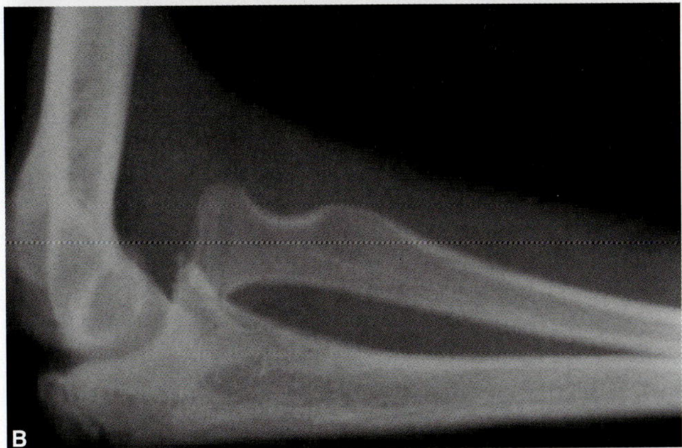

Figs. 19A and B: X-rays showing ulnar bow sign.

Additional Tests

Mill's maneuver (Fig. 23):

- Flex the elbow and fully pronate the hand
- Now extend the elbow
- Pain over the lateral epicondyle is almost diagnostic of tennis elbow
- As an alternative, pain may be sought by pronating the arm with the fully extended elbow (Fig. 24).

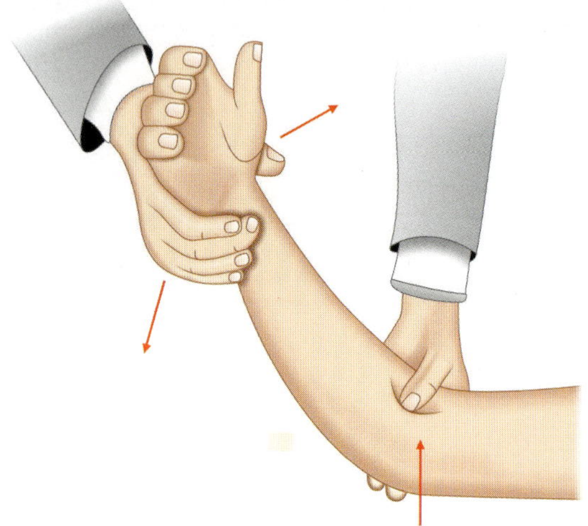

Fig. 20: Demonstrating the ulnar bow sign.

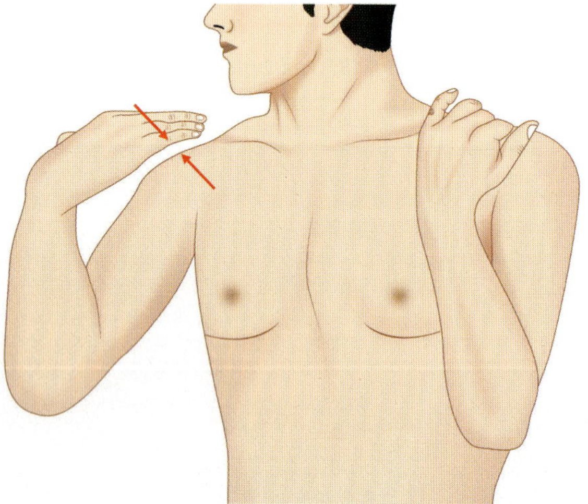

Fig. 21: Flexion movement of elbow joint.

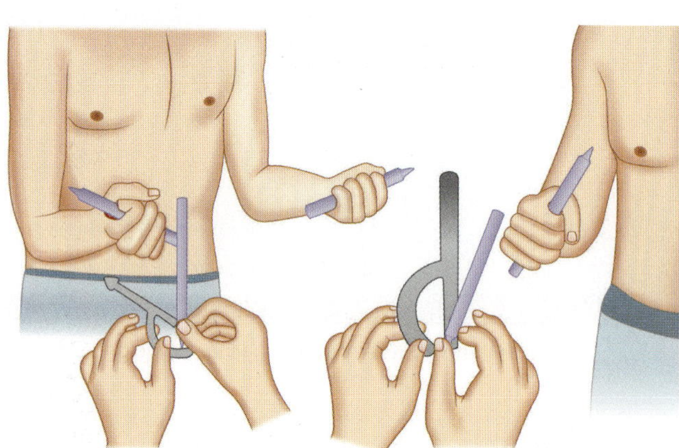

Fig. 22: Supination and pronation movements of elbow.

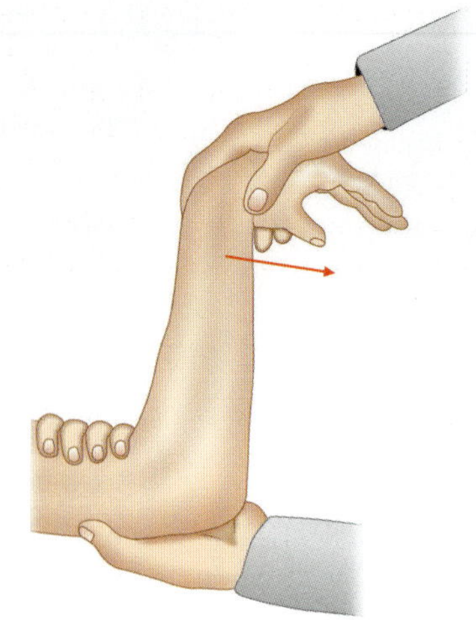

Fig. 23: Mill's maneuver.

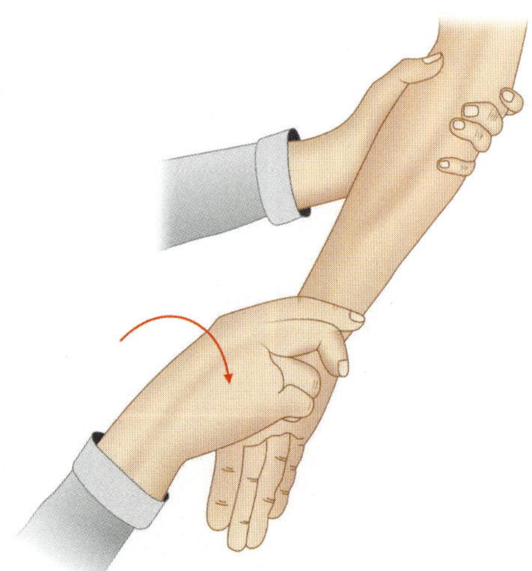

Fig. 24: Pronation of arm with fully extended elbow.

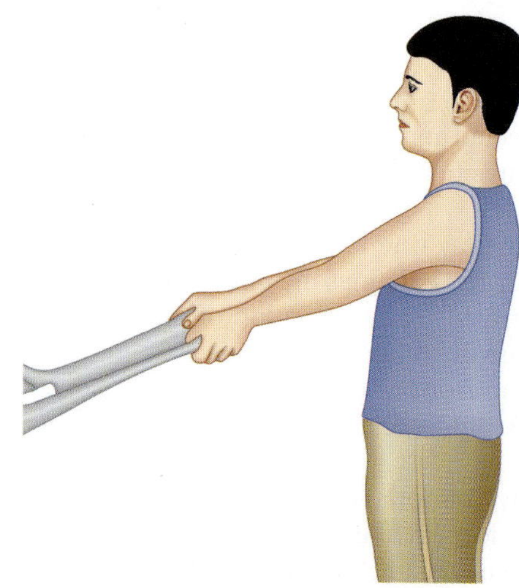

Fig. 25: Chair test.

Chair test (Fig. 25):
- Ask the patient to attempt to lift the chair (3.5 kg) with the elbows extended and the shoulders flexed to 60°.
- Difficulty in performing this maneuver, with complaint of pain on the lateral aspect of the elbow is suggestive of tennis elbow.

Thomsen's test or Cozen's test (Fig. 26):
- Ask the patient to clench the fist, dorsiflex the wrist, and extend the elbow.
- Try to force the hand into palmar flexion, while the patient resists.

- Severe pain over the lateral epicondyle is suggestive of tennis elbow.
- Also repeat the test, this time attempt to flex the extended middle finger rather than the wrist.

Golfer's elbow (Fig. 27):
- Flex the elbow, supinate the hand, and then extend the elbow.
- Pain over the medial epicondyle is very suggestive of golfer's elbow.

Ulnar Nerve Palsy (Fig. 28)
- Inspect the medial side of the joint carefully, while the patient flexes and extends the elbow.
- The nerve is visible in thin patients and displacement on movement may be visible.
- Palpate again and note the extent of any tenderness or thickening (Fig. 28).
- Look for any evidence of ulnar nerve palsy.

Elbow Instability (Figs. 29 and 30)
- Both valgus and varus instability may be elicited by stressing the joint in extension and 30° of flexion.
- Any gap or opening up of the joint space is noted, as shown in Figure 29.

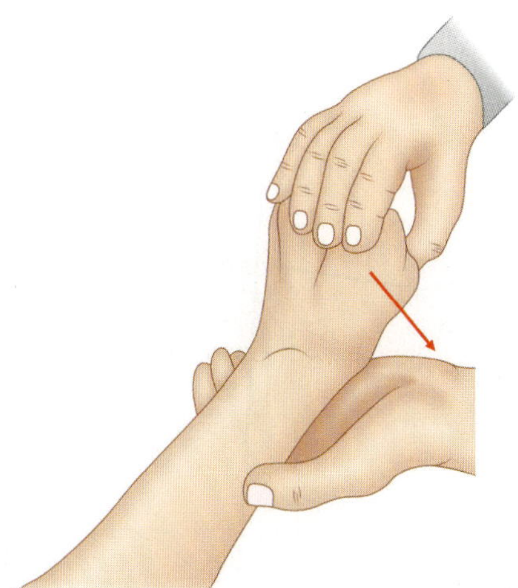

Fig. 26: Thomsen's test (Cozen's test).

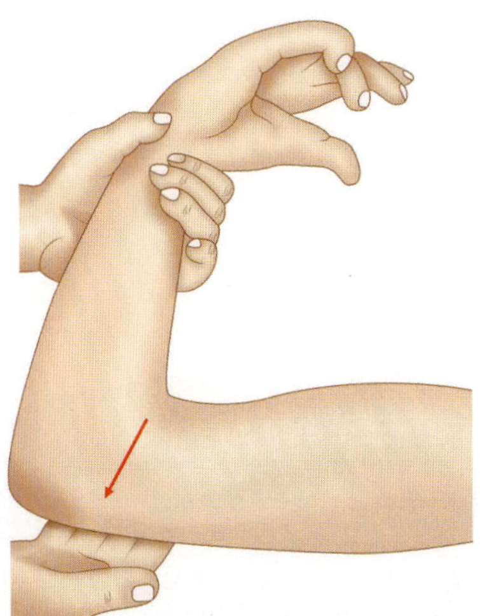

Fig. 27: Test of golfer's elbow.

- Another method for finding joint instability mainly carried out in children where extension is not possible due to pain is shown in Figure 30.

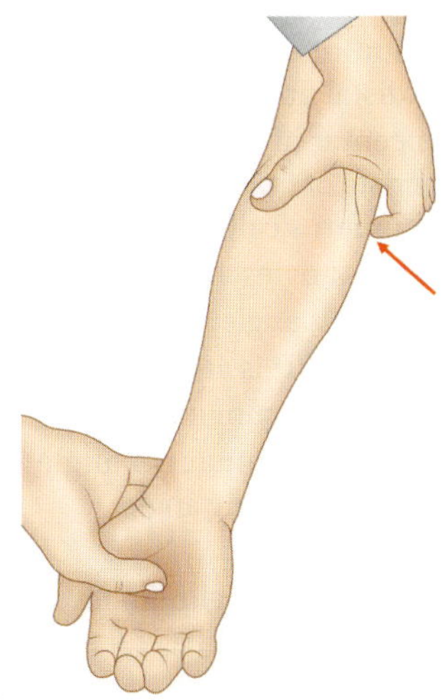

Fig. 28: Palpating ulnar nerve on the medial aspect of the joint.

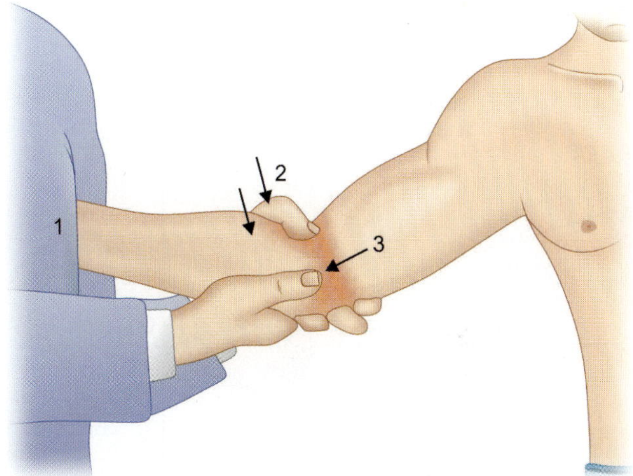

Fig. 29: Test for elbow instability: (1) The fixed arm; (2) The valgus force; (3) Opening up of the medial joint space.

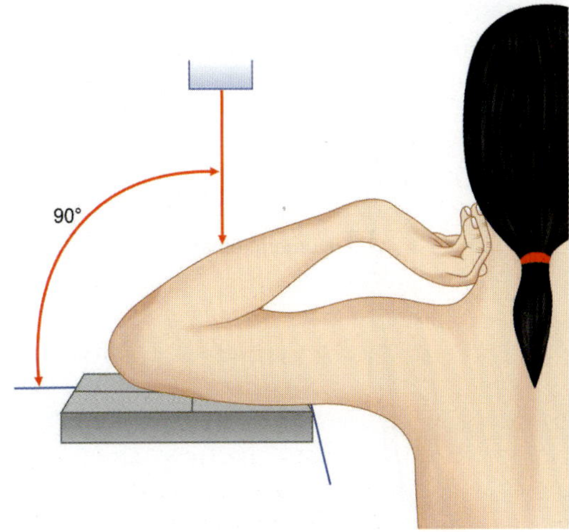

Fig. 30: Procedure for testing elbow instability, when extension is not possible.

- The radius or ulna and their relation to each other are seen.
- The humerus is overlapped, but the supracondylar fractures can be visualized with the displacements.

Angles around Elbow

Baumann's angle (Fig. 31):

- It is the angulation of the physeal line between the lateral condyle and the distal humeral metaphysis.
- The ossification center of the lateral condyle extends into the radial or lateral crista of trochlea. This line forms an angle with long axis of the humerus called the Baumann's angle.
- Different Baumann's angles and its significance:
  - Normal Baumann's angle is 72°
  - Angle greater than 81° is cubitus varus
  - Angle less than 61° is cubitus valgus
  - A change in 5° of Baumann's angle corresponds to 2° change in clinical carrying angle.

Humeral-ulnar angle (Fig. 32):

- It is determined by lines longitudinally bisecting the shaft of humerus with shaft of ulna.
- Normal value is 12–18°. A greater value signifies a valgus abnormality and a lesser value signifies a varus abnormality.

Metaphyseal-diaphyseal angle (Fig. 33):

- It is determined by a line that longitudinally bisects the shaft of the humerus, with a line that connects the widest points of the metaphysis of the distal humerus.
- Normal angle is 90°. Angle greater than 90° indicates varus inclination and angle less than 90° indicates valgus inclination.

Teardrop of distal humerus (Fig. 34):

- The lateral projection of the distal humerus presents a teardrop-like shadow above the capitulum.
- On a true lateral film, the teardrop should be well defined.
- *Significance:* Teardrop is disturbed in fractures of distal end of humerus.

Shaft-condylar angle:

- On lateral X-ray, there is angulation of 40° between the long axis of humerus and long axis of lateral condyle.
- *Significance:* It defines extension and flexion type of injury.

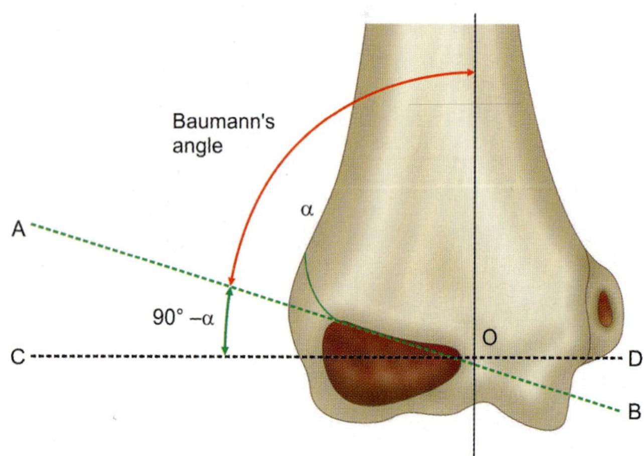

Fig. 31: Baumann's angle.

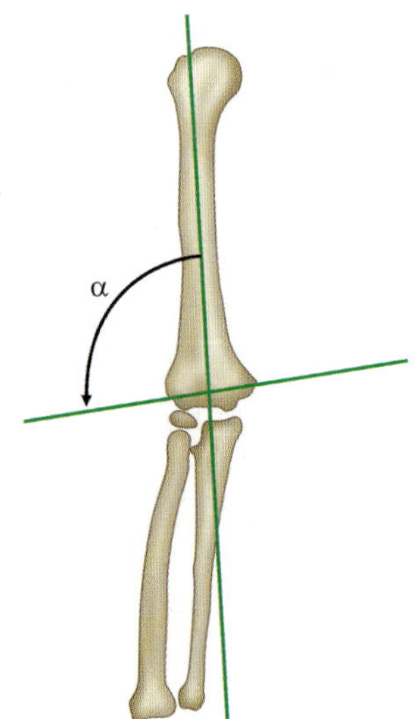

Fig. 33: Metaphyseal-diaphyseal angle.

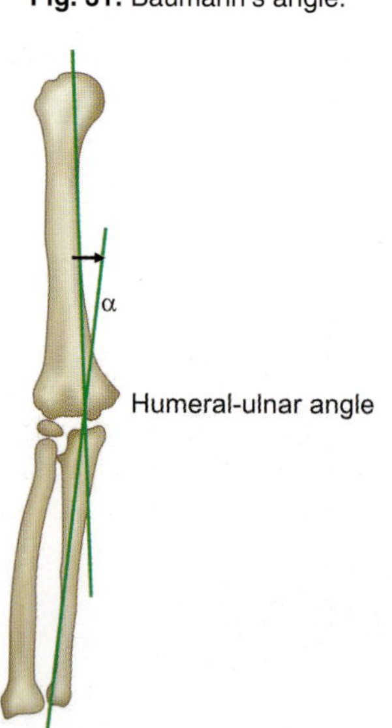

Fig. 32: Humeral-ulnar angle.

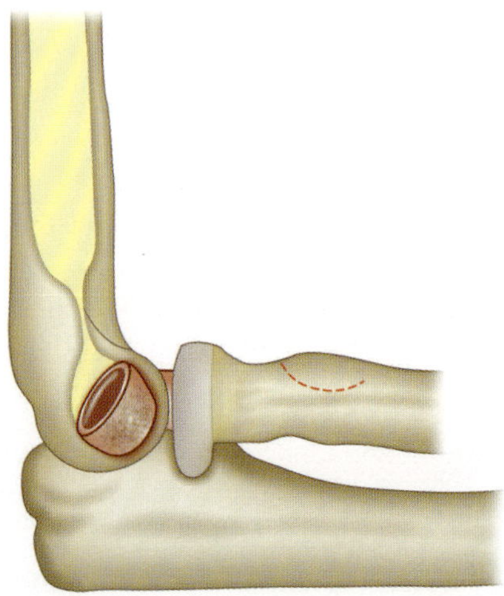

Fig. 34: Teardrop of distal humerus.

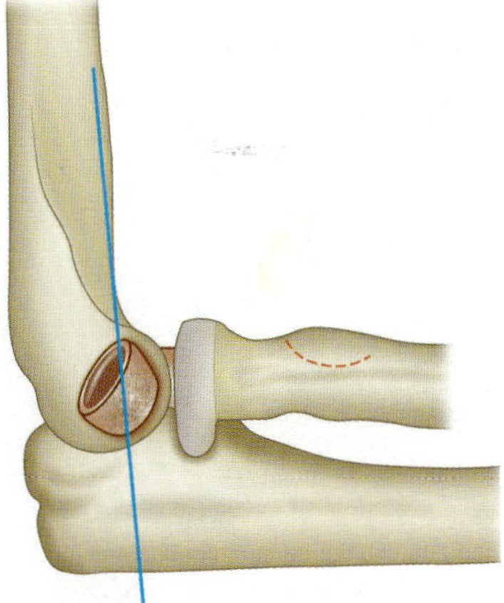

Fig. 35: Anterior humeral line.

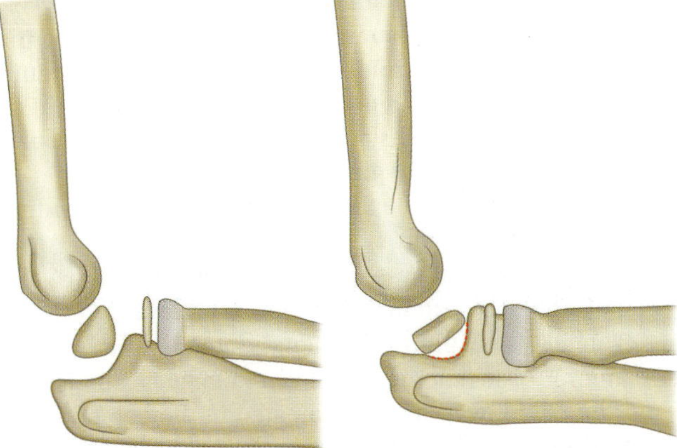

Fig. 37: Crescent sign.

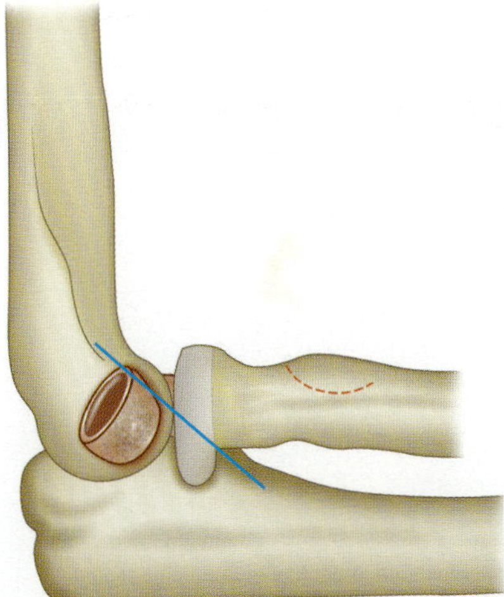

Fig. 36: Coronoid line.

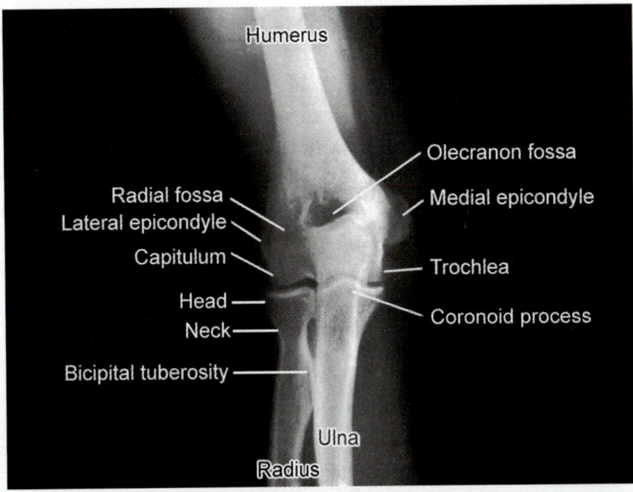

Fig. 38: X-ray of the elbow.

- If angle is less than 40°, extension deformity is present. If angle greater than 40°, flexion deformity is present.

Anterior humeral line (Fig. 35):

- If a line is drawn along the anterior border of the distal humeral shaft, it should pass through the middle-third of ossification center of the capitulum.
- If it passes anterior to this landmark, there is posterior angulation and vice versa.

Coronoid line (Fig. 36):

- A line directed proximally along the anterior border of the coronoid process should barely touch the anterior portion of the lateral condyle.
- Posterior displacement of the lateral condyle projects the ossification center posterior to this coronoid line.

Crescent sign:

In varus deformity, part of ulna overlies distal humeral epiphyses producing crescent sign. This is shown in Figure 37.

Radiological Findings

Normal lateral X-ray of the elbow (Figs. 38 and 39).

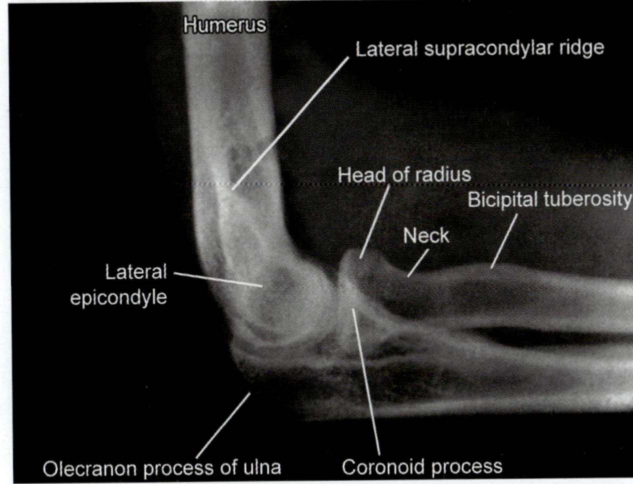

Fig. 39: Normal lateral X-ray of the elbow.

CONGENITAL ANOMALIES AROUND THE ELBOW JOINT

Congenital Radial Head Dislocation

- Congenital dislocation of the radial head was described by McFarland. The direction of the displacement of the radial head may be anterior, posterior, or lateral.

- Condition is often unilateral.
- The abnormality is usually not detected at birth, but is diagnosed later on in childhood when the elbow is examined following some minor injury.
- Usually the elbows are asymptomatic. A complaint of stiffness may be reason of visit to physician in some cases.
- The ulna is bowed in the direction of convexity depending on the type of dislocation:
  - Anterior dislocation—ulnar bow is forward
  - Posterior dislocation—ulnar bow is backward
  - Lateral dislocation—ulnar bow is lateral.
- In anterior dislocations, the range of elbow flexion is limited and the radial head may be palpated in the cubital fossa. In posterior dislocations, the elbow will not fully extend and the prominent radial head may be palpated posteriorly.

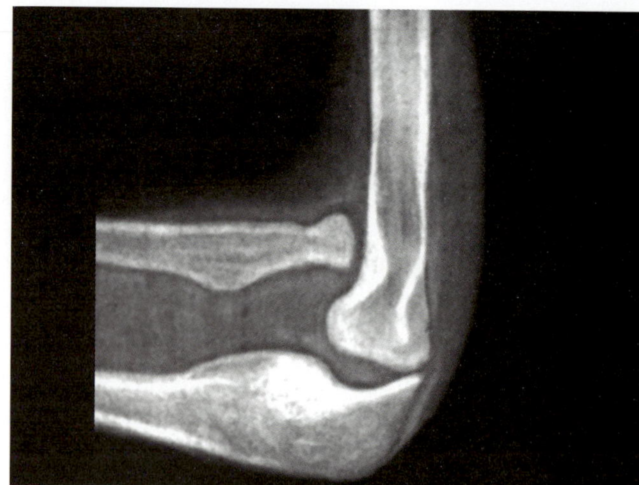

Fig. 40: Diagrammatic representation of the superior surface of dome-shaped head of the radius.

Radiographs

- In a normal elbow, a line drawn through the longitudinal axis of the radial shaft bisects the capitulum of the humerus. This normal finding is absent in this condition. The head of the radius is dome shaped on its superior surface (Figs. 40 and 41).
- It is important to distinguish traumatic dislocation from congenital dislocation. The types of injury that cause traumatic dislocation of the radial head are missed Monteggia fracture dislocations, fracture of the radial neck, pulled elbow, and occasionally a primary traumatic dislocation of the radial head with other associated injury.
- In the newborn and infant, arthrography of the elbow is helpful in the definitive diagnosis of radial head dislocation.

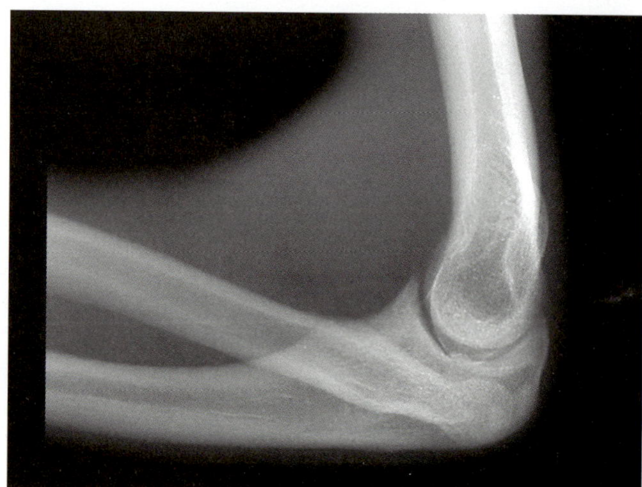

Fig. 41: X-ray of the elbow joint, showing dome-shaped head of the radius on its superior surface.

Treatment

- When the diagnosis is made in the newborn or young infant, closed reduction may be attempted.
- The posteriorly dislocated radial head is reduced by supination of the forearm and extension of the elbow.
- The anteriorly dislocated radial head is reduced by flexion of the elbow.
- Reduction is maintained in an above elbow cast for 4–6 weeks.
- Closed reduction is often unsuccessful.
- In children up to 3 years of age, open reduction should be carried out.
- In the older children, it will be impossible to reduce the radial head.
- The dislocation is left alone until late adolescence, when if symptoms warrant, the radial head is excised.

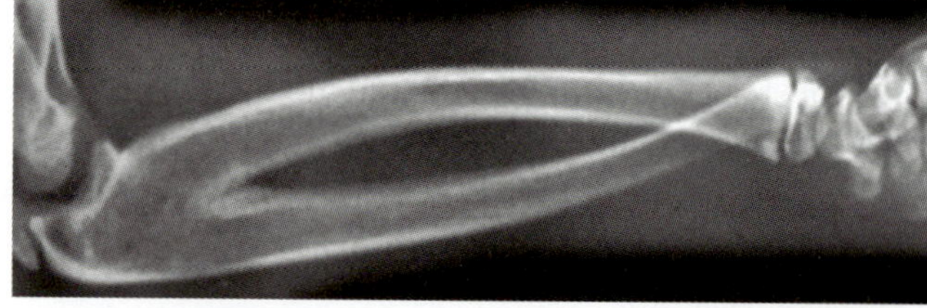

Fig. 42: Congenital radioulnar synostosis.

Congenital Radioulnar Synostosis

- Synostosis, or osseous union, of any two adjacent bones can involve any part of the upper extremity. Synostosis between the radius and ulna can take two forms:
  1. Congenital (Fig. 42)
  2. Post-traumatic (Fig. 43)
- The degree of fusion in radioulnar synostosis varies and may or may not involve the radial head.

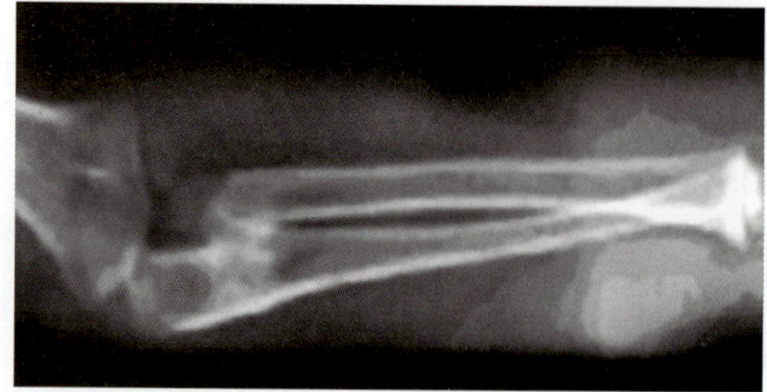

Fig. 43: Post-traumatic radioulnar synostosis.

Etiology

Congenital:

- In 1793, Sandifort provided the initial description of congenital radial-ulnar (radioulnar) synostosis.

- This condition is caused by a failure of segmentation between the radius and ulna.
- Embryologically, the upper limb bud arises from the unsegmented body wall between 25 days and 28 days.
- The elbow becomes visible in 34 days and the humerus, radius, and ulna become visible in 37 days.
- Initially, the three cartilaginous analogs of the humerus, radius, and ulna are connected before segmentation. Therefore, for a short time, the radius and ulna share a common perichondrium.
- Abnormal events at this time can lead to a failure of segmentation.
- The duration and severity of the insult can determine the degree of subsequent synostosis.
- Endochondral ossification then proceeds and the cartilaginous synostosis ossifies, either partially or completely, in the longitudinal or transverse plane.
- In the forearm, congenital radioulnar synostosis usually occurs between the proximal radius and ulna.
- Although the condition is present at birth, it usually is not discovered until early adolescence, when the patient presents with a lack of pronation and supination.
- Initially, the union may be more of a synchondrosis, but as the skeleton matures, the osseous bridge between the radius and ulna becomes more apparent.
- Usually, motion between the two adjacent bones, if existent, is minimal.

Post-traumatic:

- It is a separate entity from the congenital form, and having a different cause, treatment, and prognosis.
- The traumatic form can occur anywhere between the radius and ulna along the length of the interosseous membrane.
- The most common cause of post-traumatic radioulnar synostosis is an operatively treated forearm fracture.
- Patients with high energy, comminuted, and open fractures appear to be more likely to develop this complication.
- Monteggia and proximal forearm fractures also appear to have a higher incidence of synostosis.
- The use of bone graft and screws protruding through the opposite cortex also increases the incidence of synostosis.
- Additionally, radioulnar synostosis is described as a consequence of soft-tissue injury, reconstructive procedures, or any trauma causing hematoma formation between the radius and ulna or injury to the interosseous membrane.
- Patients with closed head injuries (skull/cranial trauma) appear to be more prone to this complication, presumably for the same reason that they develop heterotopic ossification.

Classification

- Wilkie described two types of congenital synostosis based on the proximal radioulnar junction:
  1. In Type 1, complete synostosis has occurred, with the radius and ulna fused proximally for a variable distance.
  2. In Type 2, there is less involvement and may exist as a partial union. Type 2 involves the region just distal to the proximal radial epiphysis and is associated with radial head dislocation.
- Cleary and Omer described four types of congenital synostosis, which are as follows:
  1. Fibrous synostosis
  2. Bony synostosis
  3. Associated posterior dislocation of the radius
  4. Associated anterior dislocation of the radius.
- Simmons and colleagues considered congenital synostosis to be a spectrum of anomalies in which the synostosis occurred in varying lengths, with or without involvement of the radial head.
- Post-traumatic radioulnar synostosis has been classified, based on location, into the following three types:
  1. *Type 1*: Least common, occurs in the distal forearm
  2. *Type 2*: Occurs in the mid forearm
  3. *Type 3*: Occurs in the proximal forearm.

Frequency

- Congenital radioulnar synostosis occurs rarely, with approximately 350 cases reported in the literature. The rarity of this condition often leads to a delayed clinical diagnosis.
- Cleary and Omer reported an average patient age at diagnosis of 6 years, with a range of from 6 months to 22 years.
- There is no sex predilection in congenital radioulnar synostosis and no particular inheritance pattern is apparent.
- 60% of cases are bilateral.
- Because congenital radioulnar synostosis is caused by an in utero insult, its association with other abnormalities is not surprising.
- About one-third of cases are associated with general skeletal abnormalities, such as hip dislocation, knee anomalies, clubfoot, polydactyly, syndactyly, Madelung deformity, ligamentous laxity, thumb hypoplasia, carpal coalition, and problems of the cardiac, renal, neurological, and gastrointestinal (GI) systems.
- Some associated abnormalities and syndromes are genetically determined, including acrocephalosyndactyly, Apert syndrome, Carpenter syndrome, arthrogryposis, mandibulofacial dysostosis, William syndrome, Klinefelter syndrome, Holt–Oram syndrome, microcephaly, multiple exostoses, and fetal alcohol syndrome. In 20% of their patients, Cleary and Omer found a genetic basis for an autosomal-dominant form (with variable penetrance) of congenital radioulnar synostosis.

Pathophysiology

- The skeletal anomaly includes varying degrees of proximal radial and ulnar fusion, with or without involvement of the radial head.
- If the radial head is involved, it may be dislocated anteriorly or posteriorly.
- A fibrous synostosis may allow limited motion.
- Regional soft-tissue hypoplasia is often present in severe cases, including when atrophy and fibrosis of the brachioradialis, pronator teres, pronator quadratus, and supinator muscles occur.
- The interosseous membrane also may be abnormal.

Presentation

- Functional deficits associated with congenital radioulnar synostosis depend on the severity of the deformity and on whether or not it is bilateral.
- In cases involving severe fixed forearm pronation deformity, the patient cannot compensate for the resulting functional limitations by using scapular and glenohumeral motion.

- The forearm usually lies in the pronated or hyperpronated position (*see* Fig. 42).
- Radioulnar synostosis occurs as either a congenital or a post-traumatic condition (*see* Fig. 43).
- Radioulnar synostosis occurs as either a congenital or a post-traumatic condition.
- The degree of fusion in radioulnar synostosis varies and may or may not involve the radial head.
- Hypermobility at the midcarpal and radiocarpal joints can disguise this lack of forearm rotation, particularly with neutral or mild pronation deformities.
- There is usually full or nearly full elbow range of motion, with flexion contractures rarely exceeding 30°.
- An abnormal carrying angle of the elbow or a shortening of the forearm may be observed.
- Pain is usually not a presenting symptom until the teenage years, when progressive and symptomatic radial head subluxation may be noted.
- This accounts for the delayed clinical diagnosis in many cases, but it also indicates that function may be satisfactory.
- The disability is most significant in bilateral cases with severe pronation.
- Children may initially have a reduced radial head and in adolescence may develop symptomatic radial head subluxation. Therefore, radiographic follow-up is necessary.

Indications for Surgical Treatment

- Indications for surgical treatment of congenital radioulnar synostosis still remain somewhat controversial but are related to bilaterality and to the degree of deformity.
- Patients with neutral rotation, mild pronation or rare supination positions can compensate somewhat with ipsilateral shoulder motion. Wrist hypermobility allows further functional compensation.
- Severe pronation deformities (specifically those >60°) cause significant functional difficulty, especially with activities requiring supination.
- Therefore, indications for surgery must be determined based more on individual functional limitations than on absolute forearm position.
- It is recommended that surgery should be performed in childhood before patients are of schoolgoing age.
- In patients with symptomatic subluxation of the radial head, the radial head may be excised at maturity.
- Appropriate workup includes plain radiography performed in orthogonal planes (e.g. posteroanterior and lateral views).

Contraindications for Surgical Treatment

The only contraindication to surgical correction is the presence of milder deformity in an older patient, if the patient has only minimal functional deficit and has already made adjustments in his/her activities to accommodate the synostosis.

Congenital Ankylosis of the Elbow Joint

Congenital ankylosis of the cubital joint is extremely rare.

- When reporting one case, *Romanus* (1933) had been able to collect only 23 cases formerly described in the literature.
- *Frostad* (1940) reported five cases of bilateral ankylosis in adults.

Anatomical Findings

- In all of the formerly reported cases, except one, the radius had been found to be the chief bone in the formation of the ankylosis, merging broadly with osseous connection directly into the humerus.
- In one case, the ulna was ankylotically joined with the humerus, while the radius articulated freely with both.
- The brachialis muscle is poorly developed. Biceps, the long head of triceps, and the muscles of the forearm originating at the humerus, are all present.
- This finding is not surprising, as these muscles also exert their effect on the shoulder and the wrist joint, respectively, and thus maintain some activity despite a stiff elbow.
- The presence of these muscles is of the greatest importance to a successful operative treatment of a congenital ankylotic elbow.

Treatment

- In schools of surgery and in textbooks, it seems to be an established rule that in cases of congenital ankylosis of the elbow, arthroplasty should be postponed until the patient reaches adult age, partly because of the close relationship between the epiphysis and the joint.
- But especially because of the difficulties connected with the after-treatment in children, there are a number of important daily tasks, which these patients cannot perform.
- For example, they cannot wash the face or neck, the upper part of the chest or back. They cannot shave, wash their teeth, or comb their hair. They cannot button their coats or upper part of the vest. They all have difficulties in eating. They have to bend the head forward in order to meet the spoon or fork.
- So, surgeons feel that operation should be performed in early childhood, before atrophy of the muscles had time to occur.

TRAUMA TO ELBOW FRACTURES AROUND ELBOW

Surgical Anatomy

Medial and lateral columns diverge from humeral shaft at 45° angle. The columns are the important structures for support of the "distal humeral triangle".

Mechanism of Injury

The fracture is related to the position of elbow flexion, when the load is applied, as shown in Figures 44A to C.

Evaluation

Physical Examination

- Soft-tissue envelope
- Vascular status, e.g. radial and ulnar pulses
- *Neurological status:*
  - *Radial nerve:* Most commonly injured
  - *Median nerve:* Rarely injured
  - *Ulnar nerve.*

Radiographic Examination

- Anteroposterior and lateral radiographs.
- Traction views are necessary to evaluate intra-articular extension and for preoperative planning. Traction removes overlap.

- Computed tomography (CT) scan is also helpful in selected cases, e.g. comminuted capitulum or trochlea.

Fractures at Distal End of Humerus

- Supracondylar fractures
- Transcondylar fractures
- Intercondylar fractures
- Fractures of the condyles (lateral and medial)
- Fractures of the articular surfaces (capitulum and trochlea)
- Fractures of the epicondyles
- Fractures of the radial head
- Fractures of olecranon
- Monteggia fracture dislocation
- Fractures at the distal end of humerus.

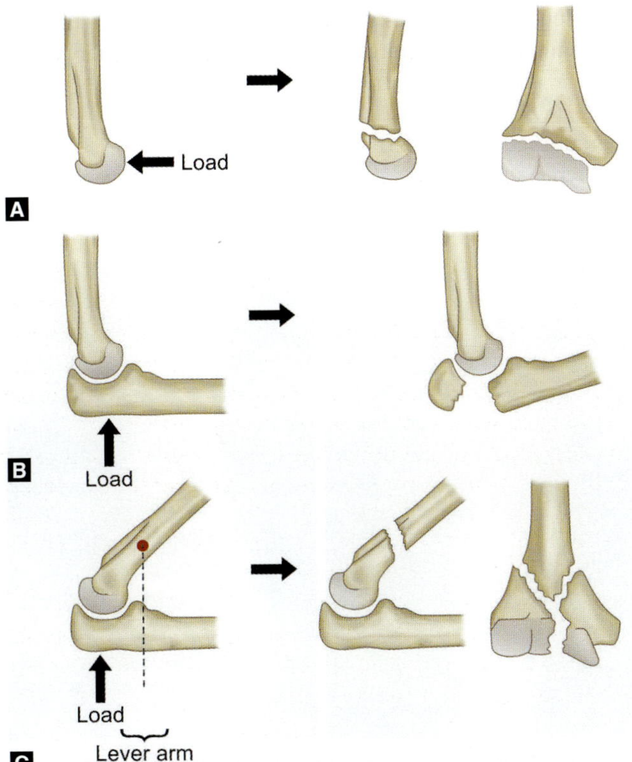

Figs. 44A to C: Different mechanisms of elbow injury.

Classifications

OTA Classification

Humerus, distal segment:

Types: These are shown in Figures 45A to C and are of the following types:

- Extra-articular fracture (A2)
- Partial articular fracture (B1)
- Complete articular fracture (C2).

Anatomical Classification

- Supracondylar fractures
- Transcondylar fractures
- Intercondylar fractures; fractures of the condyles (lateral and medial)
- Fractures of the articular surfaces (capitulum and trochlea)
- Fractures of the epicondyles.

Treatment Principles

- Anatomic articular reduction
- Stable internal fixation of the articular surface
- Restoration of articular axial alignment
- Stable internal fixation of the articular segment to the metaphysis and diaphysis
- Early range of motion of the elbow.

Technical Objectives for Fixation of Distal Humerus Fractures

- Every screw should pass through a plate.
- Every screw should engage a fragment on the opposite side that is also fixed to a plate.
- As many screws as possible should be placed in the distal fragments.
- Each screw should be as long as possible.
- Every screw should engage as many articular fragments as possible.
- Plates should be applied such that compression is achieved at the supracondylar level for both the columns.
- Plates used must be strong enough and stiff enough to resist breaking or bending before union occurs at supracondylar level.
- AO implants.

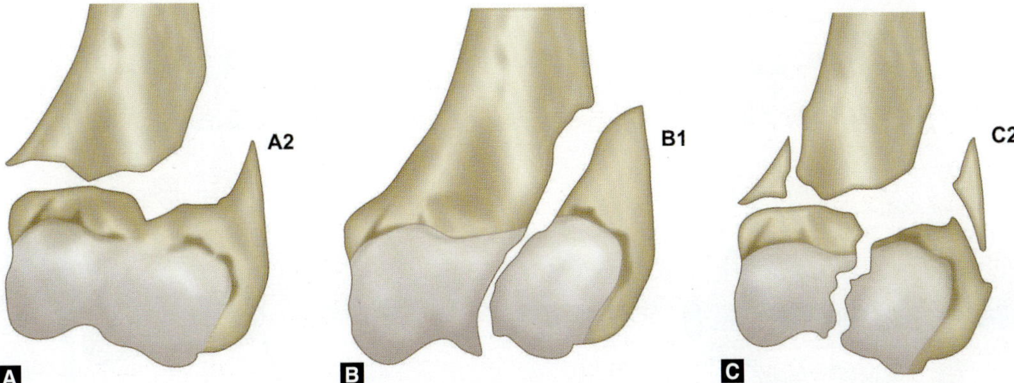

Figs. 45A to C: Orthopedic Trauma Association classification of distal humerus: (A) Extra-articular fracture; (B) Partial articular fracture; (C) Complete articular fracture of distal humeral segment.

Supracondylar Fractures

Careful neurovascular examination of the arm is essential, especially in extension-type (apex anteriorly angulated) supracondylar fractures. The brachial artery may be lacerated by the proximal fracture fragment, either at the time of injury or during reduction and a compartment syndrome may develop. All three major nerves that cross the elbow can be injured, but the radial and median nerves are those most commonly affected.

Treatment

Conservative:
- Hanging arm cast
- Overhead olecranon skeletal traction.

Open reduction and internal fixation:
They are used as a rule only in the presence of neurovascular damage or when a satisfactory position of the fracture is not obtained by closed methods.
- *Crossed screws or crossed threaded pins (Fig. 46)*: The screws or pins should be placed in the medial and lateral pillars and should engage the posterior cortex of the bone. Overdrilling of the distal fragment may be done, to allow compression, when the screws are tightened.
- *Hand-contoured plates (Fig. 47)*: When one or both columns are comminuted, hand-contoured plates can be used to reconstruct the humeral pillars.
- *Precontoured plate fixation*: It is illustrated in Figures 48A and B. Goal should be to stabilize rigid internal fixation, as shown in Figure 49.
- *Olecranon pin traction (Fig. 50)*: If operative treatment is postponed because of severe swelling, trauma, contused skin, or the patient's overall condition, displaced supracondylar fractures, side arm, or overhead olecranon pin traction should be done until operative treatment can be performed.

Transcondylar Fractures

They are often grouped with supracondylar fractures. Rare injury requires special consideration. The fracture line usually extends transversely across the condyles and often is intra-articular. They are quite unstable and unite slowly when treated conservatively.

Implant Options

- Percutaneous threaded Steinmann pins.
- AO type lag screws, as shown in Figure 51.

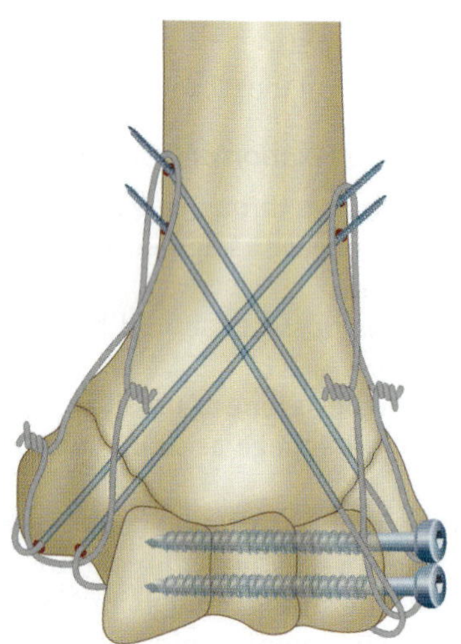

Fig. 46: Crossed screws or crossed threaded pins.

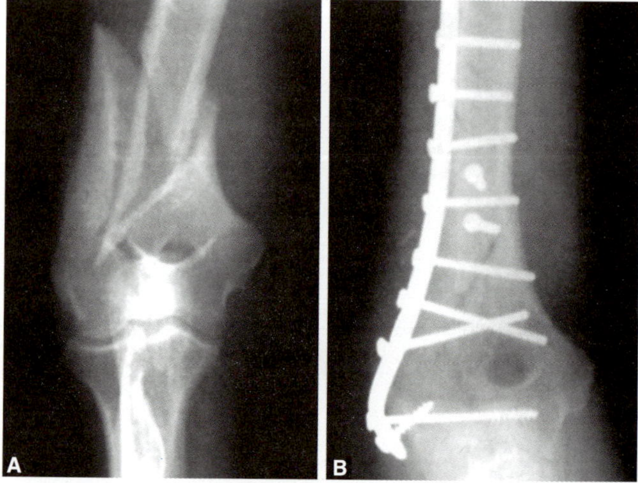

Figs. 48A and B: X-rays showing precontoured plate fixation.

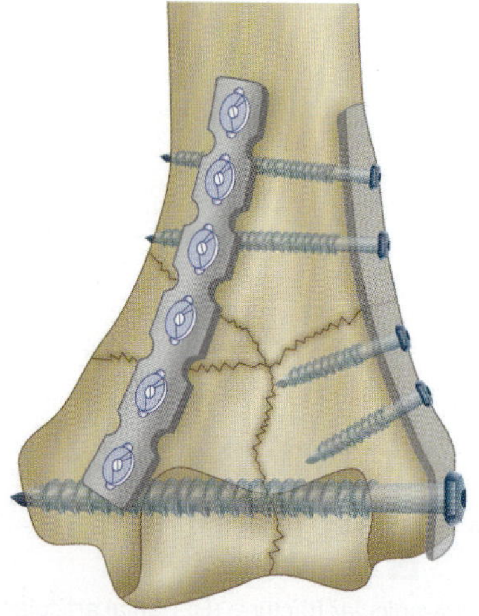

Fig. 47: Hand-contoured plates.

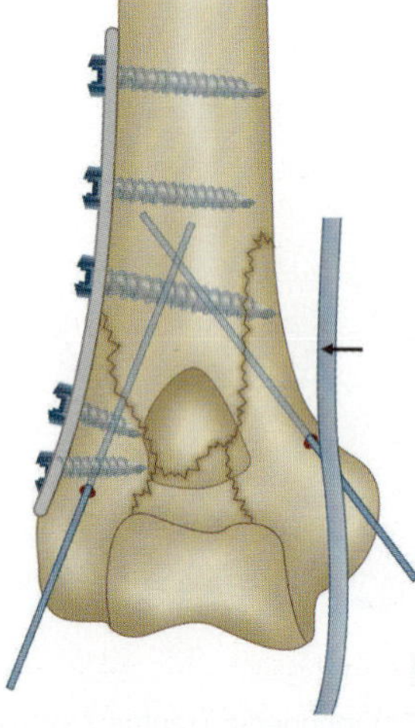

Fig. 49: Precontoured plate fixation used to stabilize rigid internal fixation.

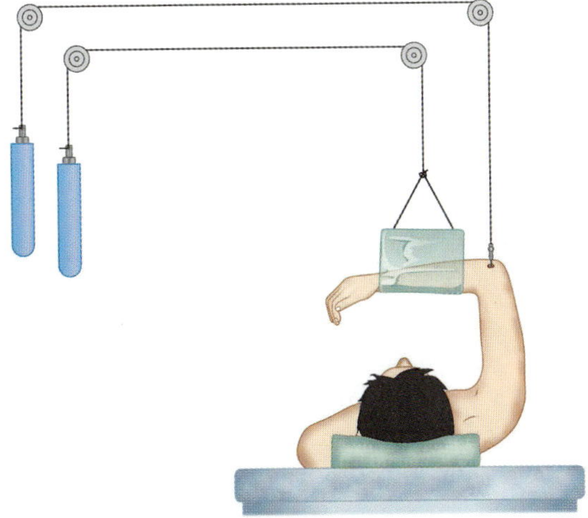

Fig. 50: Olecranon pin traction.

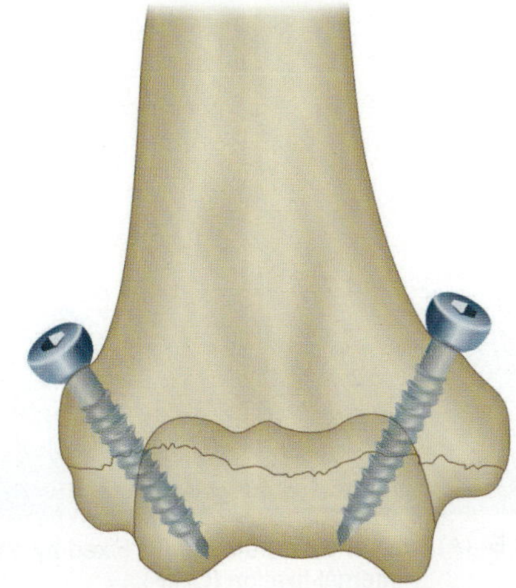

Fig. 51: AO type lag screws.

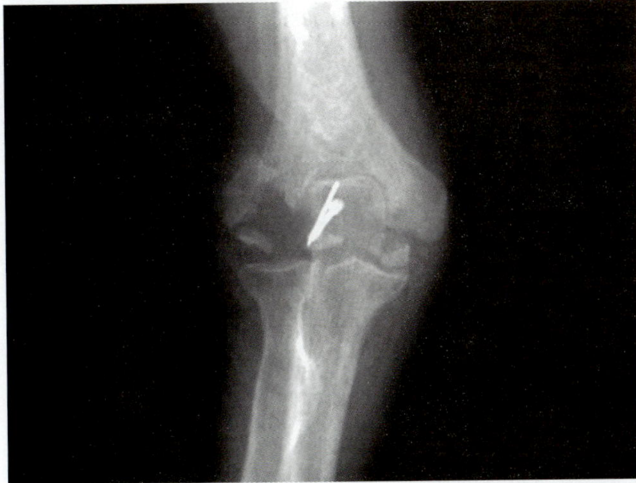

Fig. 52: Avascular necrosis in case of intra-articular fracture, with loss of fracture fixation.

- Newer cannulated screw systems allow provisional percutaneous pin fixation, followed by screw fixation without removal of the provisional pins.
- This injury, especially if it is intra-articular with loss of fixation of the fracture, can be complicated by avascular necrosis, as illustrated in Figure 52.

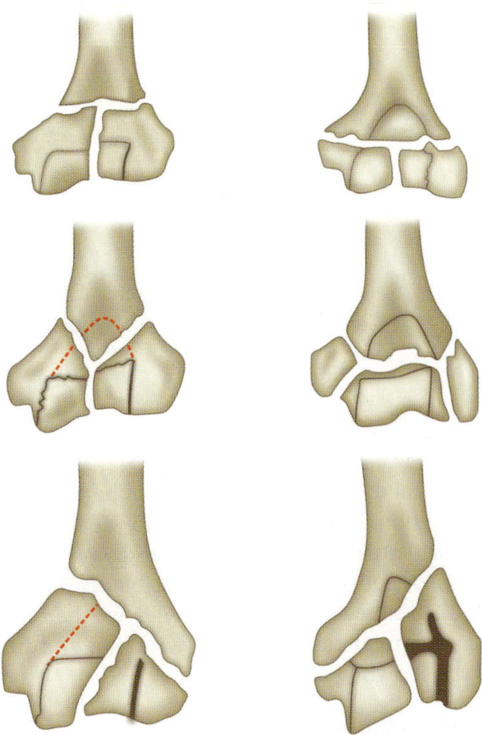

Fig. 53: Mehne and Matta classification system.

Intercondylar Fractures

Most difficult challenge of the fractures is of the lower end of the humerus.

Classification

Mehne and Matta classification system (Fig. 53):

- According to pattern of fracture line in the distal humerus.

Classification of Riseborough and Radin (Fig. 54):

- *Type I:* Fractures involving minimally displaced articular fragments.
- *Type II*: Fractures involving displaced fragments that are not rotated.
- *Type III*: Fractures involving displaced and rotated fragments.
- *Type IV*: Fractures involving comminuted fracture fragments.

Treatment

Type I fractures:

- Plaster splint immobilization, with gradual motion being permitted, once sufficient healing has occurred.

Types II and III fractures:

- Open reduction internal fixation (ORIF), especially when patient is young and active.
- Open fractures up to Gustilo type II
- Surgery is best performed within the first 24–48 hours.

Type IV fractures "a bag of bones" (Figs. 55A and B):

- Usually treated nonoperatively by:
  - Sling and early motion, if the patient is elderly
  - Skeletal traction through an olecranon pin, if the patient is younger
- When the patient is young, ORIF of two or three of the major articular fragments, as shown in Figure 55B, is done followed

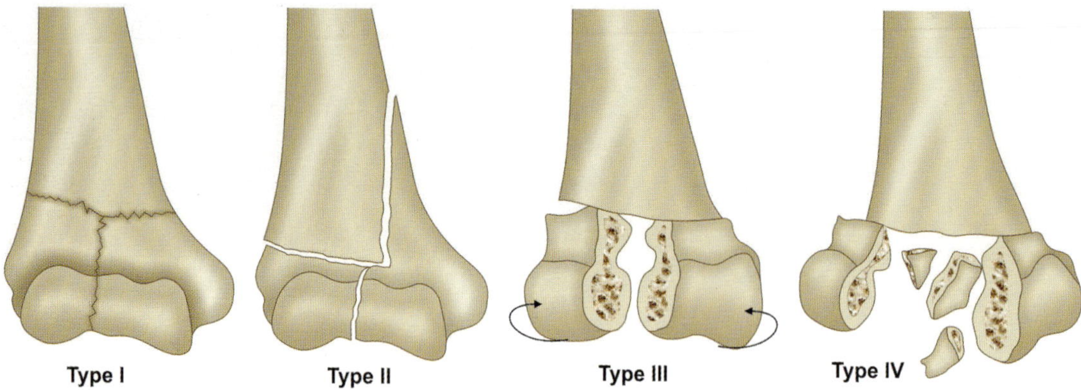

Fig. 54: Riseborough and Radin classification.

by skeletal traction and early motion may be preferred. Hinged-type distraction external fixator that allows early motion can be a satisfactory treatment option for intercondylar fractures, for which total reconstruction is not possible, as shown in Figures 56 and 57, besides it is more cost-effective than traction, and may yield similar results. Open reduction and fixation of Y fracture is shown in Figure 58.

Comminuted Fractures

If there is comminution of pillars hand contoured, one-third tubular plate is applied to the medial edge of the medial humeral pillar and a contoured reconstruction plate may be applied to the posterior aspect of the lateral humeral pillar, as illustrated in Figure 59.

Lateral Comminution (Figs. 60 to 63)

If the medial pillar is not severely comminuted, a rigid and prebent plate can be applied alone to the lateral pillar.

Minifragment

After treatment:

- Light posterior plaster splint is applied from the posterior axillary fold to the palm of the hand.
- At 7 days, the posterior plaster splint is removed periodically and gentle active and active-assisted exercises are carried out.
- By 3 weeks, the posterior plaster splint can be removed and arm is supported by a sling with active motion in the elbow as pain permits.
- Vigorous stretching by a therapist, forced motion, whether active or passive, and manipulation under anesthesia are contraindicated, as it may result in increased periarticular hemorrhage and fibrosis, heterotrophic calcification, increased joint irritability, and decreased rather than increased motion.

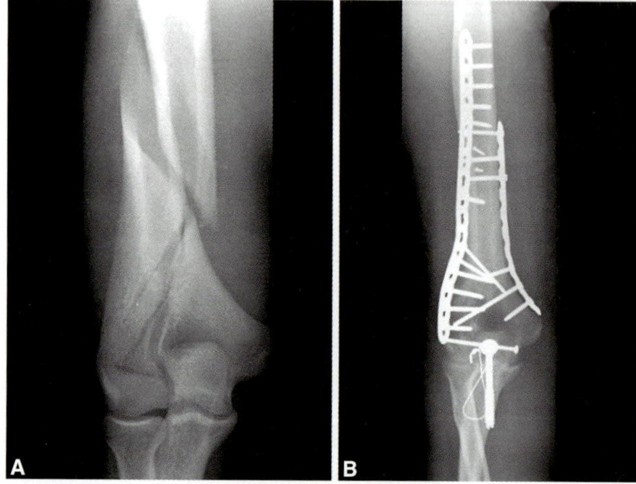

Figs. 55A and B: (A) Intercondylar fracture; (B) Fixed by open reduction internal fixation (ORIF).

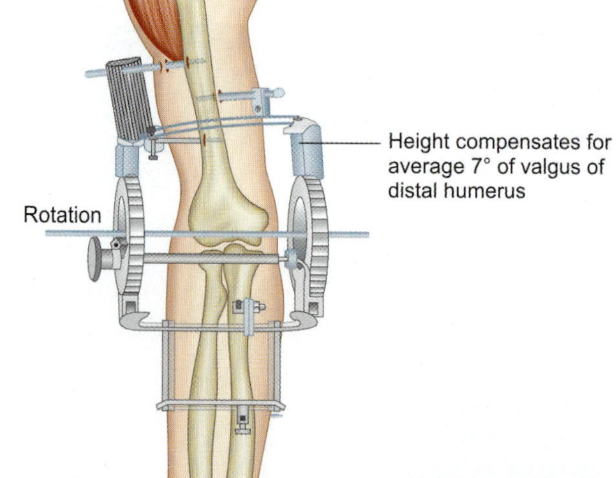

Fig. 56: Hinged-type distraction external fixator.

Fractures of Condyles of Humerus (Medial or Lateral)

Isolated fractures of the medial or lateral condyle of the humerus in adults are uncommon. When the condyle is displaced, ORIF is the best treatment. Lateral condylar fractures are more common than medial. Mechanism of injury is abduction or adduction of forearm with elbow in extension.

- Medial condyle fractures include trochlea and medial epicondyle fractures, as shown in Figure 64.
- Lateral condyle fracture includes lateral epicondyle and capitulum fractures.

Classification

Milch classification:

- *Type I*: In the type I fracture, the fracture line courses medially to the trochlea through and into the capitellar-trochlear groove. This type of fracture is rare because of the location of the fracture line. It is a true Salter-Harris type IV fracture, but is frequently stable.

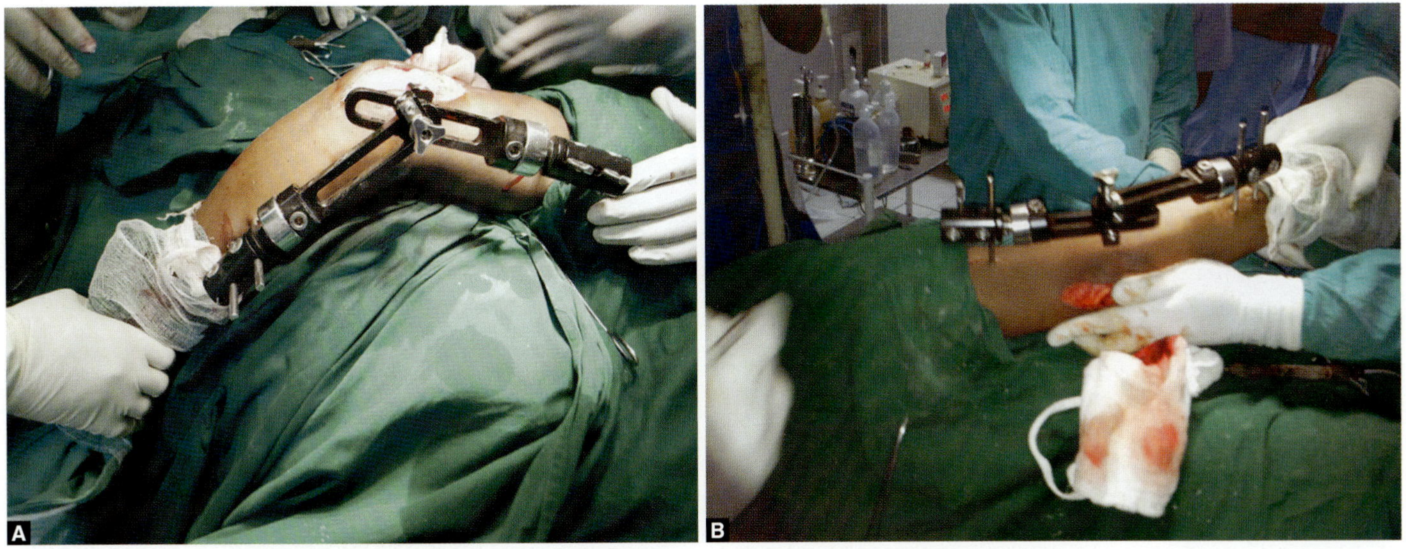

Figs. 57A and B: AO elbow hinge fixator: (A) Elbow at flexion; (B) Extended elbow.

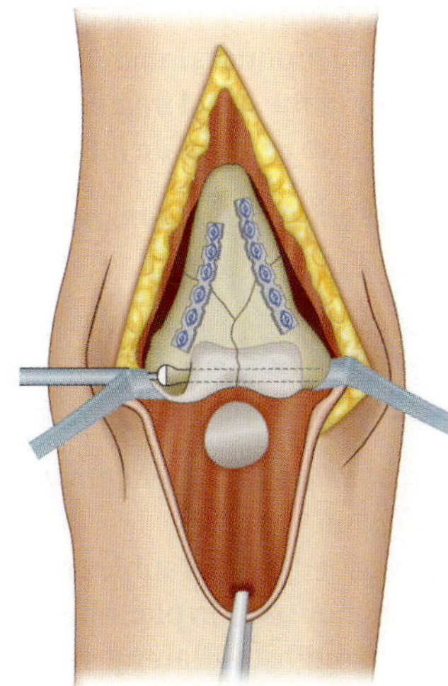

Fig. 58: Open reduction internal fixation of Y fracture of distal humerus.

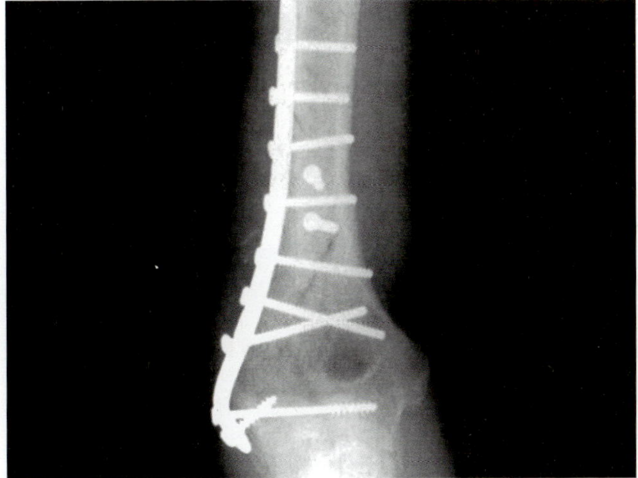

Fig. 60: Precontoured DuPont plate fixation.

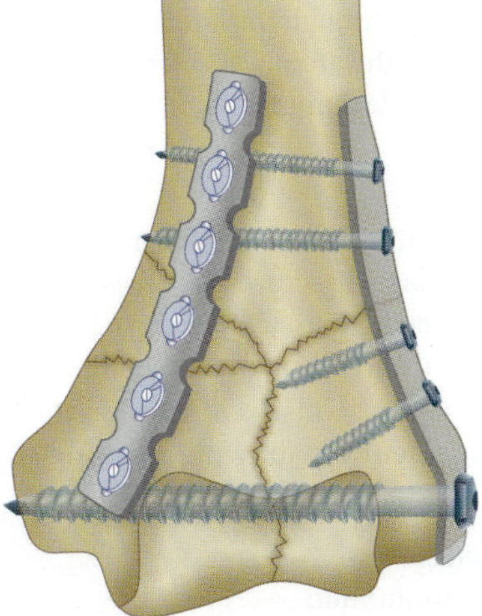

Fig. 59: Contoured reconstruction plate is applied to the posterior aspect of lateral humeral pillar.

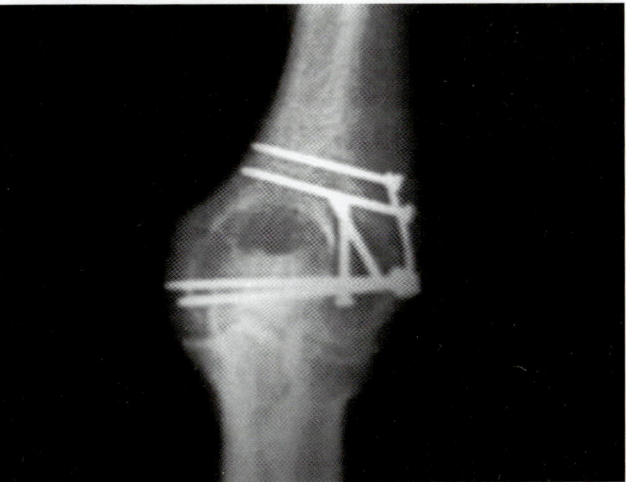

Fig. 61: Anteroposterior (AP) view showing precontoured plate applied to lateral pillar.

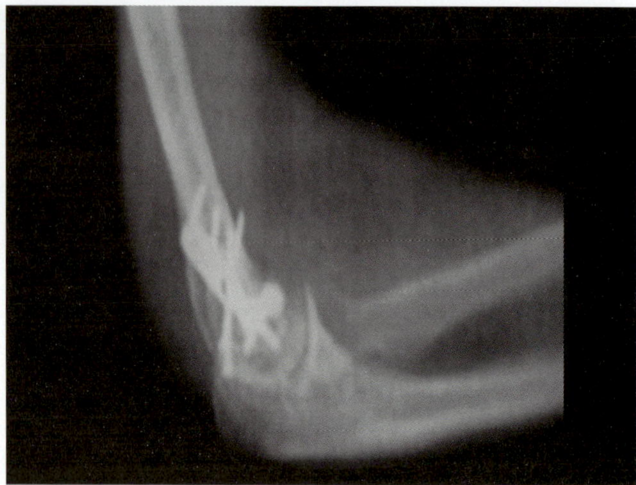

Fig. 62: Lateral view showing precontoured plate applied to lateral pillar.

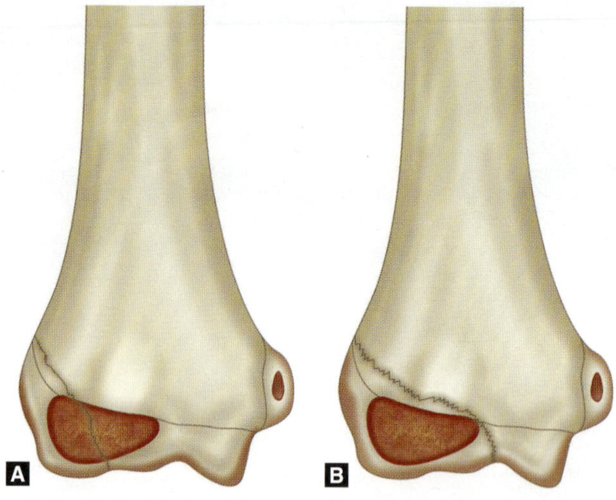

Figs. 65A and B: (A) Type I fracture of lateral condyle according to Milch classification; (B) Type II fracture.

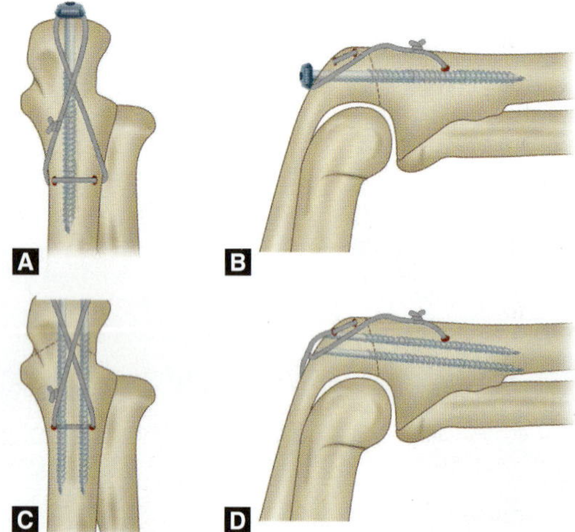

Figs. 63A to D: Tension band wiring and screw.

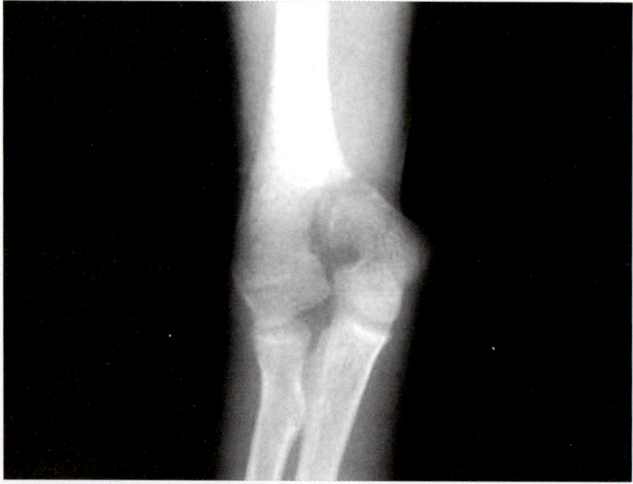

Fig. 64: X-ray showing medial condyle fracture including lateral epicondyle and capitulum fractures.

- *Type II (Figs. 65A and B)*: In the type II fracture described by Milch, which is more common, the fracture line extends into the area of the trochlea and produces inherent instability of the elbow because of the ability of the distal fragment and the forearm not only to angulate, but also to translate into a lateral position.

Classification of lateral condylar fractures according to the amount of displacement:

- Undisplaced
- Moderately displaced
- Completely displaced and rotated.

Radiographic criteria of determining fracture stability according to Finnbogason et al. (Figs. 66A to C):

Finnbogason et al. described radiographic criteria for determining fracture stability, which they used in planning the initial treatment.

- *Type I*: Fracture through the lateral humeral condyle with minimal lateral gap—a stable fracture.
- *Type II*: Fracture through the lateral humeral condyle to the epiphyseal cartilage with a lateral gap—a fracture with undefinable risk.
- *Type III*: Fracture through the lateral humeral condyle with the fracture gap as wide laterally as medially—a fracture with high risk of lateral displacement.

Treatment

- Nonoperative treatment is indicated in nondisplaced or minimally displaced fractures. It consists of posterior splinting with elbow in 90° flexion, with forearm in supination in lateral condylar fracture and pronation in medial condylar fractures.
- Operative treatment consists of screw fixation with or without collateral ligament repair, with attention to rotational axis restoration.

Prognosis depends on:

- Degree of comminution
- Accuracy of reduction
- Stability of internal fixation (Figs. 67 and 68).

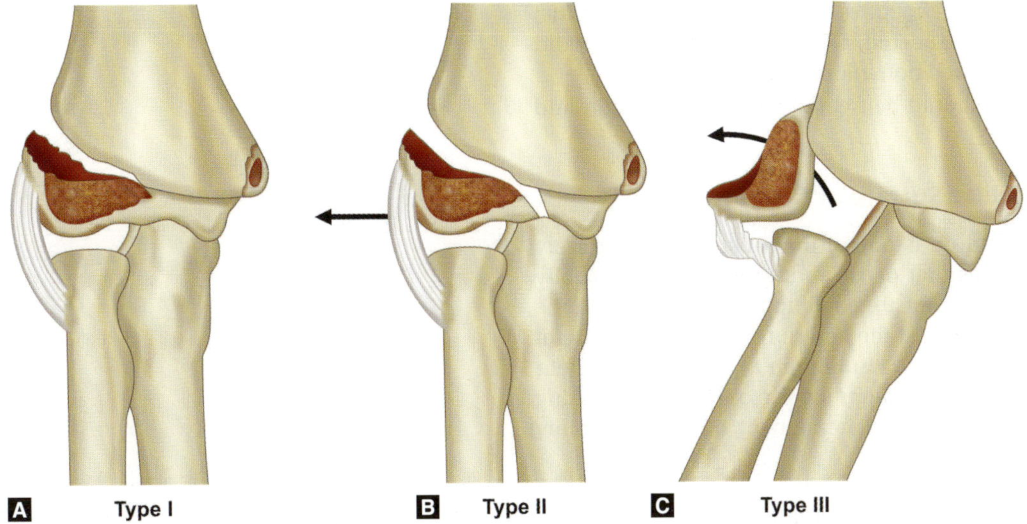

Figs. 66A to C: Radiographic criteria of determining fracture stability.

Complications

Improper reduction in failure of fixation may result in cubitus valgus and tardy ulnar palsy in lateral condyle fractures.

Medial condyle fractures:

- Post-traumatic arthritis, especially in fractures involving the trochlea groove.
- Ulnar nerve symptoms with excess callus formation in malunion.
- Cubitus varus.

After treatment:

- Usually fixation is sufficiently rigid to permit early active motion.
- After treatment is similar to that described for intercondylar fractures, but usually rehabilitation advances at a more rapid pace.

Medial Condyle Fractures

Fractures of the medial humeral condyle in adults and children are among the least common injuries of the elbow. Diagnosis of a medial condylar fracture can be difficult because the trochlea ossifies much later than the capitulum and does not become completely ossified until about age of 9 years. Oblique radiographic views, arthrography, or MRI may be helpful in establishing the diagnosis and angle of displacement.

Classification

Kilfoyle described three types:

1. *Type I*: A greenstick or impacted fracture.
2. *Type II*: A fracture through the humeral condyle into the joint with little or no displacement.
3. *Type III*: It is an epiphyseal fracture (intra-articular) and involves the medial condyle with the fragment displaced and rotated.

Treatment

- Type I and undisplaced type II fractures can be treated by observation and posterior splinting with elbow in 90° flexion.

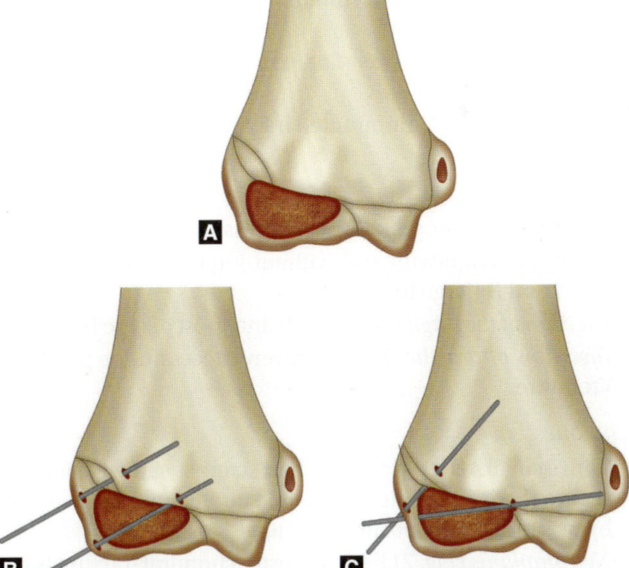

Figs. 67A to C: Stability of internal fixation.

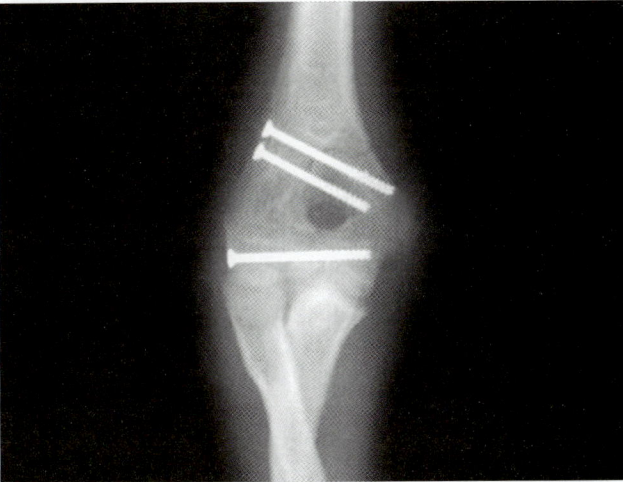
Fig. 68: X-ray showing securing of fractured condyle to uninvolved condyle with lag screws.

- Displacement of type II fractures can be difficult to determine; if displacement is suspected, ORIF is appropriate to avoid growth disturbance and nonunion.
- Type III fractures should be treated by open reduction and internal fixation.

Fractures of Articular Surface of Distal Humerus

Fracture of the capitulum is one of the most common purely intra-articular fractures that occur about the elbow. It usually is caused by a fall on the outstretched upper extremity with the radial head impacting against the anterior portion of the lateral humeral condyle (capitulum), resulting in a varying sized shear fracture. Fractures of the capitulum involve only the articulating surface, producing an intra-articular fragment, but elbow stability is maintained.

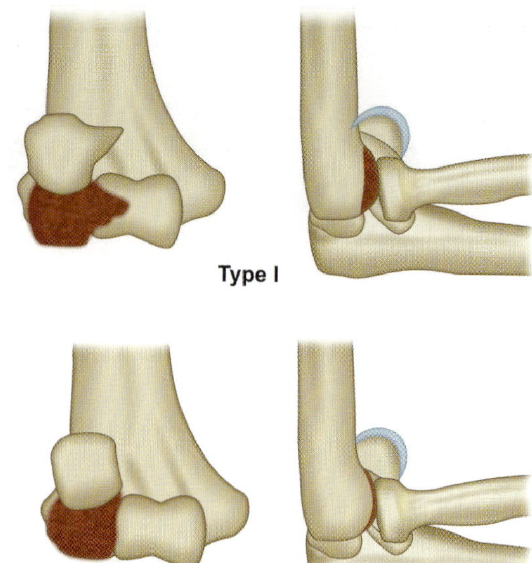

Fig. 69: Type I and type II capitulum fractures.

Classification of Fractures of the Capitulum

Classification depends on the size of the articular fragment and its comminution; this is shown in Figure 69.

- *Type I fracture (Hahn-Steinthal):* A large fragment of bone and articular cartilage.
- *Type II fracture (Kocher-Lorenz):* A small shell of bone and articular cartilage.
- *Type III fracture:* Comminuted fracture.

Treatment

- Closed reduction, usually not successful
- Open reduction with and without internal fixation, done for type I and II (large fragment)
- *Excision of the fragments*: Type II and most of type III fractures.
- *Insertion of prosthesis*: Not proven successful or practical in literature.

Technique:

- With a small AO lag screw/Herbert screw as shown in Figure 70, secure the fragment in place and countersink the screw head by overdrilling the posterior cortex.
- *New implants (Fig. 71)*: A small osteochondral fracture is being fixed with absorbable screws.

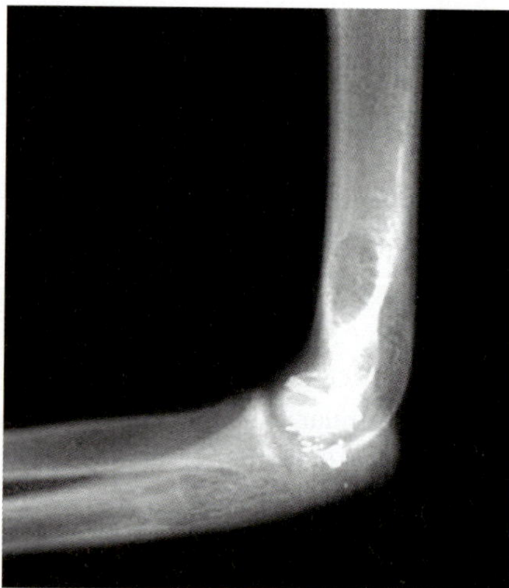

Fig. 70: Osteochondral fracture, fixed by absorbable screws.

Outcomes: Outcomes are based on pain and function. Flexion is the first to return usually, within the first 2 months. Extension usually takes 4–6 months to return. Supination/pronation is usually unaffected.

Complications

Painful retained implant is the most common complaint. Common locations are olecranon and medial implant. Implant removal is done after fracture union. One plate at a time in bicolumnar fractures. Removal of both plates with a single surgery is a fracture risk.

Ulnar nerve palsy:
It can be due to:

- Operative manipulation
- Hardware prominence
- *Inadequate release:* Prevention is the best treatment.

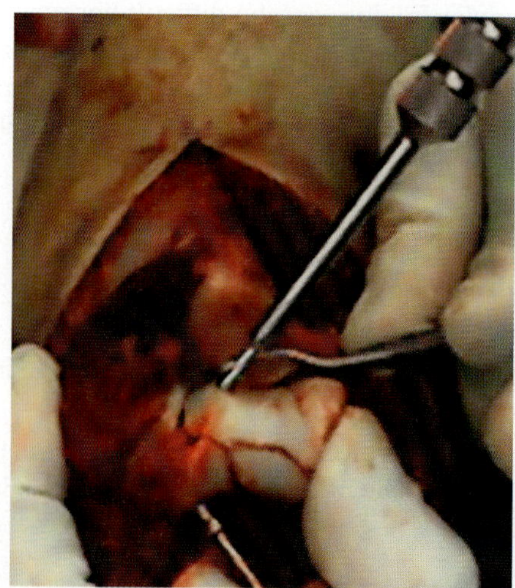

Fig. 71: Osteochondral fracture fixation with screws.

Heterotopic ossification:

- It occurs in up to 50% of cases after treatment of distal humerus fractures.
- *Hastings and Graham functional classification system:*
  - *Class I:* These fractures are associated with no functional limitations.
  - *Class II:* These can further be classified into following types:
    - *IIA:* Functional limitation of flexion and extension
    - *IIB:* Functional limitation of supination and pronation.
- *Class III*: These fractures are associated with ankylosis that eliminates elbow range of motion (ROM).

Preventive measures:

- Early operative treatment (24–48 hours)
- Nonsteroidal anti-inflammatory drugs (NSAIDs)
- Low-dose radiation therapy
- Continuous passive ROM exercises.

Treatment:

- *Indomethacin*: Recommended dose is 75 mg orally BD for 3 weeks.
- Low-dose radiation therapy, single doses of 600–700 cGy. The timing of the irradiation (preoperative vs postoperative) does not seem to affect operative outcomes.

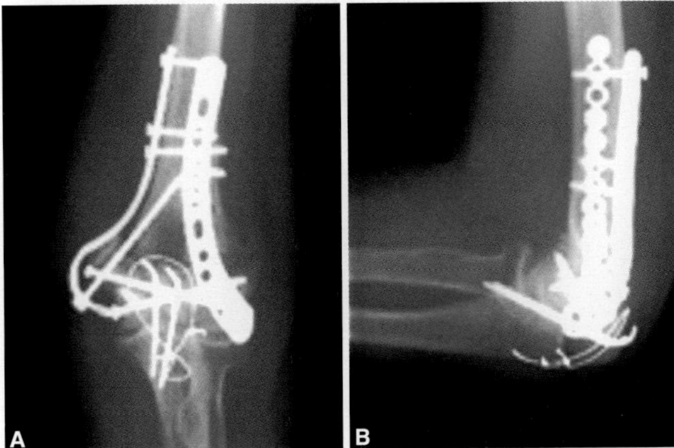

Figs. 72A and B: Bone graft with revision plating.

- Operative excision of heterotopic ossification is recommended 12 months after the injury.

Failure of fixation:

- Associated with stability of operative fixation
- K-wires fixation alone is inadequate
- If diagnosed early, revision fixation indicated
- Late fixation failure must be tailored to radiographic healing and patient symptoms.

Nonunion of distal humerus:

Nonunion of distal humerus is uncommon and is usually a failure of fixation. Symptomatic treatment is required. A bone graft with revision plating is generally used to correct it as shown in the Figures 72A and B.

Nonunion of olecranon osteotomy:

- Rates as high as 5% or more
- Treated with bone graft and revision tension band technique
- Excision of proximal fragment is salvage
- 50% of olecranon must remain for joint stability.

Infection:

Highest for open fractures, no style of fixation has a higher rate than any other.

Lateral Epicondyle and Capitulum Fracture (Figs. 73 to 75)

Lateral approach (Figs. 74A and B)

- *Capitulum*: Posterior-to-anterior lag screws.
- *Epicondyle:* Screw and buttress plate healed.

Tension band screw and ORIF for medial column fracture are shown in Figures 75A and B.

Distal, Two Column Fracture (Figs. 76 to 79)

Prognosis: Healed lacks 20° flexion and extension. Osteotomy healed without complications.

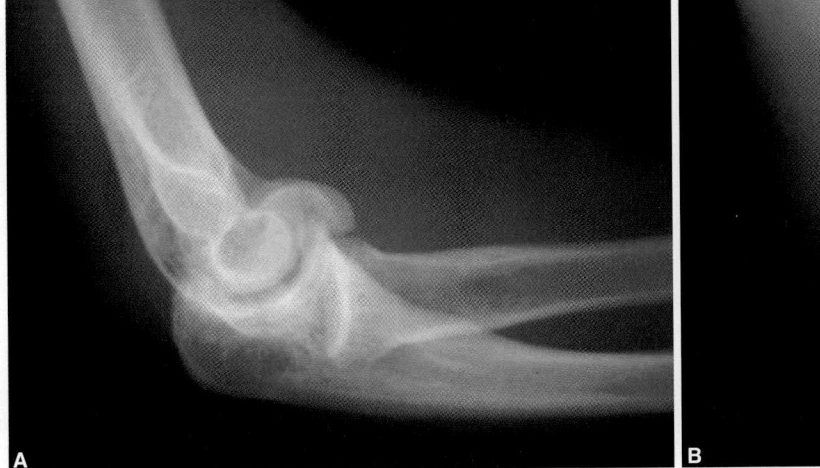

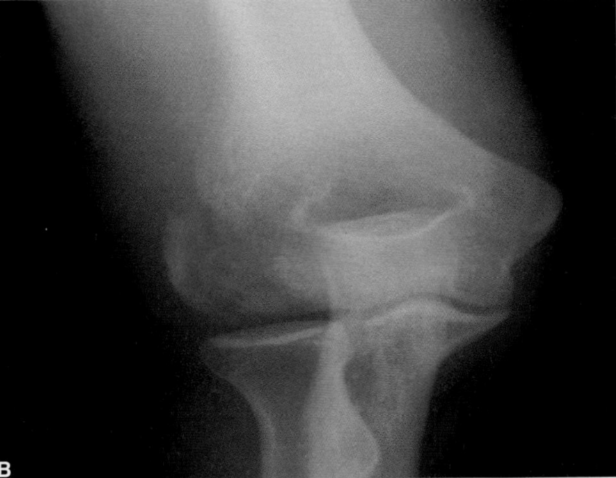

Figs. 73A and B: Lateral epicondyle and capitulum fracture: (A) Lateral view; (B) Anteroposterior view.

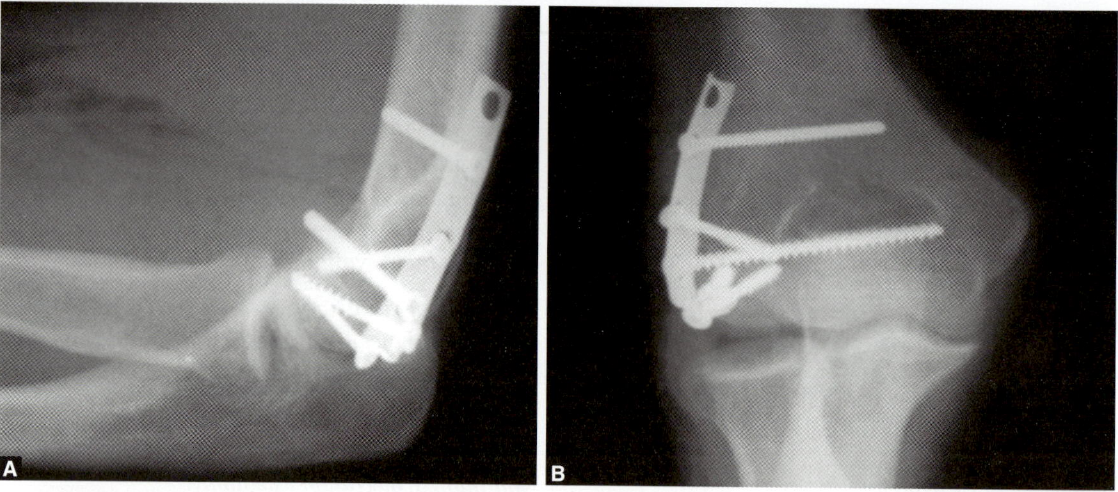

Figs. 74A and B: Lateral approach for treating lateral epicondyle and capitulum fracture: (A) Lateral view; (B) Anteroposterior view.

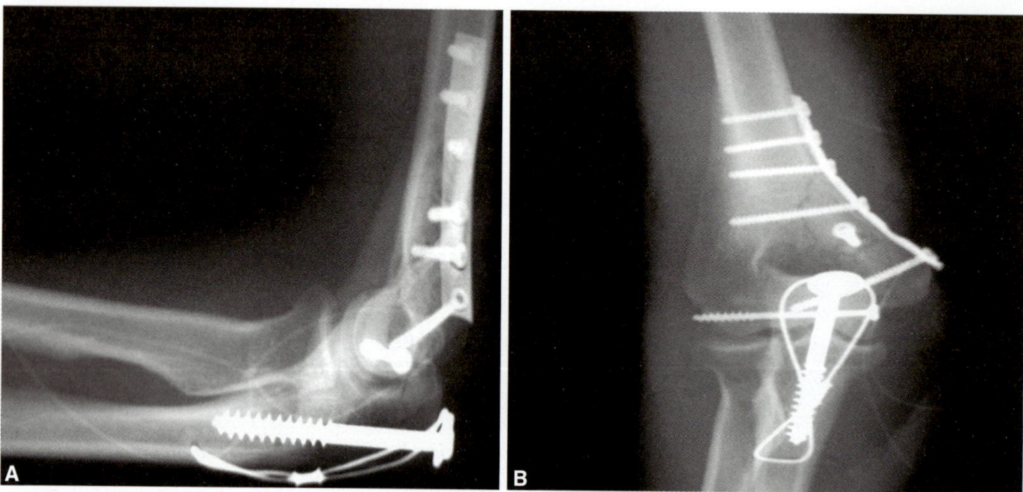

Figs. 75A and B: Tension band screw and open reduction internal fixation (ORIF) medial column fracture: (A) Lateral view; (B) Anteroposterior view.

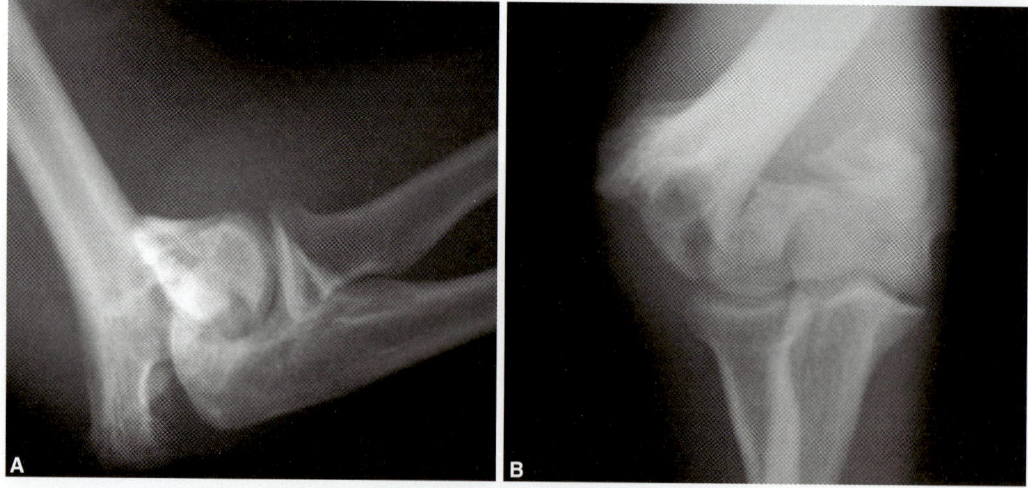

Figs. 76A and B: Distal, two column fracture.

Radial Head Fractures (Figs. 80A and B)

Mode and Mechanism of Injury (Fig. 81)

The radial head fracture, when it collides with the capitulum. This can occur with a pure axial load (Essex-Lopresti injury), a valgus load with a posterolateral rotatory (elbow dislocation) type of load or as the radial head dislocates posteriorly as part of a posterior Monteggia fracture or posterior olecranon fracture-dislocation.

Signs and Symptoms

- It is painful because the elbow joint is usually distended with blood.

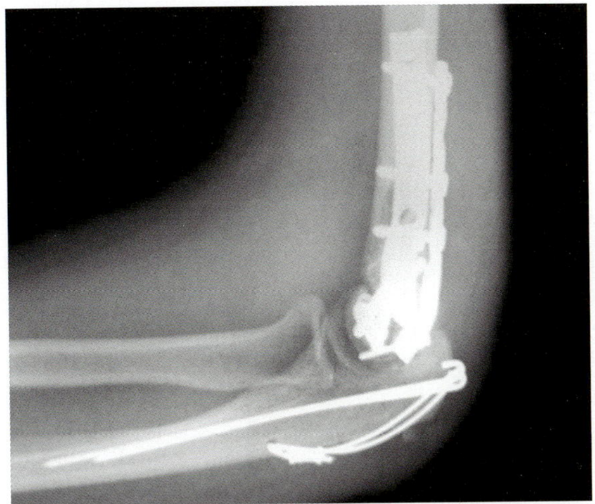

Fig. 77: Transverse intra-articular approach.

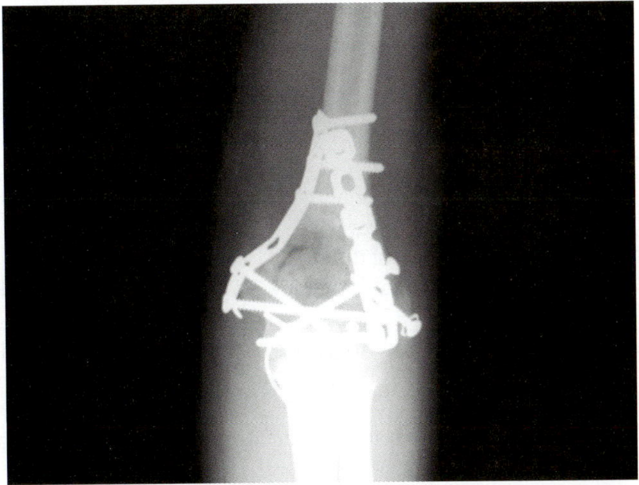

Fig. 78: Lag screw and bicolumn plating.

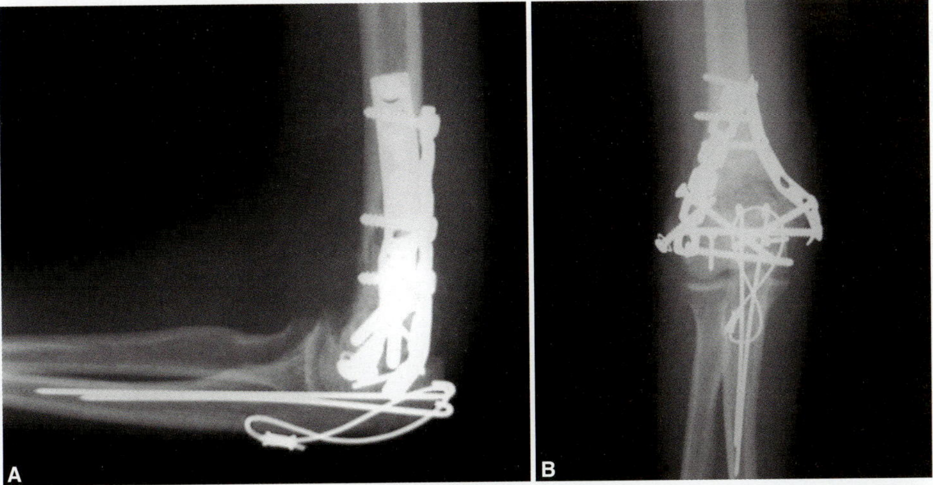

Figs. 79A and B: Tension band wire with cable: (A) Lateral view; (B) Anteroposterior view.

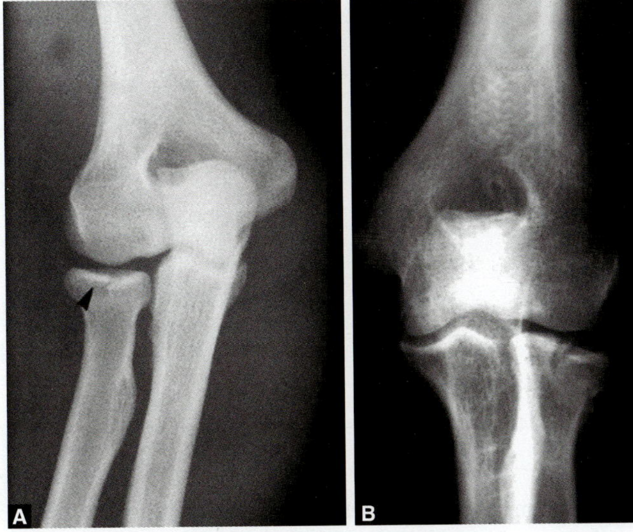

Figs. 80A and B: Radial head fracture.

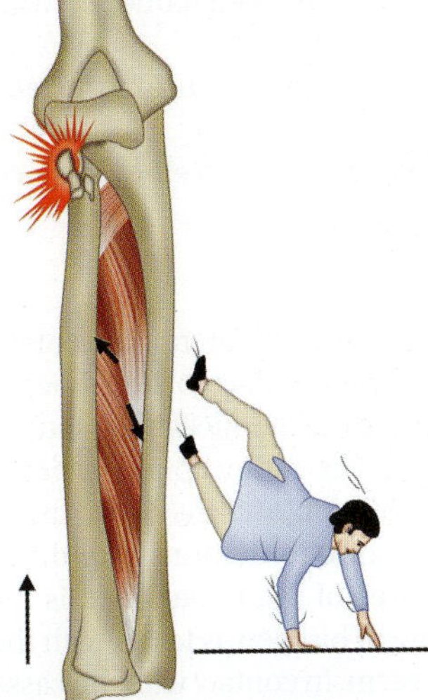

Fig. 81: Mechanism of radial head injury due to collision of radial head with capitulum.

- Variable amount of swelling and ecchymosis, which may correspond with the degree of associated ligament injury.
- There is often crepitation of the radial head with forearm rotation and occasionally a fracture fragment will block forearm rotation.

Associated Injuries

- Fracture of the radial head associated with rupture of the medial collateral ligament (MCL).
- Concomitant fracture of the radial head and capitulum.
- Posterior dislocation of the elbow with fracture of the radial head.
- Posterior dislocation of the elbow with fracture of the radial head and the coronoid process (the so-called terrible triad of the elbow).
- Posterior Monteggia fractures, including posterior olecranon fracture-dislocations.
- Essex-Lopresti lesions and variants.

Classification

- In 1924, speed proposed a classification based on the amount of radial head involvement, marginal or complete, and the degree of displacement.
- In 1954, Mason further subdivided the classification into three groups:
  1. *Type I*: Small or marginal fractures with minimal displacement.
  2. *Type II:* Marginal fractures with displacement.
  3. *Type III*: Comminuted fractures.

Modified Mason's classification:

- *Type I (Fig. 82)*:
  - Nondisplaced or minimally displaced fracture of head or neck.
  - Forearm rotation (pronation/supination) is limited only by acute pain and swelling.
  - Intra-articular displacement of the fracture is less than 2 mm.
- *Type II (Fig. 83):*
  - Displaced fracture of the head or neck.
  - Motion may be mechanically limited with or without significant joint incongruity.
  - It can be repaired by open reduction with internal fixation.
- *Type III (Fig. 84):*
  - Severely comminuted fracture of the radial head and neck.
- *Type IV:*
  - Comminuted fracture with elbow dislocation.

Radiographic Examination

Plain films:

X-rays in the anteroposterior, lateral, and oblique planes of the elbow are usually sufficient to diagnose the fracture. However, if a fat pad sign is present without a noticeable fracture, a radiocapitellar view may be helpful. The radiocapitellar view is taken with the forearm in neutral rotation and the X-ray tube angles cephalad. An alternative technique to demonstrate difficult minimally or nondisplaced fractures of the radial head is the modified radial head capitellum view. This view is taken with the posterior aspect of the supinated forearm, in contact with the cassette and the elbow slightly flexed. The beam is directed 45° mediolateral.

CT scan:

CT scans of the radial head in axial, sagittal, and coronal cuts can be quite helpful in estimating the fracture size, degree of fragmentation, and displacement. For fractures under consideration for ORIF, a CT scan often provides better visualization. The use of the CT scan has also dissuaded us from operating because the displacement was less than expected from the plain X-rays. Reconstructed images may also be helpful. 3D reconstruction CT is shown in Figure 85.

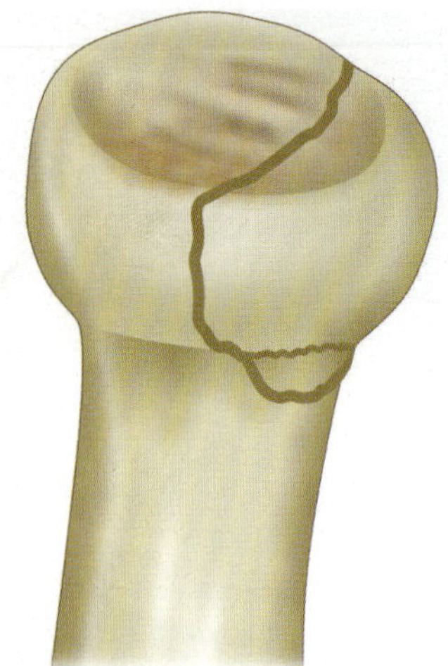

Fig. 82: Modified Mason's type I fracture of radial head.

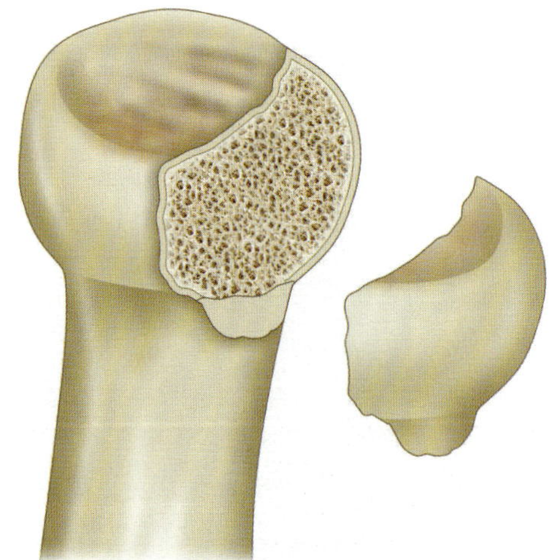

Fig. 83: Modified Mason's type II fracture of radial head.

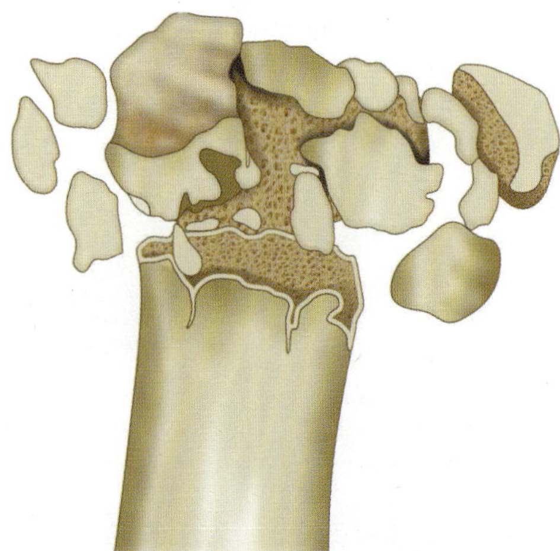

Fig. 84: Modified Mason's type III fracture of radial head.

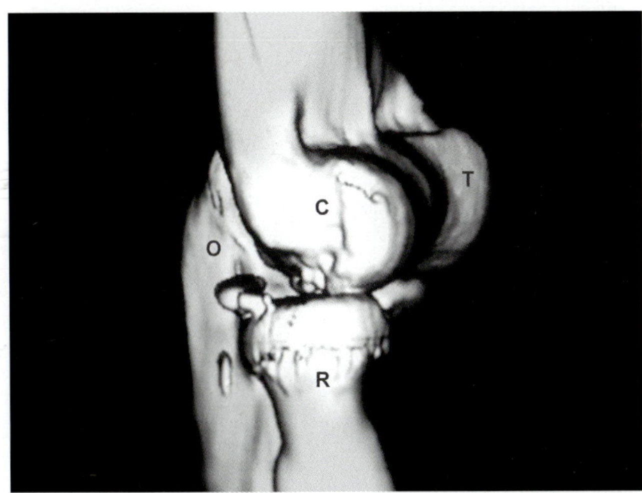

Fig. 85: Radial head comminuted fracture.
(R: radius; C: capitulum; T: trochlea; O: olecranon)

Factors Influencing Choice of Treatment

Depends on high- or low-demand elbow:

An ideal high-demand patient is typically considered young and athletically active, as compared to a low-demand patient, who would be elderly and less likely to stress the elbow physically. For low-demand patients excision without prosthetic replacement is often well tolerated. If replacement is needed in the low-demand elbow, to obtain acute instability, there is less likely to be a problem of long-term wear.

In the younger, high-demand patient, metallic radial head replacement poses more potential for long-term failure. In considering radial head arthroplasty, the patient must be counseled carefully about the risks of loosening the radiocapitellar wear and ultimate removal.

Treatment Modalities

Type I:

Relief of pain can be provided by aspirating the hematoma and injecting a local anesthetic into the joint, thus aiding in the initial physical examination. The patient is given a sling or the arm can be splinted, but for no longer than 3–4 days. Active forearm rotation is started as soon as tolerated.

Type II:

- *Without mechanical block:* Type II fractures that have no mechanical block, crepitus and incongruity of less than 2 mm can be treated similarly to type I. Close follow-up is required and X-rays should be taken at 1, 2, 4, and 6 weeks, as displacement can occur.
- *With mechanical block*: The decision to be made in this situation is ORIF versus excision. As there is no evidence of associated interosseous injury, radial head arthroplasty is not a consideration. Patient selection is crucial.
- *With associated injury:* Associated injury can be interosseous ligament tear. In that case, preservation of the radial head (or radial head function with a prosthesis) is crucial in this setting. Excision of the radial head may lead to symptomatic proximal migration of the radius.
- *Elbow dislocation (with or without coronoid fracture)*: In most instances, the combination of elbow dislocation and radial head fracture does not result in gross instability or recurrent dislocation. If radial head fracture displacement requires open treatment, it is preferable to preserve the radial head, if technically possible.

Type III (unrepairable):

Fractures of the radial head and neck with extensive comminution and displacement, but without concomitant elbow dislocation or longitudinal dissociations, should undergo early excision as the treatment of choice. These patients do not require radial head replacement. They should begin early active motion.

- *With associated injury:* With interosseous ligament tear, the fractured native radial head must be excised to permit early motion, and a metallic radial head must be implanted to stabilize the forearm.

Open Reduction and Internal Fixation

There are three major technical challenges:

1. Reassembling the fractured radial head
2. Securing the fractured radial head to the radial neck
3. Ensuring that the implants do not interfere with pronation and supination.

The radial head should be approached laterally, just anterior to the anconeus. The structure at risk is the posterior interosseous nerve. Once the fracture is thoroughly exposed, the pieces should be repositioned to reconstruct the radial head, small Kirschner wires can be used to temporarily hold the fracture.

Safe Zones for ORIF (Figs. 86A to C)

Based on anatomic dissections, there is a safe zone of hardware placement, comprising approximately 90°, and centered about the equator in the neutral position. If this zone is used, normal headed screws and plates can be placed without fear of impinging in the proximal radioulnar joint. If the fracture is limited to the radial head, without extension to the radial neck, the Herbert screw can be used and placed below the chondral surface. Absorbable pins have also been used.

Screw Fixation

Figure 87 shows screw fixation.

Plate Fixation

Figure 88 represents plate fixation.

Prosthetic replacement:

A metal prosthesis is inserted, when there is elbow or forearm instability in most young and active patients.

Excision:

The fragments are excised and the neck is smoothed off. In the setting of an olecranon fracture-dislocation or posterior Monteggia injury, it may be useful to seal the end of the radius with bone wax. The lateral collateral ligament (LCL) complex should be repaired, if injured. There are various designs of prosthesis available—vitallium, silastic, metallic, bipolar.

Complications:

- Laceration or permanent injury to the posterior interosseous nerve during open reduction and internal fixation of a radial head fracture
- Infection
- Malunion
- Nonunion (rare)
- Pain
- Pronation—supination restriction.

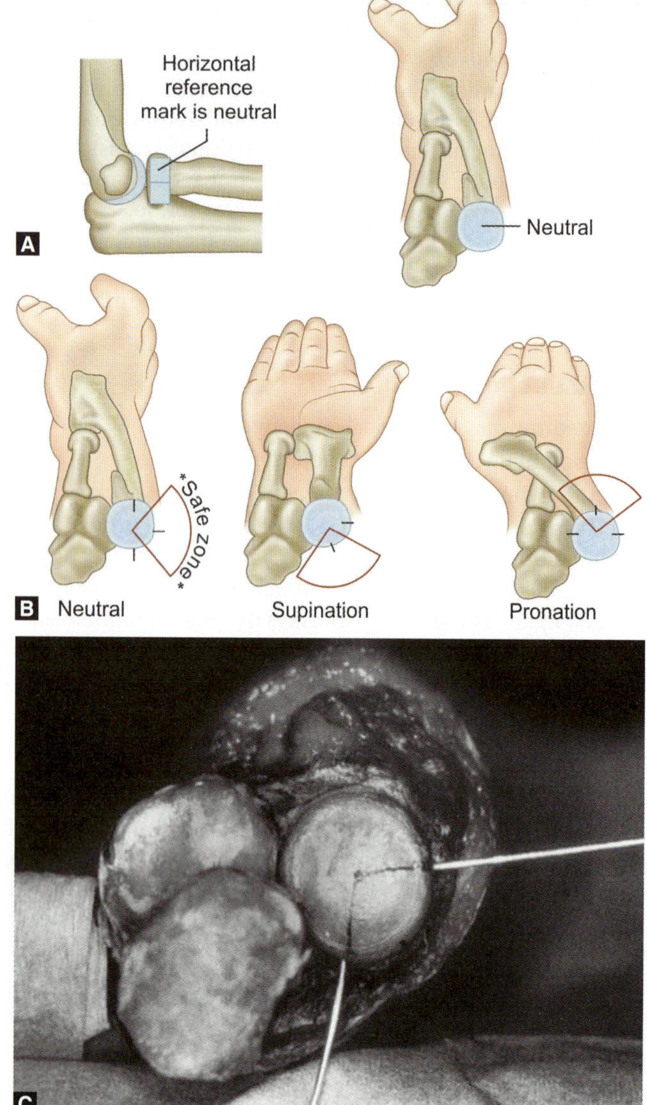

Figs. 86A to C: Safe zones for open reduction internal fixation (ORIF), approximately 90° centered about the equator in the neutral position.

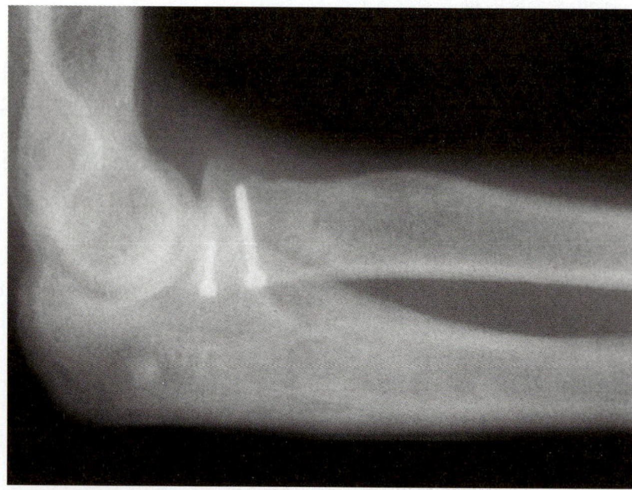

Fig. 87: Correcting radial head fracture by screw fixation.

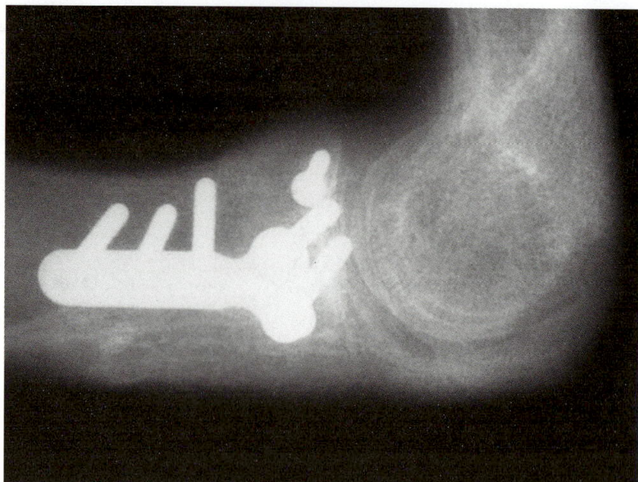

Fig. 88: Plate fixation for fixing radial head fracture.

Olecranon Fractures (Figs. 89A and B)

Fractures of the olecranon can be caused either by direct trauma, such as falling on the tip of the elbow, or by indirect trauma, such as falling on a partially flexed elbow, with indirect forces generated by the triceps muscle avulsing the olecranon.

Clinical Features

- Swelling due to hemorrhagic effusion of the elbow joint
- Pain on movement
- Tenderness
- Palpable defect may be noted at the fracture site
- Inability to extend the elbow actively against gravity.

Radiological Studies (Figs. 90A and B)

Classification:

- *Mayo classification (Fig. 91)*: It distinguishes three factors that have an influence on treatment. These are:
  1. Fracture displacement
  2. Comminution
  3. Ulnohumoral stability.
  - *Type I:* Nondisplaced or minimally displaced:
    - Noncomminuted (type IA)
    - Comminuted (type IB)
  - *Type II:* Fractures have displacement of proximal fragment, without elbow instability.
    - Noncomminuted (type IIA)
    - Comminuted (type IIB)
  - *Type III:* Fractures feature instability of ulnohumoral joint and require surgical treatment.
- *Colton classification:*
  - *Type I (nondisplaced):*
    - Less than 2 mm of displacement
    - No increase in displacement with flexion of 90°
    - Patient able to extend their arm against gravity.
  - *Type II (Displaced):*
    - Type IIA = Avulsion
    - Type IIB = Oblique and transverse
    - Type IIC = Comminuted
    - Type IID = Fracture-dislocation

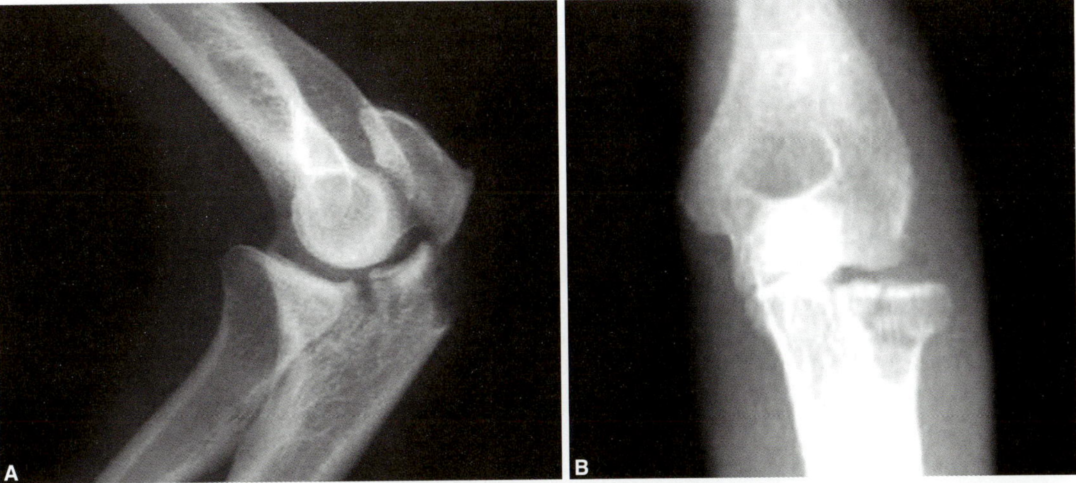

Figs. 89A and B: X-rays showing olecranon fracture.

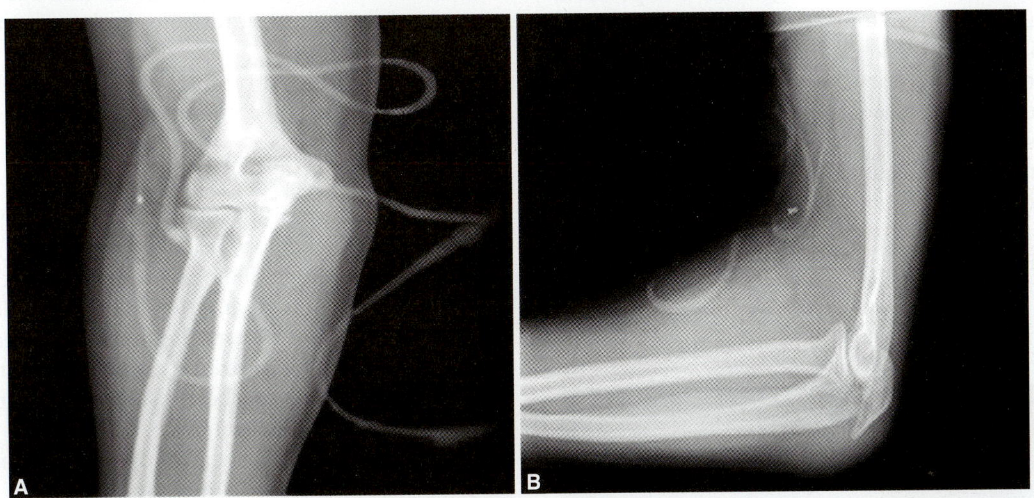

Figs. 90A and B: X-rays showing olecranon fractures: (A) Anteroposterior view (B) Lateral view.

- *Fractures were classified by Schatzker, based on fracture pattern and mechanical considerations, as to the type of internal fixation required for repair:*
  - Transverse
  - Transverse impacted
  - Oblique
  - Comminuted
  - Oblique distal
  - Fracture dislocation.

Operative Treatment

The methods of operative treatment commonly used are:

- Open reduction and fixation with a figure-of-eight wire loop
- Medullary fixation
- A combination of intramedullary pin or screw and tension bands
- Contoured plate and screws
- Excision of the proximal fragment.

Open reduction and internal fixation and excision of the olecranon fragments have their advocates. Advocates of ORIF claim that this method provides an anatomical reduction of the bony fragment and a congruous articular surface, rigid fixation allows for an early range of motion, elbow stability is preserved, and the extensor power of the triceps muscle is maintained.

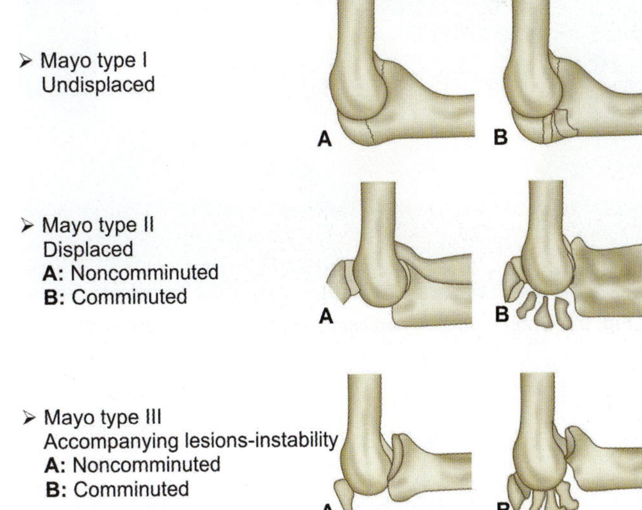

Fig. 91: Mayo classification of olecranon fracture.

Open reduction and fixation with figure-of-eight wire loop (Fig. 92): Open reduction and fixation with figure-of-eight wire loop is applicable to fractures of the olecranon that are not comminuted and that are well proximal to the coronoid process. This fixation is used most commonly for avulsion and transverse fractures, but may be combined with intramedullary fixation in comminuted fractures and fracture-dislocations.

Intramedullary fixation:
Displaced olecranon fractures fixed with intramedullary Kirschner wires and tension band wiring or long intramedullary cancellous screw fixation combined with a figure-of-eight wire.

Plate fixation:
If comminution with bone loss prevents use of a tension band compression technique because of the possibility of shortening of the olecranon, hand-contoured plates and screws provide rigid fixation, applied most easily on the posterior surface, and unicortical screws are used near the articular surface.

Excision of proximal fragment:
Excision of a proximal fragment has several advantages. First, the possibility of nonunion is eliminated and only the triceps tendon must become anchored to the distal fragment. The possibility of traumatic arthritis resulting from irregularity of the articular surface is minimized. This method can be used only if enough of the olecranon is left to form a stable base for the trochlear excision of olecranon fragments, we consider it the method of choice in the following circumstances:

- In severely comminuted fractures, in which open reduction and internal fixation are not technically possible.
- In nonarticular fractures
- After failed ORIF
- In nonunions

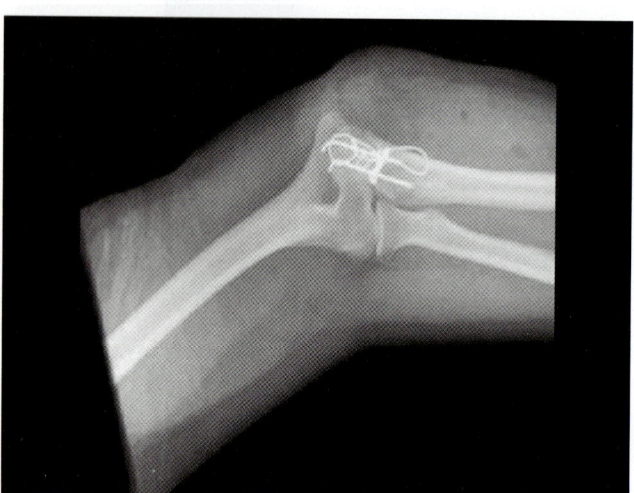

Fig. 92: Open reduction and fixation with figure-of-eight wire loop.

- In type III open fractures, or if local soft-tissue conditions are precarious and the subcutaneous location of the internal fixation devices might present a problem.

Fractures of the Coronoid Process (Figs. 93A to C)

Classification by Regan and Morrey

- *Type I*: A small chip fracture
- *Type II*: A fracture involving less than 50% of the process
- *Type III*: A fracture involving more than 50% of the process.

Type III and some Type II fractures render the elbow extremely unstable, especially if there is an associated fracture of the radial head.

Treatment

- Type I and Type II coronoid fractures are fixed with heavy suture woven into the brachialis and coronoid insertions, passed through two drill holes in the proximal ulna, and tied securely.
- Type III coronoid fractures are fixed with a screw, using interfragmentary techniques or a coronoid plate.

Olecranon Fracture-dislocations

Olecranon fracture-dislocations are complex injuries, involving a fracture of the olecranon (usually comminuted) and subluxation or dislocation of the radial head or the coronoid process or both. The dislocation is in an anterior or posterior direction (anterior fracture-dislocations disrupt the humeral-olecranon articulation and usually leave the proximal radioulnar joint intact. Posterior fracture-dislocations can be considered variants of Bado type II Monteggia fracture-dislocations.

Fractures of the radial head and coronoid process are common in olecranon fracture-dislocations and need to be treated, if they compromise elbow stability, when the olecranon fracture is repaired. Repair of the lateral collateral or medial collateral ligament or both also may be necessary, if residual instability is present.

Monteggia in Adults (Fig. 94)

Monteggia is fractures of the proximal third of the ulna with dislocation of the radial head. The combination of injuries known as a Monteggia fracture–dislocation is an often treacherous condition to treat. This combination of fracture of the ulna with dislocation of the proximal end of the radius, with or without fracture of the radius, usually can be treated conservatively in children, but routinely requires open reduction in adults.

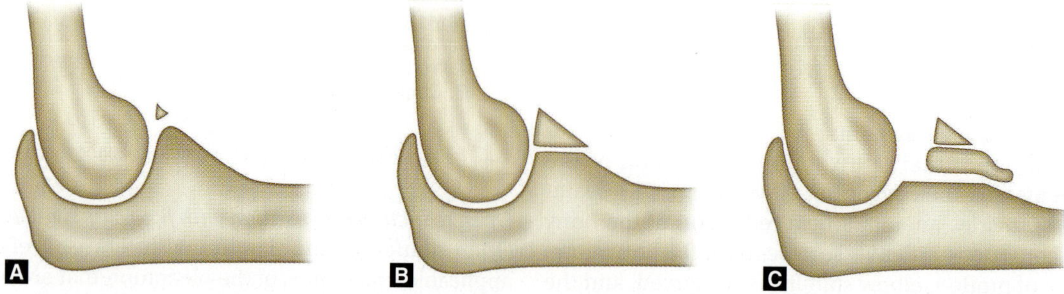

Figs. 93A to C: Fracture of coronoid fracture: (A) Type I fracture; (B) Type II fracture; and (C) Type III fracture.

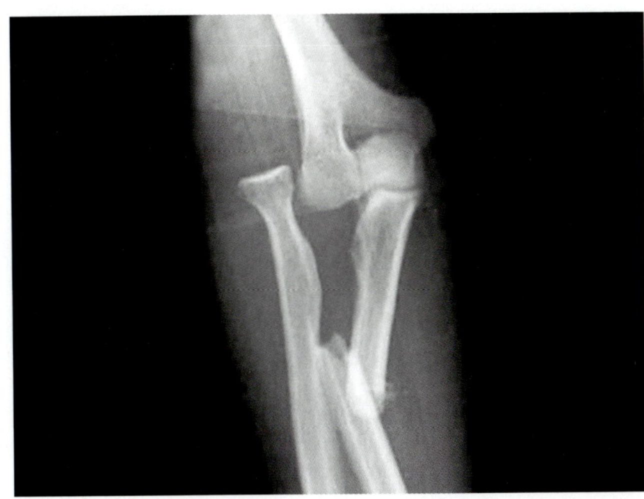

Fig. 94: Monteggia fracture dislocation.

Classification

Bado suggested classification of Monteggia fracture-dislocation into four types:

1. *Type 1*: Fracture of the middle or proximal third of the ulna with anterior dislocation of the radial head and characteristic apex anterior angulation of the ulna.
2. *Type 2*: Fracture of the middle or proximal third of the ulna (the apex usually is posteriorly angulated) with posterior dislocation of the radial head and often a fracture of the radial head.
3. *Type 3*: Fracture of the ulna, just distal to the coronoid process with lateral dislocation of the radial head.
4. *Type 4*: Fracture of the proximal or middle third of the ulna, anterior dislocation of the radial head and fracture of the proximal third of the radius below the bicipital tuberosity.

Type 1 far exceeds all others in frequency. Several mechanisms of injury probably exist, including direct blows to the ulnar aspect of the forearm and a fall with hyperpronation or hyperextension, with the strong supinating force of the biceps pulling the radial head anteriorly as the fracture of the ulna is produced by the compression forces of the fall.

Most of Type 1 injuries can be treated by rigid fixation of the fracture of the ulna, and closed reduction of the radial head and immobilization of the elbow for 6 weeks in a position of flexion above 90° with the forearm supinated. Nonunions of the ulna, synostosis, and limitation of elbow motion are the factors primarily responsible for poor results, head can be reduced by closed methods, open reduction of the dislocation is not indicated, but the fracture of the ulna is rigidly fixed. In the proximal third of the ulna, where the medullary canal is large, a compression plate is used. In the middle third, where the medullary canal is small, either a compression plate or a triangular intramedullary nail is used.

Fractures in Children

- Extremely common, 15% of all fractures in pediatric patients.
- Most common fractures in children are supracondylar fractures, lateral condyle fractures, medial epicondyle fractures, and transphyseal fractures.
- Evaluation of pediatric patient.
- A gentle approach with parent and child is always best.
- Cubital fossa must be checked for any tenting of skin that would indicate that fracture has punctured the brachialis, which would be difficult for reduction (Figs. 95A and B).

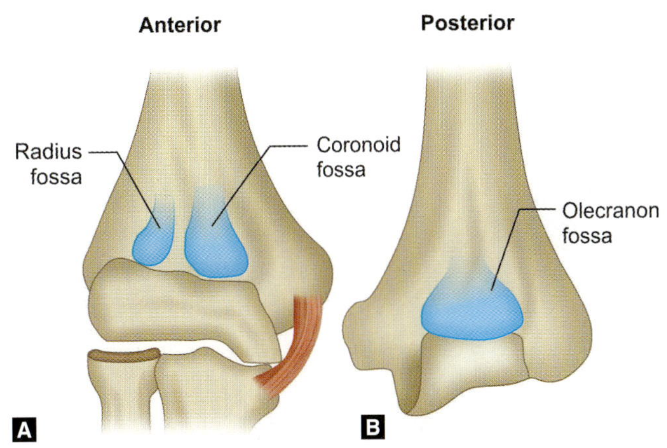

Figs. 95A and B: (A) Anterior view of elbow joint showing radial and coronoid fossa; (B) Posterior view of elbow joint showing olecranon fossa.

- Signs and symptoms of compartment syndrome must be ruled out.
- Finger flexion must be assessed for anterior interosseous nerve palsy.
- If a child has a warm hand with a good capillary refill, a vascular injury is unlikely.

Supracondylar Fractures

It is most common elbow fracture in children. Mechanism of injury is an extension on distal humerus, causing an extension-type fracture. A flexion-type fracture may occur with a direct blow to the elbow with elbow flexed.

Gartland classification for extension type supracondylar humerus fractures:

- *Type 1*: Fracture is a nondisplaced fracture and difficult to detect on X-rays.
- *Type 2*: Fracture has the posterior periosteum intact, connecting the distal fragment and humeral shaft.
- *Type 3*: Fracture has a complete displacement of distal fragment relative to humeral shaft with fractures of both cortices.

Treatment

- Type 1 fracture should be splinted with a long arm posterior splint or cast in neutral rotation and in 90° of elbow flexion.
- Preferred treatment of Type 2 and Type 3 is closed reduction and percutaneous pinning.

Complications

- Early complications are attributable to neurovascular compromise.
- Compartment syndrome
- Volkmann's ischemic contracture
- Malunion, usually cubitus varus due to rotational malrotation
- Stiffness is rare.

Radial Head and Neck Fractures

Children with radial neck fractures usually are 4–14 years old, primarily because ossification of the radial head usually does not begin before 5 years of age. The normal anatomical angulation of the radial neck in children has been erroneously diagnosed as a buckle fracture in this area. Most fractures in children are of the radial neck and not the radial head. Fractures of the epiphysis of the radial head are usually Salter–Harris type IV fractures. Most radial

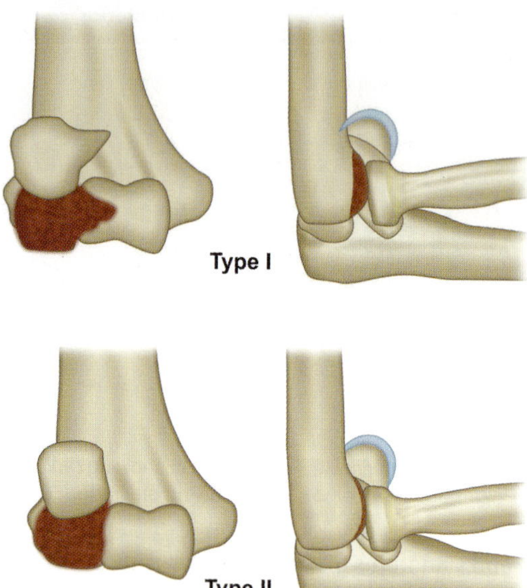

Fig. 96: Types of capitellar fractures.

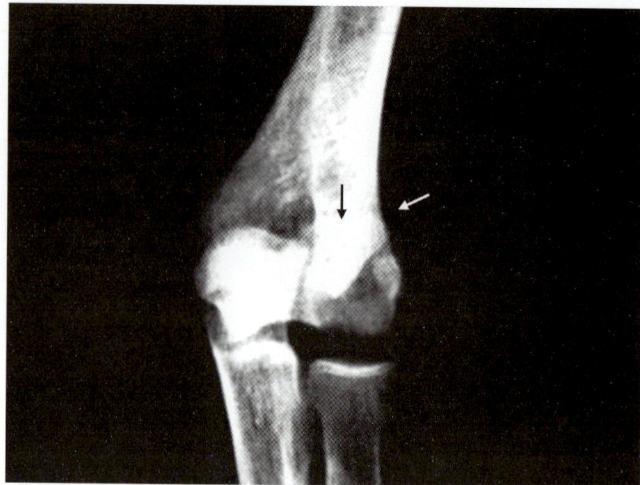

Fig. 97: Double-arch sign.

neck fractures occur through the metaphysis, but they can occur through the physis, with a metaphyseal spike of bone producing a characteristic Salter–Harris type II epiphyseal injury.

- *Type A*: Salter–Harris Type I and II injuries of the proximal radial epiphyses
- *Type B*: Salter–Harris Type IV injuries of the proximal radial epiphysis
- *Type C*: Fractures involving only the proximal radial metaphysis
- *Type D*: Fractures occurring when a dislocated elbow is being reduced
- *Type E*: Fractures occurring in conjunction with the elbow dislocation.

Capitellar Fractures

This fracture was first described in 1853 by Hahn. This fracture has only one portion of lateral column and not epicondyle or metaphysic. It is an uncommon fracture, not many reports are presented. A small series was presented by Johnsson.

Morphology

Basically, it is a terminal intra-articular fracture. It can be due to a fall on hand, either extension or flexion.

Two types (Fig. 96):

1. Hahn–Steinthal (Type I)
2. Kocher–Lorentz (Type II).

- *Hahn–Steinthal:* Injury in extension is more common. A large portion of capitellum with a small piece of trochlea attached.
- *Kocher–Lorentz:* It is articular chip fracture, with small subchondral bone. It may be associated with ulnar collateral injury.

Clinical features:

- X-rays anteroposterior (AP) and lateral views are important
- Restricted elbow movements
- Tenderness
- Loss of rotatory movements
- Fractured chip generally migrates anteriorly and superiorly
- Double arch sign (Fig. 97).

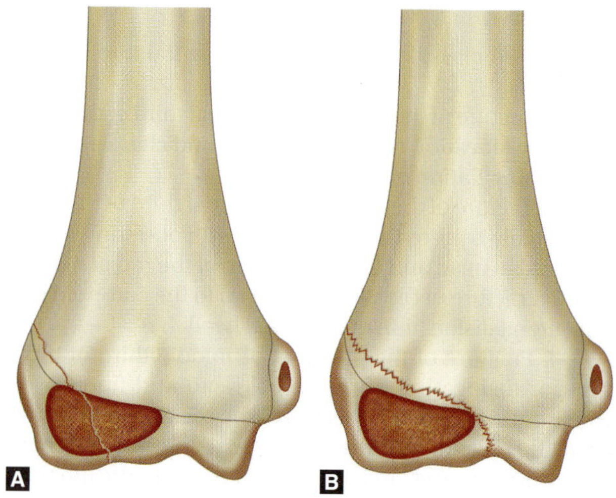

Figs. 98A and B: (A) Milch Type I lateral condylar fracture; and (B) Type II fracture.

Fractures of Lateral Condyle of Humerus

These are most common distal humeral epiphyseal fracture (16–18%). Approximate average age is 6 years.

The pertinent anatomical considerations in lateral condylar fracture include:

- Capitulum, lateral epicondyle, and soft tissue attached to it namely extensors and supinators.
- Difficult to diagnose and have propensity for late displacement.

Mechanism of Injury

- Pull-off or avulsion theory (most common)
- Elbow forced in varus along with extensor
- Muscles and lateral collateral ligaments apply an avulsion force to the lateral condyle (Milch Type II)
- Push-off theory (less common)
- Fall on palm with elbow flexed, the radial head is forced against the capitulum and may cause Milch Type I fracture.

Classification

Milch classification (Figs. 98 and 99):

- Milch Type I lateral trochlear ridge is left intact.
- Milch Type II (more common).

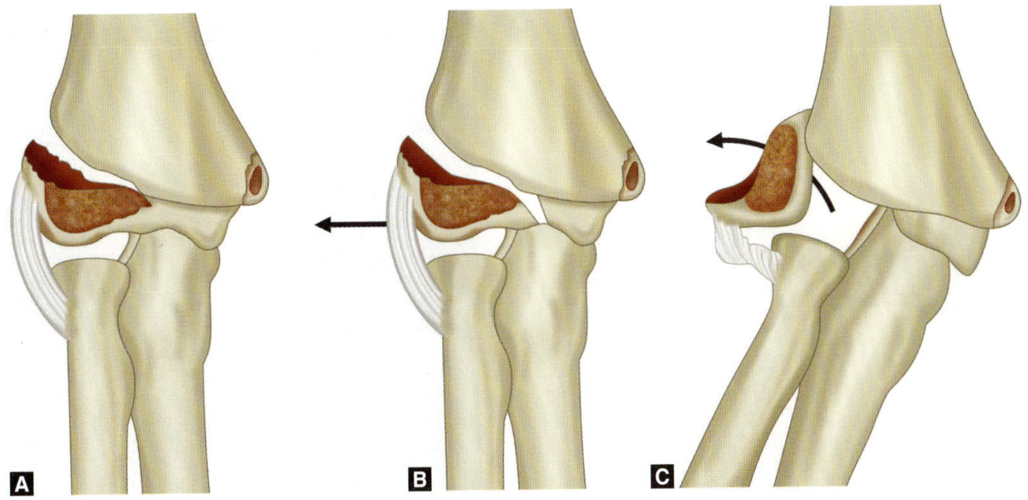

Figs. 99A to C: Different types of lateral condylar fractures.

Anatomical location:
- Salter–Harris Type II (Milch Type II)
- Salter–Harris Type IV (Milch Type I).

Signs and Symptoms

- Distortion of elbow is less due to hematoma
- Location of soft tissue swelling concentrated over lateral aspect of distal humerus
- Undisplaced fractures, produce local tenderness
- *Displaced and rotated fracture*: Some amount of crepitus with the movement of fragment.

Radiography

Finnbogason et al. described roentgenographic criteria for determining fracture stability, which they used in planning and initial treatment.
- *Type A (Fig. 100A)*: Fracture through the lateral humeral condyle with minimal lateral gap—a stable fracture.
- *Type B (Fig. 100B)*: Fracture through the lateral humeral condyle to the epiphyseal cartilage with a lateral gap—a fracture with undefinable risk.
- *Type C (Fig. 100C)*: Fracture through the lateral humeral condyle, as shown in Figures 100A to C with the fracture gap as wide laterally as medially—a fracture with high risk of later displacement.

Magnetic resonance imaging:
- Diagnosis of minimally displaced fracture
- Used to distinguish between this fracture and fracture of entire distal humeral physis.

Arthrogram:
It determines the stability of nonossified articular cartilage of trochlea.

Treatment

Immobilization:
- If fracture is minimally displaced on X-ray (i.e. metaphyseal fragment is less than 2 mm from the proximal fragment on AP and lateral views) and clinically limited soft-tissue integrity.
- Above elbow (A/E) posterior splint with elbow in 90° and forearm in neutral rotation.
- Check X-ray, 3–5 days without splint and elbow in extension and taken again after 3–5 days.

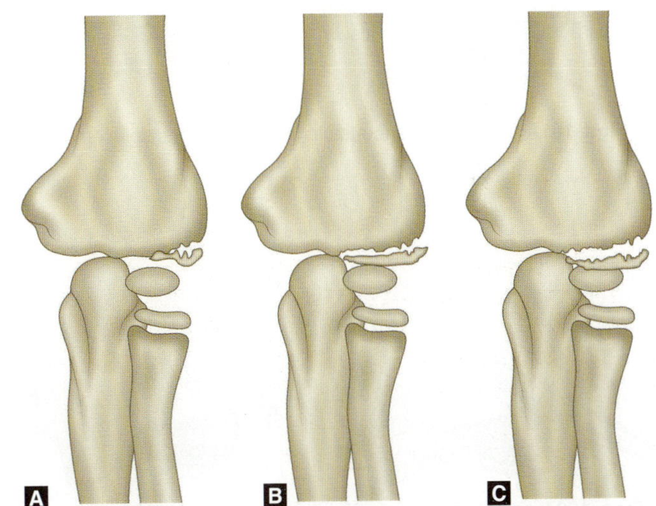

Figs. 100A to C: Roentgenographic criteria for determining fracture stability. (A) Type A stable fracture with minimal lateral gap; (B) Type B fracture through the lateral humeral condyle to the epiphyseal cartilage with a lateral gap; (C) Unstable type C fracture.

- If no displacement A/E cast for at least 3 weeks or until fracture union is apparent.

Percutaneous pinning:
- Stage II displacement (2–4 mm), with varus stress views under anesthesia by arthrography, as shown in Figures 101A to C.
- If fracture is stable then percutaneous pinning is indicated.

Open reduction internal fixation:
- All fracture with stage III displacement
- *Approach:* Kocher's lateral "J"
- *Fixation*: Suture fixation, which is inadequate
- Smooth pin fixation, preferably with two pins, either through the epiphysis or through the metaphyseal spike, as shown in Figures 102A and B.
- Screw fixation, preferably through the metaphyseal area.

Complications

Biological problems:
- Lateral spur formation
- Cubitus varus
- Cubitus valgus (Fig. 103).

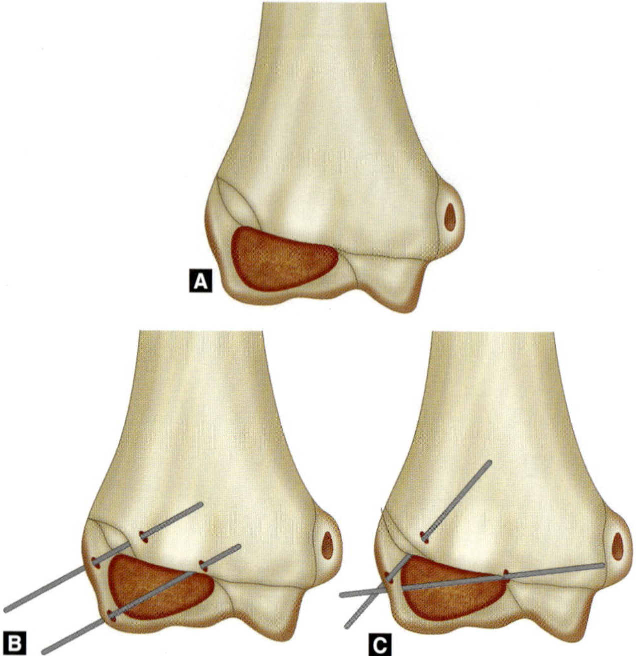

Figs. 101A to C: Percutaneous pinning of stage II displacement.

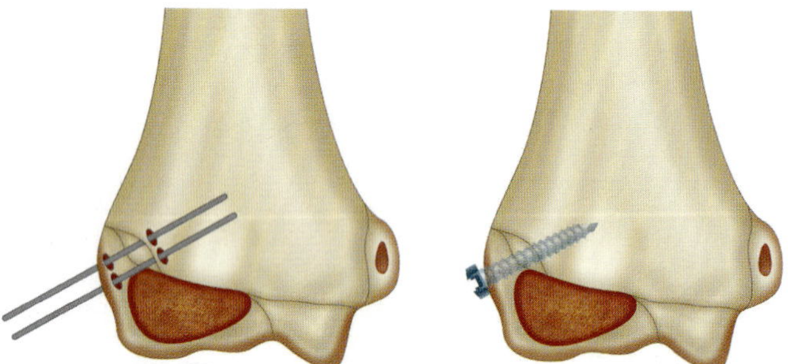
Figs. 102A and B: Open reduction internal fixation. (A) Pin fixation; (B) Screw fixation.

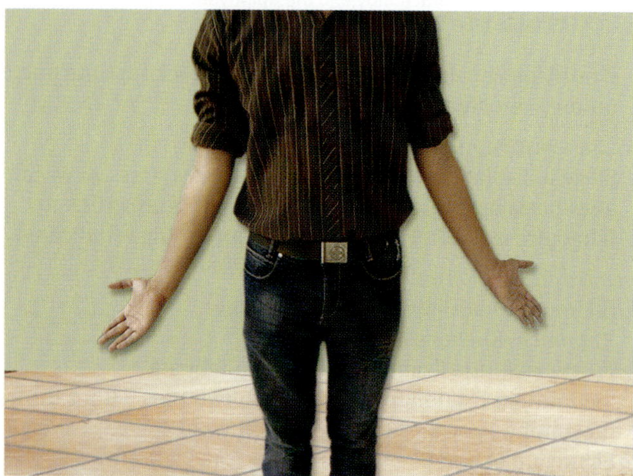
Fig. 103: Cubitus valgus.

Technical problems (Fig. 104):
- Nonunion/delayed union
- Fishtail deformity
- Tardy ulnar nerve palsy

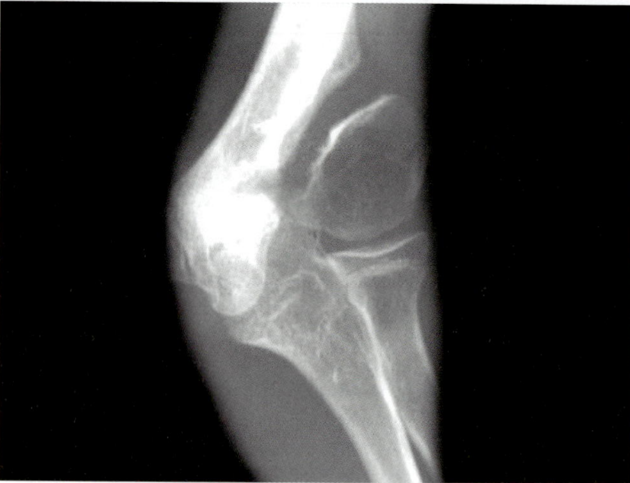
Fig. 104: Nonunion of lateral condylar fracture.

- Myositis ossificans
- Osteonecrosis of condylar fragment.

Nonunion: Flynn et al. criteria, if fracture has not united by 12 weeks, it is classified as nonunion. Criteria outlined by Flynn et al. for surgical treatment include:
- A large metaphyseal fragment
- Displacement of less than 1 cm from joint surface
- An open viable lateral condyle physis.

Open reduction and internal fixation with bone grafting for nonunion or delayed union of minimally displaced fractures is the main line of treatment for these fractures.

Monteggia in Children

Introduction

The eponym Monteggia fracture is most precisely used to refer to a dislocation of the proximal radioulnar joint in association with a forearm fracture. These injuries are relatively uncommon, accounting for less than 5% of all forearm fractures. The ulna fracture is usually clinically and radiographically apparent. Findings associated with the concomitant radial head dislocation are often subtle and can be overlooked.

The keys to successful diagnosis of a Monteggia fracture are clinical suspicion and radiographs of the entire forearm and elbow. Properly assessing the nature of this injury in a timely fashion is imperative, in order to prevent permanent disability or limb dysfunction.

History

In 1814, Giovanni Battista Monteggia of Milan first described this fracture, as a fracture to the proximal third of the ulna with associated anterior dislocation of the radial head. Interestingly, he described this injury pattern in the pre-Roentgen era, based solely on the history of injury and on physical examination findings. However, this particular fracture pattern only accounts for about 60% of these types of injuries. More than 150 years later in 1967, Bado coined the term Monteggia lesion and classified the injury into four types.

Classification by Bado

1. *Type I*: Fracture of the proximal or middle-third of the ulna with anterior dislocation of the radial head.

2. *Type II*: Fracture of the proximal or middle-third of the ulna with posterior dislocation of the radial head.
3. *Type III*: Fracture of the ulnar metaphysis with lateral dislocation of the radial head.
4. *Type IV*: Fracture of the proximal or middle-third of the ulna and radius with anterior dislocation of the radial head.

The basis of the Bado classification is in the recognition that the apex of the fracture is in the same direction as the radial head dislocation. The first challenge is correctly assessing the extent and nature of the injury. The ulna fracture is usually noted, commonly in the proximal third of the ulna. The olecranon, mid and distal shafts may be involved. Some injuries associated with radiocapitellar dislocation (such as the transolecranon fracture-dislocation of the elbow) are mislabeled as Monteggia lesions, when in fact the proximal radioulnar joint remains intact. The Monteggia lesion is most precisely characterized as a forearm fracture in association with dislocation of the proximal radioulnar joint.

The radial head dislocation may not be apparent and may be missed, if the elbow is not included in the radiograph. Whenever a fracture of a long bone is noted, the joints above and below should be evaluated using radiographs in orthogonal planes (planes at 90° angles to each other). If one of the forearm bones is injured, look for injury in the other bone and associated joints of the forearm, elbow, and wrist. This principle also applies to Galeazzi fractures, the eponym used to refer to a fracture of the distal radius and concomitant dislocation of the distal radioulnar joint. Separate radiographs should be taken of the elbow. The radial head should point toward the capitellum on all radiographs of the elbow. Unrecognized dislocations may result from reduction of the dislocated radius prior to presentation. This may occur in the field spontaneously or as a result of manipulation by emergency responders. The treating physician may reduce an unrecognized dislocation, while reducing or immobilizing the ulna fracture.

Frequency

Fixation to stabilize the ulna and prevent further displacement forces on the radiocapitellar joint. Closed Monteggia fractures in pediatric patients are generally treated in a closed fashion. A posterior long-arm splint with the elbow in 90° of flexion and full supination is the immobilization method of choice for types I, III, and IV. Type II injuries (posterior lesions) are best splinted in Monteggia fractures comprise less than 5% of forearm fractures, with published literature supporting 1–2%. Of the Monteggia fractures, Bado type I is the most common (59%), followed by type III (26%), type II (5%), and type IV (1%). Monteggia fractures are one-third as common as the more familiar Galeazzi fractures.

Etiology

Monteggia fractures are primarily associated with falls on an outstretched hand with forced pronation. If the elbow is flexed, the chance of a type II or III lesion is greater. In some cases, a direct blow to the forearm can also produce similar injuries. Penrose considered type II lesions as variation of posterior elbow dislocation. Bado believed that the type III lesion, the result of a direct lateral force on the elbow was primarily observed in children. In essence, high-energy trauma (e.g. motor vehicle collisions) and low-energy trauma (e.g. a fall from standing) can result in the described injuries. A high index of suspicion, therefore, should be maintained with any ulna fracture.

Pathophysiology

The forearm structures are intricately related, and any disruption to one of the bones affects the other. The ulna and radius are in direct contact with each other only at the proximal and distal radioulnar joints. However, they are unified along their entire length by the interosseous membrane. This allows the radius to rotate around the ulna. When the ulna is fractured, energy is transmitted along the interosseous membrane, displacing the proximal radius. The end result is a disrupted interosseous membrane proximal to the fracture, dislocated proximal radioulnar joint and dislocated radiocapitellar joint.

Clinical Features

- Elbow pain
- Elbow swelling
- Deformity
- Crepitus
- Paresthesia or numbness
- Some patients may not have severe pain at rest, but elbow flexion and forearm rotation is limited and painful.
- The dislocated radial head may be palpable in the anteroposterior or anterolateral position.
- In Type I and IV lesions, the radial head can be palpated in the antecubital fossa.
- The radial head can be palpated posteriorly in Type II lesions and laterally in Type III lesions.
- The skin should be closely inspected to ensure an open fracture is not present.
- Pulses and capillary refill should be documented.
- A negligible hematoma may be present at the site, if no direct trauma is associated.
- Monteggia fractures in children based on type of ulnar injury are as follows:
  - Plastic deformation
  - Incomplete (greenstick or buckle) fracture
  - Complete transverse or short oblique fracture
  - Long-oblique or comminuted fracture.

Treatment

Indications for treatment of Monteggia fractures are based on the specific fracture pattern and the age of the patient (i.e. pediatric or adult). Most pediatric fracture patterns can be managed conservatively with closed reduction and long-arm casting. However, most adult fractures require open reduction and internal fixation techniques. The radial head dislocation should be reduced emergently. Closed reduction under sedation should be performed within 6–8 hours of the injury. This is usually achieved with supination of the forearm, but it may require traction and direct pressure on the radial head.

If closed reduction is unsuccessful, the patient should be taken to the operating room within this same time frame for open reduction. Delay in reduction of the radius may lead to permanent articular damage, further nerve injury, or both. An open fracture requires emergent operative intervention. In closed injuries, once the radial head is reduced, the forearm is splinted and operative fixation of the ulna fracture may be carried out in an elective fashion for closed injuries. Adults usually require operative internal 70° elbow flexion with supination.

Imaging Studies

Plain radiography (Figs. 105 to 107):
Views of the forearm in AP and lateral are needed with the wrist and elbow joints included. The evaluating physician should also obtain separate radiographs of the elbow to assess the proximal radioulnar joint, ulnohumeral articulation, and the radiocapitellar joint.

The ulna fracture is usually obvious, but the findings associated with the radial head dislocation may be subtle and overlooked. To assess the radiocapitellar joint, draw a line parallel to the long axis of the radius. This line should point directly at the capitulum on any projection of the elbow.

The radial head dislocation almost always points in the same direction as the apex of the ulna fracture. In children, recognizing a plastic deformation of the ulna, which may also lead to radial head dislocation, is important.

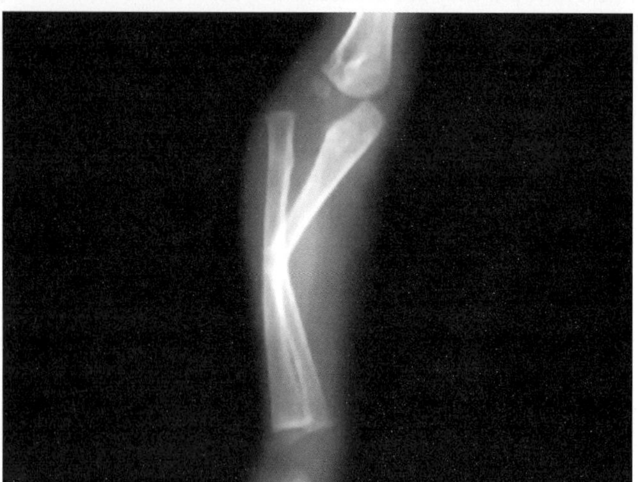

Fig. 105: X-ray showing Monteggia fracture dislocation.

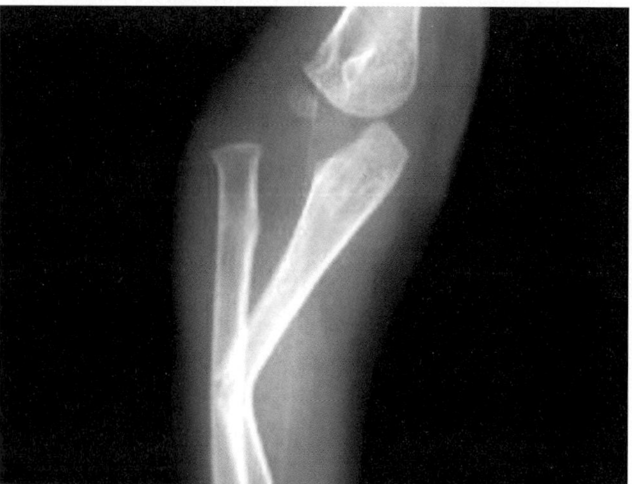

Fig. 106: Magnified view of Figure 105.

Nonoperative Management

Nonoperative treatment is successful for most Monteggia injuries in children because the majority of the fractures are inherently stable, they require a shorter time for both the osseous and the ligamentous injuries to heal, they can be immobilized for the duration of the initial healing period (3–6 weeks) with little trouble regaining motion lost through stiffness and they may have the potential for remodeling of mild residual angular deformities (less than 10°).

Surgical Management

Open fractures require emergent surgical consultation. The initial treating physician may reduce the radial head dislocation and splint this fracture. Unless the fracture is open, surgical treatment is performed on an elective basis. While, most adults require operative treatment and most pediatric fractures are treated closed. Operative fixation of complete fractures of the ulna with proximal radioulnar joint dislocation is recommended in children. The complete disruption of bone continuity is likely to be associated with substantial soft tissue trauma in these injuries. Shortening and angulation of complete fractures after cast immobilization are common. Anatomic reduction of the ulnar fracture and radial head often requires operative treatment.

Transverse and short oblique fractures are adequately treated with intramedullary wire fixation. Intramedullary wires, however, cannot be relied on to maintain reduction of complete fractures that are either long oblique in pattern or comminuted. These fractures are likely to displace or even shorten and, therefore, should be fixed with a plate and screws, as shown in Figures 108A and B.

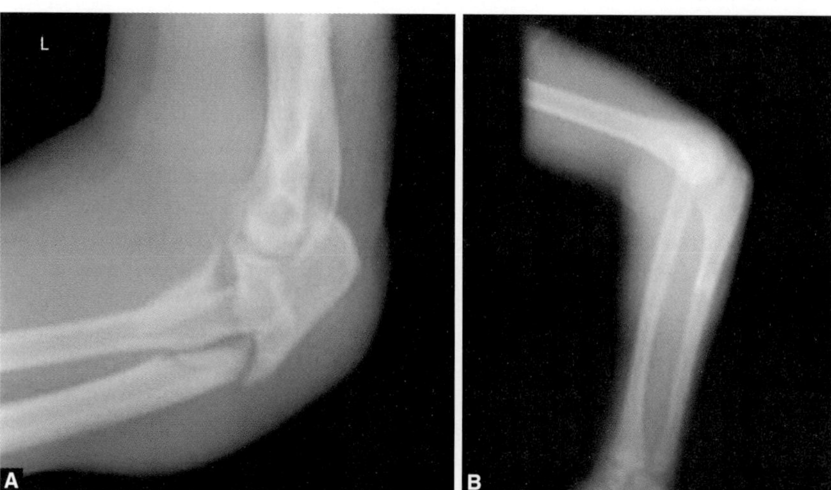

Figs. 107A and B: Lateral X-ray taken, showing Monteggia fracture dislocation.

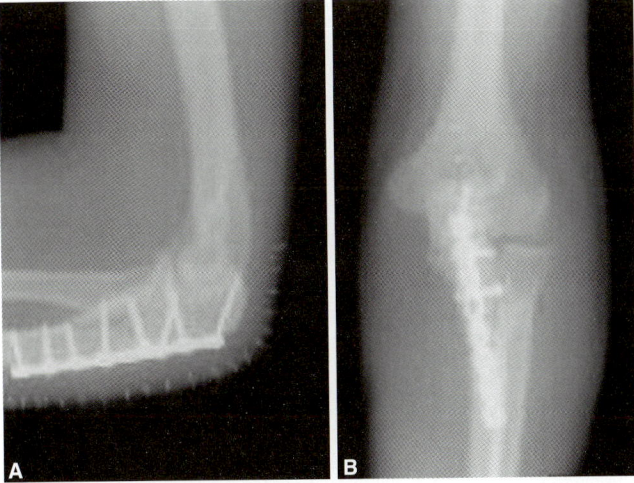

Figs. 108A and B: Plate and screw fixation of Monteggia fractures.

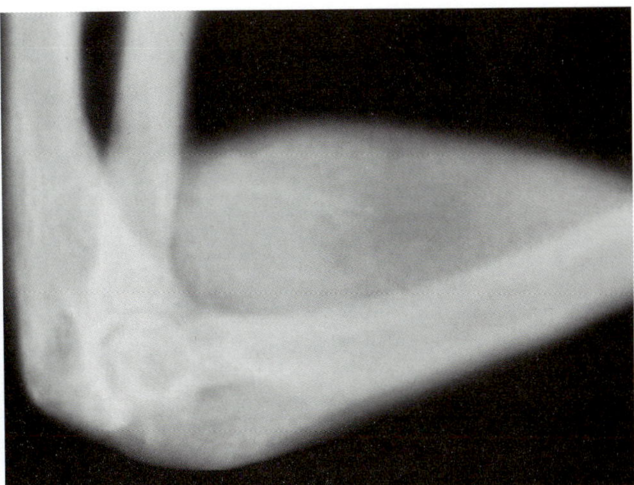

Fig. 109: Myositis ossificans traumatica.

Complications

- Infection
- Bleeding
- Malunion
- Nonunion
- Nerve injury
- Redislocation of the radial head
- Radioulnar synostosis
- Chronic pain.

Many of the complications listed are significantly reduced with timely diagnosis, adequate reduction, stable surgical fixation, and appropriate postoperative care. Most nerve injuries are neurapraxia, and function usually returns within 1–6 months. Baseline electrodiagnostic studies are obtained early. If nerve function does not return within 2–3 months, surgical exploration may be indicated. If the nerve injury results from reduction or operative treatment, it should be addressed immediately.

Prolonged or complete nerve dysfunction requires early splinting and therapy and may result in the need for tendon transfers. If the radial head dislocates after surgery, improper ulnar reduction must be considered. If this is the case, the hardware should be removed and a proper reduction of the ulna should take place. If dislocation of the radial head is recognized more than 6 weeks after the surgery, a radial head excision should be performed. A nonunion or malunion complication can be considered for bone grafting.

MYOSITIS OSSIFICANS

Introduction

- Myositis ossificans refers to bone formation in atypical location.
- Three terms that are used interchangeably are ectopic bone, heterotopic bone, and myositis ossificans.
- The first two terms have similar connotation, but myositis ossificans usually refers to bone formation in muscle itself.
- Heterotopic ossification involves tendons, fascia periosteum, and muscle.

Calcification versus Ossification

- Calcific deposits do occur in tendons, articular cartilages, and synovium; articular capsule typically consists of calcium pyrophosphates.
- These are radiodense but have no trabecular structure, and no true bone matrix is formed.
- Ectopic calcification as opposed to ossification affects tissues including skin, brain, kidneys, and conjunctiva.
- Ectopic calcification occurs when there is an increase in serum calcium level, such as hyperparathyroidism, renal failure, dermatomyositis, scleroderma, and following tuberculosis infection.

Types of Myositis Ossificans

There are two types of myositis ossificans:

1. Myositis ossificans traumatica
2. Myositis ossificans progressiva.

Myositis Ossificans Traumatica

It is a reactive lesion occurring in the soft tissues and at times in bone periosteum. It is characterized by fibrous, osseous, and cartilaginous proliferation of the subperiosteal hematoma and followed by metaplasia (Fig. 109).

Patients who are at risk of developing myositis ossificans are suffering from:

- *Elbow trauma*:
  - Open elbow dislocations, which require multiple debridements
  - Elbow dislocations associated with fractures requiring ORIF
  - Radial head fractures treated with surgery more than 24 hours after injury
  - Failed internal fixation about the elbow, requiring revision fixation within 3 months.
- Distal biceps tendon repair
- Traumatic brain and spinal cord injury
- *Burn patients*:
  - Third-degree burns over 20% of total body area
  - Third-degree burns over the elbow
  - Long periods of bed confinement
  - A hematoma seems to be a necessary prerequisite for myositis ossificans
  - The muscles most often involved are—brachialis, anticus, quadriceps femoris, and adductor muscles of thigh. It is significant that these muscles gain attachment to the

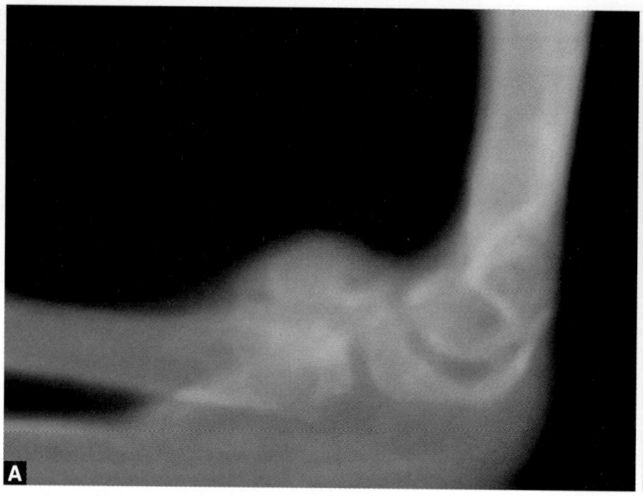

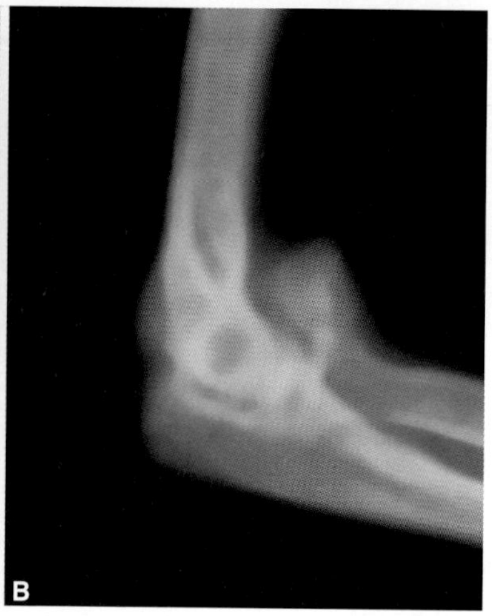

Figs. 110A and B: Radial head fracture with dislocation develops a typical pattern of myositis ossificans.

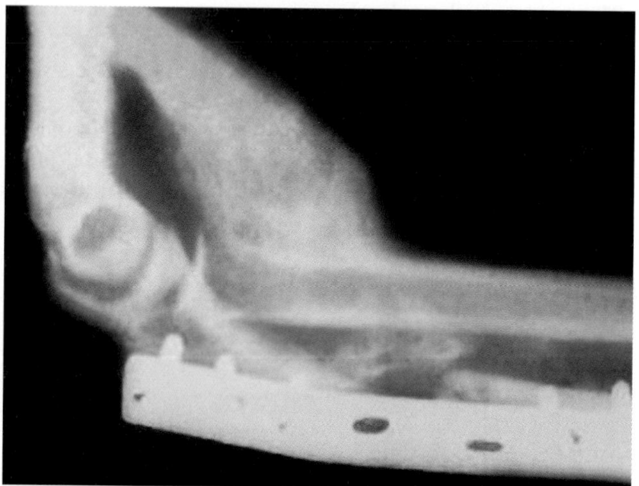

Fig. 111: Myositis ossificans in a patient with elbow dislocation proximal ulna fracture.

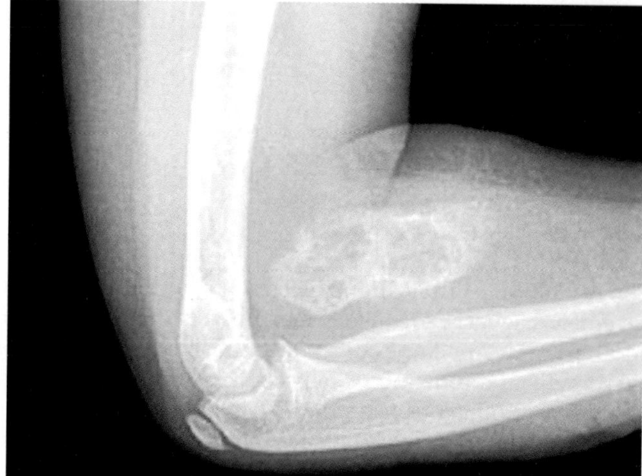

Fig. 112: Myositis ossificans in a third-degree burn patient.

bone over a wide area suggesting that the periosteum participates to some extent in the process.

- The region of elbow is a favorite site, ill-advised forcible manipulation to increase elbow movement will cause a widespread involvement (Fig. 110). Radial head fracture with dislocation develops a typical pattern of myositis ossificans (Figs. 110A and B). Myositis ossificans in a patient with elbow dislocation proximal ulna fracture (Fig. 111).

  Entire brachialis muscle has been replaced after head injury without elbow trauma.
- Myositis ossificans in a patient's third-degree burn (Fig. 112).

Pathogenesis

- The process is alteration within the ground substance of connective tissue with a striking proliferation of mesenchymal cells.
- Degeneration and necrosis of the tissue, disrupted muscle fibers retract followed by histiocytic invasion for removal of necrotic debris.
- Fibroblasts from endomysium invade the damaged area and rapidly form broad sheets of immature fibroblasts, at the same time, mesenchymal cells proliferate within the injured connective tissue and this histological picture may erroneously diagnose as fibrosarcoma.
- Sarcolemmic nuclei at the ends of the damaged muscle fibers begin to proliferate, and chains and columns of plump polyhedral cells appear followed by production of sarcoplasm, which extends as buds, the sarcolemmic nuclei cluster within the center of these sarcoplasmic masses.
- The ground substance increases in amount and encloses more mesenchymal cells, and this material becomes homogeneous or waxy.

  This is followed by mineralization and bone is formed mineralization occurs periphery to center.

Microscopic appearance

- Zone phenomenon is of great diagnostic importance.
- The central highly cellular region is surrounded by a second zone of fibroblastic tissue and this is in turn enveloped by a third zone of mature well-oriented bone.
- This zonal phenomenon, which is not present in soft-tissue sarcomas, classifies the lesion as benign and obviates the need for radical measures.
- When ossification has developed, the "tumor" is at least 3–4 weeks old.
- The cellular inner zone illustrates numerous cells with occasional atypical mitotic figures and variations in size and

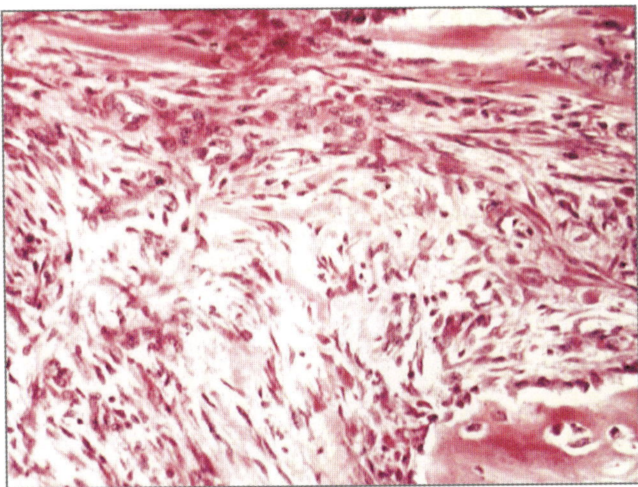

Fig. 113: Histological appearance of myositis ossificans.

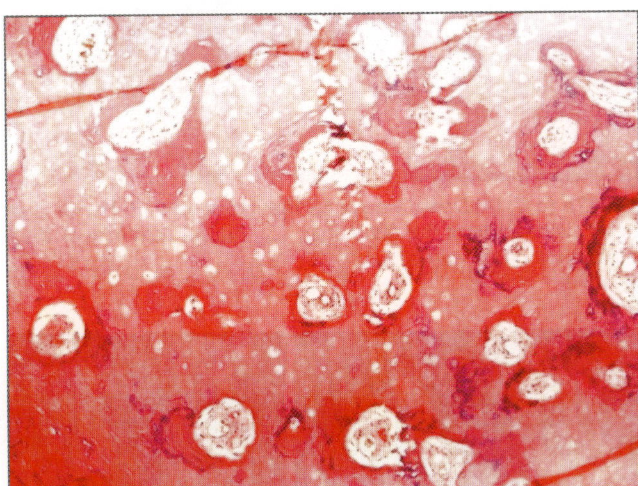

Fig. 114: Osteoid formation with fibrovascular background.

shape of the cells. The histological appearance is sarcomatous (Fig. 113).

- The middle zone shows osteoid formation with a fibrovascular background (Fig. 114).
- The outer zone illustrates mature fairly well-oriented peripheral bone. The fibrous stroma appears more mature than at the center of the lesion (Fig. 115).

Clinical picture

- Pain and loss of range of motion are the common presenting complaints during the evolution of ectopic bone formation.
- On physical examination, there may be swelling, erythema, and local warmth of the affected joint.
- During formation of extraosseous mass, the elbow area is quite swollen and tender, so active and passive movements are reduced.
- As pain and swelling are reduced, a circumscribed indurated later hard tumor mass is palpable over the elbow.
- Active extension of the joint is limited by virtue of inelasticity of the muscle and flexion is prevented by obstruction offered by the mass.
- Aggressive physical therapy, with passive stretching beyond the pain-free arc of motion, only exacerbates the formation of ectopic bone.

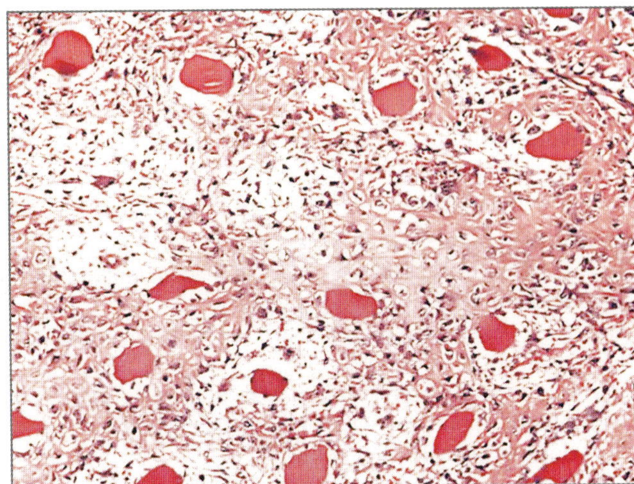

Fig. 115: Fibrous stroma appearing more mature at the center of lesion.

- Presentation can be confused with cellulitis, deep infection, thrombophlebitis, and reflex sympathetic dystrophy.

Physical examination

- *X-ray* shows findings between 4 weeks and 5 weeks
- Biopsy
- Serum alkaline phosphatase
- Technetium bone scan is markedly positive during the formation of ectopic bone and usually remains positive for a prolonged period of time
- An increased incidence of the human leukocyte antigen (HLA)-B18 in a group of central nervous system (CNS) injury has been reported.

Treatment

- *Acute stages:* Conservative treatment is the method of choice and consists of following:
  - Immobilization of elbow by splints
  - *Drugs:* Diphosphonate therapy, calcitonin, and NSAIDs
  - *Physiotherapy:* Active physiotherapy is encouraged and passive stretching is avoided
  - *Manipulation is done under general anesthesia:* Adhesions should be snapped abruptly and should not be broken gradually.
- *Chronic stages:* Surgery is the treatment of choice:
  - Not all ectopic bone formation about the elbow requires surgical treatment. The goal of surgery is to restore functional motion.
  - Careful clinical evaluation should be performed to ensure, if ectopic bone itself is blocking motion.
  - In traumatic conditions, tomograms are necessary to know the congruency of joint surfaces. If joint surfaces are not congruent, total elbow arthroplasty or distraction arthroplasty may be required.
  - In general, it is better to wait for 9–12 months after injury to allow maturation of the ectopic bone. Maturation is judged by plain radiographs.
- *Principles of surgery:*
  - Remove ectopic bone at its narrowest portion and with least risk of articulation
  - Atraumatic handling of all tissues should be done
  - Careful homeostasis
  - Suction drainage of the wound

- Postoperative compressive dressing
- Avoiding the creation and deposition of bone dust in the joint by use of osteotomes rather than saws and meticulous lavage
- Avoid injury to cartilage by excision of enough bone to initiate some motion and define joint line; once some motion is initiated, additional bone is resected as necessary.

Postoperative management

- In case of myositis ossificans, surgical field is treated with 700 cGy radiation
- Otherwise, 75 mg of indomethacin is prescribed 3 weeks before and 8 weeks after surgery.
- Elbow is managed with continuous motion and splints.
- When motion goals are not met, examination under anesthesia is performed 6 weeks after surgery.

Myositis Ossificans Progressiva

Myositis ossificans progressiva; Munchmeyer disease (Fig. 116): Progressive and diffused myositis ossificans was the term applied to this disease by Munchmeyer in 1869. This is a rare congenital condition in autosomal dominant. It is characterized by progressive ossification within the muscles and certain specific skeletal abnormalities.

Skeletal abnormalities include (Figs. 116 to 118):

- Monophalangeic great toe
- Short first metacarpal bone
- Microdactyly
- Malformation of little finger
- Reduction defects of all limbs
- Abnormalities of cervical vertebrae.

Clinical features

- Progressive ossification occurs in discrete episodes is often precipitated by minor trauma such as knock or IM injection.
- The region becomes swollen, tender, and inflamed. Patient may be pyrexial. As the swelling subsides, muscle mass is replaced by bone.
- As the disease progresses, there is interface with the function of the affected muscle leading to progressive immobility.
- Ossification characteristically involves the muscles of head and back in early childhood followed by shoulder and arms and hips (Fig. 119).

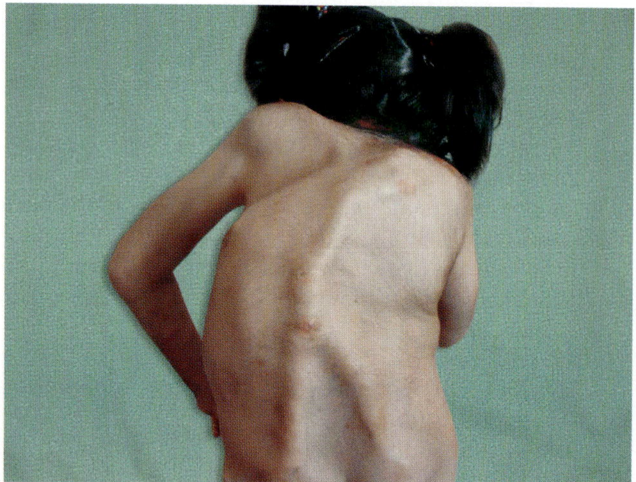

Fig. 116: Myositis ossificans progressiva.

- There is characteristic sparing of muscles of facial expression, diaphragm, laryngeal muscles, tongue, and the small muscles of hand and feet.

Pathology

- The striking feature of the disease is the replacement of muscle, tendon, and aponeurosis by masses of bone.
- Study of early lesions shows that actual bone deposits are not laid down within the actual muscle fiber, but in the

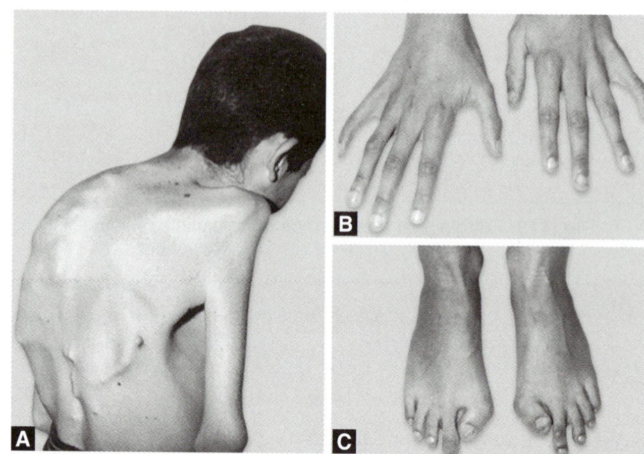

Figs. 117A to C: (A) Dorsal view of 13 year-old patient; (B) Hands to show bilateral clinodactyly of the fifth finger; (C) Typical deformity of the feet (bilateral short hallux valgus).

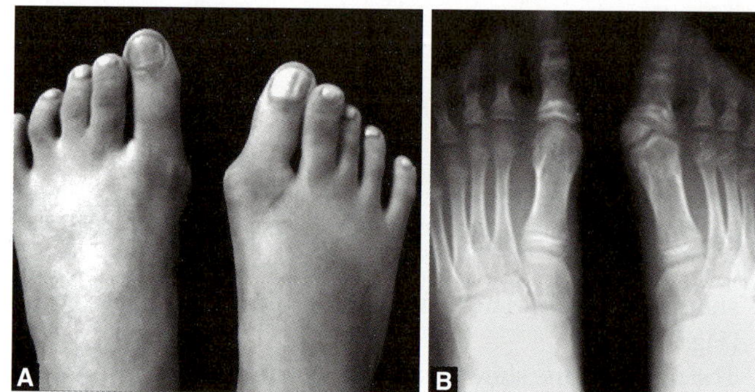

Figs. 118A and B: Hallux valgus bilateral. (A) Clinical; (B) Radiological view.

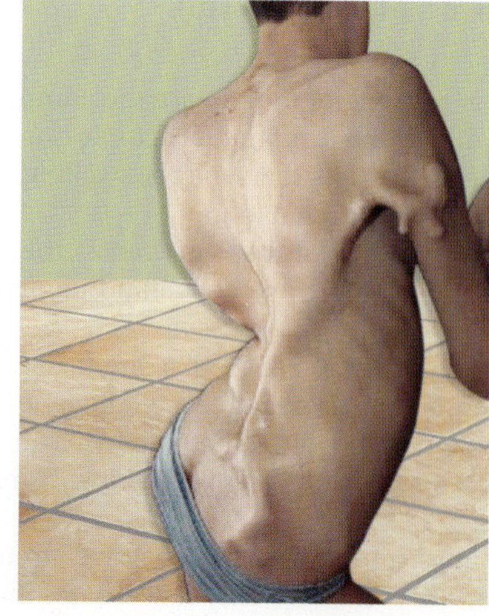

Fig. 119: Ossification involving muscles of head and back in early childhood.

connective tissue between fibers, this leads to alternative name fibrodysplasia ossificans progressiva.
- The only laboratory finding is raised eosinophil count.

Treatment
- There is no effective treatment, which prevents episodes of ossification.
- Diphosphonates have been used but proved disappointing.
- Corticotropin seems to have an effect of decreased eosinophil count and joint motion may increase.

Ulnar Neuropathy

- Ulnar neuropathy may occur as a result of compression in the cubital tunnel from ectopic bone.
- Ulnar neuropathy is more common in myositis ossificans followed by brain injury. It also occurs after burns and trauma as well.
- Treatment consists of ulnar nerve transposition anteriorly. Simple subcutaneous translocation is necessary.

VOLKMANN'S ISCHEMIC CONTRACTURE

Introduction

- In 1875, Volkmann described a contracture of muscles of the wrist and fingers, which followed tight bandaging of the arm in the treatment of fractures about the elbow.
- Volkmann's contracture (Fig. 120) results from acute ischemia of the muscles of the forearm.

Etiology

- Fractures (supracondylar fracture)
- Crush injuries
- Sympathetic causes (intimal tear, sympathetic stimuli, vessel constriction, and mechanical block ischemia)
- Other causes, which result in compartment syndrome and lead to Volkmann's ischemic contracture, are:
  - External compression (e.g. tight bandaging)
  - Internal bleeding (e.g. hemophilia)
  - Burns
  - Excessive exercise
  - Snake bites
  - Intra-arterial injections of drugs or sclerosing agents
  - Infections.

Pathology

Ischemia necrosis/infarct fibrosis contracture

Eaton and Green's traumatic ischemia-edema cycle in Volkmann's contracture:
- Any situation that causes a decrease in compartment size or increase in compartment pressure can initiate compartment syndrome.
- As the intracompartmental pressure increases, capillary blood perfusion is reduced to a level that cannot maintain tissue viability.
- The increase in interstitial pressure overcomes the intravascular pressure of the small vessels and capillaries, causing the walls to collapse and impeding local blood flow.
- The local tissue ischemia leads to local edema, which increases intracompartmental pressure.
- Traumatic ischemia-edema cycle in Volkmann's contracture is shown in Figure 121.
- Volkmann's contracture is the result of infarction produced by a segmental arterial spasm of the main artery to an extremity with reflex spasm of the collateral circulation (Fig. 122).
- Ischemia is produced and the muscle bellies demand the greatest amount of blood and therefore the most vulnerable tissues to its loss are first affected.
- The infarct takes the form of an ellipsoid with its axis in the line of the anterior interosseous artery and with its central point, a little above the middle of the forearm.
- The greatest damage is at the center and usually falls most heavily on flexor digitorum profundus and flexor pollicis longus, which are often necrotic.
- The median nerve runs near the center of the ellipsoid and may exhibit profound ischemia.
- The ulnar nerve tends to be less severely affected. It gets involved when extensive fibrosis of the surrounding muscles occurs.
- The most extensive degeneration occurs in the center of the muscle sequestrum and cellular activity, and fibrosis takes place only at the periphery, which is surrounded by a sheath of dense fibrous tissue.

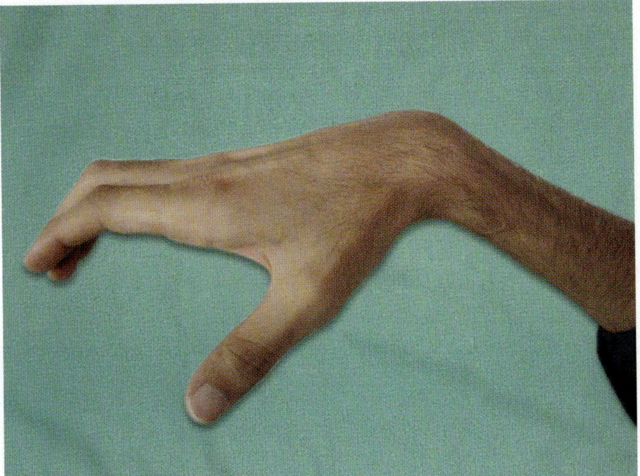

Fig. 120: Volkmann's contracture.

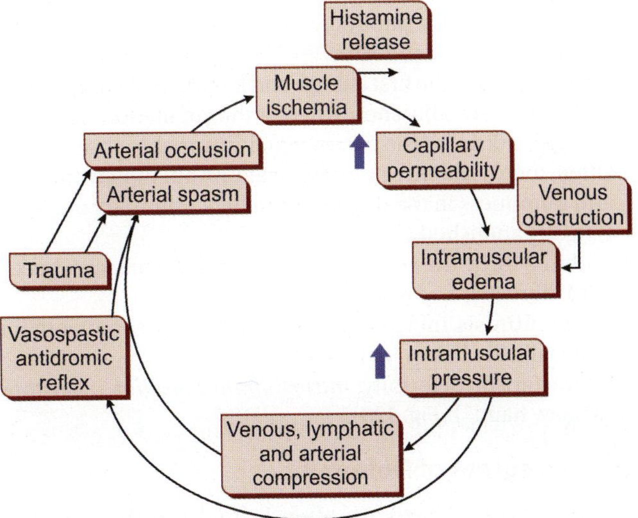

Fig. 121: Traumatic ischemia–edema cycle.

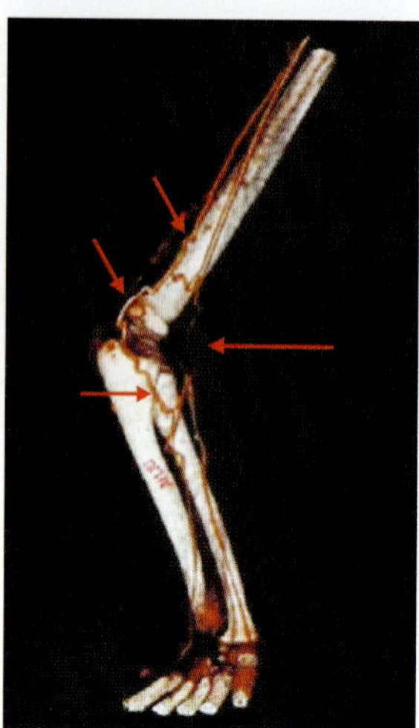

Fig. 122: A 6-year-old girl with Volkmann's ischemic contracture. Upper extremity volume-rendered multidetector computed tomography (MDCT) angiogram shows occlusion of distal brachial artery and reconstitution of ulnar and radial arteries, mainly by recurrent branch of deep brachial artery (short arrows) and small antecubital collaterals (long arrow).

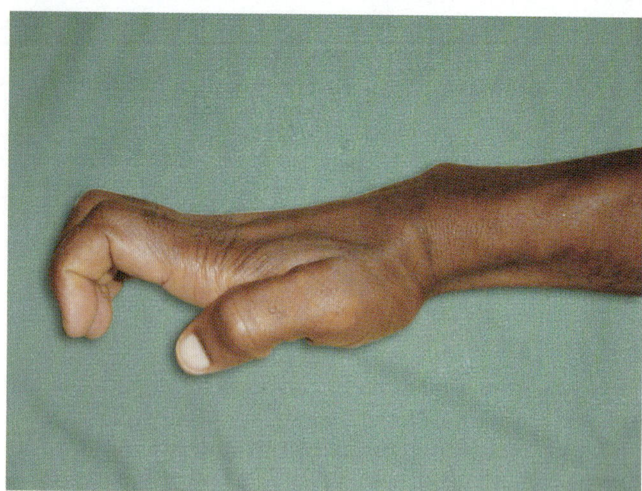

Fig. 123: Claw hand deformity [fingers extended at metacarpophalangeal (MCP) joint and flexed at interphalangeal (IP) joints].

- In the center of the mass, the muscle fibers lose their nuclei along with cross-striations and fuse into a homogeneous mass. As the periphery is approached, some signs of function are preserved and there is an area of intense cellular activity, both fibroblastic and phagocytic.
- This picture is in contrast to muscle degeneration from all other causes, such as denervation and sepsis, in which the appearance is one of diffuse interfibrillar fibrosis.
- This entity has also to be differentiated from the compression compartment syndrome of the forearm, due to lying on a limb for a long period of time, poisoning by drugs, e.g. alcohol, etc. or in hemophilia with bleeding into the forearm.
- The succeeding phases are those of replacement— fibroblasts appear and deposit fibrous tissue at first in thin threads and later more densely.
- The whole process thus seems to be one of absorptions and replacements by fibrosis of dead muscular tissue.

Clinical Features

- The symptoms usually begin within 1–24 hours after injury.
- Severe pain, pallor, paralysis, and pulselessness are all present in a greater or lesser degree.
- Pallor is usually the first change and it is often striking; pressure on a nail will readily show whether the circulation is impaired.
- The pulse distal to the obstruction is invariably absent.
- Often, there is intense pain, especially on attempted movement and numbness in the fingers; ultimately, voluntary movement is totally abolished.
- Within 2 days, the swelling reduces and the muscles become hard, fibrosed, and resistant.
- As the fibrosis increases, the deformity becomes obvious, especially the flexion of fingers.
- Characteristic deformity: *Intrinsic minus position* (also known as "claw hand") (Fig. 123).

Various Degrees of Deformity

- *Mild degrees*: These are often brought to the consultant several years after the injury to the elbow. The patient may be unable to extend the fingers completely but yet may possess a considerable range of movement when the wrist is flexed. It is usually possible to straighten the fingers completely with the wrist fully flexed.
- *Severe type*: Fully developed deformity with characteristic attitude.
- Severe type complicated by nerve involvement, either a median or ulnar nerve, which is coincidentally involved:
  - In the absence of direct damage, however, either nerve may be implicated in the actual ischemic contracture.
  - The median nerve is frequently compressed, where it passes between the two heads of pronator teres and the ulnar nerve may suffer from the contraction of the fibrous tissue, which surrounds it; in each case, the signs are those of an incomplete nerve lesion—usually partial anesthesia and paralysis of the small muscles of the hand.
  - In addition, the nutrition of the limb is impaired, the hand is cold and blue, and trophic ulceration occurs.

There are three levels of severity in Volkmann's contracture:

1. *Mild*: Flexion contracture of two or three fingers only with no or limited loss of sensation.
2. *Moderate*: All fingers are flexed and the thumb is stuck in the palm; the wrist may be stuck in flexion and there is usually loss of some sensation in the hand.
3. *Severe*: All muscles in the forearm that both flex and extend the wrist and fingers are involved; this is a severely disabling condition:
   - When the damage is reversible, a limited number of muscle fibers die and they are gradually replaced by new ones growing longitudinally, along the surviving sarcolemmal tubes.
   - When the damage is irreversible, all grades of fibrosis are present up to almost complete fibrous replacement.

Prognosis

- Early intervention produces good results.
- Outlook is grave in severe types and in cases with accompanying nerve involvement.

Prophylaxis

- In all cases of elbow injury, look out for pain, stiffness, swelling, cyanosis or lividity of the fingers, or obliteration of the radial pulse.

- First step, if the event has followed a fracture, is to see that the fragments are displaced or not. If they are displaced, a further reduction should be carried out at once. Even if they have not moved, it is wise to extend the limb slightly because this is followed occasionally by relief of the spasm. Failure of the pulse to return within a few minutes is an indication for immediate operation.

Treatment

Acute Stage

- The goal of treatment is to restore adequate circulation before irreparable damage is done and thus to avert contracture deformities.
- Time is a major factor. The condition is a progressive one in which more and more damage is done.
- All measures favoring circulation generally are of great value, e.g. elevation of the part, removal of any splint or circular bandage, and application of mild external warmth. The contralateral limb or other limbs may be warmed.
- Emergency fasciotomy is required to prevent progression to Volkmann's ischemic contracture. Decompression is performed via volar or dorsal approach. Medial nerve decompression throughout its course is essential, especially in high-risk areas, including deep to the lacertus fibrosus; between the humeral and ulnar heads of the pronator teres, the proximal arch and deep fascial surface of the flexor digitorum superficialis; and in the carpal tunnel.
- The next logical step is the interruption of the sympathetic reflex supply by ganglion injection or arteriectomy. The appearance of Horner's syndrome is the evidence of a successful cervical sympathetic block.
- If the circulation does not improve immediately, the artery should be exposed (preferred method nowadays).
- Two percent Papaverine test.
- Segmental resection of the spasmodic artery at the fracture site results in interruption of the sympathetic reflex, which in turn leads to vasodilation of the collaterals.
- If fracture fragments are not reduced perfectly (as shown on X-ray), attempt should be made to complete the reduction by open operation with wire external fixation.

Fully-developed Stage

Physiotherapy:

The first step in treatment is to prevent contractures and maintain a supple joint with a full range of movements and so a splint is applied, which makes use of elastic traction to prevent the muscles contraction, while at the same time, permitting the joints of the fingers and wrist to be moved, if necessary, passively to prevent them from becoming stiff.

Operative treatment:

- A great variety of operations has been recommended for this condition, from tenoplasty, bone section, and excision of elbow joint to muscle sliding operation described by Max Page.
- In every case, operation should be preceded by a course of thorough stretching (physiotherapy).
- Max Page described a muscle slide operation in which a straight incision is made from just above the medial epicondyle downward for about 10 cm on the medial aspect of the forearm; and the flexor muscles, arising from the medial epicondyle of the humerus and upper ends of the radius and ulna, are erased from their origins by a periosteal elevator. The hand and fingers are then hyperextended and, in this way, the muscle origin is dragged downwards. The muscles obtain, in time, a new origin lower down the forearm. Watch out for ulnar nerve during operation. The after treatment consists of careful splinting of hand and fingers and physiotherapy.
- Littlewood recommended lengthening of all the shortened tendons. But lengthening of the tendons weakens the power of the muscles. It should be attempted only if the contraction is limited to one or two of the forearm muscles.
- Shortening of bones of the forearm by resection of 2–2.5 cm from each bone is liable to be followed by nonunion due to trophic changes in the arm.
- Seddon achieved a good results by completely excising the belly (or the scar representing it) of every muscle that had been completely destroyed, except for flexor carpi ulnaris, because of the danger to the ulnar artery. Reconstructive procedures were carried out by transplanting living muscles to replace the dead ones.
- Tendon transfers or tenotomies appear to be most rational, but they have the risk of recurrence because of contractures.
- In very severe deformity cases, arthrodesis of the wrist can be done, particularly where it has been necessary to use extensors for giving flexion to various digits.

Treatment of Nerve Complications

Neurolysis and Grafting

- When there is clinical evidence of nerve involvement, which does not show any sign of improvement, after a reasonable period of 2 or 3 months of physiotherapy, the nerves should be exposed at the sites where they are more likely to be compressed.
- The median nerve should be free from the callus of the fracture and also released from compression as it passes under the superficial head of pronator teres.
- The ulnar nerve is freed throughout the length the flexor muscle bellies.
- If the nerves have suffered irreversible damage, they should be dealt with grafts.
- General physiotherapy should afterwards be carefully carried out, the muscles at the same time being protected from overstretching by adequate splints.

OSTEOCHONDRITIS DISSECANS OF ELBOW

Osteochondritis

Definition

It is a derangement of the normal process of bone growth, which occurs at various ossification centers during the period of greatest activity.

Etiology

Vascular changes:

Interruption of the blood flow occurs by infarction, occlusion, or malformation of vessels, which leads to osteochondrosis. For example, Perthes disease, Friedberg infarction of metatarsal head, and OCD of capitulum.

Trauma:

In small proportion of cases, history of significant trauma should be elicited, for example, Osgood-Schlatters and OCD of capitulum.

Hormonal features:

Hormone changes during periods of altered growth give rise to increased osteogenic proliferation, these rapidly dividing cells are more susceptible to trauma or ischemia, e.g. severely affected dyschondrotic epiphysis such as capital femoral epiphysis in Gaucher's disease when exposed to normal weight-bearing.

- Traction epiphysis of 5th metatarsal base (Iselin disease)
- Osteochondritis of metatarsal head (Freiberg infraction)
- Osteochondritis of navicular bone (Kohler's disease).
- Osgood-Schlatter disease
- OCD knee
- OCD patella
- Legg-Calvé-Perthes syndrome.

Osteochondritis of Elbow

- It is also known as little Leaguer's elbow.
- Overuse and resultant chronic lateral impaction will lead to OCD capitulum, radial head, or medial epicondyle.
- *Age group*: Adolescent 12–16 years. Commonly in baseball pitchers and gymnasts.
- It is bilateral in 20%.
- It accounts for 6% of all cases of OCD.

Pathology

- Repeated valgus stress and tenuous blood supply within the capitulum are the reason for frequent occurrence of OCD in this location.
- Increased rotatory, compressive, or axial loads generated during the acceleration and deceleration phases will cause radiocapitellar compressive and shearing forces.

Clinical Presentation

- Pain
- Impaired range of motion elbow
- Radiographic signs (Figs. 124 and 125).

X-ray elbow AP and lateral AP in 45° flexion:

- Degenerative changes in elbow
- Diameter of radial head increased
- Loose body.

ICRS Classification

- *International Cartilage Repair Society (ICRS) OCD I*: It indicates a stable lesion with a continuous but softened area covered by intact cartilage.
- *ICRS OCD II*: A lesion with partial discontinuity that is stable when probed.
- *ICRS OCD III*: A lesion with a complete discontinuity that is not yet dislocated.
- *ICRS OCD IV*: An empty defect as well as a defect with a dislocated fragment or a loose fragment lying within the bed.

Although routine anteroposterior radiographs (Figs. 126 and 127) show only slight radiolucency (arrowheads in Fig. 127) in the capitulum, and anteroposterior radiographs of the elbow in 45° of flexion (Figs. 128A and B) clearly show nondisplaced fragments (arrowheads in Fig. 128B) of the capitulum and avulsion (arrow in Fig. 128B) of the medial epicondyle.

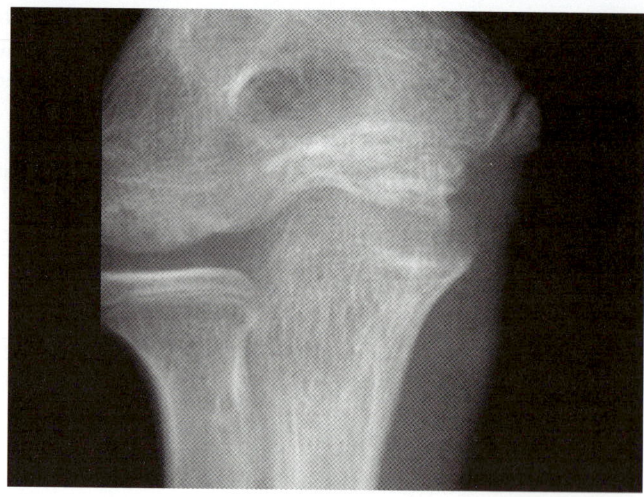

Fig. 124: Radiological sign in anteroposterior view.

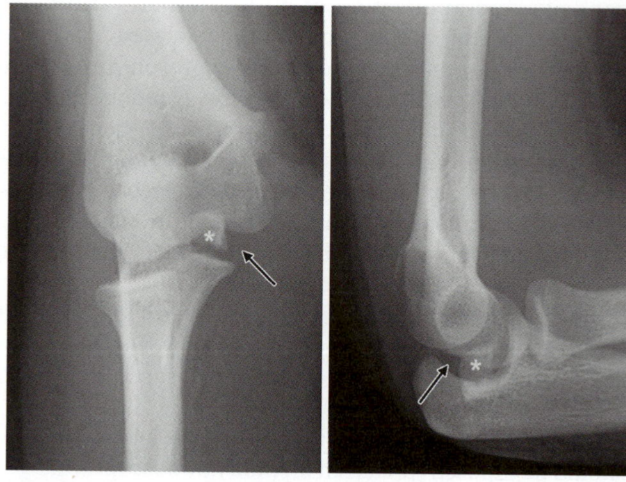

Fig. 125: Osteochondritis dissecans (OCD) of elbow, arrows showing osteochondral fragment.

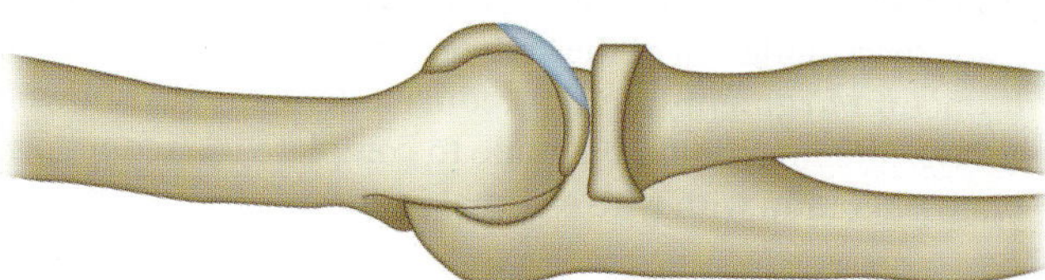

Fig. 126: Blue color showing osteochondral defect in extension.

MRI is gold standard for diagnosing OCD (Fig. 129)

Grading system (Figs. 130 to 133):

- *Grade 1*: Hyaline cartilage covering lesion remains intact.
- *Grade 2*: Enhancing zone of separation but they are stable.
- *Grade 3*: Fluid in zone of separation, unstable.
- *Grade 4*: Loose body.

Treatment

- Conservative
- Operative.

Conservative:

- Indications:
  - Stable lesion
  - No loose body

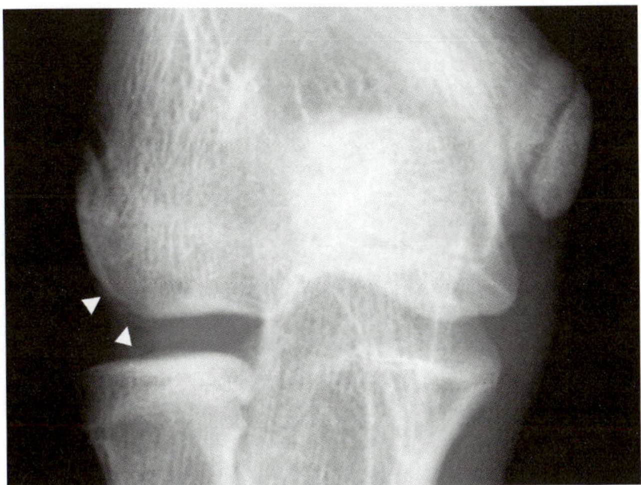

Fig. 127: X-ray showing osteochondral defect in full extension.

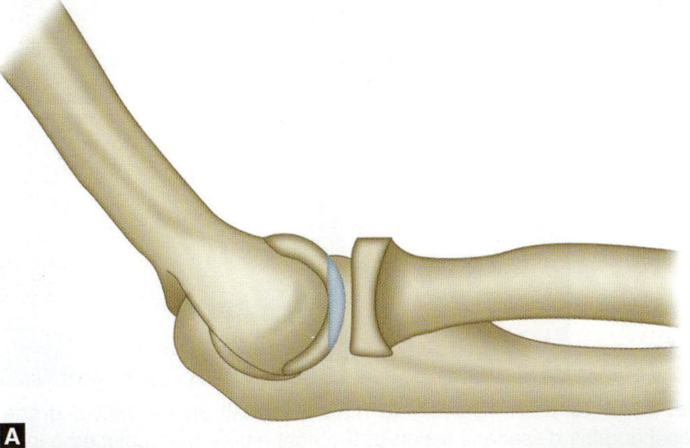

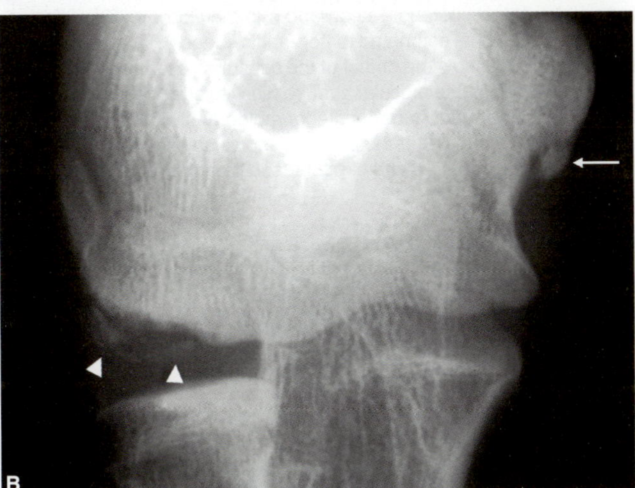

Figs. 128A and B: (A) Blue color showing osteochondral defect in 45° flexion; (B) X-ray showing osteochondral defect in 45° flexion.

- Mode of treatment:
  - Rest
  - Splinting
  - Symptomatic treatment.

Operative:
- Indications:
  - Unstable lesions
  - Loose body.

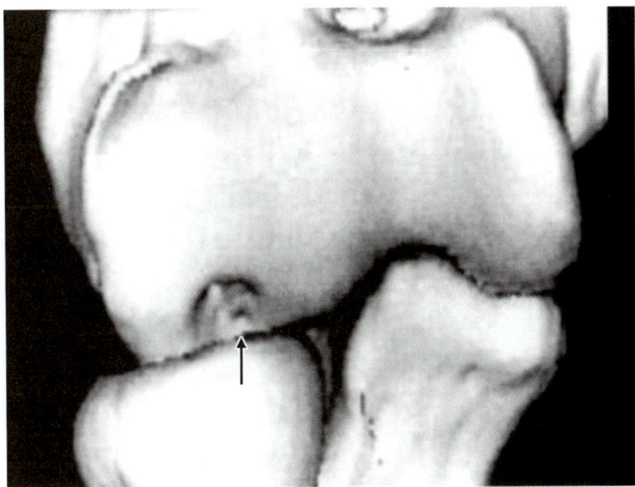

Fig. 129: Magnetic resonance imaging (MRI) showing osteochondritis dissecans.

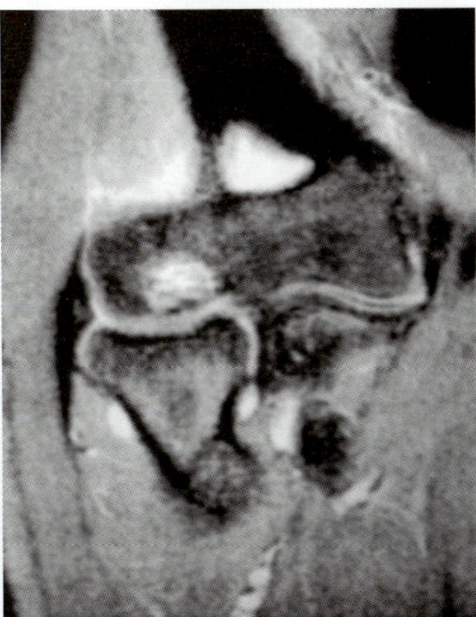

Fig. 130: Grade 1 osteochondritis.

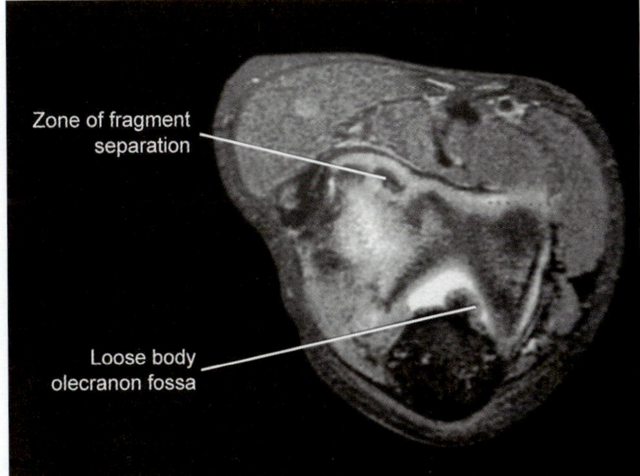

Fig. 131: Grade 2 osteochondritis.

- Mode of treatment:
  - Treated with internal fixation of unstable fragment with Herbert screw or using pull-out wires

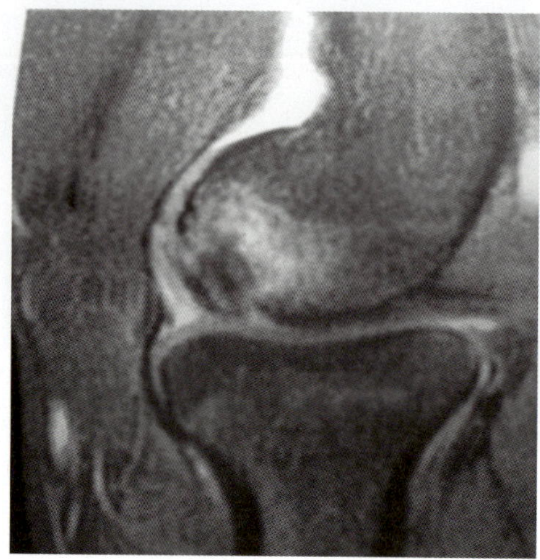

Fig. 132: Grade 3 osteochondritis.

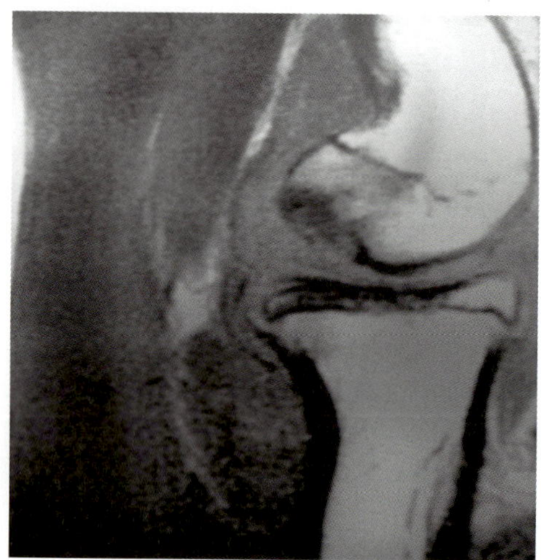

Fig. 133: Grade 4 osteochondritis.

- Bone grafting
- Arthroscopy.

- Arthroscopic procedures are the following:
  - Partial synovectomy
  - Excision of loose body
  - Drilling the crater
  - Fixing unstable viable fragment
  - Osteotomy of capitulum.
- *Proposed treatment:* Proposed treatment of osteochondritis is given in Table 2.
- *Case with Pictorial Description (Figs. 134A to E).*

TENNIS ELBOW AND GOLFER'S ELBOW

Tennis Elbow

Introduction

Lateral epicondylitis (Fig. 135) *(tennis elbow)* is a familiar term used to describe myriad symptoms around the lateral aspect of the elbow, and it occurs more frequently in nonathletes than athletes, with a peak incidence in the early 5th decade and a nearly equal gender incidence:

- Lateral epicondylitis can occur during activities that require repetitive supination and pronation of the forearm with the elbow in near full extension (Fig. 136).

TABLE 2: Proposed treatment of osteochondritis.

ICRS classification	*Capitular growth plate*	*ROM*	*Preferred treatment*
1 (Stable)	Open	Normal	Elbow rest
2 (Stable)	Closed	Restricted	Fixation and bone peg graft
3 (Unstable)			Fixation/bone peg/ iliac bone graft
4 (Unstable)			Fragment removal and reconstruction for large defect

(ICRS: International Cartilage Repair Society; ROM: range of motion)

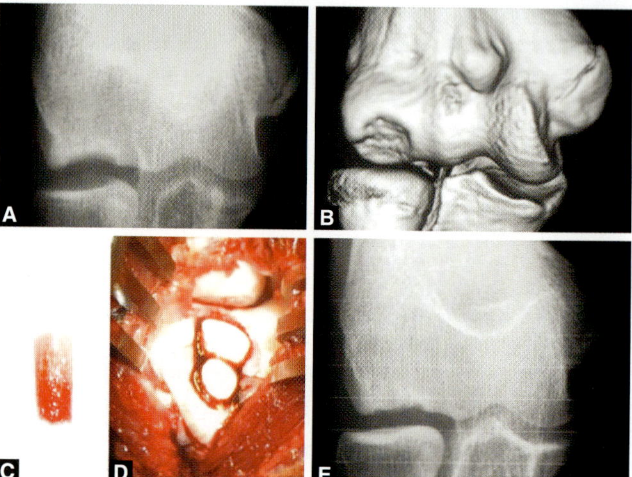

Figs. 134A to E: A 12-year-old male baseball player with a grade III osteochondritis dissecans lesion of the right elbow with a closed capitellar growth plate. Anteroposterior radiograph with the elbow in 45° of flexion (A) and three-dimensional computed tomographic image (B) made at the time of initial presentation show the defect of the capitulum. Removal of free bodies and reconstruction of the articular surface (D) with use of osteochondral plug grafts (C) are performed. Anteroposterior radiograph with the elbow in 45° of flexion, made 5 months after the surgery, shows union of the osteochondral plug grafts and flattening of the capitular subchondral bone (E).

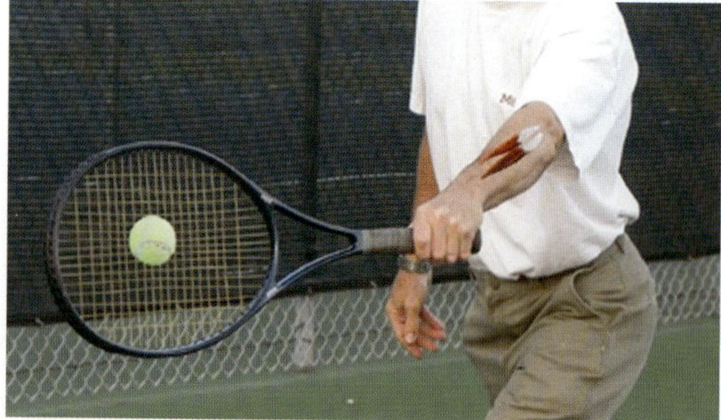

Fig. 135: Tennis elbow.

- Although originally described as an inflammatory process, the current consensus is that lateral epicondylitis is initiated as a microtear, most often within the origin of the extensor carpi radialis brevis (ECRB). Microscopic findings show immature reparative tissue that resembles angiofibroblastic hyperplasia (Fig. 137).

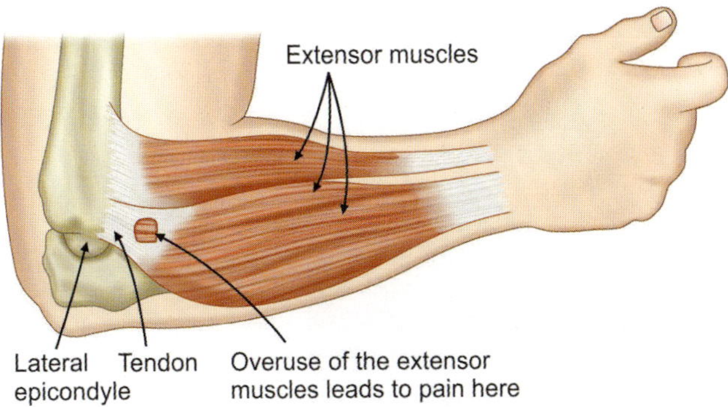

Fig. 136: Mechanism causing tennis elbow.

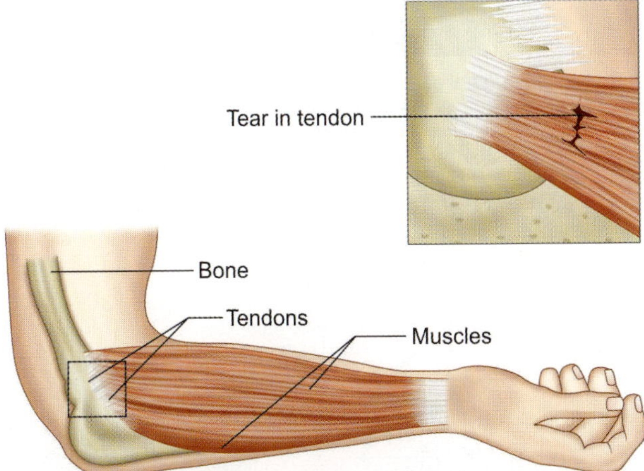

Fig. 137: Diagrammatic representation of microscopic findings show immature reparative tissue that resembles angiofibroblastic hyperplasia.

Pathology

The pathological process mainly involves the origin of the ECRB, but can involve the tendons of the extensor carpi radialis longus and the extensor digitorum communis (EDC).

Diagnosis

The diagnosis of tennis elbow is made by localizing discomfort to the origin of the ECRB. Tenderness is present over the lateral epicondyle approximately 5 mm distal and anterior to the midpoint of the condyle. Pain usually is exacerbated by resisted wrist dorsiflexion and forearm supination.

Thomsen's test or Cozen's test:

Refer text page number 421 and *See* Figure 26.

Investigations

Plain radiographs usually are negative; occasionally, calcific tendinitis may be present. MRI shows tendon thickening (Fig. 138).

Differential Diagnosis

Other entities that can produce pain in this general vicinity are:

- Osteochondritis dissecans of the capitulum
- Lateral compartment arthrosis
- Varus instability
- *Radial tunnel syndrome*: It is a compressive neuropathy of the posterior interosseous nerve caused by any of four different anatomical structures in the radial tunnel, including a fibrous band near the anterior aspect of the radial head, a vascular leash of the recurrent radial artery, the distal ECRB tendon margin, or the supinator margin at the arcade of Frohse.
- The pain of radial tunnel syndrome is located 3–4 cm distal to the lateral epicondyle and may be reproduced with long finger extension against resistance.

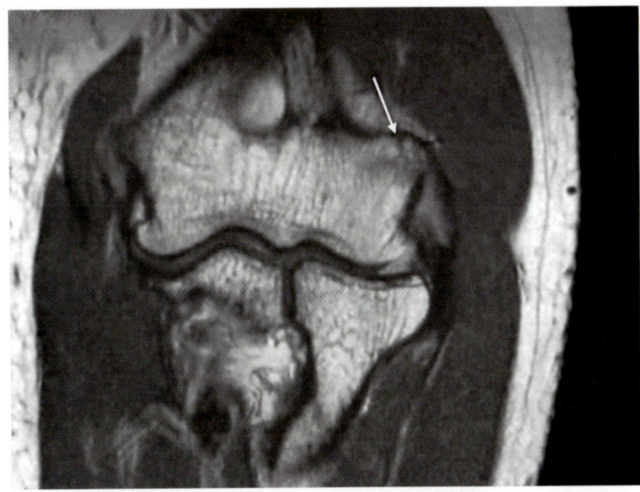

Fig. 138: Arrow showing tendon thickening and bone edema.

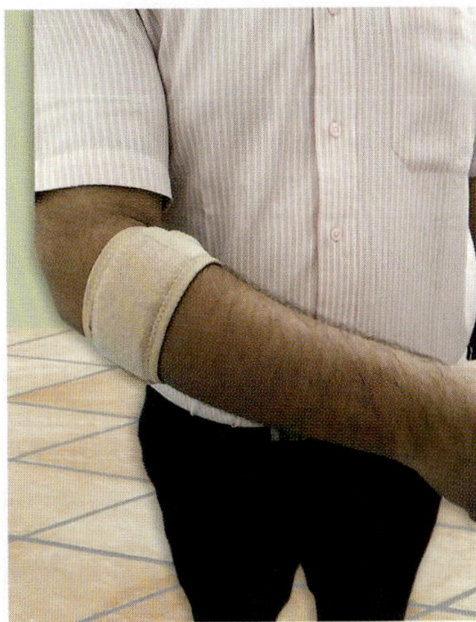

Fig. 139: One or two local injections of a steroid preparation with local anesthetic like lignocaine to the area of maximal tenderness are helpful.

Treatment

Conservative:

- Regardless of the underlying cause, nonoperative treatment is successful in 95% of patients with tennis elbow.
- Initial nonoperative treatment includes rest, ice, injections, and physical therapy with ultrasound, iontophoresis, electrical stimulation, manipulation, soft-tissue mobilization, friction massage, stretching, and strengthening exercises along with counterforce bracing. One or two local injections of a steroid preparation with local anesthetic like lignocaine to the area of maximal tenderness are helpful (Fig. 139).
- If prolonged (6–12 months) nonoperative treatment is ineffective, operative treatment may be considered; it is effective in 90% of properly selected patients.

Surgical treatment:

Numerous surgical procedures have been described for the treatment of tennis elbow:

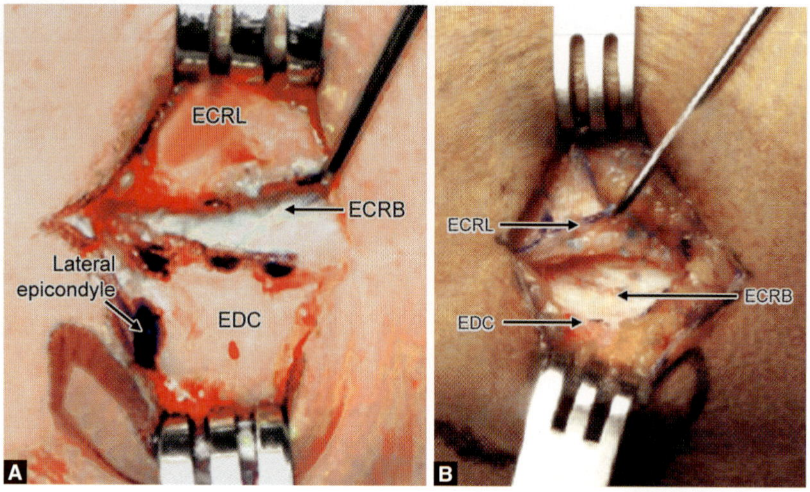

Figs. 140A and B: Tennis elbow according to Nirschl and colleagues. (ECRB: extensor carpi radialis brevis; ECRL: extensor carpi radialis longus; EDC: extensor digitorum communis).

- Mills and, later, Wadsworth advocated manipulation under anesthesia, especially in patients with concomitant flexion contractures. The technique involves sudden, forcible, and full extension of the elbow with the wrist and fingers flexed and the forearm pronated to place the ECRB and extensors under tension. An audible and palpable snap frequently can be elicited.
- Almquist et al. described epicondylar resection with anconeus muscle transfer for chronic lateral epicondylitis.
- Nirschl and colleagues described lateral tennis elbow as angiofibroblastic hyperplasia (AF hyperplasia) of the ECRB and, on occasion, a small area of the anteromedial border of EDC (Figs. 140A and B).
- Make a gently curved incision 5 cm long centered over the lateral epicondyle.
- Incise the deep fascia in line with the incision and retract it. Identify the extensor carpi radialis longus and the origin of the EDC, which partially obscures the origin of the deeper ECRB.
- Elevate the brevis portion of the conjoined tendon at the mid-portion of the lateral epicondyle toward the elbow joint.
- As normal-appearing Sharpey's fibers are elevated, excise abnormal-appearing tendon. The diseased tissue may appear fibrillated and discolored and may contain calcium deposits.
- Decorticate a small area of the lateral epicondyle with a rongeur or osteotome, taking care not to enter the joint and damage the articular cartilage (Fig. 141).
- Suture the remaining normal tendon to the fascia or periosteum, or attach it with nonabsorbable sutures through drill holes in the epicondyle. The use of suture anchors has been reported to be successful in attaching the tendon.
- Close the extensor carpi radialis longus and EDC interval with absorbable sutures. Close the skin incision with subcuticular nylon 4-0 sutures and adhesive strips.
- Apply a dressing and a posterior splint with the elbow in 90° of flexion and palmar flexion.

Rehabilitation

- A long-arm splint that includes the wrist is applied and worn for 7 days.
- The elbow is flexed at 90°. After 7 days, passive range of motion is started and done three times daily by the patient.

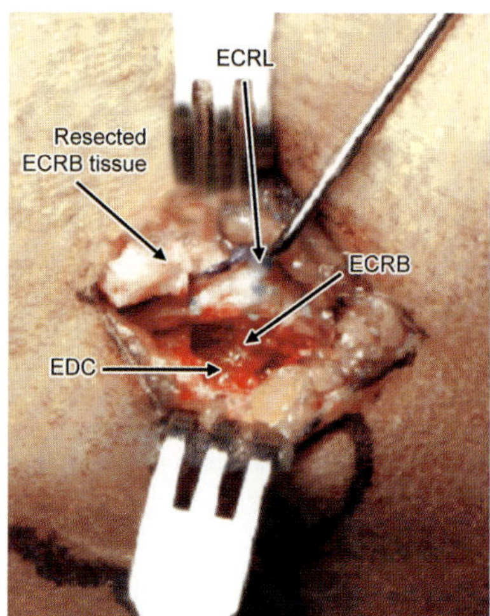

Fig. 141: Decortication of a small area of the lateral epicondyle with a rongeur or osteotome.

- Between the passive exercise periods, the arm is held at rest in a long-arm elbow splint.
- The splint is removed at 4 weeks and the patient begins mild nonresistive ROM exercises, progressing to resistive range of motion at 6 weeks.
- The patient may resume full activities as soon as tolerated, although heavy or strenuous activities should be delayed for 10–12 weeks.
- The rehabilitation protocol is not time dependent, but rather goal dependent, with patients passing from one phase to the next after certain goals have to be met.

Rehabilitation protocol for epicondylitis:

Phase 1—Acute:

- *Goals:*
  - To reduce inflammation and pain
  - To promote tissue healing
  - To retard muscular atrophy.

Phase 2—Subacute:

- *Goals:*
  - To improve flexibility
  - To increase muscular strength and endurance
  - To increase functional activities and return to function.

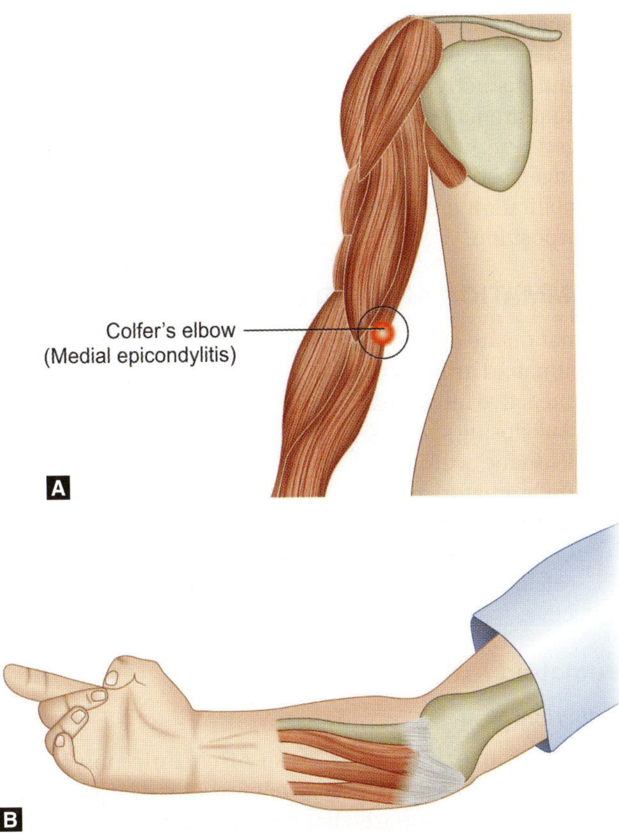

Figs. 142A and B: Golfer's elbow.

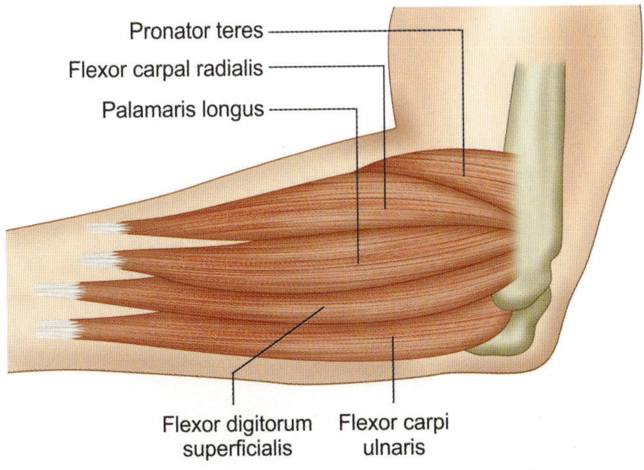

Fig. 143: Common muscles involved in golfer's elbow.

Phase 3—Chronic:

- *Goals:*
  - To improve muscular strength and endurance
  - To maintain and enhance flexibility
  - Gradually return patient to sport or high-level activities.

Golfer's Elbow (Medial Epicondylitis)

Golfer's elbow is shown in Figures 142A and B.

Introduction

- Medial epicondylitis is similar to lateral epicondylitis, although much less common and more difficult to treat.
- The origin of the flexor carpi radialis and pronator teres (flexor pronator mass) are commonly involved and less typically, the flexor digitorum superficialis and flexor carpi ulnaris (Figs. 142 and 143).
- Medial epicondylitis frequently occurs in overhead athletes, including athletes involved in racket sports and others who participate in activities that create a valgus force at the elbow (Figs. 144 and 145).

Clinical Features

- Physical examination usually reveals pain along the medial elbow that becomes worse on resisted forearm pronation or wrist flexion.
- The area of maximal tenderness is approximately 5 mm distal and anterior to the midpoint of the medial epicondyle.
- Loss of range of motion and a flexion contracture may be present.

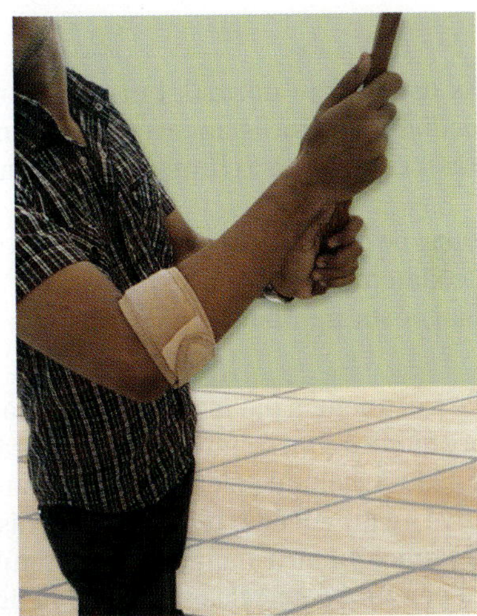

Fig. 144: Medial epicondylitis frequently occurs in activities that create a valgus force at the elbow.

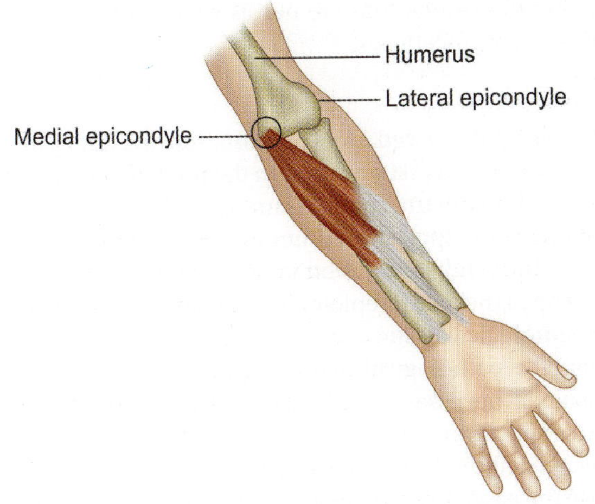

Fig. 145: Medial epicondylitis occurring after a valgus force at the elbow.

Diagnosis

Test for diagnosing golfer's elbow (Fig. 146):

Flex the elbow, supinate the hand, and extend the elbow. Pain over medial epicondyle is definitively suggestive of golfer's elbow.

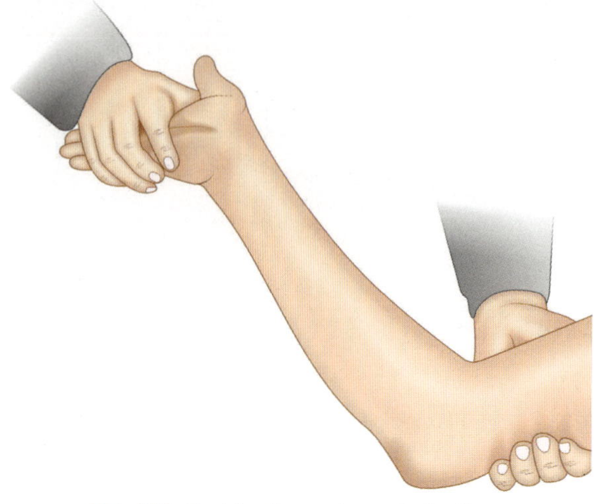

Fig. 146: Test for diagnosing golfer's elbow.

Investigations

- Radiographs usually are normal, but medial ulnar traction spurs and medial collateral ligament calcifications may be seen and may be associated with a chronic ulnar collateral ligament injury.
- This entity must be differentiated from ulnar nerve neuropathy and medial collateral ligament instability.
- MRI is the diagnostic approach.

Treatment

- Conservative treatment is the mainstay of management. Anti-inflammatory medication, splinting, and an occasional steroid injection provide sustained relief in most patients.
- If nonoperative treatment fails, excision of the diseased tendon origin and reattachment usually are successful. Techniques range from a percutaneous release to open debridement with or without release of the flexor pronator origin.
- Vangsness and Jobe described the release of the flexor pronator origin, excision of the pathological tissue, and reattachment of the flexor pronator origin to bleeding bone. Nirschl preferred excising the results that are not as successful as with lateral epicondylar procedures.

Nirschl Technique

- Make a slightly curved 5-cm incision, starting approximately 1 cm proximal and just posterior to the medial epicondyle.
- Retract the subcutaneous tissue and skin over the medial epicondyle to expose the common flexor origin.
- Make a longitudinal incision in the tendon origins, beginning at the tip of the medial epicondyle, distally for 3–4 cm to expose the pathological tissue.
- Excise the pathological tissue elliptically, including the joint capsule, if necessary, while leaving the normal tissue of the attachment to the medial epicondyle intact.
- Close the elliptical defect with absorbable suture.
- Close the subcutaneous tissue with absorbable suture and the skin with a running subcuticular suture.
- Apply a dressing and a posterior splint with the elbow in 90° of flexion.

Rehabilitation

- The splint is removed 1 week after surgery and elbow ROM exercises are initiated.
- Strengthening exercises are started when full ROM is achieved, typically 3 weeks after surgery.
- Strenuous activity can resume when the patient achieves normal strength without pain, which is typically 3 months after surgery.
- A longer period of immobilization and slower progression of rehabilitation are indicated in patients who had ulnar nerve transposition.

INFLAMMATION AROUND ELBOW

Inflammation are of following three types:

1. Rheumatoid arthritis (RA)
2. Seronegative inflammatory arthritis:
   - Ankylosing spondylitis
   - Psoriatic arthritis
   - Inflammatory bowel disease
   - Reactive arthritis (Reiter's syndrome)
   - Crystalline arthropathies (metabolic)—gout, pseudogout, calcium hydroxyapatite crystal arthritis.
3. Infective.

Rheumatoid Arthritis

Introduction

Rheumatoid arthritis is a disease of chronic polyarticular inflammation that leads to joint swelling, joint deformity, loss of joint function, and extra-articular manifestations.

This disease occurs worldwide and has a prevalence of about 0.5–2%.

Etiopathogenesis

- The etiology is unknown
- The genetic predisposition, the involvement of activated immune cells, the clonal expansion of the cells in the pathologic lesions, and the response to immunosuppressive therapy suggest that this disease is immune mediated (*MHC class II DR-4 gene*, people, who are HLA-DRB4 positive, are more likely to develop erosive, disabling disease but only one-third of RA patients are DRB4 positive).
- Nongenetic factors include infections (*Streptococci, Parvovirus, Epstein–Barr virus, Proteus mirabilis*), pregnancy, smoking, and others.
- Endocrinal (adrenocortical steroids)
- Cross-reaction to self-antigens (in synovial tissues) triggers autoimmune response.
- In the early stages, edema, microvascular proliferation, and T-lymphocyte infiltration occur in the subsynovial tissues.
- Followed by synovial lining cell proliferation.
- Synovial infiltration by B-cells, macrophages, and fibroblasts.
- B-cells develop into plasma cells and reside in the synovium chronically, producing *rheumatoid factor*, and leading to complement activation.
- The lymphocytes produce hydrolases, deoxyribonuclease (DNase), and proteinases, which accumulate in the synovial fluid and articular cartilage and lead to destruction of tissues.
- In chronic RA, this proliferative granulation tissue called pannus advances across the joint surface, destroying marginal articular cartilage and invading subchondral bone.
- Pannus attached to the joint capsule, ligament, and tendons results in joint deformity.

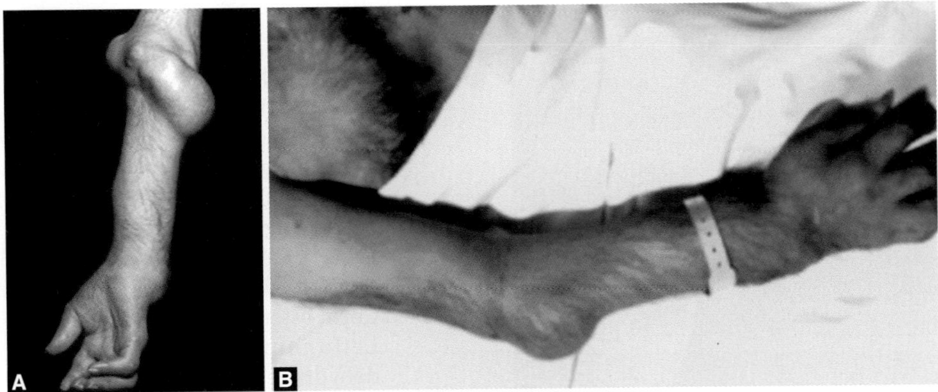

Figs. 147A and B: Clinical features of rheumatoid arthritis.

- Active inflammation is accompanied by attempted repair and collagen production may become dominant, leading to fibrosis and joint contractures.

Clinical Features

Clinical features of RA are shown in Figures 147A and B.

- The presentation of RA can be variable.
- Patients present with a symmetric polyarthritis, and can present with a single joint swelling (21%), a few swollen joints (44%), or a more typical polyarthritis (35%).
- The onset may be acute (days or weeks) in about half of the patients and insidious in the other half.
- The joint reacts to an insult in a limited number of ways (stiffness, pain, tender, swelling, and loss of function).
- Stiffness and pain in the morning, which last for 1 or more hours and improve with low-grade activity.
- The hands and wrist are the most common joints involved. Elbow involvement has been reported in 20–65% of patients with RA.
- The earliest change noted in the elbow is loss of extension.
- There is loss of the groove on either side of the olecranon.
- Large cystic swellings can occur.
- The inflammation in RA goes through intermittent exacerbations and remissions.
- In chronic cases, fatigue, malaise, fever, weight loss, and lymphadenopathy may be present.
- In long-standing cases, nodules may occur, typically along the olecranon border, spine, occiput, Achilles tendon, or extensor surfaces of the hands and feet and other areas are exposed to mechanical pressure.
- Nodules can be observed in tendon sheaths, heart (arrhythmias and heart blocks), lungs (pleural effusion and fibrosis), liver, eyes, and the meninges.

American College of Rheumatology classification criteria for rheumatoid arthritis:

- Morning stiffness in and around joints lasting at least 1 hour.
- Arthritis of three or more joint areas proximal interphalangeal (PIP), MCP, wrist, elbow, knee, ankle, and MTP joints of either or same side.
- Arthritis of joints of the hands, at least one joint area is involved.
- Symmetric arthritis symmetric involvement of the two sides (PIP, MCP, and MTP joint involvements do not require absolute symmetry).
- Rheumatoid nodules observed by a physician.
- Serum rheumatoid factor in levels above the normal population.
- X-ray changes should include typical erosions and/or juxta-articular osteoporosis.

Criteria for diagnosis:

- *Classic*: Any seven criteria for at least 6 weeks
- *Definite*: Any five criteria for at least 6 weeks
- *Probable*: Any three criteria for at least 4 weeks.

Routine Investigations

- Anemia
- Raised erythrocyte sedimentation rate (ESR)
- C-reactive protein (CRP) is positive in active inflammatory stages
- Increased serum alkaline phosphatase
- Decreased serum albumin
- Increased platelets
- Serological
- Renal function (RF) tests are positive in about 80% of patients with RA
- Positive antinuclear antibody (ANA) occurs in 40%
- Anticitrullinated cyclic peptide (anti-CCP) antibody can be positive early in RA when the rheumatoid factor is negative.
- *Synovial fluid analysis*:
  - Sugar—normal
  - Proteins—slightly decreased
  - Increased counts
  - Positive rheumatoid factor
- Histology (Fig. 148)
- Lymphoid proliferation
- Inflammatory granulation tissue (pannus)
- Pannus invades into articular cartilage, subchondral region
- X-ray (Fig. 149)
- Juxta-articular osteoporosis
- Erosion of joint margin
- Joint space is decreased
- Deformities of joints
- Subchondral erosion and cyst formation
- Fibrous and bony ankylosis develops in late stages.

Criteria for Diagnosis

- Morning stiffness
- Pain on motion or tenderness in at least one joint
- Swelling (soft-tissue thickening or fluid; not bony outgrowth alone) in at least one joint continuously for not less than 6 weeks

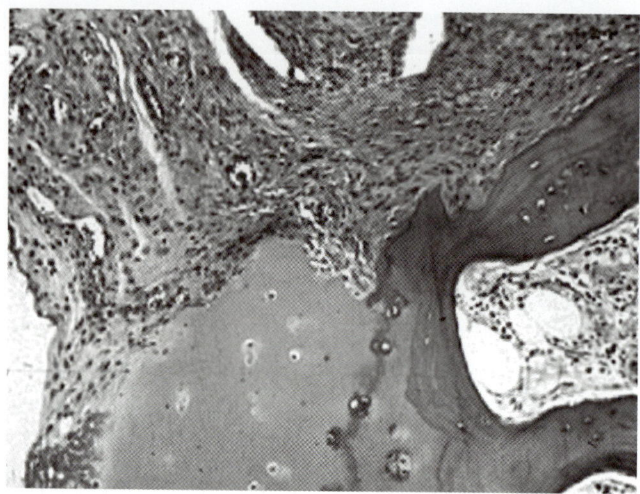

Fig. 148: Histology.

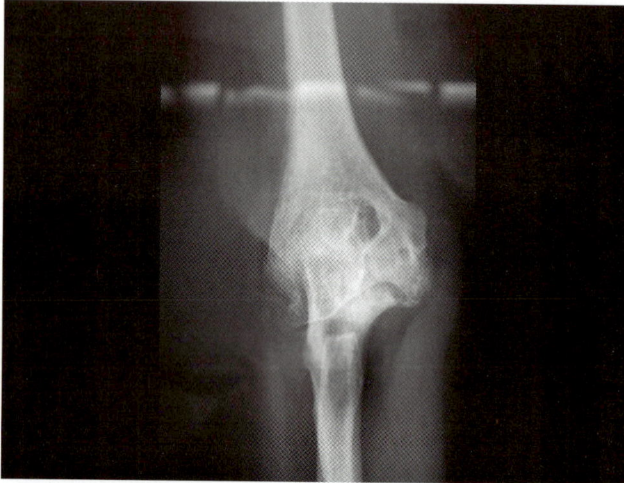

Fig. 149: X-ray showing rheumatoid arthritis.

- Swelling of at least one other joint
- Symmetrical joint swelling
- Subcutaneous nodules
- X-ray changes typical of RA
- Positive latex fixation test
- Poor mucin clot
- Characteristic histological changes in synovial membrane
- Characteristic histological changes in nodules.

Management

Aims of treatment:

- To keep inflammatory treatment to minimum
- To keep constitutional symptoms to minimum
- Appropriate splinting to prevent deformities
- Surgical measures to correct deformity.

Circumstances in which a more aggressive clinical course of RA should be suspected:

- Positive rheumatoid factor and anti-CCP antibodies in high titer
- Elevated inflammatory markers (ESR and CRP)
- Presence of shared epitope alleles (HLA-DRB1*0401 and HLA-DRB1*0404)
- Presence of bony erosions (plain X-rays or MRI)
- Degree of functional disability.

Drug therapy:

- *Analgesics and anti-inflammatory*: NSAIDs—aspirin/ibuprofen/diclofenac sodium
- *Disease-modifying antirheumatic drugs (DMARDs)*:
  - Injectable gold and oral gold (sodium aurothiomalate)
  - D-penicillamine (T-cell suppressor)
  - Sulfasalazine antimalarials (interference with antigen processing)
  - Dapsone and levamisole
  - Methotrexate (inhibits dihydrofolate reductase)
  - Corticosteroids
  - Leflunomide inhibits the enzyme dihydroorotate dehydrogenase, thus leading to inhibition of pyrimidine synthesis. This inhibition, in turn, inhibits both T-cell and B-cell function.
- *Immunomodulators*:
  - Etanercept and anakinra.
- Physiotherapy and occupational therapy
- *Surgery*:
  - Synovectomy
  - Osteotomy
  - Arthrodesis
  - Arthroplasty.

Seronegative Inflammatory Arthritis

- It refers to a group of conditions in which clinical evidence of noninfectious and active inflammation is noted in the joints, but serum autoantibodies, such as rheumatoid factor (RF) or anticyclic citrullinated peptide antibodies (anti-CCP), are absent.
- They present with pain, limited motion and swelling of the affected joint, in the absence of trauma.

They are classified for descriptive propose as:

- *Spondyloarthropathies:*
  - Ankylosing spondylitis
  - Inflammatory bowel disease
  - Psoriatic arthritis
  - Reactive arthritis (Reiter's syndrome).
- *Crystalline arthropathies:*
  - Gout
  - Pseudogout
  - Calcium hydroxyapatite crystal arthritis.

Spondyloarthropathies

- They share an increased prevalence of the HLA class I B-27.
- Classically, the spondyloarthropathies manifest as an inflammatory arthritis of the spine and sacroiliac joints, but an asymmetric peripheral arthritis can occur.
- A key clinical feature distinguishing SpA from RA is the presence of *enthesitis* (inflammation that is located at the sites of ligamentous insertion into bone, such as the Achilles tendon or plantar fascia).
  - Clinical differences between spondyloarthropathies and rheumatoid arthritis.

Elbow involvement in spondyloarthropathies (Table 3):

Management:

- NSAIDs reduce pain and inflammation
- Synovial fluid aspiration and local corticosteroid injection
- Systemic corticosteroid therapy in severe cases and extra-articular involvement

TABLE 3: Elbow involvement in spondyloarthropathies.

Spondyloarthropathy	*Frequency of elbow involvement*
Ankylosing spondylitis	12%
Psoriatic arthritis	25%
Inflammatory bowel disease	35%
Reactive arthritis	Uncommon

- Sulfasalazine and methotrexate
- Anti-tumor necrosis factor (TNF) therapy (etanercept, infliximab, and adalimumab) in severe cases.
- Cutaneous psoriasis frequently responds to topical preparations and especially well to weekly pulse methotrexate.

Crystalline Arthropathies

- Crystalline arthropathies are a group of inflammatory arthritides, which are associated with crystal deposition in the synovial space.
- Patients frequently present with an acute painful monoarthritis, which often is indistinguishable from septic arthritis.

Gout:

- It is metabolic disorder, manifesting in the primary and secondary forms, and characterized by hyperuricemia and joint lesions.
- Gout is a common condition associated with the deposition of monosodium urate (MSU) crystals in the synovial fluid, synovial tissue, and surrounding soft tissues. MSU crystals are by-products of an aberrant uric acid metabolism.

Etiopathogenesis:

- The actual cause is unknown
- Hereditary
- Risk factors for gout include hypertension, renal insufficiency, obesity, type 2 diabetes mellitus, ethanol intake, lead exposure, and use of diuretics, particularly thiazide diuretics.
- *Age:* 2nd and 4th decade
- *Sex:* Males are more affected
- Adrenocortical insufficiency (ACTH precipitates attacks)
  Secondary gout—it occurs due to renal insufficiency, hematological disturbances, etc.
- MSU crystals deposited in articular cartilage
- The crystals enter the joint space and synovial fluid
- They erode the cartilage and subchondral bone leading to punched out lesions
- Urate crystals stimulate inflammatory reactions resulting in further damage
- Crystals are deposited in synovium and other soft tissues like bursa and subcutaneous tissue forming tophi.
- Elbow is involved in 17–33% cases of gout.

Clinical features:

- It occurs mostly in men, in 3rd or 4th decade
- The condition may present clinically as an acute attack or chronic gout
- The most commonly affected joint in gout is the MCP joint of big toe
- The attack is characterized by sudden onset of excruciating pain at night with marked swelling and redness of joint of big toe.

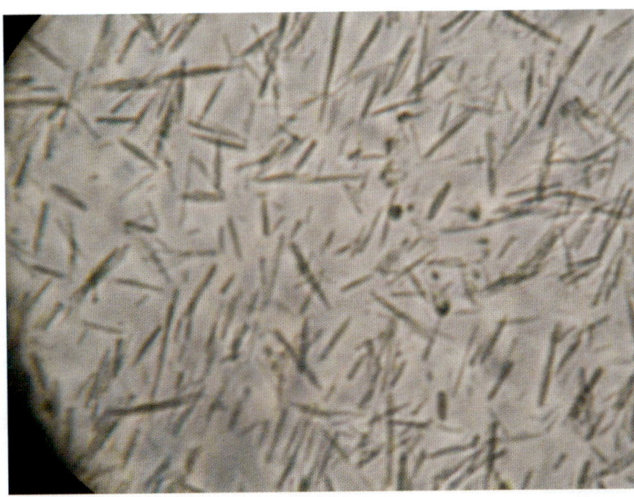

Fig. 150: Needle-shaped negatively birefringent monosodium urate (MSU) crystals.

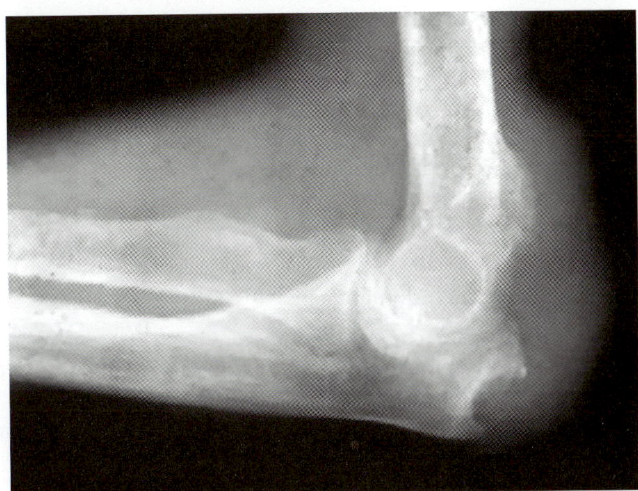

Fig. 151: X-ray showing gout of elbow joint.

- The attack may subside in a week.
- The arthritis shows remission and exacerbation and gradually becomes chronic.
- In chronic stage, there is deposition of urate salts in the juxta-articular tissue of the involved joint or the subcutaneous tissue of the ear or in olecranon bursa.
- These lumps are called gouty tophi.
- After certain attacks, the joint develops features of secondary osteoarthritis.

Laboratory investigations:

- *Raised ESR:*
  - Leukocytosis
  - Raised serum uric acid (>7 mg/dL), sometimes the levels may be normal
  - Synovial fluid analysis
- Needle-shaped negatively birefringent MSU crystals (Fig. 150)
- Synovial membrane shows deposition of crystals, leukocyte infiltration with crystals, and occasional pannus formation.
- X-ray (Fig. 151)
- In chronic stage, the characteristic punched out appearance of the periphery of the articular cartilage in the metatarsophalangeal joints.

- Tophi may be seen as radiopaque shadow in the juxta-articular tissue.
- In late stages, degenerative changes with narrowing of joint space and sclerosis.

Treatment:
- Anti-inflammatory drugs like indomethacin in high doses are given
- Colchicine is the specific drug for acute gout. It is both analgesic and diuretic. Its dose is 1 mg/2 hourly.
- Uricosuric drugs like probenecid are given in conjunction with colchicine, dose is 0.5–1 g daily.
- Allopurinol is given to inhibit the synthesis of uric acid. Dose is 300 mg daily.
- Surgical procedures for excision of tophaceous deposits can be done.

Pseudogout:

It is a form of arthritis due to deposition of crystals of calcium pyrophosphate dihydrate (CPPD) in the synovium or the articular cartilage or menisci.

Clinically, the acute attack resembles gout but the serum uric acid is normal.

Synovial fluid analysis shows positively birefringent CPPD crystals, which are rhomboid shaped and exhibit positive birefringence undercompensated polarized light, appearing blue. The condition responds to indomethacin.

Radiograph shows calcified spots in articular cartilage (Fig. 152).

Treatment:
- NSAIDs
- Responds well to indomethacin.

Hydroxyapatite crystal deposition disease:
- It may present as primary crystal-induced arthropathy or secondary to trauma or degenerative joint disease.
- Hydroxyapatite crystals are deposited in soft tissue of joint space, rotator cuff tendons, or bursa.
- Shoulder and knee are commonly involved.
- Hydroxyapatite crystals are nonbirefringent
- Radiologically, the disease appears as radiopaque calcification in a local tumor mass like fashion.
- Treatment is with NSAIDs, colchicine and oral as well as intra-articular corticosteroids with physiotherapy.
- Large tumor mass-like deposits may sometime need excision.

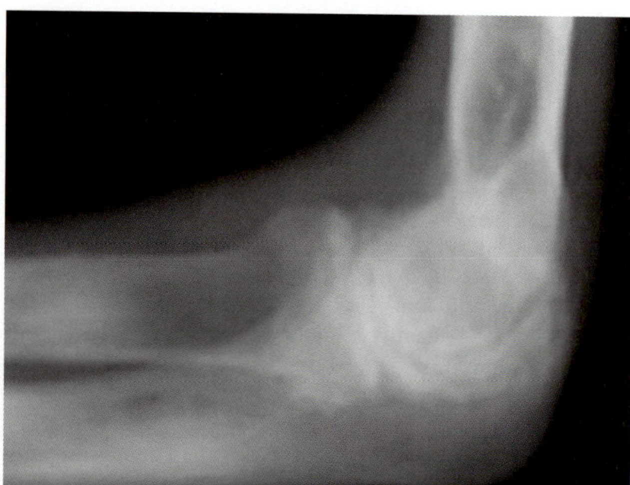

Fig. 152: X-ray showing calcified spots in articular surfaces.

Infections

- Osteomyelitis
- Septic arthritis
- Septic olecranon bursitis
- *Bone infection occurs:*
  - Hematogenously
  - By direct inoculation after open fracture or surgery
  - By contiguous spread from a local process.

Hematogenous Infections

- Hematogenous infection is the most common type of osteomyelitis.
- In the growing child, the end-arterial loop of the metaphyseal bone causes sluggish bone blood flow. The lack of phagocytic activity in these loops allows maturation of a septic thrombus at the arterial site. The abscess spreads through the Haversian system into the subperiosteal space.
- As the metaphysis is not intra-articular in the elbow, the abscess does not spread to the joint.
- Acute hematogenous osteomyelitis is most common in children younger than 3 years and older than 7 years of age.
- The first group is vulnerable owing to the lack of acquired host immunity; the second age group corresponds to the time of rapid growth.
- Elbow is involved in 8% of the cases.
- The most common pathogen causing acute hematogenous osteomyelitis is *Staphylococcus aureus*.
- Opportunistic organisms are isolated in the debilitated patient and *Pseudomonas aeruginosa* is most commonly associated with drug addiction or chronic draining wounds.

Direct Inoculation

- Direct inoculation is a relatively common cause of infection of the elbow joint.
- The thin soft tissue coverage predisposes to compound fractures that may become secondarily infected.
- Elective nonprosthetic surgery of the elbow region has been associated with an infection rate of about 2–4%, significantly greater than the commonly quoted 1% for elective orthopedic procedures.

Spread from a Contagious Focus

- Infection, spread from a contiguous focus, occurs at the elbow from a septic joint or from an infected olecranon bursa.
- These circumstances are most commonly noted in a patient with RA.

Clinical Features and Diagnosis

- Local pain, warmth and swelling
- Irritability, restlessness, headache, vomiting, convulsion, chills, and fever.
- In children, a predisposing and traumatic event is common, remote septic foci identification is difficult.
- Afebrile in a few cases.
- Overlying skin becomes shiny, red, and edematous.
- Discharging sinus may be present.
- The elbow is held in flexion and pseudoparalysis or reflex inhibition may be present.

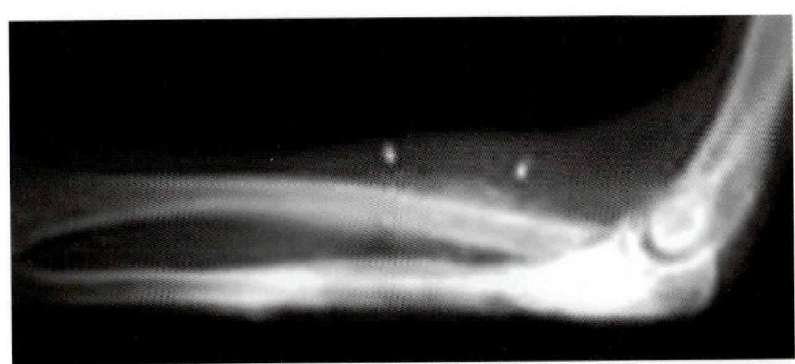

Fig. 153: Plain X-ray.

Physical Examination

- The specific point of maximal tenderness should be determined by gentle palpation. The focus of the septic process can often be accurately localized in this way, even before radiographic changes are apparent.
- Gentle passive motion of the joint should be done. With joint infections, all motion is resisted; with metaphyseal osteomyelitis, gentle and supported passive motion is possible.

Laboratory Studies

- Complete blood count, including differential and erythrocyte sedimentation rate, is a more sensitive tool raised in about 80% cases (markedly raised in joint infections than bone).
- C-reactive protein.
- Blood culture.
- Pus culture sensitivity.
- Synovial fluid analysis (if joint infection is suspected).
- Plain X-ray is not helpful in early detection. After 7–14 days, osteoporosis may be present, which is followed by periosteal elevation or erosions (Fig. 153).
- Computed tomography scan helps to document the presence of sequestra.
- Magnetic resonance imaging, for detection of the septic process, is most helpful to determine the extent of damage.
- Bone scan (99mTc).
- Leukocyte scanning technique.
- Ultrasonography is an effective and noninvasive method to assess soft-tissue involvement.
- Polymerase chain reaction (PCR).

Treatment

- Prolonged immobilization is to be strictly avoided. In the acute phase of treatment, the joint should be splinted, elevated, and put to rest. As the process resolves, gentle active motion is encouraged as soon as possible. Continuous passive motion may prove to be beneficial in some patients to avoid ankylosis or adhesions.
- In cases that are diagnosed early, antibiotics alone may be adequate.
- Surgery is indicated when there is no response to parenteral antibiotic therapy after 36–48 hours.
- Intravenous antibiotics should be continued for about 3 weeks. Oral agents can be used for an additional 4 weeks.
- Infection involving bone may become subacute or chronic; and in this instance, incision and drainage with limited bone debridement and secondary soft-tissue healing may be necessary.
- An extensive debridement of bone severely impairs function because the joint becomes dysfunctionally unstable.
- If soft-tissue coverage is a problem, the flexor carpi ulnaris muscle pedicle flap may be used for coverage of the proximal ulna and elbow. Flap brings improved blood supply as well as soft tissue coverage.

Septic Arthritis of the Elbow

- Elbow septic arthritis occurs in 12–18% diagnosed cases of septic joints.
- Peak incidence is at extremes of life.
- The frequent association of elbow septic arthritis with RA is well recognized.
- About 33% of septic joints in patients with RA are involved the elbow.
- *Staphylococcus aureus* is more common (60–80%), *Streptococcus* (20%), *Pneumococcus* (10%), *Gonococcus, Escherichia coli,* and *Haemophilus influenzae* is common in children less than 2 years of age.
- *Predisposing factors*: Trauma, diabetes, steroid therapy, malignancy, HIV (drug addicts and hemophilics), etc.

Routes of Entry

- Primary focus is in respiratory system, GIT, urinary system, etc.
- Pyogenic osteomyelitis
- Punctured wound
- Pneumonia, typhoid, etc.
- Primary focus in joint.

Pathogenesis

- The presence of bacteria in the joint initiates local reaction.
- The synovial membrane becomes hyperemic and edematous and proliferates.
- Infiltration by the leukocytes, producing mediators of inflammation and proteolytic enzymes.
- The articular cartilage and bones are destroyed leading to fibrosis and ankylosis.

Clinical Features

- Constitutional symptoms are chills, fever, sweats, malaise, anorexia, and in infants refusal to feeds, vomiting, etc.
- Pain gradually increases in intensity over several hours and becomes excruciating.
- Pain accentuates on movement of joints and thus limits the movement.
- Swelling and redness around elbow.
- Local raise in temperature and tenderness present.
- The patient holds the limb in position of maximum capacity to reduce the intra-articular pressure and thus minimizes pain (50–80° of flexion).
- White blood cells (WBCs) (polymorphs 80%) are raised to 50,000–100,000.
- Erythrocyte sedimentation rate is raised.
- Hemoglobin (Hb) is decreased.
- Blood culture is positive in 35–50% of cases.
- C-reactive protein is positive.
- *Synovial fluid aspiration* is critical for diagnosing and treatment of septic arthritis (Figs. 154A and B).
- X-ray shows increased joint space (ballooning), anterior or posterior fat pad sign, juxta-articular osteopenia, articular

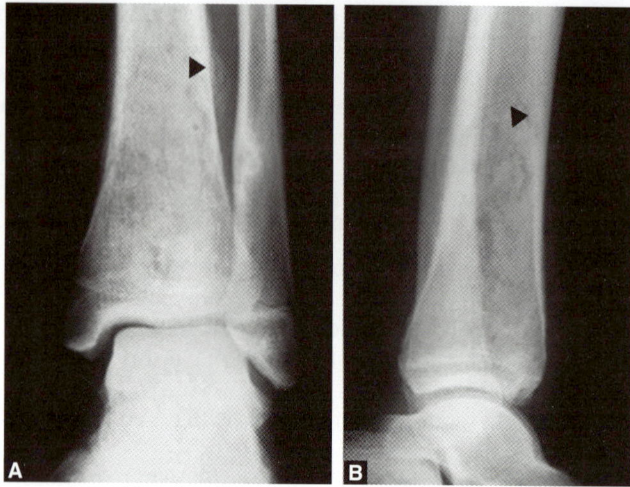

Figs. 154A and B: X-ray showing periosteal reaction.

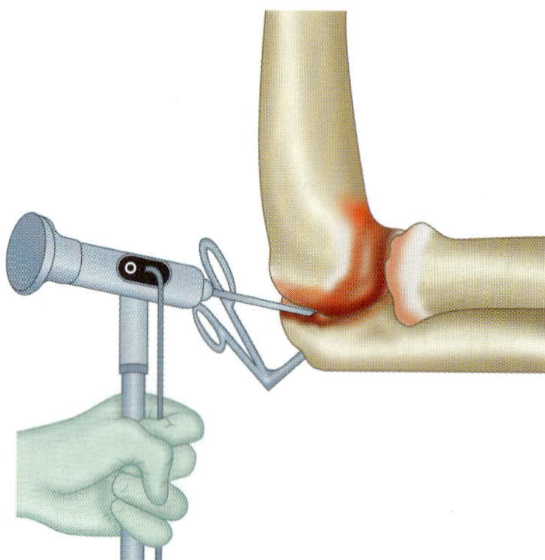

Fig. 155: Arthroscopic debridement.

cartilage destruction, and fibrous and bony ankylosis in later stages.
- Gallium or labeled white cell scans may be more specific than technetium scans.
- Magnetic resonance imaging lacks the specificity of distinguishing septic from nonseptic fluid but can assist in the diagnosis of a contiguous osteomyelitis.

Treatment

- Initial specific antibiotic treatment is first based on the gram stain.
- Immobilization in initial period with splint/slab. Early mobilization is recommended.
- If infection is suspected and no organism is isolated, initial antibiotic treatment should be based on age and presentation.
- In initial stages, joint fluid aspiration and lavage are followed by local antibiotic (cefazolin) injection.
- Arthroscopic/arthrotomy debridement is done in those who are not responding immediately to the initial aspiration, lavage, and antibiotic injection.
- Infections that are subacute, postoperative, or due to direct inoculation, adequate clearance by aspiration is not reliable and drainage by arthroscopy is preferred (Fig. 155).

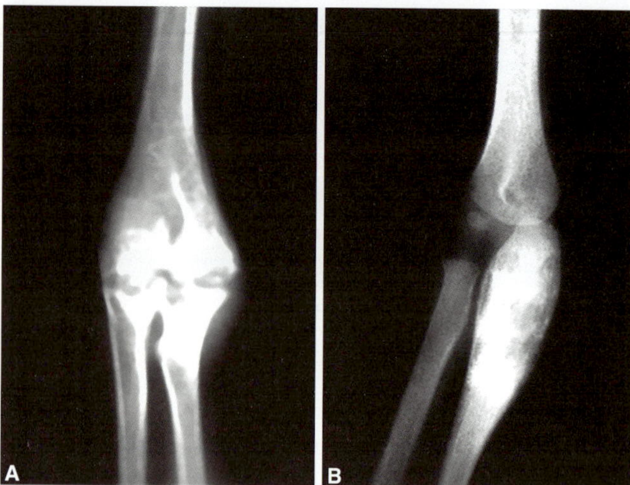

Figs. 156A and B: Radiology.

- If extra-articular involvement is present, arthrotomy may be necessary, so that early motion may begin.

Early motion helps in:
- Preventing adhesions and pannus
- Improving nutrition of cartilage
- Enhancing clearance of exudates including lysosomal enzymes
- Stimulating the living chondrocytes.

Tuberculosis of Elbow

Introduction

Tuberculosis of the elbow is rare and constitutes nearly 2–5% of all skeletal tuberculosis.
The sites are:
- Olecranon
- Humerus
- Synovium of radius
- Pulmonary tuberculosis is present in only about half of the cases
- Atypical *Mycobacterium* infection, e.g. *Mycobacterium kansasii*, may also occur, both from direct inoculation and from lung involvement, and may become slowly progressive over many years.

Clinical Features

- Pain
- Swelling
- Limitation of movements
- Wasting of arm and forearm muscles
- Lymphadenopathy
- Sinus.

Radiology (Figs. 156 A and B)

- Destruction commonly in olecranon/humerus
- Generalized demineralization and fuzziness of joint margins
- Articular cartilage is usually spared
- Subperiosteal new bone formation on the ulna, resembling spina ventosa or humerus
- Pathological posterior dislocation.

Treatment

- Chemotherapy is the mainstay of treatment.
- Plaster in 90° of flexion and mid-prone position of the forearm is advisable.

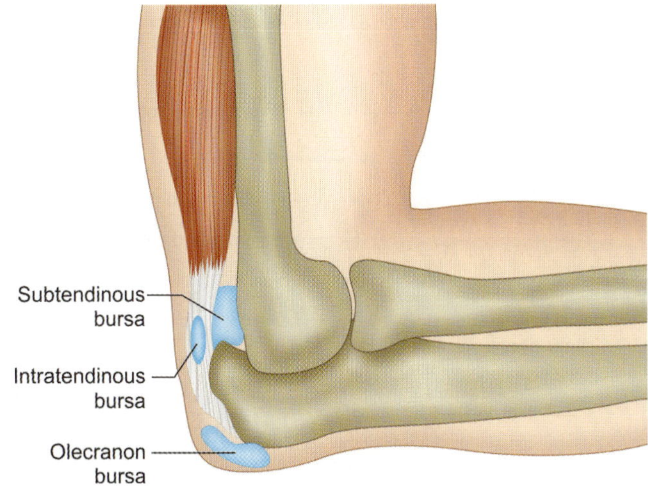

Fig. 157: Olecranon bursitis.

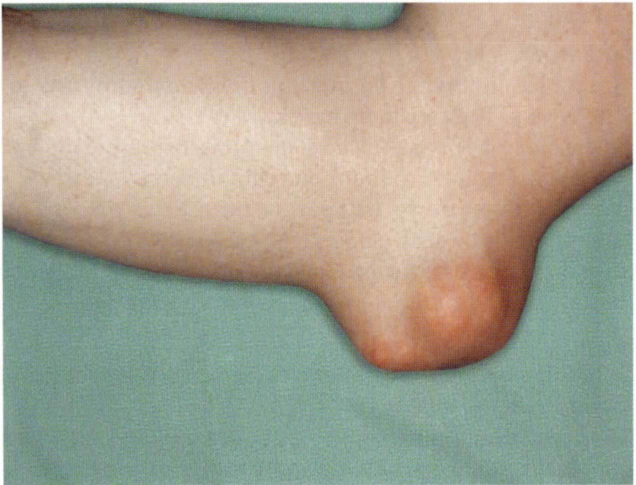

Fig. 158: Distended olecranon bursa.

- As pain reliefs, splint is advisable for 6–9 months.
- For residual dysfunction, synovectomy with or without radial head excision.
- Excision arthroplasty in advanced arthritis/ankylosis.
- Rarely, arthrodesis of elbow is justified for heavy manual work.

Nonbacterial Infections

- Coccidioidomycosis caused by *Coccidioides immitis* has been reported in the elbow infections.
- The treatment recommended is synovectomy with intravenous amphotericin B for the disseminated disease.

Bursitis

- Olecranon bursitis (Fig. 157) is the most commonly involved site followed by the bicipital radial bursa. Inflamed medial epicondylar bursa is associated with chronic subluxation of the ulnar nerve.
- Olecranon bursa is not present at birth and has been shown to develop after the 7th year.
- Olecranon bursitis is caused by a number of pathologic conditions that are traumatic (overuse or direct impact), inflammatory (RA, gout, or pseudogout), infectious, or noninfectious.
- It has been associated with dialysis in the ipsilateral extremity.
- Inflammation of the superficial olecranon bursa can also result from direct trauma or repetitive stress—*miner's elbow* or *student's elbow*.
- Use of anticoagulants increases the possibility of hemobursitis.

Clinical presentation:

- A distended olecranon bursa is usually painless unless it is associated with a septic or crystalline inflammatory process (Fig. 158).
- The bursa may rupture and dissect proximally, presenting as triceps swelling.
- In patients with RA, the bursa may also communicate with the joint, dissect anteriorly and distally into the forearm or even rupture, and present as a subcutaneous fullness over the subcutaneous border of the ulna.
- When the bursitis is symptomatic, flexing elbow to more than 90° causes most symptoms (Fig. 159).
- In acute septic olecranon bursitis, diffuse swelling is noted about the distal arm and the proximal forearm.

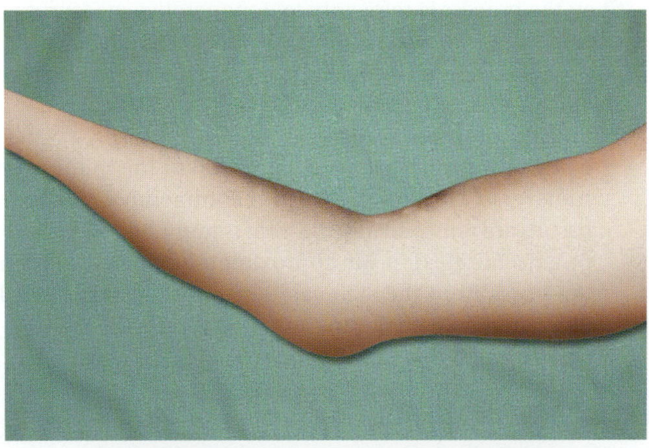

Fig. 159: In symptomatic bursitis, elbow cannot be flexed to more than 90°.

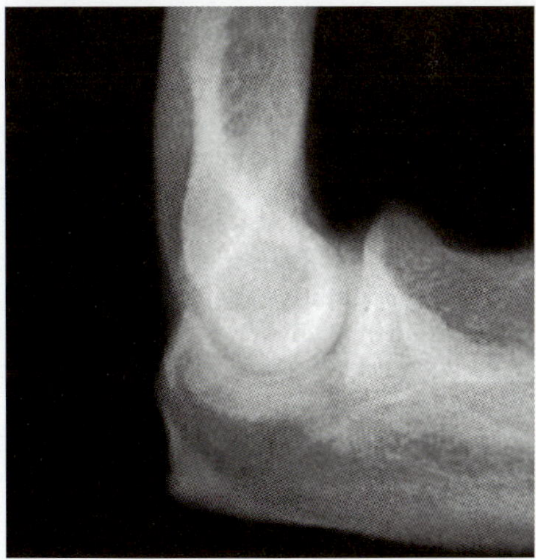

Fig. 160: X-ray showing olecranon spur in chronic cases.

Laboratory investigations:

- Raised ESR in septic and inflammatory conditions
- Synovial fluid aspiration
- Crystals
- In subacute and chronic nonspecific cases, total leukocyte count (TLC) is 800–900 cells (monocyte predominance)
- X-ray olecranon spur in chronic cases, punched out bony erosions in gout (Fig. 160).

Treatment

Acute bursitis:

- Control of any underlying systemic or inflammatory process is the obvious first step in treatment.
- If the bursa is not painful, local measures to prevent injury are all that is required (splinting and compression).
- Acute traumatic or idiopathic bursitis is also treated symptomatically with elbow pads.
- If pain in the bursa prevents daily or occupational activity, aspiration and corticosteroid injection are indicated.

Chronic bursitis:

- Chronic recurrent or painful olecranon bursitis may require more definitive measures.
- A 16-gauge indwelling needle/suction irrigation system, which maintains drainage with a compressive dressing for about 3 days, has been cited as being effective in reducing recurrence of bursal swelling.
- When the process is refractory to nonoperative measures and is interfering with occupational or daily activities, operative intervention should be considered.
- *Operative*:
  - Endoscopic procedures
  - *Open:* A longitudinal incision medial to the midline or a transverse incision has been recommended. All bursal tissues are removed and the joint is immobilized in flexion or extreme flexion for approximately 2 weeks. Freeing the bursa from the skin can devitalize the skin over the olecranon process or can cause problems with healing. Quayle and Robinson method (Figs. 161A and B).

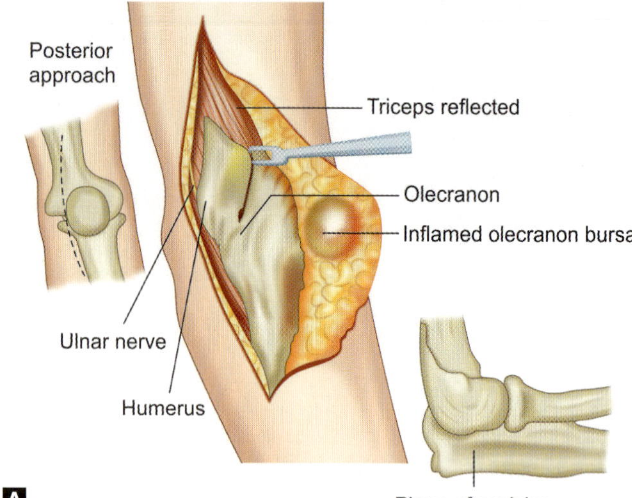

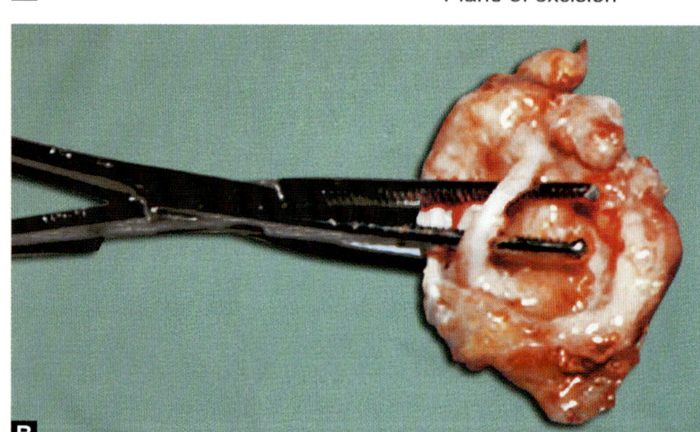

Figs. 161A and B: Quayle and Robinson method.

ELBOW ARTHRODESIS

Introduction

- It is designed to produce bony ankylosis of a diseased joint. It often is a satisfactory solution for infection, tumors, trauma, paralytic conditions, and for certain patients with osteoarthritis and RA.
- Arthrodesis often results in stiffness in adjacent joints; and in the lower extremity, energy requirements for ambulation usually are increased.
- Arthrodesis can be intra-articular, extra-articular, or combined.
- Extra-articular techniques are especially useful in treating children, since much of children's joint surfaces are cartilage and in treating patients who have large amounts of necrotic bone or active infection, as in tuberculosis.
- Intra-articular techniques permit greater correction of deformity and are satisfactory, if adequate areas of healthy bone surfaces can be apposed.
- If adequate bone is not available locally, bone grafts, preferably autogenous and cancellous bone, should be added.

Indications

- Reserved for patients with *painful arthritis* who are not candidates for total elbow arthroplasty, especially those who place high demands on the upper extremities, such as manual laborers.
- Persistent infection, including tuberculosis, which historically was the main indication for this procedure.
- Severely comminuted intra-articular fractures of the distal humerus are not amenable to repair and may be indicated *after failed total elbow arthroplasty*.
- Bilateral elbow arthrodesis is rarely indicated because of resultant functional limitations. If indicated, one elbow should be placed in 110° of flexion to permit the patient to reach the mouth and the other should be placed in 65° to aid in personal hygiene.
- Unilateral elbow arthrodesis is to be performed *with 90° of flexion at the elbow*, although many surgeons simulate the position of arthrodesis by splints before actual surgery.

Technique

Technique shown by Steindler (Fig. 162)

- Posterolateral incision from a point 10 cm above the elbow to a point 2.5 cm below the olecranon.
- Dissect the triceps tendon from its insertion on the olecranon process.
- Then excise the articular cartilage of the semilunar notch of the olecranon and the trochlear surface of the humerus and "fish scale" the subchondral bone.
- Before entering the elbow, obtain a graft from the upper half of the tibia, approximately 1.5 cm wide and 9 cm long.
- With the elbow in flexion, fit the graft into the olecranon cleft and then, after extending the elbow to the position of fusion, place it in its humeral bed.

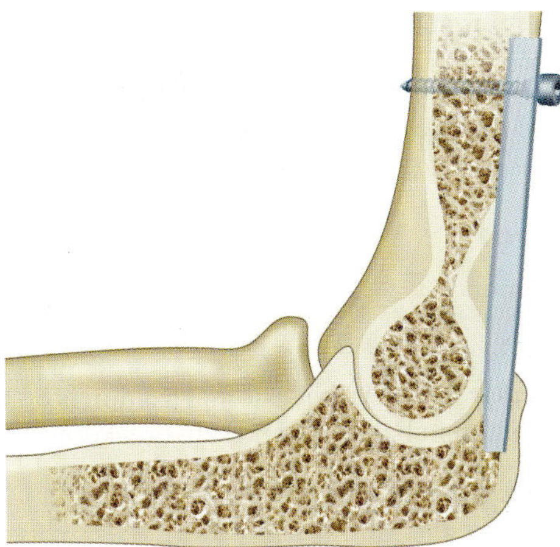

Fig. 162: Steindler technique.

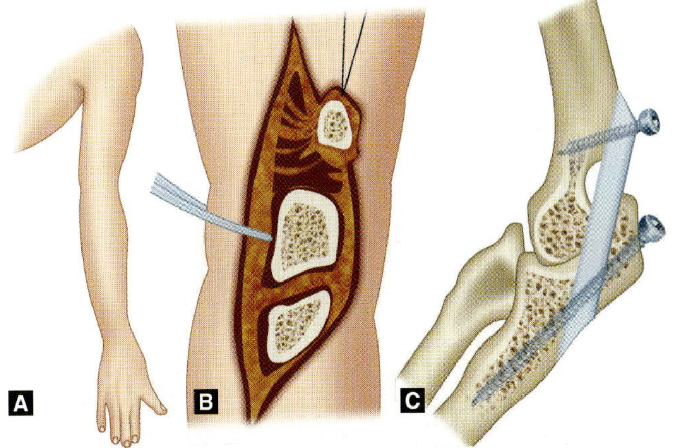

Figs. 164A to C: Technique shown by Staples.

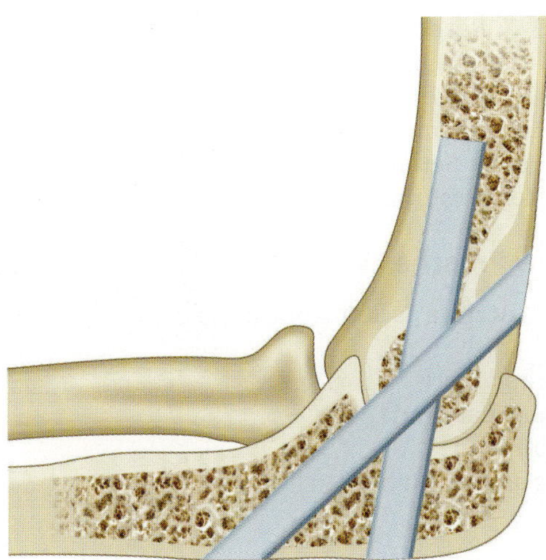

Fig. 163: Technique shown by Brittain.

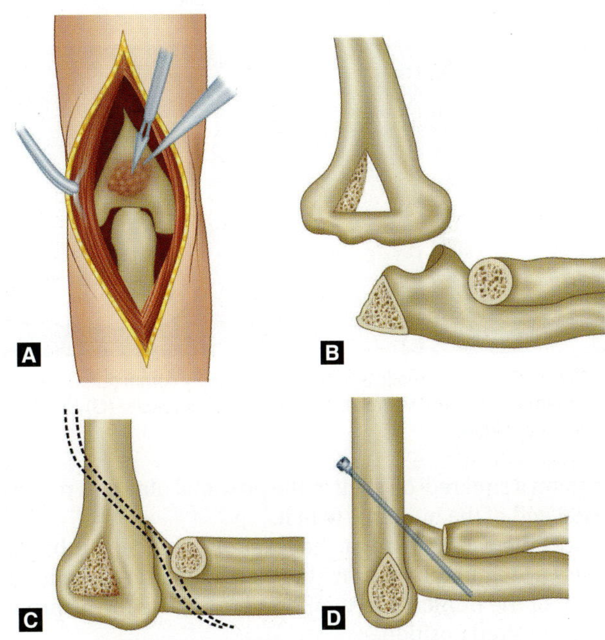

Figs. 165A to D: Technique shown by Arafiles.

- Insert one or two screws through the graft into the humerus to make it secure and pack the ulnohumeral joint with cancellous bone from the proximal end of the tibia.
- After treatment (Steindler).
- Above-elbow cast with forearm in neutral rotation for 8 weeks.
- Corset till osseous union.

Technique shown by Brittain (Fig. 163)

- Two tibial grafts crossed in shape of letter "X"
- No important anatomical structure encountered
- Considerable latitude possible as elbow in flexion, the vessels and nerves in cubital fossa displaced forward.

Technique shown by Staples (Figs. 164A to C)

- Posterior longitudinal incision and isolate and retract the ulnar nerve. Osteotomize the olecranon.
- Denude the elbow joint of cartilage and cut the distal posterior surface of the humerus. Pack iliac bone chips in the joint.
- Anchor the graft above with one screw. Then replace the olecranon process and fasten it with a second screw that passes through the olecranon and the lower end of the graft and into the upper end of the ulna.

Technique shown by Arafiles (Figs. 165A to D)

- Technique for fusion in tuberculous arthritis of elbow.
- Isolation of ulnar nerve, splitting and release of triceps tendon from olecranon and posterior synovectomy.
- Excision of radial head and anterior synovectomy; shaping of olecranon and creation of triangular hole through distal end of humerus.
- Insertion of olecranon through hole in distal end of humerus, screw fixation, medial and lateral epicondylectomy, and anterior transposition of ulnar nerve. Resulting bone chips are used to fill any ground stump of olecranon.
- Completed fusion with screw fixation.
- After treatment (Arafiles).
- The elbow is immobilized in a long-arm cast for 3 months and in a removable splint for another month.
- Hand and shoulder exercises are begun soon after surgery.

Technique shown by Müller et al. (Fig. 166)

- Expose the elbow posteriorly as described in previous techniques.

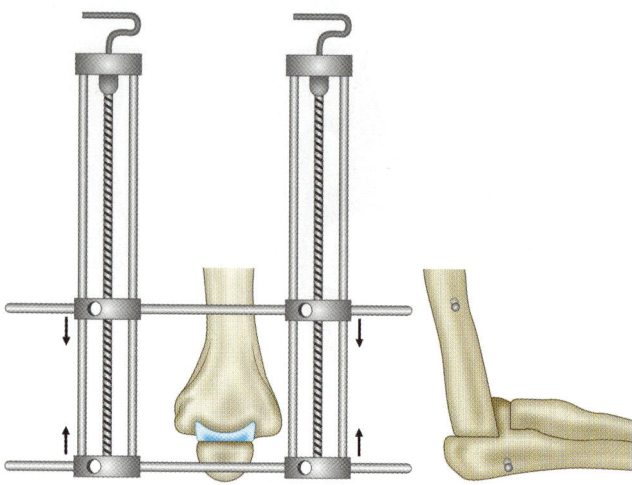

Fig. 166: Technique shown by Müller et al.

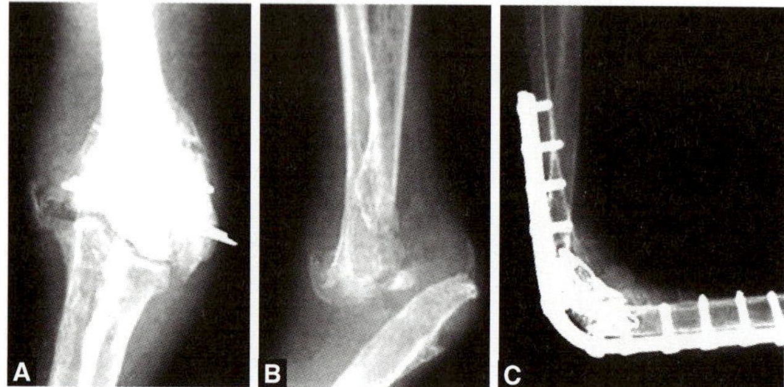

Figs. 167A to C: (A) Traumatic arthritis after severely comminuted fracture of distal humerus; (B) After two failed attempts at arthrodesis; (C) Solid fusion after Spier technique.

- Fashion a squared-off shelf in the proximal ulna and resect the distal end of the humerus to fit it.
- Resect the radial head at the level of the biceps tuberosity. Insert a Steinmann pin from the olecranon into the medullary canal of the humerus to temporarily stabilize the arthrodesis in the desired position.
- Then, insert a Steinmann pin transversely through the olecranon in line with the anterior cortex of the humerus.
- Remove the transfixing medullary pin and replace it with a cancellous screw and washer.
- Insert another transverse Steinmann pin through the humerus and use an external fixator to apply compression across the arthrodesis. Close the wound in layers overdrains.
- The fixator and pins are removed at 6–8 weeks and a long-arm cast is worn until the arthrodesis is solid.

Technique shown by Spier (Figs. 167A to C)

- Expose the elbow posteriorly. Osteotomize the olecranon and humerus to fit as in the AO technique.
- Contour an 8–12 hole AO plate to achieve the desired degree of flexion at the elbow and secure it to the humerus posteriorly by the standard AO technique.
- Secure a tensioning device to the ulna and the distal end of the plate and apply compression to the arthrodesis site.
- Accessory cancellous screws may be used for additional stability, if needed.
- Apply bone graft about the fusion.
- As shown in Figures 167A to C, A is traumatic arthritis after severely comminuted fracture of distal humerus, B is after two failed attempts at arthrodesis, and C is solid fusion after Spier technique.
- Long-arm cast is applied. The sutures are removed at 2 weeks and the cast is changed. Support is continued until the arthrodesis is solid.

Complications

- Delayed union
- Nonunion
- Malunion
- *Neurovascular injury*: When external fixation is done
- Painful prominent hardware and skin breakdown.

ELBOW ARTHROPLASTY

Introduction

Arthroplasty is an operation to restore stability and pain-free motion to a joint and function to the muscles, ligaments, and other soft-tissue structures that control the joint.

History

- *1885–1947*: Resection and anatomical arthroplasty with or without interposition.
- *1947–1970*: Hinge arthroplasty.
- *1970–1975*: Polymethylmethacrylate fixation technique from 1975 till date: Semiconstrained and unconstrained metal to polyethylene resurfacing.

Ideal Elbow Prosthesis

- It should sacrifice as little bone as possible
- Stable
- Durable and inert
- Leave minimal dead space
- Easy to implant
- Carrying angle with built in laxity
- No pain
- Mobile.

Types of Arthroplasty

- Interpositional (fascial) arthroplasty
- Resection arthroplasty
- Debridement arthroplasty
- Implant arthroplasty
- Constrained metal on metal
- Semiconstrained metal to high-density polyethylene with a locking pin or a snap-fit device.
- Unconstrained/resurfacing arthroplasty—metal on high-density polyethylene without a locking pin or a snap-fit device.

Resection Arthroplasty (Figs. 168A and B)

- Verneuil was the first who used this technique in 1860.
- Resection of distal humerus, ulna, and radius.
- It is used for ankylosis of elbow after refractory sepsis and RA.
- It is used to treat instability of elbow joint.
- Salvage procedure.

Functional Arthroplasty (Figs. 169A and B)

- It was advocated by Hass.
- It is a variation of resection arthroplasty.
- Wedge-shaped section of humerus is taken.

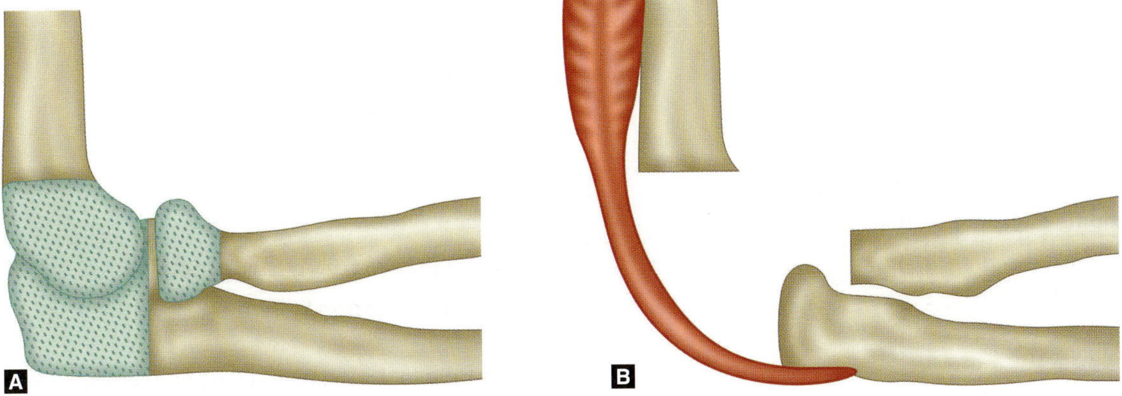

Figs. 168A and B: Resection arthroplasty.

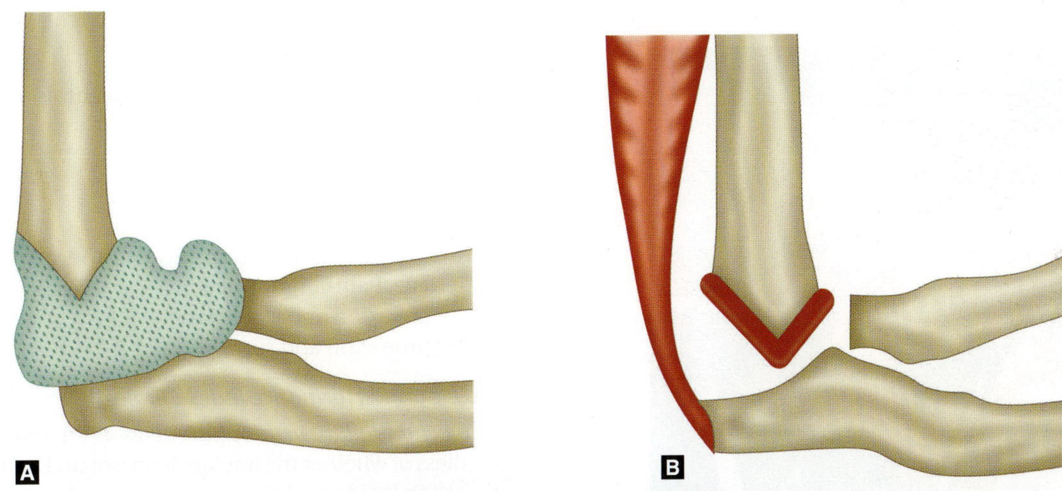

Figs. 169A and B: Functional arthroplasty.

- It is used in painful ankylosis of elbow without sepsis and as a salvage procedure after infection or failed arthroplasty.

Interposition Arthroplasty (Figs. 170 and 171)

- Murphy, in 1902, described interposition arthroplasty using fascia lata and fat.
- Lexer, in 1909, described fascia lata and vastus externus as interposition material.
- Campbell described the use of other material like tin, zinc, silicone, celluloid, linoleum rubber, and skin.
- It is used in painful ankylosis of elbow without sepsis.
- After myositis ossificans.
- Septic arthritis after a period of 6 months to 1 year.

Debridement Arthroplasty

Debridement arthroplasty of elbow is shown in Figures 172A to G.

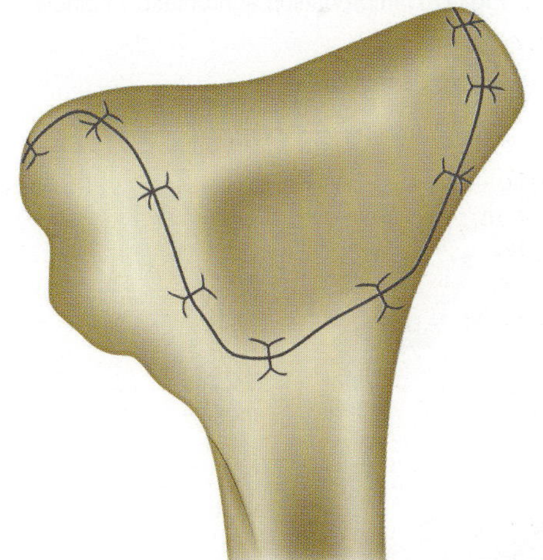
Fig. 170: Interposition arthroplasty.

Implant Arthroplasty

Indications:
- Pain, instability, and bilateral elbow ankylosis
- Bony/fibrous ankylosis with elbow in poor functioning position
- Failed elbow arthroplasty of any type
- Loss of bone stock due to trauma, tumor, or infection
- Painful and disabling RA.

Hinged prosthesis: Constrained (Fig. 173):
- Skin breakdown
- Triceps tendon rupture
- Failure due to implant loosening
- Used as salvage procedure.

New designs (Fig. 174):
- Semiconstrained
- Totally unconstrained or snap fit.

Unconstrained prosthesis (Fig. 175):
- Two-part device
- Without pin and link

- Anatomical design
- Requires intact ligaments and capsules.

Contraindications:
- History of previous sepsis
- Ankylosis of the ipsilateral shoulder
- Presence of a neuropathic joint
- Excessive loss on either side of the joint
- Poor functioning flexor and extensor mechanism.

Implant arthroplasty—complications:
- Rarely requiring surgery
- Nerve paresthesias
- Wound problems
- Fracture humerus
- Fracture ulna
- Usually requiring surgery

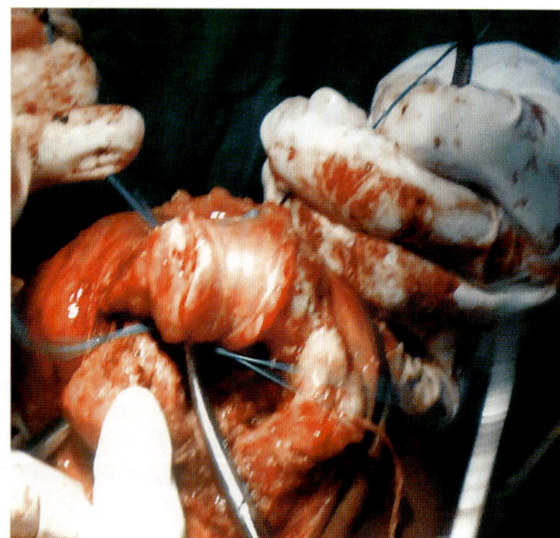

Fig. 171: Interposition arthroplasty of elbow.

- Nerve entrapment
- Triceps problems
- Ankylosis
- Usually requiring revision
- Loosening (semiconstrained)
- Instability (unconstrained)
- Infection
- Fracture and loosening.

Rating System for Arthroplasty

Morrey Classification System

Good results:
- No radiological change at the bone cement–prosthesis interface
- No pain
- > 90° flexion
- 60° of pronation and supination.

Fair result:
- 1 mm widening of bone cement–prosthesis interface
- Mild pain
- 50–90° flexion
- < 40° pronation and supination.

Poor result:
- More than 2-mm widening of bone cement–prosthesis interface. Pain-limiting activity
- < 50° of flexion and extension
- < 40° pronation and supination.

Mayo Elbow Performance Index (Table 4)

Radial head implant arthroplasty (Figs. 176A and B):
Regardless of whether the fracture is an isolated injury or associated with other lesions, internal fixation is the preferred option, providing that stable anatomical reduction can be achieved, so as to enable an exercise regime to be instituted immediately.

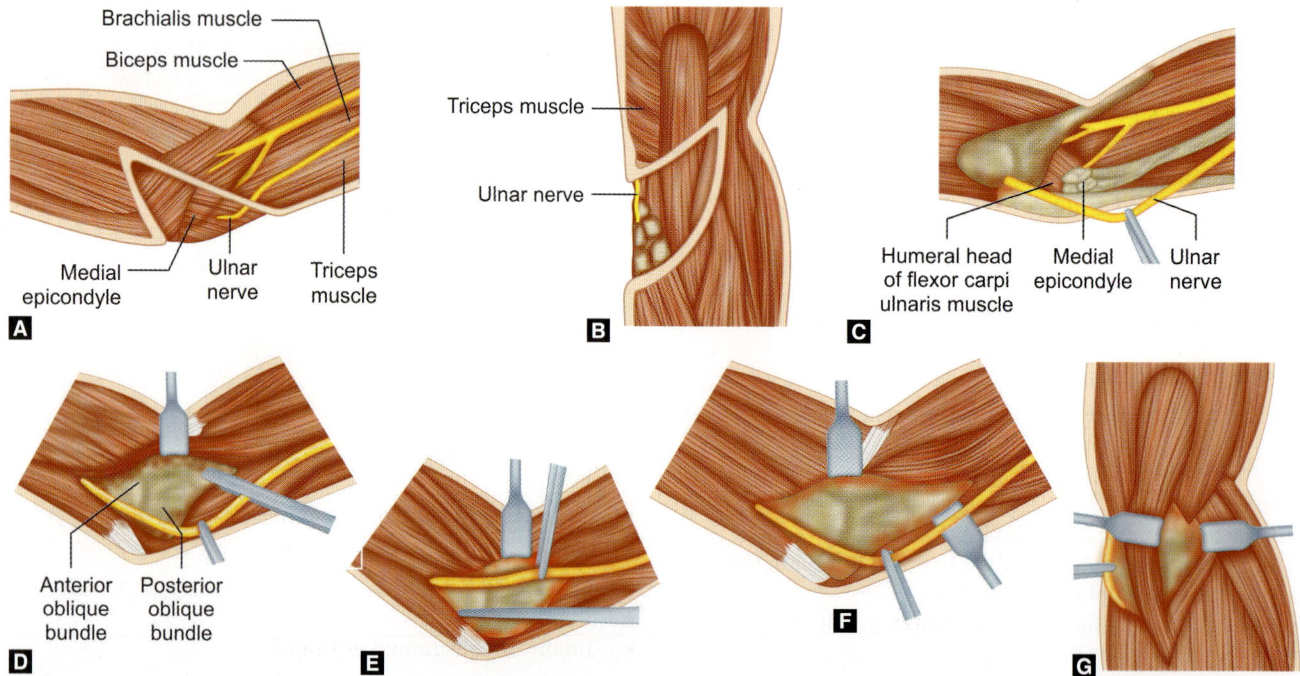

Figs. 172A to G: Debridement arthroplasty of elbow: (A and B) Incision; (C) Elevation of flexor pronator origin; (D) Exposure of anterior elbow compartment; (E) Excision of posterior oblique bundle and posterior capsule; (F) Exposure of anterior, medial, and posterior aspects of ulnohumeral joint; (G) Exposure and excision of osteophytes on lateral aspect of olecranon fossa.

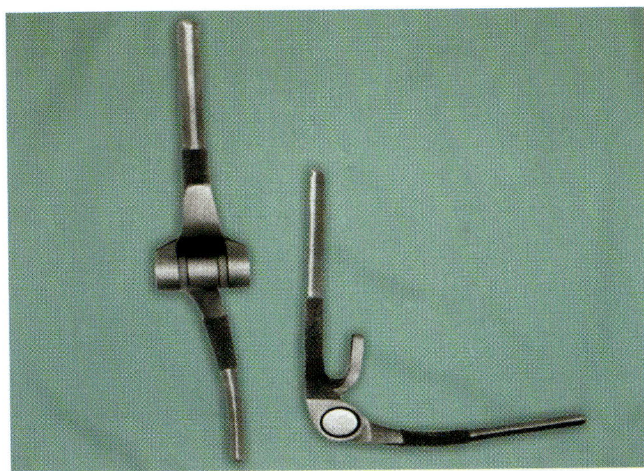

Fig. 173: Hinged prosthesis—constrained.

TABLE 4: Mayo elbow performance index.

Function	*Points*	*Definition*	*Points*
Pain	45	None	45
		Mild	30
		Moderate	15
		Severe	0
Motion	20	Arc >100°	20
		Arc 50–100°	15
		Arc <50°	5
Stability	10	Stable	10
		Moderate instability	5
		Gross instability	0
Function	25	Comb hair	5
		Feed	5
		Hygiene	5
		Shirt	5
		Shoe	5
Total	100		
Excellent result	>90		
Good result	75–89		
Fair result	60–74		
Poor result	<60		

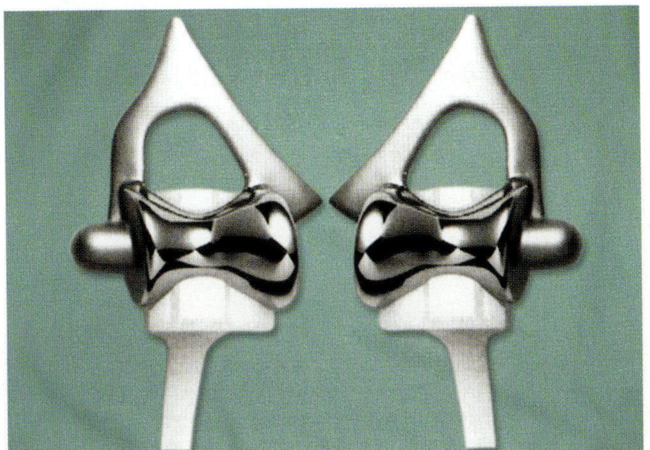

Fig. 174: Newer designs.

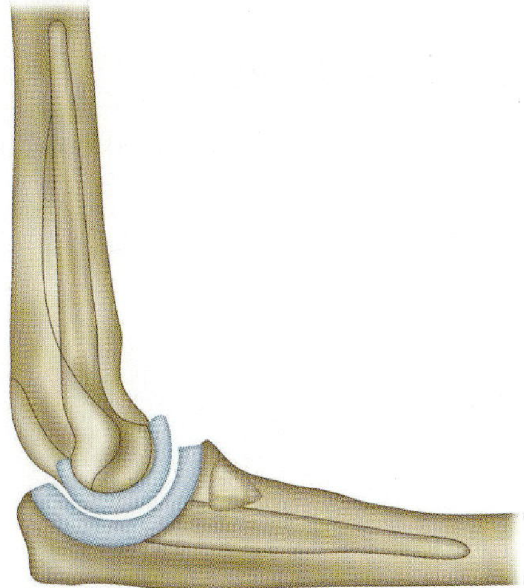

Fig. 175: Unconstrained prosthesis.

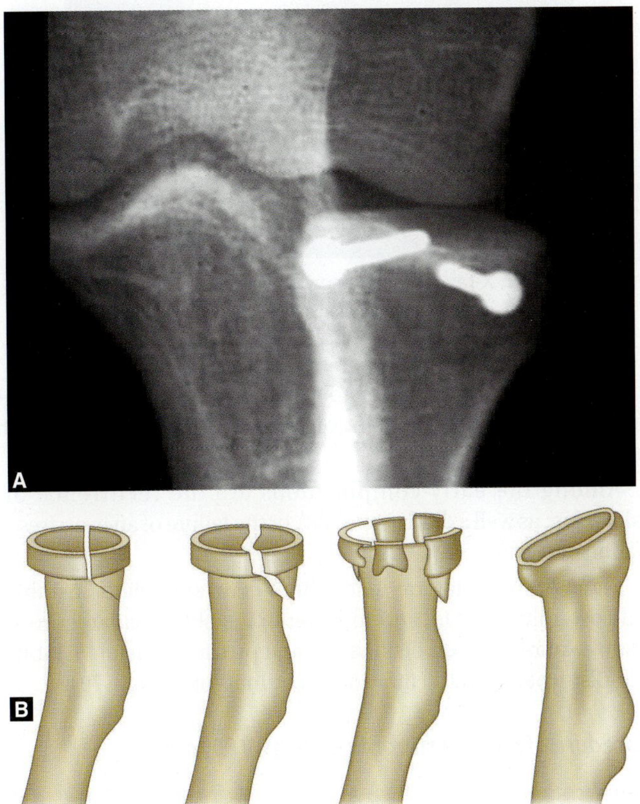

Figs. 176A and B: Radial head implant arthroplasty.

If internal fixation is not possible or if a successful outcome is uncertain, it should not be considered. The patient is not helped by IF that does not restore the anatomical pattern or which requires protective immobilization.

Resection or replacement (Fig. 177):

If the radial-head fracture is definitely isolated, resection should give satisfactory medium- and long-term results, as documented in the literature (Fig. 178).

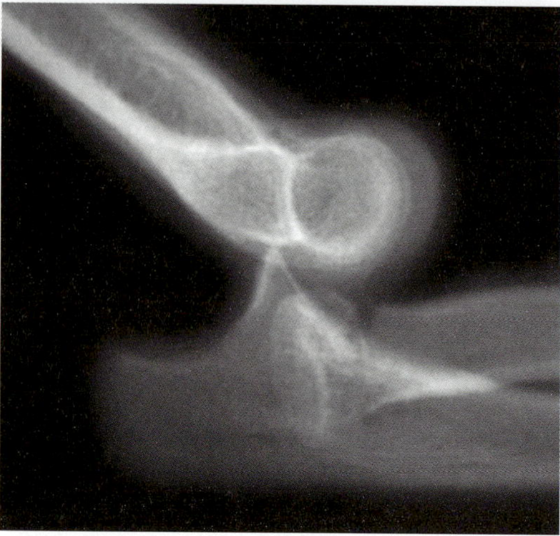

Fig. 177: Resection or replacement.

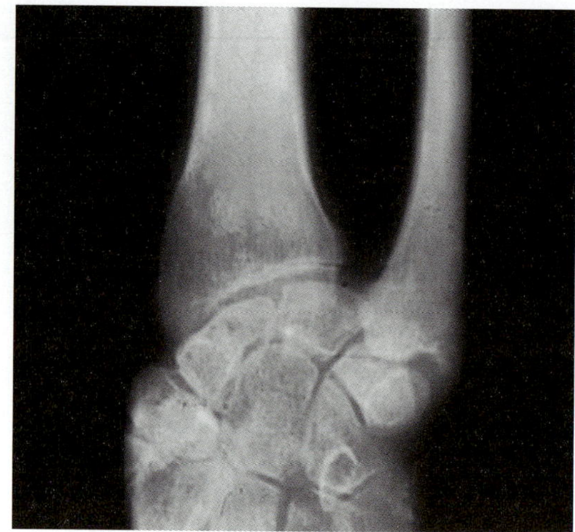

Fig. 179: Disturbed inferior radioulnar joint.

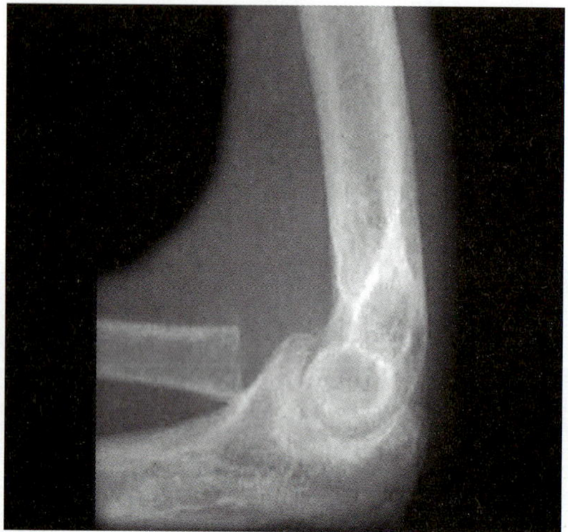

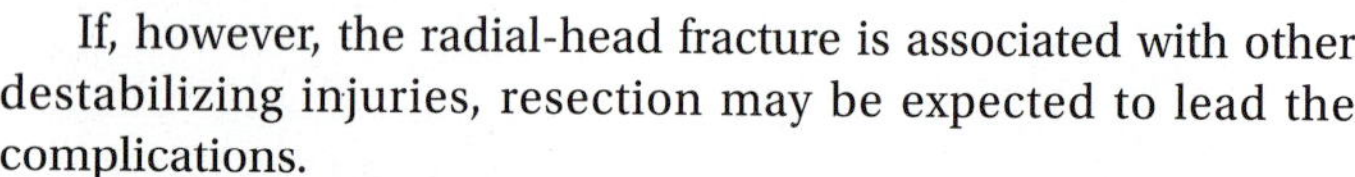

Fig. 178: X-ray showing elbow after radial head resection.

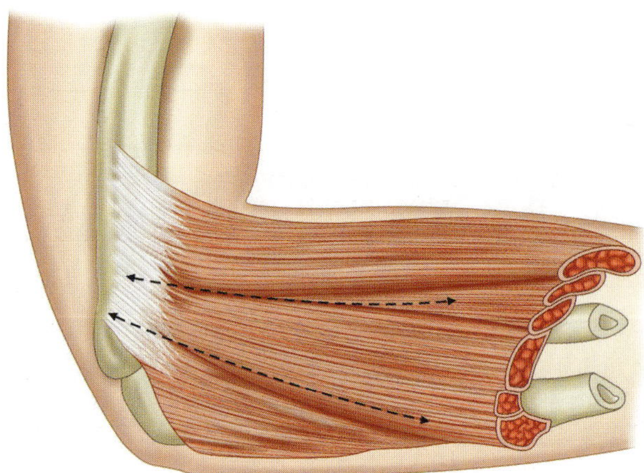

Fig. 180: Internervous plane for exposure of radius plane between extensor carpi radialis brevis and extensor digitorum communis.

If, however, the radial-head fracture is associated with other destabilizing injuries, resection may be expected to lead the complications.

Among the early complications are the recurrence of a dislocation, as well as early instability or the failure of an overstressed fixation construct.

Signs of mediolateral instability, recurrent valgus instability and posteromedial OA, anteroposterior instability with recurrence of subluxation or even dislocation and proximal-distal instability, with disturbance of the inferior radioulnar joint (Fig. 179).

Procedure of Elbow Arthroplasty (Figs. 180 to 190)

Complications

- Stiffness
- Valgus instability
- Recurrent dislocation
- Cartilage damage
- “Floating radial head prosthesis” is seen when the implant is sitting too high.

TUMORS AROUND THE ELBOW

Tumors around the elbow are broadly divided into three categories:

1. Bone tumors
2. Soft-tissue tumors
3. Metastatic tumors.

Bone Tumors

They are classified into two categories:

- Benign
- Malignant.

Benign Bone Tumors

Osteoid osteoma:

- This small benign bone tumor occurs in patients of any age, most commonly children and young adults.
- It shows predilection for male sex.

Clinical features:

- Unremitting pain is a usual symptom for which the patient seeks medical attention.

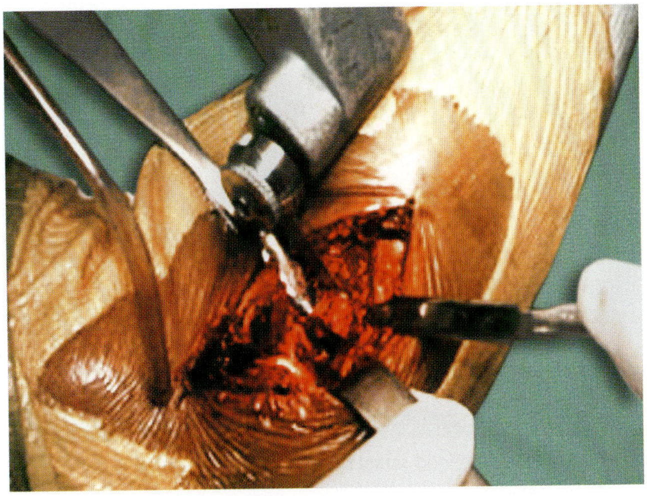

Fig. 181: Cutting the remaining part of radial neck.

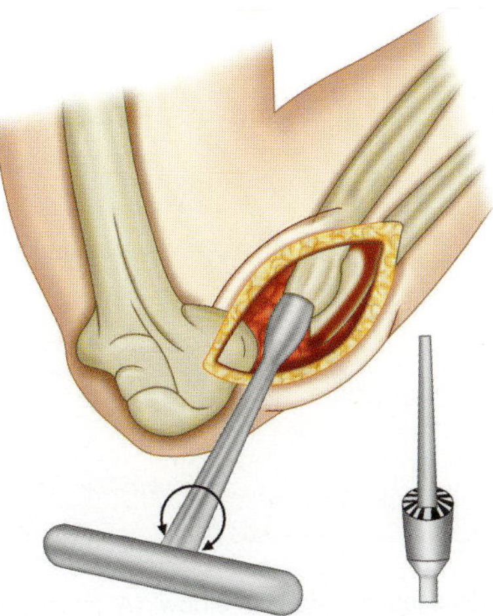

Fig. 182: Reaming of proximal radius.

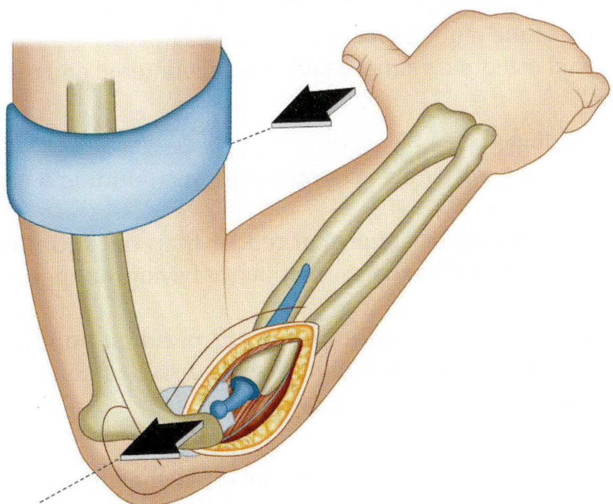

Fig. 183: Introducing the trial prosthesis.

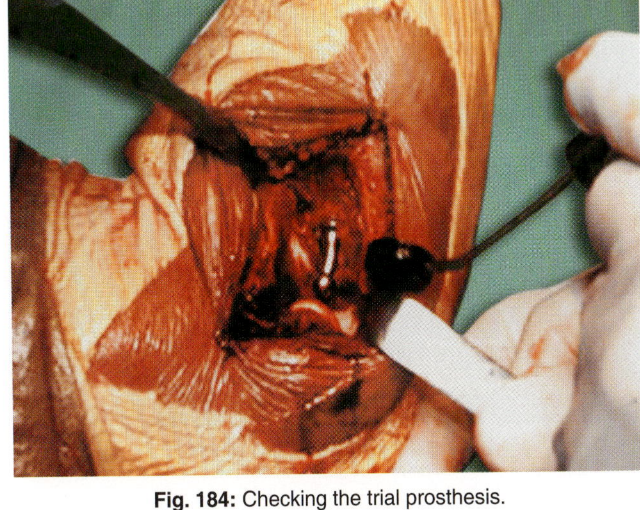

Fig. 184: Checking the trial prosthesis.

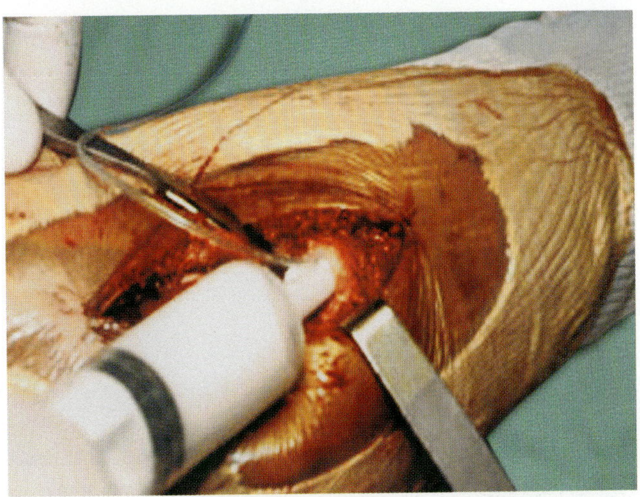

Fig. 185: Cementing of proximal end of radius.

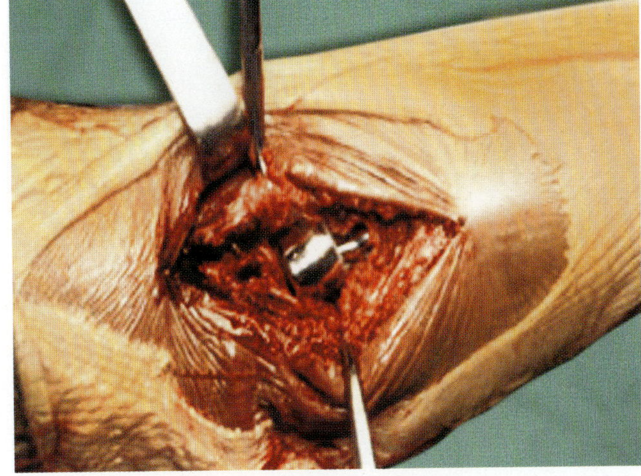

Fig. 186: Implanting the prosthesis.

- Progressive loss of motion may also be a characteristic feature.
- Pain during the night is particularly prominent.
- Aspirin may afford very dramatic relief of pain, a fact that may even suggest the diagnosis of osteoid osteoma.
- Occasionally, the pain may be experienced at a site remote from the lesion.
- Another peculiar feature of this tumor is its occasional association with atrophy of the adjacent soft tissues. Common sites of lesion in elbow are shown in Figure 191.

Pathoanatomy:

- The osteoid osteoma, by definition, is small, usually no more than 1.5 cm in diameter.

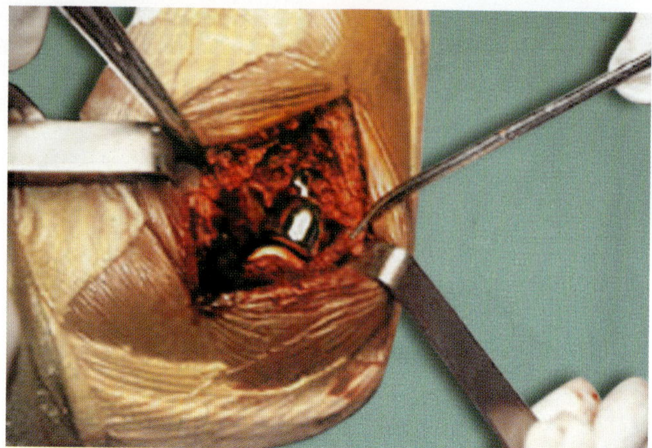

Fig. 187: Prosthesis after reduction.

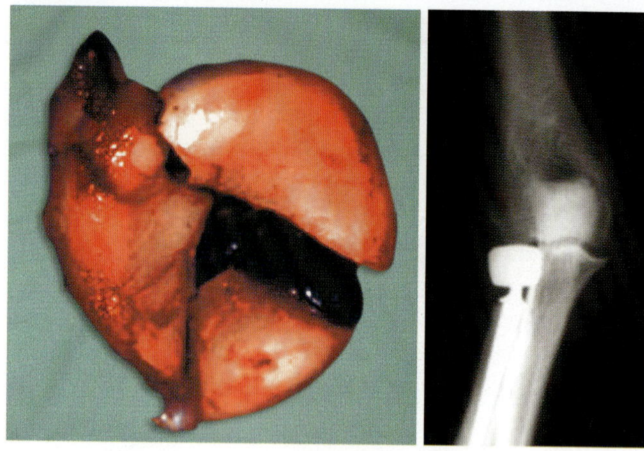

Fig. 190: Excised radial head and postoperative X-ray.

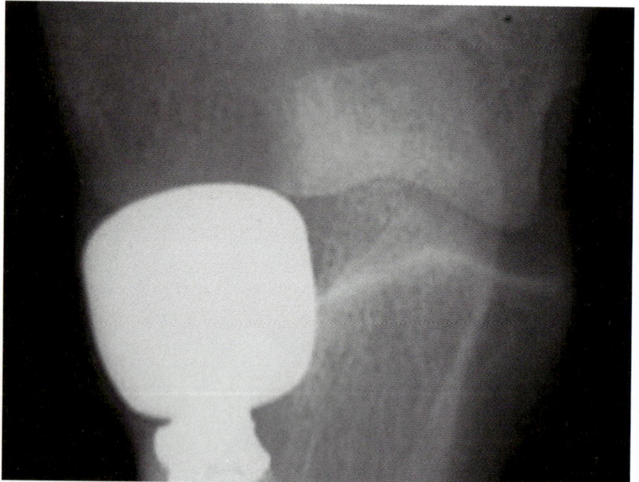

Fig. 188: Conforming the position of the prosthesis with X-ray.

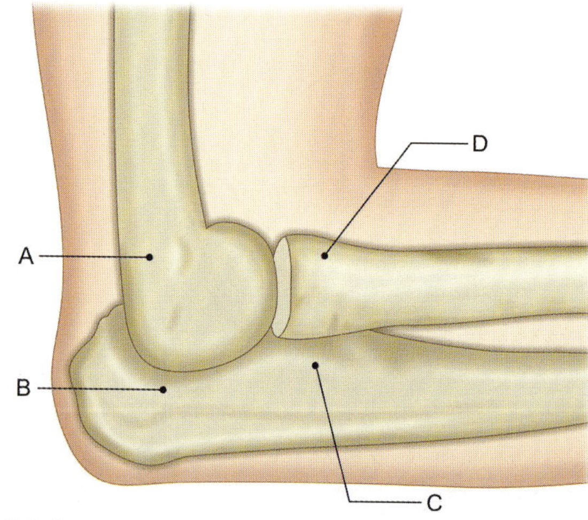

Fig. 191: Common sites of lesions in elbow. (A: lower end of humerus; B: olecranon process; C: coronoid process; D: radial head).

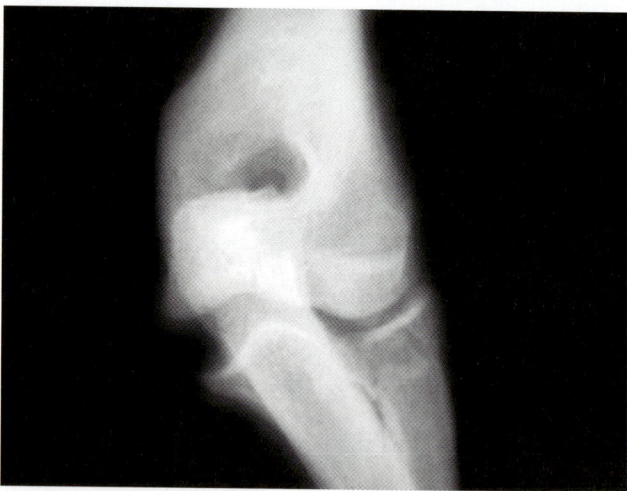

Fig. 189: Preoperative X-ray of radial head fracture.

- When osteoid osteoma occurs at or near the elbow joint, there is characteristic loss of some flexion or extension, but pronation and supination are preserved.
- In addition, there may be a synovial reaction that may further confuse the diagnosis.
- The most striking feature of these tumors is the prolonged average time required for making the diagnosis.
- Osteoid osteoma is small when first encountered and remains small.

Histopathology:
- There is usually some sclerotic bone surrounding a central nidus.
- This nidus may be somewhat redder than the surrounding cortical bone and has been described as having the appearance of a small cherry.
- Microscopic examination of the surrounding bone shows no unusual features; the nidus itself consists of a network of osteoid trabeculae.

Imaging:
- *Plain radiograph:* It may or may not reveal the presence of the tumor.
- The lesion typically appears as a central small nidus (Fig. 192), which is a radiolucent area usually surrounded by an area of sclerosis, it is the sclerosis that is usually seen; the central area of the nidus is more difficult to identify.
- When the lesion is located on the surface of the bone, there may be periosteal new bone formation that further obscures the nidus.

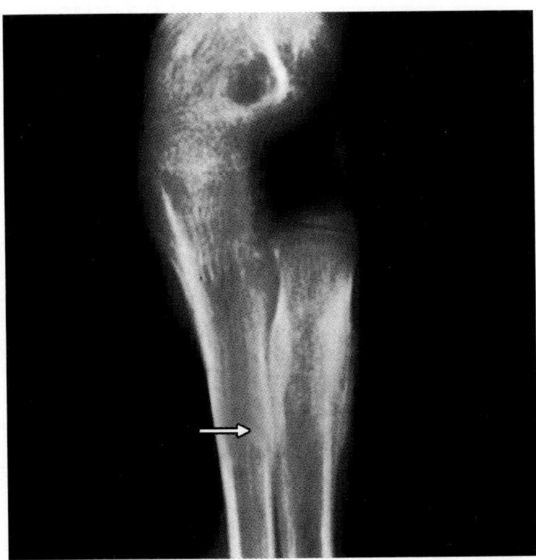

Fig. 192: Tumor lesion seen as a small nidus in X-ray film.

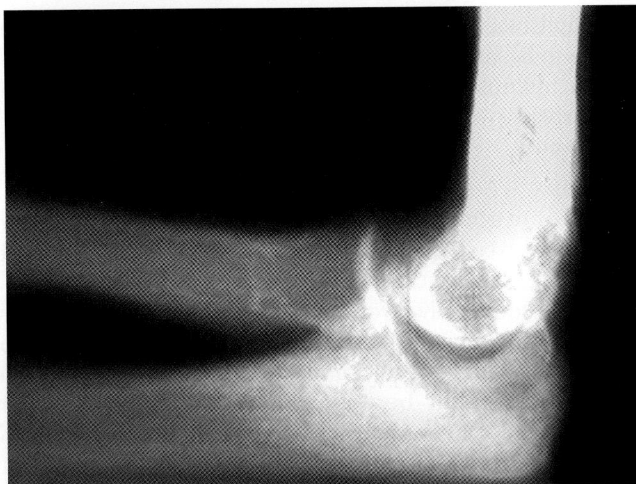

Fig. 193: An osteoid sarcoma in the distal end of humerus exhibiting periosteal new bone formation.

- Cronemeyer and colleagues described an unusual radiographic feature of osteoid osteoma in the elbow joint—subperiosteal new bone formation in adjacent bones; for example, an osteoid osteoma in the distal end of the humerus that exhibits periosteal new bone formation in the proximal radius and ulna. These authors concluded that "awareness of this association will prevent misdiagnosis of the benign neoplasm as an inflammatory arthritis" (Fig. 193).
- *Bone scan:* Technetium-99m scintigraphy has been helpful in locating these lesions.
- CT scan is today's diagnostic standard.

Treatment:
- In the past, the treatment of osteoid osteoma was surgical excision of the nidus.
- It is not necessary to remove all of the sclerotic bone.
- The main problems with this type of surgery are identification of the lesion and confirmation of its removal by the pathologist, which may be difficult.
- Ghelman and associates have described a method for localizing an osteoid osteoma intraoperatively by using a scintillation probe.
- This technique may simplify the localization of the lesion at the time of surgery.

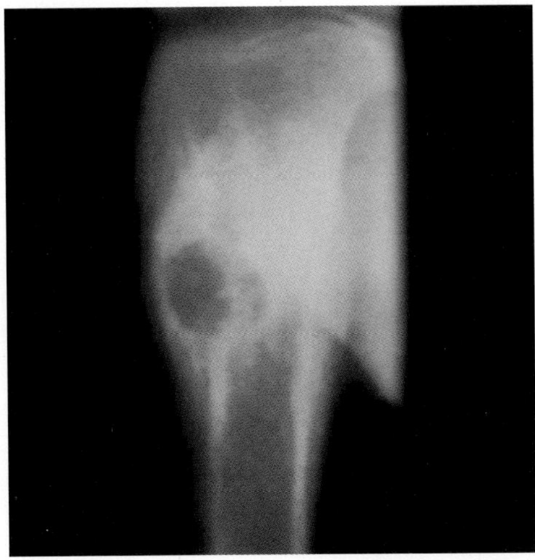

Fig. 194: X-ray showing radiolucent lesion, surrounded by a thin margin of reactive bone.

- Patients, whose lesions are not completely excised, will probably continue to have the same pain and will probably require a second operation.
- The authors have observed that the loss of motion, so characteristic of this lesion at the elbow, resolves with removal of the nidus. Hence, capsular release is not necessary as an adjunctive procedure.
- At present, the treatment of choice for most lesions is radiofrequency obliteration performed under CT direction.

Osteoblastoma:
- Osteoblastoma is an uncommon osteoid tissue-forming primary neoplasm of the bone, categorized as a benign bone tumor.
- It resembles osteoid osteoma in some respects but it is larger (>2 cm).
- *Unlike osteoid osteoma*:
  - Osteoblastoma occurs in older adolescents and young adults.
  - Osteoblastoma usually does not cause localized night pain; and when pain occurs, it is usually not relieved by salicylates (aspirin).
  - Intense bony reaction that is seen with osteoid osteoma does not occur with osteoblastoma.
  - Osteoblastoma is more often located in the posterior elements of vertebra.
  - Osteoblastoma will not resolve spontaneously.
- If the lesion is superficial, the patient may have localized swelling and tenderness.
- In rare cases, malignant transformation is possible.

Histopathology:
- It reveals scattered mitotic figures.
- Proliferation of immature plump osteoblasts
- Prominent vascular and stromal tissue component; giant cells and broad osteoid seams.

Imaging:
- X-rays show radiolucent lesion, which is surrounded by a thin margin of reactive bone that may have expanded—aneurysmal appearance (Fig. 194).
- Bone scan shows intense radioisotope uptake that helps to localize the lesion.

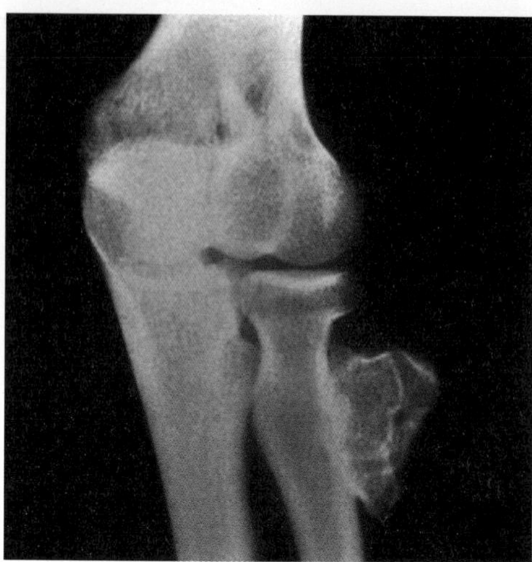

Fig. 195: Osteochondroma in a 23-year-old woman showing radial shaft with cortical and medullary bone extending into tumor.

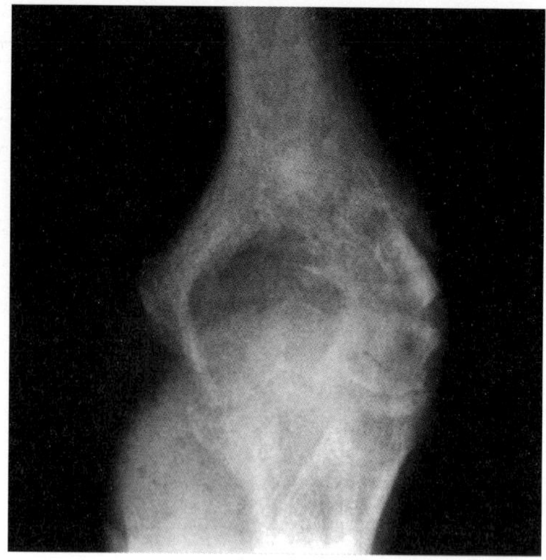

Fig. 196: Giant cell tumor.

- The CT scan confirms preoperative diagnosis and helps to determine surgical approach.
- Angiography is used for staging of aggressive tumors.

Treatment:
- En bloc marginal excision is treatment of choice.
- Active tumors are likely to recur, if intracapsular resection is performed.
- Risk of recurrence after marginal excision of aggressive stage 3 is 30–50%
- Radiation therapy or chemotherapy is not effective.

Osteochondroma:
- Osteochondroma is probably the most common benign bone tumor, but it is not very commonly encountered in the elbow.
- The tumor may be found in a patient of any age, but it usually stops growing when skeletal maturity is reached.
- An osteochondroma may arise from the surface of any bone but most commonly does so in the metaphyseal region of long bones.
- The tumor tends to project away from the joint along the direction of attached muscles.

Clinical features:
- The osteochondroma is not inherently painful but causes symptoms by pressure on adjacent structures.
- Osteochondromas (Fig. 195), in the region of the elbow, may cause mechanical difficulties; specifically, interference with the motion of the elbow joint.
- In addition, the cartilage cap may impinge on important neurovascular structures.

Histopathology:
- The tumor may be pedunculated on a stalk or may be sessile and may have a broad base.
- The tumor is covered by a cartilage cap, which, if becomes markedly thickened, suggests the possibility of sarcomatous transformation.
- If it is more than 1 cm thick, the risk of secondary chondrosarcoma is relatively high.
- In children, the cartilage cap is normally thicker than in adults.
- Probably less than 1% of osteochondromas ever become malignant.
- Multiple osteochondromas sometimes occur, a condition that tends to be familial.
- When multiple bones are involved, there may be some element of dysplasia with the deformity and the elbow can be severely involved.

Treatment:
- If there are symptoms or mechanical or cosmetic difficulties, complete excision of the osteochondroma, together with the overlying cartilage cap, is performed.
- Excision commonly involves the use of an osteotome to shave the lesion level with the underlying cortical bone. Such simple excision generally results in cure, although local recurrence may occasionally be noted, indicating that part of the cartilaginous cap was left behind.
- If the cap is thicker than 1 cm in an adult, the lesion must be carefully studied histologically to exclude the possibility of a sarcoma.

Giant cell tumor (Fig. 196):
- Benign giant cell tumor is occasionally encountered in the region of the elbow.
- It shows predilection for female sex.
- It occurs commonly in persons older than 20 years (differentiate from aneurysmal bone cyst).
- Giant cell tumors nearly always occur in the epiphyseal region and may extend to the articular surface of the bone.

Classification by Campanacci et al.:
- *Grade I*: Tumors are radiologically indolent.
- *Grade II*: Radiologically aggressive but the tumor has not yet broken through cortical bone.
- *Grade III*: Radiologically aggressive with breach in the cortex.

Histopathology:
- Grossly, the tumor consists of a red soft tissue that typically extends up to the subchondral bone at the articular surface.
- Microscopically, a giant cell tumor shows a combination of giant cells and mononuclear cells, with a more or less uniform distribution of the giant cells.

Treatment:
- The extent of surgery required to eradicate giant cell tumors is somewhat controversial.

- *Distal end of humerus*:
  - Excision by curettage will suffice in grade I lesion.
  - In other grades, total excision of the distal end of humerus with allograft replacement is considered (creates a very serious problem for the reconstructive surgeon).
  - Excision by curettage in other locations results in a local recurrence rate of approximately 25%. It is probably reasonable to accept this risk and to try curettage for the first treatment because the alternative of resection of the distal end of the humerus is so drastic.
  - However, if the tumor has already broken through the cortex into the surrounding soft structures, curettage is unlikely to be effective.
- *Proximal end of ulna*:
  - Curettage might be more reasonable because there is more bone to work with; hence, a larger margin of normal bone can be included in the resected specimen, whether resection is done by curettage or actual excision.
  - Whenever possible, packing the tumor cavity with methyl methacrylate has proven to be effective.
- *Radial head*:
  - Simple excision (especially in cases of small tumors).
- Radiation therapy for benign giant cell tumors should be avoided, if possible, because of significant risk of subsequent malignant transformation.

Aneurysmal bone cyst:

- An aneurysmal bone cyst typically contains abundant benign giant cells in scattered zones.
- It is different from giant cell tumor because it, nearly always contains blood-filled spaces, is somewhat fibrogenic and usually has zones with osteoid formation and trabeculae of bone.
- It occurs usually in persons younger than 20 years of age.
- The lesion is usually metaphyseal in location.

Clinical features:

- Pain
- Swelling.

Histopathology:

- An aneurysmal bone cyst contains anastomosing cavernous spaces that usually constitute the bulk of the lesion.
- The spaces are usually filled with unclotted blood, which may well up into but does not spurt from the tumor, when it is unroofed.
- The most important factor to recognize histologically is the benign quality of the constituent cells.

Imaging (Fig. 197):

- *Plain radiographs*: The disease area consists of a zone of rarefaction, which is usually well circumscribed, eccentric, and associated with an obvious soft-tissue extension of the process.
- Classically, the soft-tissue extension is produced by bulging of the periosteum and a resultant layer of radiographically visible new bone that delimits the periphery of the tumor.
- Fusiform expansion may be produced, especially when small bones are affected.

Treatment:

- Curettage and bone grafting are usually required.
- 25% of these cases will recur and require additional surgery.

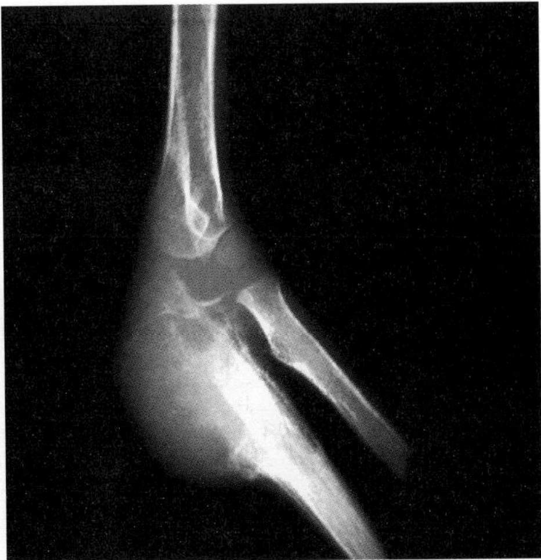

Fig. 197: Radiograph image of aneurysmal bone cyst.

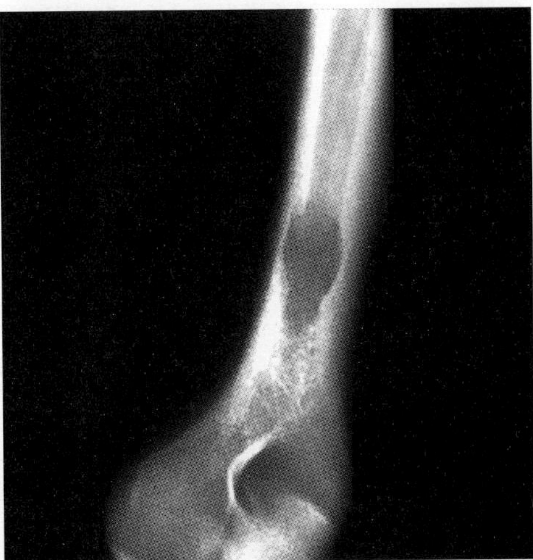

Fig. 198: Histiocytosis X-ray producing a well-defined rarefaction of the humeral shaft. This completely benign lesion is associated with a good prognosis, especially if it is solitary.

Other benign bone tumors and tumor simulators (Figs. 198 to 202):

- A number of lesions may occur in any bone and may simulate or mimic a primary bone tumor.
- Benign cartilage tumors are very rare at the elbow.

Malignant Bone Tumors

Lymphoma:

- Lymphoma tends to occur in middle-aged or elderly adults (Fig. 203).
- The tumor may arise primarily in any bone, including bones in the region of the elbow.

Clinical features:

- Patients with lymphoma generally present with pain and swelling in the region of the lesion.

Radiographic features:

- Diffuse, destructive, and mottled appearance with indistinct margins.
- Variable degrees of sclerosis may be present in the lesion; the cortical bone is usually eroded and the tumor may extend into the adjacent soft tissues.
- Periosteal new bone formation usually is not a prominent feature.

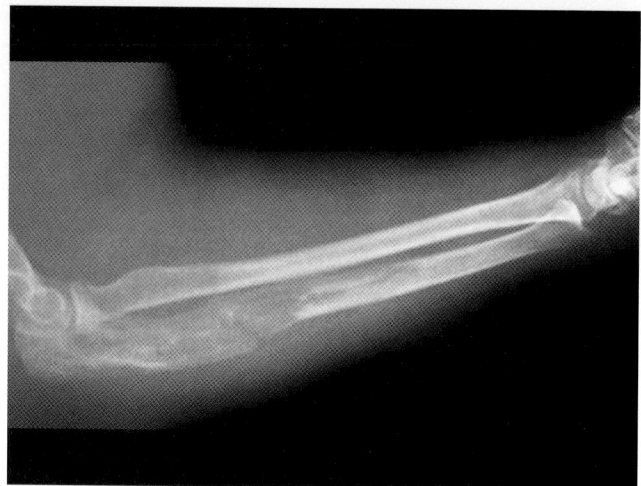

Fig. 199: Paget's disease of the proximal two-thirds of the ulna. This classic lesion is associated with pathologic fracture and extends to the end of the bone. Paget's disease of the bone is very rare in patients younger than 40 years of age.

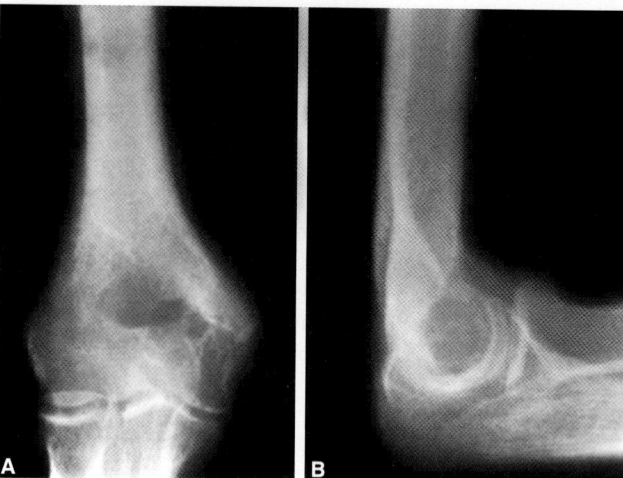

Figs. 202A and B: Benign chondroblastoma of the distal end of the humerus in a 25-year-old man. Note the discrete zone of rarefaction. Such lesions are more innocuous than giant cell tumors.

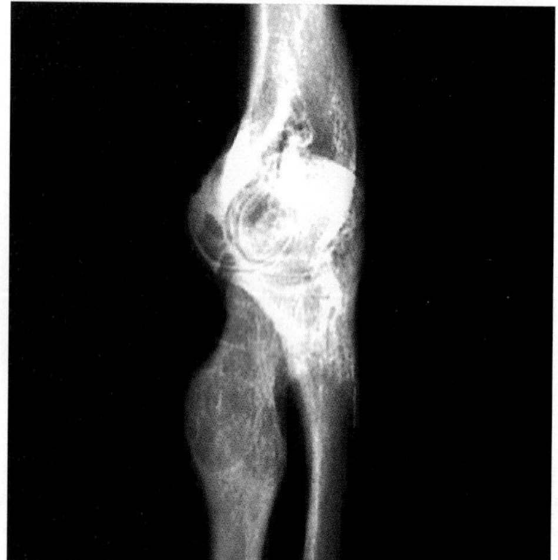

Fig. 200: Fibrous dysplasia producing extensive changes on both sides of the joint.

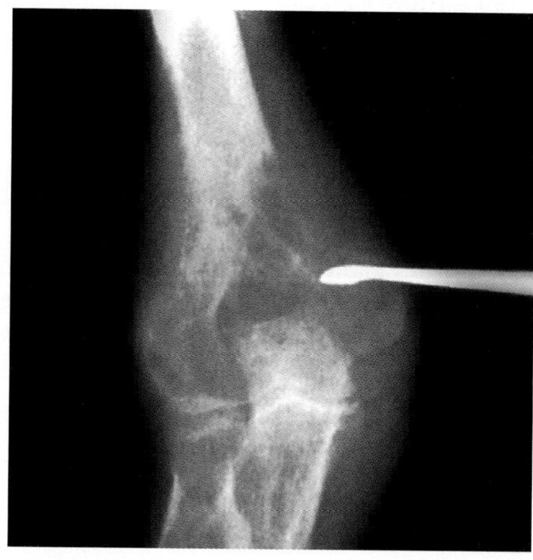

Fig. 203: Malignant lymphoma producing malignant-appearing destruction of the distal part of the humerus in a 60-year-old woman.

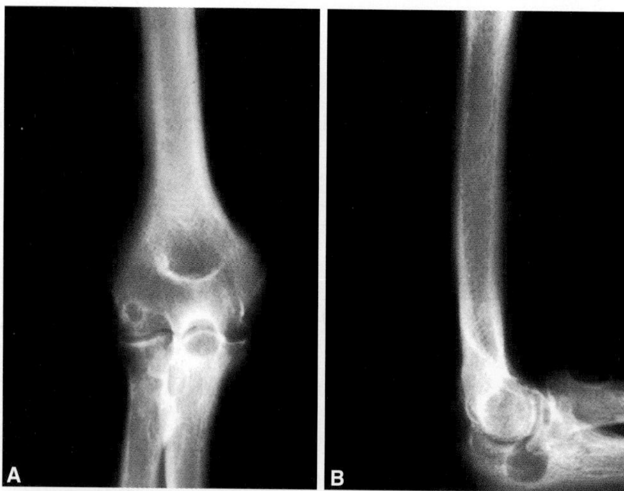

Figs. 201A and B: Cyst of upper part of the ulna secondary to degenerative joint disease at the elbow.

Histopathology:

- Grossly, lymphoma tissue is usually gray or white and very soft.
- *Microscopically*:
  - Malignant lymphomas fit into the group of small round cell tumors
  - Under low power, the tumor shows a permeative pattern
  - The infiltrate tends to fill up the marrow cavity without destroying medullary bone.

Treatment:

- Lymphoma is generally treated with radiation therapy, if there is only a solitary lesion of bone.
- Radiation therapists generally try to avoid circumferential treatment of an extremity to allow some normal lymphatic channels to remain open. Failure to do so may result in significant swelling distal to the treatment area.
- It may be difficult or impossible to avoid treating the entire circumference of the extremity in the region of the elbow.

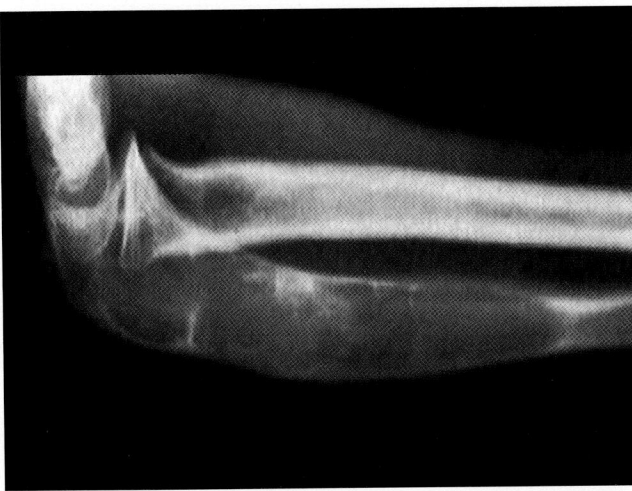

Fig. 204: Recurrent Ewing's sarcoma with a cyst-like lesion of the upper half of the ulna in a 21-year-old woman. The original tumor had been treated 10 years previously.

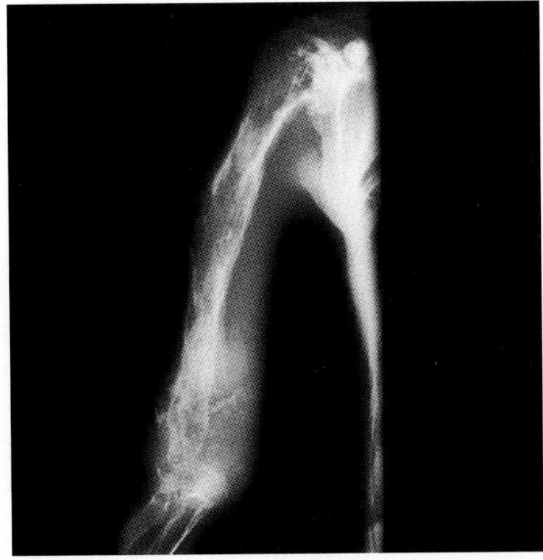

Fig. 205: Grade IV osteosarcoma of the distal end of the humerus in a patient with Paget's disease of the entire bone.

- In addition, when radiation exceeds approximately 4,000 rad, radiation therapists generally try to direct treatment away from the articular surface.
- There is no clear-cut or obvious advantage to the use of adjunctive chemotherapy at the time of initial treatment, if only a solitary lesion is present.

Prognosis:
- If the disease is localized to one site, the prognosis is excellent.
- About a fourth of patients will have multiple bones involved
- If there are other sites, such as liver, spleen, or lymph nodes, the survival rate decreases dramatically.

Ewing's sarcoma:
- Ewing's sarcoma may arise in any bone, including those in the region of the elbow.
- Children are more frequently affected than adults (Fig. 204).

Clinical features:
- Pain
- Swelling
- Fever
- Raised ESR.

Radiographic features:
- Mottled or moth-eaten destructive lesion that may contain both lytic and blastic areas.
- There is frequently periosteal reactive new bone, which may form layers, forming the "onion skin" appearance that is reported to be typical of this disease.
- The radiographic appearance combined with the presence of fever and an elevated erythrocyte sedimentation rate may lead to the erroneous diagnosis of osteomyelitis.

Histopathology:
- Grossly, Ewing's sarcoma may be very soft or even semiliquid; indeed, the appearance may simulate the purulence of infection.
- Microscopically, Ewing's sarcoma is very cellular and composed of small round cells that are remarkably similar to one another.

Treatment:
- The local lesion is generally treated with radiation therapy and systemic combination chemotherapy is generally used in an attempt to prevent micrometastases.
- Resecting malignant tumors in the region of the elbow is generally avoided because it is difficult to achieve adequate margins in this region without damaging important normal structures.
- Even if an adequate resection could be achieved, satisfactory reconstruction would be difficult or impossible.
- Therefore, the treatment for Ewing's sarcoma is radiation therapy.
- A major side effect is soft-tissue fibrosis, causing a stiff joint.

Osteosarcoma:
- Osteosarcoma (Fig. 205) is the most common bone malignancy except for myeloma.
- About one-half of these tumors are predominantly fibrous or cartilaginous and others are predominantly bone forming. *Hence, they are subclassified into*:
  - Fibroblastic
  - Chondroblastic
  - Osteoblastic
- This subclassification may be important because the osteoblastic subtype appears to have a worse prognosis than the other two subtypes.

Diagnosis:
- *Radiographically:*
  - Osteosarcoma appears to be aggressive, with evidence of cortical destruction and reactive periosteal new bone formation.
  - In the distal humerus, the classic "sunburst" appearance may be evident.
  - The precise extent of the lesion may not be apparent on plain radiographs.
  - The tumor can usually be more accurately assessed with a technetium or gallium bone scan.
  - *CT scan*: It determines the extent of soft-tissue involvement.
  - *MRI*: It determines both the extent of soft tissue involvement and the extent of intramedullary involvement.
- *Biopsy:*
  - The reactive new bone formation at the periphery of the lesion should not be sampled for biopsy because this will simply lead to confusion in the interpretation of the histological findings.

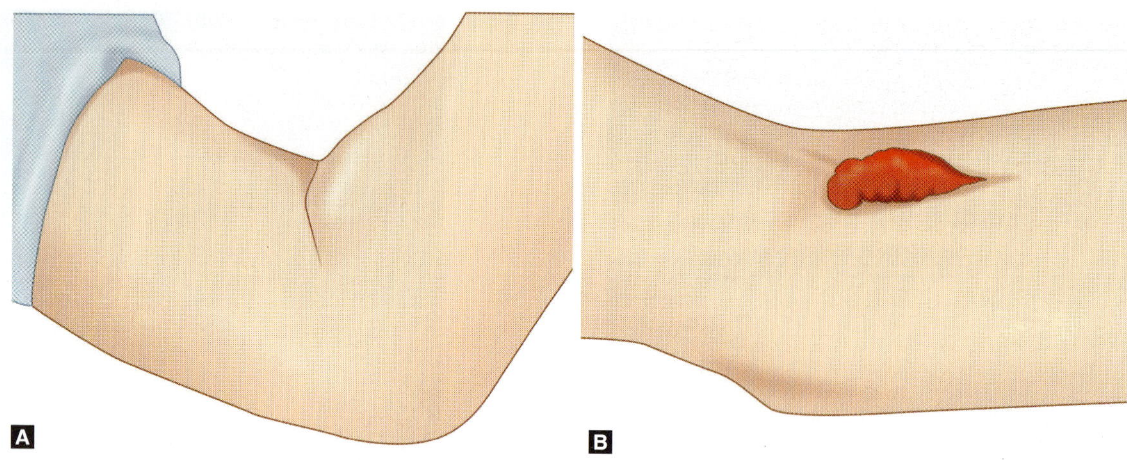

Figs. 206A and B: (A) Expanding and prominent soft-tissue mass in the cubital space and (B) was found to be a benign lipoma.

- If there is a soft-tissue extension of the tumor, this is the area, which is best for biopsy because it is usually the most malignant and the easiest to process in the pathology laboratory.

Treatment:
- It is a radioresistant malignant bone tumor.
- Hence, the usual treatment of osteosarcoma is surgical ablation.
- In the past, for many years, amputation was carried out.
- Today, the majority of patients with osteosarcoma can be managed with various limb salvage procedures.
- Neoadjuvant chemotherapy is generally employed before one proceeds with surgery and additional chemotherapy is usually offered after surgery.

Prognosis:
Today, the prognosis for patients with osteosarcoma is much improved; 70–90% of such patients may be long-term survivors.

Metastatic Tumors

- There is no particular predilection for metastatic disease to involve the elbow.
- Yet, extensive destruction is observed on occasion from several tumor types.
- Treatment is most commonly joint replacement.
- Patients do well in general with this palliative treatment.
- Complications relate to nerve dysfunction and stiffness.

Soft-tissue Tumors

They are classified into:
- Benign
- Malignant.

Benign Soft-tissue Tumors

Lipoma:
- Lipoma is probably the most frequently encountered benign soft-tissue neoplasm and is the most common tumor in the elbow region.
- It is usually solitary but multiple lipomas have occurred.
- The tumor is simply a localized collection of adipose tissue that is histologically and chemically similar to ordinary fat.

Clinical features:
- Most lipomas are small, asymptomatic, and relatively dormant in that they seem to remain approximately the same size.
- Occasionally, however, the tumor may grow and become symptomatic.
- If there is trauma to the area, necrosis may develop within the lipoma and this is usually symptomatic.
- Most lipomas consist almost entirely of adipose tissue; however, there may be increased vascularity, in which case the lesion is referred to as angiolipoma.

Diagnosis:
- Mainly on clinical examination.
- Some lipomas (Figs. 206A and B), which do not have the clinical characteristics of the usual subcutaneous lipoma, may require further diagnostic modalities.

Treatment:
Surgical excision should be considered for lipomas that:
- Increase in size
- Symptomatic or cosmetically undesirable
- Interfere with function
- In situations when the diagnosis is not certain.
- Simple marginal excision should be carried out
- The vulnerability of the neurovascular structures is of particular concern for lipoma of the antecubital space.
- When a lipoma is located within the belly of a muscle, it may be necessary to sacrifice some normal muscle tissue on all aspects to minimize the risk of local recurrence.
- At the elbow, this can cause permanent stiffness.

Ganglion:
- A ganglion is a cystic lesion generally found in the hands, wrists, and feet, but it may be found less commonly in the region of the elbow.
- The lesion may occur within a tendon, in a muscle, or even on occasion in bone.

Treatment:
- Symptomatic treatment (not all ganglia require excision)
- Simple excision.

Myxoma:
- A myxoma occasionally occurs in the soft tissues at the elbow.
- It is soft, well-circumscribed, and myxoidal.
- A myxoma is relatively small and is usually encountered in the superficial soft tissues.

Histologically:
- The lesion is hypocellular and contains stellate cells in a myxoid stream.

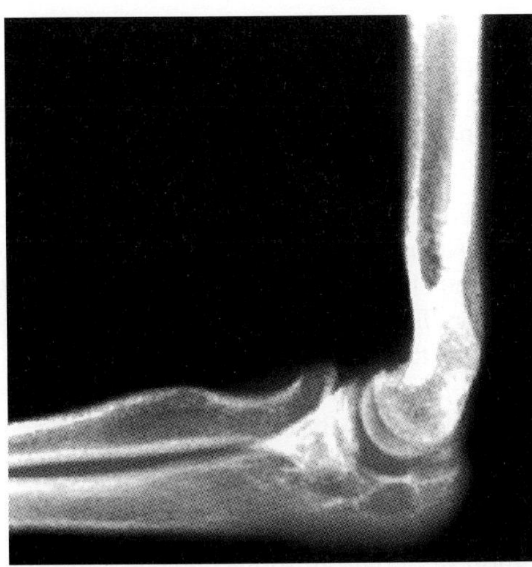

Fig. 207: Pigmented villonodular synovitis in a 17-year-old girl, with a 3-year history of pain and swelling. Note cystic erosions.

Treatment:
- Wide excision (because marginal resection tends to recur).

Pigmented villonodular synovitis:
- Pigmented villonodular synovitis (PVNS) (Fig. 207) is a locally destructive fibrohistiocytic proliferation, characterized by many villous and nodular synovial protrusions, which affect joints, bursae, and tendon sheaths.
- The PVNS was first described by Jaffe, Lichtenstein, and Sutro in 1941, who used this name to identify the lesion because of its yellow-brown, villous, and nodular appearance.
- The yellow-brown pigmentation is due to excessive deposits of lipid and hemosiderin.
- It shows predilection for female sex with 2:1 ratio.
- Clinically, there are two forms of the disease:
  1. Nodular (or) localized
  2. Diffuse.
- When a discrete intra-articular mass is present, the condition is called "localized pigmented villonodular synovitis". (In European literature—"pigmented giant cell tumor of articulations").
- When the entire synovium of the joint is affected and there is a major villous component, the condition is referred to as "diffuse pigmented villonodular synovitis".
- The diffuse form usually occurs in the knee, hip, elbow, or wrist.
- The nodular or localized form is most often seen in the fingers and is the second most common soft-tissue tumor of the hand, exceeded only by the ganglion.
- One of the most characteristic findings in PVNS is the ability of the hyperplastic synovium to invade the subchondral bone, producing cysts and erosions.

Clinical features at the elbow:
- Mild pain
- Joint swelling
- Increased thickening of the synovium
- Restriction of joint motion
- Knee joint is most commonly affected and patients present with bloody joint effusion. In fact, the presence of a serosanguinous synovial fluid in the absence of a history of recent trauma should strongly suggest the diagnosis of PVNS. The synovial fluid contains elevated levels of cholesterol and fluid reaccumulates rapidly after aspiration.

Imaging:
- *X-ray*: Cystic erosions on either side of the joint.
- When erosions are found and there is no loss of joint space and no demineralization of the surrounding bone, the diagnosis should be suspected.
- In most cases of pigmented villonodular synovitis, however, there is no bony erosion, but there is evidence of lobular swelling of the soft tissues.
- *Arthrography*: It reveals multiple lobulated masses with villous projections, which appear as filling defects in the contrast-filled suprapatellar bursa.
- *CT scan*: It demonstrates the extent of the disease.
- *MRI*: Useful in making the diagnosis (also in defining the extent of the disease).

Histopathology:
- Microscopic study shows a stromal background of reticulin and collagen fibers, in which various different cells may be found.
- The firm, nodular lesions have more collagenous stroma, whereas the soft villous lesions have less stroma.

Treatment:
- Nodular form—the nodule may be simply excised.
- Diffuse form—simple excision is likely to be followed by local recurrence.
- Radiation therapy has been attempted (but there is no convincing evidence that such treatment will actually eliminate the disease and prevent local recurrences. High doses of radiation are avoided at the elbow joint.)
- *Synovectomy is the treatment of choice:*
  - Open procedure reported incidence of 33% recurrence
  - Arthroscopic procedure—less recurrence (hence, today's treatment of choice)
- If synovectomy leads to symptomatic local recurrence, arthrodesis is considered in most joints.
- At the elbow, however, because this joint does poorly with an arthrodesis, replacement arthroplasty would appear to be the treatment of choice.

Synovial chondromatosis:
- Synovial chondromatosis (also known as synovial osteochondromatosis or synovial chondrometaplasia) is a benign, tumorous, multifocal, chondromatous, or chondro-osseous metaplastic proliferation involving the subsynovial connective tissue of joints, tendon sheaths, or bursae.
- Knee is the most commonly affected joint, but the process can involve any joint.
- It is almost invariably monoarticular; rarely, multiple joints may be affected.
- The average age of the patients is about 40 years.
- Men are affected more often than women.

Clinical features:
- Pain
- Swelling
- Joint effusion
- Tenderness
- Limited range of motion in the joint
- Soft-tissue mass.

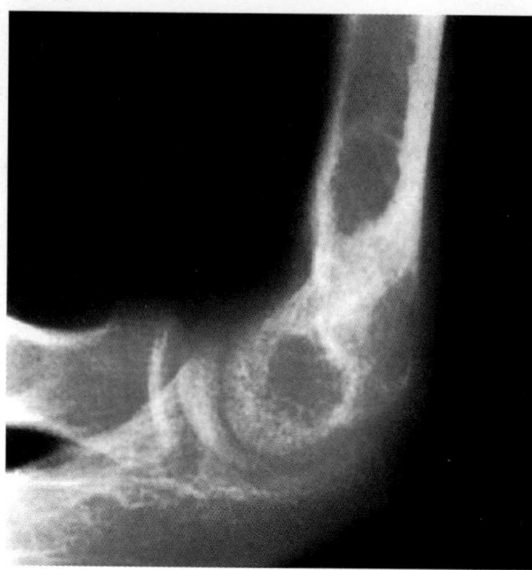

Fig. 208: Synovial chondromatosis of the elbow. Note that a small mineralized focus is evident in the antecubital fossa.

Imaging:

- *On X-ray (Fig. 208):* Radiopaque joint bodies, which are calcified cartilaginous bodies (may/may not reveal on X-ray—depend upon the degree of calcification).
- CT and MRI scans are useful in visualizing even noncalcified bodies and these also help in location and extent of the disease process (bony erosion).
- Diagnostic arthrotomy or arthroscopy is indicated when the radiographic diagnosis is indefinite and symptoms persist without any other obvious cause.

Joint loose bodies:

Fibrous, bony, cartilaginous, and osteocartilaginous fragments in a synovial joint. Major causes are OCD, synovial chondromatosis, osteophytes (degenerative arthritis), fractured articular surfaces, and damaged menisci.

Histopathology:

- Microscopically, many cartilaginous nodules are observed as they form beneath the thin layer of cells that line the surface of the synovial membrane.
- These nodules are highly cellular and the cells themselves may exhibit a moderate pleomorphism, with occasional plump and double nuclei.
- Although such cytologic atypia mainly indicates an actively growing cartilaginous focus, an erroneous diagnosis of malignancy may sometimes be considered. [However, evidence of aggressive growth (invasion) and lack of attachment of a lesion to the synovial lining support the diagnosis of malignancy.]
- The cartilaginous nodules, which often are undergoing calcification and enchondral ossification, may detach and become loose bodies.
- The loose bodies continue to be viable and may increase in size, as they receive nourishment from the synovial fluid.
- Synovial chondromatosis may undergo malignant change to chondrosarcoma.

Treatment:

- Treatment consists of removing any loose osteochondromatous bodies and the involved synovium, from which they arise.
- Arthroscopic complete synovectomy is today's choice of treatment.
- If the condition recurs, due to left out nests of synovium, revision arthroscopic synovectomy or may be even arthrotomy can be done.
- Long-standing synovial osteochondromatosis creates secondary osteoarthritis.

Other non-neoplastic benign conditions mimicking tumors:

- *Myositis ossificans (heterotopic or ectopic ossification):* It may occur near the elbow, either in muscle or in other soft tissue. In its early or "florid" stage, there may be such pronounced cellular activity that it may be mistaken for sarcoma.
- *Proliferative fasciitis*: Poorly defined small mass showing prominent mitotic activity; has been mistaken for entities such as liposarcoma or fibrosarcoma. The rapidly proliferating cells again do not show true anaplasia.
- *Proliferative myositis:* There is a tumefactive and intramuscular proliferation of benign fibroblastic cells, but no discernible osseous metaplasia. Mitotic activity may be pronounced, making it possible to mistake this lesion for a malignant tumor.

Malignant Soft-tissue Tumors

Synovial sarcoma:

- Synovial sarcoma, or synovioma, is a malignant soft-tissue tumor that usually arises near but not in a joint; about 70% of lesions involve the lower extremity, most commonly the thigh, but this tumor does occur in the region of the elbow.
- Despite its name, it does not arise from synovium, although it may originate from any other structure, including joint capsules, bursae, and tendon sheaths.
- Because of the similarity between cells of this tumor and primitive synoviocytes, the term synovial cell sarcoma has been used.
- Young or middle-aged adults seem to be most commonly affected.

Clinical features:

- Diffuse or discrete soft-tissue swelling or mass
- Progressive pain
- Tenderness.

Imaging:

- On plain radiographs, synovial sarcoma shows evidence of calcification.
- When calcification is found in a soft-tissue tumor, synovial sarcoma should be included in the differential diagnosis.
- A periosteal reaction may also be observed.
- This tumor can invade the bone occasionally.
- CT and MRI scans effectively demonstrate the extent of the soft-tissue mass, calcifications, and bone invasion.

Histopathology:

- The tumor is lobular, circumscribed, and gray; it may contain areas of calcification, hemorrhage, necrosis, or cyst formation.
- Several subtypes of synovial sarcoma have been recognized. Among them are biphasic or bimorphic (fibrous and epithelial), monophasic, and poorly differentiated types.
- Classically, synovial sarcoma has a bimorphic histologic pattern; that is, a combination of slender spindle cells and larger epithelial-appearing cells that may form glands or even show squamous change.
- The monophasic synovial sarcoma is composed of interdigitating fascicles and "ball-like" structures formed by the spindle cells.

Treatment:
- In the past, local excision of the tumor was done resulting in local recurrence.
- Today, the treatment of choice is combination of radiation therapy and surgery. (With this approach, local recurrence occurs in only about 5% of cases).

Liposarcoma:
- Liposarcomas may arise in any part of the body and are occasionally found at the elbow.
- Older adults are more commonly affected than younger persons.
- A lipoma that shows evidence of growth should be suspected of being malignant.

Imaging:
- X-rays are not as diagnostic for liposarcoma as they are for lipoma, but the combination of more dense and less dense tissues may be characteristic of liposarcoma.
- CT scan is very helpful not only in defining the extent of the lesion but also in showing relative densities.

Histopathology:
- The pathologic diagnosis of liposarcoma may be difficult, especially when the lesion is histologically of low-grade.
- Microscopically, liposarcomas are recognized because of their component of malignant lipoblasts.
- The diagnostic procedure of choice for liposarcoma is open biopsy. (With superficial, small, and fatty tumors, excisional biopsy is recommended for diagnosis. In large, more than 3 cm, and deep tumors, diagnosis and treatment may involve open incisional biopsy followed by definitive resection).
- Fine-needle aspiration or biopsy should be followed by histologic and immunohistochemical examination. (Immunohistochemical examination aids in excluding other sarcomas).

Treatment:
- For liposarcomas, radiation therapy may be a valuable adjunct to surgery, especially in those of the myxoid variant.
- Although surgical resection is the mainstay of curative treatment, patients with large high-grade liposarcomas may benefit from multimodality treatment with chemotherapy and radiation.
- This is difficult to do with tumors in the region of the elbow and amputation may be necessary.

Malignant fibrous histiocytoma:
- Malignant fibrous histiocytoma (MFH), described by O'Brien and Stout in 1964, is the most common soft-tissue sarcoma of late adult life.
- It is now the most commonly encountered malignant soft-tissue tumor of the extremities.
- This tumor can arise in any age group.

Clinical features:
- Painless enlarging soft-tissue mass.

Imaging:
- Radiographs may reveal a nonspecific soft-tissue mass, often greater than 5 cm in diameter.
- It can be detected by MRI, but a biopsy is required for definitive diagnosis.
- Central necrosis is often evident, especially on larger masses.

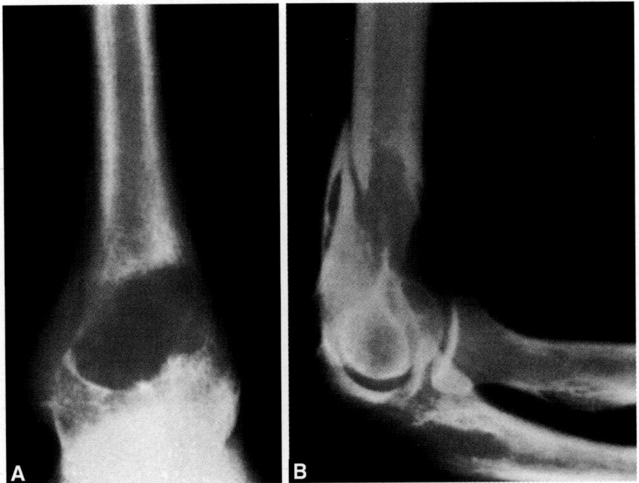

Figs. 209A and B: Epithelioid sarcoma that has eroded into and destroyed much of the distal part of the humerus in a 27-year-old woman.

Histopathology:
- Grossly, this tumor is usually soft and pink or yellow.
- Microscopically, the tumor contains both fibroblast like and histiocyte-like cells in varying proportions, with spindled and rounded cells exhibiting a storiform arrangement.
- *Several histological subtypes have been described*:
  - Storiform/pleomorphic MFH (current WHO classification: undifferentiated high-grade pleomorphic sarcoma)
  - Myxoid MFH (current WHO classification: myxofibrosarcoma)
  - Giant cell MFH (current WHO classification: undifferentiated pleomorphic sarcoma with giant cells)
  - Inflammatory MFH (current WHO classification: undifferentiated pleomorphic sarcoma with prominent inflammation)
  - Angiomatoid fibrous histiocytoma (formerly known as angiomatoid MFH) is now classified by the WHO as a tumor of uncertain differentiation.

Treatment:
- Relatively, small tumors may be excised with a margin of normal tissues on all aspects.
- Larger lesions or those that are histologically higher grade require a more aggressive approach—a course of preoperative radiation therapy using approximately 5,000 rad, followed after several weeks by excision of the lesion with a margin of normal tissue on all aspects.
- Chemotherapy remains controversial in MFH.
- The usual site of metastatic disease is the lungs, and metastases should be resected if possible.

Epithelioid sarcoma:
- Epithelioid sarcoma is a rare, slowly growing malignant tumor that usually begins in the superficial tissues of the hand or forearm and may occur at the elbow (Figs. 209A and B).
- This rare malignant tumor occurs in adolescents and young adults.
- The tumor spreads along fascial and neurovascular structures with formation of satellite nodules.
- Multiple recurrences are known to occur in this tumor.

- Lymphatic or hematogenous metastasis to the scalp, lymph nodes, and lungs occurs frequently.

Histopathology:
- The tumor is made up of small and poorly defined tumor nodules composed of epithelioid cells or histiocytic aggregates.
- Sometimes, central necrosis in these aggregates of cells suggests that the disease is a granulomatous infection.
- Rarely, the tumor erodes into underlying bones.

Treatment:
- Marginal or intralesional excision almost always results in tumor recurrence and subsequent disease progression.
- Treatment for cure requires wide excision.
- Regional lymph node dissection should be included as lymph node metastasis is common in epithelioid sarcoma.
- Surgical excision is combined with radiotherapy.

Hematopoietic involvement:
- Although certainly not characteristic, the elbow may be involved from hematopoietic neoplastic processes.
- The key feature is having a level of suspicion.
- A history of pain, often at night, without an easily identified or explained cause is almost always present for infection or neoplasm.
- Diagnosis may be made by open biopsy or arthroscopy.
- Treatment is as for the underlying pathology.

CHAPTER

Shoulder

29

OBJECTIVES

- Normal Anatomy and Biomechanics of Shoulder Joint
- Examination of Shoulder
- Congenital Anomalies of Shoulder
- Fractures around Shoulder and Epiphyseal Injuries
- Shoulder Dislocation
- Rotator Cuff Tears
- Shoulder Arthrodesis
- Shoulder Arthroplasty
- Inflammations around Shoulder
- Tumors around the Shoulder
- Brachial Plexus Injury and its Management
- Thoracic Outlet Syndrome

NORMAL ANATOMY AND BIOMECHANICS OF SHOULDER JOINT

INTRODUCTION

Knowledge of normal anatomy and biomechanics of the shoulder joint provides a foundation for evaluation and treatment of shoulder disorders.

SHOULDER GIRDLE

Shoulder girdle is described in Figures 1A and B.

- Glenohumeral (GH) joint
- Acromioclavicular (AC) joint
- Sternoclavicular (SC) joint
- Scapulothoracic (ST) joint
- Subacromial space

SCAPULOHUMERAL MUSCLES

Muscles of anterior and posterior shoulder girdle are shown in Figures 2A and B, respectively.

Intrinsic Muscles

- Rotator cuff (RC) muscles
- Deltoid
- Pectoralis major

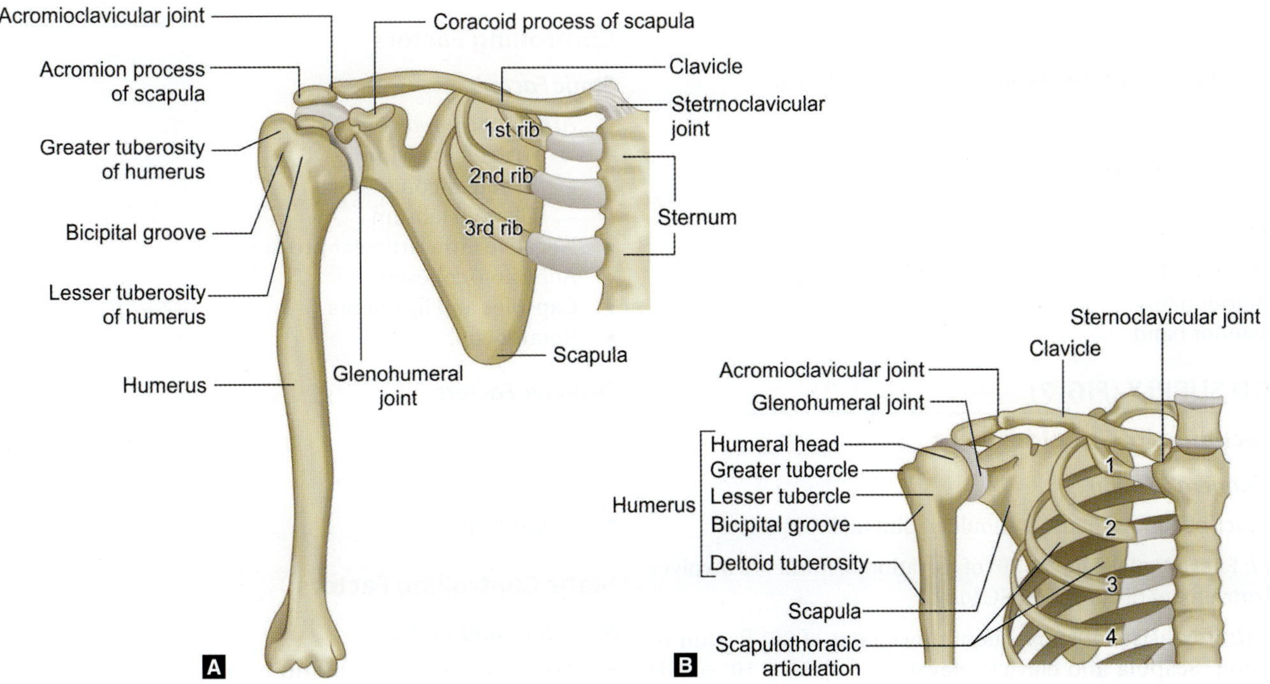

Figs. 1A and B: Anatomy of shoulder girdle.

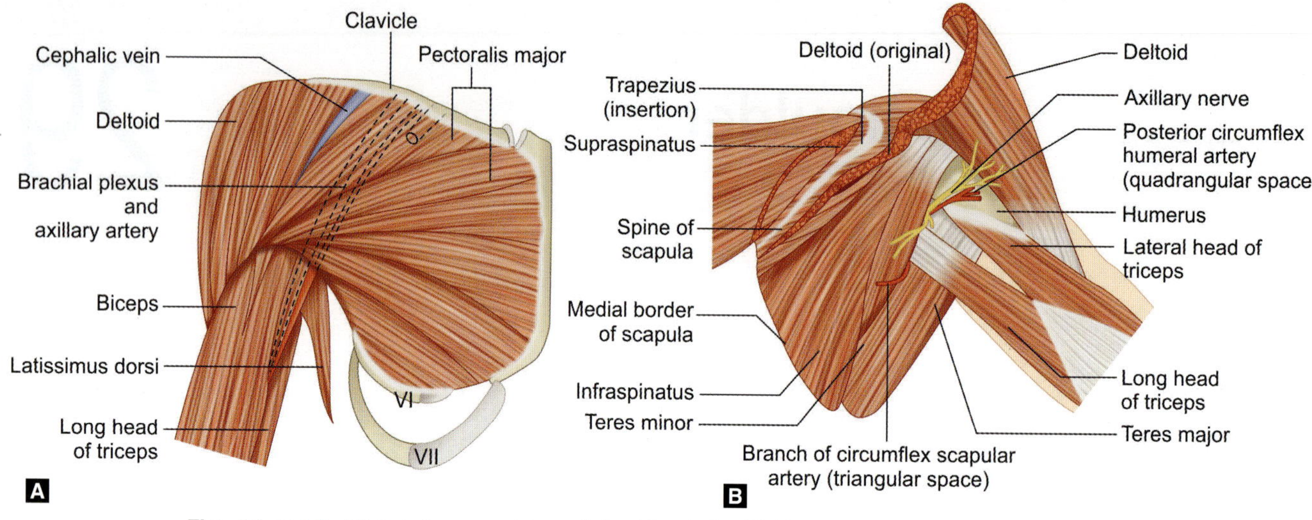

Figs. 2A and B: (A) Anterior musculature of shoulder girdle; (B) Musculature of posterior shoulder girdle.

- Teres major
- Latissimus dorsi
- Biceps brachii

Extrinsic Muscles

Origin, insertion, nerve supply, and action of extrinsic muscles are illustrated in Table 1. Important extrinsic muscles of the shoulder girdle are:

- Rhomboids major and minor
- Levator scapulae
- Trapezius
- Serratus anterior.

CAPSULOLIGAMENTOUS STRUCTURES (FIGS. 3 TO 6)

Glenohumeral Ligaments

- Superior glenohumeral ligament (SGHL)
- Middle glenohumeral ligament (MGHL)
- *Inferior glenohumeral ligament complex (IGHLC)*:
  - Anterior band
  - Posterior band
  - Axillary pouch.

Coracohumeral Ligaments

Coracohumeral ligaments are shown in Figures 5 and 6.

- Anterior band
- Posterior band.

BLOOD SUPPLY (FIG. 7)

Biomechanics of Shoulder Joint

Glenohumeral Motion

Saha described movements at shoulder joint in three phases:

Phase I: First 60° of flexion or 30° of elevation of humerus involves 15° of movement of clavicle at SC joint.

Phase II: It consists of subsequent movement of 90° flexion or abduction. Scapula and clavicle elevate 5° for every 10° of GH movement.

Phase III: This phase completes movement of humerus to elevated position; elevation of scapula is now twice that of GH joint, without further elevation of clavicle. Clavicle rotates along its long axis to permit elevation of scapula.

Normal Movements at Shoulder Joint

- *Abduction*: 0–170°
- *Adduction*: 0–50°
- *Flexion*: 0–165°
- *Extension*: 0–60°
- *External rotation at 90° abduction*: 100°
- *Internal rotation at 90° abduction*: 70°
- Circumduction.

Normal arthrokinematics: Combines rotation and translation, to keep humeral head centered on glenoid.

Capsular tightness: Resulted in abnormal arthrokinematics.

Controlling Factors

Static Factors

- *Articular component*:
  - Articular version
  - Articular congruence
  - Glenoid labrum
- Negative intra-articular pressure
- Adhesion-cohesion
- Capsules and ligaments
- Rotator cuff.

Dynamic Factors

- Rotator cuff
- Biceps brachii
- Scapular rotators
- Proprioception.

Static Controlling Factors

Articular Components

- *Articular version:* With arm hanging at side in an adducted position, the scapula faces 30° anteriorly on the chest wall and

TABLE 1: Origin, insertion, nerve supply and action of extrinsic muscles.

Muscle	*Origin*	*Insertion*	*Nerve supply*	*Action*
Trapezius	Medial 1/3rd of superior nuchal line of occipital bone, spinous process and supraspinous ligaments of T1–T12	Upper fibers into lateral third of clavicle; middle and lower fibers into acromion and spine of scapula	Spinal accessory nerve	Upper fibers elevate the scapula; middle fibers pull scapula medially; lower fibers pull medial border of scapula downward
Rhomboid minor	Ligamentum nuchae and spines of seventh cervical and first thoracic vertebrae	Medial border of scapula	Dorsal scapular nerve	Raises medial border of scapula upward and medially
Rhomboid major	Second to fifth thoracic spines	Medial border of scapula	Dorsal scapular nerve	Raises medial border of scapula upward and medially
Levator scapulae	Transverse processes of first four cervical vertebrae	Medial border of scapula	C3 and C4 and dorsal scapular nerve	Raises medial border of scapula
Serratus anterior	Upper eight ribs	Medial border and inferior angle of scapula	Long thoracic nerve	Draws the scapula forward around the thoracic wall; rotates scapula
Subscapularis	Subscapular fossa	Lesser tuberosity of humerus	Upper and lower subscapular nerves	Medially rotates arm and stabilizes shoulder joint
Teres major	Lower third of lateral border of scapula	Medial lip of bicipital groove of humerus	Lower subscapular nerve	Medially rotates and adducts arm and stabilizes shoulder joint
Teres minor	Upper two-thirds of lateral border of scapula	Greater tuberosity of humerus; capsule of shoulder joint	Axillary nerve	Laterally rotates arm and stabilizes shoulder joint
Supraspinatus	Supraspinous fossa of scapula	Greater tuberosity of humerus; capsule of shoulder joint	Suprascapular nerve	Abducts arm and stabilizes shoulder joint
Infraspinatus	Infraspinous fossa of scapula	Greater tuberosity of humerus; capsule of shoulder joint	Suprascapular nerve	Laterally rotates arm and stabilizes shoulder joint
Deltoid	Lateral third of clavicle, acromion, spine of scapula	Middle of lateral surface of shaft of humerus	Axillary nerve	Abducts arm; anterior fibers flex and medially rotate arm; posterior fibers extend and laterally rotate arm
Pectoralis major	Clavicle, sternum and upper six costal cartilages	Lateral lip of bicipital groove of humerus	Medial and lateral pectoral nerves from brachial plexus	Adducts arm and rotates it medially; clavicular fibers also flex arm
Latissimus dorsi	Iliac crest, lumbar fascia, spines of lower six thoracic vertebrae, lower three or four ribs and inferior angle of scapula	Floor of bicipital groove of humerus	Thoracodorsal nerve	Extends, adducts and medially rotates the arm
Biceps brachii short head	Tip of coracoid process	Posterior part of radial tuberosity	Musculocutaneous nerve	Supination, flexor of elbow
Long head	Supraglenoid tubercle of scapula			Long head keeps humeral head in glenoid cavity during abduction

tilts 3° upwards relative to transverse plane and 20° forward to the sagittal plane (Fig. 8). Scapular inclination may have a contributory role in controlling inferior instability. Retroversion averages 30° relative to transepicondylar axis of distal humerus. Neck shaft angle is 130–140° (Fig. 9).

- *Articular congruence:* Congruence can be defined as the difference in the radii of humeral head and glenoid articulating surfaces; GH articulating surfaces are shown in Figure 10. Closer the difference is to 0°, the more congruent is the joint. This congruent articulation provides the foundation for the RC to establish a concavity-compression effect, as it dynamically compresses the convex humeral head into the matched concavity of the glenoid. The glenoid surface is "pear-shaped", similar to inverted comma. The GH joint has been compared to a "golf-ball sitting on a tee", as shown in Figure 11.
- *Glenoid labrum:* Labrum enhances stability by deepening the concavity of the glenoid socket to an average of 9 mm to 5 mm, in superoinferior and anteroposterior planes, as demonstrated in Figure 12.

  Loss of labrum decreases the depth of socket by 50% in either direction. Functionally, it acts as "chock-block", preventing the head from slipping over the edge of the glenoid. Labrum acts to increase the surface area of contact, acting as a load-bearing structure.
- *Negative intra-articular pressure:* In normal shoulder, relative vacuum exists as a result of high osmotic pressure in the interstitial tissue, causing water to be drawn out of the GH joint. As articular surfaces are pulled apart, a suction effect develops to resist further displacement. It becomes important when the

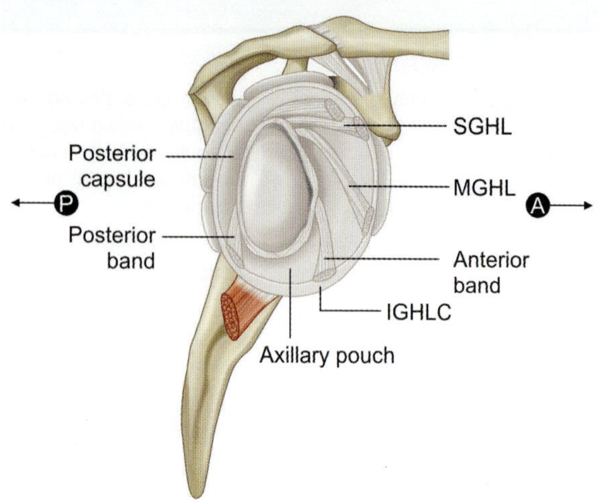

Fig. 3: Capsuloligamentous structures (MGHL: middle glenohumeral ligaments; IGHLC: inferior glenohumeral ligament complex; SGHL: superior glenohumeral ligament).

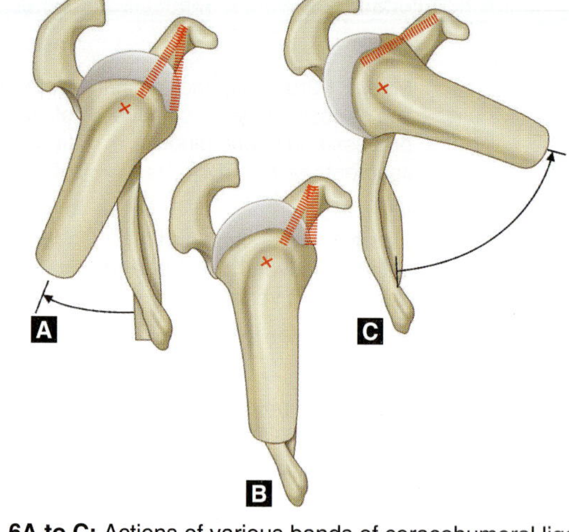

Figs. 6A to C: Actions of various bands of coracohumeral ligaments.

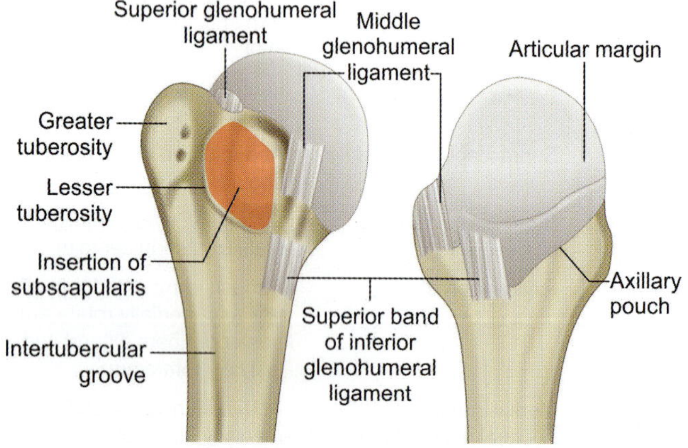

Fig. 4: Ligaments of shoulder joint showing various attachments of glenohumeral ligaments.

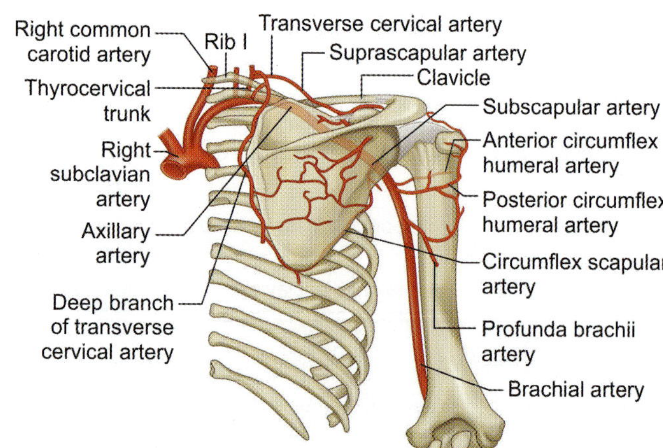

Fig. 7: Blood supply of the shoulder joint.

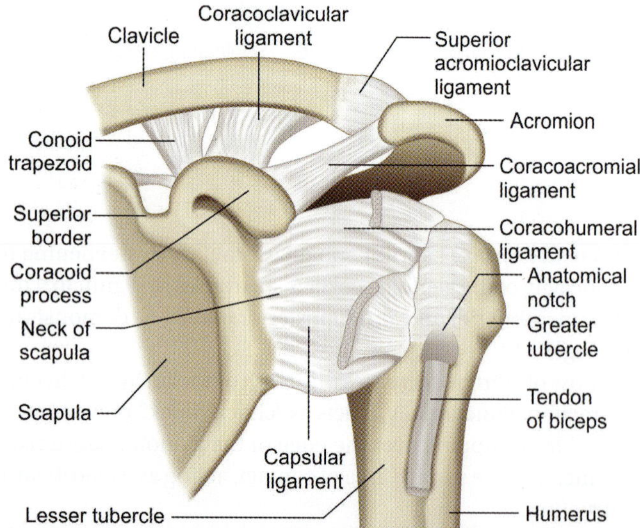

Fig. 5: Ligaments of shoulder joint showing attachments of coracohumeral ligaments.

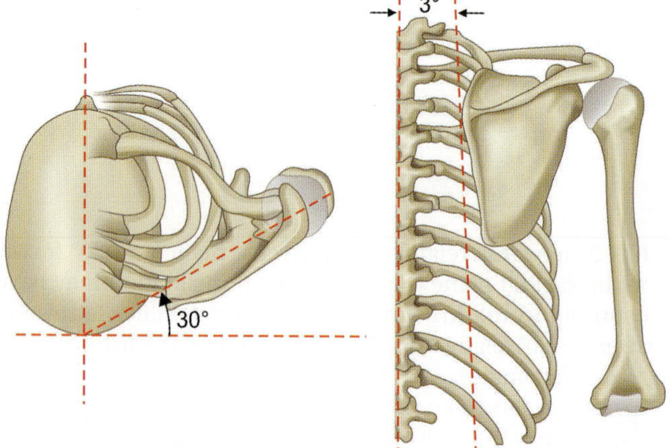

Fig. 8: Humeral articular version.

RC is not contracting or when tension has not developed in the superior and coracohumeral ligaments.

- *Adhesion-cohesion:* Glenohumeral joint contains 1 mL of synovial fluid that provides articular nourishment through diffusion and lubrication through several mechanisms. Viscous and intramolecular forces help to create this adhesion-cohesion effect. Negative intra-articular pressure and adhesive

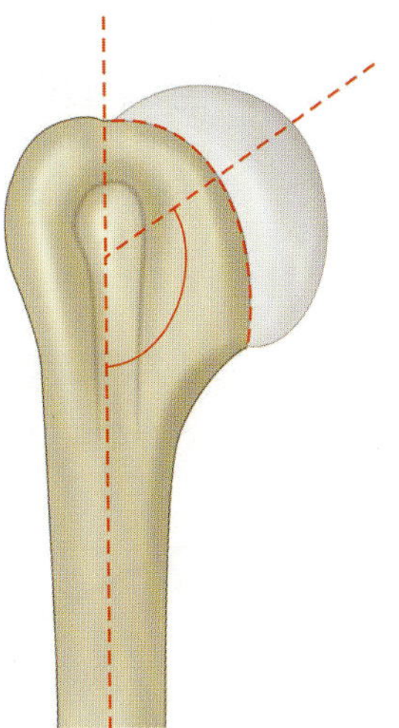

Fig. 9: Retroversion averages 30° relative to transepicondylar axis of distal humerus.

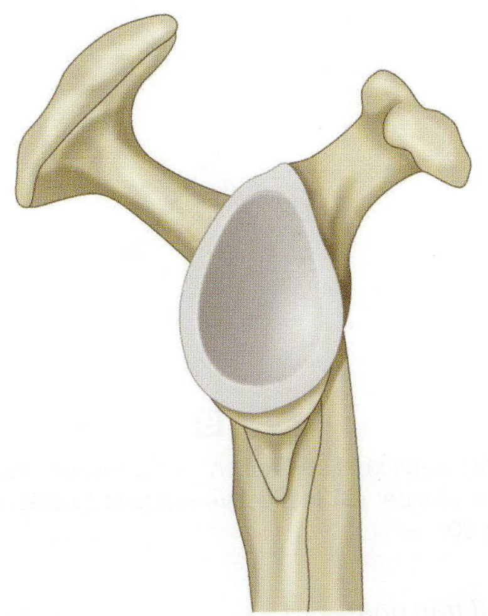

Fig. 10: Articular surface of glenohumeral joint.

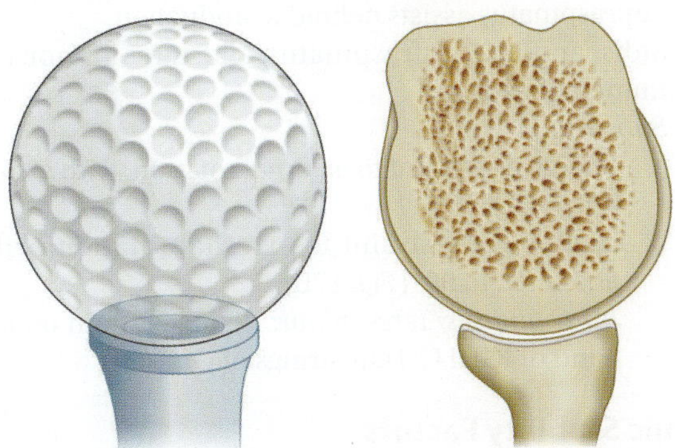

Fig. 11: Glenohumeral joint, compared to a golf ball sitting on a tee.

forces resulting from presence of synovial fluid between the articular surfaces, contribute static restraints when capsule is lax and muscles are inactive.

- *Capsuloligamentous structure:* Various capsuloligamentous structures are shown in Figure 13. Restraints to various movements, by these capsuloligamentous structures are described here:
  - *Restraints to external rotation (Fig. 14)*: Dependent on arm position; this is illustrated in Table 2.

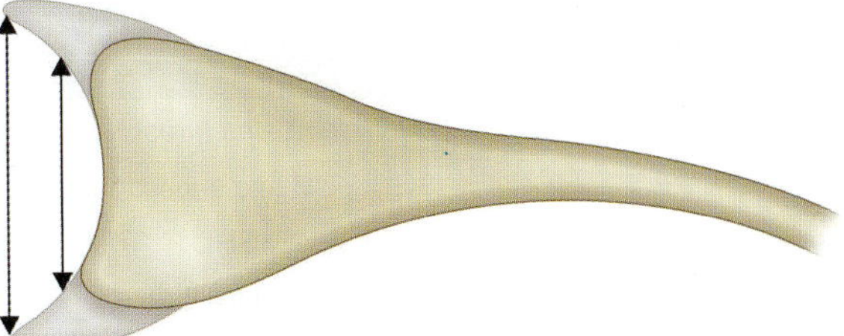

Fig. 12: Deepening of concavity of glenoid socket by glenoid labrum.

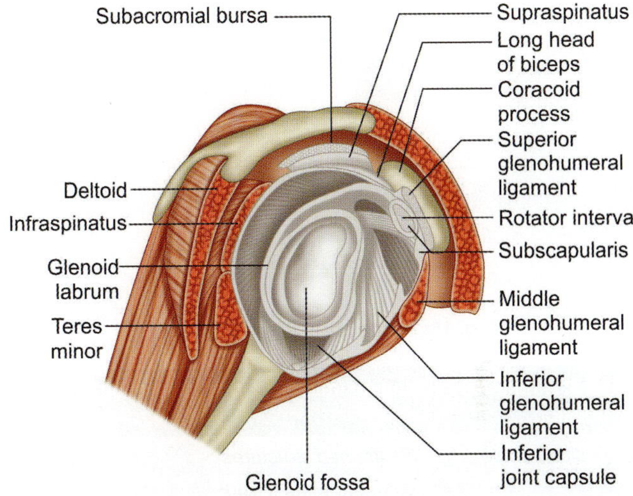

Fig. 13: Capsuloligamentous structure of glenohumeral joint.

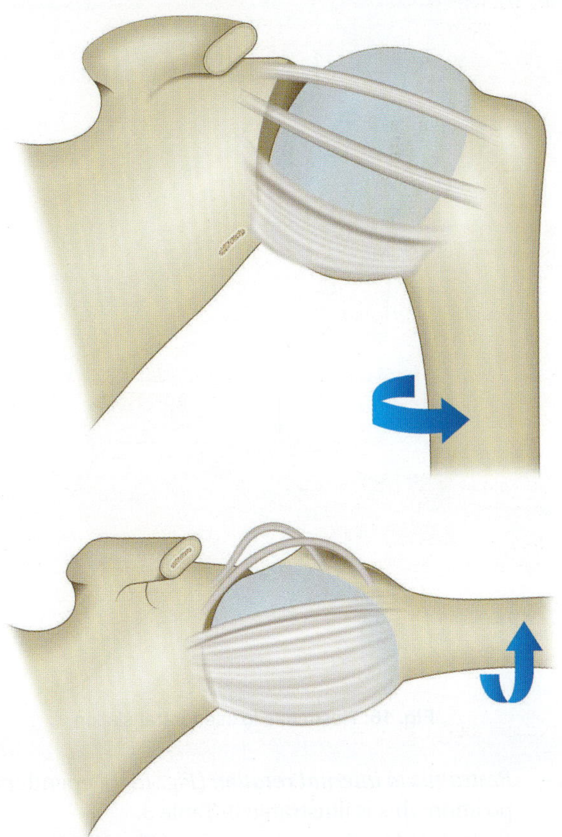

Fig. 14: Restraints to external rotation.

TABLE 2: Structures causing restraining to external rotation at different arm position.

Arm position/angle	*Restrained structures*
At 0°	SGHL, CH and subscapularis
45°	SGHL and MGHL
90°	Anterior band IGHLC

(CH: coracohumeral; IGHLC: inferior glenohumeral ligament complex; MGHL: middle glenohumeral ligament; SGHL: superior glenohumeral ligament)

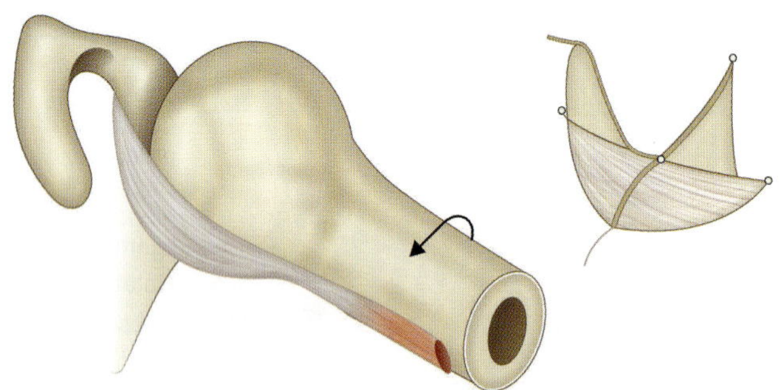

Fig. 15: Restraints to internal rotation.

TABLE 3: Structures causing restraining to internal rotation at different arm position.

Arm position/angle	*Restrained structures*	
At 0°	Posterior band IGHLC	
At 45°	Anterior and posterior band	IGHLC
At 90°	Anterior and posterior band	IGHLC

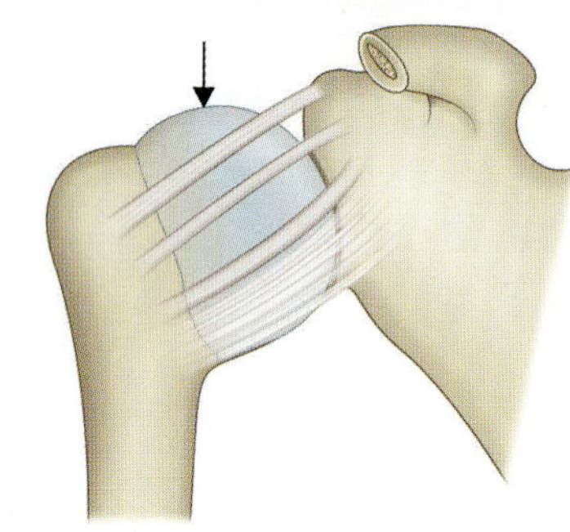

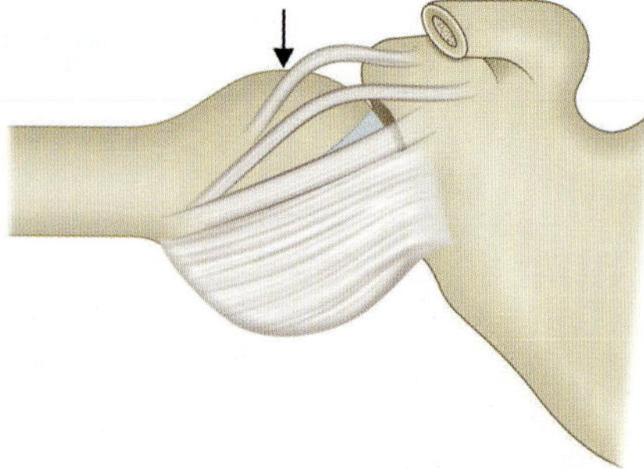

Fig. 16: Restraints to inferior translation.

- *Restraints to internal rotation (Fig. 15)*: Dependent on arm position; this is illustrated in Table 3.
- *Restraints to inferior translation (Fig. 16)*: Dependent on arm position; this is illustrated in Table 4.

TABLE 4: Structures causing restraining to inferior translation at different arm position.

Arm position/angle	*Restrained structures*
At 0°	SGHL and CH
90°	IGHLC

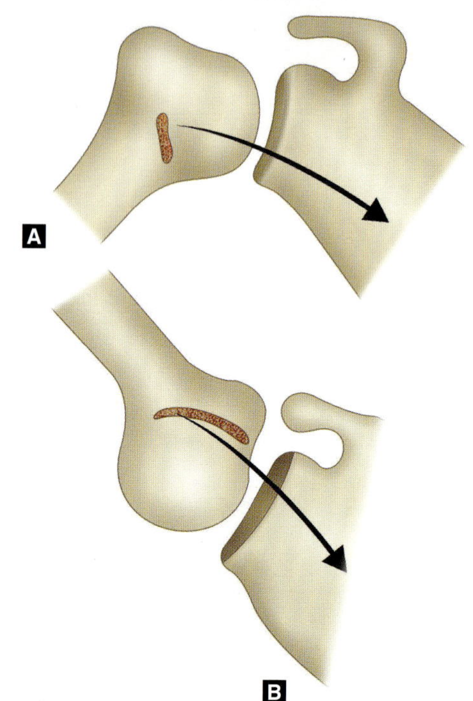

Figs. 17A and B: Subscapularis action: (A) Effective restraint to external rotation, with arm at side; (B) Ineffective restraint to external rotation, with arm abducted to 90°.

- *Rotator cuff function:*
  - Approximates humerus, to function
  - Supraspinatus assists deltoid in abduction
  - Subscapularis, infraspinatus and teres minor depress humeral head
  - *Subscapularis*:
    a. Effective restraint to external rotation, with arm at side (Fig. 17A).
    b. Ineffective restraint to external rotation, with arm abducted to 90° (Fig. 17B).
    Infraspinatus/Teres minor: Reduces strain on anterior band of IGHLC. Hamstrings of GH joint.

Dynamic Stability Factors

Long Head of Biceps Brachii (Fig. 18)

- Biceps tendon force increases torsional rigidity to external rotation.
- No effect on strain of IGHLC.
- Effect lost with SLAP (Superior labral tear from anterior to posterior) lesion.
- Biceps becomes more important anterior stabilizer as capsuloligamentous stability decreases.
- Biceps tended to stabilize the shoulder (Fig. 19) joint anteriorly, when the arm was internally rotated and served as a posterior stabilizer when humerus is externally rotated.

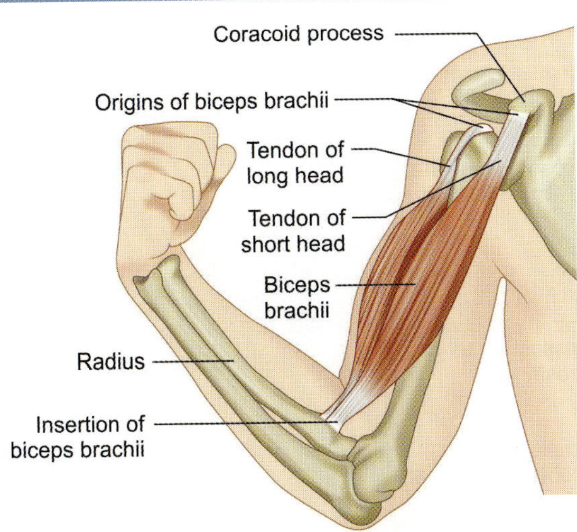

Fig. 18: Attachments of the long head of biceps brachii.

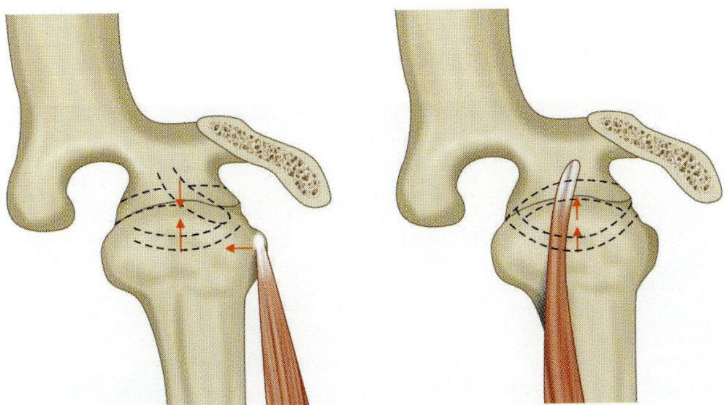

Fig. 19: Action of biceps as dynamic stabilizer of shoulder joint.

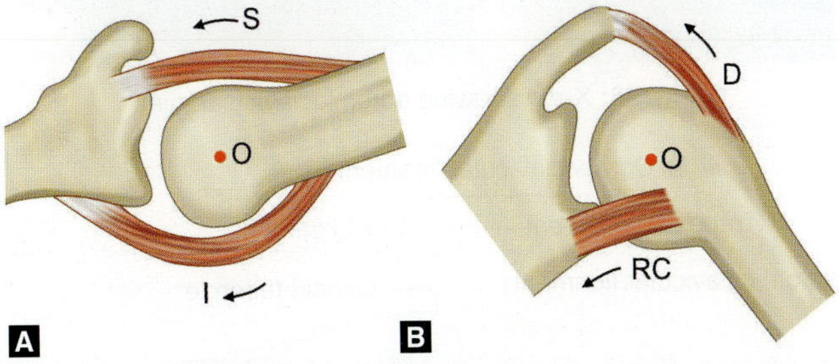

Figs. 20A and B: Force couples acting on glenohumeral joint: (A) Subscapularis versus infraspinatus; (B) Deltoid versus inferior RC muscles.

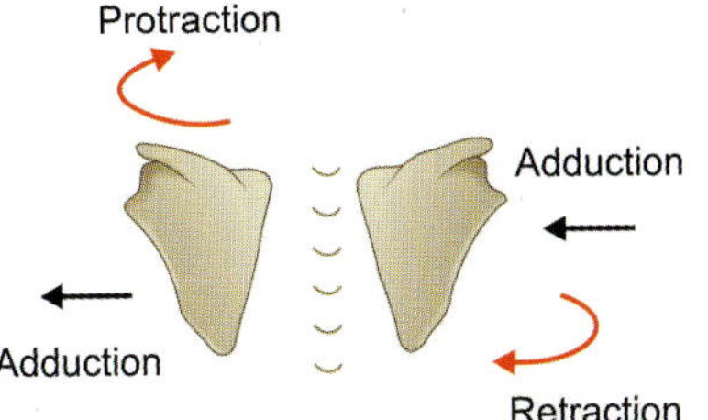

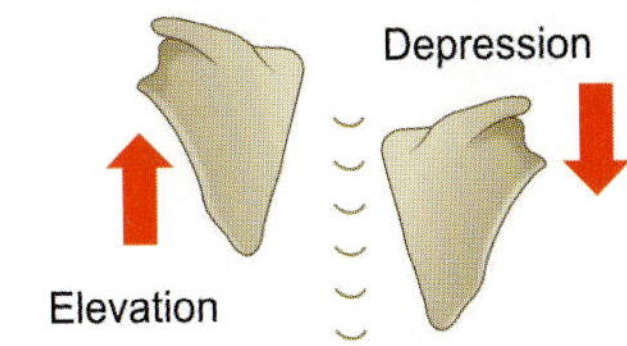

Fig. 21: Scapulothoracic motions.

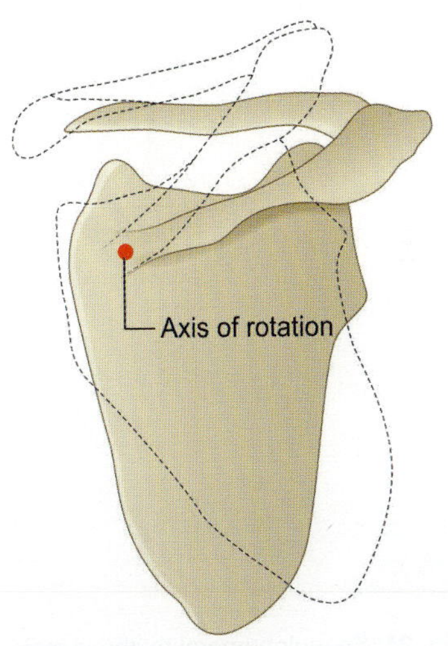

Fig. 22: Scapular rotation—Phase I.

Force Couples

Force couples acting on GH joint are:

- *Transverse plane:* Subscapularis versus infraspinatus (Fig. 20A)
- *Coronal plane:* Deltoid versus inferior RC muscles (Fig. 20B).

Scapulothoracic muscles

- Trapezius
- Serratus anterior
- Rhomboids
- Levator scapulae
- Pectoralis minor
- Subclavius
- Scapulothoracic motions (Fig. 21) are:
  - Elevation/depression
  - Protraction/retraction
  - Upward/downward rotation.

Biomechanics of Scapular Rotation

- Scapulothoracic motion occurs as part of closed kinetic chain involving:
  - Acromioclavicular joint
  - Scapuloclavicular joint
- *Scapular rotation*: Different phases of scapular rotation are:
  Phase I: Upper and lower portions of trapezius and serratus anterior produce upward rotatory force on scapula. Motion at AC joint is prevented by coracoclavicular (CC) ligament. Rotation of scapula occurs as elevation of clavicle at SC joint (Fig. 22).
  Phase II: Further motion at SC joint prevented by costoclavicular ligament. Continued upward rotation of scapula pulls on costoclavicular ligament, causing posterior rotation of clavicle. Posterior rotation of clavicle allows further upward rotation of scapula (Fig. 23).
- *Scapular rotation is necessary to*:
  - Enhance GH stability
  - Elevate acromion to avoid impingement
  - Maintain effective length tension relationship of scapulohumeral muscles.
- *Proprioception:* The perception of the joint position and joint motion is termed as proprioception. Proprioceptive

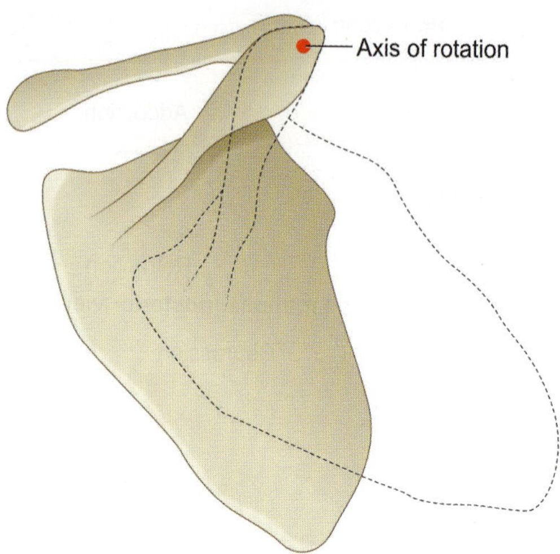

Fig. 23: Scapular rotation— Phase II.

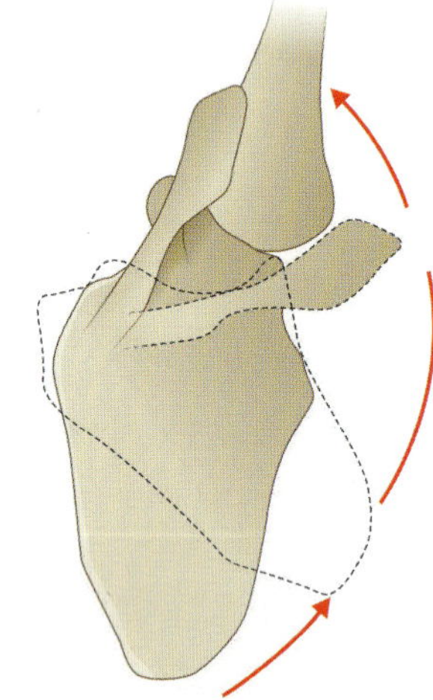

Fig. 24: Scapulohumeral rhythmic motion.

interaction between ligaments and muscles mediate a protective mechanism against capsular failure and instability. Mechanoreceptors are specialized nerve endings that transduce mechanical deformation into electric signals that transmit information about joint position and motion.

- *Force couple at ST joint:*
  - Serratus anterior produces anterolateral movement of inferior angle.
  - Upper trapezius pulls scapula medially.
- *Scapulohumeral rhythm:* Total elevation is 120° at GH joint and 60° at ST joint (Fig. 24).

ACROMIOCLAVICULAR JOINT

It is shown in Figures 25 and 26, and consists of:

- Joint capsule
- AC ligaments
- Intra-articular disk
- *Coracoclavicular ligaments*:
  - Conoid (medial)
  - Trapezoid (lateral)
- Diarthrodial joint between medial facet of acromion and the lateral (distal) clavicle
- Contains intra-articular disk of variable size

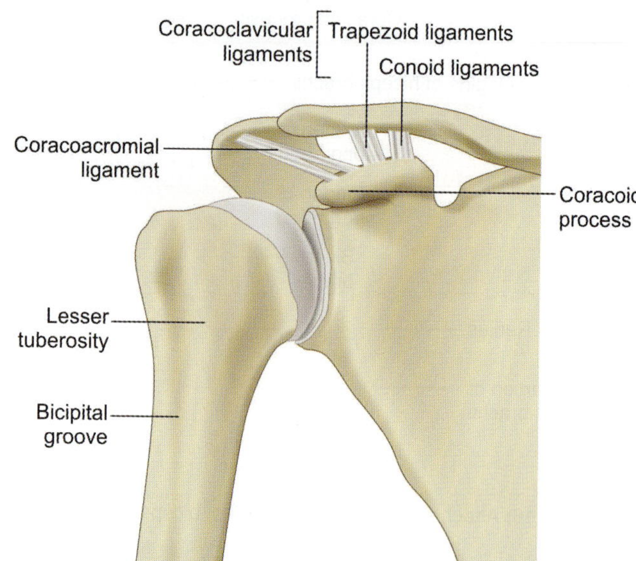

Fig. 25: Acromioclavicular joint and adjoining structures.

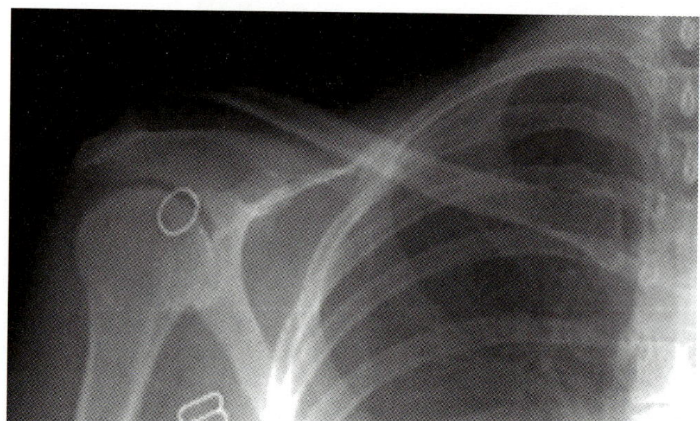

Fig. 26: X-ray showing acromioclavicular joint.

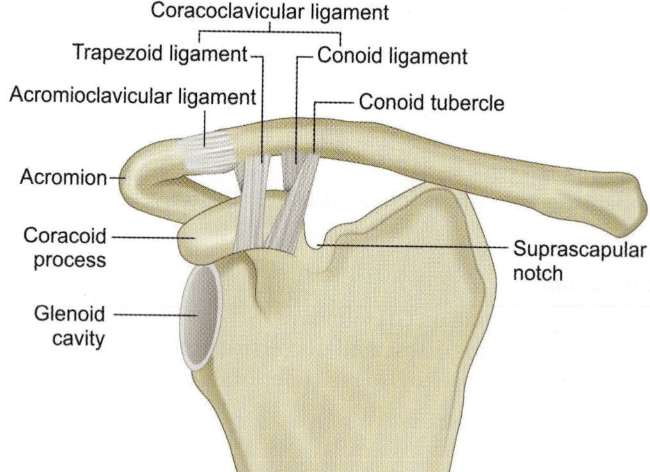

Fig. 27: Normal anatomy of AC joint.

- Thin capsule stabilized by ligaments on all sides:
  - AC ligaments control horizontal (anteroposterior) displacement
  - Superior AC ligament is most important
- Normal anatomy of AC joint, shown in Figure 27
- Normal inclination of AC-SC joint is shown in Figure 28.

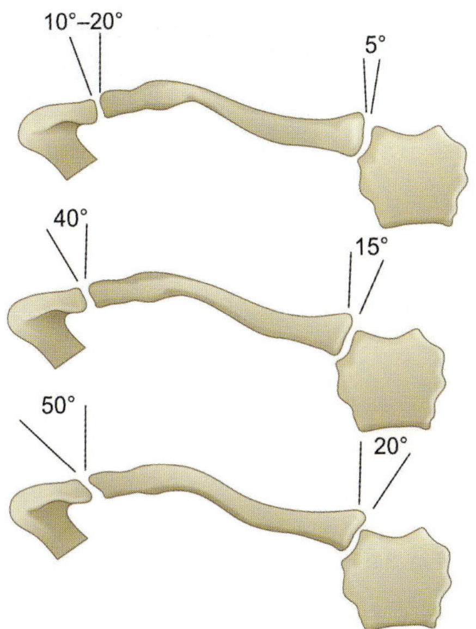

Fig. 28: Different inclination of AC-sternoclavicular joint.

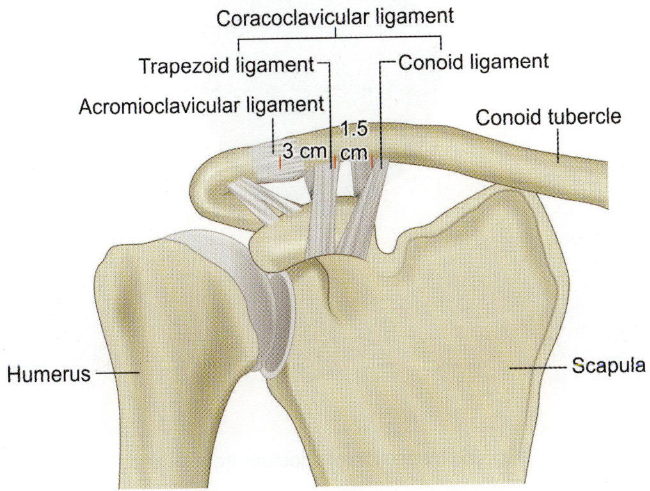

Fig. 29: Stability provided by ligaments.

- *Stability provided by ligaments* (Fig. 29):
  - Horizontal stability controlled by AC ligament
  - Vertical stability controlled by CC ligament
- *Movements*:
  - Axial rotation of clavicle (spin)
  - Angulation between scapula and clavicle.

STERNOCLAVICULAR JOINT

Sternoclavicular (SC) joint is shown in Figure 30 and SC joint consists of following structures:

- Joint capsule
- Anterior and posterior SC ligaments
- Intra-articular disk
- Interclavicular ligament
- Costoclavicular ligament.

Anatomy of Sternoclavicular Joint

- The anatomy of the SC joint is shown in Figure 31.
- It is a diarthrodial joint.
- It is a saddle-shaped joint.

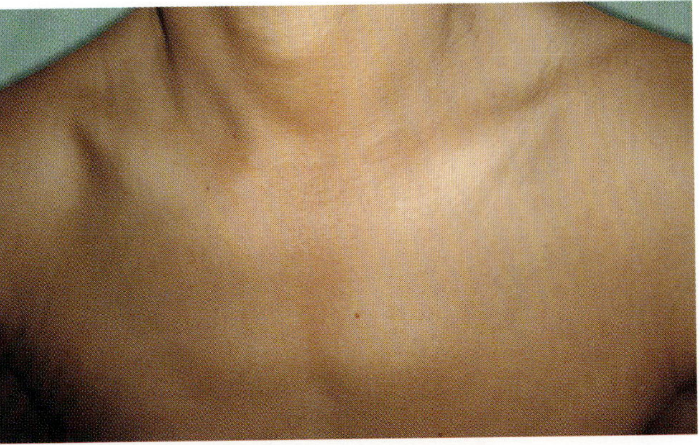

Fig. 30: Sternoclavicular joint.

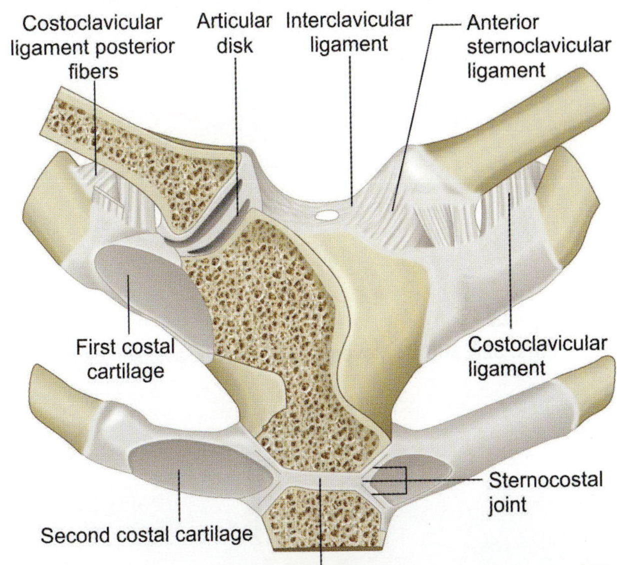

Fig. 31: Anatomy of sternoclavicular joint.

- Poor congruence.
- *Intra-articular disk ligament:* It divides SC joint into two separate joint spaces.
- *Costoclavicular ligament (rhomboid ligament):* Short and strong and consist of an anterior and posterior fasciculus.
- *Interclavicular ligament:* Connects the superomedial aspects of each clavicle with the capsular ligaments and the upper sternum.
- *Capsular ligament:* Covers the anterior and posterior aspects of the joint and represents thickenings of the joint capsule. The anterior portion of the ligament is heavier and stronger than the posterior portion.
- *Movements (Figs. 32A and B):* Different SC joint movements are:
  - Protraction/retraction
  - Elevation/depression
  - Axial rotation (spin).

EXAMINATION OF SHOULDER

INSPECTION

From Front

- Prominent SC joint, e.g. subluxation
- Deformity of clavicle, e.g. old fracture

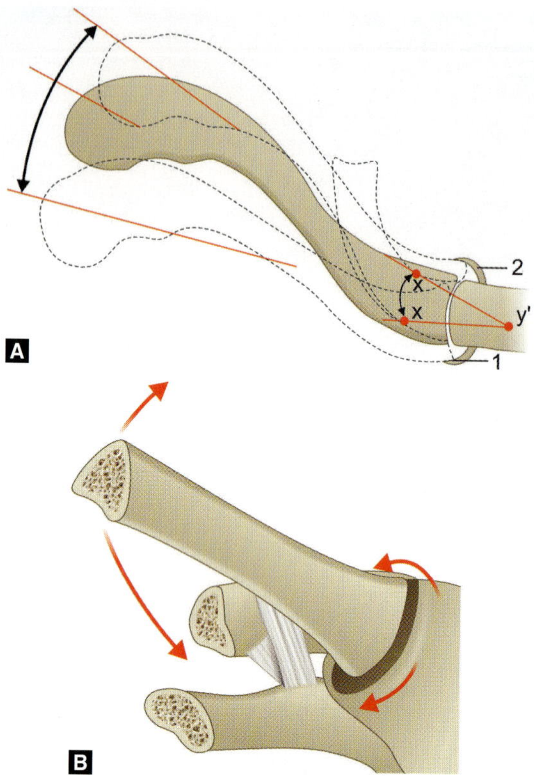

Figs. 32A and B: Movements of sternoclavicular joint.

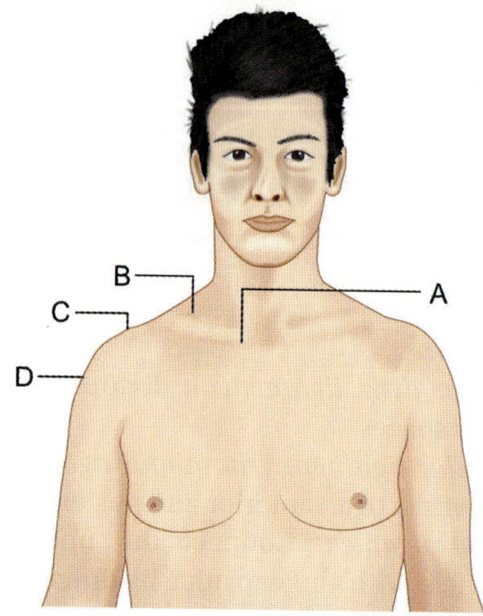

Fig. 33: Inspection of shoulder joint from front: A. Prominent sternoclavicular joint; B. Clavicular deformity; C. Prominent acromioclavicular joint; D. Deltoid wasting.

- Prominent AC joint, e.g. subluxation or osteoarthritis (OA)
- Deltoid wasting, e.g. disuse/axillary nerve palsy.

Methods of inspection of the shoulder joint from front are shown in Figure 33.

From Side (Fig. 34)

Any swelling of the joint suggesting infection or inflammatory reaction.

From Behind (Fig. 35)

While inspecting the shoulder from behind, one needs to answer the following questions:

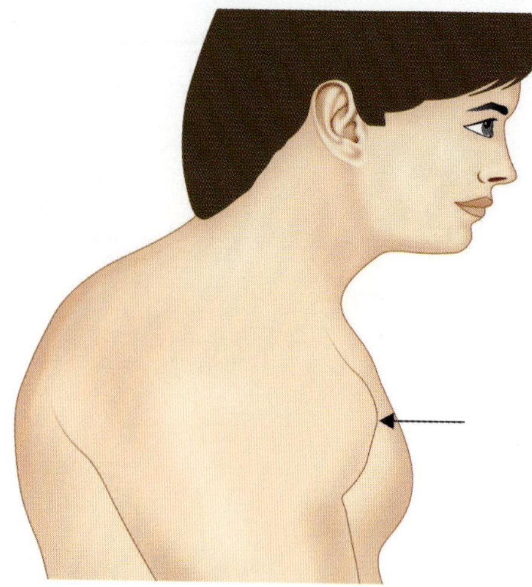

Fig. 34: Inspection of shoulder from side.

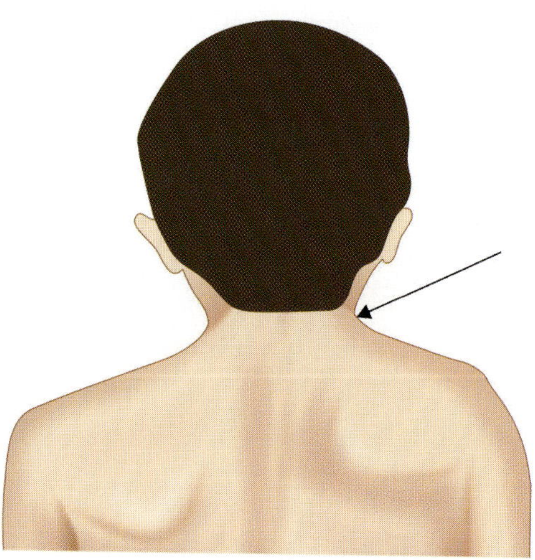

Fig. 35: Inspection of shoulder from behind.

- Is the scapula normally shaped and situated?
- Is it small and positioned high?

From Above (Fig. 36)

While inspecting the shoulder from above, one has to take note of the following:

- Swelling of the shoulder
- Deformity of the clavicle
- Asymmetry of supraclavicular fossa.

Palpation

- Palpate the anterior and lateral aspects of GH joint (Fig. 37). Diffuse tenderness is suggestive of infection or calcifying supraspinatus tendinitis.

  Tenderness over the AC joint is found after recent dislocation and osteoarthritis (OA) of the joint, as shown in Figure 38. Lipping is palpable and crepitus may be detected when arm is abducted.
- Press acromion and abduct the arm as illustrated in Figure 39. Tenderness is present in cases of tear and inflammatory lesions involving RC.

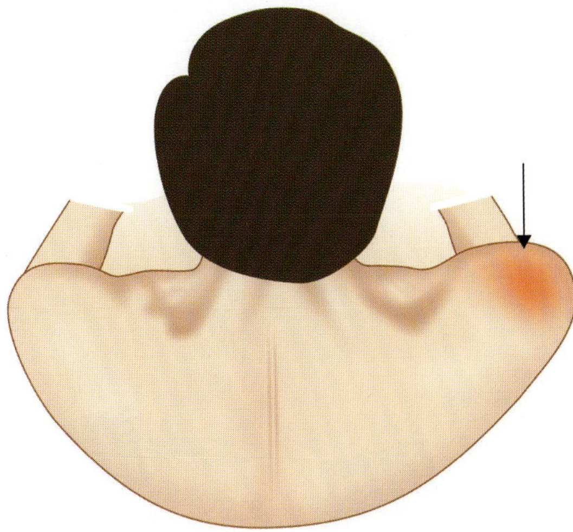

Fig. 36: Inspection of shoulder from above.

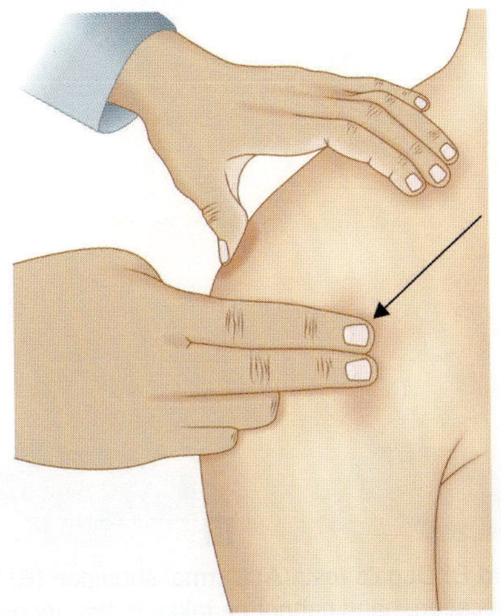

Fig. 37: Palpating the anterolateral aspect of glenohumeral joint.

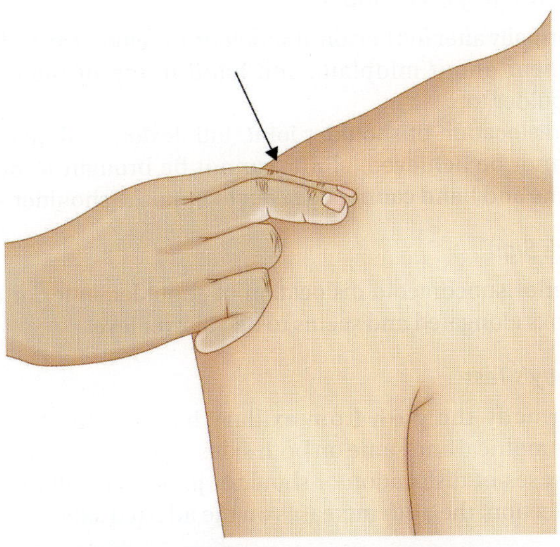

Fig. 38: Acromioclavicular joint palpation.

Movements

- Abduct both the arms; observe the smoothness of movement and range achieved (Fig. 40).

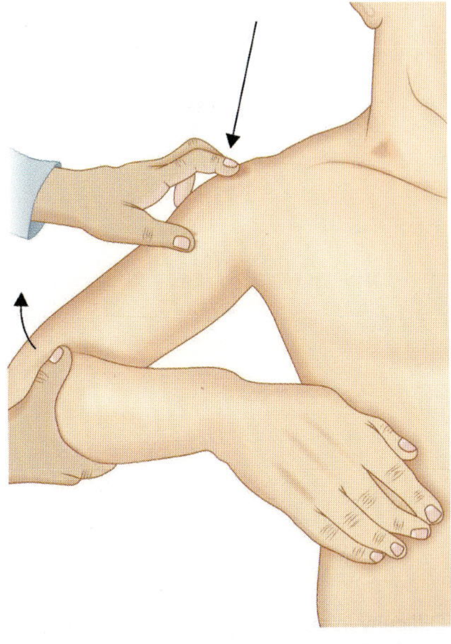

Fig. 39: Pressing acromion while simultaneously abducting the arm.

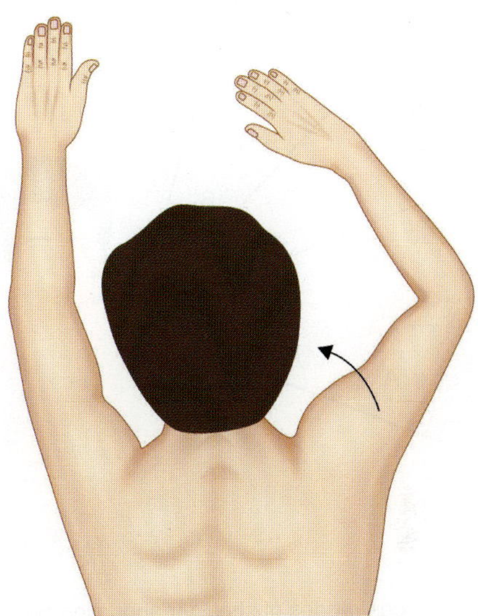

Fig. 40: Both arms abducted.

- Difficulty in abducting the arm is suggestive of shoulder cuff tear (Fig. 41).

Pain During Abduction (Fig. 42)

- Pain during arc of 70–120° suggests shoulder cuff impingement in region of acromion.
- Pain during later phase of abduction (above 120°) suggests shoulder cuff impingement in region of AC joint or coracoacromial (CA) ligament.

SHOULDER EVALUATION

Active Range of Motion (ROM)

- Flexion of 180°
- Extension of 50°
- Abduction of 180°
- Adduction of 40°
- Internal rotation of 90°
- External rotation of 90°.

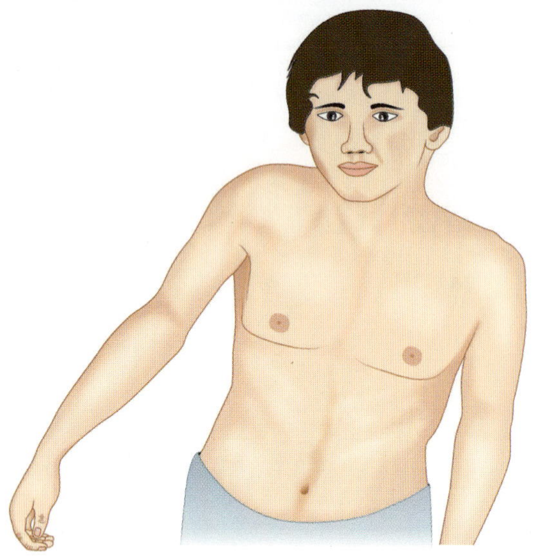

Fig. 41: Difficulty in abducting arm due to shoulder cuff tear.

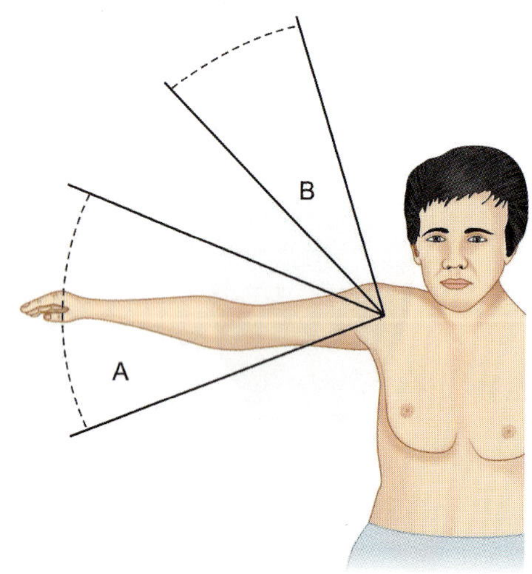

Fig. 42: Pain at various ranges of shoulder abduction suggests different joint involvement.

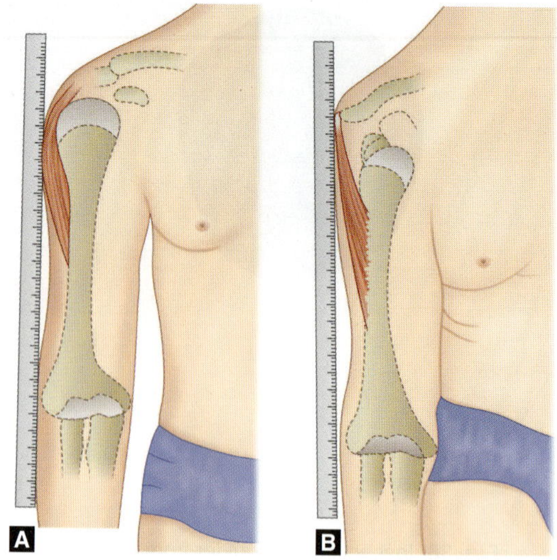

Figs. 43A and B: Hamilton ruler test.

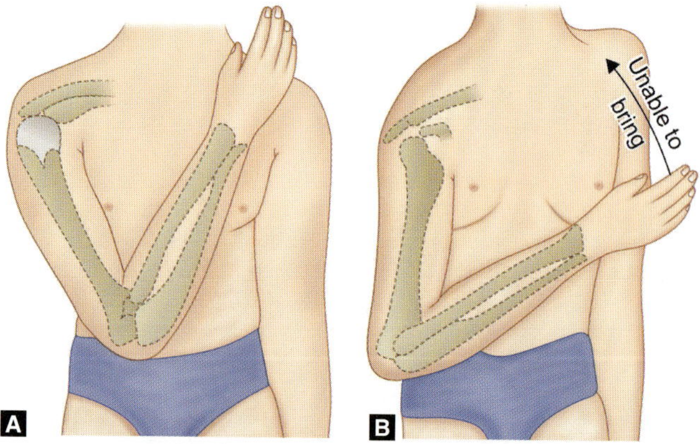

Figs. 44A and B: Duga's test: (A) Normal shoulder; (B) With anterior shoulder dislocation, hand cannot be taken to the opposite shoulder.

Manual Muscle Testing

Five points Grading System

- Grade 5 = Complete ROM against gravity, with full resistance
- Grade 4 = Complete ROM against gravity, with some resistance
- Grade 3 = Complete ROM against gravity, with no resistance
- Grade 2 = Complete ROM, with gravity omitted
- Grade 1 = Some muscle contractility with no joint motion
- Grade 0 = No muscle contractility.

Special Tests

Hamilton Ruler Test (Figs. 43A and B)

- In normal shoulder ruler cannot touch acromial process, and lateral epicondyle of humerus because of prominence of bulge of deltoid supported by head of humerus.
- Ruler touches both the points in dislocation of shoulder, absence of head, polio paralysis, and dissolution of humeral head in septic arthritis.

Duga's Test (Figs. 44A and B)

- Normally after full flexion at shoulder, the elbow can be brought to near about midplane and hand to top of the opposite shoulder top.
- In dislocation of shoulder joint, full flexion of shoulder joint cannot be achieved; elbow cannot be brought to midbody plane and hand cannot be taken to opposite shoulder.

Bryant's Sign

In anterior subcoracoid dislocation of shoulder, anterior axillary fold looks elongated and seems to be at lower level.

Callaway's Test

- Normally the girth from axillary base to shoulder top is symmetrical and same on both sides.
- In cases of dislocation of shoulder joint and axillary abscess collection, the girth increases on the affected side.

Sulcus Test for Inferior Instability of the Shoulder

- With the patient in the sitting position, downward traction is placed on the adducted arm (Fig. 45A).
- With a positive test (Fig. 45B), excessive inferior translation produces a dimple (arrow) on the lateral aspect of the acromion.

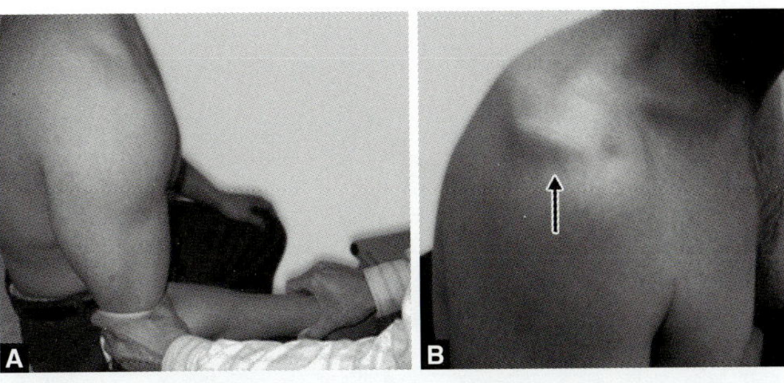

Figs. 45A and B: Sulcus test for inferior instability of the shoulder: (A) In the sitting position, a downward traction is placed on the adducted arm; (B) Positive test produce dimple (arrow) on the lateral aspect of the acromion due to excessive inferior translation.

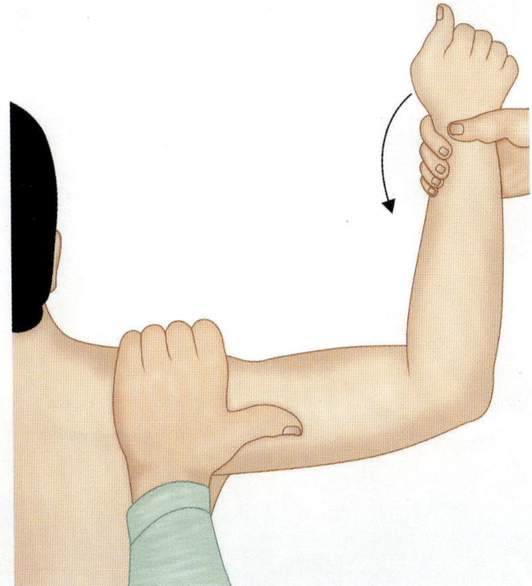

Fig. 46: Apprehension test.

- By performing this test with the arm in external rotation, the maneuver can also be used to test the integrity of the rotator interval structures.

Apprehension Test (Fig. 46)

- Stand behind the patient; abduct the shoulder to 90°.
- Externally rotate shoulder and push head of the humerus forward.
- Apprehension, fear, refusal is evident of chronic anterior instability of shoulder.
- Pain felt in minor subluxation.

Relocation Test (Fig. 47)

Apprehension test done in recumbent position:

- Abduct and externally rotate the shoulder.
- Press down on upper arm if pain is present, this stabilizes head of humerus in glenoid. When subluxation is imminent, this relieves the pain.
- Release of downward pressure with return of pain is confirmatory to anterior instability.

Drawer's Test of Gerber and Ganz (Anterior Glenohumeral Instability) (Fig. 48)

- Patient rests in supine position and arm relaxed with shoulder in 90° of abduction, slight flexion and external rotation.

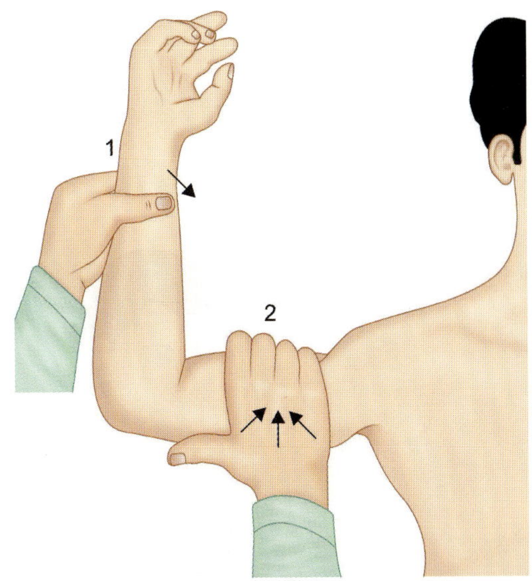

Fig. 47: Relocation test performed to detect shoulder instability—(1) Abduct and externally rotate the arm with one hand; (2) Apply downward pressure on arm and look for relief of pain.

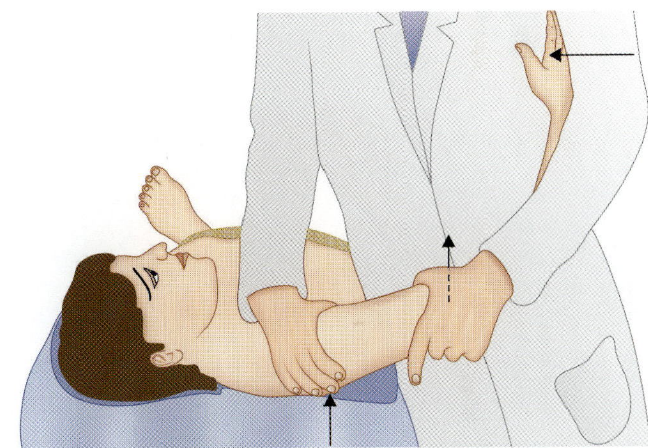

Fig. 48: Drawer's test of Gerber and Ganz.

- Scapula is steadied on coracoid then the humeral head is moved.
- Any movement or click confirms instability. Axial X-ray should be taken.

Neer's Test (Fig. 49)

- With the patient seated, the examiner raises the affected arm in forced forward elevation while stabilizing the scapula, causing the greater tuberosity to impinge against the acromion. This maneuver produces pain with impingement lesions of all stages.
- It also produces pain in many other shoulder conditions, such as adhesive capsulitis, OA, calcific tendinitis, and bone lesions.

Hawkins-Kennedy Test (Fig. 50)

The test is performed by forward flexing the humerus to 90° and forcibly internally rotating the shoulder. This maneuver drives the greater tuberosity farther under the CA ligament, reproducing the impingement pain.

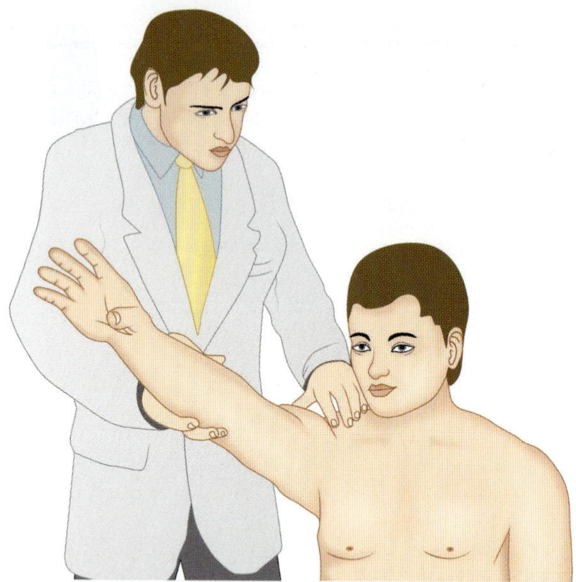

Fig. 49: Neer's test.

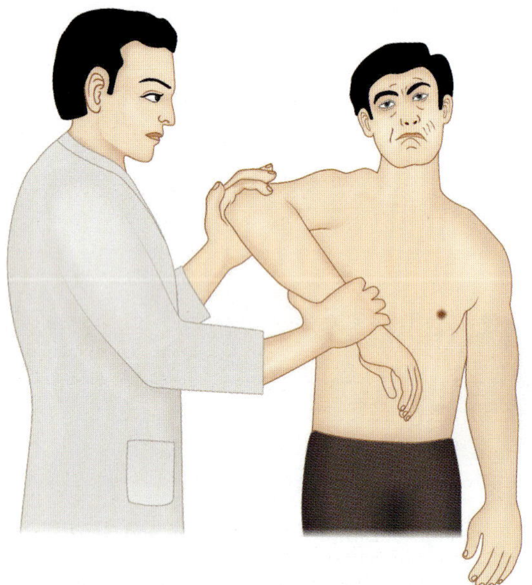

Fig. 50: Hawkins-Kennedy test.

SUPRASPINATUS WEAKNESS

Jobe's Test (Fig. 51)

- The test is performed by placing the shoulder in 90° of abduction and 30° of forward flexion and internally rotated so that the thumb is pointing towards the floor.
- Muscle testing against resistance shows weakness or insufficiency of the supraspinatus owing to a tear or pain associated with RC impingement.

BICEPS TENDON IRRITATION

Yergason's Test (Fig. 52)

The elbow is flexed to 90°, and the forearm is pronated. The patient attempts to supinate the forearm actively against resistance applied by the examiner at the patient's wrist. Pain localized to the bicipital groove indicates inflammation of the long head of the biceps.

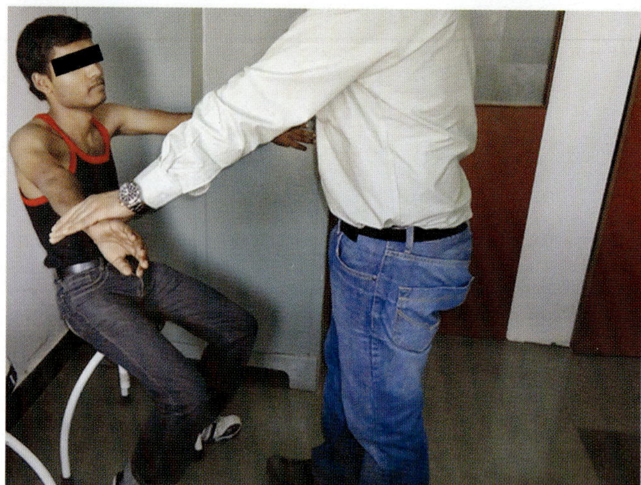

Fig. 51: Jobe's test.

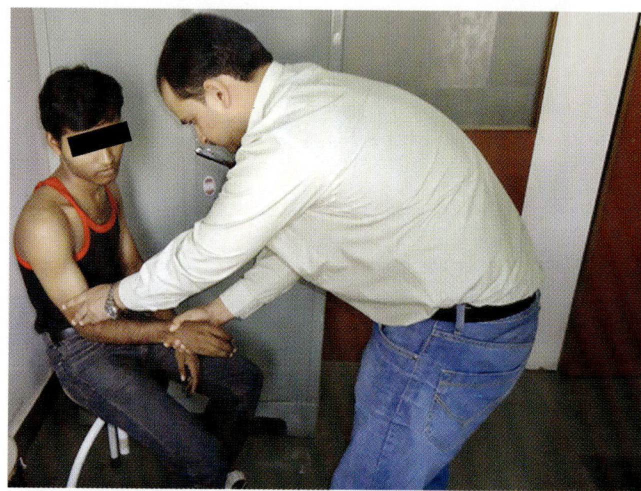

Fig. 52: Yergason's test.

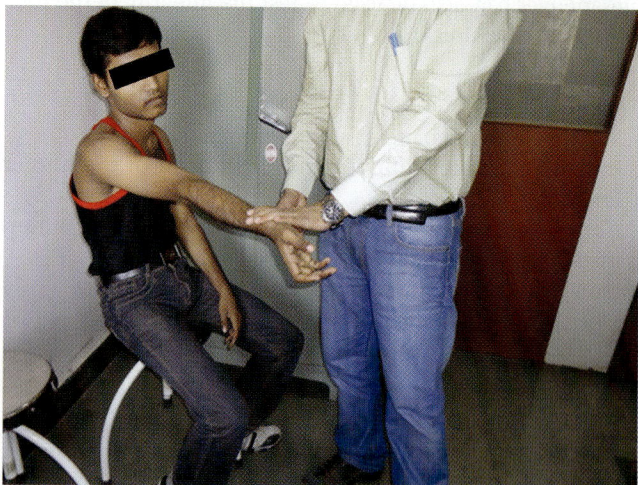

Fig. 53: Speed's test.

Speed's Test (Fig. 53)

The Speed's test is performed by having the patient forward flexed the shoulder to 90° with the elbow extended and the forearm supinated. Resistance is applied to the forearm, and a positive result produces pain localized to the bicipital groove.

TESTS FOR EVALUATING ROTATOR CUFF INTEGRITY

Lift-off Test (Fig. 54)

Patient sitting or standing, arm is internally rotated and dorsum of hand is placed against the lower back. If patient is unable to lift the dorsum of hand from the back, the test is positive.

Belly-press Test (Fig. 55)

Patient presses the abdomen with the flat of the hand and attempts to keep the arm in maximum internal rotation. If active internal rotation is strong, elbow does not drop backwards.

In case of weakened subscapularis, maximal internal rotation cannot be maintained and elbow drops behind the trunk.

Drop Sign (Fig. 56)

Patient is sitting with his/her back to the examiner.

Affected arm is held at 90° of elevation in scapular plane and in almost full external rotation with elbow flexed at 90°. Patient is asked to maintain this position actively as the examiner releases the wrist, while supporting the elbow, which is a function of infraspinatus. Sign is positive if *lag or drop* occurs.

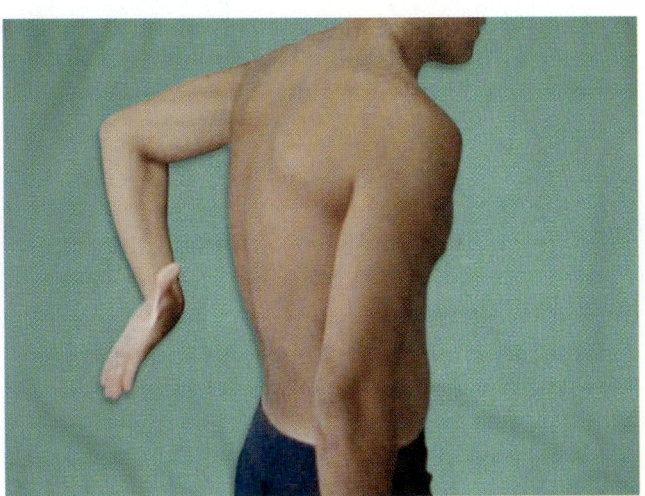

Fig. 54: Lift-off test.

CONGENITAL ANOMALIES OF SHOULDER

Congenital anomalies of shoulder are classified into two subgroups: (1) Common malformations of the shoulder, and (2) Rare anomalies.

CLEIDOCRANIAL DYSOSTOSIS

- Cleidocranial dysostosis is a hereditary disorder that affects bones formed by intramembranous ossification.
- The skull, clavicles, ribs, teeth, and pubic symphysis are most commonly affected.
- Enlarged head and forward-sloping shoulders are the typical clinical features.
- The range of shoulder function in this condition is vast.
- Patients with this syndrome have been reported to work as heavy laborers without shoulder complaints, whereas others report GH instability.
- The outer third of the clavicle is the most commonly affected portion, and the medial aspect is usually normal.
- The middle part of the clavicle can also be absent with spared medial and lateral portions.
- In either scenario, the missing portion of clavicle is replaced by fibrous tissue.
- Bilateral shoulder involvement is found in 82–90% of patients. Although uncommon, normal clavicles do not exclude this diagnosis.
- Two separate reports of families with this condition included members with normal clavicles.

Treatment

Patients do well with this condition and rarely require other than dental treatment. Surgery is indicated for those with neurological or vascular compression secondary to the clavicular malformation or to prevent skin breakdown.

CONGENITAL PSEUDARTHROSIS OF THE CLAVICLE

- Easily mistaken for a fracture of the clavicle anomaly does not show evidence of callus formation.
- No or minimal resulting loss of function is thought to occur.

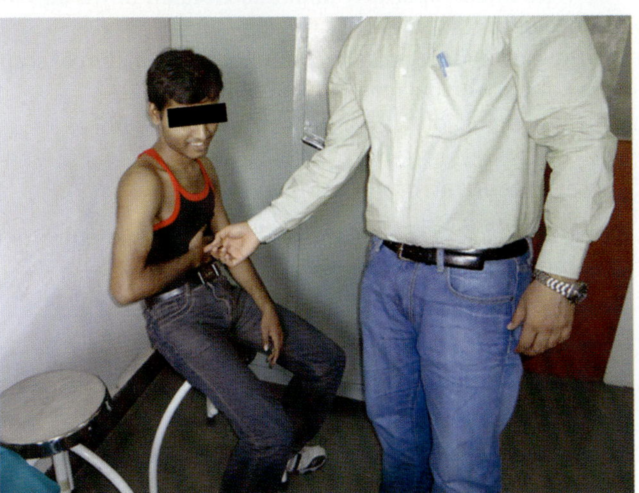

Fig. 55: Belly-press test.

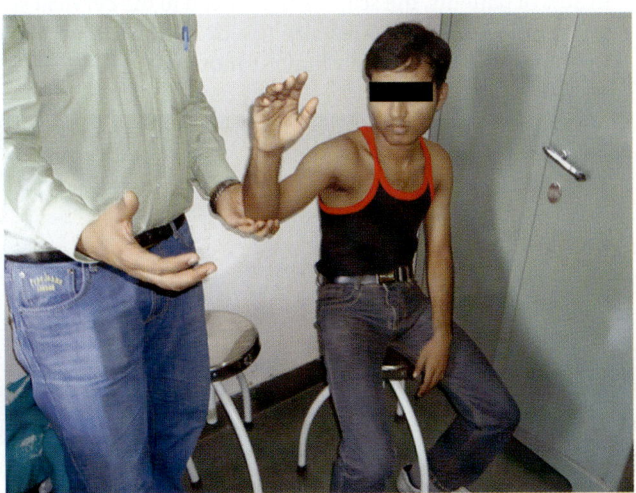

Fig. 56: Drop sign.

- The abnormality occurs unilaterally on the right side, however, left-sided and bilateral pseudarthrosis have also been reported.
- A bump in the midclavicular region is palpable and grossly seen, and smooth ends are apparent on radiographs.
- Thoracic outlet syndrome has been reported to be secondary to the pseudarthrosis.

Treatment

Benign neglect has generally been accepted as treatment of this entity. Due to reports of thoracic outlet syndrome, some authors have proposed early excision and bone grafting in younger patients (Figs. 57A and B).

SPRENGEL'S SHOULDER

History

- *1863:* Eulenberg first described three cases of congenital elevated scapulae.
- *1880:* Willett and Walsham described the first case involving an omovertebral bone.
- *1891:* Sprengel described four cases.
- *1891:* Kolliker reported several cases and labeled the deformity after Sprengel.

Etiology

Sprengel's deformity is a failure of descent of the scapula caused by:
- Too great an intrauterine pressure
- Abnormal articulations of scapula with the spine (omovertebral bone)
- Defective musculature of the ST region
- Arrest of development due to ineffective muscular tension.

Introduction

This is an uncommon congenital anomaly which arises from interruption of normal caudal migration of the scapula.

Characteristics

- Deformity is characterized by elevation and medial rotation of inferior scapula.
- Involved scapula is both smaller and more cephalad than normal.
- In 30% of patients, the scapula is attached to the cervical spine by an omovertebral bone, cartilage or fibrous tissue, which, when present, can severely limit ST motion.

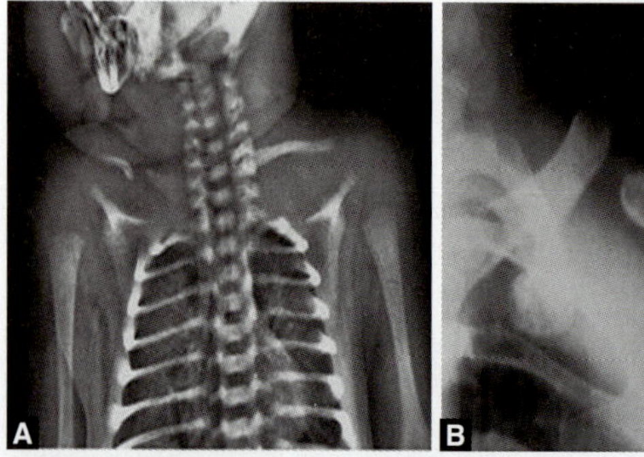

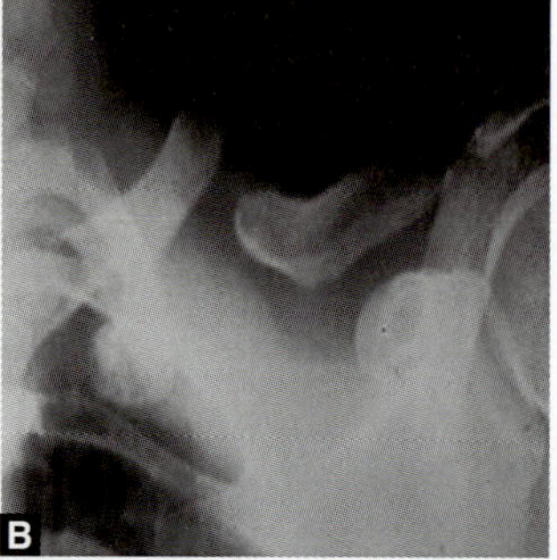

Figs. 57A and B: (A) The right side is most commonly involved in congenital pseudarthrosis of the clavicle; (B) Note the anterosuperiorly displaced sternal fragment that can manifest as a palpable lump.

Associated Anomalies

- Absence/Fusion of ribs
- Cervical ribs
- Klippel-Feil syndrome
- Congenital scoliosis with hemivertebrae
- Cervical spina bifida
- Syringomyelia
- Paraplegia
- Platybasia
- Situs inversus
- Mandibulofacial dysostosis
- Clavicular abnormalities
- Cardiac anomalies such as atrial septal defect, ventricular septal defect, etc.
- Kidney malformations.

Pathology

- The scapula appears at the 5th week of gestation at C5–T1. It then migrates to the adult position by birth to T2–T7.
- Some have bony articulations with the spine via omovertebral bones.
- *Others have defective musculature:* Trapezius, rhomboids, levator scapula are the most commonly affected while others, like pectoralis major/minor, latissimus dorsi, sternocleidomastoid, serratus anterior, are less commonly affected.
- The affected muscles undergo degeneration, necrosis, fibrosis, and secondary contracture.
- Also the scapula is hypoplastic on the affected side.

Clinical Features

- Most common congenital deformity of the shoulder.
- Asymmetry of shoulder (in unilateral cases).
- Female : male ratio is 3 : 1.
- Left scapula is more commonly affected than right scapula.
- Neck appears fuller and shorter on the affected side.
- Clavicle tilted superiorly about 25° rotated down and away from spine.
- Decreased abduction, lateral motion, and rotation of scapula are limited with decreased ST motion.
- Glenohumeral joint is normal with normal ROM.

Clinical Presentation (Fig. 58)

- Deformity tends to be painless, and many patients are not diagnosed until adolescence.
- Due to scapular asymmetry, some patients are mistaken for having scoliosis.
- Minor asymmetries commonly seen between right and left scapula should not be designated as having Sprengel's deformity.
- Look for loss of shoulder abduction and forward flexion.
- If an omovertebral bone is present, abduction of the shoulder is commonly limited to less than 90°.

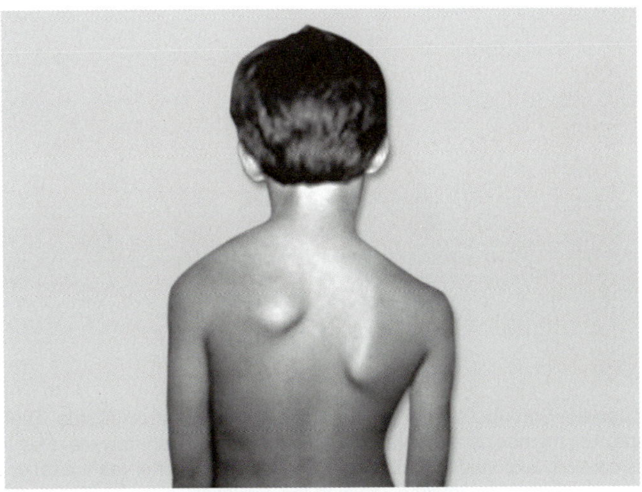

Fig. 58: Clinical presentation of Sprengel's deformity.

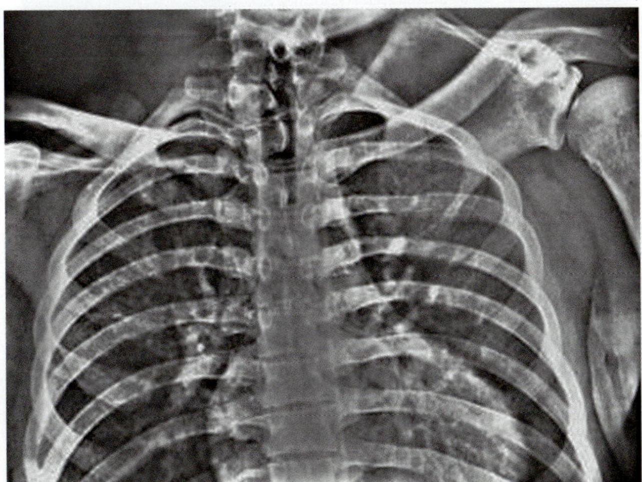

Fig. 59: X-ray showing elevated scapula in case of Sprengel's deformity.

Radiographic Findings

Associated radiographic findings for Sprengel's shoulder are summarized here:

- Elevated scapula (Fig. 59)
- Associated bony deformities
- *Best views:* AP of both shoulders with arms abducted and adducted maximally
- Lateral cervical and thoracic spine to look for other abnormalities
- Oblique and lateral of scapula to show omovertebral bone (one-third of cases) (Fig. 60).

Cavendish Classification

- *Grade I:* Very mild
  - Shoulders appear symmetrical when clothed.
- *Grade II:* Mild
  - Superomedial angle of scapula is visible as a lump in the web of the neck.
- *Grade III:* Moderate
  - Shoulder joint is elevated by 2–5 cm.
  - Deformity is easily visible.

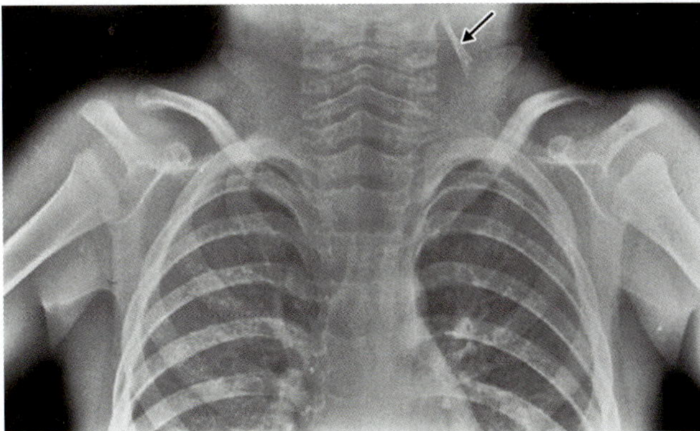

Fig. 60: On the left side, an omovertebral bone (arrow) connects the transverse process of the lower cervical spine of C6 with the superomedial angle of the scapula.

- *Grade IV:* Severe
  - Superior angle is near the occiput.
  - Severe webbing of the neck.

Treatment

Goals

- Correct deformity
- Improve function
- Improve cosmesis
- Physical-therapy to maintain ROM preoperative and improve strength.

Factors in Considering Surgical Correction

- *Cosmesis:*
  - Cavendish Grade III or IV
- *Functional:*
  - Omovertebral bone or ST fibrous adhesions have better outcomes and improve function with resection.
- *Associated anomalies:*
  - To treat scoliosis at the same time
- *Age of patient:*
  - Although somewhat controversial, most agree 3–8 years of age.

Nonsurgical Treatment

As passive stretching exercises advocated in the past are not successful, treatment is primarily surgical.

Surgical Treatment

- *Timing:*
  - Surgery is indicated for children between 3 and 8 years of age without significant deformities, both functional and cosmetic.
  - Patients older than 8 years of age are not good candidates for scapular displacement procedures.
- *Options:*
  - Detachment of medial and superior scapular muscles, repositioning scapula caudal and subsequently re-attaching the muscles to lowered scapula.

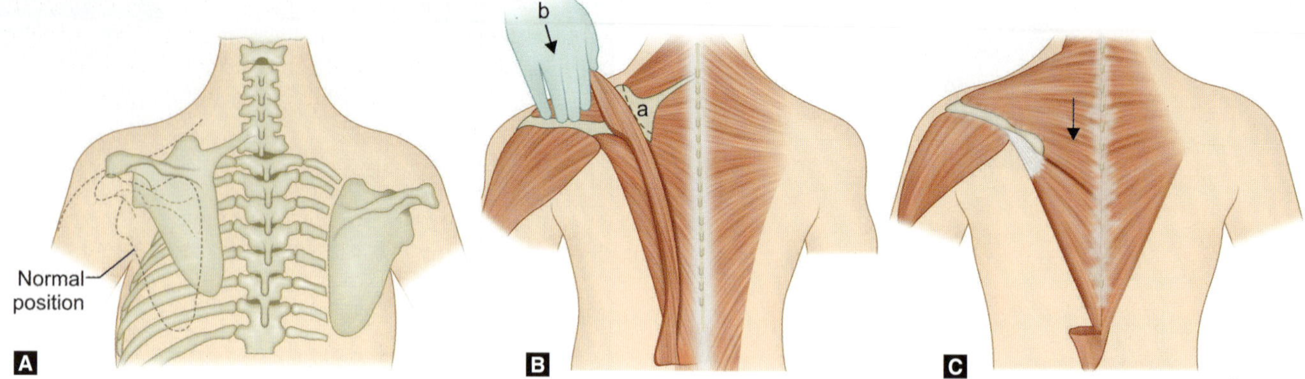

Figs. 61A to C: Essential steps of the Woodward procedure: (A) Position of the scapula in Sprengel's deformity as it relates to the unaffected side. There is tethering of the superior angle of the scapula to the cervical vertebrae; (B) The trapezius, rhomboids and levator scapulae origins are sharply elevated from the spinous processes and retracted laterally. The superior angle of the scapula is carefully exposed and all tethers to the cervical vertebrae are resected. The scapula is reduced into its anatomic position and (C) The free fascial edge is sutured distal to proximal, holding the reduction (arrow).

Woodward Procedure

- Procedure has 80% satisfactory functional and cosmetic results.
- Increase shoulder abduction following surgery, ranges from 34° to 60°.
- Child's age at operation and differing methods of measurement play the largest role in accounting for these differences.
- Younger patients obtain better motion and postoperative correction.
- Caudal displacement of scapula is reported to be 1.9 times vertebral body heights in one series and 4 cm in another.

Technique (Figs. 61A to C)

- Involves resection of omovertebral bone and division of vertebral attachments of trapezius, rhomboids, and levator scapula.
- Scapula is subsequently rotated and translated caudally.
- Detached muscle's origins are then sutured to more inferior vertebral spinous processes.

Postoperative Phase (Figs. 62A and B)

- Three weeks of postoperative immobilization is required.
- Osteotomy of clavicle may be required to prevent compression of nerve/vein (N/V) structures against first rib.
- Postoperative improvement in shoulder abduction is maintained, although some loss of scapular translation can occur in first four months postoperatively.
- One third of patients will have widening of their surgical scars, which can be cosmetically disturbing.
- X-ray taken, demonstrates:
  - Elevated left scapula worse than right
  - No evidence of omovertebral bone on either side.
- Thoracic kyphosis—no other spinal abnormalities.

Modified Woodward Procedure with Clavicular Osteotomy and Morcellation on Left Side is shown in Figure 63.

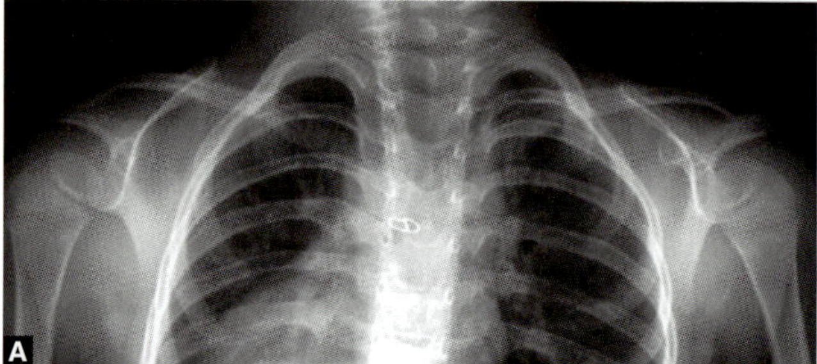

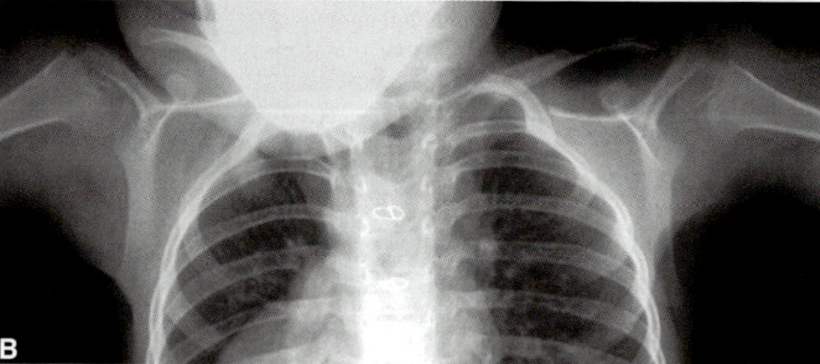

Figs. 62A and B: Postoperative X-rays demonstrate elevated left scapula, no evidence of omovertebral bone on either side.

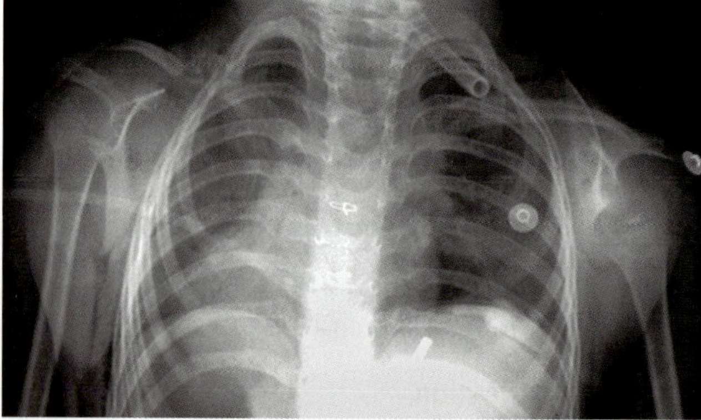

Fig. 63: Postoperative X-ray modified Woodward procedure with clavicular osteotomy and morcellation on left side.

Conclusion

- In a recent article from the Alfred I, duPont Institute reviewing the long-term results (with average follow-up period of 8 years) of the modified Woodward procedure in 15 patients, there was improved cosmesis with a decrease of at least one Cavendish grade in all patients.
- Average scapular lowering of 2.7 cm, and an average improvement in shoulder abduction by 35°.
- There were only minor complications noted, including one transient brachial plexus palsy, one widened scar, and one scapular winging.

OS ACROMIALE (FIG. 64)

- Failure of the acromion process to fuse.
- It is more common in black patients and in male patients.
- The acromion is formed from three ossification centers. Failure of any of these centers to unite causes an os acromiale.
- The most common site of persistent cartilage is between the meta-acromion and the mesoacromion.
- It has been suggested that a more posteriorly situated AC joint in relation to the anterior acromial edge is a predisposing factor to the development of an os acromiale.
- The acromion process should get fully ossified by 25 years of age.
- Os acromiale is bilateral in 33–62% of cases.
- Most often the abnormality is asymptomatic and is an incidental discovery.
- The acromion has three separate ossification centers. The most common site of os acromiale is between the mesoacromion and the meta-acromion. Basic-acromion (BA), meso-acromion (MSA), meta-acromion (MTA), and pre-acromion (PA) are shown in Figure 65.

Treatment

- Symptomatic os acromiale falls into two categories:
  - *First group:* Those associated with pain at the unstable segment
  - *Second group:* Those associated with symptoms of impingement.

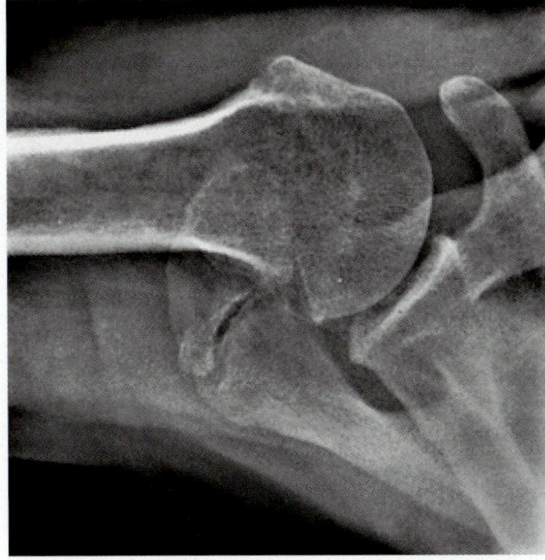

Fig. 64: An os acromiale is best seen in an axillary radiograph.

- The first group of patients must be managed conservatively with a sling, if seen acutely after trauma, followed by early mobilization. Persistent pain that lasts longer than 3 months and limits work or activities of daily living (ADLs) is an indication for surgery.
- The second group of patients undergoes a more complex treatment protocol.
- Initially, treatment of the impingement does not vary much from that in patients without this finding. Nonsteroidal anti-inflammatory medication and tendon-gliding exercises are used for the treatment.
- If the patient has evidence of a RC tear or does not have pain relief, surgical intervention is considered.
- A small pre-acromion is excised and the deltoid is repaired.
- For larger pieces, a decision to perform fusion or subacromial decompression must be made.

All acromioplasties and RC repairs are done via an open approach and evaluation of the stability of the os is performed. If the os acromiale is stable to palpation, a standard acromioplasty is performed. If the segment has motion with palpation, a *fusion operation* is undertaken.

Steps followed in repair of an unstable os acromiale (Figs. 66A to C):

- Guidewires for two 4 mm cannulated screws are placed in the free fragment in an anterior-to-posterior direction (top). The fragment is reduced and the guidewires are advanced across nonunion site (bottom).
- Two distally threaded screws are inserted to compress the reduction.
- Cancellous bone graft obtained from the hip is placed on the superior surface of the acromion. Large nonabsorbable suture is placed through each screw and secured in a figure-of-eight manner.

GLENOID HYPOPLASIA

- Glenoid hypoplasia (Fig. 67) results from failure of the inferior glenoid to develop.
- The true incidence is uncertain, and the diagnosis is often made on the basis of routine chest radiographs.
- Patients might complain of pain and limited abduction in the second through fifth decades of life.
- Instability of the GH joint is reported to be found in a subgroup of patients.
- Glenoid hypoplasia is most commonly bilateral and noted commonly in men.

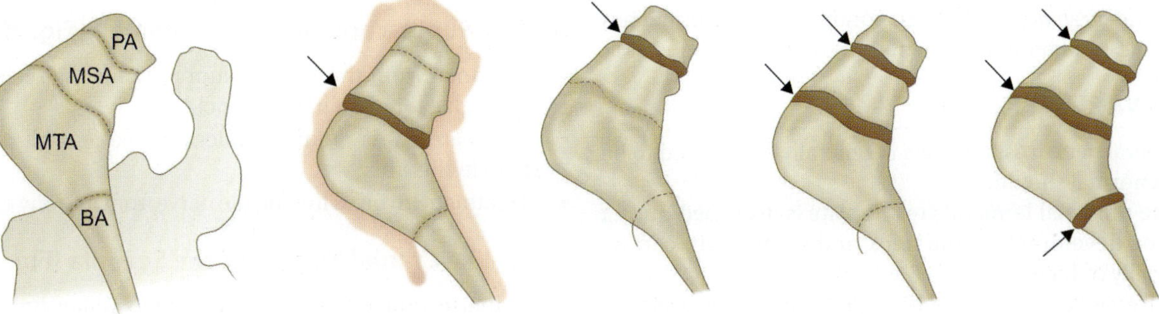

Fig. 65: Separate ossification centers of os acromiale (arrows).

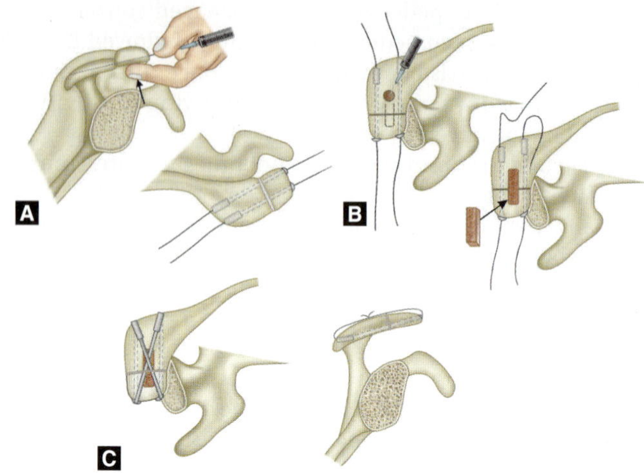

Figs. 66A to C: Different steps followed in repair of an unstable os acromiale (arrows).

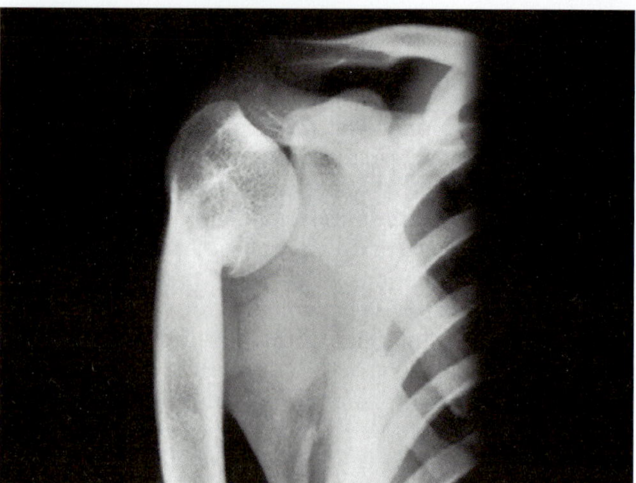

Fig. 68: X-ray showing a typical appearance of humerus varus.

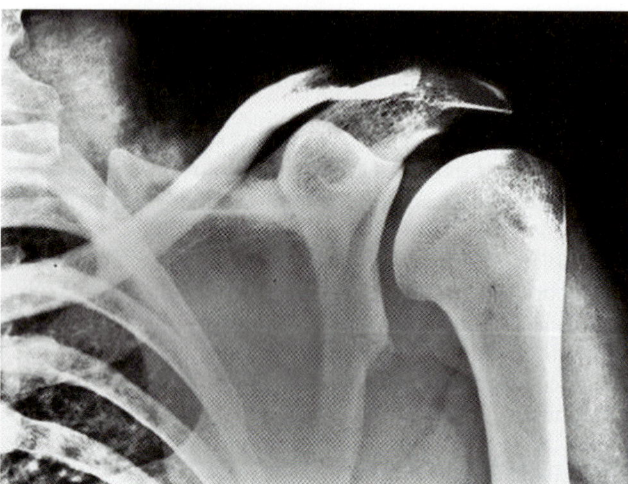

Fig. 67: Varying degrees of glenoid flattening are seen in glenoid hypoplasia.

Treatment

- In these types of patients, avoidance of manual labor and overhead activities are commonly suggested.
- Arthroscopic debridement of the ragged articular cartilage to alter symptoms.
- Arthroplasty as treatment of the secondary degenerative arthritis but its having a limited result.
- In hemiarthroplasty, it requires revision of total shoulder or bipolar arthroplasty due to pain.
- *Total shoulder replacement:* When nonoperative treatment has failed, total shoulder replacement is the only treatment.

HUMERUS VARUS (FIG. 68)

- The humeral neck-to-shaft angle is generally considered to be 140° in a normal shoulder.
- When the proximal humeral growth plate is disturbed during growth or development, the neck and shaft angle can be dramatically reduced.
- Premature closure of the medial growth plate results in a differential growth of the lateral and medial humeral lengths.
- Kohler defined a neck-to-shaft angle less than 90°, elevation of the greater tuberosity above the top of the humeral head and reduction of the distance between the articular surface and the lateral cortex as the radiographic criteria for diagnosis of humerus varus.
- Patients have either a decreased ability to perform overhead activities or pain from impingement.
- Compensation by the unaffected shoulder can result in overuse tendinitis as another complaint.
- Trauma during birth or early life may be the underlying cause of idiopathic humerus varus. It occurs unilaterally.
- Several other processes can be responsible for humerus varus, including thalassemia, skeletal dysplasia, neoplasm, osteomyelitis, cerebral palsy, arthrogryposis, and brachial plexus injuries.

Therefore, the underlying cause of humerus varus must be investigated before treating the deformity.

RARE ANOMALIES

Duplicated and Bifurcated Clavicle (Fig. 69)

- Duplication of the clavicle has been described in the literature with some variation.
- Complete duplication of the clavicle has been described once and caused no symptoms in that patient.
- In a few cases, bifurcation of the clavicle has also been described in which there is duplication of either the lateral or medial side. Duplication of the clavicle is an extremely rare abnormality.

Middle Suprascapular Nerve Foramen (Fig. 70)

- A branch from the middle suprascapular nerve might pass through a foramen in the clavicle.
- No treatment is required unless the patient has neurogenic pain in this area.
- Treatment involves freeing the nerve from its bony entrapment.

Clasp-like Cranial Margin of the Scapula (Fig. 71)

The superior margin of the scapula looks like the handle of a bucket. But this anomaly has no clinical significance.

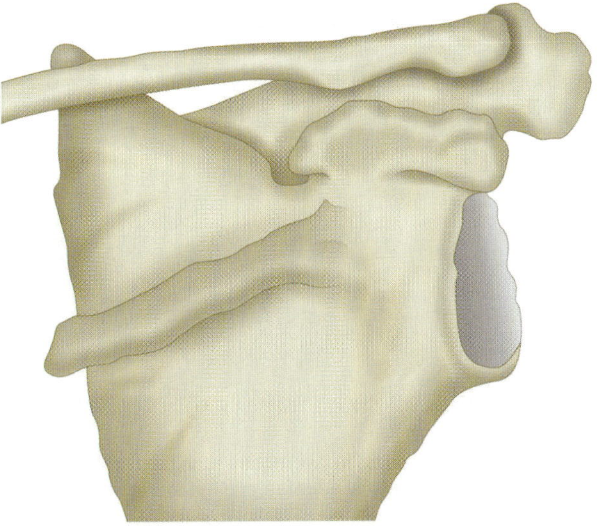

Fig. 69: The lateral end of the extraclavicle attaches to the base of the coracoid process.

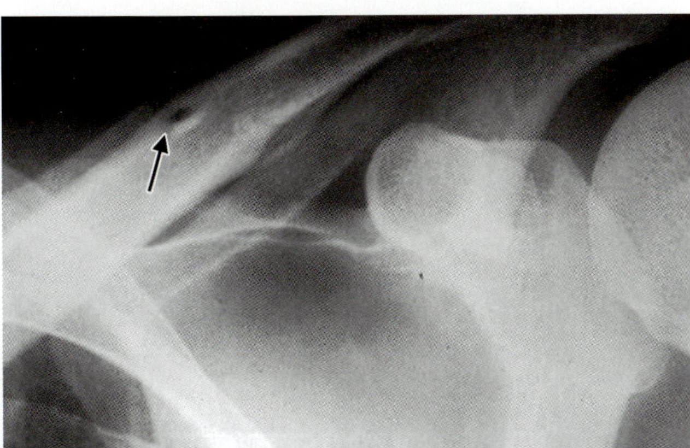

Fig. 70: This clavicle has a large foramen (arrow) through which supraclavicular nerve passes.

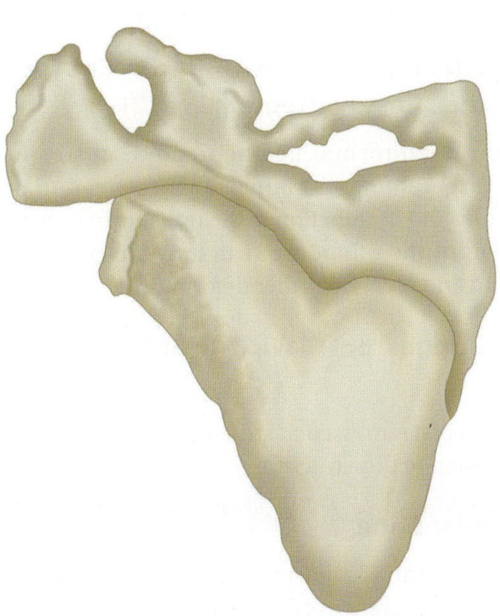

Fig. 71: Clasp-like cranial margin of the scapula.

Double Acromion and Coracoid Process (Fig. 72)

Reported only once, this malformation restricted motion of the shoulder but required no treatment.

Duplicated Scapula (Fig. 73)

- Multiple humeri and forearm bones are commonly associated.
- Fusion of the two scapulae has been reported to be successful in patients whose motion is restricted.

Coracoclavicular Joint or Bar (Figs. 74 to 76)

- The CC ligaments may be replaced by an articulation or a bony bar.
- Symptomatic patients might complain of neurovascular compression, restriction in ROM, or pain from arthritis of the joint.
- When symptomatic, the articulation or bar may be excised.

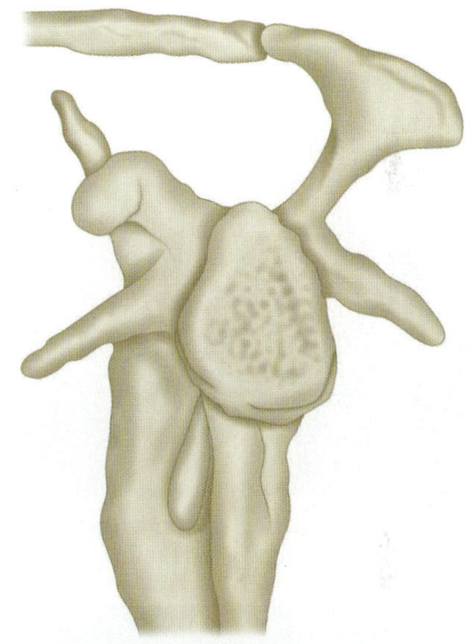

Fig. 72: The double acromion and coracoid processes shown here have been identified only once.

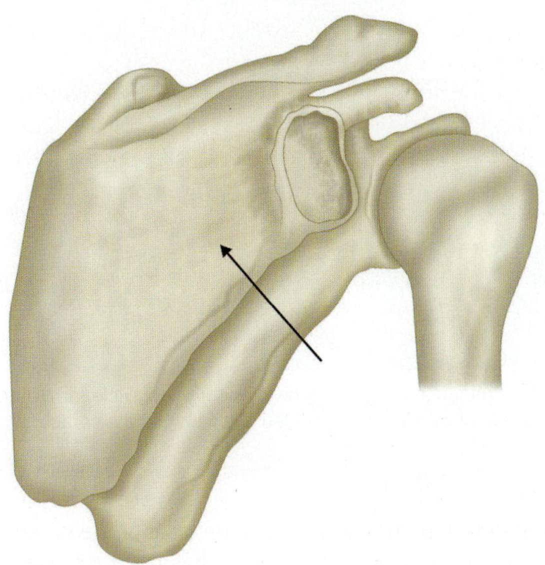

Fig. 73: Arrow showing duplicated scapulas (reported only thrice).

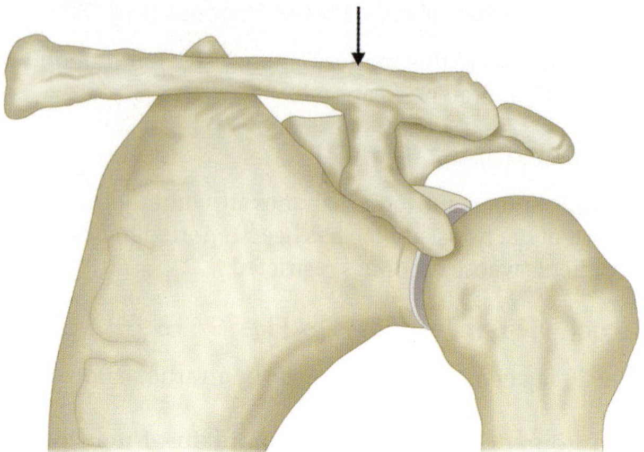

Fig. 74: Rarely, a solid bony strut (arrow) connects the coracoid to the clavicle.

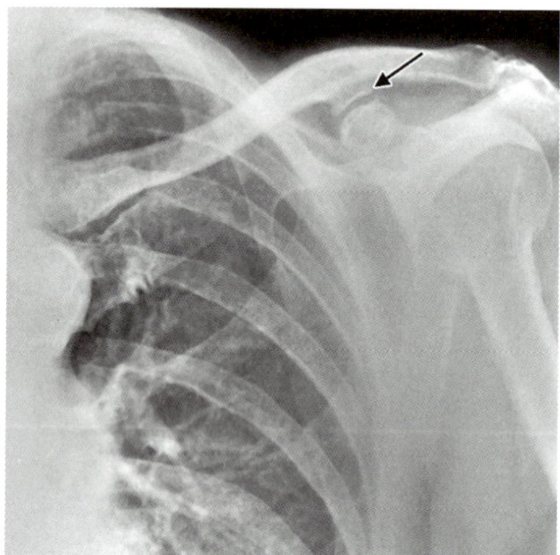

Fig. 75: Both the coracoid and the clavicular projections may be covered with cartilage and form a true diarthrodial joint (arrow) with an articular capsule.

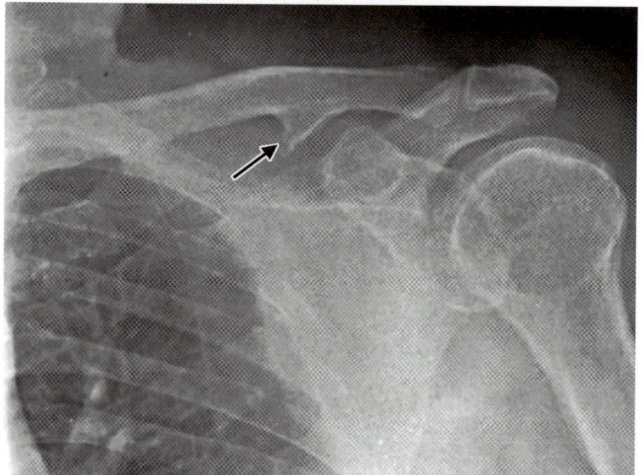

Fig. 76: A triangular bony overgrowth under the clavicle (arrow) may be present with its apex directed down toward the coracoid.

Coracosternal Bone

- A bony bridge originating from the base of the coracoid and extending cephalad and medially has been reported in one patient with Sprengel's deformity.

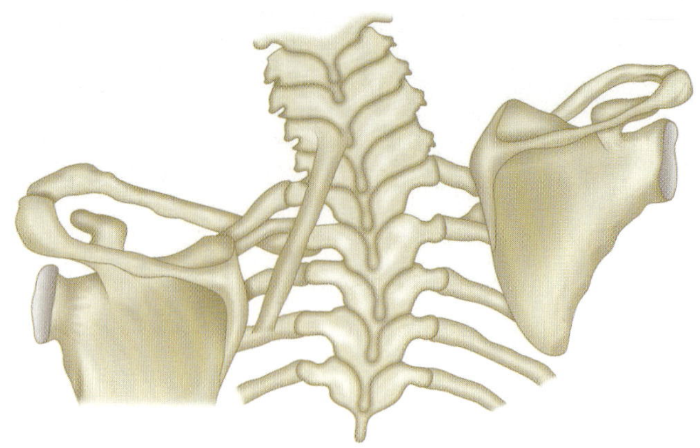

Fig. 77: The costovertebral bone ties together the bifid spinous process of the sixth cervical vertebra and the fourth rib.

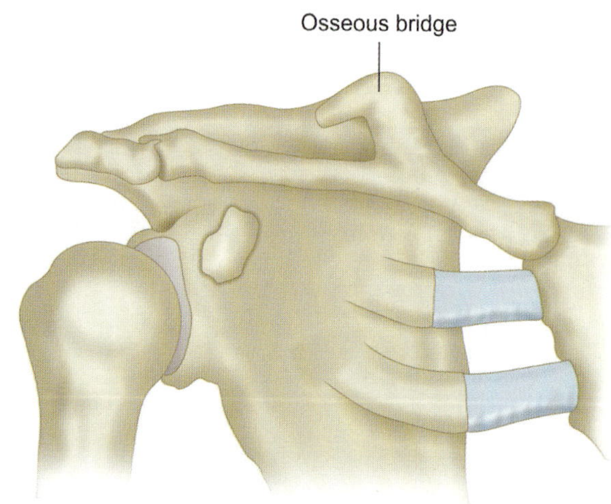

Fig. 78: An osseous bridge can extend from the midportion of the clavicle to the spine of the scapula.

- It was thought to be the persistence of a mesenchymal coracosternal connection normally seen in an early embryologic stage.

Ligamentous Connecting Bands: Costocoracoid, Costosternal, Costovertebral (Fig. 77)

- The three abnormal costocoracoid, costosternal, and costovertebral fibrous connections can lead to progressive deformity and dysfunction of the upper extremity.
- Excision of the offending structure can provide improved function and prevent further deformity.

Osseous Bridge from Clavicle to Spine of Scapula (Fig. 78)

Compression of neurovascular structures and restriction of motion require excision of this structure.

Infrascapular Bone

Infrascapular bone is a normal variant of scapula ossification; represents the attachment of the teres major muscle; and may be misinterpreted as a fracture (Fig. 79).

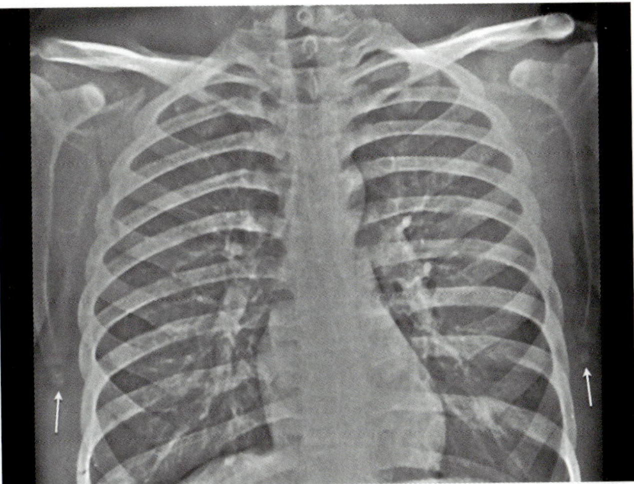

Fig. 79: An infrascapular bone (arrows) is present bilaterally in this patient.

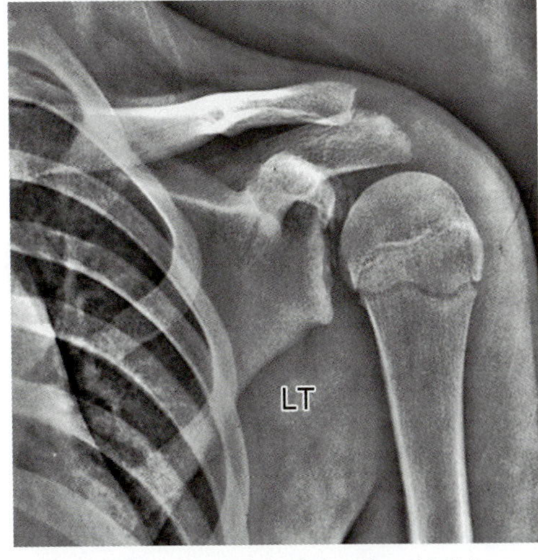

Fig. 81: The epiphyseal annular ring of the glenoid; it has not fused and appears to be rippled or dentated (the letters LT indicate that the radiograph is of the left shoulder).

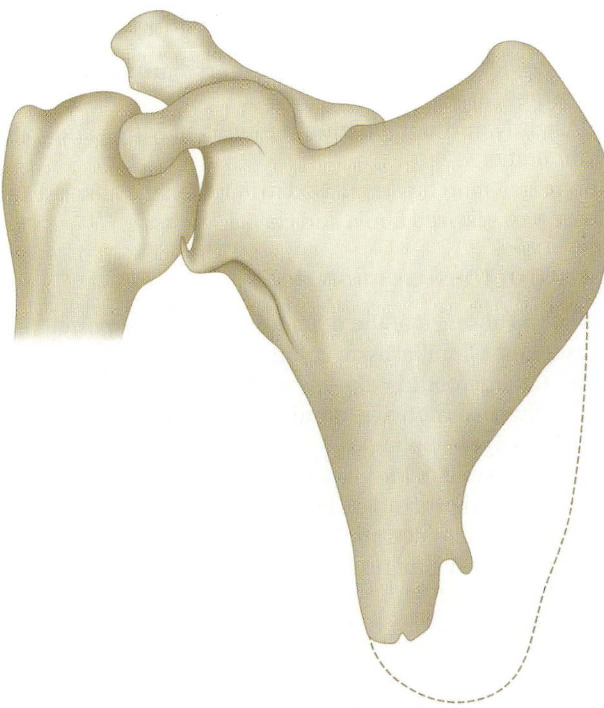

Fig. 80: A notched inferior angle of the scapula probably represents an absence of the ossification nucleus of the inferior angle of the scapula.

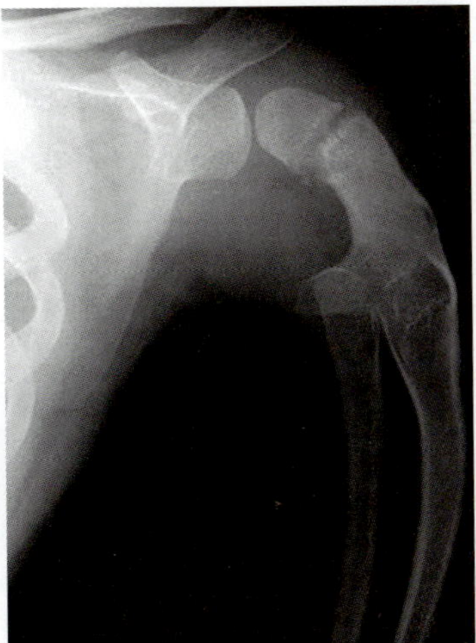

Fig. 82: This child with phocomelia has a fairly well-developed shoulder with a small humerus and fused elbow.

Notched Inferior Angle of the Scapula (Fig. 80)

Incomplete development of the inferior scapula results in a misshapen scapula.

Dentated Glenoid (Fig. 81)

- Incomplete development of the inferior glenoid results in a rippled appearance of the glenoid.
- Fusion of the growth plates usually resolves this appearance, but it can continue to be present in adulthood.

Phocomelia (Figs. 82 to 87)

- Absence of the entire upper extremity or severe shortening of the limb with absent portions was a major health catastrophe

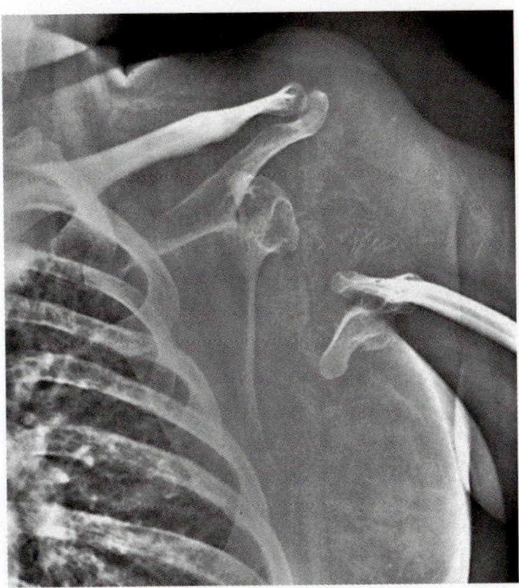

Fig. 83: An abnormal glenoid articulates with only a deformed, short distal end of the humerus and a one-bone forearm in this patient with phocomelia.

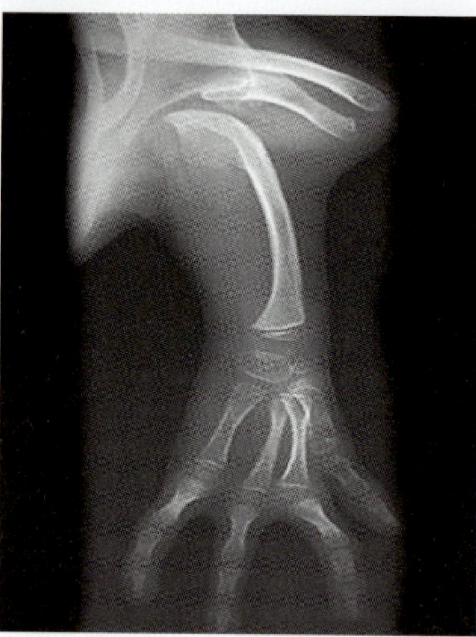

Fig. 84: This child has a poorly formed scapula with part of an elbow articulating inside the shoulder joint and only a radius in the forearm.

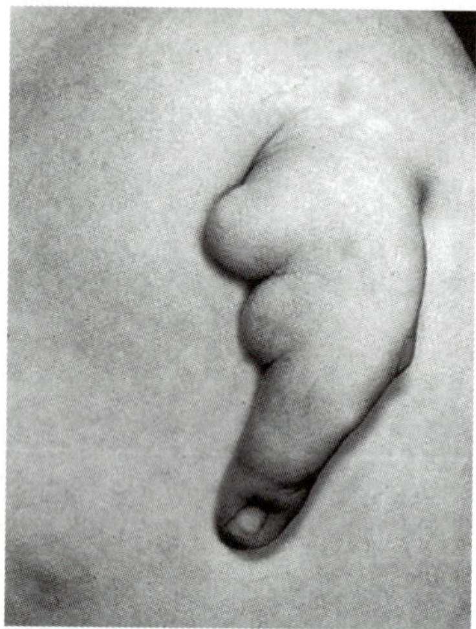

Fig. 85: In an extreme case of phocomelia, sometimes only a finger attaches to the trunk.

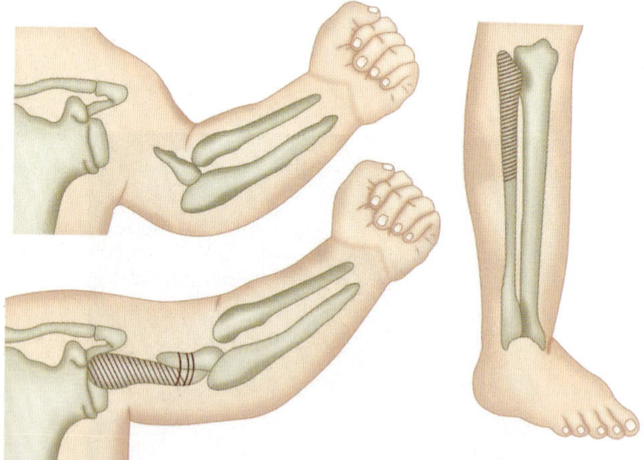

Fig. 86: The fibula may be transplanted to the upper part of the arm by placing the epiphysis in the glenoid fossa and attaching the distal end to the humeral remnant.

during the 1950s with the use of thalidomide in pregnant women.

- Currently, phocomelia is rare.
- The function of the remnant limb dictates intervention.

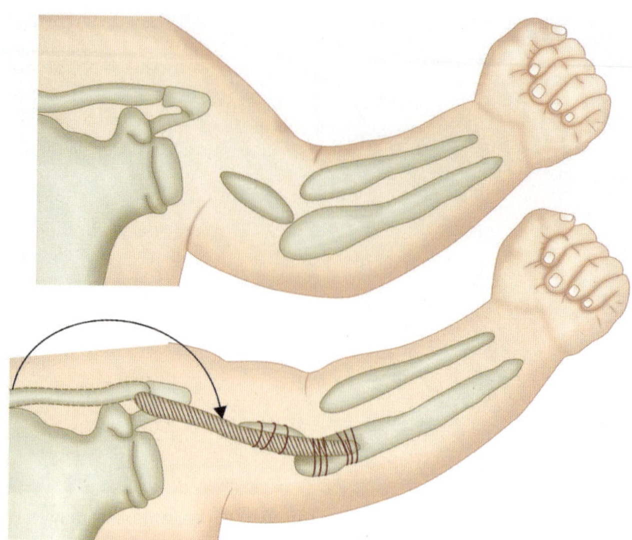

Fig. 87: Transposition of the clavicle is accomplished by exposing it subperiosteally and using the sternal end to lengthen the humerus.

- Preservation of functional fingers can allow improved prosthetic use.
- Unsightly and nonfunctioning limbs may be candidates for amputation.
- Bone transport has been used to lengthen the affected limb, as have vascularized fibula and clavicle grafts.

Absence of the Acromion Head

- Bilateral absence of the acromion has been reported in a few cases and a familial association has been identified.
- The CA ligament is absent, and the deltoid origin and the trapezius insertion are found both on the lateral clavicle and on the scapular spine.
- The lateral end of the clavicle is blunted, and both the clavicle and coracoid process are hypertrophied.
- Clinical appearance and ROM of the shoulders were normal, although mild superior translation of the humeral head was noted in one patient.
- Congenital absence of the humeral head has been reported twice.

Holt-Oram Syndrome

- The condition involving multigenerational cardiac and upper extremity congenital anomalies is termed Holt-Oram syndrome.
- These scapular abnormalities are similar to Sprengel's deformity and are the most common shoulder manifestation.
- Misshapen clavicles, acromia, and humeral heads have also been reported.
- Inheritance is autosomal dominant.

Nail-Patella Syndrome (Fig. 88)

- This autosomal dominant syndrome is a relatively common entity in England.
- Nail-Patella syndrome is also known as onycho-osteodysplasia.
- The main features of Nail-Patella syndrome are:
  - Absent or hypoplastic nails, typically more severe on the radial side of the hand

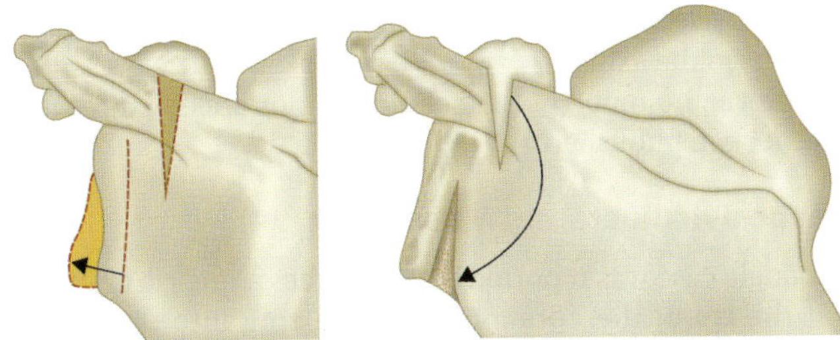
Fig. 88: For correction of the shoulder deformity in the Nail-Patella syndrome, an opening wedge osteotomy of the inferior glenoid with bone from the spine of the scapula works well.

- Dysplasia of the patella and lateral femoral condyle of knee
- Dysplasia of the capitellum and radial head of the elbow
- Dysplasia of the iliac crests.

- Although not the main abnormality of the disease, the scapula and the humerus are often misshapen.
- The proximal end of the humerus is often small and directed superiorly.
- The glenoid is often small and directed laterally or inferiorly.
- A small acromion, a prominent lateral clavicle, and a small coracoid complete the bony abnormalities often found.
- Some patients complain of impingement-like pain with use of the extremity.
- On examination, glenohumeral (GH) joint is prominent anteriorly and unstable.
- Double osteotomy of the scapula that successfully relieved the pain of a patient, when nonoperative treatment has failed.

Oto-onychoperoneal Syndrome

- This rare syndrome is characterized by dysmorphic facial features with characteristic ear abnormalities, nail hypoplasia, absent or hypoplastic fibulae and shoulder anomalies. It is thought to be an autonomic recessive disorder.
- Shoulder abnormalities include straight clavicles, fibrous fusion of the distal clavicle and the scapular spine, and an abnormal AC joint.

Apert's Syndrome (Figs. 89 and 90)

- Apert's syndrome is typically thought of for the hand manifestation, acrocephalosyndactyly.
- However, several authors have reported that the shoulder is often affected.
- The shoulder is reduced but subluxates anteriorly.
- The humeral head and glenoid are dysplastic, and the acromion is sometimes enlarged.
- The function and pain typically worsen with age as the joint surfaces degenerate and the joint continues to subluxate.

Multiple Epiphyseal Dysplasia (Fig. 91)

- A defect in the ossification center of the epiphysis results in multiple joint involvement with this disease.
- Patients commonly have shoulder manifestations that fall into two categories:
  1. Mild abnormalities that lead to GH arthritis
  2. Severe failure of epiphyseal development.

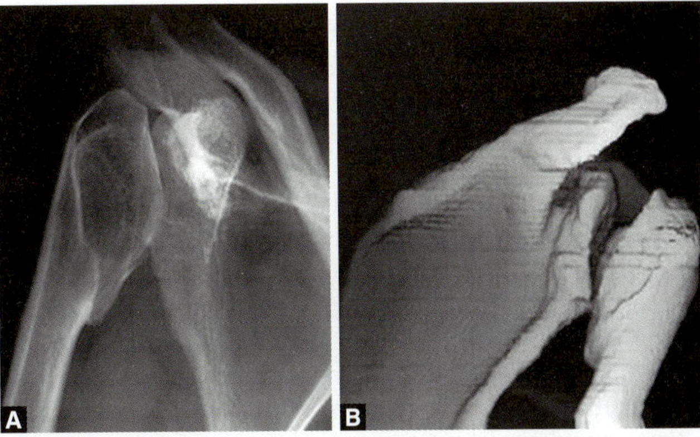
Figs. 89A and B: (A) This 23-year-old man with Apert's syndrome has flattening of the humeral head with arthropathy; (B) CT scan with three-dimensional reconstruction shows the abnormalities even more dramatically.

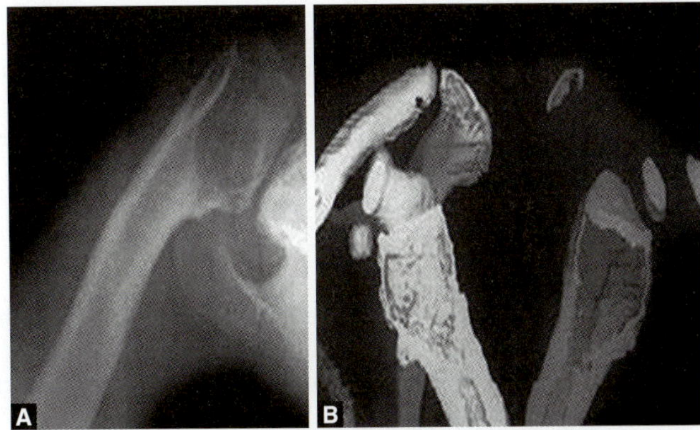
Figs. 90A and B: (A) The left shoulder of a man with Apert's syndrome; (B) CT scan with three-dimensional reconstruction.

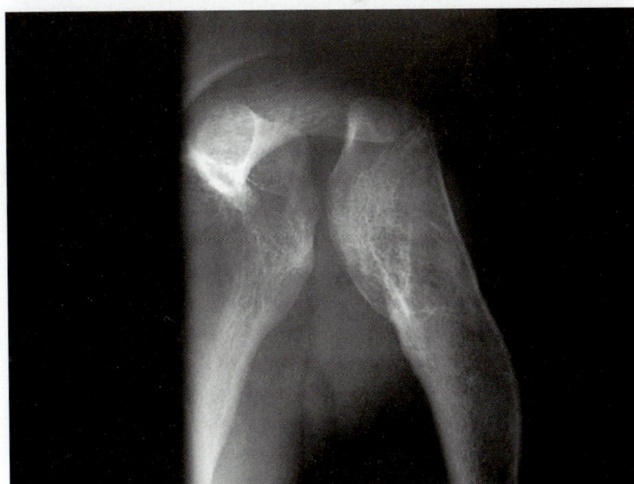
Fig. 91: Typical hatchet head shoulder.

- Both the groups typically have pain in the fifth and sixth decades of life.
- The ROM and function of the two groups are vastly different.
- Mildly affected shoulders have nearly normal motion initially but lose motion and become painful over time.
- Severely deformed shoulders lack motion from an early age but are not painful until later in life.

Pelvis-shoulder Dysplasia

- Pelvis-shoulder dysplasia, also known as scapuloiliac dysostosis or Kosenow's syndrome. It is an autosomal dominant condition characterized by extreme hypoplasia of the scapulae and ilea.
- The scapular body and glenoid display severe hypoplasia, and the acromion and coracoid may be normal.
- The clavicles many times appear elongated but can also be hypoplastic. Cases without shoulder girdle involvement have been reported.
- Anomalies of the eyes, ears, vertebrae, ribs, and upper and lower limbs, along with severe lumbar lordosis and hip dislocation have been reported.

Congenital Dislocation of the Shoulder

- Whether congenital dislocation of the shoulder is a real entity or is controversial.
- The presence of a dislocated shoulder in a child is often associated with brachial plexus injury or arthrogryposis multiplex congenital.
- If a congenital shoulder dislocation is confirmed, closed reduction is the preferred treatment.
- Failure of closed reduction can necessitate open reduction.

Chondroepitrochlearis Muscle (Fig. 92)

- Reports of this muscle have come mainly from examining the remains of fetuses that died of multiple anomalies.
- The muscle arises from the pectoralis major fascia and inserts into the medial brachial fascia.
- The chondroepitrochlearis muscle is thought to represent an abnormal insertion of the pectoralis major muscle because of its innervation by the pectoral nerves.
- In those rare patients who have this muscle and suffer from restricted ROM, excision is warranted. As a secondary gain, improved appearance of the axilla should also occur.

Subscapularis-teres-latissimus Muscle (Fig. 93)

- This anomalous muscle arises from the lateral border of the scapula, subscapularis or latissimus dorsi and inserts into the lesser tuberosity with the tendon of the subscapularis.
- The muscle may be responsible for compression of the brachial plexus in the axilla.
- However, no reports of the clinical importance of this muscle have been published.

Coracoclaviculosternal Muscle (Fig. 94)

- A single case was reported that describes a muscle originating at the tip of the coracoid and inserting into the anterior clavicular facet.
- The patient was asymptomatic.

Deltoid Muscle Contracture

- Fibrosis and subsequent contracture of the deltoid most commonly follow intramuscular injection.
- Numerous drugs have been implicated.
- A rarer condition is a development of a deltoid contraction without an antecedent history of injection.
- In either case, ROM does not improve greatly with physical therapy.

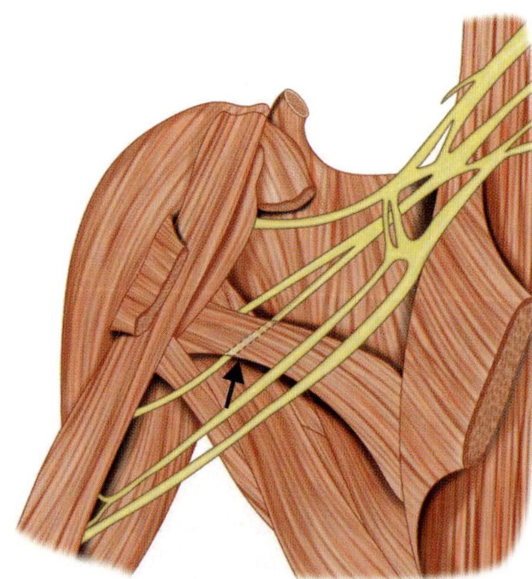

Fig. 93: The subscapularis-teres-latissimus muscle (arrow) penetrates the brachial plexus and can lie on top of the axillary, lower subscapular, thoracodorsal or radial nerves.

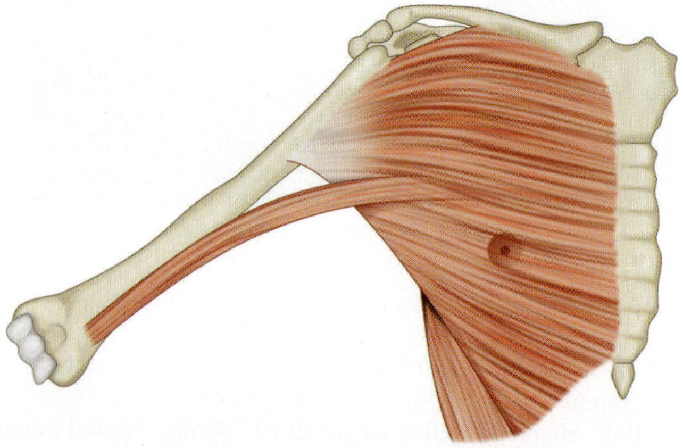

Fig. 92: The chondroepitrochlearis muscle originates on the anterior chest wall and inserts along the medial epicondyle.

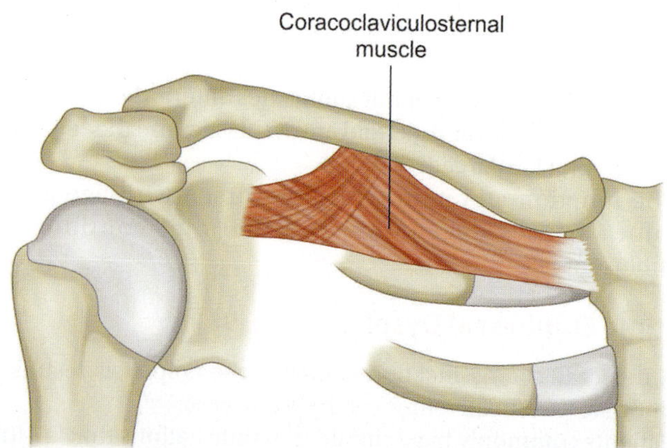

Fig. 94: The coracoclaviculosternal muscle originates from the anterior margin of the coracoid process and inserts into the clavicular facet of the sternum.

- Surgery is indicated for patients who have an abduction contracture greater than 25° and have experienced progressive deformity.
- Release of the fibrotic bands with or without transfer of the posterior deltoid has been recommended.

Poland's Syndrome (Figs. 95 and 96)

- Absence of the pectoralis major muscle causes relatively little disability.
- The remnant pectoralis major tendon can form an axillary web that can limit shoulder motion.
- Excision of the aberrant tendon and Z-plasty lengthening can greatly benefit a patient in this instance.
- The term Poland's syndrome should be reserved for patients with an absent pectoralis major and ipsilateral syndactyly.
- The underlying ribs, fascia, or breast might also be abnormally formed.
- Breast reconstruction may be of cosmetic benefit for female patients.
- Shoulder dysfunction is unusual unless it is associated with an axillary web, but associated conditions are common.

Pectoralis Minor Insertion into the Humerus (Fig. 97)

- The pectoralis minor usually inserts into the coracoid process.

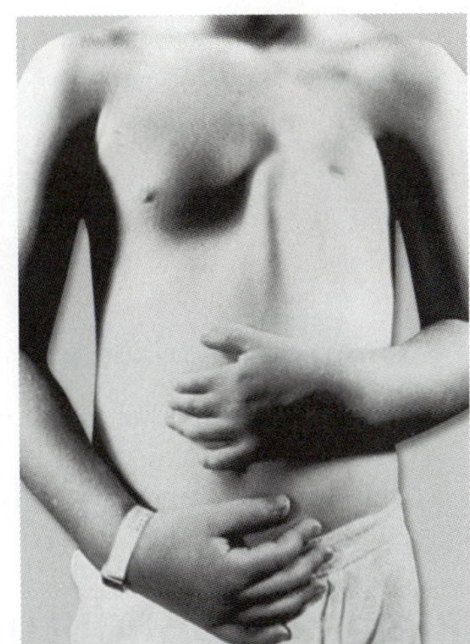

Fig. 95: A typical patient with Poland's syndrome.

- However, it occasionally passes the coracoid process, travels with the coracohumeral ligament, and inserts onto the humeral head.
- The abnormal slip has been identified as a site of compression for neurovascular structures, as well as a possible cause of impingement.
- When the pectoralis minor inserts abnormally and causes dysfunction, excision or transfer of the tendon to the coracoid process may be warranted.

Multiple Insertions of the Coracobrachialis (Fig. 98)

- The coracobrachialis is usually composed of a single muscle belly. However, up to three separate muscle bellies may be present.
- No clinical significance is attached to this variation.

Dorsal Epitrochlearis Muscle (Fig. 99)

- The latissimus dorsi muscle often has an associated muscle that originates from the tendon of the latissimus dorsi and inserts into the brachial and forearm fascia, the humerus and the lateral epicondyle.
- In contrast to the chondroepitrochlearis muscle, the dorsal epitrochlearis muscle is innervated by the radial nerve and occurs in 18–20% of people.
- No clinical significance has been identified for this muscle.

Axillopectoral Muscle (Fig. 100)

- Langer's armbogen, Langer's arm arch and axillo-pectoral muscle are names attributed to the anomalous portion of the latissimus dorsi.
- The slip of the latissimus dorsi courses along the inferior border of the axilla and inserts into the pectoralis major muscle.
- The muscle, which becomes tight with abduction and external rotation, overlies the neurovascular structures in the axilla.
- The muscle is innervated by the pectoral nerve.
- The anomaly occurs in 4–7.7% of the population and is usually asymptomatic.

Sternalis Muscle (Fig. 101)

- The sternalis is a long thin muscle that extends from the sternocleidomastoid to the rectus abdominis along the sternum.

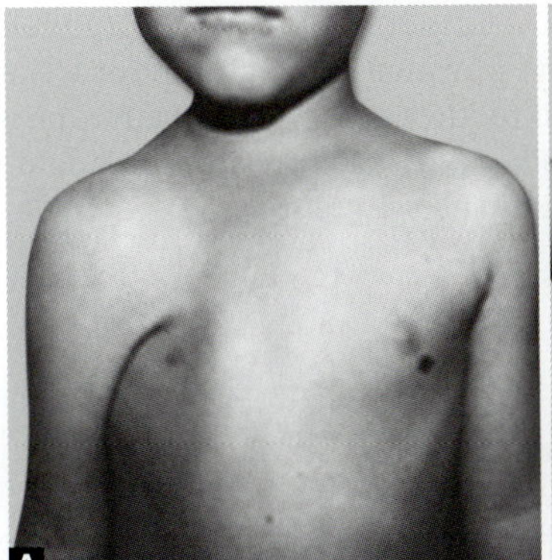

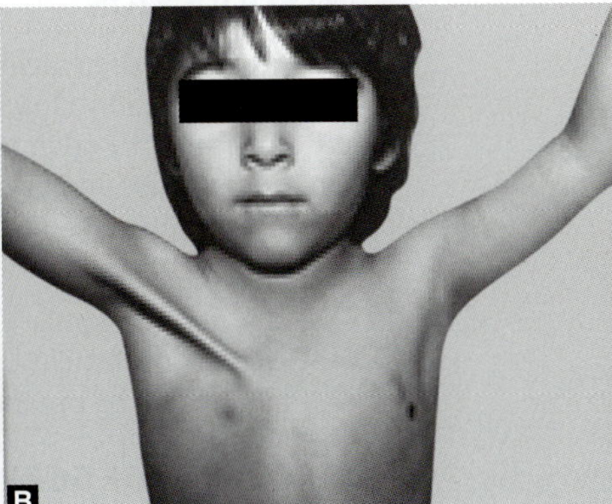

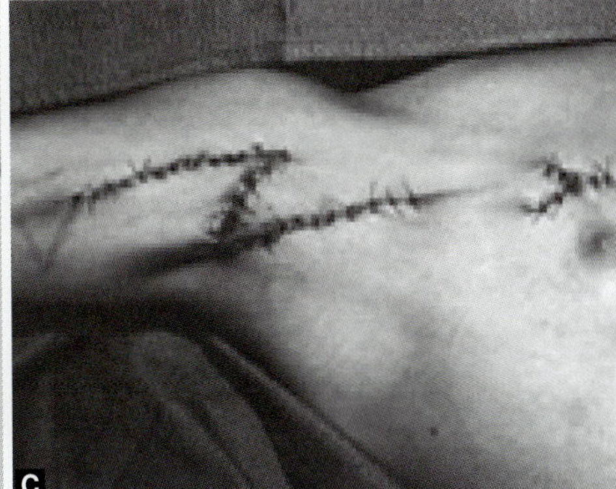

Figs. 96A to C: (A) This boy has an axillary fold contracture; (B) The axillary fold limited abduction and extension of the shoulder; (C) The contracture was easily corrected by excising the fibrous remnant and closing with a Z-plasty.

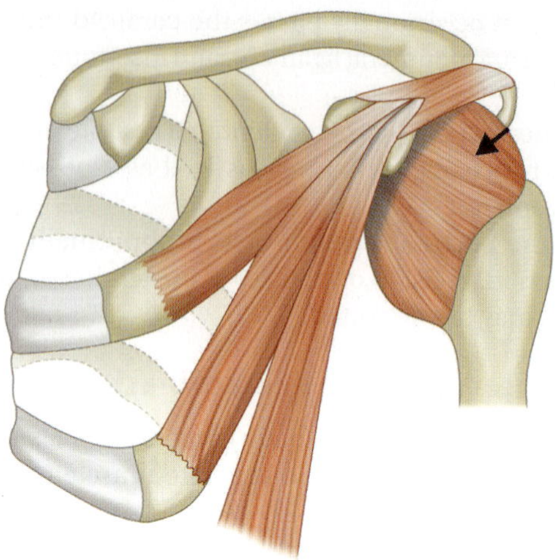

Fig. 97: The tendon of the pectoralis minor can pass over the coracoid process and insert into the humeral head (arrow). A bursa can form under the tendon and cause an impingement syndrome.

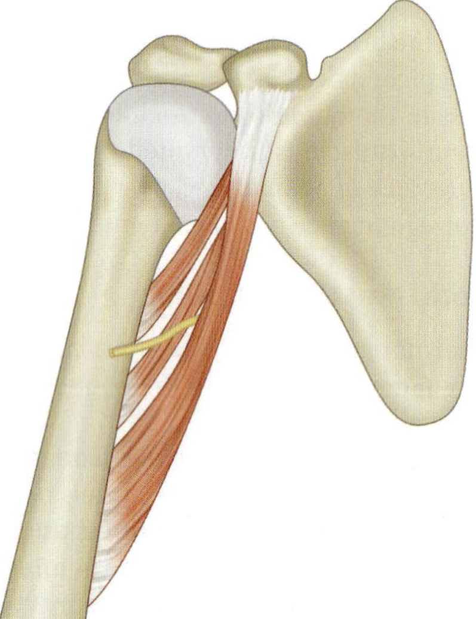

Fig. 98: The coracobrachialis can contain two or three muscle bellies through which the musculocutaneous nerve must pass.

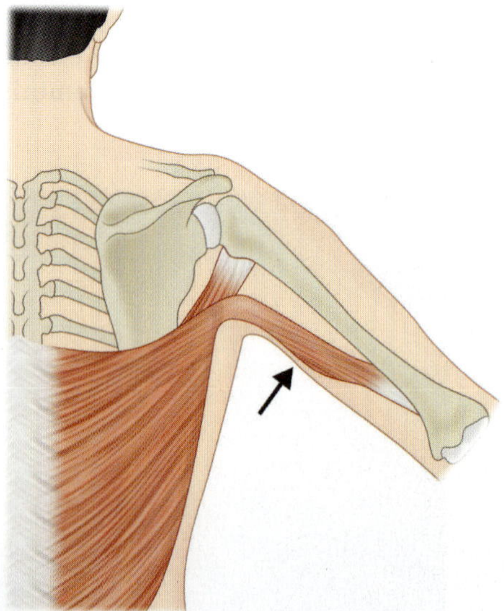

Fig. 99: The dorsal epitrochlearis muscle (arrow) originates from the tendon of the latissimus dorsi and inserts into the brachial and forearm fascia, the humerus, the lateral epicondyle, and the olecranon.

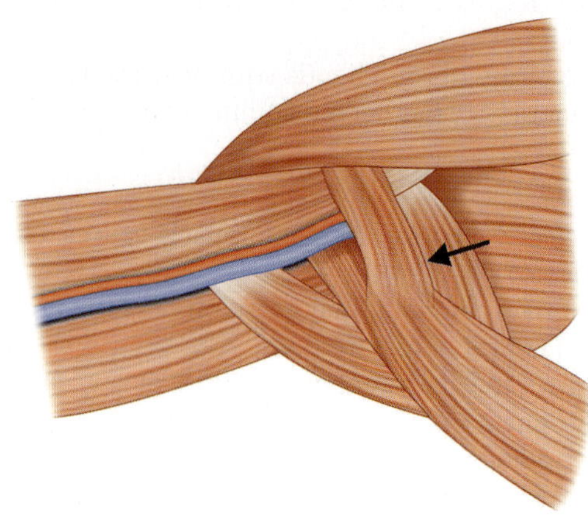

Fig. 100: The axillopectoral muscle (arrow) extends from the latissimus dorsi and inserts into the pectoralis major. It overlies the neurovascular bundle in the axilla.

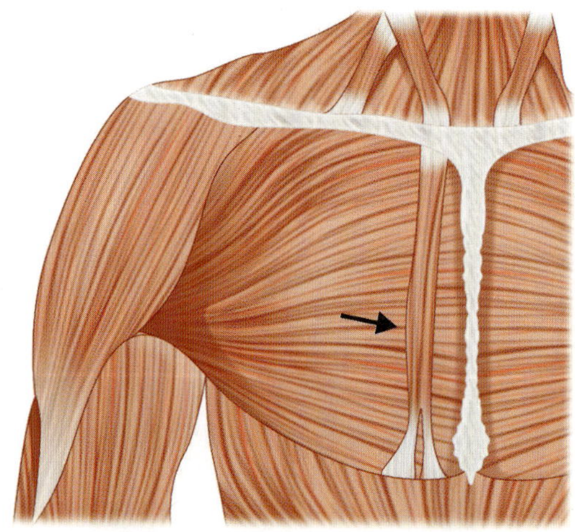

Fig. 101: The sternalis muscle (arrow).

- The muscle is superficial and medial to the pectoralis major muscle.
- The sternalis is twice as commonly unilateral as bilateral, and occurs equally in male and female patients.

FRACTURES AROUND SHOULDER AND EPIPHYSEAL INJURIES

INTRODUCTION

Fractures in children involve proximal humeral epiphysis. They are mostly managed by closed reduction and conservative measures and sometimes by open reduction. Fractures around shoulder are common injuries and occur in all age groups.

Classification

- Fractures of scapula
- Fractures of clavicle
- Fractures of the proximal humerus.

FRACTURES OF SCAPULA (FIG. 102)

Injury to the scapula is rare because it is well protected by multiple layers of muscle and other soft-tissues. Only 1% of all fractures involve scapula. However, when scapular injuries occur, they

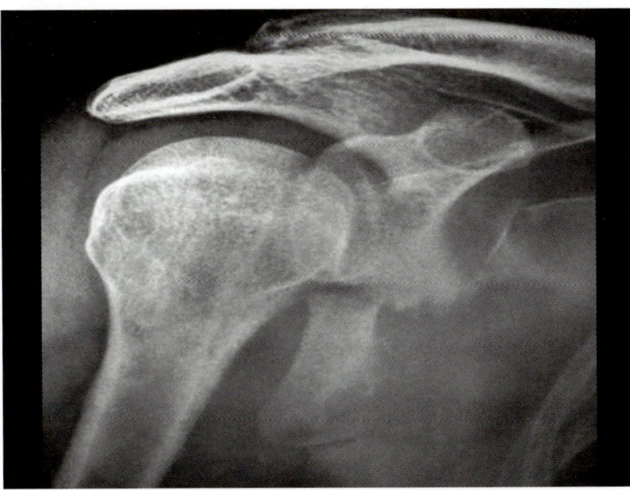

Fig. 102: X-ray showing fractured scapula.

are almost certainly a result of high energy trauma and may be associated with significant injuries to other major organ systems. Therefore, all children with apparently isolated scapular fractures should be evaluated for the presence of potentially life-threatening visceral injuries that require further intervention.

Classification of Fractures of Scapula

Idenberg's Classification

Fractures of the scapula are described by anatomic area for ease of discussion, i.e. body and spine, glenoid (scapular) neck, intra-articular glenoid, coracoid and acromion. The neck and the body are the most commonly involved areas. Skull fractures may also occur.

Acromial Fracture

- *Type I:* Minimally displaced
- *Type II:* Displaced but does not reduce subacromial space
- *Type III:* Displaced with narrowing of the subacromial space.

Coracoid Fracture

- *Type I:* Fracture proximal to coracoclavicular (CC) ligaments
- *Type II:* Fracture distal to CC ligaments.

Extra-articular Glenoid Neck Fracture

- *Type I:* Extra-articular glenoid neck fracture without associated clavicle fracture or AC separation
- *Type II:* Extra-articular glenoid neck fracture with associated clavicle fracture and with AC separation.

Intra-articular Glenoid Neck Fracture

- *Type I:* Fracture of the glenoid rim
  - *Type IA:* Anterior
  - *Type IB:* Posterior
- *Type II:* Transverse or oblique fracture through the glenoid fossa, with an inferior triangular fragment displaced with the subluxated humeral head
- *Type III:* Oblique fracture through the glenoid, exiting at the mid superior border of the scapula, often associated with AC fracture or AC dislocation
- *Type IV:* Horizontal exiting through medial border of the scapula
- *Type V:* Combination of type IV and with the fracture separating the inferior half of glenoid
- *Type VI:* Severe comminution of the glenoid surface.

Mechanism of Injury for Scapular Fracture

- The scapula is subject to indirect injury through axial loading on the outstretched arm involving scapular neck, glenoid and intra-articular space through direct trauma, often of high energy, like from blow or fall (body) and through direct trauma to the point of the shoulder, involving acromion or coracoid
- Glenohumeral dislocation may also cause glenoid fracture. Traction by muscles or ligaments may cause avulsion injuries.

Mechanism of Injury for Glenoid Fractures

- Fractures of glenoid typically occur with fall on the upper extremity.
- This drives the humeral head into the glenoid causing its fracture.
- Depending on the direction of force, the fracture may injure the rim of glenoid or the entire glenoid fossa.

Mechanism of Injury for Body of Scapula

- Fractures of the body of scapula occur via direct impact or avulsion mechanisms.
- The direct impact mechanism is typically of high energy and rarely an isolated injury.
- The avulsion type fractures may occur at any point of the several muscle attachments on the scapula.
- Child abuse must be excluded as a cause for scapular injury when no clear traumatic cause is evident.

Signs and Symptoms of Fractured Scapula

- The typical presentation is with the arm held adducted against chest wall and protected from all movements, abduction is especially painful.
- Local tenderness is present.
- With a displaced scapular neck or acromial fracture, the shoulder may appear flattened.
- Ecchymosis is less than what might be expected from the degree of bony injury present, especially compared with the fracture of the upper humerus.
- With deep inspiration, pain may be caused by the pull of attached muscles with a coracoid fracture (pectoralis minor) or due to body fracture (serratus anterior).
- The clinician should always be aware of the possibility of an associated pneumothorax either, immediate or delayed.
- With body fractures especially, deep swelling may be quite painful, producing "pseudorupture of the rotator cuff".
- In this syndrome, there is weak rotator cuff (RC) function and loss of active arm elevation, which is probably due only to inhibition of muscle contractions from intramuscular hemorrhage, it usually resolves within few weeks.
- This syndrome can be differentiated from a true RC tear by identifying the fracture radiographically and noting that swelling present with this pseudorupture syndrome exceeds that normally seen with a cuff tear.

Associated Injuries (Fig. 103)

- Pneumothorax, ipsilateral rib fractures, etc.
- Pulmonary contusion can be present, which is a life-threatening problem
- Fracture clavicle is frequently present with glenoid or glenoid neck
- Brachial plexus injury, which is usually a supraclavicular type with poor prognosis.

Treatment

- Most scapular fractures are treated by supporting the upper extremity in a sling and by providing an early active motion
- Open reduction with or without internal fixation is rarely required for fractures of the scapula
- Computed tomography (CT) scan is often necessary for accurate assessment of these injuries.

Following fractures of scapula require open reduction and internal fixation:

Fractures of the Acromion and Lateral Scapular Spine

These are significantly displaced fractures of the acromion and lateral scapular spine, with retraction of the fragment and encroachment on the subacromial space. These fractures are extremely rare.

If the subacromial space is significantly compromised, causing impingement of the tuberosities during abduction, open reduction and internal fixation using K-wires or screws and plates may be indicated.

Fractures of Coracoid with Acromioclavicular Separation

When fracture of coracoid occurs with dislocation of outer end of clavicle, open reduction internal fixation (ORIF) of coracoid with screw or heavy suture and repair of AC ligament should be done.

Glenoid Rim Fractures (Figs. 104 to 107)

They are generally associated with traumatic dislocation of the shoulder. If a glenoid rim fracture involves one fourth of the articulating surface, open reduction and internal fixation are required to prevent recurrent dislocation or subluxation. This is illustrated in Figures 107A and B. Small glenoid rim fractures after a dislocation should be treated by nonoperative measures. Fracture of anterior glenoid rim is usually produced by medially directed blow to humeral head, shown in Figures 105 and 106. Other fractures of the glenoid and scapular neck usually can be treated by sling support and early active motion.

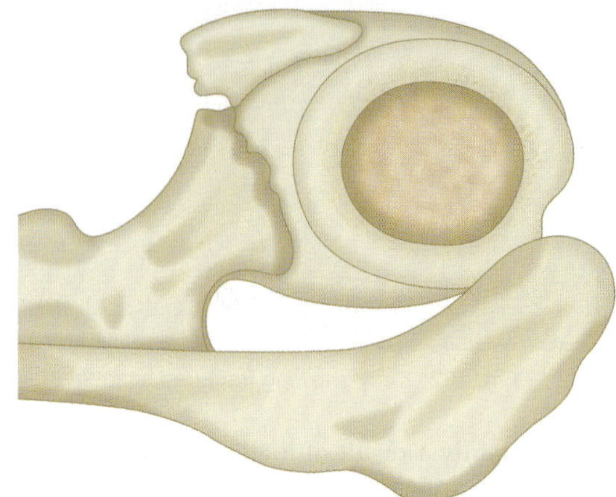

Fig. 104: Fracture of anterior glenoid rim.

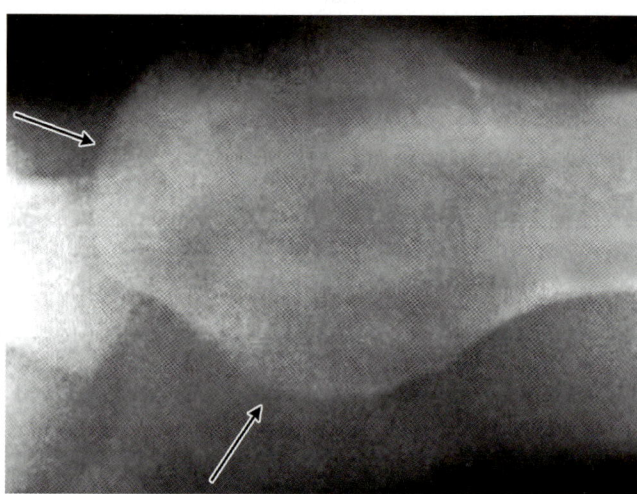

Fig. 105: Large anterior glenoid rim fractures with associated posterior Hill-Sachs lesion (arrows).

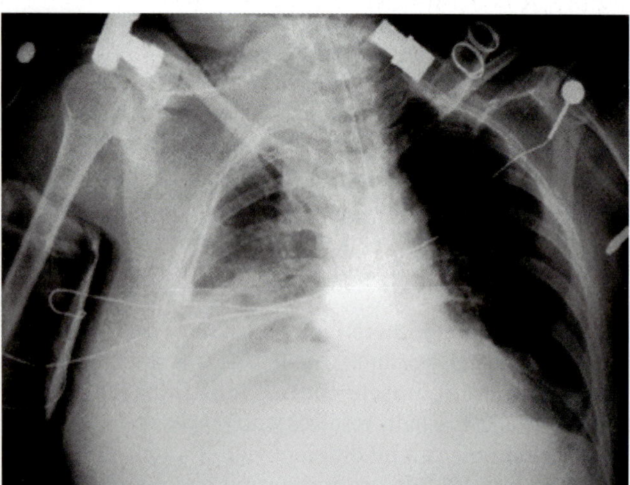

Fig. 103: Radiograph of multiple trauma patient with a fractured scapular neck, associated with upper extremity fractures and pulmonary contusion.

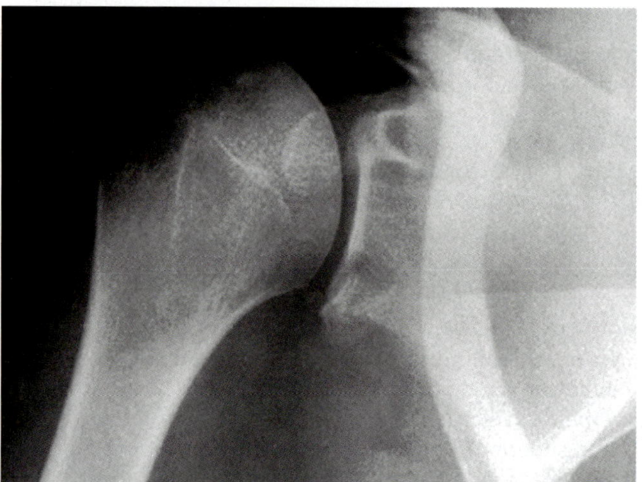

Fig. 106: Anteroposterior (AP) view of the glenoid showing an anteroinferior glenoid fracture.

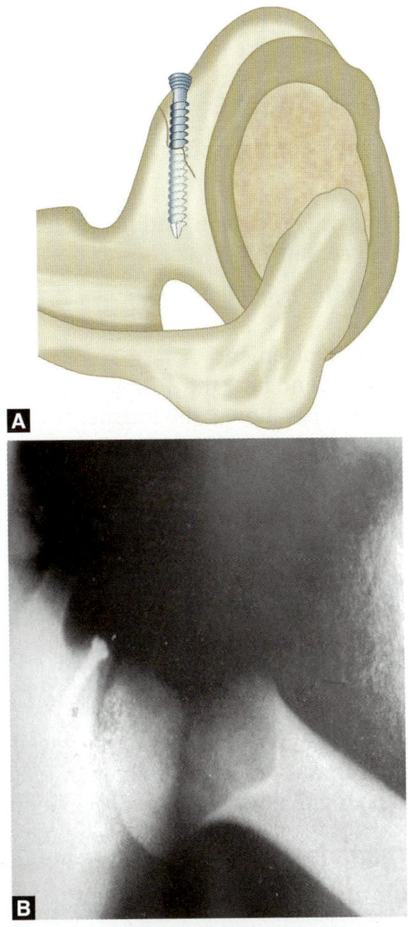

Figs. 107A and B: Open reduction and internal fixation of glenoid rim fractures with single screw.

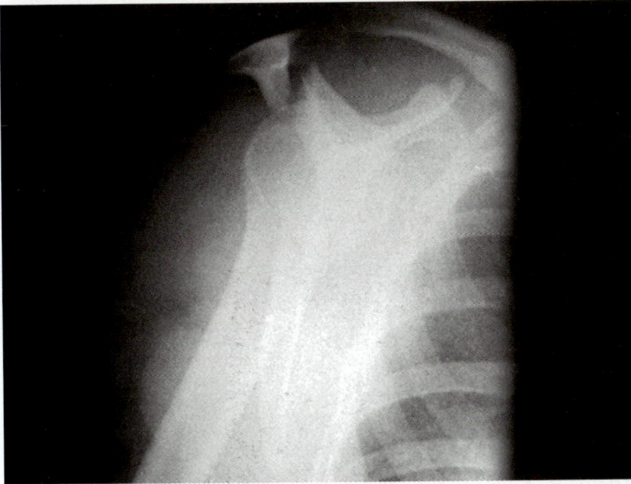

Fig. 108: A displaced acromial fracture.

Acromial Fracture

Acromion commonly absorbs direct blows, and AC separation is much more common than the fracture of the acromion. Most acromial fractures are minimally displaced. Commonly the fracture line is little lateral to AC joint, causing confusion with os acromiale. The fractured base of acromion is well seen on a true (tangential) scapular lateral view. A displaced acromial fracture is a candidate for an open reduction (Fig. 108).

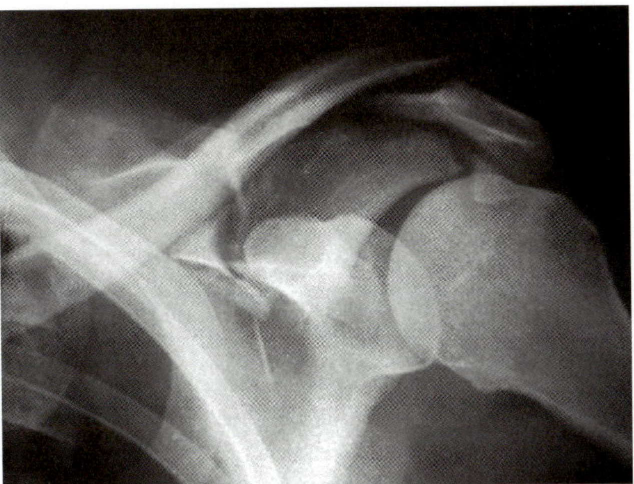

Fig. 109: Superior displacement of the humeral head due to some trauma.

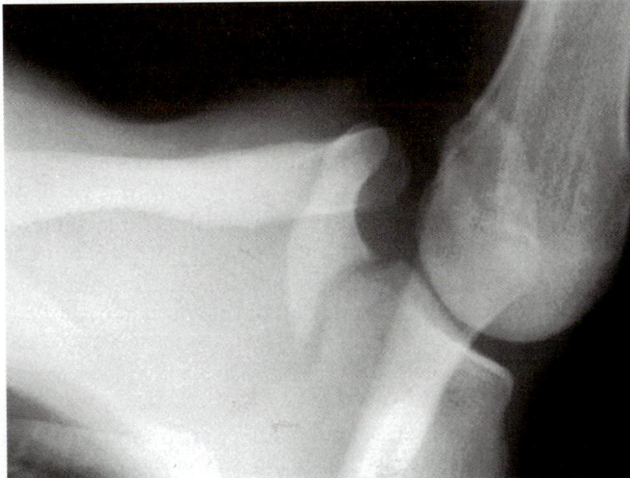

Fig. 110: Stryker notch view, showing fracture of the base of coracoid.

Another mechanism of an acromial fracture is traumatic superior displacement of the humeral head; this is shown in Figure 109. This mechanism often also results in an associated extensive RC tear. If the humeral head is displaced upward into the subacromial space (acromiohumeral distance reduced), a RC tear should be suspected. A nondisplaced fracture of the acromion responds well to initial symptomatic treatment and the use of the sling for three weeks. Displaced fractures require reduction and fixation with tension band wire technique or screws to eliminate impingement or to reduce the AC joint.

Coracoid Fracture

Fractures of the coracoid may be isolated, occurring from direct blow to it or to the point of the shoulder. Coracoid fracture may also occur in association with AC dislocation. The coracoid tip may be avulsed by muscle pull of the biceps and coracobrachialis or from direct contact from a dislocating humeral head. A fracture of the base of coracoid is best seen on Stryker notch view; shown in Figure 110.

Coracoid fracture occurs most commonly through the coracoid base and is minimally displaced unless significant AC separation occurs. For an isolated coracoid fracture no specific treatment is needed because anatomic alignment is not essential for either of adequate function or healing.

Indications for surgery with coracoid fracture:
- For a displaced coracoid fracture with third degree AC separation, AC fixation should be done.
- If there is obstruction to the reduction of anterior shoulder dislocation.
- Displaced fracture of coracoid involving the glenoid fossa.
- Third degree AC separation associated with coracoid fracture is an indication for open reduction and threaded Steinmann pin fixation of the AC joint.

Scapular Body Fracture (Fig. 111)

Direct violence and sudden contraction of divergent muscles may cause fractures of the body of the scapula. Other causes include electrical shock treatments and seizures. In the immediate treatment of these fractures, no reduction is attempted. Restoration of the normal bony anatomy is not necessary for good function in a healed scapular body fracture. A true scapular lateral view showing displaced scapular body fracture is shown in Figure 111.

Symptomatic treatment with ice and immobilization for comfort is all that is needed initially. Cross strapping with adhesive, to immobilize the scapula may be needed in some cases. Pendulum exercises, use of overhead pulleys and a further passive or active assisted ROM program should be started within 1 week after injury. Earlier there was a case report published for symptomatic scapular body malunion, in which removal of rib prominences and portion of scapula relieved symptoms and improved ROM. Operative fixation with bone graft has been reported in some cases of nonunion.

Glenoid Neck (Extra-articular) Fracture

A fracture of the neck of scapula is the second most common pattern of scapular fracture, occurring from direct trauma; a fall on the point of shoulder; or a fall on the outstretched hand. True AP, tangential scapular lateral and axillary lateral radiographs and often CT scans are necessary to confirm the extra-articular nature of the fracture and verify the reduced position of the humeral head. Reduction of scapular neck fracture and restoration of the glenoid to its anatomic position is not necessary. Sling immobilization for comfort is probably enough.

FRACTURES OF CLAVICLE

This is one of the most common bony injuries, which rarely require an open reduction.

Mechanism of injury: Direct blow and fall on outstretched hand. Mostly treated conservatively.

This may require ORIF in following cases:
- Nonunion
- Neurovascular involvement
- Fracture of lateral end near the AC joint in an adult
- Persistent wide separation of the fragments with interposition of soft tissue
- Floating shoulder.

Nonunion of Clavicle

This is the most frequent indication for an open reduction. Internal fixation with an intramedullary pin or a plate and bone grafting are required.

Neurovascular Involvement in Fractured Clavicle

Neurovascular compromise is not easily resolved by reduction of the fracture. It requires an immediate open reduction and the fracture should be internally stabilized, if open reduction is done.

Fracture of the Lateral End of Clavicle Near the Acromioclavicular Joint in an Adult

Neer's classification of clavicle fractures: Neer identified five types of lateral clavicular fractures:
- *Type I:* Is minimally displaced and lateral to CA ligament
- *Type IIA:* Unstable lateral clavicular fractures, CA ligaments and AC joint capsule are intact (Fig. 112)
- *Type IIB:* Unstable lateral fracture with disruption of CA ligament but AC joint capsule is intact (Fig. 113)
- *Type III:* Fractures involve extension into AC joint
- *Type IV:* Fractures involve a distal fracture with periosteal sleeve disruption

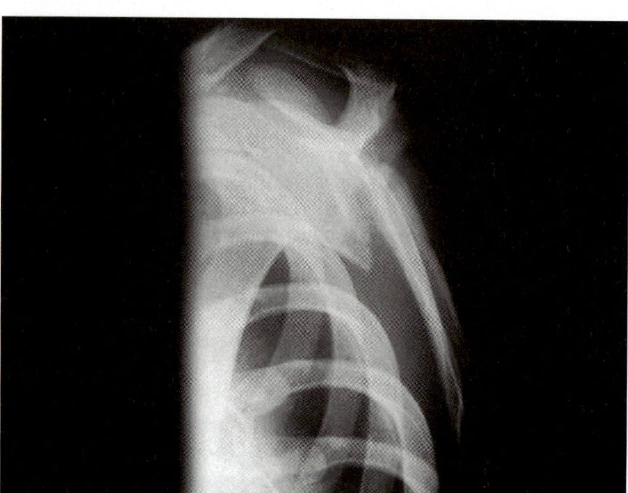

Fig. 111: X-ray of scapular lateral view showing displaced scapular body fracture.

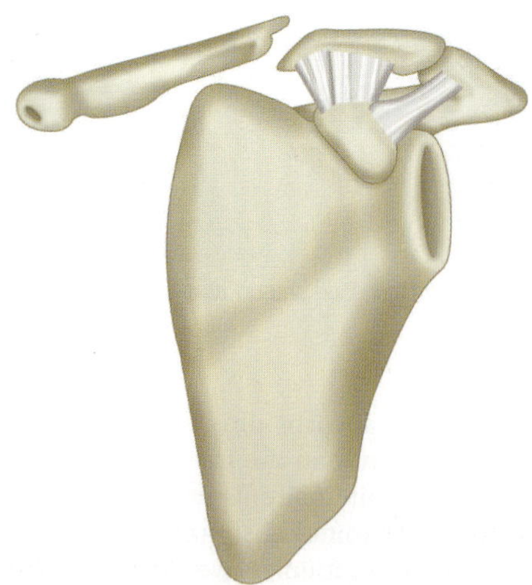

Fig. 112: Neer's type IIA, unstable lateral clavicle fracture. Coracoacromial ligaments and joint capsule are intact.

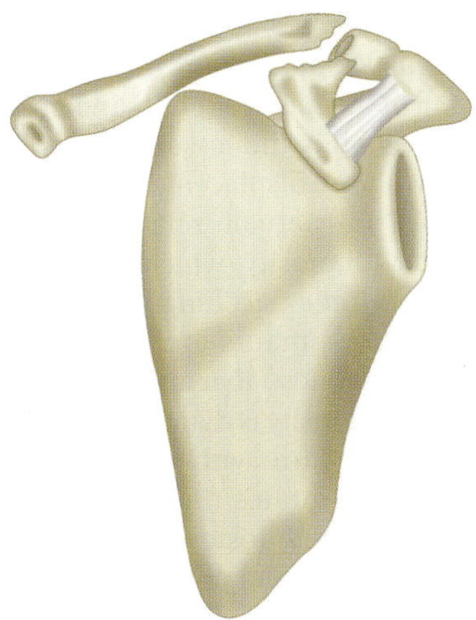

Fig. 113: Type IIB unstable lateral fracture with disruption of coracoacromial ligament. Acromioclavicular joint capsule is intact.

- *Type V:* Fractures are similar to type II fractures and involve an avulsion, leaving only an inferior cortical fragment attached to the CC ligaments.

Surgical techniques used for displaced lateral clavicular fractures:
- Plate and screw fixation for more medial fractures.
- Transacromial K-wires and tension band wires.
- Horizontal figure of eight wires or polydioxanone suture (PDS), ethicon.
- Single transacromial Knowles pin.
- Coracoclavicular ligament reconstruction with Mersilene tape, Dacron arterial graft material, or PDS bands.
- Internal fixation of a fracture is often combined with CC ligament reconstruction to improve the chances of good result.

Floating Shoulder

Fracture of the clavicle and surgical neck of scapula make the scapular fractures unstable. The weight of the arm and shoulder girdle muscles that insert into the proximal humerus rotate the glenoid fragment anteromedially. In this case, open reduction and internal fixation of clavicular fractures with a 3.5 mm plate and screws to prevent malunion of the scapular fracture and drooping of shoulder is recommended. This can be illustrated in Figures 114A to D.

Intramedullary compression clavicular nail used for widely displaced middle-third of clavicle as shown in Figure 115. For intramedullary fixation of the clavicle, the pin must be strong enough to withstand unsupported weight of the upper extremity without bending or breaking. It should be threaded or lateral end should be bent to 90° to prevent medial migration to vital structures. Rockwood developed an intramedullary clavicular nail with a lateral compression nut. When tightened, the nut allows compression across the fracture site. Precontoured clavicle plate, which is used for widely displaced middle-third clavicle fractures, is illustrated in Figure 116.

Intramedullary Fixation of Clavicle

- Over the fracture site make a 2.5 cm long incision.
- Pass Steinman pin of 3.2 mm into the medial fragment.
- Remove the pin and pass it laterally into the lateral fragment to emerge in till conoid tubercle.

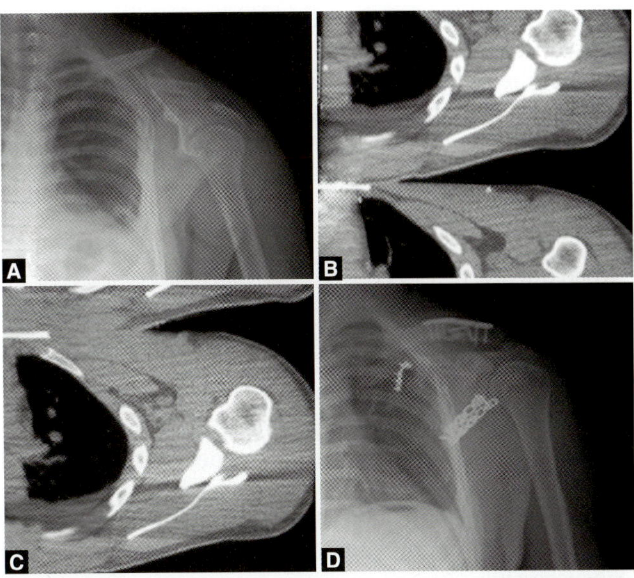

Figs. 114A to D: X-ray and CT scan images of floating shoulders: (A) Widely displaced floating shoulder injury; (B and C) CT scans showing anteromedial displacement of glenoid fragment; (D) Clavicular and scapular fractures after repair.

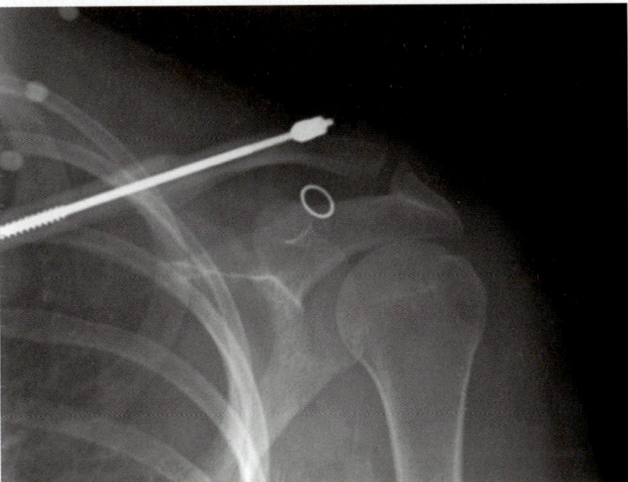

Fig. 115: Intramedullary compression clavicular nail used for reducing widely displaced middle-third of clavicle.

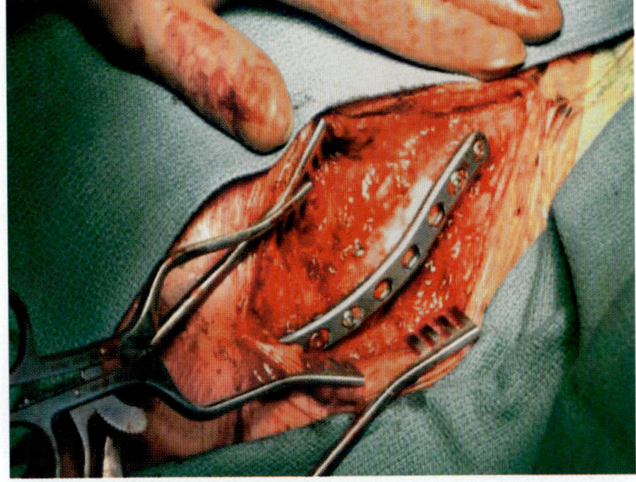

Fig. 116: Precontoured clavicle plate, used for widely displaced middle-third clavicle fractures.

- Now take a threaded Steinman pin and drill it retrogressively into the lateral fragment.
- Reduce the fracture and drill the pin into the medial fragment.
- Alternatively 2 mm K-wires can be used.
- Method of pin fixation in case of external fixation of clavicle fractures is depicted in Figure 117.

Indications for External Fixation in Clavicle Fractures

- Open fractures
- Closed fractures with major displacement and overlying skin damage
- Multiple trauma
- Painful delayed union or nonunion
- Fractures with accompanying thoracic outlet syndrome
- A persistent wide separation of the fragments with interposition of soft tissue
- If deltoid or trapezius muscle is impaled by the sharp spike of one of the major fragments, closed reduction may be unsuccessful
- In this case, open reduction and internal fixation should be done
- At open reduction interposed soft tissue should be removed, and fracture should be fixed with plates or screws or with intramedullary pins.

PROXIMAL HUMERAL FRACTURES (FIG. 118)

Pathomechanics

Most fractures of the proximal humerus are a result of indirect force, such as a fall on the outstretched hand rather than a direct blow to the shoulder. The origin of a proximal humeral fracture is due to combination of factors, which include relatively osteoporotic bone (in the elderly), direct contact against the adjacent acromion or glenoid rim and forceful pull of the RC muscles and extrinsic muscles, such as the pectoralis major. The muscular pull of adjacent tendon attachments on humeral fracture fragments determines the patterns of displacement, as shown in Figure 119.

The pectoralis major pulls the humeral shaft anteriorly and medially. The supraspinatus and infraspinatus pull the greater tuberosity posterosuperiorly, depending on the integrity of their tendinous insertion. Displacement of the fracture fragments depends on the pull of the muscles of RC and pectoralis major.

The subscapularis pulls the lesser tuberosity medially. In a three-part fracture with the displacement of the lesser tuberosity, the humeral head will be externally rotated away from the glenoid by the pull of greater tuberosity, which remains attached to the articular segment. Top three-part fracture with greater tuberosity remaining intact, supraspinatus and infraspinatus externally rotate the articular fragment so that articular segment is oriented anteriorly and lesser tuberosity is displaced medially.

Bottom three-part fracture with lesser tuberosity intact, the subscapularis internally rotates the articular segment so that articular segment is oriented posteriorly. The greater tuberosity fragment is pulled superiorly and posteriorly.

Classification

Classification is based on four-part anatomy of proximal humerus:
1. The humeral head
2. The lesser tuberosity
3. The greater tuberosity
4. The proximal humeral shaft.

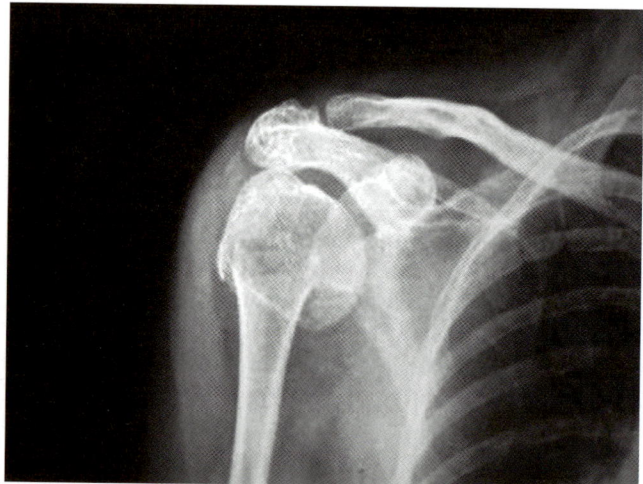

Fig. 118: X-ray depicting proximal humeral fracture.

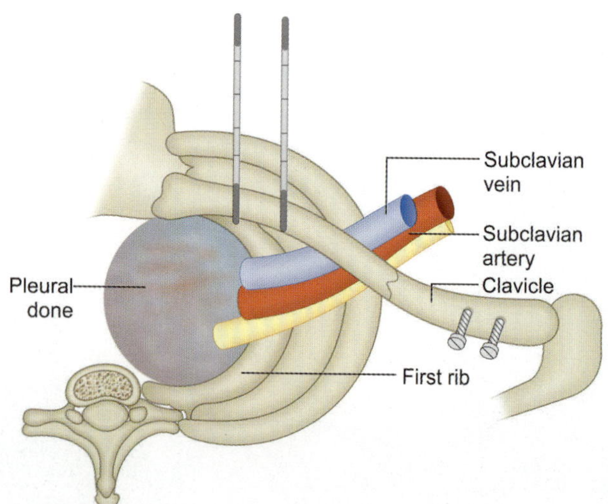

Fig. 117: Pin fixation in external fixation of clavicle.

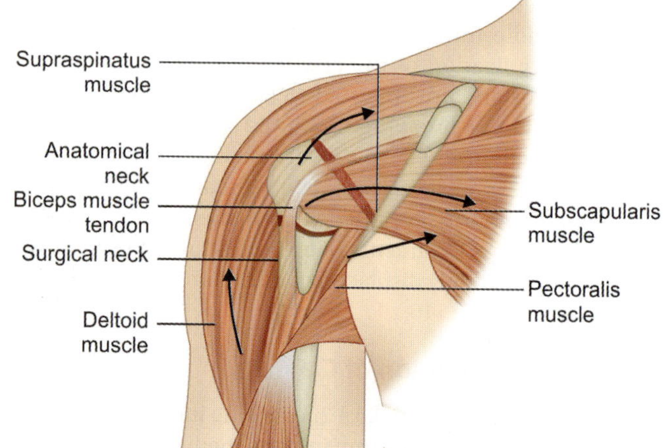

Fig. 119: Muscular pull of adjacent tendon attachments on humeral fracture fragments determines the patterns of displacement as shown by the arrows.

Criteria for displacement: Greater than 1 cm of separation of a part or angulation of 45°. Osteonecrosis is most likely displaced after four-part fractures (Fig. 120).

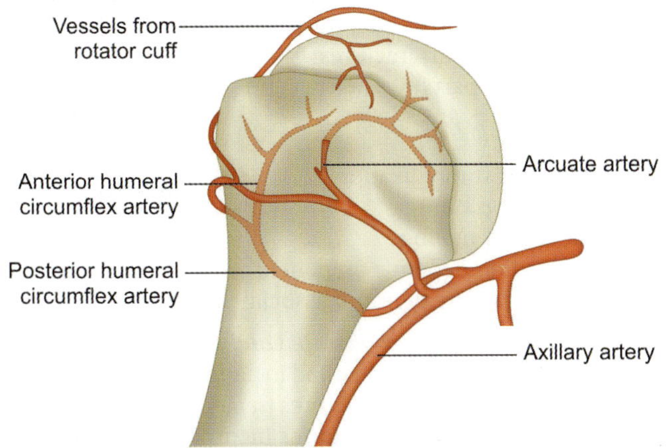

Fig. 120: Blood supply of the humeral head.

Neer's classification of proximal humeral fractures (Fig. 121): He described that the fracture can be two-part, three-part, or four-part. He also described the key segment displaced in each two-part pattern, segment named is one which is displaced. Two-part surgical neck fractures can be:

- Impacted
- Unimpacted
- Comminuted.

All three-part patterns have displacement of the shaft segment. In four-part pattern, all segments are displaced. Fracture dislocations are identified by the anterior or posterior position of articular segment. Large articular surface defects require separate recognition.

Signs and Symptoms

- In most cases of proximal humeral fractures, there is significant swelling and pain. It may be associated with ecchymosis.

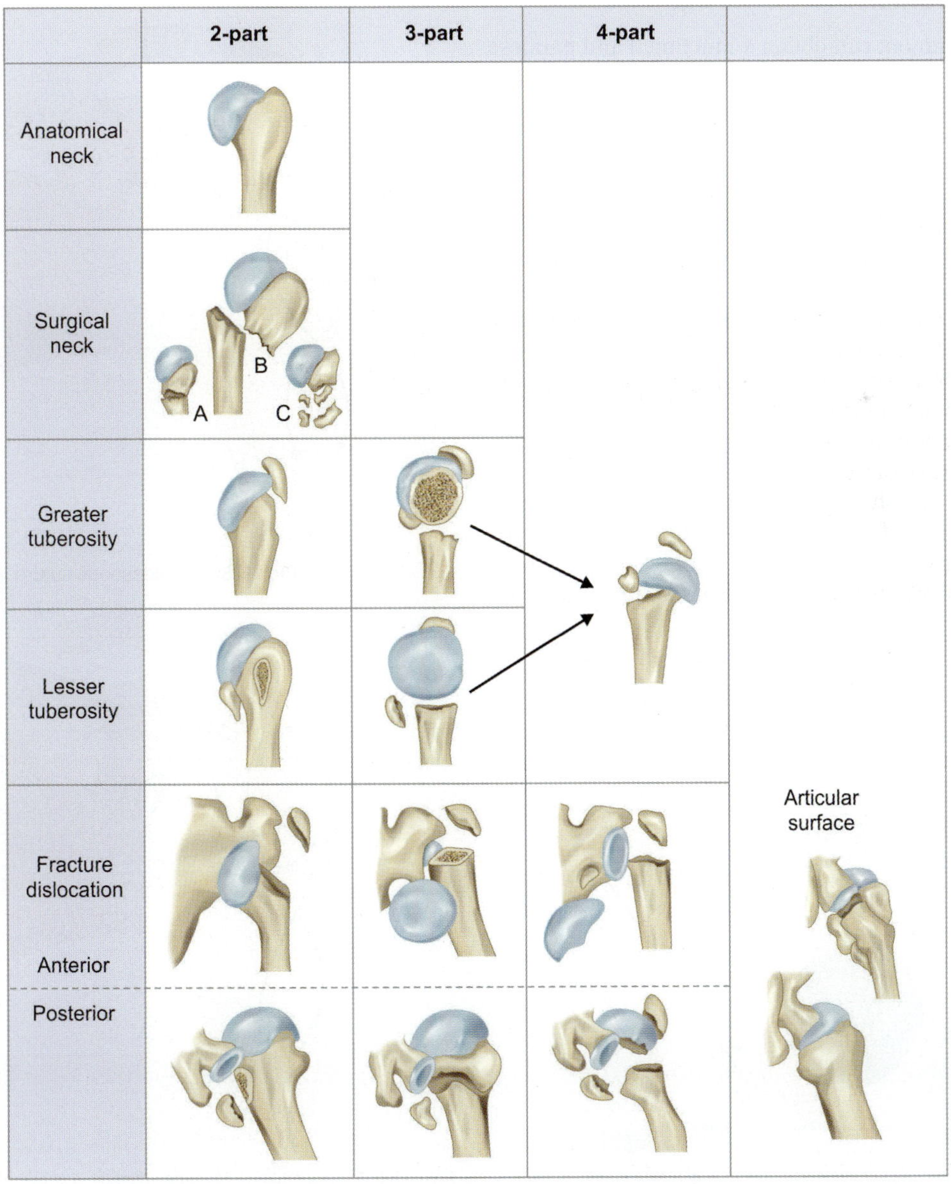

	2-part	3-part	4-part	
Anatomical neck				
Surgical neck	A B C			
Greater tuberosity				
Lesser tuberosity				
Fracture dislocation Anterior				Articular surface
Posterior				

Fig. 121: Neer's terminology of four segment classification of displaced fractures.

- As the swelling subsides over the first 2–4 weeks, ecchymosis changes from the classic blue bruising to green and then yellow and may move distally down the arm.
- Patients may occasionally note tingling or numbness in the extremity, which may be related to brachial plexus stretch.

Physical Findings

Initially other injuries of the neck or chest wall should be excluded, since this association is common with proximal humeral fractures, especially if high energy trauma, such as motor vehicle accident has occurred. Neurovascular evaluation is the next step.

Radiographic Evaluation

Special radiographic view perpendicular to the plane of scapula, to show GH joint in profile, is illustrated in Figure 122.

Radiographic view parallel to the plane of scapula is taken to show anterior and posterior displacement.

Nonoperative Treatment

- Nonoperative treatment can obtain a functional and painless extremity in most proximal humeral fractures.
- The ROM of the shoulder joint accommodates moderate angular deformity without significant functional loss.
- Neer described acceptable angulation as less than 45° and less than 1 cm of displacement.
- The first step in treatment decision making is to determine if displacement and angulation are acceptable for a particular patient.
- The second step is to determine if humeral head and shaft move as a unit.
- If both of these conditions are present, then fracture is stable and is in an acceptable position.
- A sling is used for comfort, and a physical therapy regimen with pendulum exercises is started.
- If humeral head and shaft do not move as a unit, physical therapy can be delayed for 2–4 weeks, in patients who are poor surgical candidates.
- In young active patients, early operative fixation should be considered.

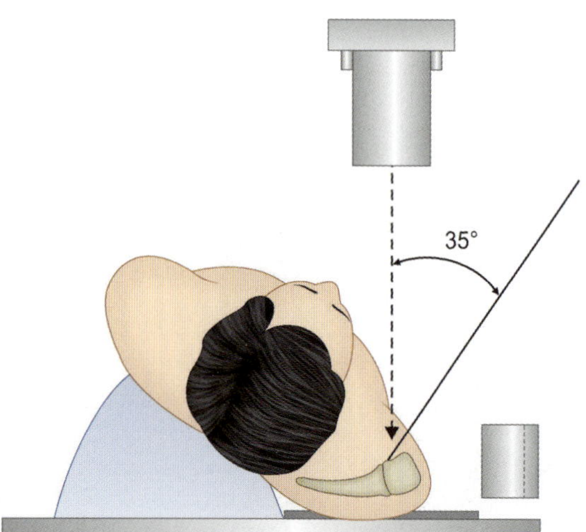

Fig. 122: Radiographic view perpendicular to the plane of scapula.

Operative Treatment

Indications

- Displaced two-part surgical neck fractures
- Displaced (> 5 mm) greater tuberosity fracture.
- Displaced three-part fractures
- Displaced four-part fractures in young patients.

Types of Fixation

- Transosseous suture fixation
- Percutaneous pinning
- Intramedullary nailing
- Type of fixation depends on patient's age, activity level, bone quality, the fracture type and associated fractures.

Transosseous suture fixation (Figs. 123 and 124): Excellent results have been obtained in patients with two part and three part proximal humeral fractures treated with suture fixation. Transosseous nonabsorbable sutures incorporate RC to increase fixation and help control tuberosity fragments. This has been illustrated in Figure 124.

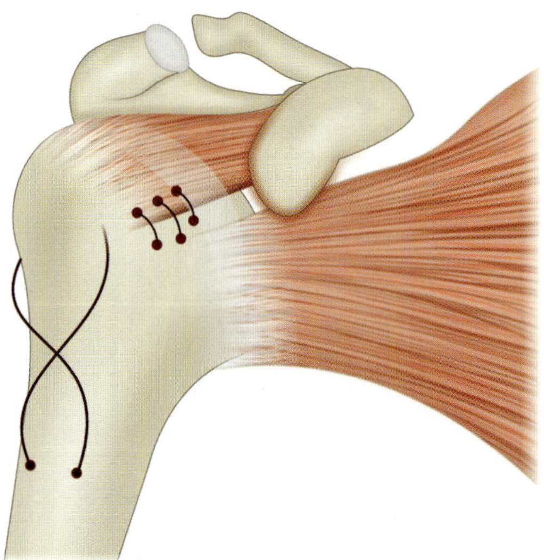

Fig. 123: Transosseous suture fixation.

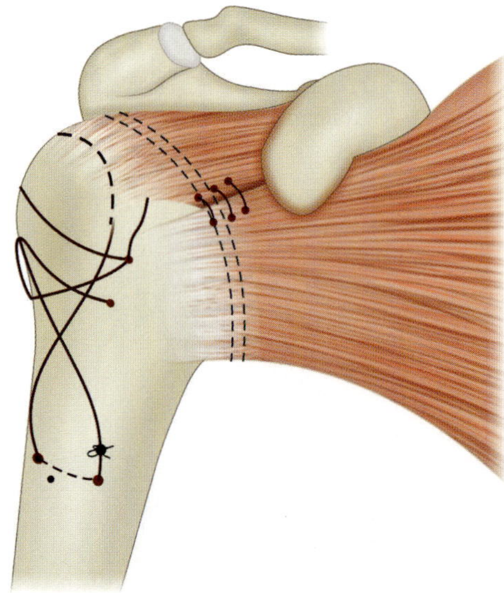

Fig. 124: Transosseous nonabsorbable sutures incorporate rotator cuff to increase fixation.

The use of strong nonabsorbable suture provides the advantage of incorporating the RC insertion to increase fixation in patients with poor bone quality. The level of soft-tissue dissection is not extensive, and osteonecrosis is low with these techniques. Since, it is a nonrigid construct, loss of reduction can occur.

Percutaneous pinning (Fig. 125):
Percutaneous pinning has the advantage of avoiding further damage to the soft tissue envelope blood supply to the humeral head. The procedure is technically challenging, loss of fixation and pin track infections are common complications. Terminally threaded Schanz pins and bicortical pins inserted from greater tuberosity to the medial humeral shaft add stability. Percutaneous pinning is contraindicated in fractures with metaphyseal comminution. Methods of placement of percutaneous pins for fracture fixation shown in Figure 126.

Intramedullary nailing (Fig. 127):
Intramedullary nailing provides more stable fixation than percutaneous pinning, but less than the locked plate fixation. Insertion of an intramedullary nail into the proximal humerus violates the RC. This can lead to postoperative shoulder pain. The advantage of this technique includes preservation of soft tissues.

Plate and Screw Constructs (Fig. 128)

This provides the most stable fixation of the three fixation methods. Locked plates add stability, especially in an osteoporotic bone. Open reduction and rigid fixation allows accurate reduction and stabilization of the tuberosities. Historically, plate fixation of the proximal humerus has many complications with malunion and nonunion caused by poor fixation in humeral head.

Extensive tissue dissection increases the possibility of osteonecrosis of humeral head, leading to a painful and functionally limited shoulder joint. Locked proximal humeral plate is the implant of choice in proximal humeral fractures. Another problem with open reduction and locked plating includes extensive exposure, required for plate application that carries risk of damage to the neurovascular structures, especially the ascending branch of lateral circumflex artery. The most frequent complication of plate fixation is infection and osteonecrosis of humeral head.

Fixation of Specific Fractures Types (Figs. 129 and 130)

Two-parts greater tuberosity fractures: They are treated operatively, when displacement is greater than 1 cm. These fractures are stabilized with transosseous sutures or occasionally with screws in larger fragments.

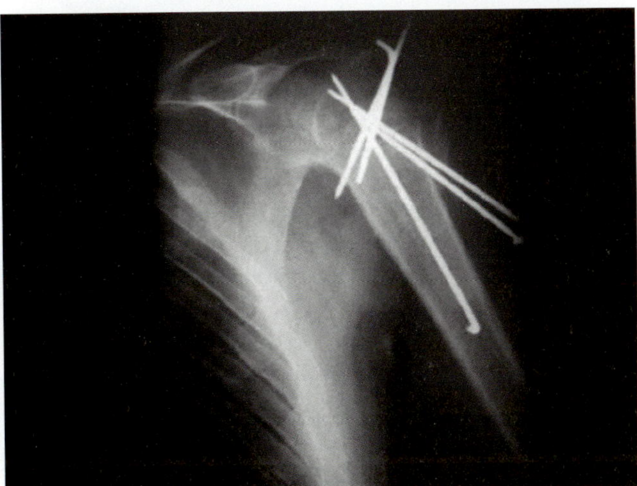

Fig. 125: X-ray showing percutaneous pinning: Two part proximal humerus fracture stabilized with pins.

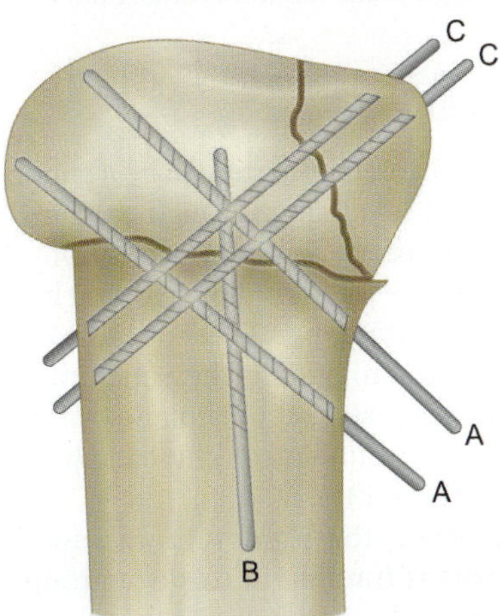

Fig. 126: Various methods of placement of percutaneous pins for fracture fixation: (A) Two are passed through lateral aspect of the shaft, just above deltoid insertion; (B) One is placed through anterior cortex; (C) Two pins are inserted retrograde, to reduce and repair this fracture component.

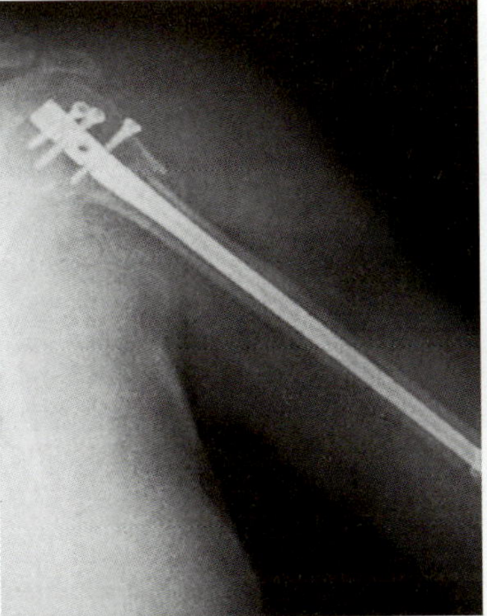

Fig. 127: Intramedullary nailing.

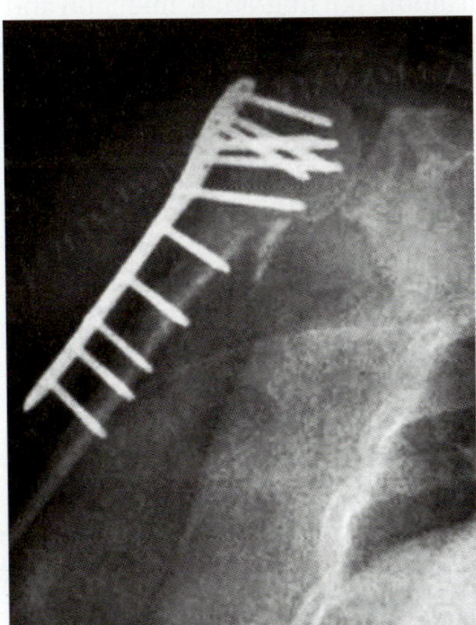

Fig. 128: Plate and screw constructs.

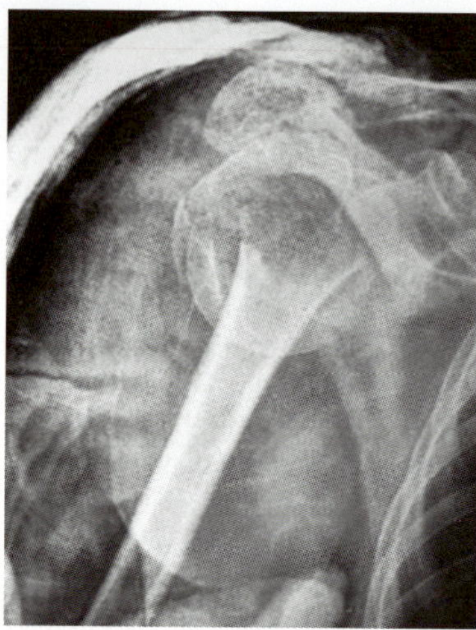

Fig. 129: Preoperative X-ray of fractured surgical neck of humerus.

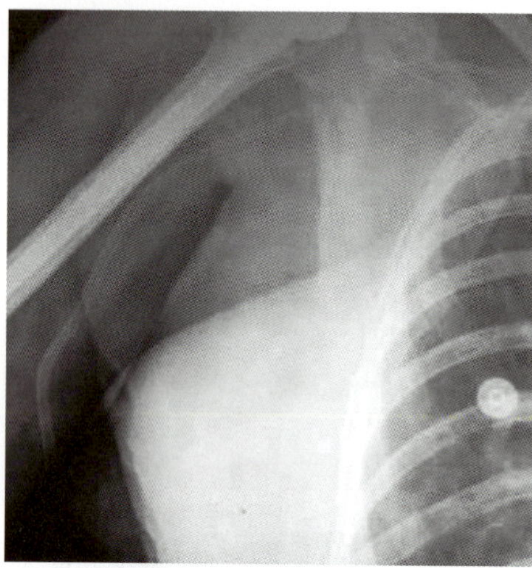

Fig. 130: Postoperative X-ray of the same patient.

Two-parts surgical neck fractures: Closed reduction and percutaneous pinning have been reported to be successful in fractures that are reducible and are not comminuted. Complications such as loss of fixation, pin migration, infection and malunion have made rigid intramedullary nailing the preferred technique. Widely displaced fractures, fractures with comminution and irreducible fractures are stabilized with the locked plate construct. Improved proximal fixation of these systems has increased stability, so that immediate postoperative ROM is allowed.

Three-parts proximal humerus fractures: These fractures in elderly patients with osteopenic bone may require hemiarthroplasty, but for most of these fractures plate fixation is the preferred procedure. The rigid fixation provided with locking plates allows early ROM which is one of the goals of operative treatment.

Four-parts proximal humeral fractures: These fractures treated nonoperatively have poor outcome. Poor bone quality make fixation difficult, vascular insult to the articular surface increases the risk of osteonecrosis of the humeral head. In young active patients, open reduction and plate fixation usually are successful, if soft tissue stripping is kept to minimum to avoid further damage to the humeral blood supply. Rigid fixation with locking plates currently is the procedure of choice for four parts proximal humeral

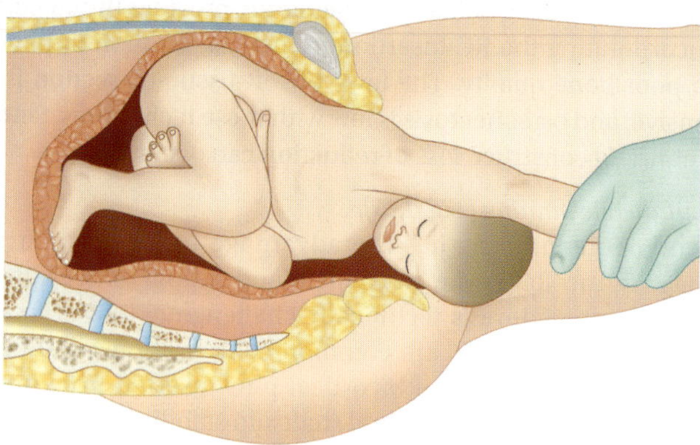

Fig. 131: Proximal humeral or physeal injury during birth due to hyperextension or rotation of the ipsilateral arm.

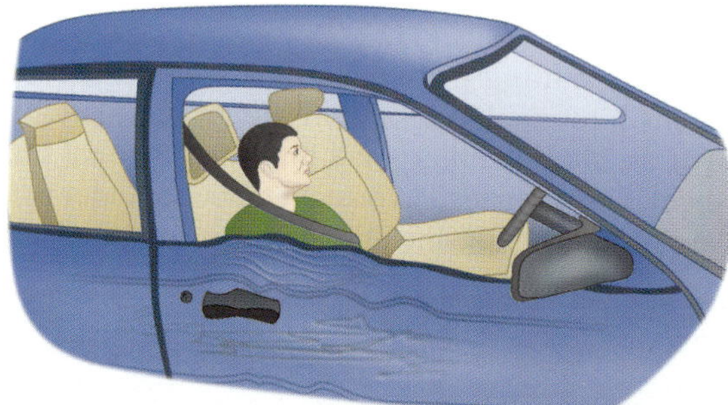

Fig. 132: Motor vehicle crashes may result in proximal humeral fractures.

fractures in young active patients. Hemiarthroplasty is a good option in elderly patients with low functional demands. Head of the humerus is removed and replaced with Neer's prosthesis.

Fractures of the Proximal Humerus in Children

Fractures of the proximal humerus are relatively uncommon injuries of childhood. Fractures in this region have enormous potential to heal and remodel, more than anywhere else in the body, mainly due to the thick periosteum at the proximal humerus and proximity to the physis.

Thus, proximal humeral fractures in children can be expected to heal without significant residual functional or cosmetic deficits in most cases.

Mechanism of Injury

Fractures of the proximal humerus can be a common birth related injury. As an infant is passing through the birth canal, the arm may be placed in a variety of abnormal positions that can result in separation through the physis of the proximal humerus.

These fractures are generally believed to be resulted from hyperextension and/or rotation of the arm during passage through the birth canal. Hyperextension or rotation of the ipsilateral arm may result in proximal humeral or physeal injury during birth this has been depicted (Fig. 131).

In older children, the predominant cause of fractures in proximal humerus is trauma. In this age group, these fractures can involve the metaphysis, the physis or both. Proximal humerus fractures are typically moderate to high energy injuries and are typically seen in motor vehicle crashes and sporting activities (Fig. 132).

Blunt trauma from contact sports may result in fracture of the proximal humerus in children, as shown in Figure 133. Less often, pediatric proximal humeral fractures in newborns result from other conditions, such as malignant or benign tumors and pituitary gigantism. This can also be a complication of radiation therapy to the shoulder region. In addition, shoulder joint neuropathy secondary to Arnold-Chiari malformation, myelomeningocele, or syringomyelia is also etiologic factor in case of proximal humeral fractures.

Signs and Symptoms

- Clinical features of proximal humeral fractures in newborns may be subtle and not readily identified.
- Infant may be irritable when there is a movement of upper extremity.
- Infant may refuse to move the arm giving appearance of paralysis called pseudoparalysis.
- Older children typically reports a history consistent with a proximal humeral fracture, immediate development of moderate-to-severe global shoulder pain exacerbated by motion of the arm.
- They also present with obvious deformity or fullness in anterior shoulder region, with the overall contour of the shoulder altered in comparison with the contralateral uninjured shoulder.
- The arm is internally rotated against the abdomen and the patient usually refuses to use the involved arm.
- Pain, swelling, and ecchymosis are present to some degree.
- The internally rotated position of the injured extremity is due to pull of the pectoralis major muscle on the distal fragment.
- Some children with the fractures of the greater tuberosity have an unusual presentation of luxatio erecta where the involved shoulder is positioned in extreme abduction.
- Fracture of the proximal humerus may result in twisting at the elbow as illustrated in Figure 134.

Associated Injuries

- In high energy trauma, fractures of the proximal humerus may be associated with concomitant dislocations of the GH joint.
- The direction of the dislocation may be anterior, posterior, or inferior.
- Neurologic injury to the brachial plexus can result from fractures and fractured dislocations of the proximal humerus.
- Typically these nerve deficits are transient and full function typically returns in less than 6 months.
- Fractures of the proximal humerus in children can also be associated with other injuries, including rib fractures and pneumothorax.

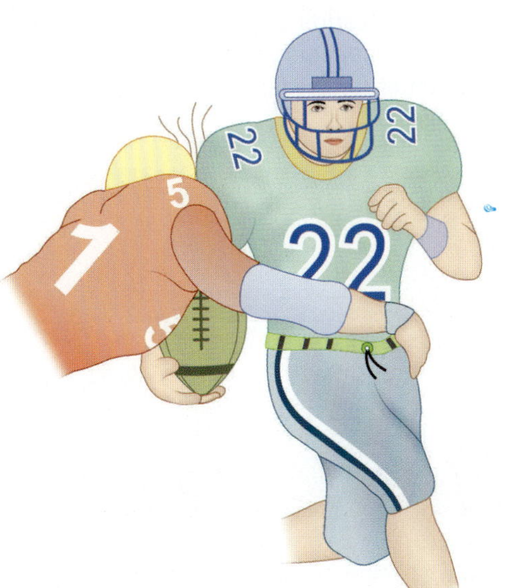

Fig. 133: High contact sports may result in fracture of the proximal humerus.

Diagnosis

The proximal humeral epiphysis is not visible on plain X-rays, until about 6 months of age. On an AP X-ray, a change in the positional relationship between the proximal humeral metaphysis and the scapula and acromion is often visible in proximal humeral fractures. A "vanishing epiphysis sign", as shown in Figure 135 is seen in posteriorly displaced physeal fractures of the proximal humerus.

On an AP X-ray, epiphysis appears to vanish when it is displaced posteriorly. Because some lesser tuberosity fractures may be visible only on axillary lateral view, X-ray of lateral view should be included whenever possible. When adequate X-rays cannot be obtained, CT is useful in evaluating proximal humeral fractures. CT may be especially useful in characterizing posterior fracture dislocations.

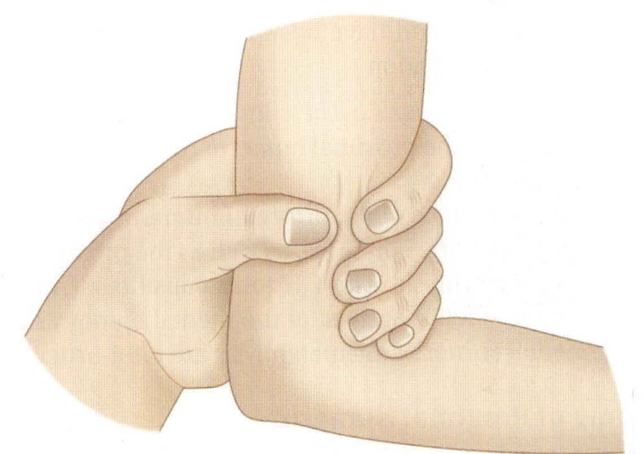

Fig. 134: Twisting at the elbow due to fracture of the proximal humerus.

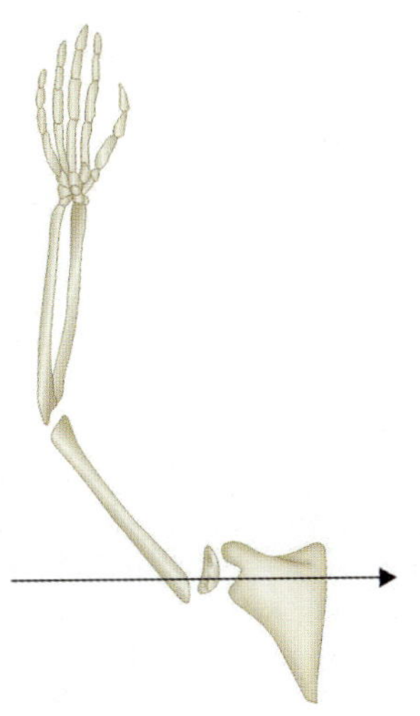

Fig. 135: Vanishing epiphysis sign.

If the child continues to report shoulder pain despite negative radiographic and CT results, an occult fracture must be ruled out. For this purpose, magnetic resonance imaging (MRI) can be diagnostic, due to its ability to identify the intramedullary signal change of edema and the fracture plane. A bone scan may also be useful in equivocal cases. However, due to the normally increased radionuclide uptake at the physis of the proximal humerus, additional uptake due to a fracture may be difficult to interpret.

Classification

Fractures of the proximal humerus in the pediatric population are categorized by their anatomic location. The fractures may involve the physis, the metaphysis, the lesser tuberosity or the greater tuberosity.

Fractures involving the physis are classified according to the Salter-Harris classification (Figs. 136A to D).

Salter-Harris type I injuries: These are associated with fractures through the physis. Occur mostly in patients under 5 years of age.

Salter-Harris type II injuries: These are associated with the fracture line, exiting through the metaphysis and are occasionally associated with an additional anterolateral bony fragment.

Salter-Harris type III injuries: These are associated with the fracture line exiting through the epiphysis. Rarely occur in the proximal humerus of children and have been reported with and without concomitant GH dislocation.

Salter-Harris type IV injuries: These involve both the metaphysis and the epiphysis of the proximal humerus, though have not been reported in children.

The articular surface of the proximal humerus covers most of the medial aspect of the epiphysis, as well as the proximal medial corner of the metaphysis. The GH joint capsule surrounds the articular surface, such that most of the medial epiphysis and the proximal medial corner of the metaphysis are intra-articular.

Anatomy of Proximal Humerus

Anatomy of proximal humerus with prominent demarcation of joint capsule and physis is being shown in Figure 137.

Fractures of the metaphysis occur mostly in children of 5–12 years of age and are categorized by their anatomic location and the degree of displacement. This rather unexpected finding has been attributed to the rapid metaphyseal growth that occurs during this age, which in turn results in a relative structural weakness of the metaphysis. The anatomic location is described in relation to the major deforming forces in the region, namely the insertions of the pectoralis major and the deltoid muscles.

Presence or absence of other fractures in the ipsilateral upper extremity must also be documented, because segmental fractures may require alternative treatments. Other isolated fractures of the proximal humerus may include the greater and the lesser tuberosities.

Physeal Fractures of the Proximal Humerus

Healing displaced fracture of proximal humerus in a 5-year old child is shown in Figure 138.

The degree of displacement in proximal humerus fractures is classified with respect to the shaft diameter of the humerus.

Grade I: There is up to 5 mm of displacement.

Grade II: In this fractures are displaced by up to one-third of humeral shaft diameter.

Grade III: Fractures are displaced by up to two-thirds of the humeral shaft diameter.

Grade IV: Displacement of greater than two-thirds of the shaft diameter is classified as a grade IV injury.

In addition to the degree of displacement, fractures in this region typically demonstrate concomitant angular deformities. Proximal humeral fractures are typically moderate to high energy injuries and are frequently seen in motor vehicle crashes and sporting activities. Approximately 50% of shoulder girdle fractures in children have been reported to be associated with sporting and playing activities.

Athletic activities associated with proximal humeral fractures, include contact sports (football, hockey), horseback riding (fall from horses), gymnastics (upper extremity impact and weight bearing) and baseball (repetitive throwing).

Surgical and Applied Anatomy

The proximal humeral ossification center cannot be seen on plain X-rays until about 6 months of age. In addition to the proximal humerus, both the greater and lesser tuberosities contain their own separate ossification centers. The ossification center for the greater tuberosity appears at around 1–3 years of age, while the ossification center for the lesser tuberosity takes form at around 4–5 years of age.

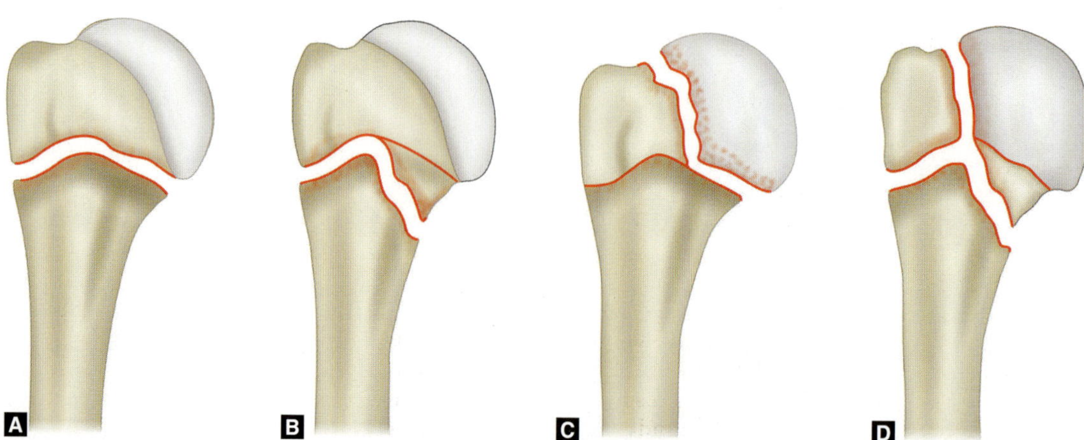

Figs. 136A to D: Salter-Harris classification: (A) Salter-Harris type I; (B) Salter-Harris type II; (C) Salter-Harris type III; (D) Salter-Harris type IV.

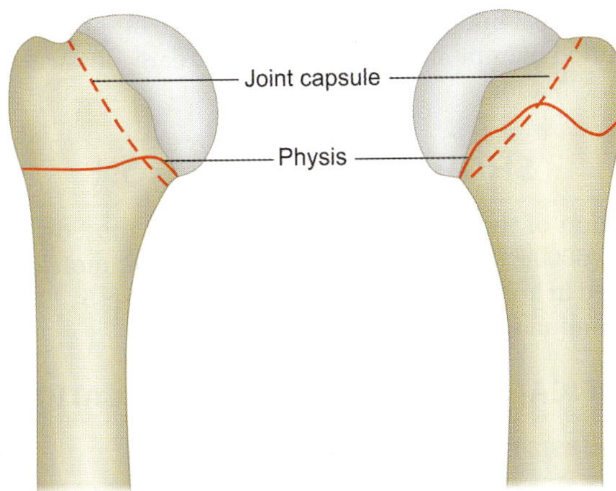

Fig. 137: Anatomy of proximal humerus.

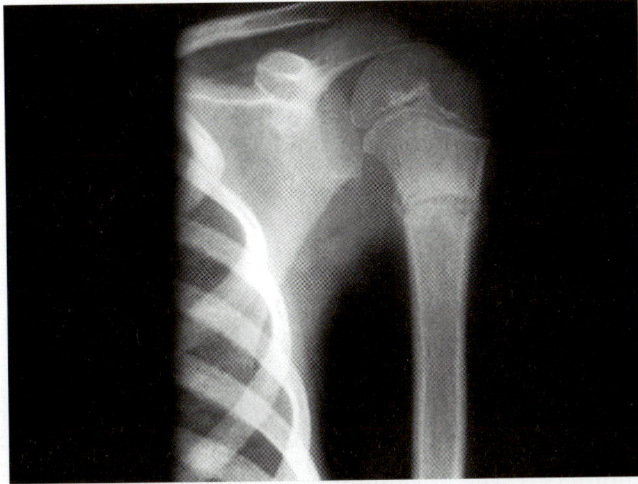

Fig. 138: Healing displaced fracture of the proximal humerus in a five-year-old child.

The two tuberosities typically coalesce between 5 years and 7 years of age and subsequently fuse with the humeral head at around 7–13 years of age. The proximal physis of the humerus continues to be active well into the teenage years and is ultimately responsible for approximately 80% of the overall humeral growth. Interestingly, longitudinal growth at the proximal humeral physis changes during development, such that it is responsible for only 75% of humeral growth before the age of two, but up to 90% of growth after the age of 11.

For girls, this growth continues until around 14 years of age, with subsequent fusion of the epiphysis with the shaft at 14–17 years of age. For boys, growth continues until about age of 16 years, after which closure of the physis begins. For most boys, the proximal humeral physis is closed by about 18 years of age. The extracapsular location of the proximal humeral physis makes this structure susceptible to injury.

Physeal fractures are thought to occur through the zone of hypertrophy and provisional calcification, while relatively sparing the cells in the resting and proliferative zones. Salter-Harris type I or II fractures in children have high remodeling potential and rarely result in growth arrest. Sling and swathe for immobilization of proximal humerus fractures.

Treatment

Current Treatment Options

As there is tremendous potential for healing and remodeling, fractures of the proximal humerus in children infrequently require operative reduction and fixation. This is especially true for obstetric proximal humeral fractures in infants. If needed, these fractures are amenable to gentle reduction with minimal anesthesia or sedation.

Proximal humeral fractures in this age group heal quite rapidly, typically within 2–3 weeks and result in no residual functional or cosmetic deficits. Nondisplaced or minimally displaced proximal humeral fractures (Neer's grades I and II) in older children and adolescents should also be treated nonoperatively. Initial management of these fractures involves sling and swathe immobilization followed by protected motion. Overall, nonoperative treatment provides excellent long-term results.

The remodeling potential of the fracture in young children is significant, but decreases with the increasing age of the child. Hence, the degree of acceptable displacement and angulation also changes with the age of the child. Generally, relative greater displacement and angulation can be accepted in younger children. For fractures in children under the age of 11, good to excellent long-term outcomes have been reported regardless of the fracture displacement. Various types of shoulder immobilization to maintain reduction have been advocated and include sling and swathe, thoracobrachial bandage (Velpeau), hanging arm cast, shoulder spica cast, salute position shoulder spica cast and Statue of Liberty cast.

Grossly displaced or angulated proximal humeral fractures (Neer's grades III and IV) in children over the age of 11 years are managed with fracture reduction and sometimes with specialized immobilization. Multiple maneuvers exist for the reduction of pediatric proximal humeral fractures. Most fractures can be reduced by applying longitudinal traction to the arm, while positioning it in abduction, flexion and external rotation.

If this maneuver does not sufficiently reduce the fracture, better reduction can be obtained by moderate abduction, flexion to 90° and external rotation. Alternatively, the fracture can be reduced by direct manual manipulation of the fragments, while the arm is placed in marked abduction of about 135°, slight flexion of about 30° and longitudinal traction. Some fractures cannot be adequately reduced because of a barrier at the fracture site. Anatomic structures that can prevent reduction of proximal humeral fractures, include the periosteum, the shoulder joint capsule and the biceps tendon. In these situations, open reduction through a small deltopectoral incision is needed to remove the obstacles to reduction. Proximal humeral fractures that have significant displacement (Neer's grades III and IV) and angulation in patients over 11 years of age are the fractures that typically undergo reduction to improve fracture alignment. General anesthesia is typically necessary for patient comfort and for adequate muscle relaxation due to the difficulties that can be encountered in obtaining and maintaining an acceptable reduction.

Reduction is performed with longitudinal traction on the injured limb, while the arm is placed in abduction, external rotation and flexion, to align the distal fragment with the epiphysis. Increasing the abduction up to 90° and flexion up to 90° of the distal fragment, may be necessary to reduce the fracture. For fractures requiring operative reduction, percutaneous Kirschner wire stabilization is routinely used. The starting point for percutaneously placed implants is at the lateral cortex of the distal fragment, near the insertion of the deltoid muscle and aimed obliquely into the humeral epiphysis. At least two pins of 0.062 or 0.078 inches and preferentially three pins are used and typically allow adequate stabilization. The Kirschner wires may be cut beneath the level of the skin or may be left through the skin and protected with Jergen's balls. The arm is placed into a shoulder immobilizer, with the arm at the patient's side, while the patient is under general anesthesia. The implants can usually be removed as early as 4 weeks after surgery after documenting healing on X-ray.

Complications

In children with multiple traumas, the diagnosis can be delayed due to the need to focus on more life or limb-threatening problems and the absence of any dramatic limb malalignment. Even after the diagnosis of proximal humeral fracture is made, full evaluation and characterization of the fracture pattern can remain incomplete because of inadequate radiographic studies. A high index of suspicion, thorough physical examination and insistence on high quality X-rays must be present to ensure prompt diagnosis and treatment of proximal humeral fractures. Neurologic injury to the brachial plexus can result from fractures and fractured dislocations of the proximal humerus.

Most nerve deficits can be diagnosed immediately because the clinical signs are readily apparent. Rarely, however, nerve deficits from proximal humeral fractures can evolve slowly and delay the diagnosis. Typically, these nerve deficits are transient and full function typically returns in less than 6 months. If the neurologic deficit persists longer than 3 months, further evaluation with electromyography is warranted. If no evidence of nerve recovery or regeneration is present, nerve exploration, repair and grafting can be considered. Salvage operations for permanent nerve deficits include proximal humeral osteotomy and muscle or tendon transfers.

Fractures of the proximal humerus in children can also be associated with other injuries, including rib fractures and pneumothorax. In adults, these fractures have been associated with disruptions and thrombosis of the axillary vessels as well. Operative fixation of proximal humeral fractures with pins and wires has been associated with hardware migration, which can be fatal. Therefore, serial radiographic monitoring of the hardware after shoulder operations is essential.

Late Complications

Humerus varus after trauma is a rare complication that typically affects neonates and children under 5 years of age. Children with humerus varus have a significant decrease in the humeral neck shaft angle and shortening of the upper extremity. Although shoulder abduction may be moderately limited, most children with humerus varus have only mild functional deficits and do not require surgical correction of the deformity. If, however, active abduction and flexion are severely limited, corrective osteotomy of the proximal humerus can produce good results.

Osteonecrosis of the humeral head after proximal humeral fractures occurs frequently in adults, but is rare in children. Even after acute disruption of the vascular supply to the proximal humeral epiphysis, subsequent remodeling and revascularization usually occur in children and that lead to excellent clinical results. Similarly, GH subluxation after proximal humeral fractures is a rare complication in the pediatric population that typically results in good clinical outcomes. These children are best treated with a short period of immobilization followed by early physical therapy and rehabilitation.

SHOULDER DISLOCATION

Dislocation of the shoulder was described in the Edwin Smith Papyrus (3000 BC). Shoulder joint is the most common joint to be dislocated in human body. Males to females ratio is 5 : 1 and is the most common in 20–30 years of age group.

CLASSIFICATIONS OF SHOULDER DISLOCATION

On the Basis of Duration

- Acute
- Chronic.

On the Basis of Occurrence

- Single
- Recurrent.

On the Basis of Mechanism

- Traumatic
- Atraumatic.

On the Basis of Direction

- Anterior
- Posterior
- Inferior (subluxation erecta)
- Transthoracic.

ANTERIOR DISLOCATION (FIG. 139)

About 95% cases of shoulder dislocation are the anterior dislocations. Depending on the location, it can be classified as:

- Preglenoid
- Subcoracoid
- Subclavicular.

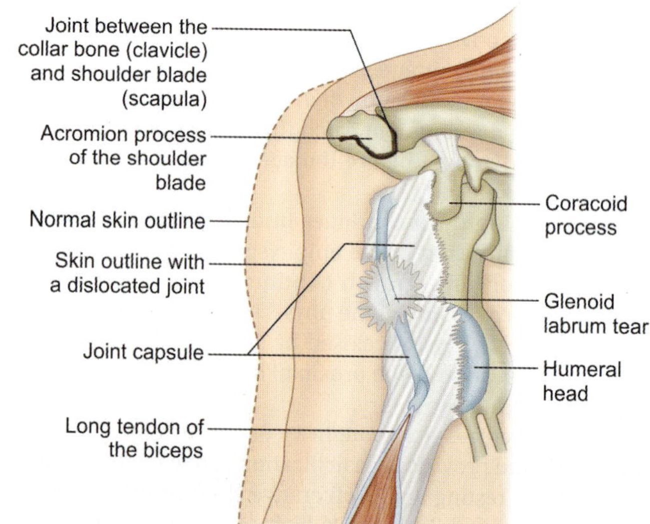

Fig. 139: Structures affected and joint position after anterior shoulder dislocation.

When the anterior capsule is torn or avulsed from the bone, the joint is dislocated. Head of humerus lies in front of glenoid fossa of scapula below the clavicle and coracoid process of the scapula. Mechanism of injury is abduction and lateral rotation or extended arm. Shoulder injury associated with fall on an outstretched hand. It may be direct, when there is a blow from behind to the shoulder. Glenoid labrum and adjoining periosteum are stripped from the front of the neck of scapula. Anterior capsule is ruptured. Anterior capsule is torn with a fragment of bone from the lesser tuberosity, as illustrated in Figures 140A to D.

Clinical Features

- Joint loses its round outline or normal contour (as the head of humerus does not occupy normal position and is displaced forward and medially).
- *Position of the arm (Fig. 141):* Patient holds the injured limb with other hand close to the trunk. The shoulder is abducted and the elbow is kept flexed.
- Loss of the contour of the shoulder may appear as a step this can be seen in Figures 142 and 143.
- Anterior bulge of the head of humerus may be visible or palpable.
- A gap can be palpated above the dislocated head of the humerus (Fig. 144).

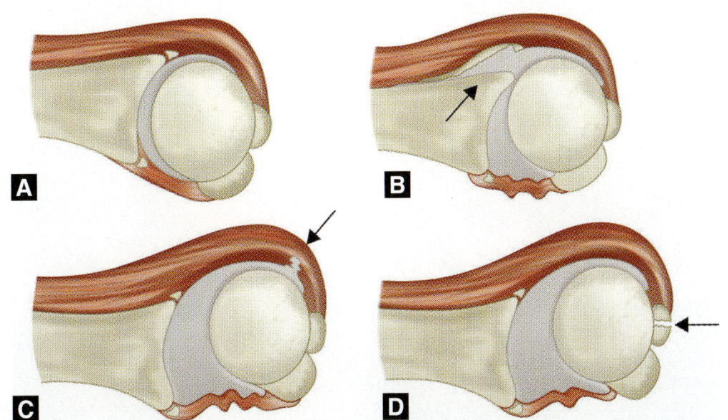

Figs. 140A to D: Structures affected due to anterior shoulder dislocation: (A) Normal; (B) Glenoid labrum and adjoining periosteum are stripped from the front of the neck of scapula; (C) Anterior capsule is ruptured; (D) Anterior capsule is torn with a fragment of bone from the lesser tuberosity.

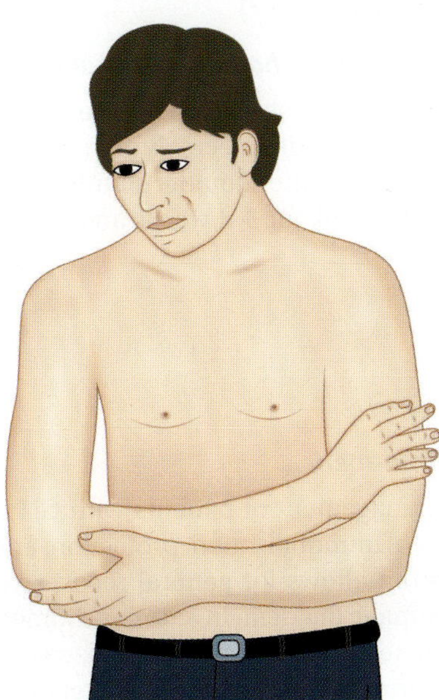

Fig. 141: A typical position of arm, held by the patient after anterior shoulder dislocation.

Special Tests

Hamilton Ruler Test

See Figure and text on page No. 500.

Duga's Test

See Figure and text on page No. 500.

Bryant's Sign

See text on page No. 500.

Callaway's Test

See text on page No. 500.

Apprehension Test

See Figure and text on page No. 501.

Relocation Test

See Figure and text on page No. 501.

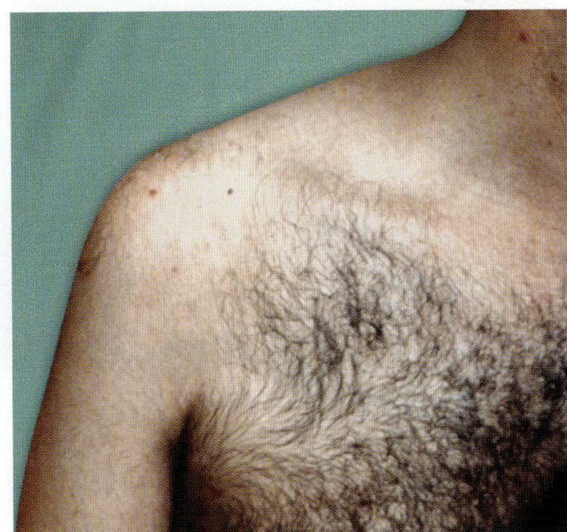

Fig. 142: Loss of the contour of the shoulder may appear as a step.

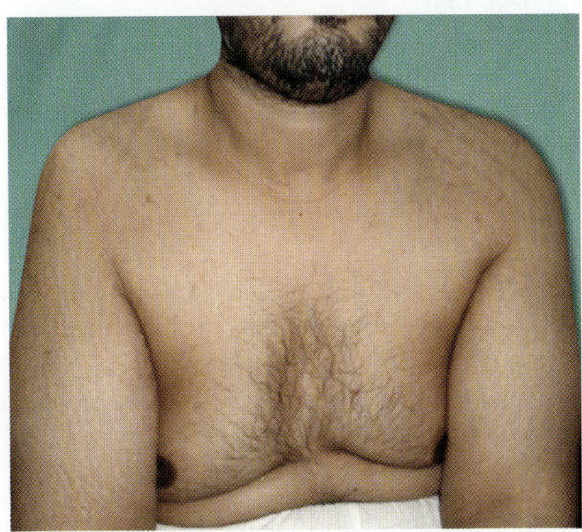

Fig. 143: Anterior bulge of the head of humerus is visible.

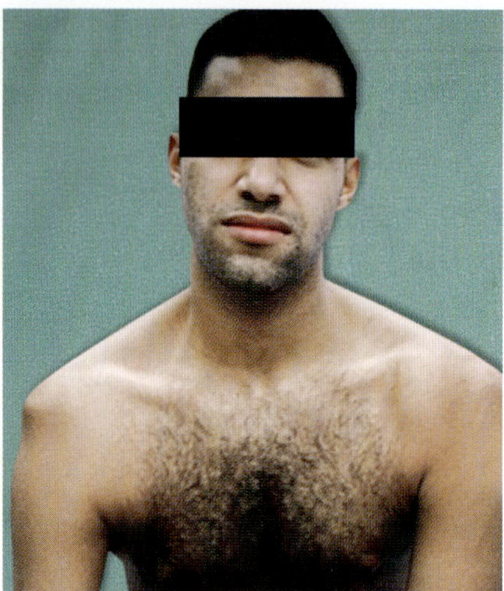

Fig. 144: Prominent acromion process and palpable gap above the dislocated head.

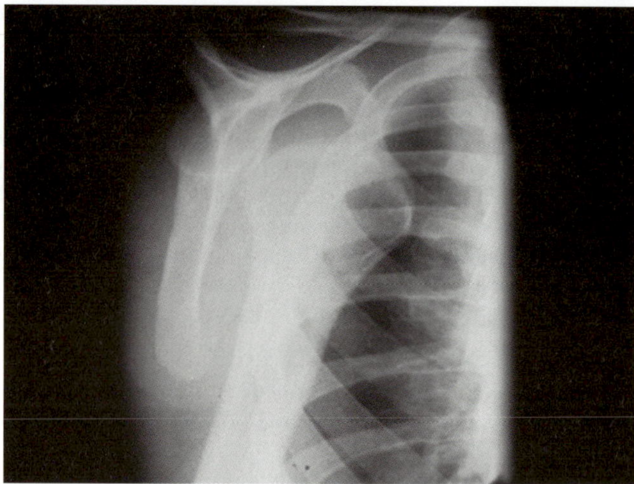

Fig. 146: X-ray shows anterior shoulder dislocation (lateral view).

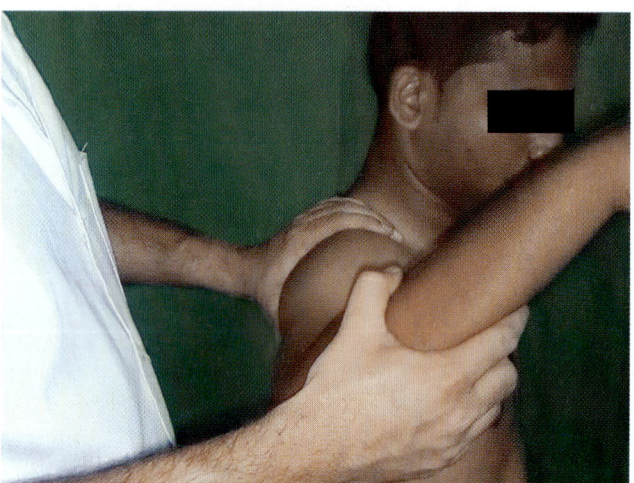

Fig. 145: Crank test.

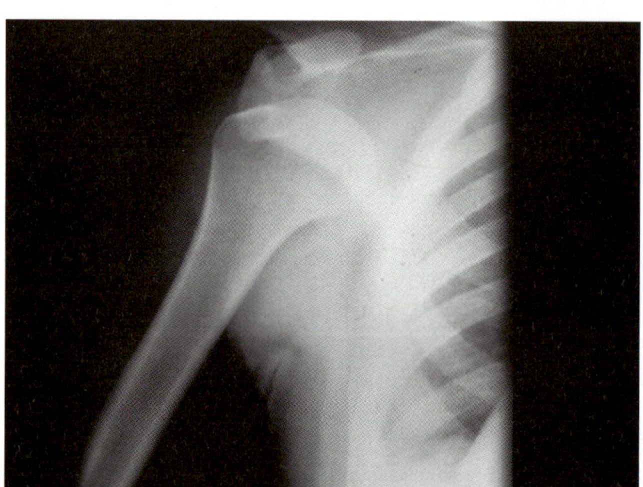

Fig. 147: X-ray shows anterior shoulder dislocation (AP view).

Drawer Test of Gerber and Ganz (Anterior Glenohumeral Instability)

See Figure and text on page No. 501.

Crank Test (Fig. 145)

The shoulder is abducted and externally rotated, such that it is in a position vulnerable to dislocation. With an anteriorly directed force on the posterior humeral head, the instability is accentuated to cause the sensation of apprehension.

Examination for Nerve and Vascular Injuries (Before and Postreduction)

Lesion of inner cord of plexus: It includes paralysis of small muscles of hand with loss of sensation of the medial side of hand and forearm.

Lesion of posterior cord of plexus: It includes paralysis of extensors of forearm with wrist drop.

Lesion of outer cord of plexus: It is difficult to recognize.

Vascular injury: Examine limb for injury to axillary vessels, which may be compressed or even ruptured.

X-rays (Figs. 146 and 147)

Management of Anterior Shoulder Dislocation

- It is an emergency and should be reduced in less than 24 hours or there may be avascular necrosis of the head of humerus.
- Following reduction, the shoulder should be immobilized and strapped to the trunk for 3–4 weeks and rested in a collar and cuff.

Treatment

- Nonoperative
- Operative.

Nonoperative Treatment

Nonoperative management of patients with GH instability relies on the principles of immobilization, protection, and rehabilitation.

- Immobilization allows for general recovery of the shoulder from the traumatic incident. In addition, immobilization allows for the initial healing of the static stabilizers.
- The second principle of nonoperative treatment is protection. A brief period of immobilization is designed to protect the shoulder from additional episodes of instability.

- The third principle of nonoperative treatment is rehabilitation. The activity level of the patient must be modified to allow for the healing of the static stabilizers. Activity patterns are altered, so that the shoulder is not placed in positions vulnerable to dislocation. Typically, this is accomplished by limiting the range of shoulder motion as well as refraining from participating in any high-risk activities.

Kocher's Manipulation (Figs. 148A to D) (Elaborated for Right-sided Dislocation)

Patient lies in supine position. The surgeon holds the patients elbow with his right hand and wrist with his left hand, gentle traction is applied to humerus in the line in which it is lying, while traction is maintained humerus is externally rotated, adducted, and medially rotated.

Hippocrates Method (Figs. 149A and B)

Use inferior traction on the arm against the counter traction provided by the foot on the thorax, as shown in Figure 149A. Do not place the foot in the axilla, as this could cause damage to the underlying neurovascular structures. A modification of this technique uses a hand-held sheet around the thorax to provide countertraction (Fig. 149B).

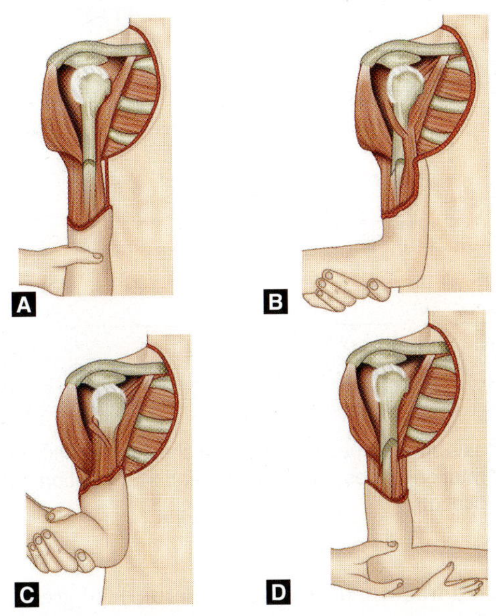

Figs. 148A to D: Kocher's manipulation, elaborated for right-sided dislocation.

Stimson Technique (Fig. 150)

It is used for closed shoulder reduction. With the patient in prone position, weight is hung from the wrist to distract the shoulder joint. Eventually, with sufficient fatigue in the shoulder musculature, the joint can be easily reduced.

Milch Technique

Another commonly used reduction maneuver is the Milch technique. Unlike some of the other maneuvers, this technique relies on shoulder position rather than distraction. The maneuver can be performed with the patient in either supine or prone position.

Upon administration of analgesia and moderate traction, the arm is abducted and externally rotated. The dislocated humeral head is then manually manipulated back into the joint. Various authors have reported that this method is associated with a high rate of success and minimal complications.

New Method

The surgeon stands behind the seated patient and inserts his flexed forearm into the axilla of the affected shoulder. His freehand applies traction on the flexed forearm of the patient. The surgeon's forearm pulls in a proximal and lateral direction and levers the head of the humerus into the socket.

The method is relatively atraumatic, provides more direct control of the limb and applies more effective forces than the Kocher, Stimson or Hippocratic maneuvers. After a successful closed reduction that is confirmed by X-rays, the arm should be immobilized for a period of time. Although most surgeons agree that a brief period of immobilization is required for patient's comfort and protection, the exact protocol for immobilization is still controversial.

Ancient Techniques of Reduction

Some of the ancient techniques for shoulder reduction are shown in Figures 151A and B.

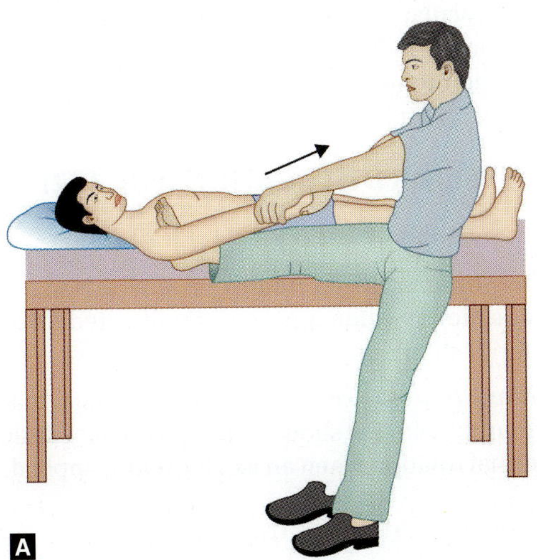

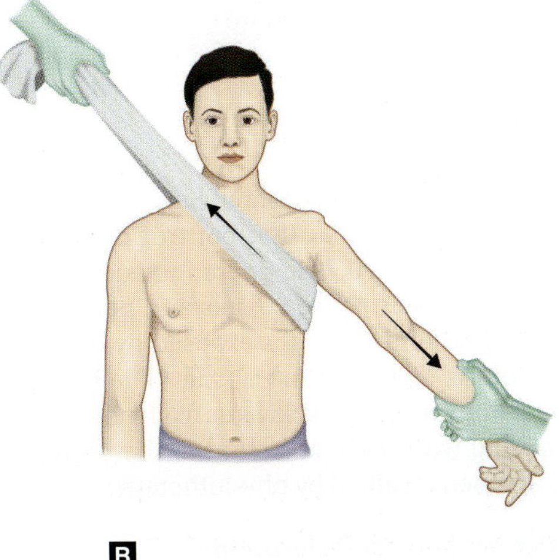

Figs. 149A and B: (A) Hippocrates method, inferior traction on the arm against the counter traction provided by the foot on the thorax; (B) Modified, hand held sheet around the thorax to provide countertraction.

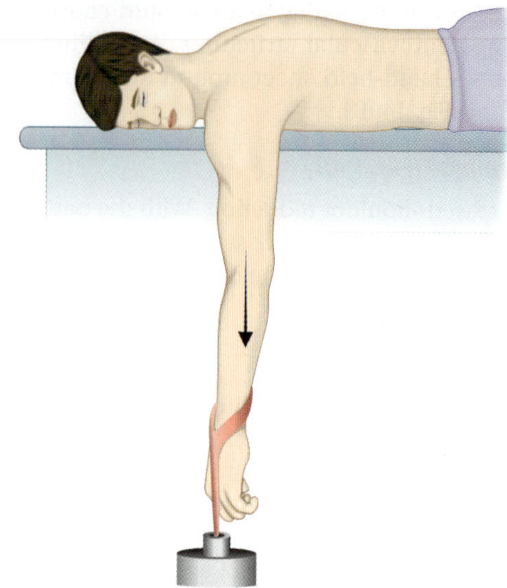

Fig. 150: The Stimson technique for closed shoulder reduction using weight hung from wrist to distract shoulder joint.

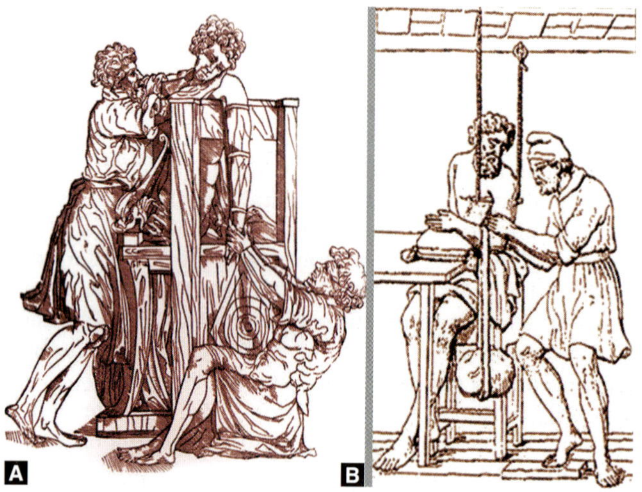

Figs. 151A and B: Ancient techniques of shoulder reduction for anterior dislocation.

Operative Procedure

Indications:
- Failed appropriate nonoperative procedure
- Recurrent dislocation at young age
- Irreducible dislocation
- Open dislocation
- Unstable reduction
- Late unreduced anterior dislocation of shoulder.

The incision must be planned so that control of vessels proximal to clavicle may be secured. The operation is designed as an exposure of axillary vessels. Once vessels and nerves are exposed and retracted, head of humerus is exposed by dividing the tightened subscapularis and anterior capsule. The head of humerus is then guided outwards and backwards to glenoid fossa. After protection in a sling with the arm bound to the body for 3 weeks, movements are then regained by physiotherapy.

Complications of Anterior Shoulder Dislocation

Early complications:
- Neurovascular injury (rare).
- Axillary nerve injury, leads to paralysis of deltoid.

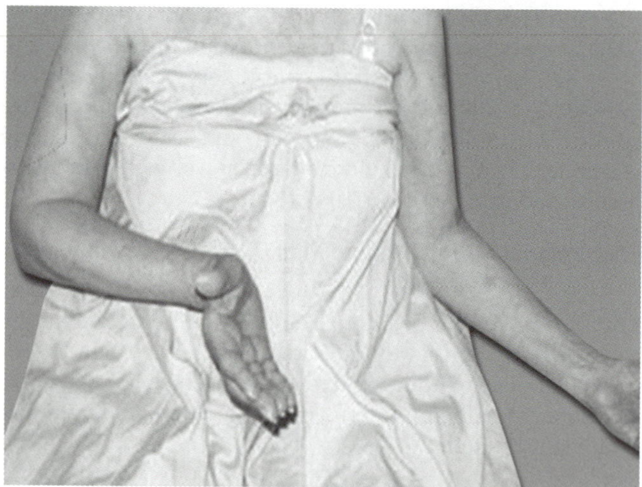

Fig. 152: Posterior dislocation of shoulder.

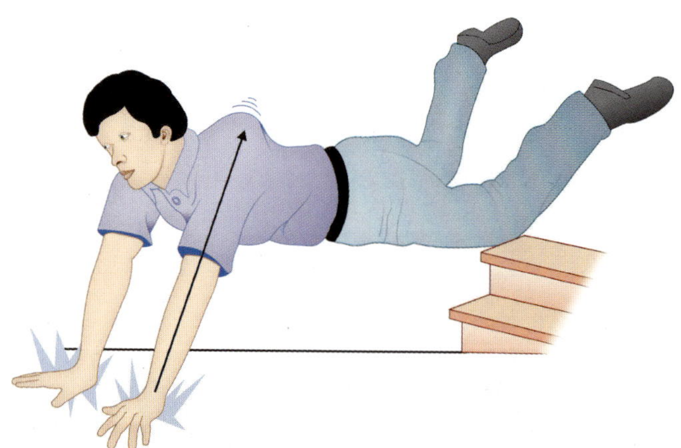

Fig. 153: An axial load to the arm, when the shoulder is in flexion, adduction and internal rotation places the humeral head in a position susceptible to posterior dislocation.

- Associated fracture of neck of humerus or of greater or lesser tuberosities.

Late complications:
- Avascular necrosis of the head of the humerus (high-risk with delayed reduction).
- Heterotopic calcification (used to be called myositis ossificans).
- Recurrent dislocations.

POSTERIOR DISLOCATION (FIG. 152)

Mechanism of Injury

Direct trauma: Direct trauma which leads to a posterior shoulder dislocation is when a posteriorly directed force is applied to the anterior shoulder.

Indirect trauma (Fig. 153): It includes axial loading to the upper extremity, with the shoulder in a position of flexion, adduction and internal rotation when an axially load is applied.

Common Causes of Injury

- *Seizures and electrocution:* These causes produce a violent muscular contraction, during which the internal rotators overwhelm the external rotators.

- *Posterior shoulder dislocations can also be associated with*:
  - Lesser tuberosity fractures of the humerus
  - Glenoid rim fractures
  - Humeral head and shaft fractures
  - Recurrent instability
  - Rarely, neurovascular injury.

Jerk Test

With the patient in either sitting (Fig. 154A) or supine (Fig. 154B) position, the arm is abducted and internally rotated. An axial load is then placed on the humerus while the arm is moved horizontally across the body. With a positive test, patients demonstrate a sudden jerk, when the humeral head slides off, of the back of the glenoid and when it is reduced back onto the glenoid. Positioning of the patient for the Velpeau axillary lateral view X-ray is shown in Figure 155.

INFERIOR DISLOCATION (FIGS. 156A TO C)

Inferior dislocations (also known as luxatio erecta) typically result from a hyperabduction force that levers the humeral head out inferiorly, as the humeral neck impinges on the acromion. Inferior shoulder dislocations can be associated with:

- Rotator cuff tears
- Proximal humerus fractures
- Neurovascular injuries
- Compressive neuropathy
- Thrombosis of the axillary artery.

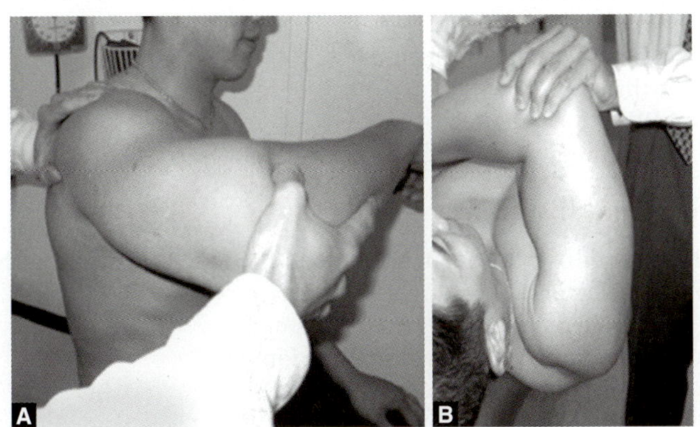

Figs. 154A and B: Jerk test for posterior dislocation of shoulder: Patient tested in sitting; (B) Supine position.

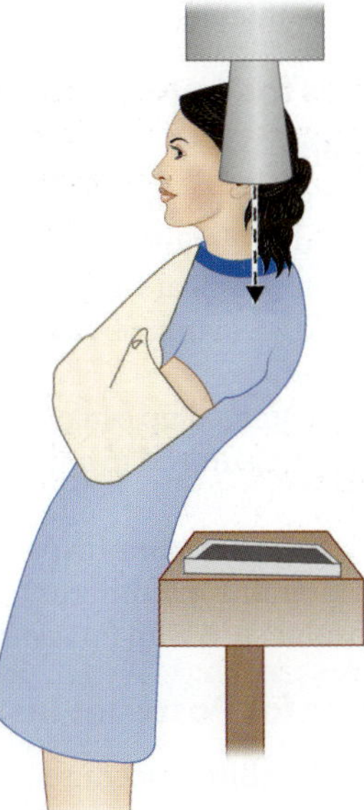

Fig. 155: Positioning of the patient for the Velpeau axillary lateral view X-ray.

Sulcus Test

The sulcus test for inferior instability of the shoulder is demonstrated in Figures 157A and B. By performing this test with the arm in external rotation, the maneuver can also be used to test the integrity of the rotator interval structures.

Possible Complications of Shoulder Dislocations

Bankart's lesion (Fig. 158): It is a permanent anterior defect of labrum.

Hill-Sachs lesion (Fig. 159): These are caused by compression of the cancellous bone against anterior glenoid rim, creating a divot in the humeral head.

X-rays (Figs. 160 to 162)

Anteroposterior View

This is a technique for obtaining anteroposterior (AP) (upper panel) and true AP (lower panel), X-rays of the shoulder. In an AP

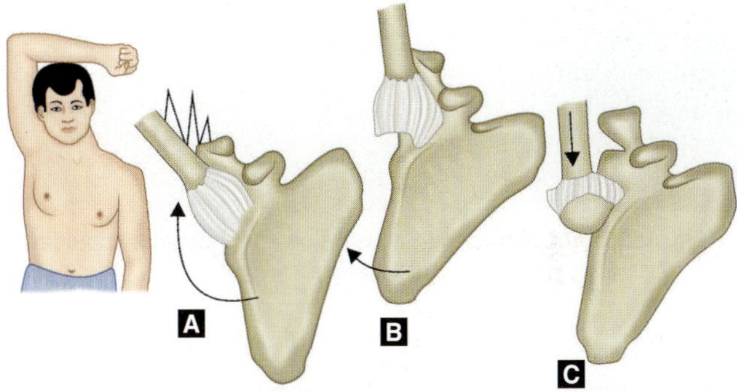

Figs. 156A to C: Locked inferior dislocation of the glenohumeral joint or luxatio erecta: (A) With hyperabduction of the arm, the lateral acromion acts as a lever against the proximal humerus to dislocate the shoulder inferiorly; (B) After dislocation; (C) The humeral head is locked inferior to the glenoid rim.

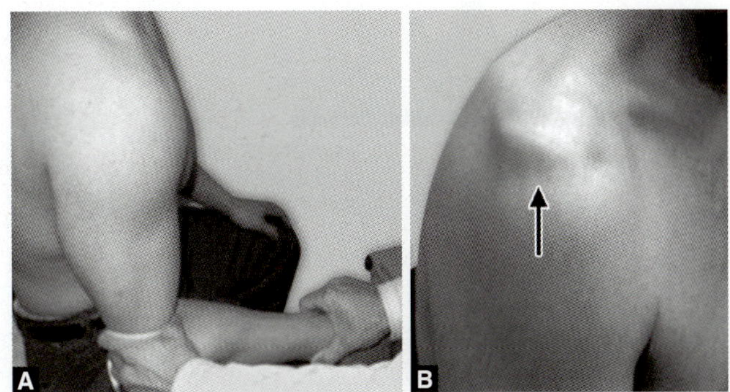

Figs. 157A and B: Sulcus test for inferior instability—(A) With the patient in the sitting position, a downward traction is placed on the adducted arm; (B) With a positive test, excessive inferior translation produces a dimple (arrow) on the lateral aspect of the acromion.

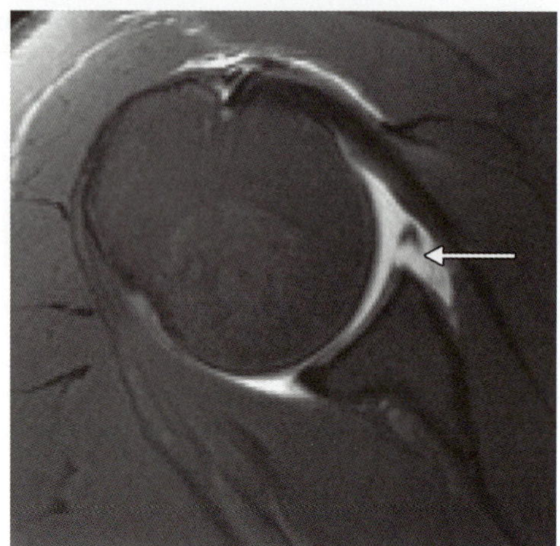

Fig. 158: Bankart's lesions in posterior dislocation of shoulder.

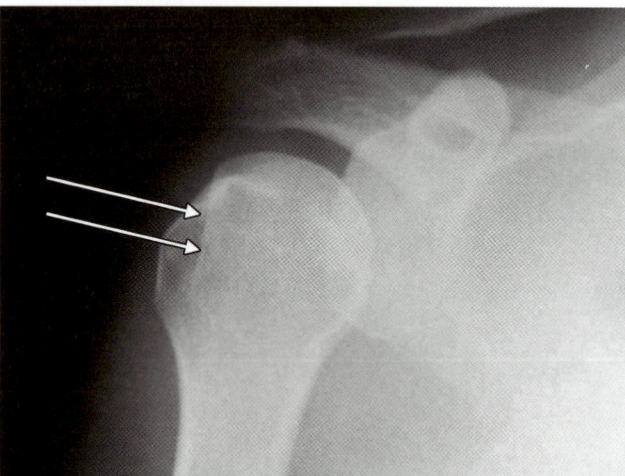

Fig. 159: X-ray shows Hill-Sachs lesion after posterior shoulder dislocation.

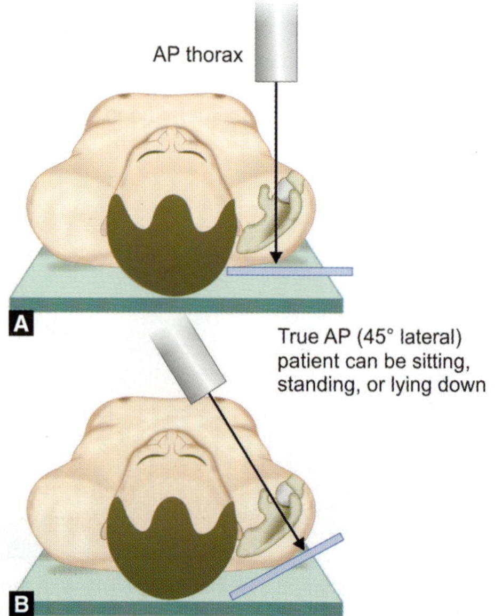

Figs. 160A and B: Positions for taking X-ray in posterior shoulder dislocation: (A) Anteroposterior (AP) view; (B) True AP view.

view, the X-ray actually represents an oblique view of the shoulder joint. In a true AP view, the X-ray beam is parallel to the joint so that there is minimal overlap between the humeral head and the glenoid surface.

Apical Oblique View

Radiographic technique for apical oblique view of shoulder has been demonstrated in Figures 163A and B. With patient seated and injured shoulder adjacent to vertical cassette, chest is rotated to 45° in oblique position. Beam is directed 45° caudally, passing longitudinally through scapula, which rests at 45° angle on thorax, while extremity is adducted.

West Point View

Radiographic technique for west point view of shoulder to show glenoid labrum lesions is shown in Figure 164. With patient prone and pillow beneath shoulder, cassette is placed superior to shoulder. 90° abduction at shoulder and cassette at 25° medial and 25° cephalad, to see anterior and posterior glenoid.

Stryker Notch View (Fig. 165)

Patient lies in supine position. Overhead abduction, with hand over forehead. Cassette is below the shoulder. This is done to see inferior glenoid.

Other investigations include:

- Arthrogram
- MRI
- Ultrasound.

Recurrent Instability

The procedure for recurrent instability should include the following factors:

- It should have a low recurrence rate.
- Accompanied with low complication rate.
- There should be low reoperation rate.
- It does not harm (arthritis).
- It helps and maintains motion.
- It should be applicable in most of the cases.
- It allows observation of the joint.
- It should correct the pathological condition.
- It should not be too difficult.

Surgical Procedures for Anterior Instability

- Bankart's operation
- Modified Bankart's repair (Montgomery and Jobe, where capsule is reattached to glenoid rim)
- Putti-Platt operation (vertical incision on subscapularis and capsule, with double breasting of subscapularis)
- Burkhart and De Beer
- Bristow procedure (coracoid tip osteotomized at base and fixed to glenoid, coracoid tip sutured to anterior portion of scapular neck)
- Magnuson and Stack operation (capsule and subscapularis muscle, attached laterally on humerus)
- O'Brien et al (capsular shift with incision adjacent to glenoid).

Surgical Procedures for Posterior Instability

- Neer inferior capsular shift procedure
- Rockwood (capsular shift reconstruction with posterior glenoid osteotomy)

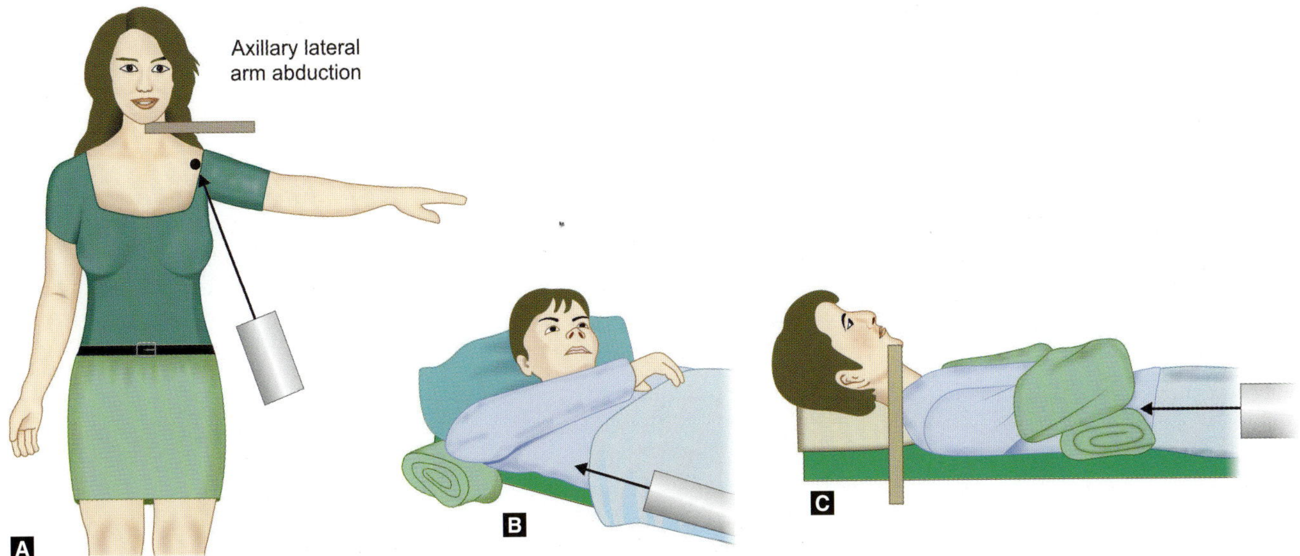

Figs. 161A to C: Techniques for obtaining axillary view X-rays: (A) Lateral view; (B and C) X-ray axillary lateral, in case of trauma.

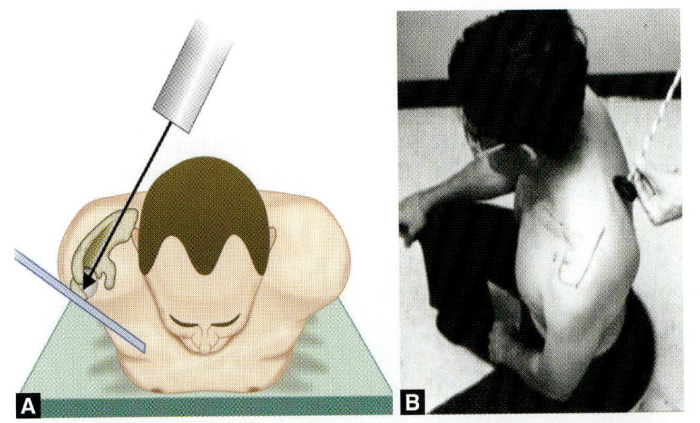

Figs. 162A and B: Technique for obtaining a scapula lateral, known as the Y-view X-ray: (A) With the cassette placed on the lateral aspect of the shoulder; (B) The X-ray beam is directed parallel to the plane of the scapula.

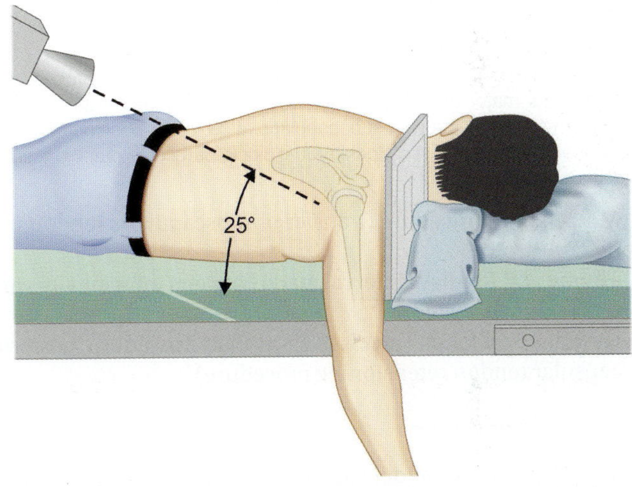

Fig. 164: Radiographic technique and positioning for west point view of shoulder, to show glenoid labrum lesions.

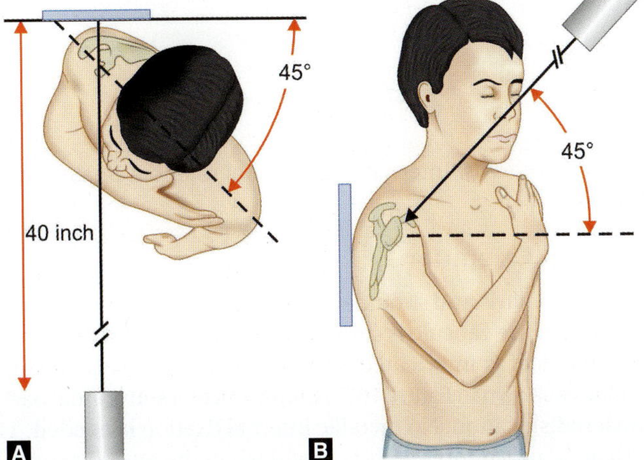

Figs. 163A and B: Radiographic technique for apical oblique view of shoulder: (A) A view from above; (B) A view from side.

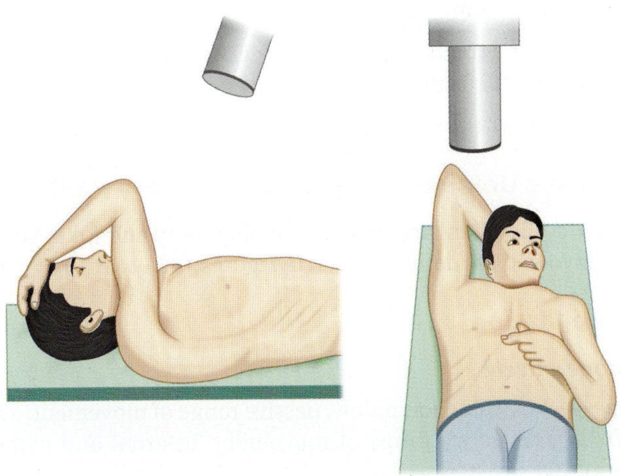

Fig. 165: Stryker notch view to see inferior glenoid.

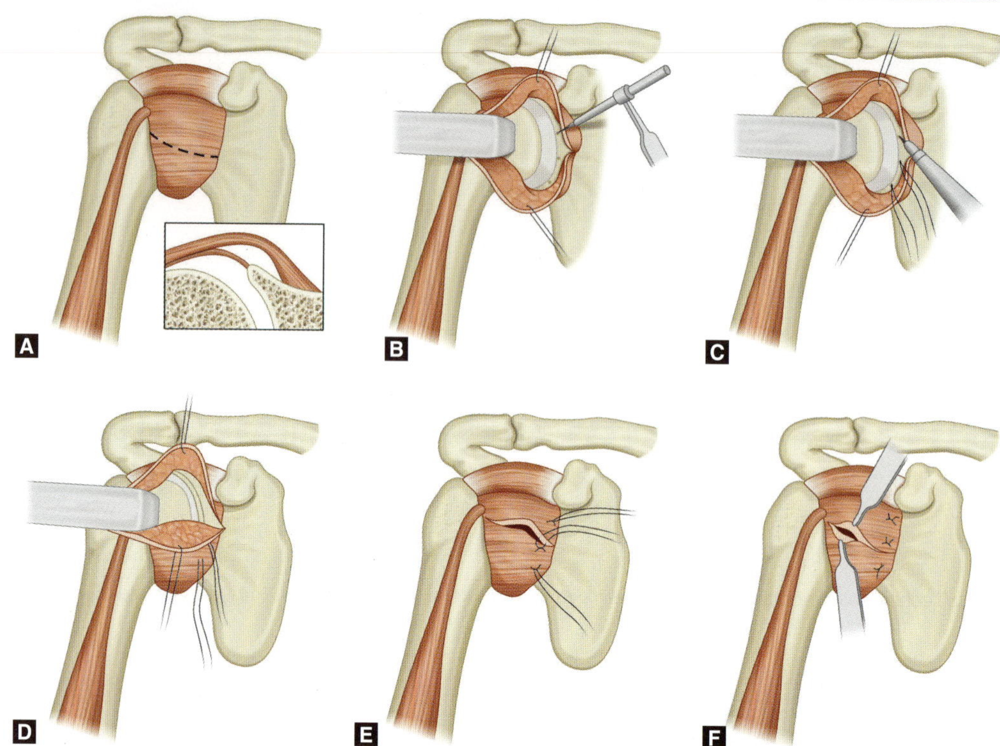

Figs. 166A to F: (A) Incision 2 cm distal and lateral to coracoid process and inferior to anterior axillary crease; (B) Retract deltoid and cephalic vein laterally, and pectoralis major muscle medially; (C) Subscapularis tendon is split at the junction of upper two-third and lower one-third; (D) Horizontal anterior capsulotomy done in line with subscapularis at 3 o'clock position of glenoid; (E) Stay sutures are taken; (F) Retract the humeral head laterally. Drill holes near glenoid at 3 o'clock, 4 o'clock, 5:30 o'clock, parallel to glenoidal surface. Maintain shoulder in 90º abduction and 60º of external rotation and shift the capsule superiorly.

- McLaughlin procedure (transfer of subscapularis tendon into defect)
- Tibone and Bradley (interval made between infraspinatus and teres minor)
- Hawkins and Janda (reversed Putti-Platt procedure, posterior capsular tendon retensioning procedure).

Bankart's Operation

Subscapularis and shoulder capsule are vertically opened. Lateral leaf of capsule reattached to glenoid rim. Medial leaf of capsule is imbricated and subscapularis is approximated.

Indication: When labrum and capsule are separated from glenoid rim/capsule is thin.

Advantage: Corrects the labral defect and imbricates capsule without internal fixation.

Disadvantage: Technical difficulty.

Traumatic Unidirectional Bankart Surgery (TUBS)

It is a modified Bankart repair, by Montgomery and Jobe. Various steps involved are demonstrated in Figures 166A to F.

Rehabilitation

Postoperatively

Three weeks: Abduction pillow, passive range of movement. *Three to six weeks:* Active range of movement, internal and external rotation.

Six weeks to three months: Active range of movement, shoulder flexion and adduction exercises.

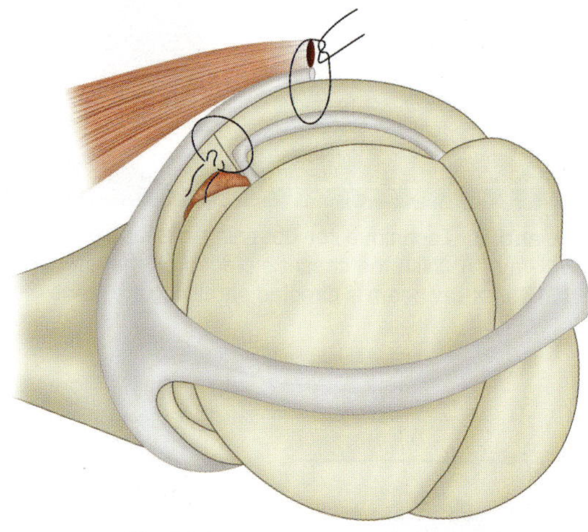

Fig. 167: Putti-Platt operation.

Three to six months: Internal and external rotation, push-ups and chin-ups.

Putti-Platt Operation

The subscapularis and shoulder capsule are incised vertically. The lateral leaf of the capsule is sutured to the capsule and the labrum, the medial leaf is imbricated and the subscapularis is advanced laterally, as shown in Figure 167. This produces a substantial barrier against redislocation. No metallic internal fixation is needed. This imbricating procedure rarely is useful when the anterior capsular mechanism is of poor quality or if a large posterior humeral head defect requires, that the surgical procedure used restricts external rotation.

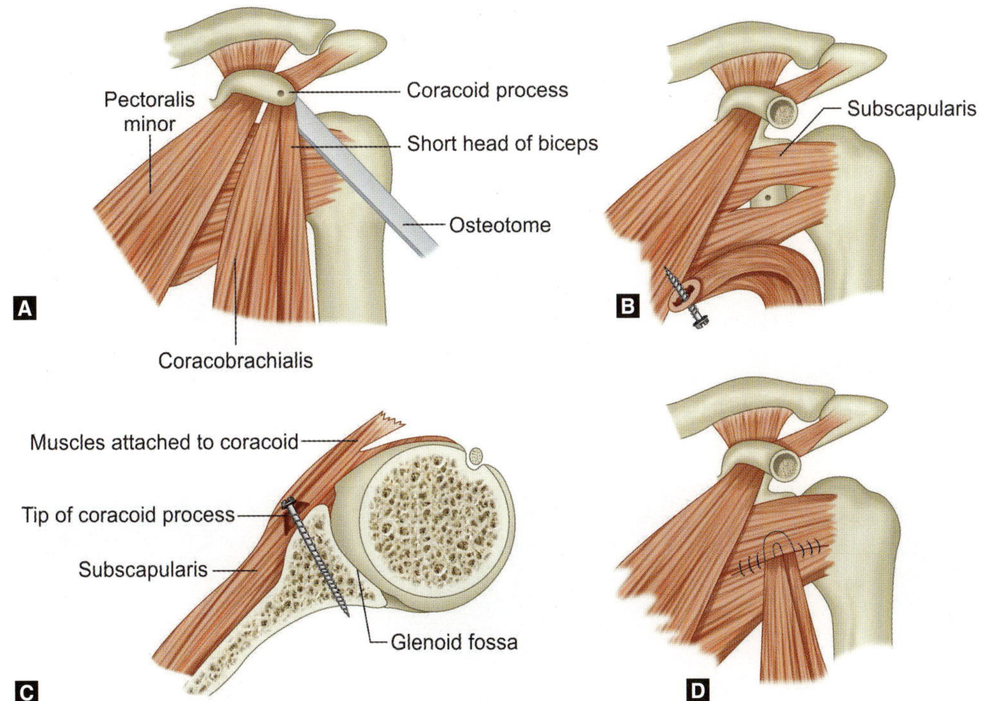

Figs. 168A to D: Bristow procedure: (A) Detachment of tip of coracoid process; (B) Method of attachment of tip of coracoid to neck of scapula anteriorly; (C) Cross-section through scapula at level of glenoid and humeral head; (D) Bristow procedure completed.

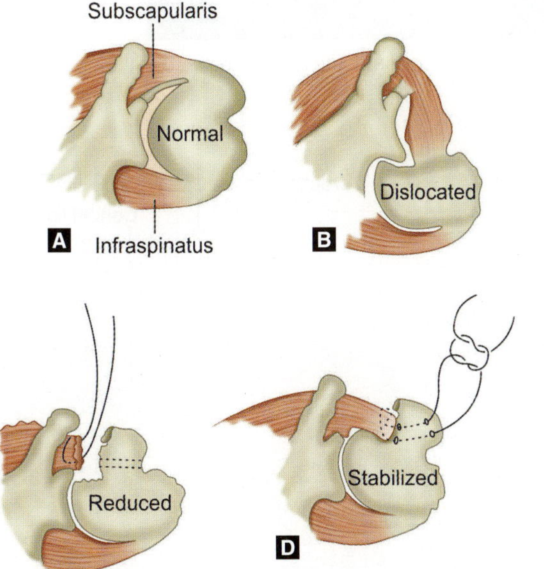

Figs. 169A to D: McLaughlin technique for posterior shoulder dislocation—(A) Normal shoulder; (B) Shoulder dislocated posteriorly; (C) Reduction of dislocated shoulder; (D) Shoulder stabilized after reduction.

Bristow Procedure

This process is illustrated in Figures 168A to D.

McLaughlin Technique for Posterior Shoulder Dislocation

This has been illustrated in Figures 169A to D. This technique is involving the following steps:

- Shoulder incised anteriorly through deltopectoral interval
- Conjoined tendons reflected medially, exposing the subscapularis muscle and transverse incision is made
- Lesser tuberosity is osteomized, the fragment of lesser tuberosity fill the defect in humeral head
- Debridement of the surface of defect is done in humeral head. Reattach the subscapularis tendon (medial transportation) to humerus into the depths of defect, by mattress sutures through drill holes in the humeral head.

Arthroscopy

For the most common types of shoulder instability or dislocation, the ligaments at the front of the shoulder, those hold the head in the glenoid socket are torn or loosen from the lip of the glenoid or labrum (Figs. 170A and 171A).

Using special implants called "suture anchors" the surgeon can repair the ligaments and labrum in place and tighten them as necessary. These anchors are buried into the bone and most are made-up of absorbable materials that will disintegrate overtime after the shoulder has healed, as illustrated in Figures 170B and 171B.

ACROMIOCLAVICULAR JOINT DISLOCATION

Acromioclavicular joint as shown in Figure 172 is a diarthrodial joint between medial facet of acromion and the lateral (distal) clavicle. It contains intra-articular disk of variable size. Thin capsule of AC is stabilized by the ligaments on all sides. AC ligaments control horizontal (anteroposterior) displacement. Superior AC ligament is most important.

Normal Anatomy of AC Joint

Anatomy of AC joint is shown in Figure 173.

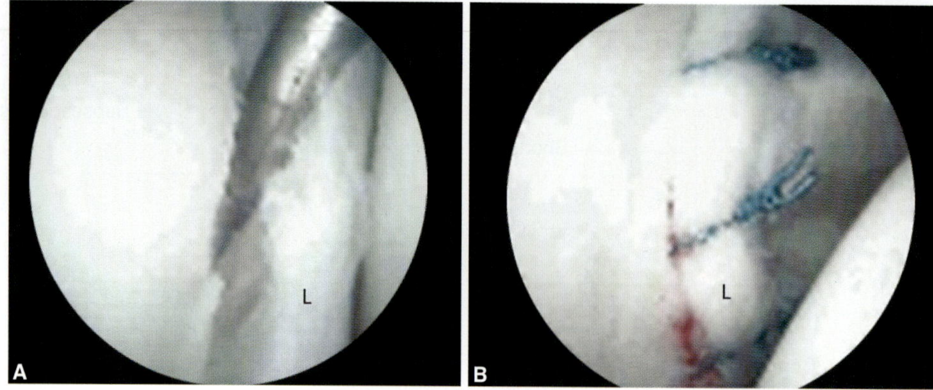

Figs. 170A and B: Arthroscopy: (A) Labrum (L) torn away from the glenoid surface; (B) Labrum (L) repaired to the glenoid using three suture anchors.

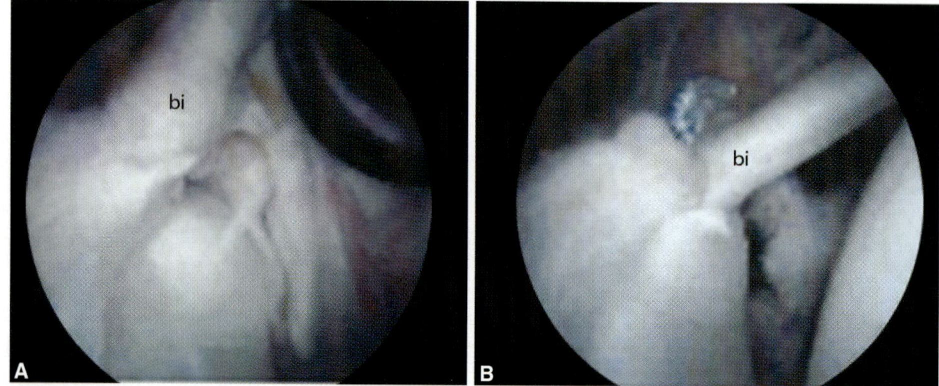

Figs. 171A and B: (A) Biceps (bi) and labrum torn away from the top of the glenoid; (B) Biceps (bi) and labrum repaired to the labrum using a suture anchor.

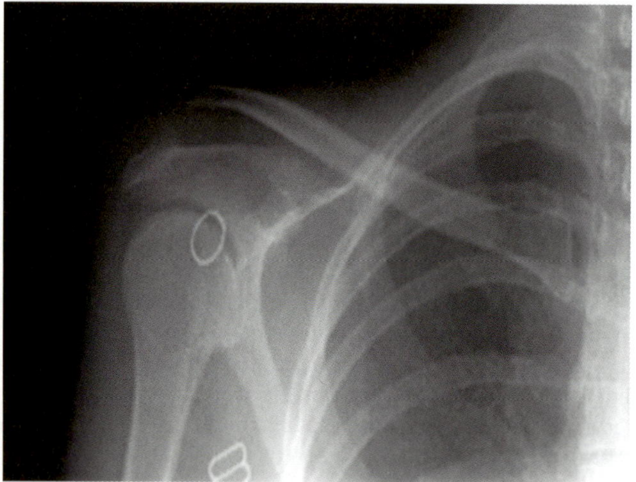

Fig. 172: X-ray shoulder shows acromioclavicular joint.

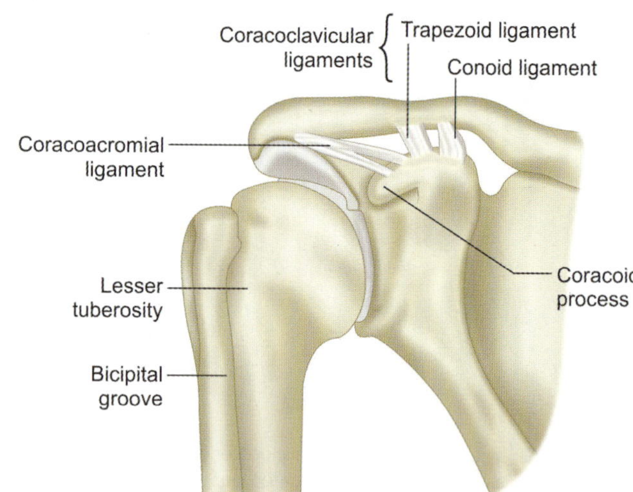

Fig. 173: Anatomy of AC joint, showing all surrounding structures.

Mechanism of Injury

- Moderate or high energy traumatic impacts to the shoulder, e.g. fall from height, motor vehicle accident and sports injury
- Blow to the point of the shoulder
- Rarely a direct injury to the clavicle. Direct force onto the superior surface of distal clavicle, with abduction of arm and retraction of scapula. This is shown in Figure 174.

Physical Examination

Inspection (Fig. 175)

Evaluate deformity and/or displacement. Beware of rare inferior or posterior displacement of distal or medial ends of clavicle. Compare with the opposite side. Find if there is normal inclination of AC and SC joint.

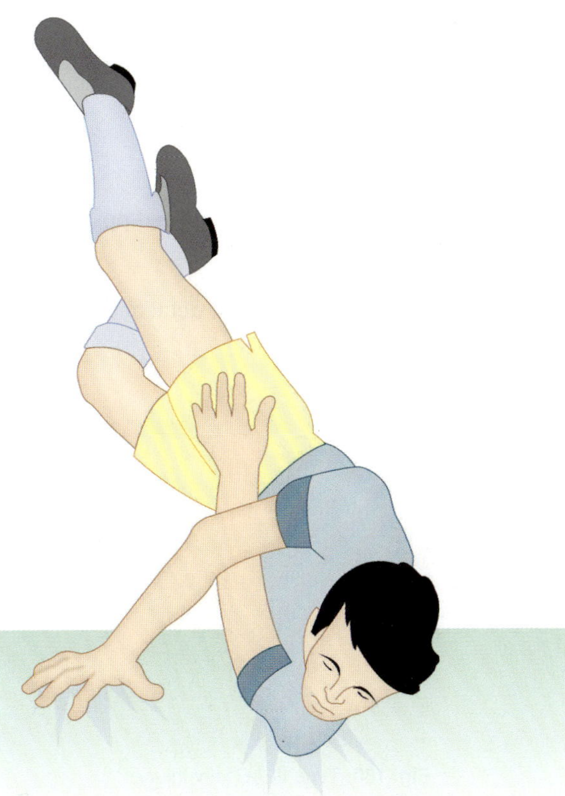

Fig. 174: Direct force or a fall on the point of shoulder.

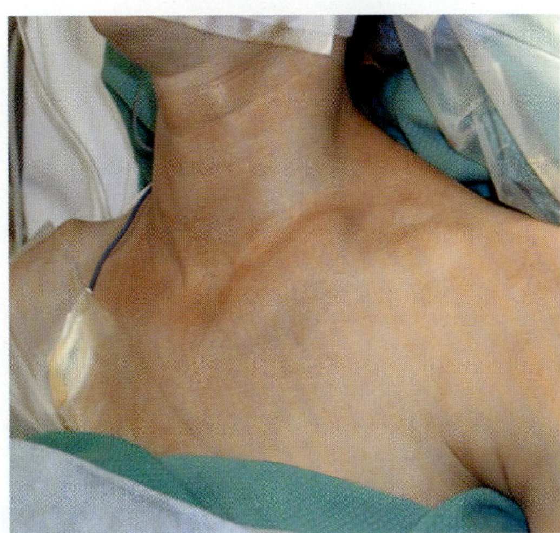

Fig. 175: Shoulder inspection in AC joint injury.

Palpation

- Evaluate pain
- Look for instability with stress.

Neurovascular Examination

- Evaluate upper extremity's motor and sensory sensation
- Measure shoulder range of motion.

Normal Inclination of AC-SC Joint

The normal inclination of acromioclavicular and sternoclavicular joint is seen in Figures 176A to C.

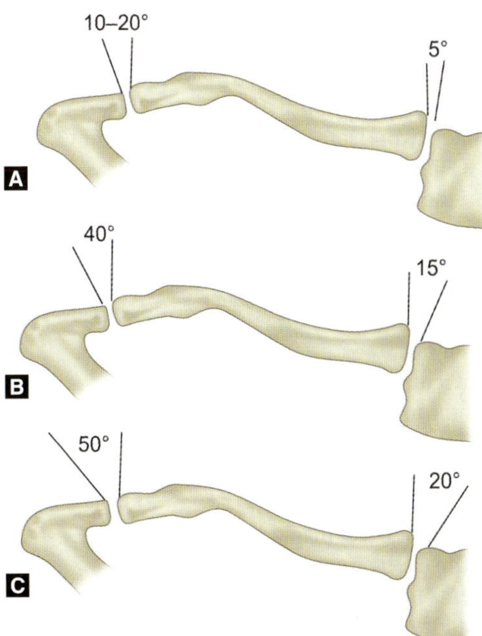

Figs. 176A to C: Normal inclination of AC and sternoclavicular joint. (A) Normal inclination of sternoclavicular and acromioclavicular joint without elevation of scapula and shoulder; (B) Normal tendency of rise of inclination of sternoclavicular and acromioclavicular joint with slight elevation of the scapula and shoulder keeping a thin sandbag under the scapula. (C) Further increase of the inclination sternoclavicular and acromioclavicular joint with further increase in elevation of scapula and shoulder.

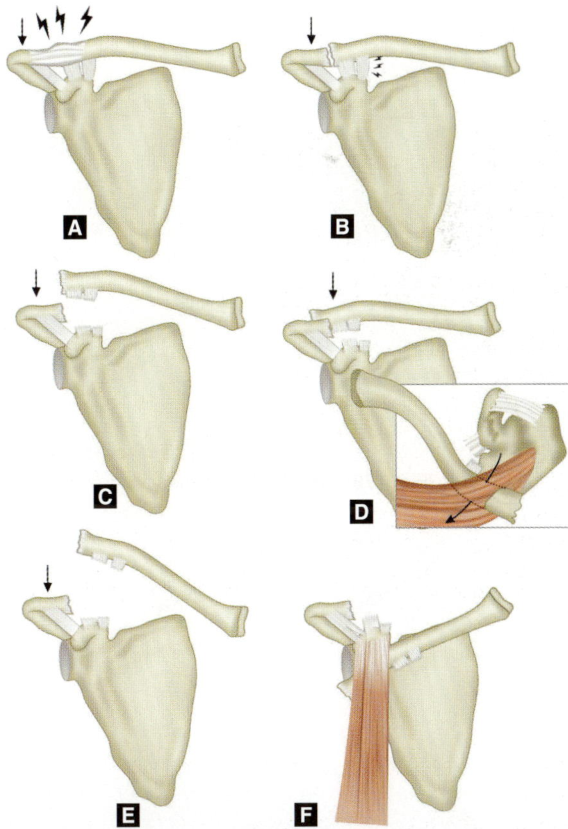

Figs. 177A to F: Different types of AC joint injuries—(A) *Type I*: With sprain of AC ligament; (B) *Type II*: With AC ligament disruption and intact CC ligament; (C) *Type III*: With both AC and CC ligament disrupted; (D to F) Dislocated AC joint.

Classification of Acromioclavicular Joint Injuries (Figs. 177A to F)

It was initially classified by both Allman and Tossy into three types (I, II and III). Rockwood later added types IV, V and VI, so that now six types of AC joint injuries are recognized. Classification varies, depending on the degree and the direction of displacement of the distal clavicle.

Type I (Fig. 178)

- There is a sprain of AC ligament
- AC joint is intact
- Coracoclavicular ligaments is intact
- Deltoid and trapezius muscles are also remain intact.

Type II (Fig. 179)

- AC joint disrupted
- Less than 50% vertical displacement
- Sprain of the CC ligaments
- CC ligaments intact
- Deltoid and trapezius muscles are also intact.

Type III (Fig. 180)

- AC ligaments and CC ligaments all disrupted
- AC joint dislocated and the shoulder complex is displaced inferiorly
- CC interspace greater than the normal shoulder (25–100%)
- Deltoid and trapezius muscles usually detached from the distal clavicle.

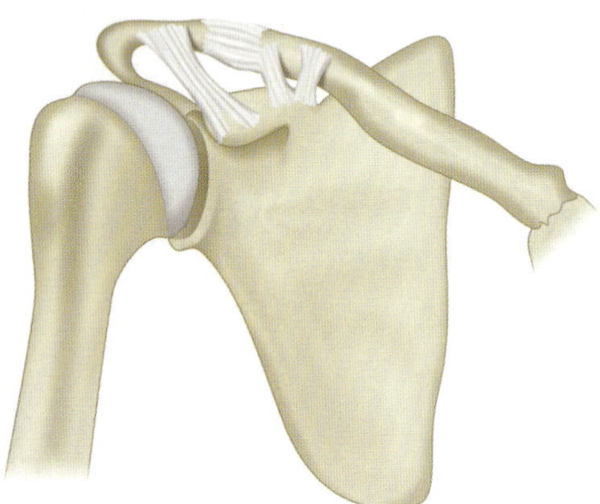

Fig. 178: Type I AC joint injury.

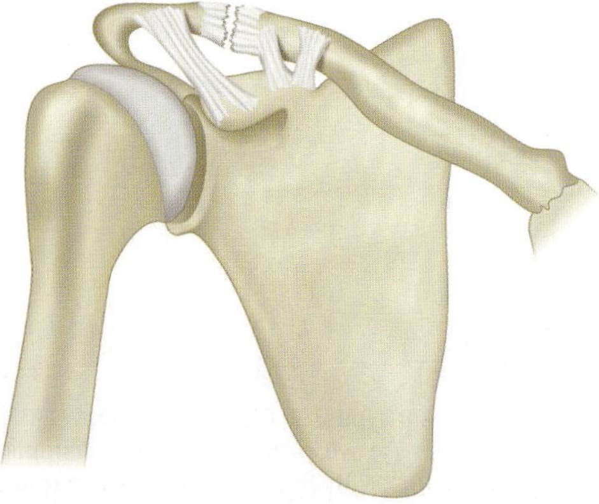

Fig. 179: Type II AC joint injury.

Type III Variants (Figs. 181 and 182)

- Pseudodislocation through an intact periosteal sleeve
- Physeal injury
- Coracoid process fractured.

Type IV (Figs. 183 to 185)

- AC joint dislocated and clavicle displaced posteriorly into or through the trapezius muscle
- AC and CC ligaments are torned
- Deltoid and trapezius muscles are detached from the distal clavicle.

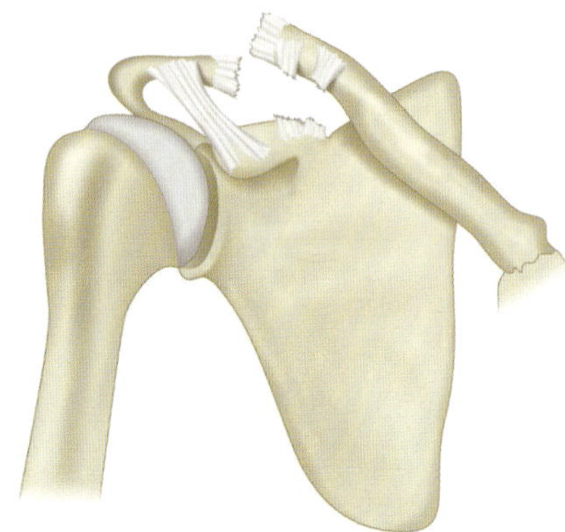

Fig. 180: Type III AC joint injury.

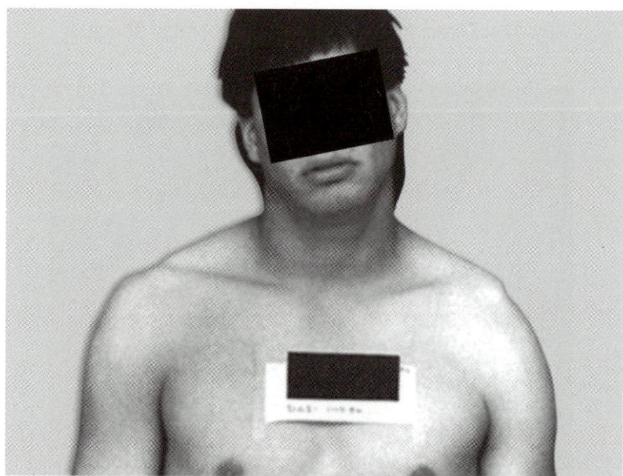

Fig. 181: Complete dislocation—type III variant.

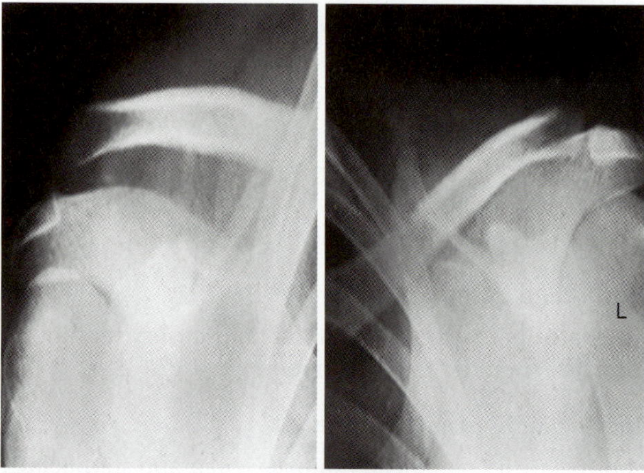

Figs. 182A and B: Type III injury—X-ray shows increase in the AC joint space.

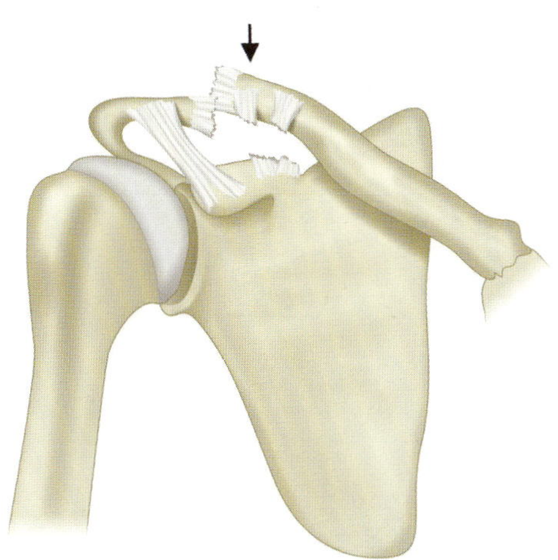

Fig. 183: Type IV AC joint injury.

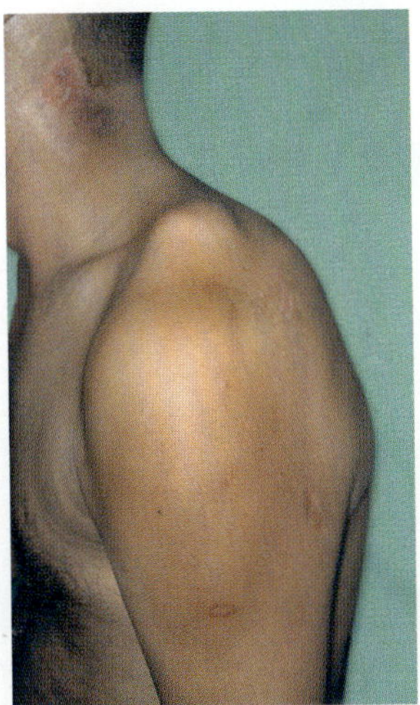

Fig. 184: Type IV injury, X-ray shows distal end of clavicle displaced posteriorly into the trapezius muscle.

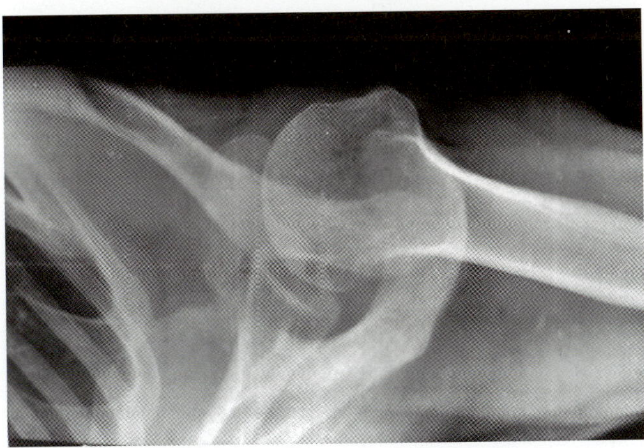

Fig. 185: Type IV injury—axillary lateral view.

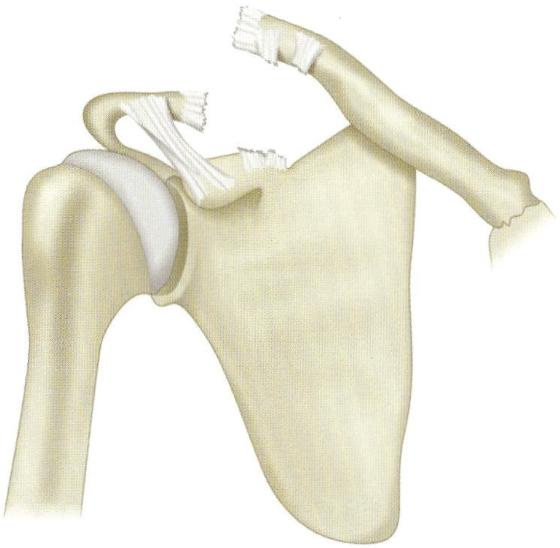

Fig. 186: Type V AC joint injury.

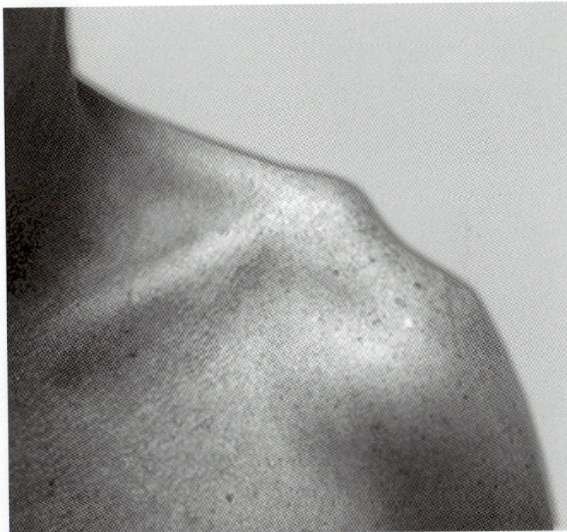

Fig. 187: Type V superior displacement of the clavicle.

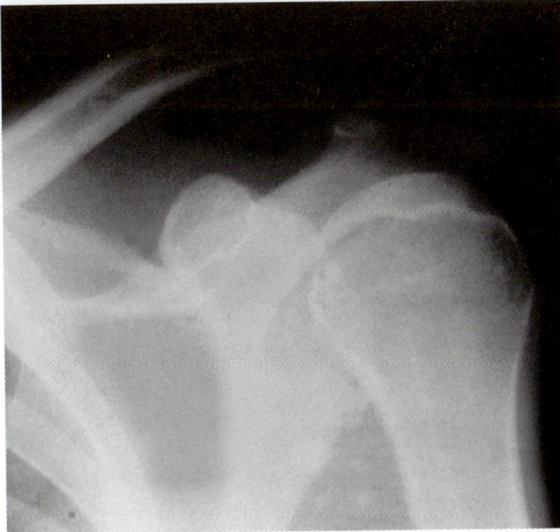

Fig. 188: Type V injury, with gross displacement of clavicle from acromion.

Type V (Figs. 186 to 188)

- AC joint dislocated and there is gross disparity between the clavicle and the scapula
- AC and CC ligaments torned
- Deltoid and trapezius muscles detached from the distal half of clavicle.

Type VI (Figs. 189 and 190)

- AC joint dislocated and clavicle displaced inferior to the acromion or the coracoid process
- AC and CC ligaments are torned
- Deltoid and trapezius muscles detached from the distal clavicle.

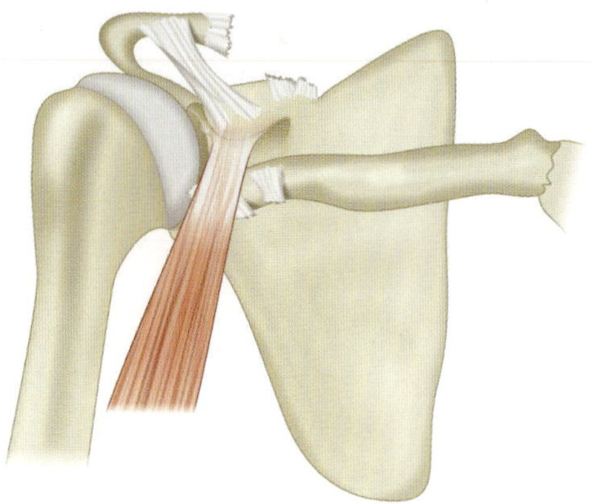

Fig. 189: Type VI AC joint injury.

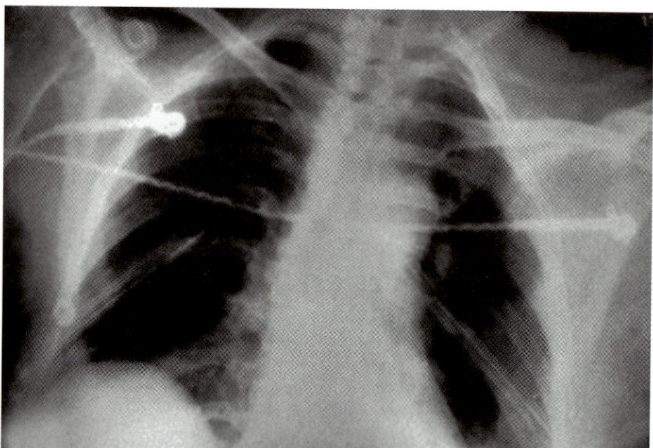

Fig. 190: Type VI injury, X-ray showing clavicle in subcoracoid position.

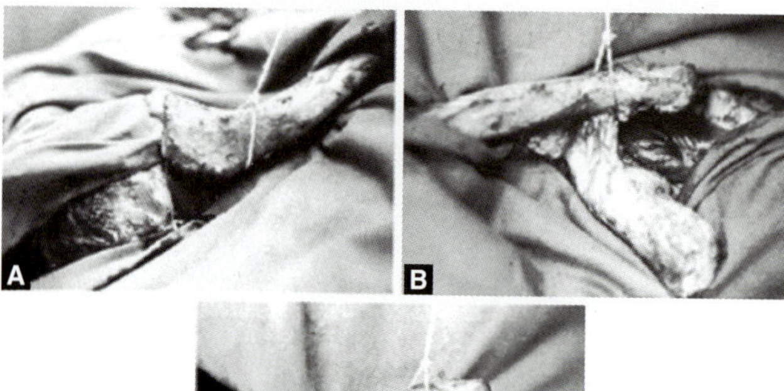

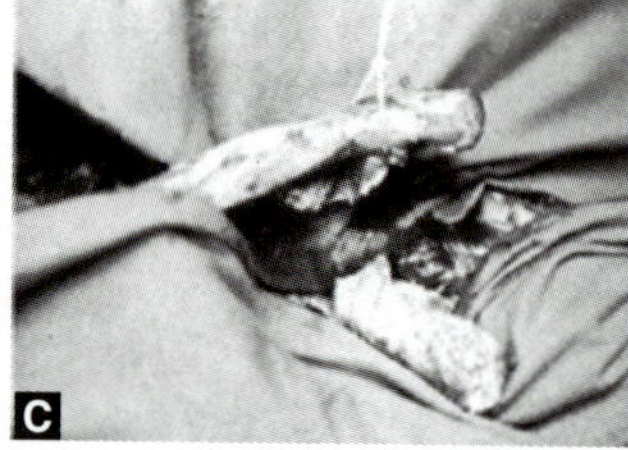

Figs. 191A to C: The importance of the AC and coracoclavicular ligaments for stability of the AC joint using a fresh cadaver.

Stability Provided by Ligaments (Figs. 191A to C)

- Horizontal stability controlled by AC ligament
- Vertical stability controlled by CC ligament.

Radiographic Evaluation of the AC Joint

Zanca's View (Figs. 192 and 193)

- AP view centered at AC joint with 10° cephalic tilt
- Less voltage than used for AP shoulder.

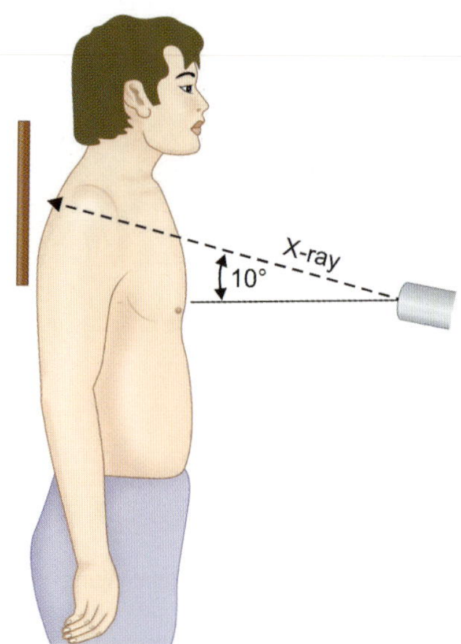

Fig. 192: Zanca's view for taking X-ray of AC joint.

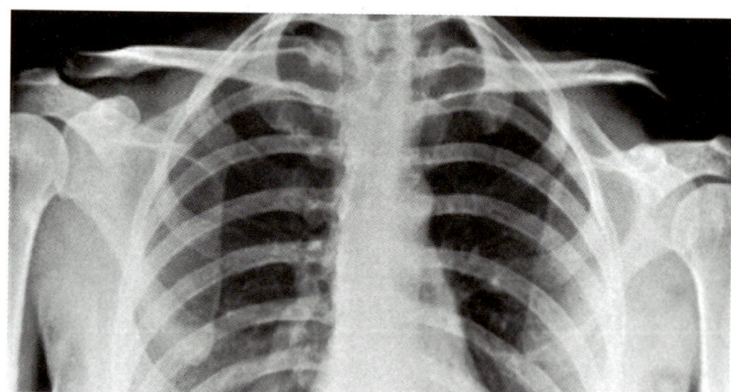

Fig. 193: AP view shows AC joint dislocation of left side.

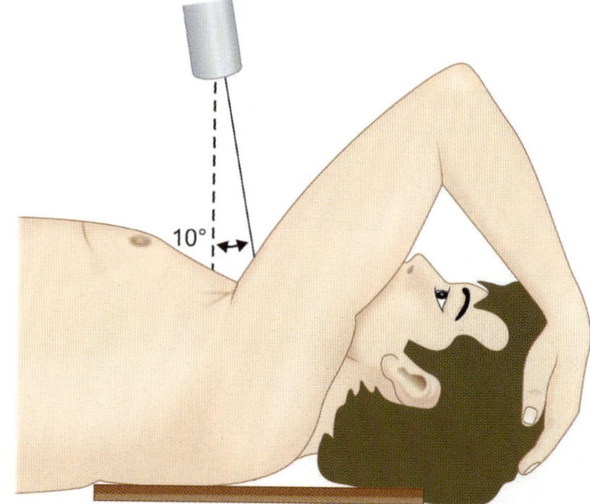

Fig. 194: Stryker notch view for taking X-ray of AC joint.

Stryker Notch View

Stryker notch view for taking X-ray of AC joint is shown in Figure 194.

Stress Views of the Distal Clavicle and AC Joint

- *Rationale:* Stress view demonstrates instability and differentiates grade III AC separations from partial Grade I and II injuries.

- Performed by having patient hold 10 lb weight with injured arm.
- Rarely used today, since most AC joint injuries treated in the same manner and management of distal clavicle fractures depends on initial displacement and location of fracture.

Treatment Options for Types I and II Acromioclavicular Joint Injuries

Nonoperative: Ice and protection until pain subsides (7–10 days). Return to sports as pain allows (1–2 weeks). No apparent benefit to the use of specialized braces.

Type II operative treatment: This is generally reserved only for the patient with chronic pain. Treatment is resection of the distal clavicle and reconstruction of the coracoclavicular ligaments.

Treatment Options for Types III to VI Acromioclavicular Joint Injuries

Nonoperative treatment: Closed reduction and application of a sling and harness to maintain reduction of the clavicle. Short-term sling and early ROM.

Operative treatment: Primary AC joint fixation, primary CC ligament fixation, excision of the distal clavicle and dynamic muscle transfers. In type III injuries, need for acute surgical treatment remains very controversial. Most surgeons recommend conservative treatment, except in the throwing athlete or overhead worker. Repair generally, avoided in contact athletes because of the risk of reinjury.

Indications for Acute Surgical Treatment of Acromioclavicular Injuries (Fig. 195)

- Type III injuries in highly active patients
- Type IV, V and VI injuries.

Surgical Options for AC Joint Instability

- Coracoid process transfer to distal transfer (dynamic muscle transfer)
- Primary AC joint fixation
- Primary CC fixation
- Distal clavicle excision with CC ligament reconstruction.

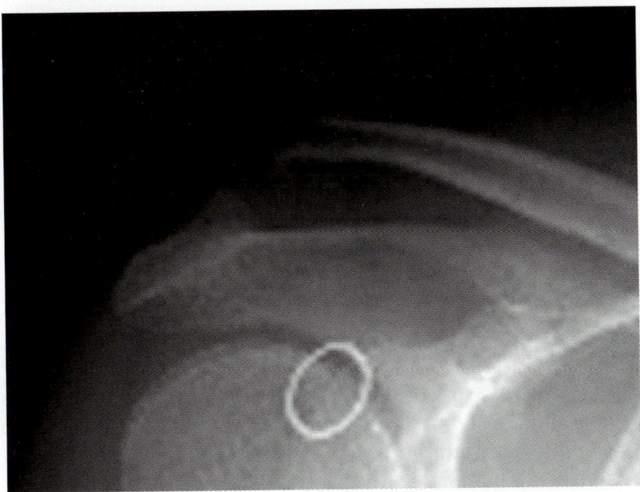

Fig. 195: Type III acromioclavicular injuries.

Operative Procedures for Injuries of AC Joint

Suturing is done between clavicle and coracoid process (Fig. 196A). Put K-wires across the AC joint (Fig. 196B) and lag screw between clavicle and coracoid process (Fig. 196C).

Surgical Repair of Chronic Type II AC Joint Injury (Figs. 197A to D)

- *Position:* Back of table, 20º short of vertical position.
- *Capsular flaps:* Small portion of anterior deltoid is reflected from acromion portion, to expose CA ligament.
- Stay suturing is done on ligament.
- Unicortical drill holes placed in distal clavicle (posterosuperior)
- CA ligament transferred to intramedullary canal.
- Sutures placed through drill holes and tied over the top of clavicle.

Postoperative phase: Arm immobilized in abduction orthosis or abduction pillow for within 1 to 3 weeks. Pendulum and passive external rotation exercises for 3-6 weeks. Active range of movements or sports activity after 4–8 months.

Operative Stabilization of Type III AC Joint (Fig. 198)

- Deltotrapezius fascia incised mediolaterally
- Two holes drilled at the base of coracoid for anchor insertion
- Sutures inserted at the base of coracoid
- Two drill holes placed through clavicle of passage sutures
- Sutures tied over bony ridges of clavicle to reconstitute CC ligament
- Deltotrapezial aponeurosis is repaired.

Postoperatively: Arm immobilized in abduction orthosis or abduction pillow for 1–3 weeks. Pendulum and passive external rotation exercises for 3–6 weeks. Active range of movements or sports activities after 4–8 months.

Repair of Type III AC Joint

Resection of Distal Clavicle and CA Ligament Transfer

- Deltotrapezius fascia incised mediolaterally superior to AC joint

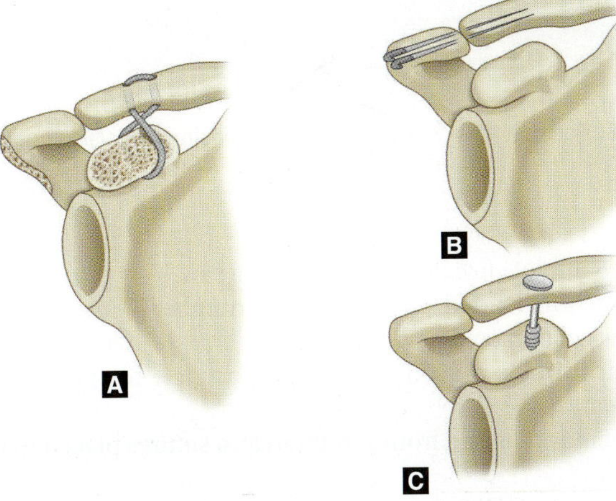

Figs. 196A to C: Operative procedures for injuries of AC joint: (A) Suture between clavicle and coracoid process; (B) Put K-wires across the AC joint; (C) Lag screw between clavicle and coracoid process.

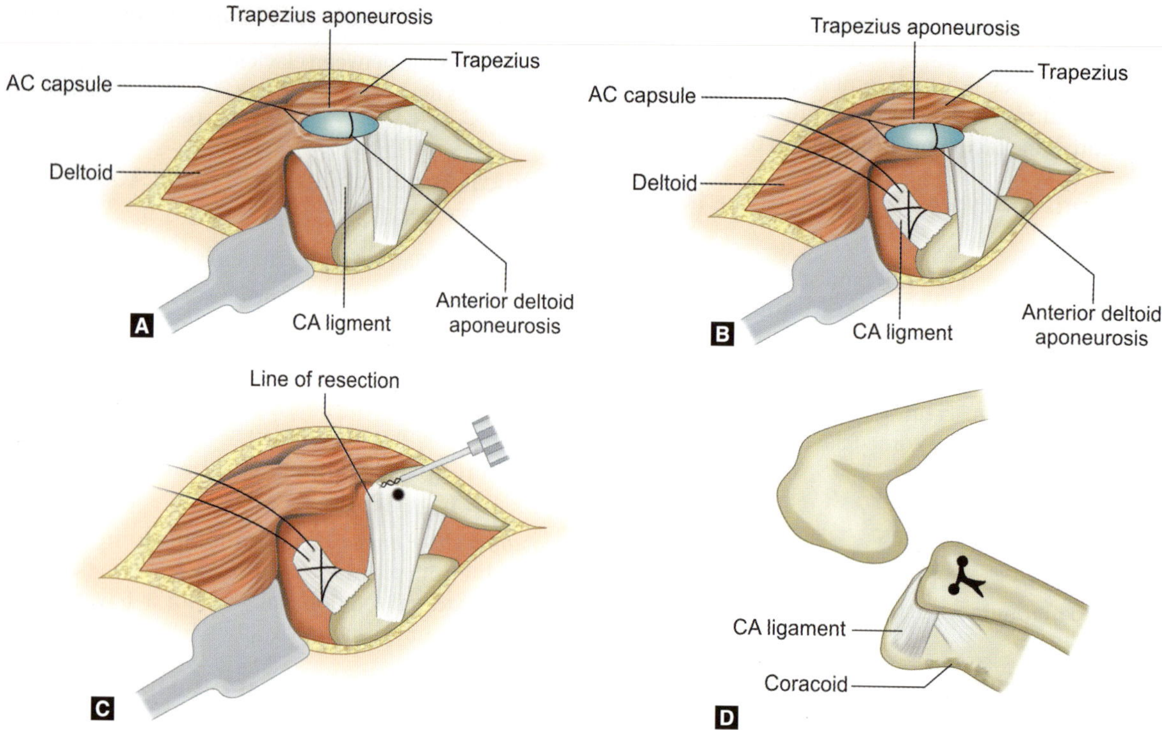

Figs. 197A to D: Surgical repair of chronic type II AC joint injury—(A and B) Incision on Langer's line medial to AC joint, deltoid muscle is reflected anteriorly and AC joint capsule incised medial to lateral; (C) Drill holes made 5 mm from articular surface and 5 mm of distal end of clavicle is excised. Drill holes placed 2 mm to resection margins; (D) Sutures placed through drill holes, capsule and muscles are then repaired.

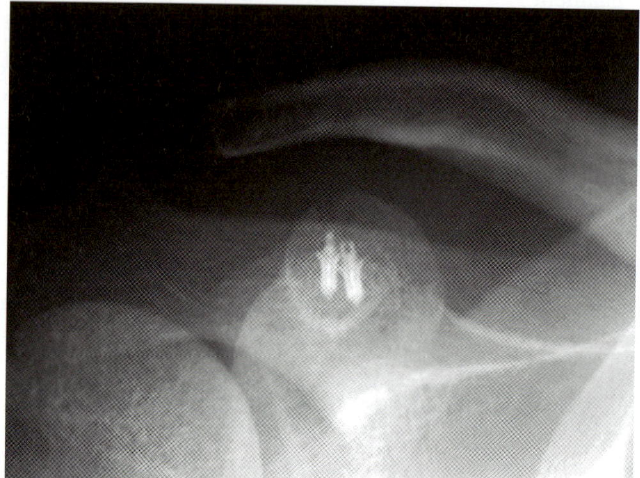

Fig. 198: Postoperative X-ray taken after reconstruction, using bone anchors of coracoid.

- Distal 5 mm of clavicle resected using a saw
- Two anchors loaded with ethibond number 5, inserted into the base of coracoid
- Two drill holes placed through the clavicle for passage of sutures
- Ligament is released from acromion and sutures placed in the end
- Coracoacromial ligaments transferred to intramedullary canal and tied through two drill holes
- AC joint capsule and deltotrapezial fascia repaired.

Indications for Late Surgical Treatment of Acromioclavicular Injuries

- Pain
- Weakness
- Deformity.

Techniques for Late Surgical Treatment of Acromioclavicular Injuries

Reduction of AC joint and repair of AC and CC ligaments. Resection of distal clavicle and reconstruction of CC ligaments (Weaver-Dunn procedure).

Weaver-Dunn Procedure (Fig. 199)

- The distal clavicle is excised
- The CA ligament is transferred to the distal clavicle
- The CC ligaments are repaired and/or augmented with a CC screw or suture
- Repair of deltotrapezial fascia.

Pros and cons of treatment options of AC joint dislocation are illustrated in Table 5.

Sternoclavicular Joint (Fig. 200)

Anatomy of the Sternoclavicular Joint

Various structures involved in the joint formation and maintenance of its stability are shown in Figure 201. The salient features and accompanied structures of the SC joint are described below:

- Diarthrodial joint
- Saddle shaped

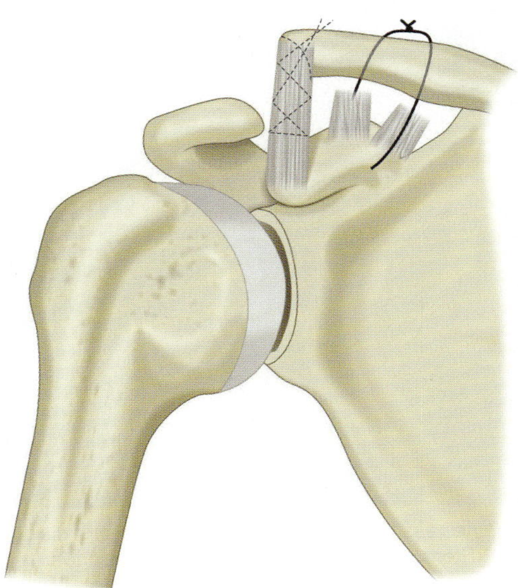

Fig. 199: Weaver-Dunn procedure, resection of distal clavicle and reconstruction of CC ligaments.

TABLE 5: Pros and cons of treatment options of AC joint dislocation.

Pros	*Cons*	
Intra-articular AC fixation	Anatomic reduction	• Hardware failure • Distal clavicle osteolysis
Extra-articular coracoclavicular repair	Superior strength of initial fixation (screw)	• Screw failure • Bone resorption
Ligament reconstruction	• Anatomic repair • No risk of metallic hardware failure	• Less initial fixation strength • Harvest coracoacromial ligament

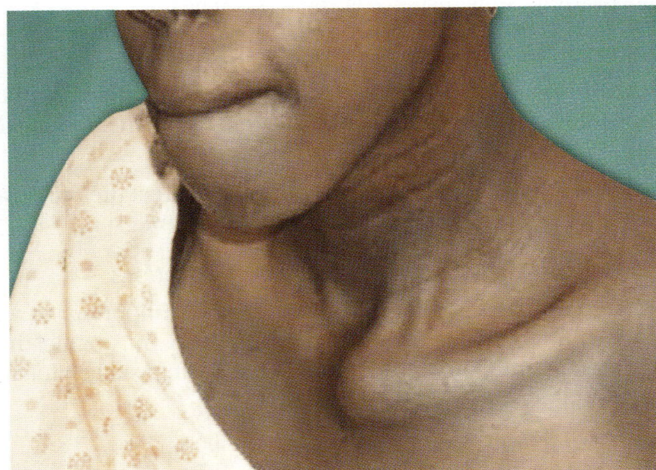

Fig. 200: Sternoclavicular joint.

- Poor congruence
- Intra-articular disk ligament divides SC joint into two separate joint spaces
- Costoclavicular ligament (rhomboid ligament) is short and strong and consists of an anterior and posterior fasciculus
- Interclavicular ligament connects the superomedial aspects of each clavicle with the capsular ligaments and the upper sternum

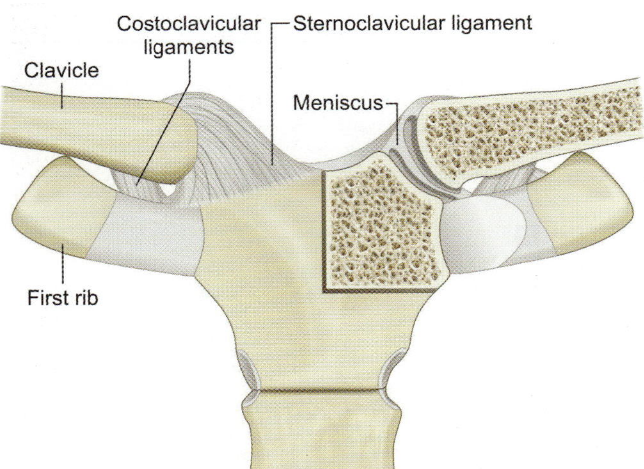

Fig. 201: The anatomy of the sternoclavicular joint and accompanying structures.

- Capsular ligament covers the anterior and posterior aspects of the joint and represents thickenings of the joint capsule. The anterior portion of the ligament is heavier and stronger than the posterior portion.

Epiphysis of the Medial Clavicle

Medial physis: Last of the ossification centers to appear in the body and the last epiphysis to close. Does not ossify until 18–20 years of age; does not unite with the clavicle, until 23–25 years of age.

Anatomical Classification of Injuries of SC Joint (Figs. 202 and 203)

Anterior dislocation: Common, medial end of clavicle displaced anteriorly or anterosuperiorly with respect to anterior margin of sternum.

Posterior dislocation: Uncommon, clavicle displaced posteriorly with respect to posterior margin of sternum.

Etiological Classification of Injuries to SC Joint

Traumatic injuries:

- *Acute dislocation:* Dislocated SC joint, with intra-articular ligaments ruptured.
- *Recurrent dislocation:* If initial dislocation does not heal, mild or moderate forces produce recurrent dislocation.
- *Chronic dislocation:* Original dislocation is unrecognized and irreducible.

Atraumatic injuries:
Spontaneous subluxation or dislocation.

Injuries Associated with Sternoclavicular Joint Dislocations (Fig. 204)

- Mediastinal compression
- Pneumothorax
- Laceration of the superior vena cava
- Tracheal erosion.

Radiographic Techniques

Radiographic techniques for assessing SC injuries include:

- *CT scan:* Best technique for SC joint problems

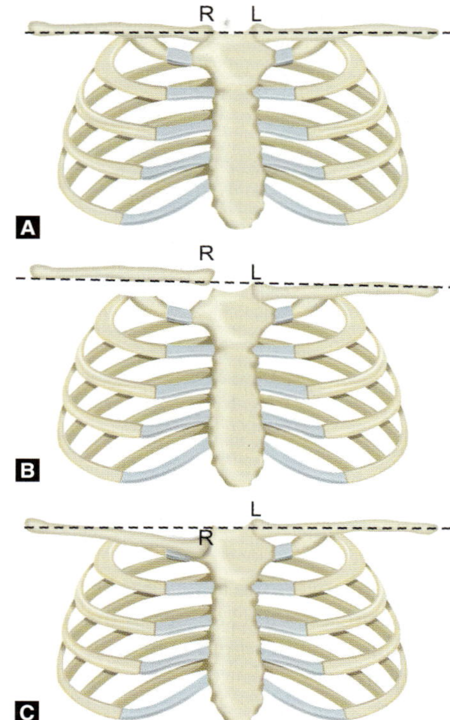

Figs. 202A to C: Injuries of SC joint: (A) Normal joint; (B) Clavicle right sided (R) dislocated anteriorly; (C) Clavicle right sided; (R) dislocated posteriorly.

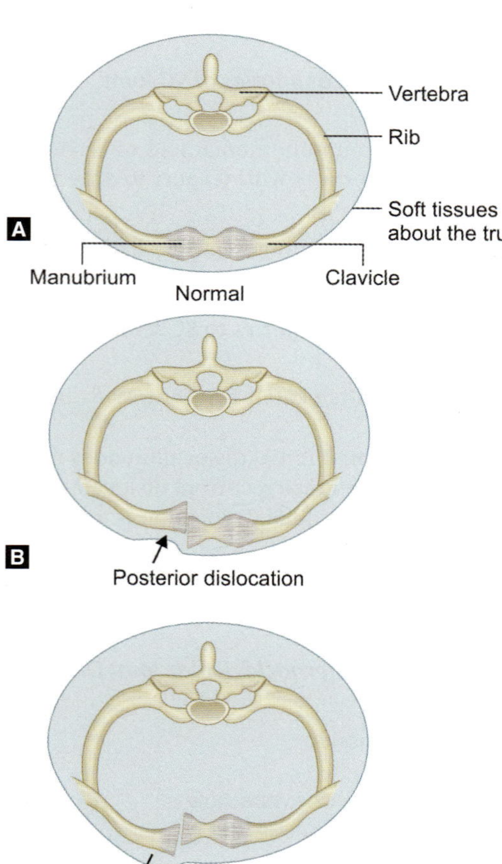

Figs. 203A to C: Cross-section through thorax, showing injuries of SC joint: (A) Normal joint; (B) Joint dislocated posteriorly; (C) Joint anteriorly dislocated.

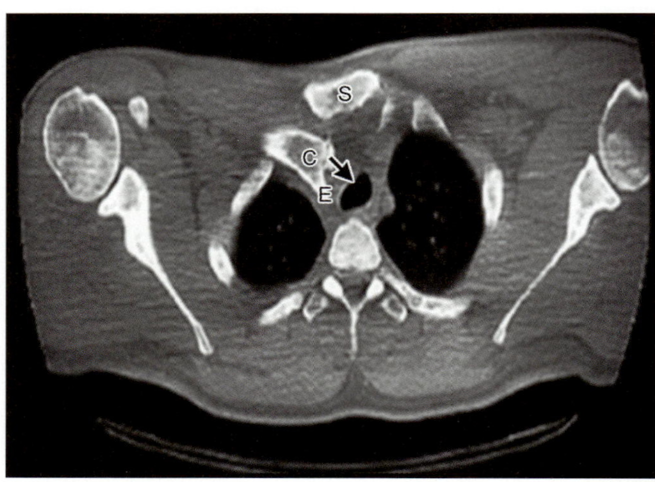

Fig. 204: Injuries associated with sternoclavicular joint dislocations—S, Sternum; C, Clavicle; E, Erosion of trachea.

- Tomograms
- MRI
- Ultrasound.

Heinig view (Figs. 205A and B):
Patient is in supine position. X-ray taken at about 30 inches, a central ray directed tangential to joint and parallel to the opposite clavicle. Cassette placed against the opposite shoulder and centered on manubrium.

Hobbs view (Fig. 206):
Patient stands and leans over the table; cassette on table and rib cage against the cassette; X-ray beam sent from above.

Serendipity view (Fig. 207):
Patient positioned in supine. Tube tilted 40° angle off vertical and centered on sternum. In children, tube distance is about 45 inches, while in adults, tube distance is about 60 inches.

Treatment of Anterior Sternoclavicular Dislocations

Nonoperative treatment: Analgesics and immobilization are main nonoperative means of treatment. Functional outcomes are usually good.

Closed reduction: Often not much successful. Direct pressure over the medial end of the clavicle may reduce the joint.

Treatment of Posterior Sternoclavicular Dislocations

Careful examination of the patient is extremely important to rule out vascular compromise. Consider CT to rule out mediastinal compression. Attempt closed reduction; it is often successful and remains stable.

Closed Reduction Techniques

This has been depicted in Figures 208 and 209. Techniques employed are:

- Abduction traction
- Adduction traction
- *Towel clip*: Anterior force applied to clavicle by percutaneously applied towel clip.

Operative Techniques

- *Resection arthroplasty:* It may result in instability of remaining clavicle unless stabilization is done. Suggest minimal resection of bone and fixation of medial clavicle to first rib.

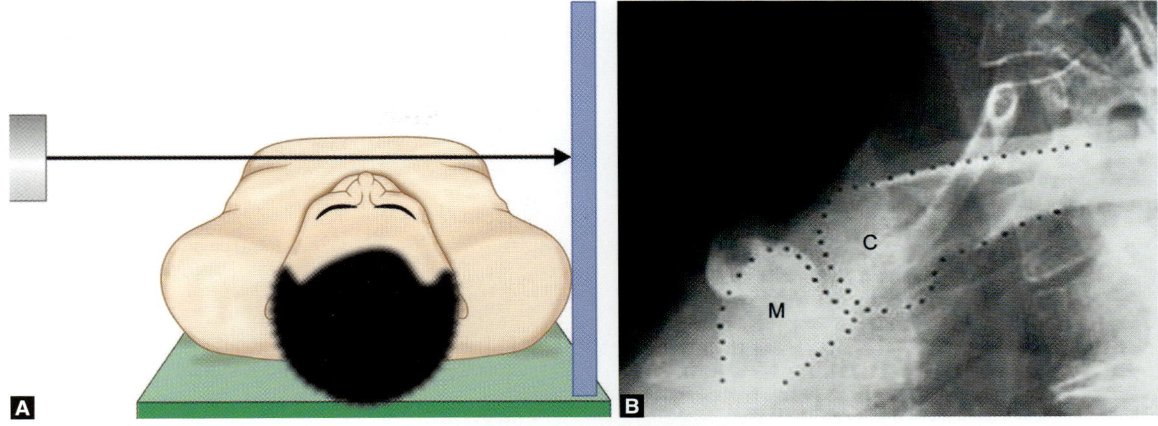

Figs. 205A and B: Heinig view.

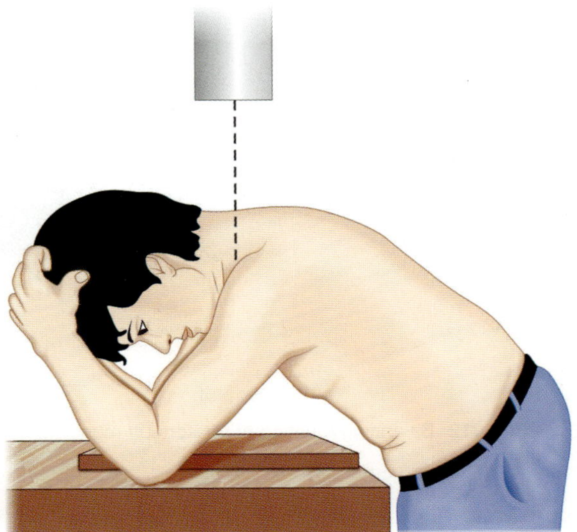

Fig. 206: Hobbs view.

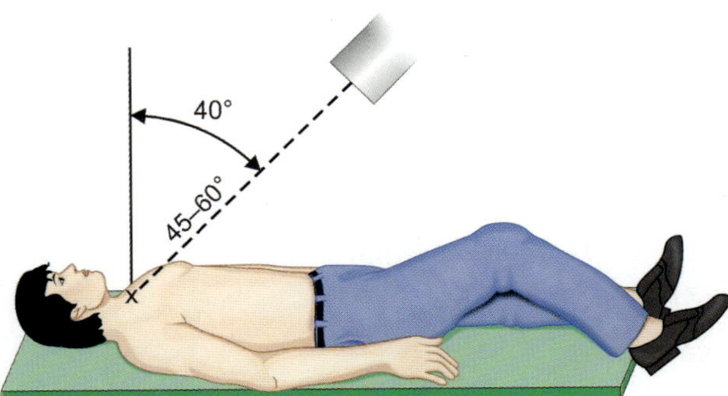

Fig. 207: Serendipity view.

- Sternoclavicular reconstruction with suture and tendon graft.
- Semitendinosus figure-of-eight reconstruction.

  The procedure is illustrated in Figures 210A to C.

Postoperatively: Figure-of-eight bandage for 4–6 weeks. Clavicular brace for 4–6 weeks. Passive movements at shoulder joint after 6 weeks. Active movements or sports at shoulder joint after 4–6 months.

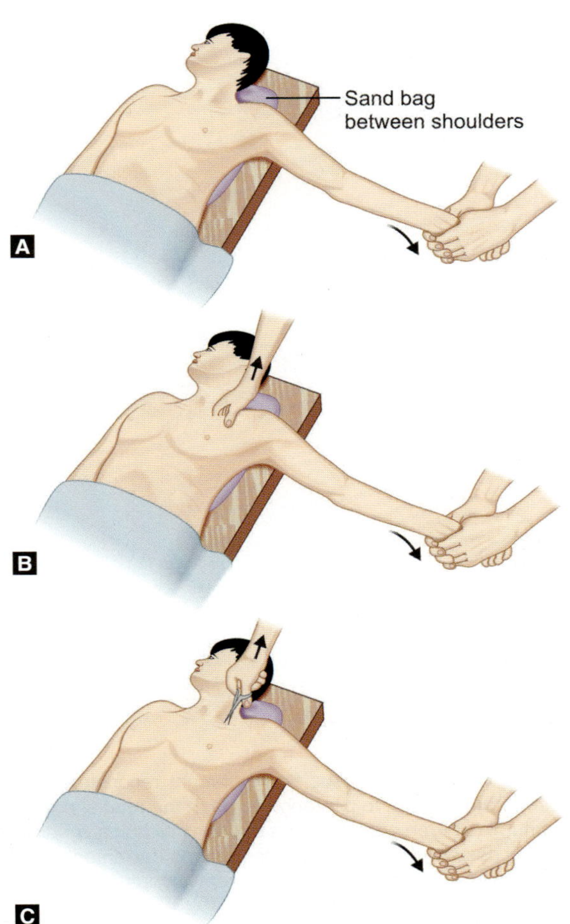

Figs. 208A to C: Closed reduction technique for dislocated SC joint.

ROTATOR CUFF TEARS

ANATOMY

The rotator cuff (RC) is a complex of four muscles that arise from the scapula and whose tendons blend in with the subjacent capsule, as they attach to the tuberosities of the humerus.

The four muscles forming RC are:

1. Subscapularis
2. Infraspinatus

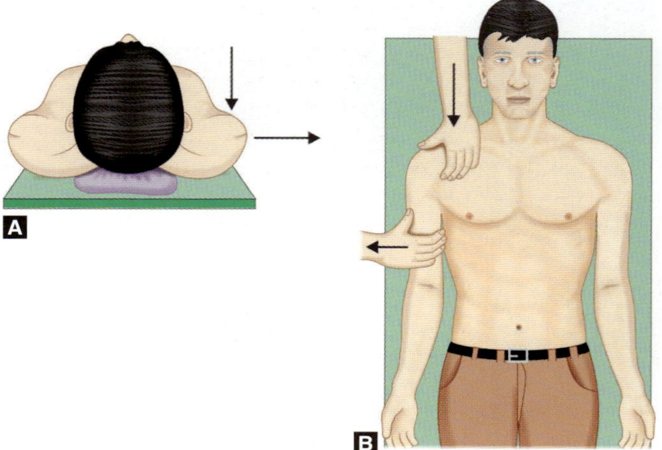

Figs. 209A and B: Buckerfield-Castle technique for SC joint reduction.

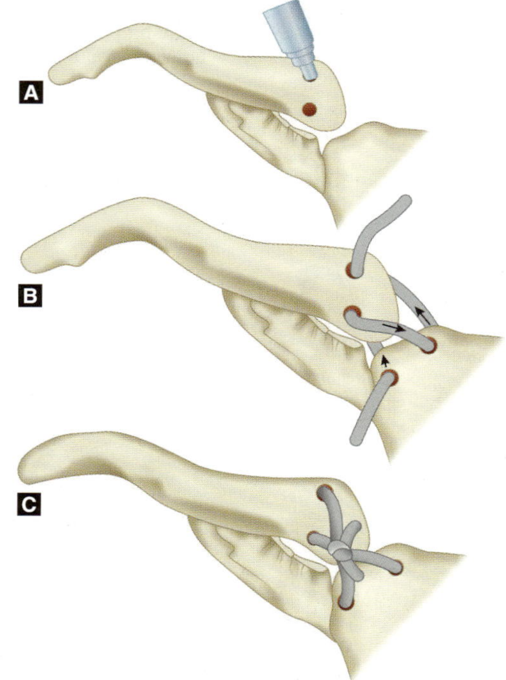

Figs. 210A to C: Semitendinosus figure-of-eight reconstruction. (A) Drill holes passed from anterior to posterior, through the medial part of clavicle and manubrium; (B) Free graft is woven through drill holes, tendons parallel to each other, posterior to joint and cross each other anterior to the joint; (C) Tendon tied in square knot and is secured with sutures.

3. Teres minor
4. Supraspinatus.

Different RC muscles and their attachments across shoulder and scapula are shown in Figure 211.

Supraspinatus

Origin: Supraspinous fossa of scapula

Insertion: Greater tubercle of humerus

Action:

- Assists deltoid muscle in abducting arm at shoulder joint.
- Initiates the first 30°–60° of abduction at which point the deltoid takes over.

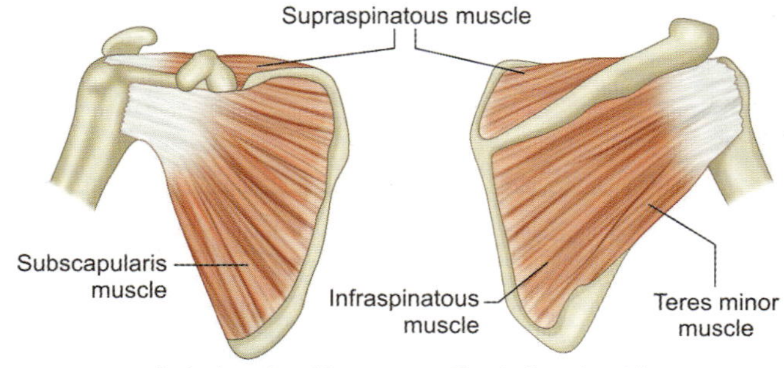

Fig. 211: Rotator cuff muscles and their attachments across shoulder and scapula.

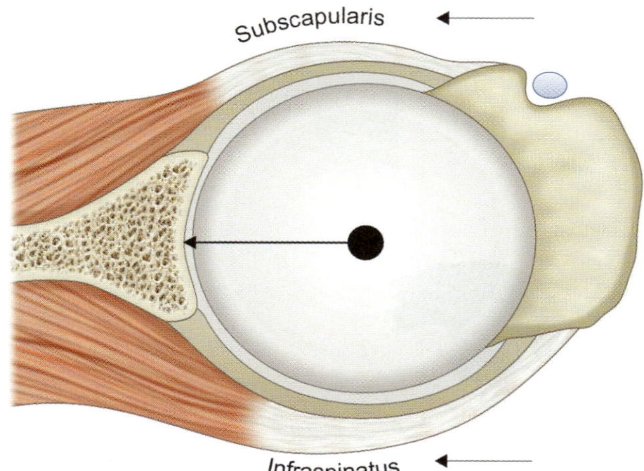

Fig. 212: Balancing function of rotator cuff muscles.

Infraspinatus

Origin: Infraspinous fossa of scapula

Insertion: Greater tubercle of humerus

Action: Laterally rotates and adducts arm at shoulder joint.

Teres Minor

Origin: Inferior lateral border of scapula

Insertion: Greater tubercle of humerus

Action: Laterally rotates, extends and adducts arm at shoulder joint.

Subscapularis

Origin: Subscapular fossa of scapula

Insertion: Lesser tubercle of humerus

Action: Medially rotates arm at shoulder joint.

FUNCTIONS OF ROTATOR CUFF MUSCLES

- They compress the head into the glenoid fossa, thereby providing a critical stabilizing mechanism to the shoulder known as concavity compression.
- They rotate the humerus with respect to the scapula.
- They provide muscular balance, a critical function, as illustrated in Figure 212.

Vascularity

They are supplied by a vascular network that receives contributions from the anterior humeral circumflex, the subscapular and the suprascapular arteries. The relative undervascularized portion is more proximal to supraspinatus insertion.

CAUSES OF INJURY TO ROTATOR CUFF MUSCLES

Chronic Tear

Found among people in occupations or sports requiring excessive overhead activity, e.g. painters, baseball pitchers, as depicted in the Figure 213. Variations in the shoulder structure causing narrowing under the outer edge of the collar bone.

Acute Tear

This is acute or sudden powerful raising of the arm against resistance, often in an attempt to cushion a fall, e.g. heavy weight lifting or a fall on the shoulder. Injury is usually associated with a significant amount of force, if person is younger than 30 years of age.

Other Causes

- Age-related degeneration
- Compromised microvascular supply.

Outlet Impingement

The RC is surrounded by the CA arch, which comprises the supraspinatus outlet and consists of the acromion, CA ligament and coracoid process. The shape of the acromion has been implicated in RC pathology.

Bigliani and Morrison Classification

Bigliani and Morrison classified three types of acromions based on cadaveric examination:

1. *Type I:* Flat
2. *Type II:* Curved
3. *Type III:* Hooked

Bigliani noted a significant increase in RC tears in curved (type II) and hooked (type III) acromions; these are shown in Figure 214.

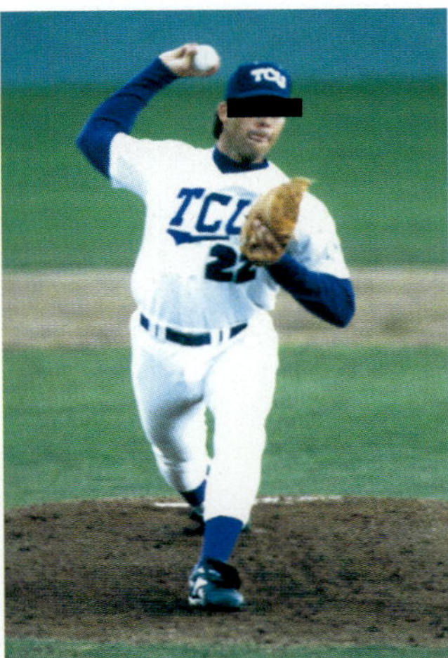

Fig. 213: Chronic causes of rotator cuff tear, due to overhead activities as in baseball players.

TYPES OF ROTATOR CUFF PATHOLOGY

- Simple tendinitis with swelling and inflammation (more commonly seen in younger patients with robust tissue).
- A partial thickness tear, involving only a portion of the RC fibers (involving less or more than 50% of the depth of the tendon).
- Full thickness tears with complete detachment from its normal insertion (as we often find in the elderly) due to severely degenerated tendons, as shown in Figure 215.

CLASSIFICATION

- Based on dimensions given by Cofield tears are classified as:
  - *Small tears:* Less than 1 cm
  - *Medium tears:* 1 to less than 3 cm
  - *Large tears:* 3 to less than 5 cm
  - *Massive tears:* 5 cm or larger
- Ellman presented a classification based on:
  - Descriptions of location, e.g. articular, bursal and interstitial
  - Grading, like grade 1 for less than 3 mm deep, grade 2 for 3 to 6 mm deep and grade 3 for more than 6 mm deep
- Third classification based on tear area (in mm^2).

CLINICAL EVALUATION

- History of trauma, occupation
- Complaints like pain (location, aggravating factors)

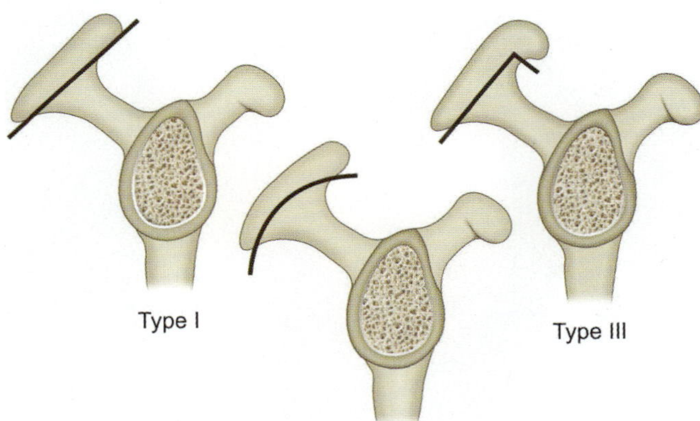

Fig. 214: Bigliani and Morrison classification of three types of acromions.

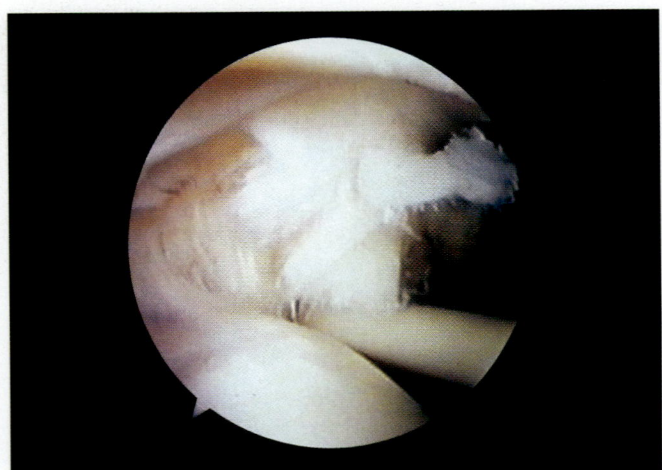

Fig. 215: Full thickness tears with complete detachment from its normal insertion.

- If there is decrease in sleep?
- Overhead weakness
- Stiffness, catching, popping of joint.

Inspection (Figs. 216 and 217)

The therapist will examine the shoulder looking for swelling, bruising, muscle wasting, postural issues, etc. It is important that the injured side is compared to the unaffected side at all times.

Palpation (Figs. 218 and 219)

- Tenderness
- Range of motion both active and passive
- Weakness
- Instability
- Roughness or crepitus.

Stiffness

Stiffness may be demonstrable as limitations in internal rotation, with the arm in abduction (measure in degrees from the neutral position) or with reaching up the back (posterior segment reached with the thumb), in cross-body adduction (measure in centimeters from the ipsilateral antecubital fossa to the contralateral acromion or coracoid), in flexion (measure in degrees from the neutral position) or in external rotation (measure in degrees from the neutral position), this is shown in Figures 220 and 221.

Weakness

Testing for weakness in abduction is done specifically for the supraspinatus tendon, which is the most common tendon that get torn out easily, as illustrated in Figure 222.

Subscapularis: Isometric internal rotation of the arm with the elbow flexed to 90° and the hand held posteriorly just off the waist.

Infraspinatus: Isometric external rotation of the arm held at the side in neutral rotation with the elbow flexed to 90°.

Subacromial Roughness

This is demonstrated in Figure 223, a test of a patient's passive range of motion (ROM) of the arm in an abducted position is done and the physician palpates for roughness underneath the acromion.

PROVOCATIVE TESTS

- Lift-off test
- Belly-press test
- External rotation stress test

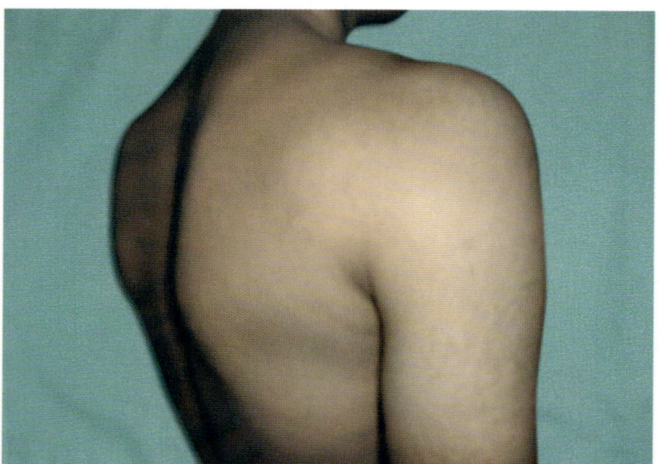

Fig. 216: Examination of the affected side of the shoulder.

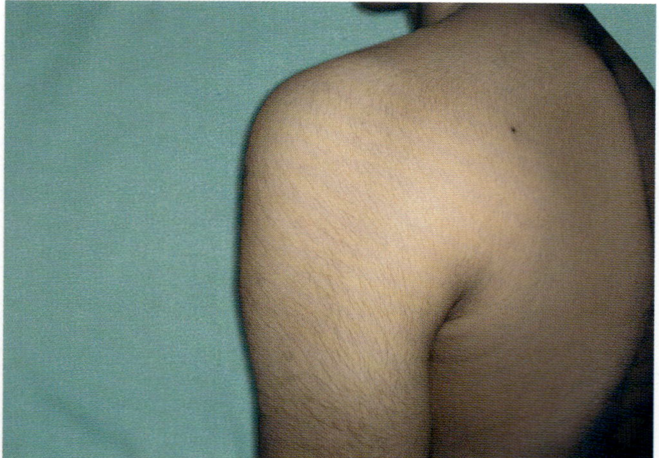

Fig. 217: Examination of the unaffected side of the shoulder compared with the affected side.

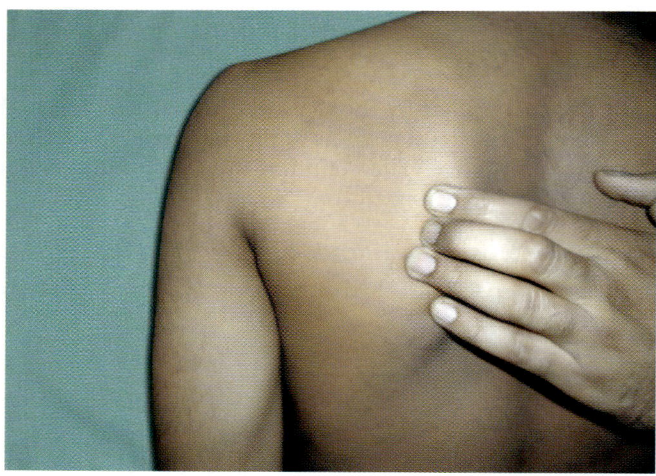

Fig. 218: Palpation done to check the roughness.

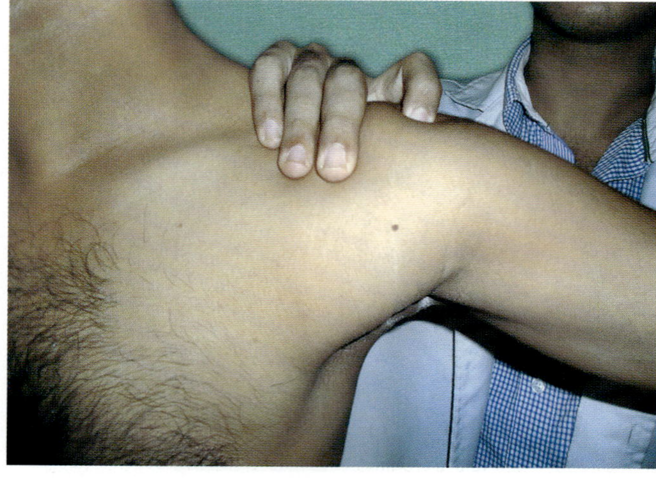

Fig. 219: Palpation done to check any crepitus.

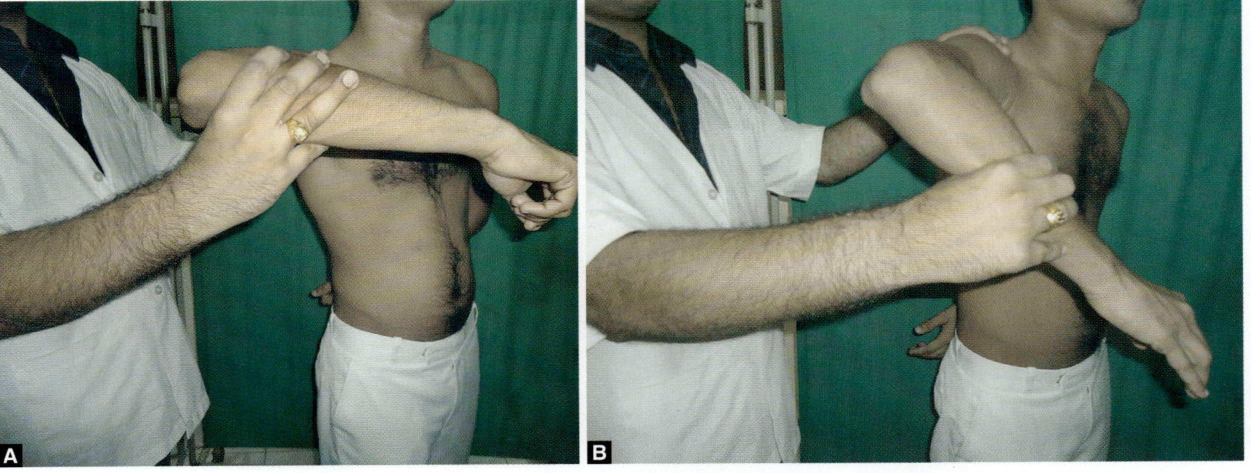

Figs. 220A and B: Arm is internally rotated, while keeping shoulder in abduction.

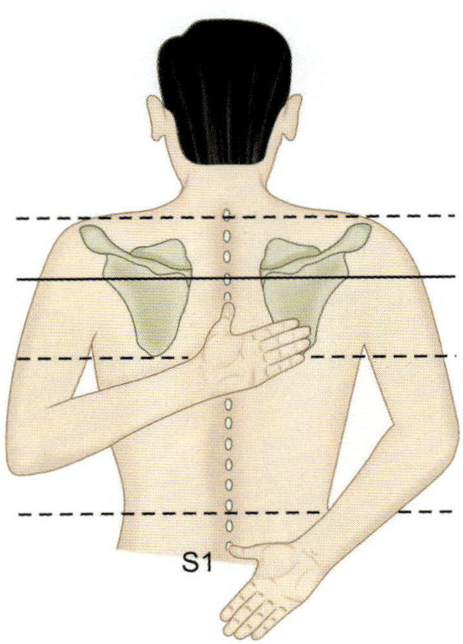

Fig. 221: With reaching up the back, measuring the posterior segment reached with the thumb.

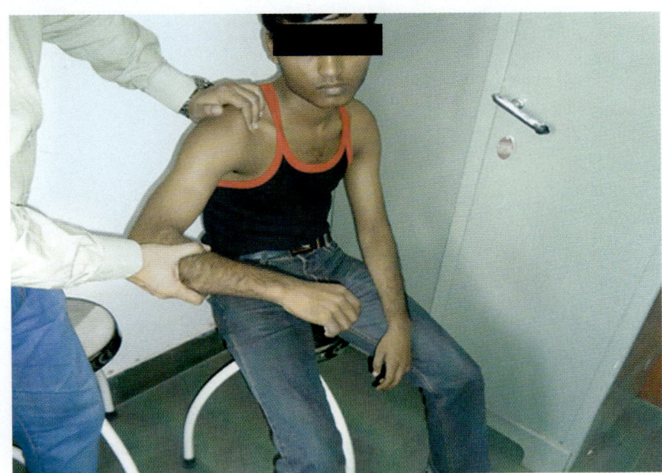

Fig. 223: Subacromial roughness is palpated while patient's arm is abducted passively.

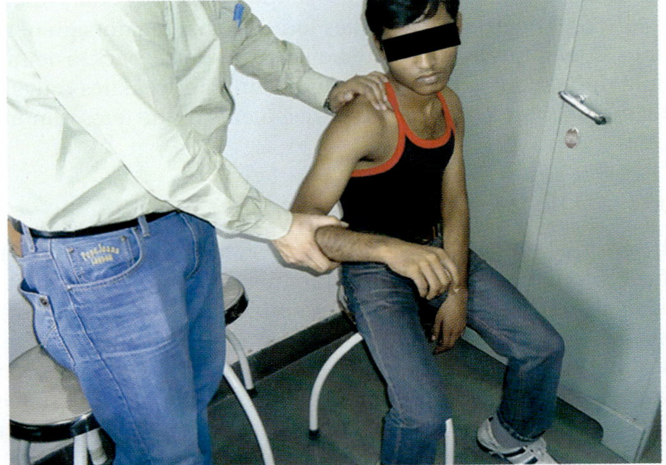

Fig. 222: Testing the weakness of rotator cuff muscles (mainly suprascapularis), while asking the patient to do shoulder abduction.

- External rotation lag sign
- Drop sign
- Internal rotation lag sign.

Lift-off Test

With the patient seated or standing, the arm is internally rotated, and the dorsum of the hand is placed against the lower back. If the patient is unable to lift the dorsum of the hand off the back, the test is positive. This test is done for subscapularis (Figs. 224 and 225).

Belly-press Test

In this test, the patient presses the abdomen with the flat of the hand and attempts to keep the arm in maximal internal rotation. If active internal rotation is strong, the elbow does not drop backward, meaning it remains in front of the trunk. If the strength of the subscapularis is impaired, maximal internal rotation cannot be maintained, the patient feels the weakness and the elbow drops back behind the trunk. The patient exerts pressure

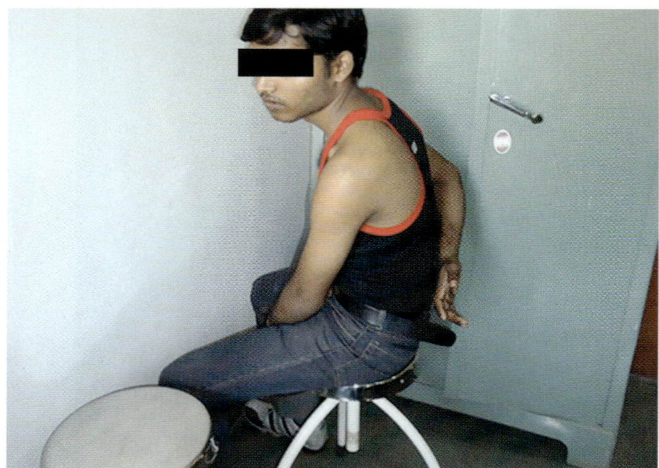

Fig. 224: Lift-off test done to check subscapularis injury or weakness.

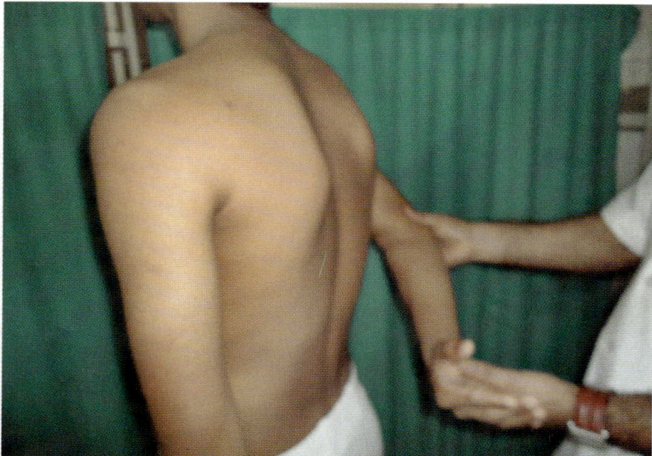

Fig. 225: Patient unable to lift off the hand, indicates positive test.

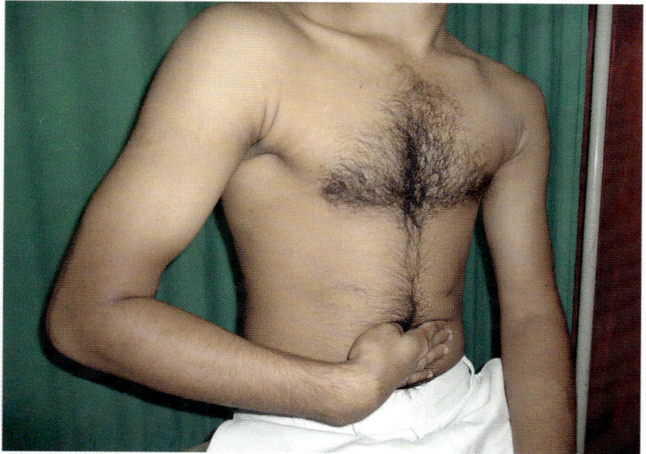

Fig. 226: Patient tends to flex the wrist to press against the abdomen, indicates subscapularis muscle being torn.

on the abdomen, by extending the shoulder, rather than by internally rotating it. Other investigators have noted that when the subscapularis tendon is torn, patients tend to flex the wrist to press against the abdomen and are unable to hold the elbow forward, as shown in Figures 226 and 227.

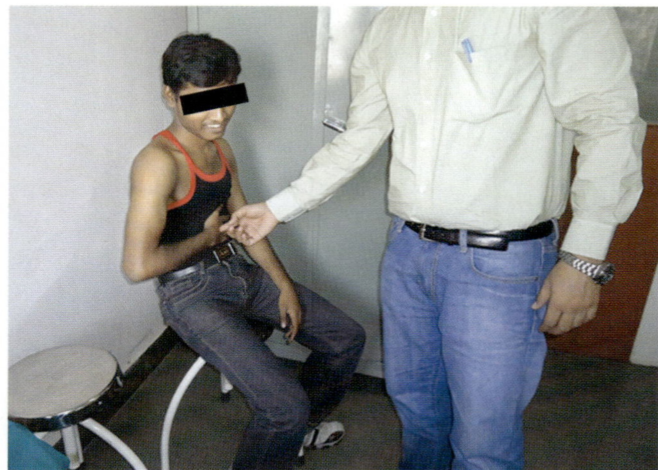

Fig. 227: Belly press test done to test the integrity of subscapularis tendon.

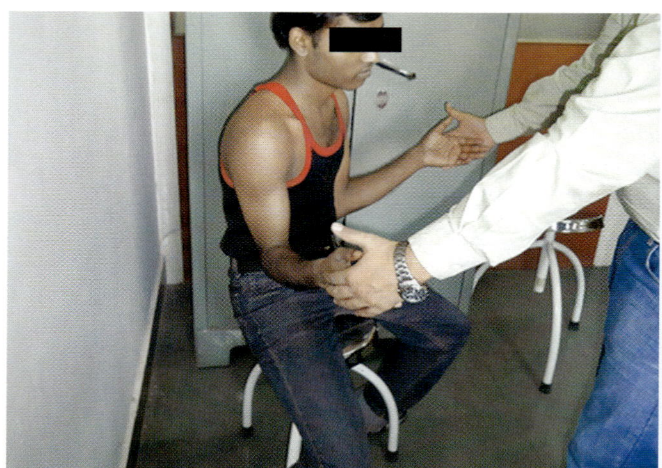

Fig. 228: External rotation stress test.

External Rotation Stress Test (Fig. 228)

The external rotation stress test is intended to test the integrity of the external rotators of the shoulder, specifically the infraspinatus and the teres minor. With the patient's arms by his or her side in neutral flexion and abduction, the shoulders are externally rotated by 45°–60°. The examiner applies force against the dorsum of the hands, attempting to rotate the shoulders internally back to neutral, while the patient is asked to resist. Pain and weakness suggest inflammation or tearing of the infraspinatus or the teres minor or both.

External Rotation Lag Sign (Fig. 229)

The external rotation lag sign test is designed to test the integrity of the supraspinatus and infraspinatus tendons. The patient is seated with his or her back to the examiner. The elbow is passively flexed to 90° and the shoulder is held at 20° of elevation and near maximal external rotation (maximal external rotation minus 5°, to avoid elastic recoil in the shoulder) by the examiner. The patient is asked to maintain the position of external rotation actively as the examiner releases the wrist, while maintaining support of the arm at the elbow. The sign is positive when a lag or angular drop is present.

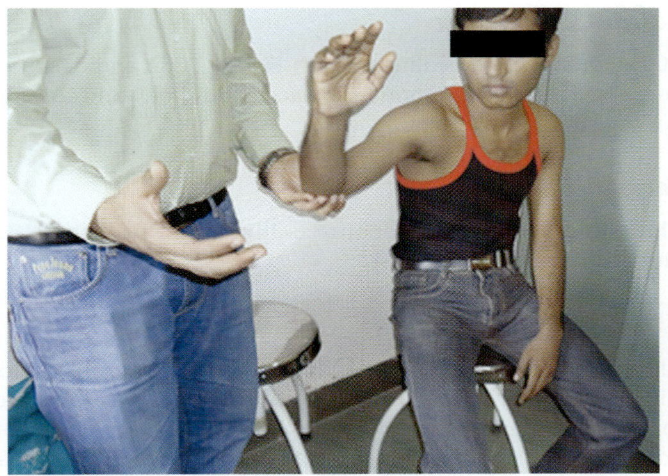

Fig. 229: The external rotation lag sign, to test the integrity of the supraspinatus and infraspinatus tendons.

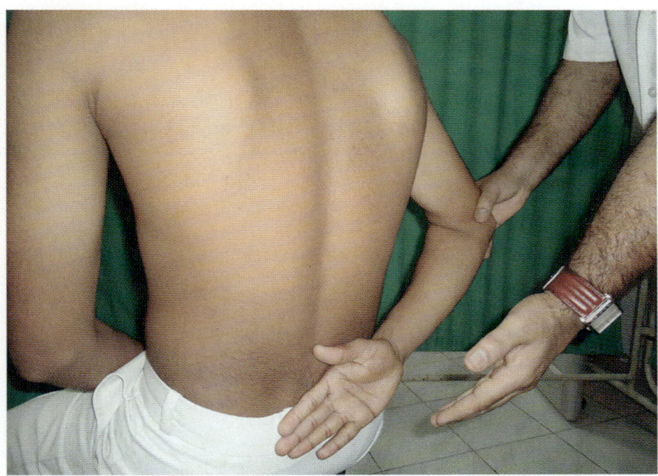

Fig. 231: Internal rotation lag sign.

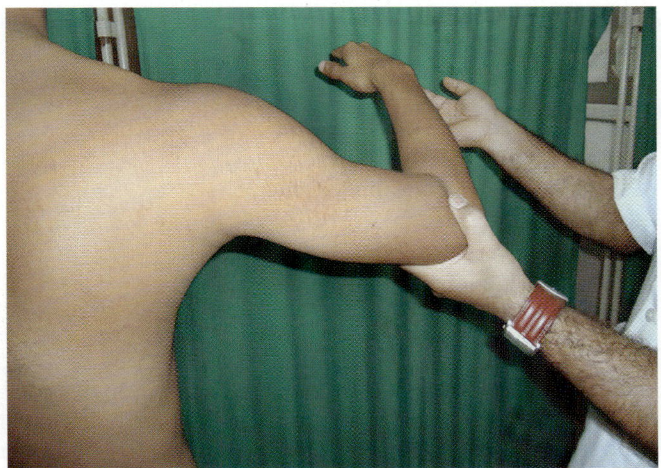

Fig. 230: The drop sign to test the integrity of the infraspinatus.

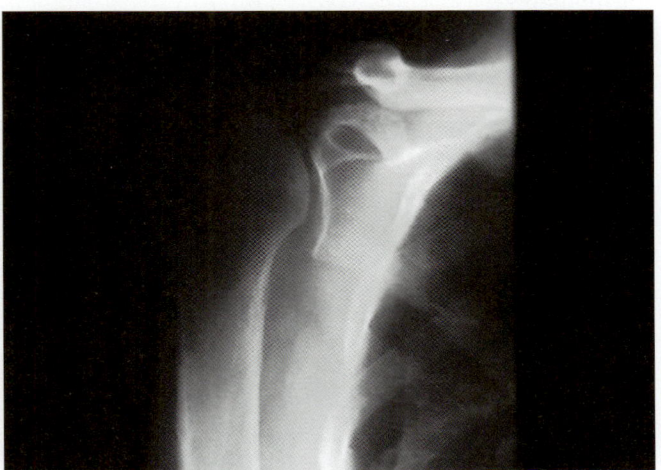

Fig. 232: X-ray findings in rotator cuff injuries.

Drop Sign (Fig. 230)

The drop sign is intended to test the integrity of the infraspinatus. The patient is seated with his or her back to the examiner. The affected arm is held at 90° of elevation in the scapular plane and at almost full external rotation with the elbow flexed at 90°. The patient is asked to maintain this position actively as the examiner releases the wrist while supporting the elbow, which is mainly a function of the infraspinatus. The sign is positive if a lag or a "drop" occurs.

Internal Rotation Lag Sign (Fig. 231)

The patient is seated with his or her back to the examiner. The affected arm is held by the examiner in almost maximal internal rotation. The elbow is flexed to 90°, and the shoulder is held at 20° of elevation and 20° of extension. The dorsum of the hand is passively lifted away from the lumbar region until almost full internal rotation is reached. The patient is asked to maintain this position actively as the examiner releases the wrist, while maintaining support at the elbow. The sign is positive when a lag occurs.

DIFFERENTIAL DIAGNOSIS

- Acromioclavicular arthritis
- Frozen shoulder
- Glenohumeral arthritis
- Herniated cervical disk
- Suprascapular nerve entrapment
- Fracture.

DIAGNOSTIC IMAGING

X-Rays

Reactive changes of the greater tuberosity on the undersurface of the acromion, sourcil or eyebrow and spur is seen, as shown in Figure 232. These occur due to failure of the cuff to keep the humeral head centered within the glenoid concavity, thus allowing it to ride higher due to unbalanced action of the deltoid and they rub on each other.

High-riding humeral head: Humeral head riding up and out of the normal glenoid concavity due to a loss of the normal compressive forces of the RC tendons, holding it into the socket.

Other Imaging Studies

- Arthrogram
- Ultrasound (Fig. 233)
- Magnetic resonance imaging (MRI) (Fig. 234)
- Computed tomography (CT) scan.

TREATMENT

Conservative Treatment

- Rest
- Nonsteroidal anti-inflammatory drugs (NSAIDs)
- Subacromial injections (Fig. 235)
- Muscle strengthening exercises.

Surgical Management

- Arthroscopic repair (Figs. 236A and B)
- Open acromioplasty (Figs. 237A to D)
- Open rotator cuff repairs
- Tendon transfers
- Humeral head replacement with maintenance of the CA arch for RC arthropathy.

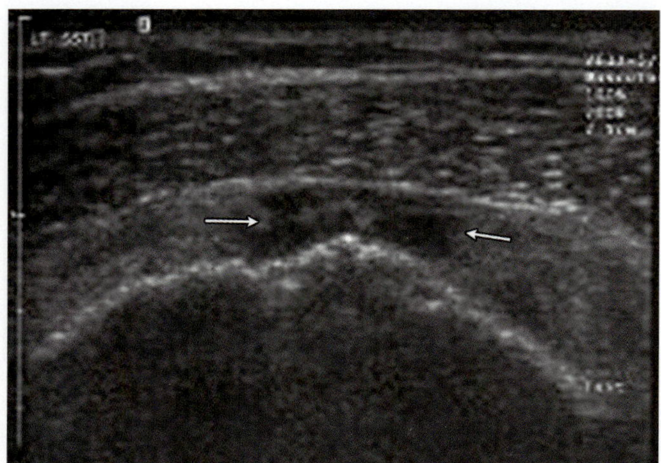

Fig. 233: Ultrasound used as a diagnostic technique to investigate about rotator cuff injuries.

Rotator Cuff Repair

McLaughlin technique illustrated in Figures 238A and B, sutures are passed through appropriately placed bony holes and cuff edge is drawn deep into trough.

Tendon Transfer

The tendon transfer procedure is illustrated in Figures 239 and 240.

After Treatment

After standard repair, an abduction pillow, a low profile pillow sling or shoulder immobilizer is worn for 6 weeks. It is removed for assisted exercises in flexion and external rotation to avoid adhesions, disuse atrophy and disruption of the repairs. The repair is weakest at 3 weeks and tendon strength is less than at the time of surgery for the first 3 months after the surgery. Empirically, we advance to isometric external rotation exercises at 6 weeks and at 12 weeks active motion is permitted. Patients are cautioned that overaggressive use of the extremity can lead to disruption of the repair for 6–12 months.

COMPLICATIONS

- Failed repairs
- Persistent subacromial impingement
- Stiffness
- Heterotropic ossification
- Deltoid insufficiency.

CALCIFIC TENDINITIS

Calcifying tendinitis (Fig. 241) of the RC is a common disorder of unknown etiology in which calcium crystals deposited in a living tendon in the course of reactive calcification usually undergone overtime with spontaneous resorption followed by healing of the tendon. Most commonly supraspinatus tendon is involved. Codman pointed out that diseases in the supraspinatus tendon tend to occur in a specific area of the tendon, i.e. about half an inch proximal to the insertion. He called this area, *the critical portion.*

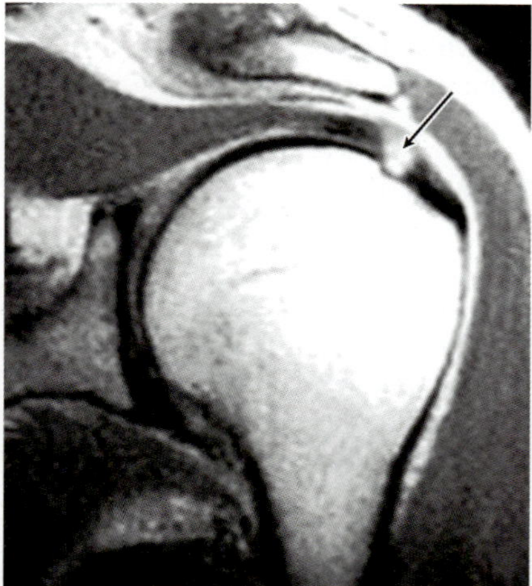

Fig. 234: MRI of shoulder showing rotator cuff injuries.

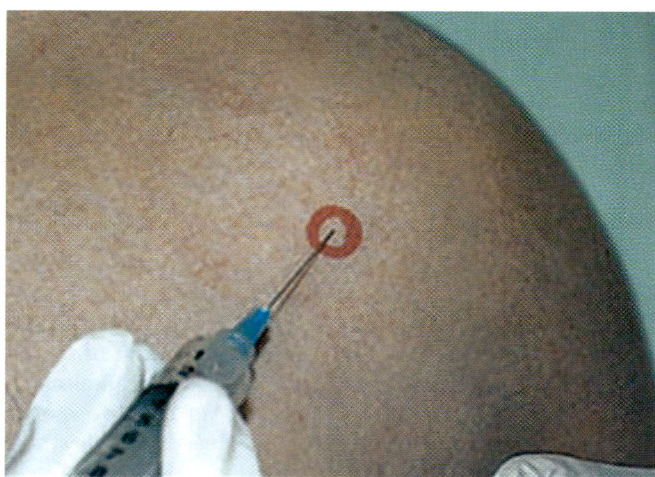

Fig. 235: Patient is given subacromial injections.

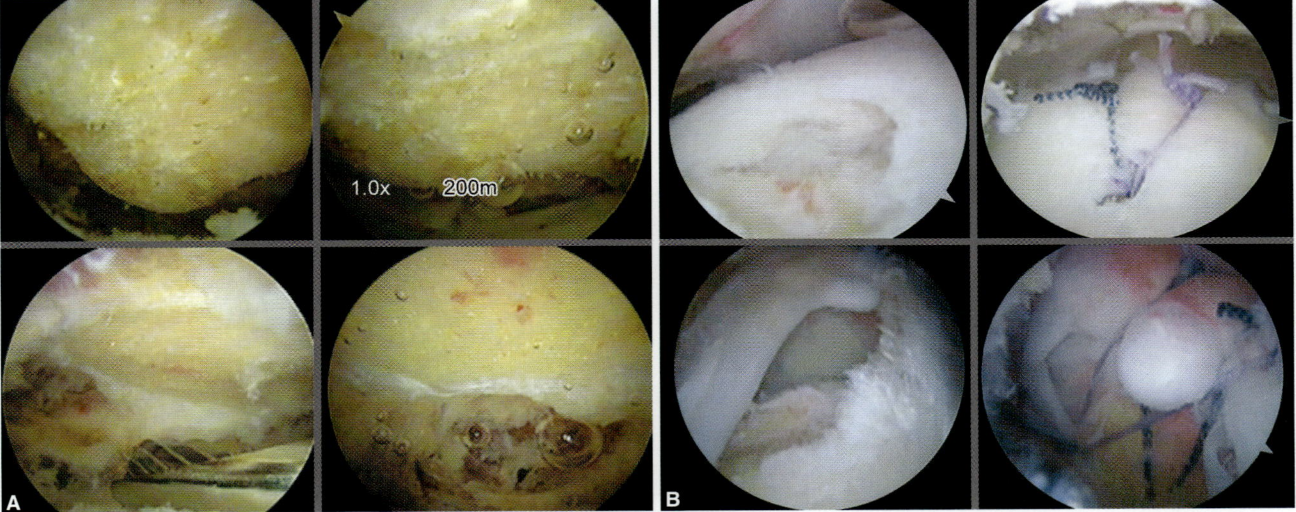

Figs. 236A and B: Arthroscopic repair.

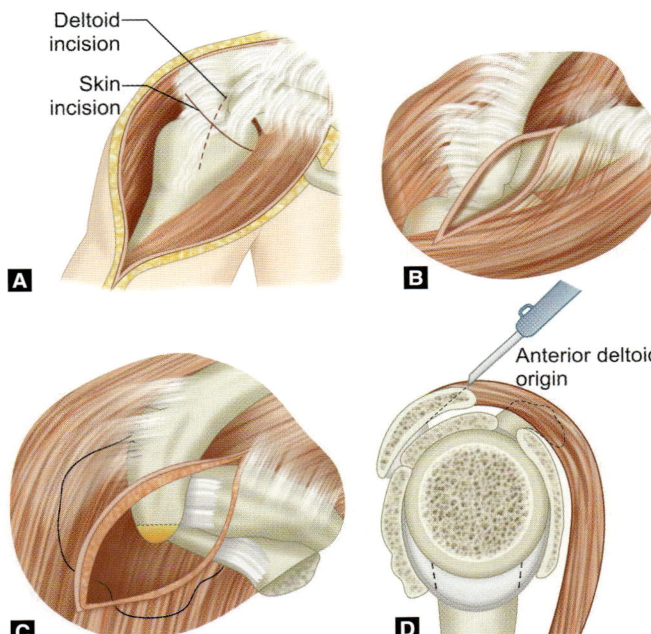

Figs. 237A to D: Open acromioplastic repair.

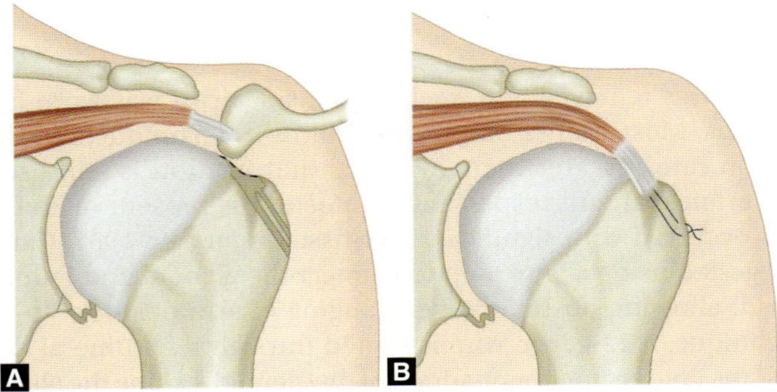

Figs. 238A and B: McLaughlin technique of rotator cuff repair.

Classification

This classification is based on the French Arthroscopic Society:

Type A: Sharply delineated, dense and homogeneous appearance.

Type B: Sharply delineated, dense and multiple fragments.

Type C: Heterogeneous appearance and fluffy.

Type D: Dystrophic calcifications at the tendon insertion.

Chronological Progression

Phase I: Precalcification stage, the site of predilection for calcification (possibly a site with a diminished blood supply) undergoes fibrocartilaginous metaplasia.

Phase II: Calcification stage, during this stage, calcium is deposited into the matrix vesicles, which are excreted by the cells and coalesce into larger calcium deposits.

Phase III: Postcalcification phase, during this phase, the granulation tissue matures into mature collagen aligned along stress lines with the longitudinal axis of the tendon, reconstituting the tendon.

Clinical Findings

- Pain is most common symptom associated with redness and swelling
- Painful arc of motion
- Range of motion decreased.

Imaging (Fig. 242)

Treatment

- Aspiration and needling of calcium deposits
- Excision of calcium deposits, as shown in Figures 243A and B.

SHOULDER ARTHRODESIS

HISTORY

Around the turn of the 20th century, shoulder arthrodesis was a relatively common procedure. Indications at that time were mainly for upper extremity paralysis, due to polio or shoulder

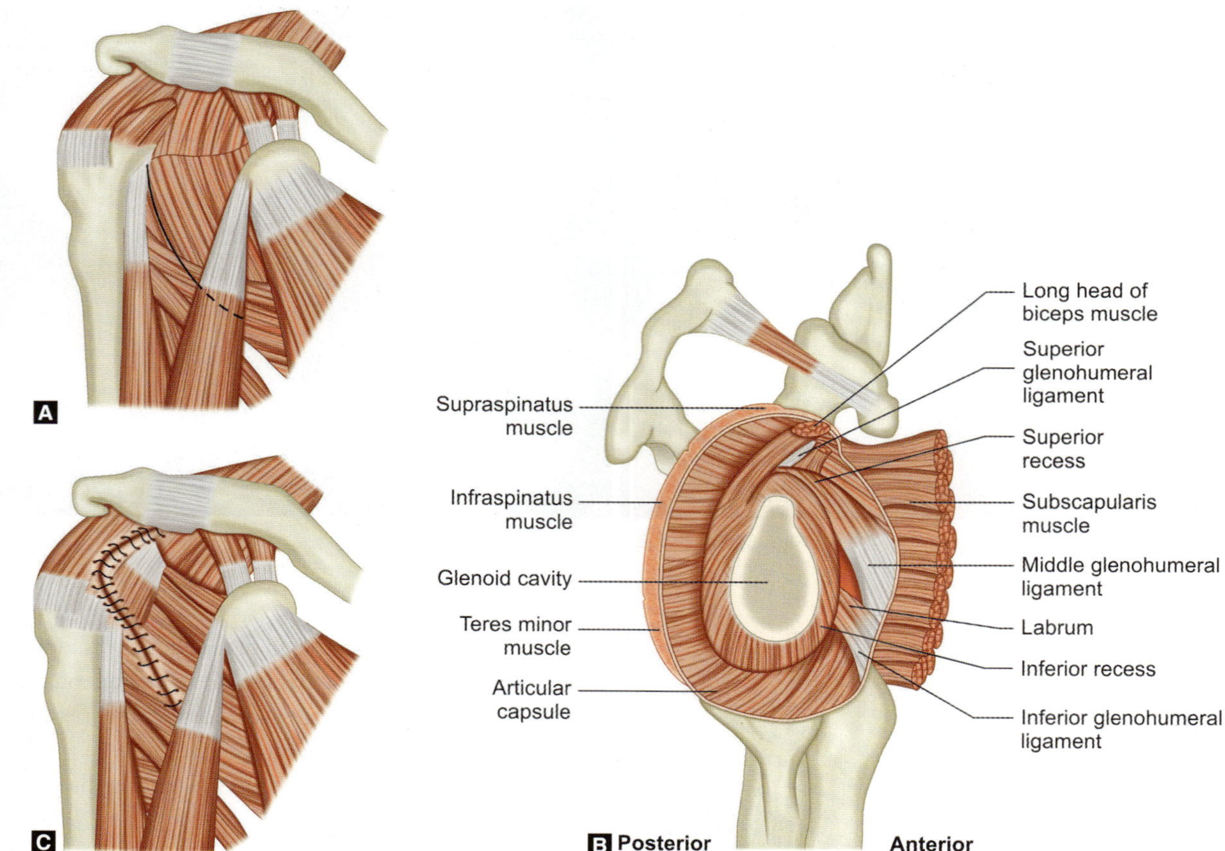

Figs. 239A to C: Technique or method employed for tendon transfer.

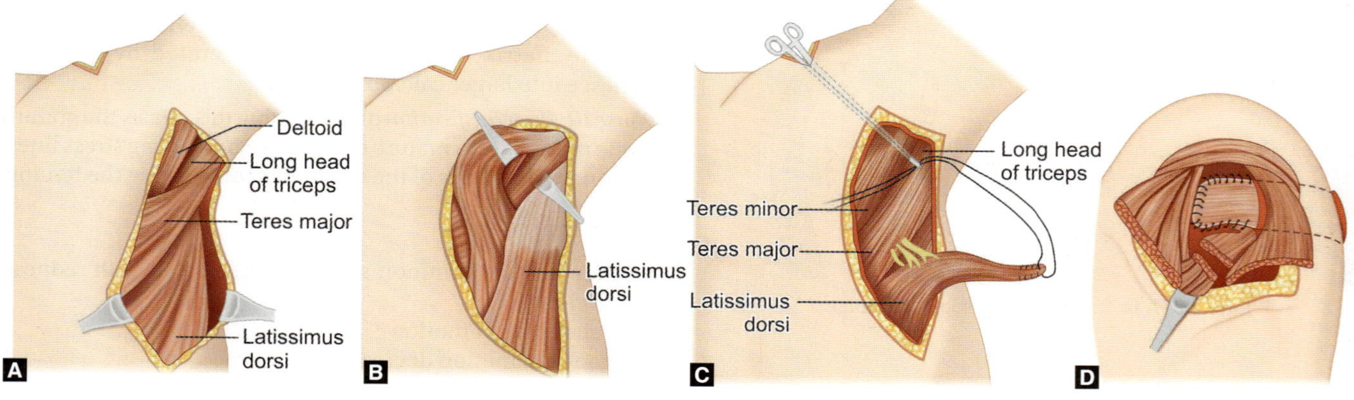

Figs. 240A to D: Tendon transfer procedure.

joint destruction, caused by tuberculosis. A purely extra-articular technique of shoulder arthrodesis was recommended for tuberculous infection, to prevent invasion from the infected joint. With the advent of antitubercular drugs, this technique became unnecessary. Later, procedures were described that placed various types of bone graft into the beds of the decorticated GH or acromiohumeral joints or both. Internal fixation is now recommended because external support alone rarely maintains complete fixation of the shoulder. Internal fixation allows better stabilization of contact surfaces and promotes fusion.

In the early 1950s, Charnley introduced the use of external fixation to apply compression across the fusion site. The external fixator was removed at 6 weeks and a spica cast was worn for 3 months. Most studies employing Charney's technique, reported fusion rates greater than 90%. External fixation is still useful in certain patients, especially if infection is present or trauma has occurred with significant soft-tissue injury. In 1957, Carroll suggested using a wire loop to connect the glenoid and humeral head, allowing postoperative changing of arm position. In this technique, a 22-gauge wire is routed through the humeral head and the anterosuperior quadrant of the glenoid, exiting the glenoid neck inferior to the coracoid process.

The 1960s saw the introduction of internal fixation for shoulder arthrodesis. Moseley and May described a technique,

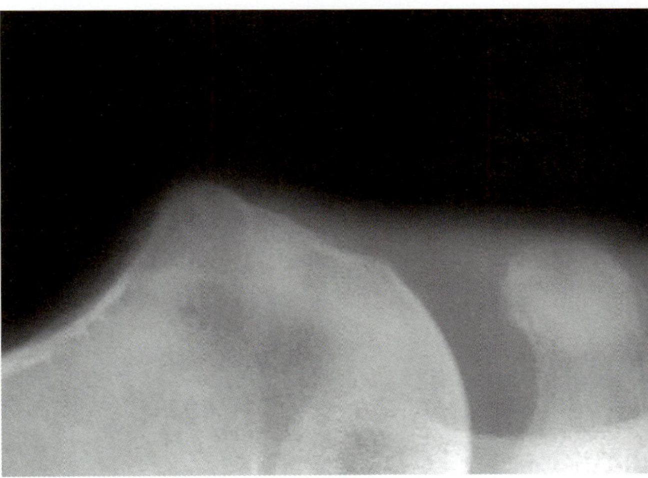

Fig. 241: Critical point for calcific tendinitis in supraspinatus.

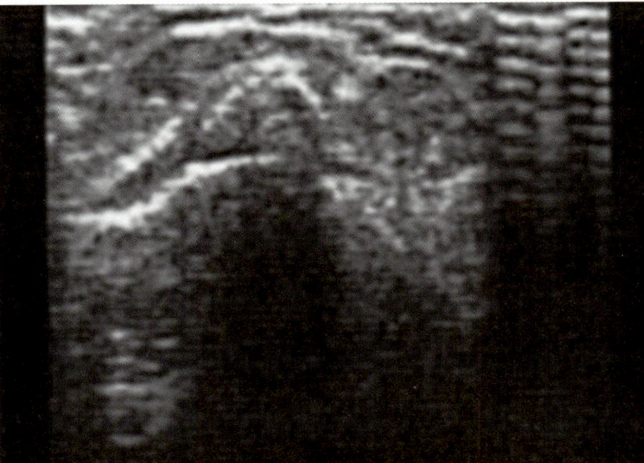

Fig. 242: Ultrasound imaging done as a diagnostic technique, to investigate about calcific tendinitis.

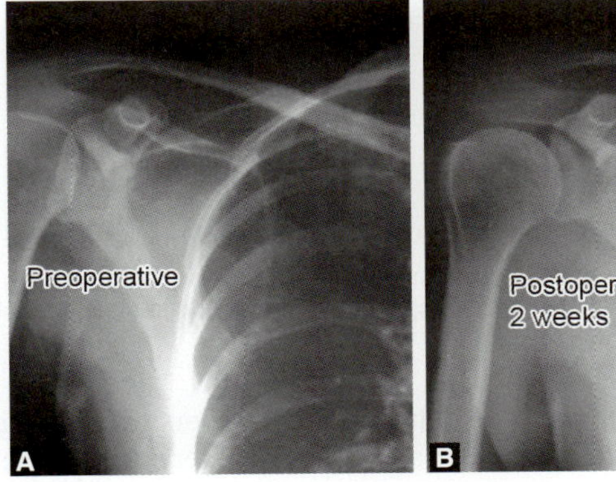

Figs. 243A and B: Radiographs showing excision of calcium deposits from tendon operatively: (A) Preoperative; (B) Postoperative view.

using internal fixation with two screws. Charnley and Houston described a technique that combined external fixation with internal fixation using screws. Disadvantages of screw fixation are a higher nonunion rate and the need for prolonged spica casting. In 1970, the Association of Orthopedics (AO) group published its technique of plate and screw fixation, to allow mobilization of the patient without a spica cast. Kostuik and Schatzker introduced the use of a second posterior buttress plate and obtained union in all 18 shoulders, they repaired using this technique. In the late 1980s, Richards et al. described a technique using a malleable pelvic reconstruction plate, without bone grafting followed by six postoperative weeks of spica casting.

INDICATIONS

Indications for GH arthrodesis are:

- Infection
- Paralytic disorders
- Unreconstructable RC tears
- Combined insufficiency of RC and deltoid
- Failed shoulder arthroplasty
- Arthritic diseases unsuitable for arthroplasty
- Recurrent dislocations
- Neoplastic lesions.

POSITION (FIGS. 244A TO D)

The proper position of the arm at the time of arthrodesis is controversial. In 1974, Rowe recognized the advantages of minimizing abduction and flexion. Cofield and Briggs found the amount of internal rotation to be the most important factor in determining the functional success of the operation. Hawkins and Neer performed a functional analysis in 17 patients, who had shoulder arthrodesis and identified a range of acceptable positions. They recommended 25°–40° of abduction, 20°–30° of flexion and 25°–30° of internal rotation. Abduction can be determined at the time of surgery, by clinically measuring the angle formed by the body and the humerus. This angle or an angle specifically determined preoperatively, can be determined by obtaining an anteroposterior radiographic view, using the spine rather than the border of the scapula as a landmark, as recommended by Ingram and Miller.

Flexion is determined, by observing the angle that the humerus forms with the horizontal plane in a supine patient. After the positions of abduction and flexion have been determined, the elbow is flexed to 90°. The hand is positioned over the ipsilateral area of the chest between the sternum and axilla, so that further flexion of the elbow allows the top of the thumb to touch the chin (Figs. 245A and B).

SURGICAL TECHNIQUES

When choosing the technique to be used, an attempt at fusion should be made between the acromion and humeral head and the GH joint. Stable internal fixation can reduce the need for bone grafting and external fixation or spica casting.

Methods

- External fixation
- Internal fixation
- Internal fixation with bone grafting.

External Fixation

Charnley described a procedure to accomplish shoulder arthrodesis, by applying external compression. In 1964, Charnley and Houston modified this technique to allow easier adjustment of arm position. Charnley and Houston technique of compression arthrodesis of shoulder involve following steps:

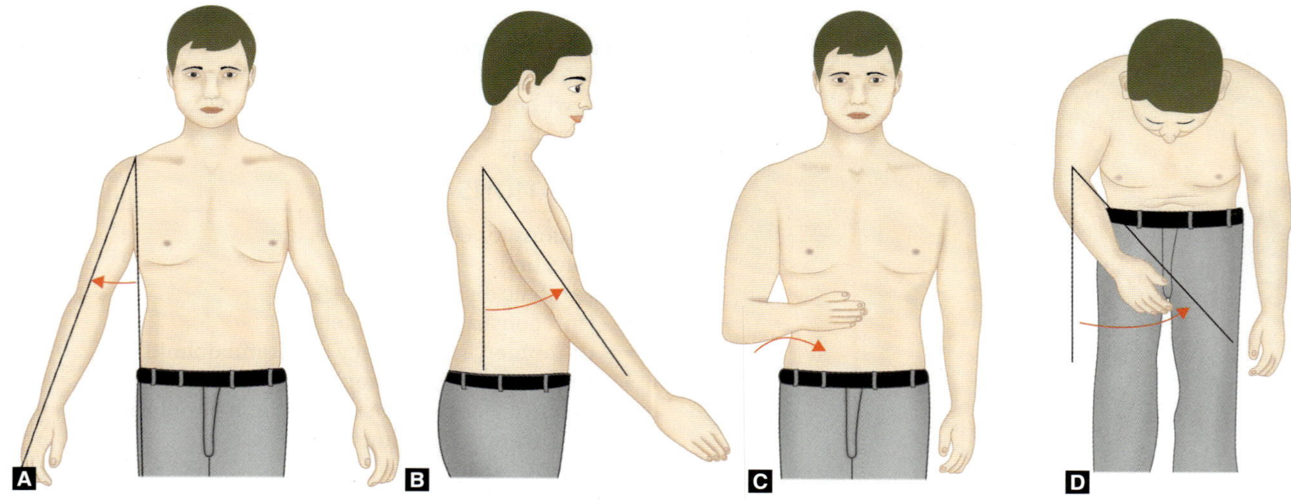

Figs. 244A to D: Various positions of arm at the time of arthrodesis.

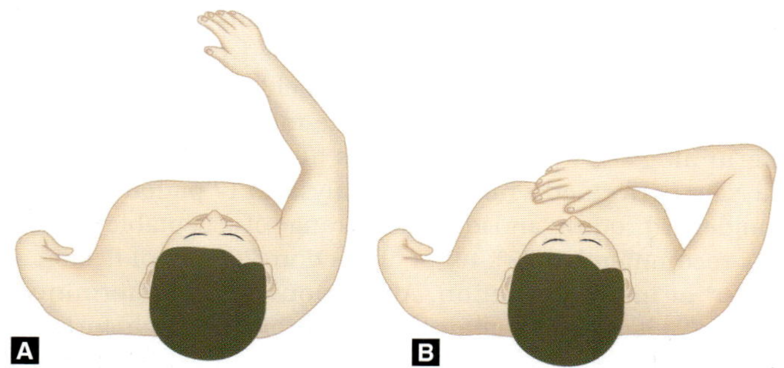

Figs. 245A and B: Recommended position of limb for shoulder arthrodesis—(A) Arm is abducted and flexed; (B) The hand is positioned over the ipsilateral area of the chest between the sternum and axilla, so that further flexion of the elbow allows the top of the thumb to touch the chin.

1. First apply the trunk portion of a shoulder spica cast with the patient awake, allow it to harden, then bivalve it and save it for later use. Position the patient in a semireclining or beach chair posture and make a saber cut incision, centered over the lateral border of the acromion.
2. Using electrocautery, take down the anterior and lateral deltoid muscle, tag and retract this muscle. Excise the soft tissue from the subacromial space. Denude the upper half of the glenoid fossa of articular cartilage and the undersurface of the acromion to bleeding bone. Remove the articular cartilage from the humeral head and reduce the joint.
3. With an osteotome, split off the greater tuberosity and resect enough bone from the humeral head, to allow it to sublux superiorly against the undersurface of the acromion and the superior part of the glenoid fossa. Use the resected bone as graft material around the fusion; this is illustrated in Figures 246A to C.
4. Insert a 4 mm pin from the posterosuperior aspect of the acromion into the scapular neck deep to the glenoid fossa, as shown in Figure 247. Another pin can be placed in the base of the coracoid process.
5. Insert a second set of similar pins into the surgical neck of the humerus posterolaterally, perpendicular to the shaft of the humerus.
6. Construct an external frame of adjustable pin clamps and bars; connect it to the pins for application of compression with the arm in the desired position for arthrodesis. Reattach the deltoid to the acromion and close the wound in layers over a drain. Apply the previously made part of the shoulder spica cast and complete it, incorporating the external fixator.

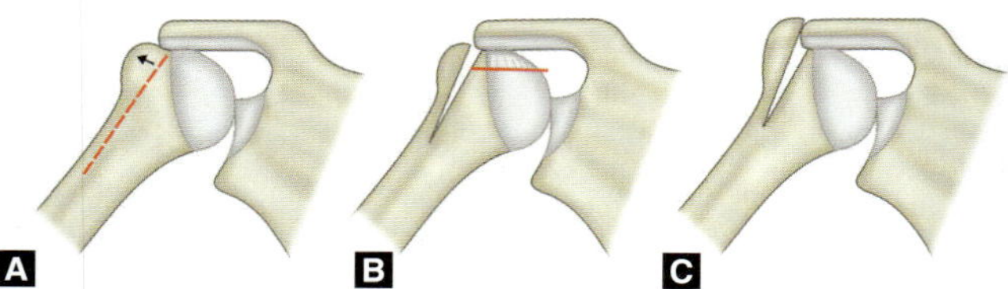

Figs. 246A to C: Various steps involved in Charnley and Houston technique of compression arthrodesis of shoulder.

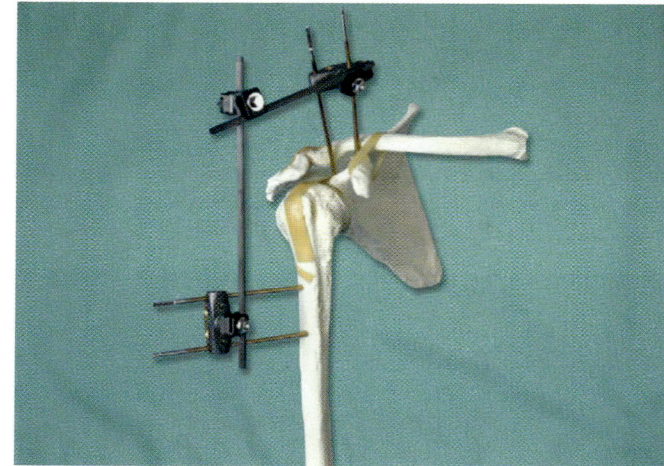

Fig. 247: Illustration showing methods employed in inserting a 4 mm pin from the posterosuperior aspect of the acromion into the scapular neck deep to the glenoid fossa.

After treatment:

The pins and external fixator are removed at 5–6 weeks and the cast is changed. The second cast is removed at 12 weeks from the time of surgery and the shoulder is examined for stability. Immobilization is continued until the arthrodesis is solid.

Screw Fixation

Cofield described a shoulder fusion technique, using screw fixation through a strap incision that may be extended posteriorly, if needed, as shown in Figure 248. The position and number of screws

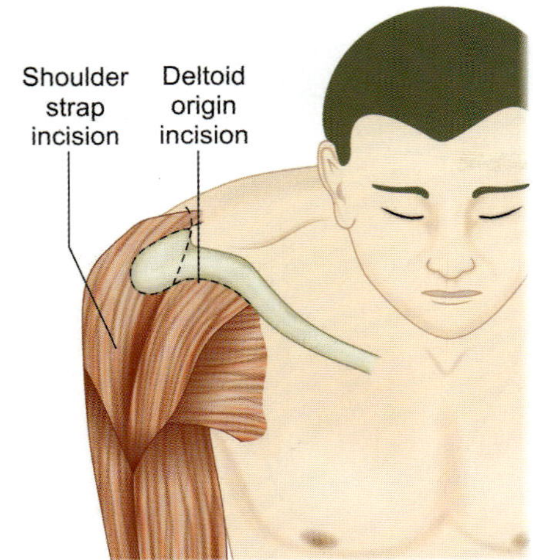

Fig. 248: Shoulder fusion technique by screw fixation through a strap incision.

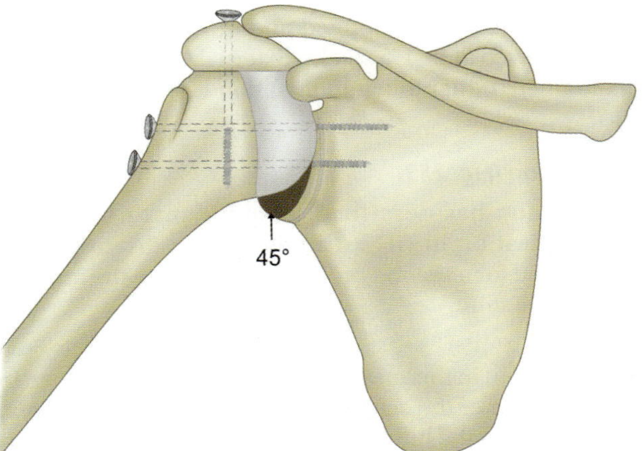

Fig. 249: Shoulder arthrodesis with screw fixation.

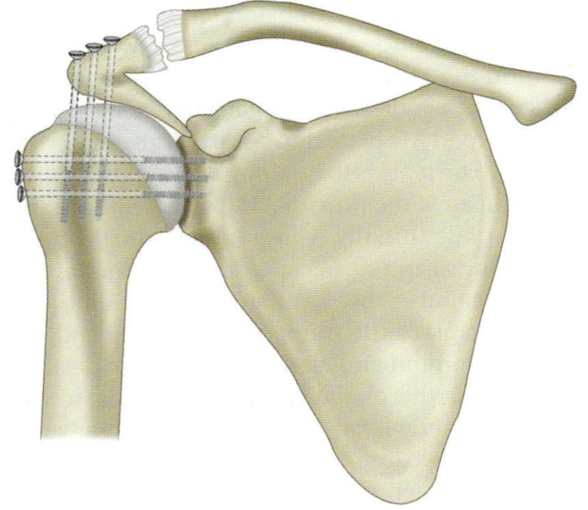

Fig. 250: Shoulder arthrodesis with screw fixation. The position and number of screws used vary, depending on the indication for arthrodesis and the condition of the bone at the time of surgery.

used vary, depending on the indication for arthrodesis and the condition of the bone at the time of surgery; this is demonstrated in Figures 249 and 250. Advantages of screw over plate fixation include, less soft-tissue dissection, lower infection rate, decreased rate of postoperative humeral fractures and lesser need to remove painful hardware. Current data still show a higher nonunion rate with screw fixation, however compared with plate fixation.

Procedure:

Place the patient in the beach chair position. Make an anterosuperior shoulder strap incision. Remove the deltoid from the anterior, lateral acromion and from the lateral clavicle. Incise the rotator cuff longitudinally in the supraspinatus and transversely from anterior to posterior. Remove the proximal biceps tendon from the superior glenoid. If the AC joint is arthritic, perform a distal clavicle excision. Position the upper extremity in 45° of abduction, flexion and internal rotation. Flexion and abduction may need to be adjusted to 30°, to allow the thumb, with the forearm in neutral, to touch the nose. Debride the bony surfaces, especially the humeral head, to increase surface contact areas.

Definitive fixation is determined by the indication for arthrodesis and by the status of bone stock. Drill two or three 0.125 inch of Steinmann pins or guidewires for cannulated screws, through the humeral head and into the glenoid, to secure the humerus to the scapula.

Assess the arm position. If it is acceptable, replace the Steinmann pins with cancellous screws over washers. Place one to three screws through the acromion and into the humeral head. Place a drain deep to the deltoid and attach the deltoid proximally to the trapezius, while covering the plate.

After treatment:

A pelvic band extending from the nipples to the pubic symphysis is applied. With the elbow flexed 90°, a cylinder cast is applied to the upper extremity. The extremity is suspended by two wooden struts or a cockup wrist splint is used. At 1–2 weeks after surgery, a plastic shoulder spica cast is applied and worn until union is achieved, 12–16 weeks after surgery.

Uematsu Posterior Approach (Fig. 251)

Position the patient on the unaffected side and make an incision 10–12 cm long, extending laterally from the middle of the scapular spine along the spine and ending 2.5 cm, distal to the acromion. Detach the deltoid and trapezius from the scapular spine and expose the supraspinatus and infraspinatus and retract them out of the way.

Make an oblique osteotomy from the lateral third of the scapular spine to the spinoglenoid notch and lateral third of the acromion, without entering the acromioclavicular joint. The osteotomized fragment may be used as a muscle pedicle bone graft, if the deltoid attachment is retained. Otherwise, it may be used as a free graft. Divide the tendinous attachments of the supraspinatus and infraspinatus, about 1.5 cm from their insertions on the greater tuberosity. Remove all articular cartilage from the glenoid fossa, humeral head and decorticate the posterior aspect of the glenoid fossa.

Position the arm in 20° of abduction, 30° of forward flexion and 40° of internal rotation. This is determined clinically with the arm at the side of the body. Insert three ASIF cancellous screws through the humeral head into the glenoid fossa and scapular neck. Check for stability and use additional screws if necessary. Fix the acromial bone graft posteriorly. Close the wound in layers over a drain, taking care to secure a tight closure of the trapeziodeltoid interval. Apply a sterile dressing and suspend the arm by overhead skin traction.

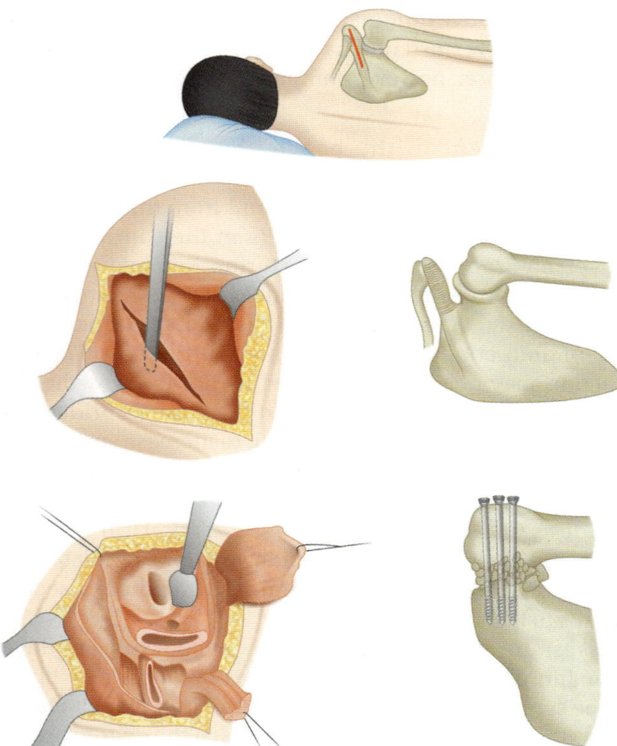

Fig. 251: Uematsu posterior approach for shoulder arthrodesis.

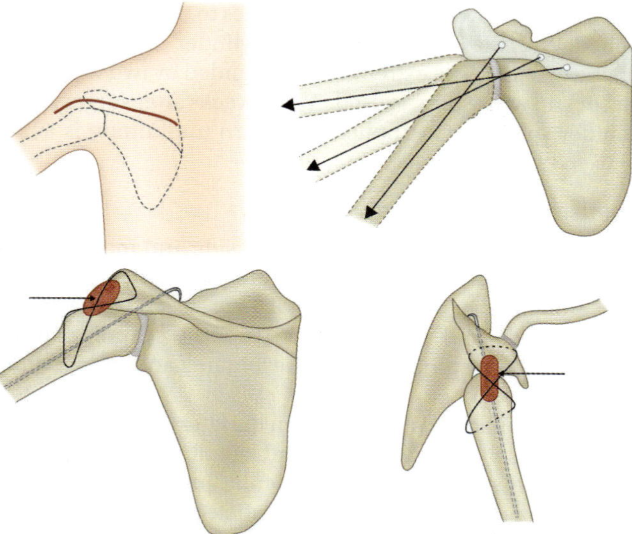

Fig. 252: Tension band wiring performed through posterior approach.

After treatment:
The dressing is changed and the drain is removed on the second day. With the patient standing, a shoulder spica cast is applied. A cast is worn for 3 months or until union become solid radiographically. Then rehabilitation of the upper extremity is begun.

Tension Band Fixation (Fig. 252)

In 1998, Mohammed reported his results of shoulder arthrodesis, using a rush rod, tension band and a muscle pedicle graft through a posterior approach.

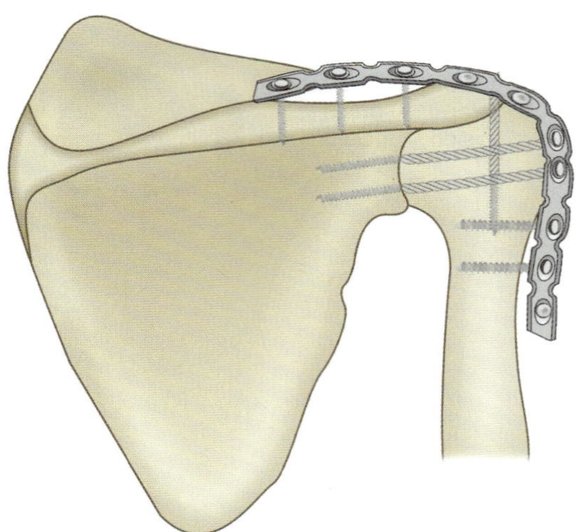

Fig. 253: Plate fixation for shoulder arthrodesis.

After treatment:
A shoulder spica cast is applied and movement of the wrist and elbow is allowed after 4–6 weeks. External support of the shoulder is maintained, until radiographic union is shown, usually at 8–10 weeks.

Plate Fixation (Fig. 253)

The AO group has described a double plating technique for rigid stabilization in GH arthrodesis. The disadvantage is the possible need for a second procedure to remove the implants after arthrodesis is solid.

Technique:
Place the patient in the lateral decubitus position. Make an incision along the spine of the scapula, over the acromion and along the proximal third of the humerus. Expose the scapular spine, glenoid fossa and proximal third of the humerus. Denude the glenoid fossa and humeral head of all cartilage. Decorticate the undersurface of the acromion and the lateral portion of the humerus for contact with the acromion. An osteotomy of the acromion may be necessary to increase surface contact between the plate and bones. Position the humeral head in the desired position in the glenoid fossa. Use a malleable template, to determine the contour for a standard broad AO plate and contour the plate with bending press and irons. The plate is to lie along the scapular spine, over the acromion and against the proximal third of the humerus.

Fasten the plate initially with a long cortical screw inserted vertically into the scapular neck. Insert the remaining proximal screws into the scapula using standard AO technique, as illustrated in Figure 254. Displace the humerus superiorly and medially to lie against the acromion and glenoid fossa in the desired position for arthrodesis. Fix the plate distally, with two screws that pass through it, the humeral head, into the glenoid fossa and scapular neck. Insert at least two more screws to fix the plate to the humerus. If the plate does not achieve complete stability at the arthrodesis site, apply a second plate posteriorly from the scapular spine to the humerus. Apply bone grafts as desired and close the wound in layers over drains.

After treatment:
A Velpeau dressing is applied. The sutures are removed at 2 weeks if nonabsorbable. Active rehabilitation of the elbow, wrist and hand is begun within the first few days after surgery, but care should

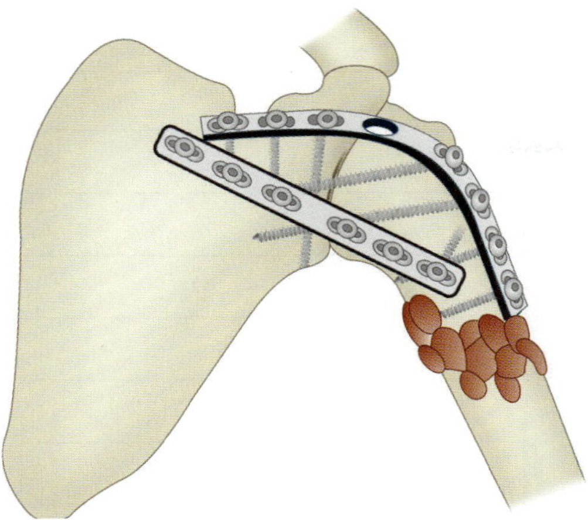

Fig. 254: The plate initially fastened with a long cortical screw inserted vertically into the scapular neck and remaining proximal screws into the scapula using standard AO technique.

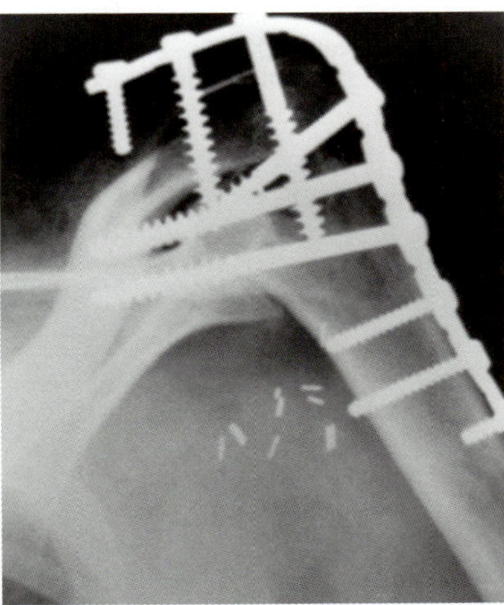

Fig. 255: Pelvic reconstruction plate, used to overcome technical difficulties of contouring the AO plate.

be taken not to place stress on the fusion site. A double plating technique can also be used.

Pelvic Reconstruction Plate (Fig. 255)

Richards et al. believe the technical difficulties of contouring the AO plate and the occasional problems caused by prominent screws can be overcome by the use of a malleable pelvic reconstruction plate.

After treatment:
The arm is supported with a pillow and a swathe. A shoulder spica cast is applied 48 hours after surgery. If there is no radiographic evidence of loosening of the internal fixation device 6 weeks after surgery, the arm is placed in a sling. Only gentle ROM exercises are allowed, until union is seen on radiograph. Strenuous activity is delayed for at least 16 weeks after surgery.

COMPLICATIONS OF GLENOHUMERAL ARTHRODESIS

- Infection
- Wound hematoma
- Skin slough
- Pressure sores under spica cast
- Pseudarthrosis/nonunion
- Painful hardware
- Malposition
- Ipsilateral humeral fracture
- Traction neuritis
- Periscapular muscle strain
- Acromioclavicular arthritis
- Epiphyseal problems or growth arrest.

SHOULDER ARTHROPLASTY

Lesions of the shoulder requiring arthroplasty are less common than lesions involving the weight-bearing joints of the body, such as hip and knee. A comparison between major joint replacement surgeries in terms of volume is shown in Figure 256.

THE SHOULDER (FIG. 257)

- Greatest ROM
- No inherent bony stability
- Relies on soft tissues for stability
- Many injuries involve the soft tissues, e.g. RC and labrum
- Little glenoid bone stock (Fig. 257).

Other anatomic variables to consider:

- Glenoid with 2° anteversion to 7° retroversion
- *Humeral offset:* Medially (coronal) of 4–14 mm, posteriorly (transverse) of 2–10 mm
- Glenoid inclination varies from 7°–20°
- Humeral head inclination of 30°–55°
- Humeral head is in 20°–40° of retroversion
- Axial computed tomography (CT scan) of the GH joint is a valuable preoperative planning tool.

BIOMECHANICS (FIG. 258)

Top of the humeral head is higher than greater tuberosity, as illustrated in Figure 259.

INDICATIONS FOR SHOULDER ARTHROPLASTY (FIG. 260)

- Osteoarthritis
- Rheumatoid arthritis
- Rotator cuff tear arthropathy
- Avascular necrosis
- Post-traumatic arthritis
- Severe proximal humeral fractures
- Neoplastic lesions.

CHOICE OF PROSTHESIS

Following points are considered before applying prosthesis:

- Patient's age
- Condition of glenoid surface and bone stock
- Axillary nerve palsy is a relative contraindication to arthroplasty.

Arthroplasty Options

Different arthroplastic techniques are illustrated in Figures 261 to 263.

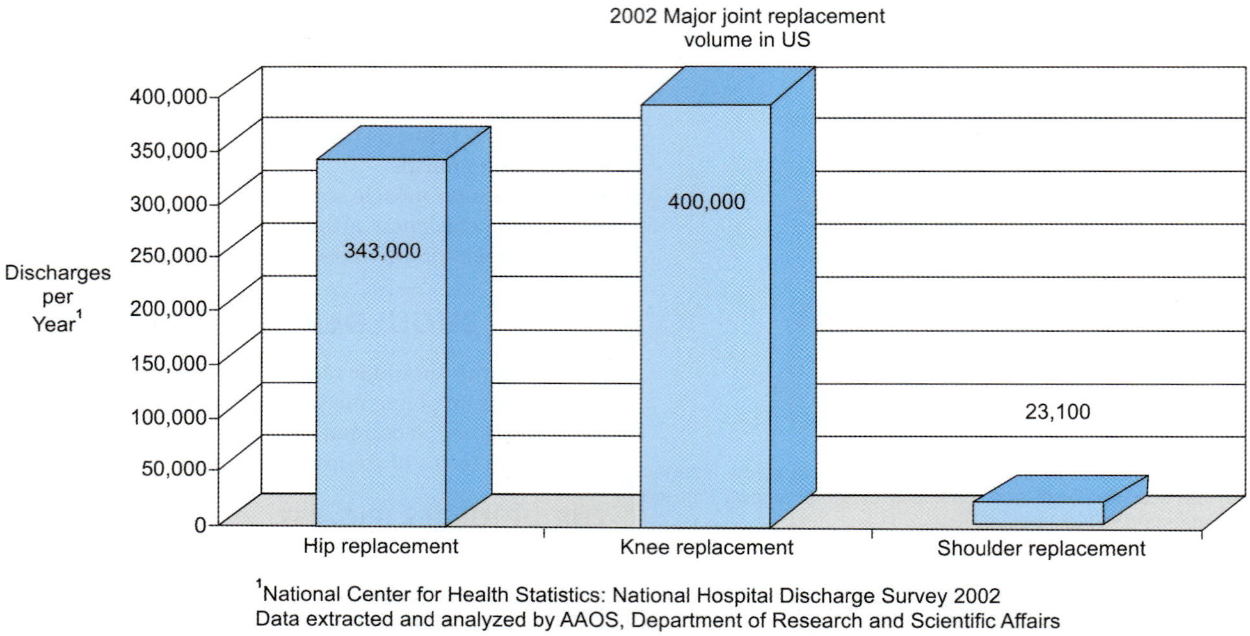

2002 Major joint replacement volume in US
400,000
350,000
300,000
250,000
200,000
150,000
100,000
50,000
0
Discharges per Year[1]
343,000
400,000
23,100
Hip replacement
Knee replacement
Shoulder replacement
[1]National Center for Health Statistics: National Hospital Discharge Survey 2002
Data extracted and analyzed by AAOS, Department of Research and Scientific Affairs

Fig. 256: Major joint replacement surgeries in terms of volume.

Glenoid
Humeral head
Humerus

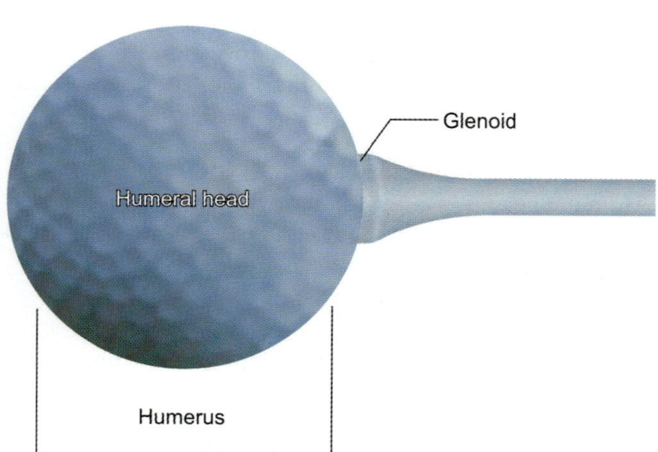

Fig. 257: Glenohumeral joint compared to a golf ball on a tee.

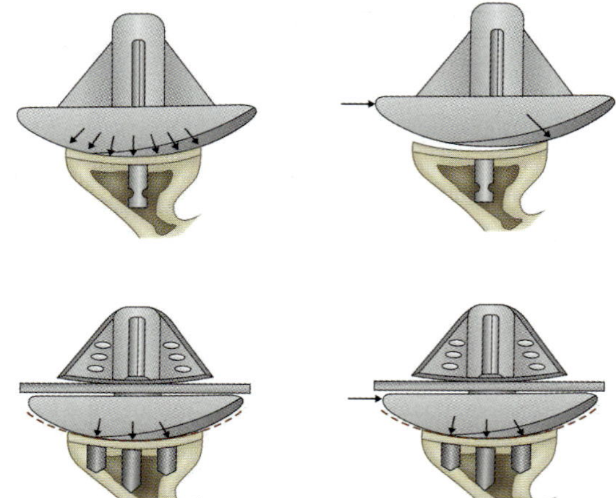

Fig. 259: Illustration showing top of the humeral head is higher than greater tuberosity.

F
G
E
D
H
C
M
A
B
o
α
N

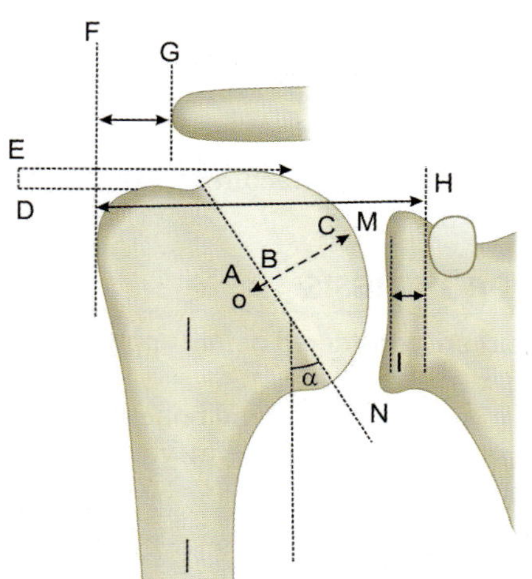

Fig. 258: Shoulder joint biomechanics: F–H = Offset; B–C = Head thickness; D–E = 8 mm.

Glenoid prosthesis
Humeral prosthesis

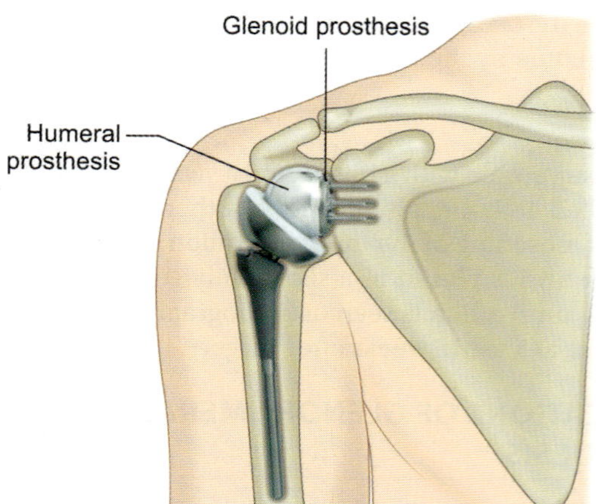

Fig. 260: Total shoulder arthroplasty.

HISTORY

1893: French surgeon Pean inserted platinum and rubber components to replace a shoulder joint destroyed by tuberculosis.

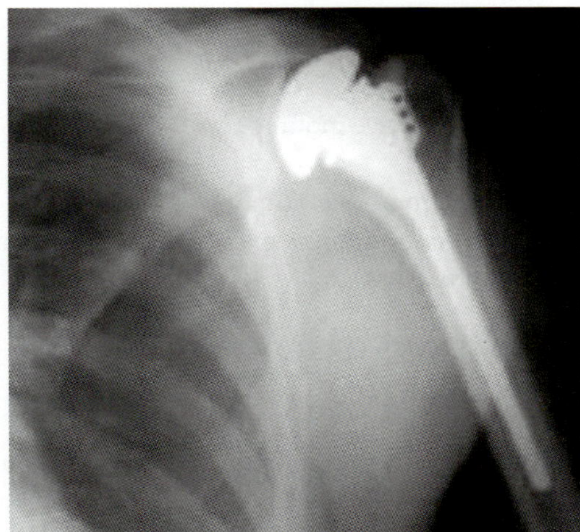

Fig. 261: X-ray taken after hemiarthroplasty.

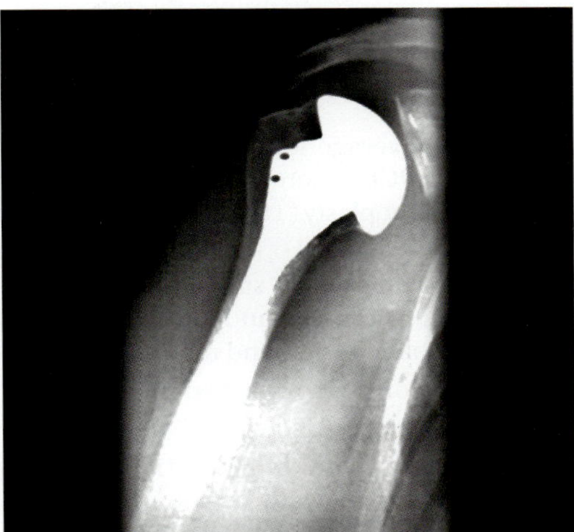

Fig. 262: X-ray total shoulder arthroplasty.

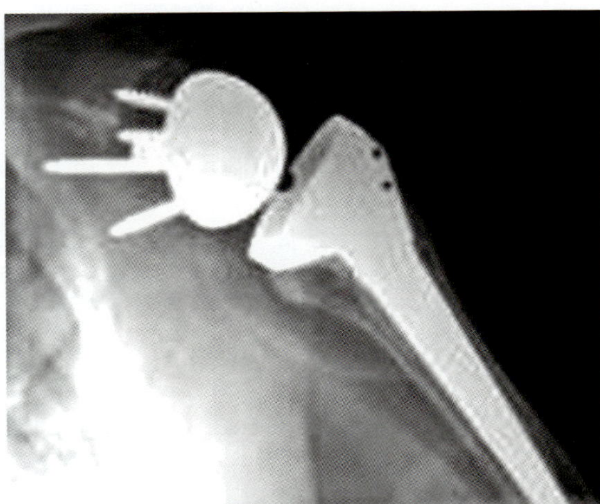

Fig. 263: Reverse total shoulder arthroplasty.

1951: Neer I prosthesis, vitallium hemiarthroplasty prosthesis which resulted in pain relief and good function compared to previous options.

1974: Neer II prosthesis (a modified Neer I prosthesis, to conform to a glenoid component). This is shown in Figure 264.

1970: Constrained components were popular, but follow-up reports demonstrated high rates of loosening, particularly of the glenoid component, as demonstrated in Figure 265.

1980: Modular humeral components were developed along with cementless glenoid fixation using polyethylene on a metal backing.

Boileau P and Avidor C, 2002

Cemented polyethylene versus uncemented metal backed glenoid components in total shoulder arthroplasty (TSA)—a prospective, double-blind, randomized study.

Forty shoulders with 3 years follow-up:
Metal-backed: 2% radiolucent lines, 100% progressive, 25% loose in 3 years. It is associated with shift and osteolysis.

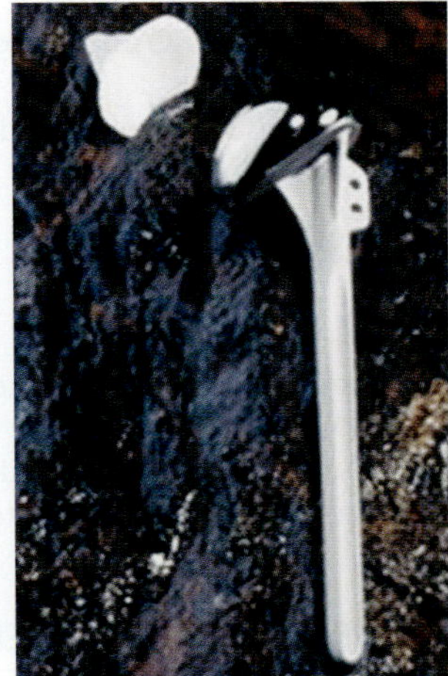

Fig. 264: Neer II prosthesis.

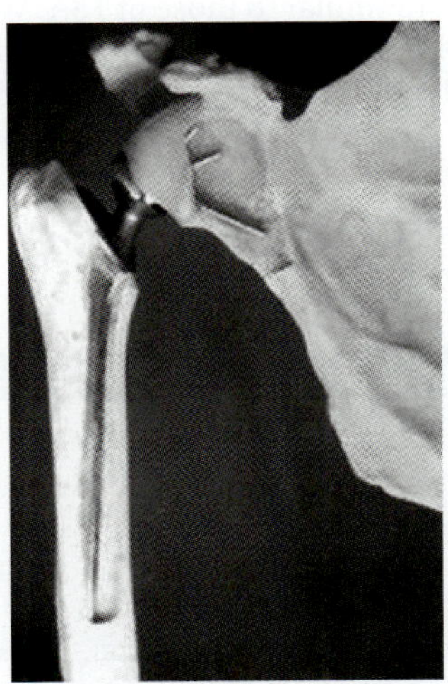

Fig. 265: A loosened prosthesis.

Cemented: 80% radiolucent lines, 25% progressive. None loose in 3 years.[1]

Other problems with metal-backed glenoid components are:

- Metal backing increased the thickness of the component and often leads to over stuffing of the joint
- To avoid over stuffing of the joint, the polyethylene thickness had to be reduced, resulting in accelerated polywear and failure
- Polymetal disassociation occurred with unacceptable frequency.

Humeral Components (Table 6)

Cemented vs press fit humeral components: Harris, Jobe, and Dai reported less micromotion with proximally cemented stems. Fully cemented stems provide no additional benefit or stability over proximally cemented stems. Sanchez-Sotelo reported a low rate of stem loosening regardless of fixation, but press fit prosthesis developed more radiolucent lines in the first 4 years.

Need for modularity: Re-establishing normal GH anatomic relationships is important to ensure optimal results.

CONTRAINDICATIONS TO SHOULDER ARTHROPLASTY

- Active or recent shoulder joint infection
- Paralysis with complete loss of RC and deltoid function
- A neuropathic arthropathy
- Irreparable RC tear is a relative contraindication to glenoid resurfacing.

SURGICAL APPROACH (FIG. 266)

Osteoarthritis (OA)

In addition to the universal features of osteoarthritic joints, shoulder can also demonstrate joint space narrowing, cysts, osteophytes, posterior glenoid erosion, flattening of the humeral head, enlargement of the humeral head. Rotator cuff tears are uncommon in OA.

RECOMMENDATIONS BASED ON EXPERIENCE

Neer, 1998

"When the articular surface of the glenoid is good, the results of hemiarthroplasty are similar to those of TSA. Wear on the glenoid has not been a problem if the articular surface was good at the time of surgery and GH motion was re- established".[2]

Hemi vs Total Shoulder

- Easy procedure
- Short operating time
- Less risk of instability
- Can be revised to TSA
- Less reliable pain relief
- Progressive glenoid erosion may cause results to deteriorate over time
- Need concentric glenoid
- More consistent pain relief
- Better fulcrum for active motion
- Difficult procedure
- Longer operation room (OR) time
- Polywear can cause loosening of both the components
- More glenoid bone loss.

TABLE 6: Different humeral components of a prosthesis.

Cemented	*Prox porous coated*	*Fully porous coated*
Good for osteopenic bone	Need good bone stock	Need good bone stock
Lower risk of intraoperative fracture	Higher risk of intraoperative fracture	Higher risk of intraoperative fracture
More stress-shielding	Less stress-shielding	Less stress-shielding
Hard to revise	Easier to revise	Hard to revise

RECOMMENDATIONS BASED ON EVIDENCE

Kirkley et al., 2000

About 42 patients, three surgeons (stratified), one year follow-up, no significant difference in Western Ontario Shoulder Instability Index (WOSI), American Shoulder and Elbow Surgeons Standardized Shoulder Assessment Form (ASES), Disability of Arm Shoulder and Hand questionnaire (DASH) constant score or ROM. Trend towards better pain relief with TSA. Two hemipatients crossed over to TSA, after one year follow-up.[3]

Gartsman, 2000

About 51 shoulders, average follow-up of 35 months show no difference in ASES or UCLA scores. Significantly better pain relief with total shoulder arthroplasty (TSA). Three patients crossed over to TSA by 35 months.[4]

This is a comparison of pain, strength, ROM, and functional outcomes after hemiarthroplasty and TSA in patients with OA of the shoulder. A systematic review and meta-analysis is as follows:

- Included four randomized controlled trials.
- On an average, two years follow-up.
- TSA resulted in significantly improved UCLA scores, pain relief and increased forward elevation by 13.

This meta-analysis concluded that at 2 years of follow-up, TSA provided a better functional outcome, however, the problems of glenoid component loosening in the TSA group and progressive

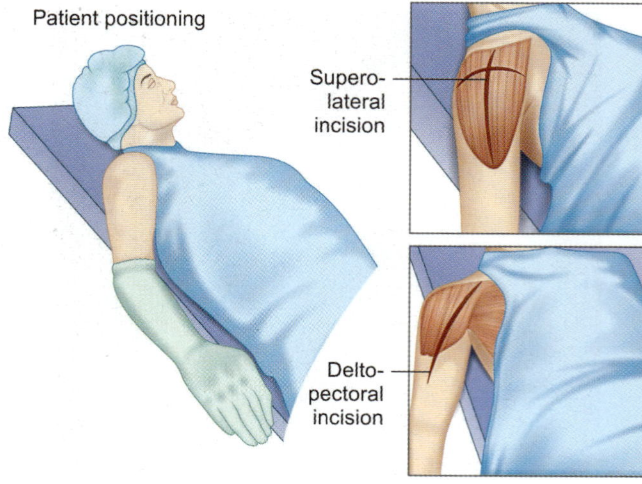

Fig. 266: Patient positioning and incisions for shoulder arthroplasty.

glenoid erosion in the hemi group may affect the eventual long-term outcome. Hence, longer follow-up is necessary.[4]

Haines JF et al., 2006

The results of arthroplasty in OA of the shoulder:
A prospective study of 124 shoulder arthroplasties for OA (Hemi and TSA) shows similar improvement in pain and function in both the groups, if RC was intact. Better results with hemi if RC tear is present. With hemi, revision at mean of 1.5 years for glenoid pain and TSA, revision at mean of 4.5 years for glenoid loosening.[5]

TECHNICAL ISSUES TO CONSIDER

Osteoarthritis tends to result in posterior glenoid wear/erosion, which if accepted, will lead to a retroverted glenoid component. Compensate by anterior reaming or placing the humeral component in lesser retroversion and failure to do so will resulted in posterior instability.

RHEUMATOID ARTHRITIS (FIG. 267)

Associated abnormalities are:

- Periarticular erosions
- Periarticular osteopenia
- Thin cortices
- Adjacent joint involvement.

Choice of prosthesis/arthroplasty includes:

- Cemented short stemmed prosthesis
- Gill, Cofield et al. recommend at least 60 mm between the cement mantles of ipsilateral shoulder and elbow arthroplasties.
- If this cannot be achieved, join both cement mantles together.
- Generally, TSA performed due to destruction of the glenoid articular surface by the disease.
- Glenoid erosion may require bone grafting. However, if glenoid is eroded to the level of the coracoid process, glenoid resurfacing is contraindicated.

ROTATOR CUFF ARTHROPATHY

This was described by Neer, Craig and Fukada in 1983. This is a distinct form of OA associated with a massive chronic RC tear. Generally, RC tears occur in less than 10% of shoulders with OA. A function of the RC is to depress the humeral head and keep it centered on the glenoid fossa. Massive RC tears result in proximal migration of the humeral head. This is a contraindication to glenoid resurfacing, as it results in an eccentric (superior) glenoid loading and early component loosening.

Surgical Options

- Hemiarthroplasty with a large head
- Repair of RC and TSA
- Reverse TSA.

Outcomes of hemiarthroplasty are:

Rockwood: About 86% satisfactory results after 4 years.

Zuckerman: About 93% adequate pain relief and 90% had improved function for ADLs.

Sanches-Sotelo: About 75% modest improvements in ROM and strength for ADLs. Good pain relief.

Field et al. and Sanchez-Sotelo reported that impaired deltoid function and previous subacromial decompression (loss of CA ligament) were significantly associated with clinical shoulder instability post-hemiarthroplasty.

REVERSE TOTAL SHOULDER ARTHROPLASTY (FIG. 268)

- Lateralizes the center of rotation and places the deltoid at a mechanical advantage
- More inherent stability prevents proximal migration of humeral head, by restoring deltoid lever arm.

Outcomes of the Reverse Total Shoulder Arthroplasty

Frankle M and Siegel S, 2005

The reverse shoulder prosthesis for GH arthritis is associated with severe RC deficiency. This is a minimum 2 years follow-up study of 60 patients.

Different outcomes are illustrated here:

- *Average age:* 70 years
- Improved ASES scores
- *Improved ROM*:
  - *Flexion*: From 55° to 105°
  - *Abduction*: From 41° to 102°

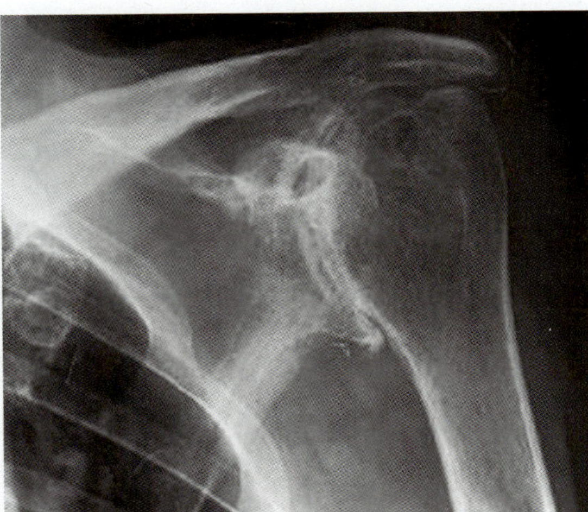

Fig. 267: X-ray shows rheumatoid arthritis of shoulder.

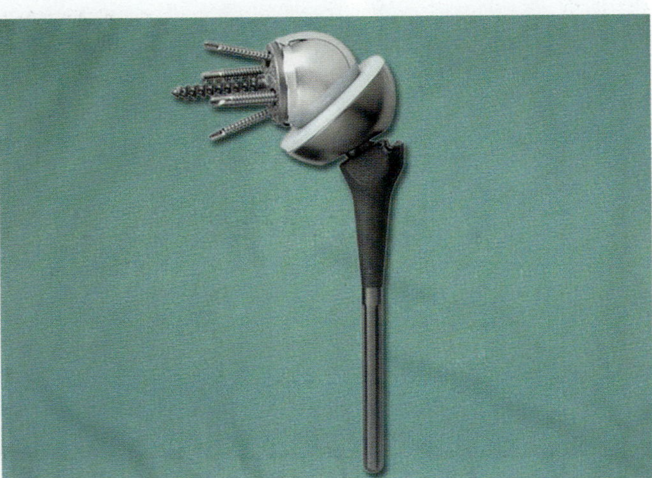

Fig. 268: Prosthesis used for reverse total shoulder arthroplasty.

- 17% complication rate
- Seven failures were reported and five out of them revised to new reverse TSA and two revised to hemiarthroplasties.[6]

Outcomes of the Reverse TSA (Delta III Prosthesis)

Treatment of painful pseudoparesis due to irreparable RC dysfunction with the delta III reverse ball and socket total shoulder prosthesis.

Werner CM and Glbart M, 2005

About 58 consecutive patients, average age is 68 years. 41 cases were revisions. Follow-up period is of 38 months. Improved constant score, pain reduction and improved ROM are:

- Flexion, from 42° to 100°, abduction, from 43° to 90°
- 50% complication rate (including minor)
- If there surgery done, to increase 1° of ROM, there is 18% reoperation rate
- If a revision surgery is done, there is about 39% of reoperation rate
- Reverse total shoulder arthroplasty is hard to revise, as little glenoid bone stock is left once component is removed, this is shown in Figure 269.[7]

OSTEONECROSIS (FIG. 270)

Causes

- Corticosteroids
- Alcoholism
- Sickle cell disease
- Lupus
- Idiopathic.

Treatment Options

Usually young patients with adequate bone stock, prefer proximally porous coated, press-fit humeral prosthesis, as it is less stress shielding and is easier to revise, if necessary. Resurface glenoid only in stage V osteonecrosis (glenoid erosion).

POST-TRAUMATIC ARTHRITIS

Due to fractures treated conservatively. This may have malunion of tuberosities, distorting normal anatomic landmarks. About 12% of patients have axillary nerve palsies (Neer). Many have soft tissue contractures and muscle weakness.

Complications

- Instability (1.2%)
- Excessive retro/anteversion
- Head too small
- Head too low (postfracture)
- Subscapularis rupture
- Rotator cuff tear (2%)
- Results in superior migration of humerus and glenoid loosening
- Infection (0.5%), e.g. *Staphylococcus aureus*. Infection is more common after revision surgery
- *Heterotopic ossification (10–45%)*:
  - Common in males
  - Diagnosis of OA
  - Low-grade
  - Nonprogressive and does not affect the outcome
- *Stiffness*:
  - Depends on indication for arthroplasty
  - Subscapularis shortening
  - Oversized components
  - Inappropriate rehabilitation
- Periprosthetic fracture
- Intraoperative (1%)
- *Postoperative (0.5%–2%)*:
  - Most common in rheumatoid arthritis (RA)
  - 85% of patients are women
  - Glenoid fractures are rare
- *Axillary nerve injury*:
  - Rare
  - Higher risk during revision surgery
  - Usually a neuropraxia.

Ultimate Bailouts

- Excision arthroplasty
- Shoulder arthrodesis.

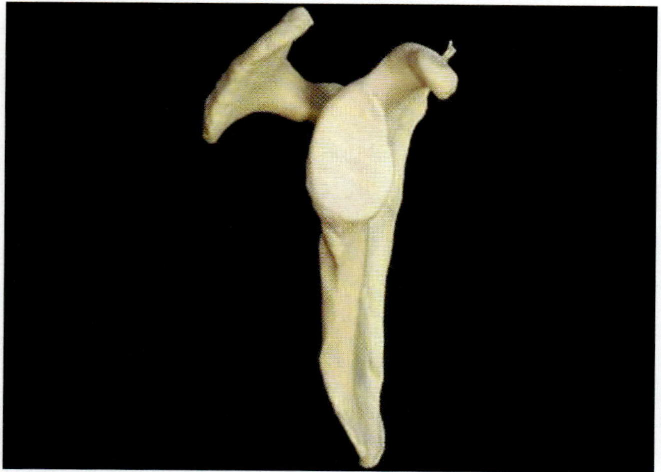

Fig. 269: Reduction in glenoid bone stock after reverse total shoulder arthroplasty.

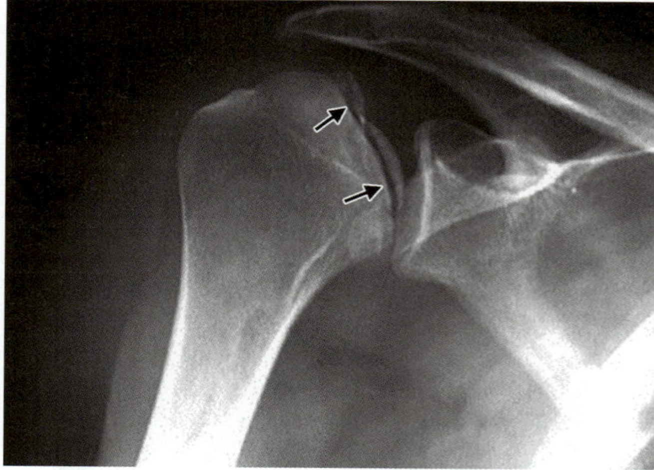

Fig. 270: X-ray shows osteonecrosis (arrows).

Revision Arthroplasty

Controlled longitudinal osteotomy for removal, revised with long stem prosthesis and cerclage wires, as illustrated in Figure 271.

INFLAMMATIONS AROUND SHOULDER

Inflammations around shoulder can be due to following factors:

AUTOIMMUNE

- Rheumatoid arthritis
- Seronegative inflammatory arthritis
- Crystalline arthropathies (metabolic), e.g. gout, pseudogout, calcium hydroxyapatite crystal arthritis.

Infective

- Septic arthritis
- Tuberculosis.

RHEUMATOID ARTHRITIS OF SHOULDER

Shoulder joint is often involved in approximately 90% patients, with longstanding RA. The pathology extends to subacromial bursa and synovial sheath of biceps tendon. The main destructive entity is inflamed and proliferating synovium.

Three Stages of the Disease

Stage I: Stage of acute synovitis

Stage II: Intermediate stage of synovial proliferation

Stage III: Final stage of destruction.

In early stages, recurring episodes of acute synovial inflammation occur associated with effusions. Eventually, inflammation spreads to subacromial bursa and bicipital sheath. The synovial tissue proliferates and destroys the capsule. Slowly, the capsule and surrounding muscles contract producing adduction and internal rotation deformity. In the last stage proliferated synovium forms *pannus* and destroys the articular cartilage, subchondral bone and biceps tendon. The RC and capsule gets weakened by synovial distension and invasion. The tendon may rupture, but may remain fixed by peritendinous adhesions in the groove.

Clinical Features

Rheumatoid shoulder assumes many forms. Acute inflammation may be limited to GH joint or it may appear as subacromial bursitis or bicipital tenosynovitis. Pertinent symptoms and findings of individual components of rheumatoid disease of shoulder are as follows:

Synovitis

- Usually occurs in early stage
- Pain with temporary limited motion
- Tender anterior joint line
- It is confirmed by aspiration.

Tendinitis of Capsule and Cuff

- Painful weak abduction
- Active abduction limited because of pain, but passive is full
- Local tenderness and supraspinatus atrophy
- Drop arm test is negative.

Rupture of Cuff

- Patient is unable to actively abduct shoulder to 90°, which is almost impossible or very weak
- Drop arm test is positive.

Tenosynovitis of Long Head of Biceps Tendon

- Tenderness over biceps tendon
- Boggy soft tissue mass may be palpable along the tendon
- Yergason's sign positive
- Pain over biceps tendon on passive maximal external rotation.

Rupture of Biceps Tendon (Fig. 272)

Usually follows trauma. When rupture is incomplete, pain is chronic until the distal end of tendon becomes adherent in its groove. If the rupture is complete tendon separation may occur and the muscle belly is palpable as a prominent mass distally in arm called popeye muscle.

Dislocation of Biceps Tendon from Groove

Groove is empty or tendon may be palpable as slipping on external rotation. Abbott-Saunders test is positive.

Subacromial Bursitis

Aspiration reveals typical fluid and later boggy swelling appears.

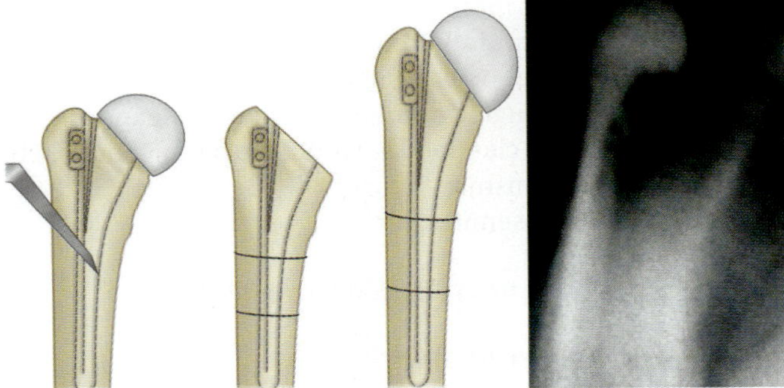

Fig. 271: Revision arthroplasty performed with longitudinal osteotomy.

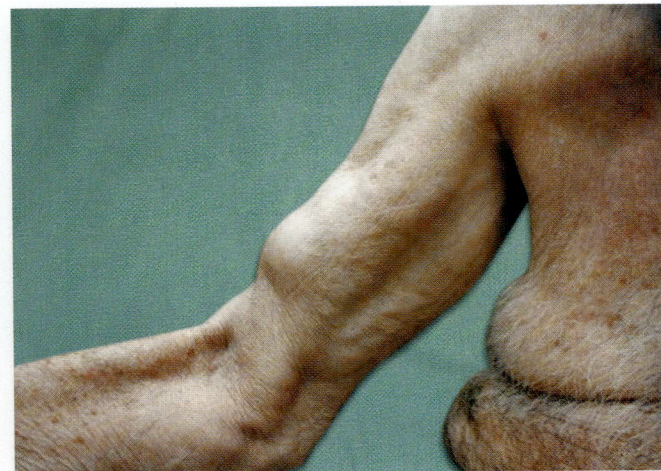

Fig. 272: *Rupture of biceps tendon*: Ruptured muscle belly is palpable as a prominent mass distally in arm called popeye muscle.

Symptoms in Later Stage of Inflammation

- Shoulder is stiff and painful.
- Range of active and passive motion is reduced.

X-ray Findings

- These include osteoporosis
- Narrowing of joint space
- Elevation of head of humerus
- Erosions, usually about the greater tuberosity and anatomical neck
- Sclerosis of greater tuberosity and subchondral cysts, as shown in Figure 273.

Arthrography (Fig. 274)

After injection of contrast medium, a typical synovial villi of the GH joint appears as filling defects. The capsular outline is replaced by patchy irregularity. When the cuff is ruptured, the dye enters the subacromial space, where the defects of villous synovial hypertrophy are revealed. Normally, the contrast enters the bicipital sheath. When the sheath is obliterated by adhesions, it fills unevenly or not at all. When the capsule is contracted, the shadow of axillary recess is reduced.

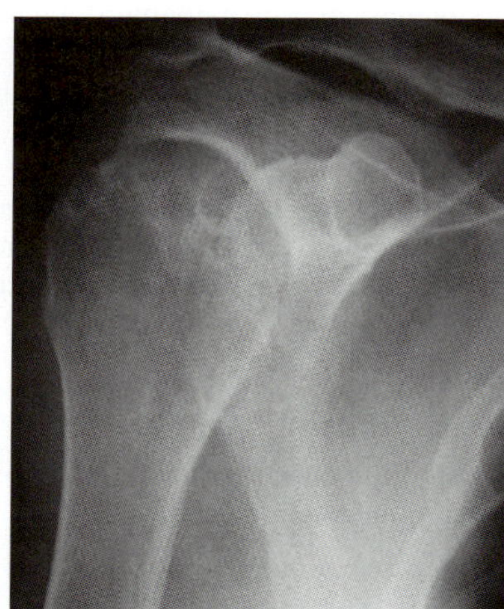

Fig. 273: X-ray showing sclerosis of greater tuberosity and subchondral cysts.

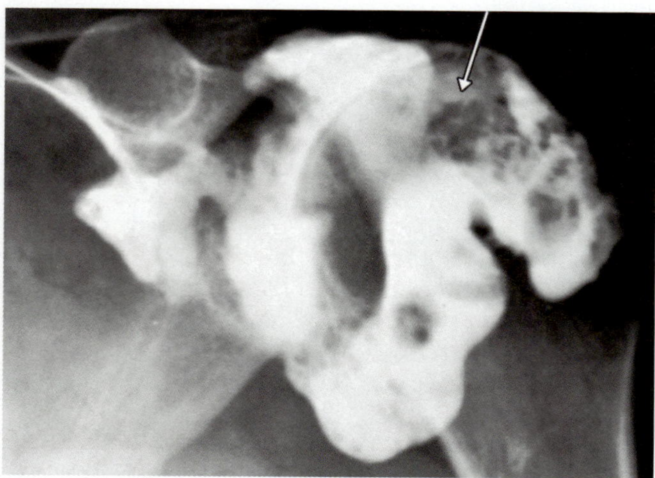

Fig. 274: Arthrography done by injecting contrast medium (arrow).

MRI

Magnetic resonance imaging (MRI) is useful in delineating the soft tissue component of the disease. The extent of synovial proliferation and joint effusion can be visualized. More importantly, the integrity of the RC can be determined with pathology, ranging from mild inflammation to full thickness tears.

CT Scan

Bone destruction and alteration in the normal osseous architecture is best evaluated with computed tomography (CT) scan.

Treatment

Initial nonsurgical management of rheumatoid arthritis, affecting the shoulder is appropriate in the early phases of disease with minimal bony destruction. Physical therapy may be helpful in maintaining active and passive motion during acute exacerbations and gradually adding resistive exercises to preserve strength. Limited trials of corticosteroid injections may be useful in reducing the symptoms of acute inflammation unresponsive to oral medications. When the medical line of nonsteroidal anti- inflammatory medications, antimetabolic drugs, steroids, and disease-modifying drugs has been exhausted, then surgical intervention should be considered.

In patients with joint swelling and pain, but relative preservation of the GH articular surfaces, bursectomy and synovectomy may be useful. Synovectomy may also help slow disease progression in aggressive cases of synovitis. In addition to synovectomy and bursectomy, a cuff defect must be repaired, the capsule is released, the intra-articular portion of the bicipital tendon is resected and the extra-articular portion is fixed in its groove. For associated acromioclavicular arthritis, the outer end of clavicle should be resected.

To overcome adduction and internal rotation contracture, subscapularis tendon is lengthened and the adductors (trapezius and rhomboids) are sectioned. Hemiarthroplasty or TSA should be considered for patients with severe pain and functional limitation, unresponsive to more conservative modalities. The indications for humeral head replacement are an irreparable RC tear or inadequate glenoid bone stock, precluding adequate fixation of the polyethylene component. Arthrodesis is rarely indicated, as it completely restricts motion and it appears to encourage deterioration of other joints of the extremity.

SEPTIC ARTHRITIS

Septic arthritis of the shoulder is an inflammation of the GH joint, involving one or more foreign pathogens that cause or are suspected of causing an inflammation. These pathogens can be bacteria, viruses, fungi or parasites. These pathogens can gain access to the joint through a number of different means.

Joint sepsis may be classified according to pathogenesis. There are three basic mechanisms:

1. Hematogenous dissemination
2. Direct inoculation
3. Contiguous spread from adjacent osteomyelitis.

Hematogenous Septic Arthritis

Hematogenous dissemination from another organ system, such as skin breakdown, urinary system infections or pneumonia is the most common. In the shoulder, branches of the suprascapular and subscapular arteries along with the medial and lateral circumflex humeral arteries form an extracapsular arterial ring, which supplies to the proximal humerus. This anastomosis gives off branches, which penetrate the capsule and form an intra-articular synovial ring. This has been termed the transition zone and is located between the synovium and the articular surface.

It is in this area that the arterioles form loop, acutely toward the periphery, causing a low flow state, making the area more susceptible to receptor specific interaction of the pathogen and the cell surface. Spontaneous shoulder sepsis is the result of joint invasion. During the abundance of the synovial vasculature and the absence of a basement membrane between the endothelial cells synovial joints, are more vulnerable to seeding by bacteria. Most patients with hematogenous nongonococcal bacterial arthritis have at least one underlying chronic medical risk factor. These factors may be local, such as prosthetic and metallic implants or systemic, such as cancer, cirrhosis, rheumatoid arthritis and intermittent bacteremic episodes from intravenous drug abuse or indwelling catheters.

Direct Inoculation

Direct inoculation may be traumatic or iatrogenic, e.g. repeated corticosteroid injections, arthroscopy and open surgical procedures, such as RC repair and arthroplasty. The existence of foreign bodies in or around the joint, such as nonabsorbable suture, stainless steel, cobalt chrome alloys, methylmethacrylate and polyethylene or devitalized bone from trauma has provided a nidus for adhesion and colonization by the bacteria. This nidus allows a glycocalyx biofilm to be expressed by the bacteria, which contributes to antibiotic resistance and limits the effectiveness of the immune response of the host.

Septic Arthritis from Contiguous Osteomyelitis

Hematogenous osteomyelitis commonly involves the metaphyseal area of rapidly growing long bones. When septic arthritis results from a contiguous infection, such as osteomyelitis, it spreads from the bone to synovium and then to the joint space. This happens most often in infancy, when there is a vascular anastomosis between the epiphysis and the metaphysis. Between the ages of 8 to 18 months, the last vestiges of the nutrient artery system close down at the growth plate, reaching sinusoidal veins and causing a low flow state. The open physis at this point provides an effective barrier to the spread of infection to the joint, by obliterating this vascular anastomosis. All synovial joints contain synovial fluid, which can act as an excellent growth medium for bacteria and have a relative lack of immunologic resistance. Type B synoviocytes are weakly phagocytic.

Bacteriology

Certain organisms such as *Neisseria gonorrhea* and *Staphylococcus aureus (S. aureus)*, seem to have avidity for the synovium, causing septic arthritis out of proportion to their incidence of bacteremia. *S. aureus* is the most common cause of adult, nongonococcal bacterial arthritis, occurring in up to 50% of patients.

Gram-negative bacilli have been increasing in incidence, ranging from 5% to 30% of all shoulder infections. *Escherichia coli* and *Proteus* species are common infecting gram-negative organisms from the urinary tract and occur in patients who are not intravenous drug abusers. *Pseudomonas* and *Serratia* are the common organisms in intravenous drug addicts. *Streptococcus pneumoniae* is the most common organism in patients with chronic alcoholism and hypogammaglobulinemia. Polymicrobial infections of the shoulder occur in 5–15% of patients, often associated with an extra-articular polymicrobial infection or penetrating trauma, especially in immunocompromised patients.

Clinical Features

The typical clinical presentation of shoulder sepsis consists of complaints of pain, warmth, and swelling. Patient may exhibit a prodromal phase of malaise, low grade fever, lethargy, and anorexia before the acute onset. The acute phase usually consists of fever and chills, with severe, incapacitating shoulder pain.

Physical examination reveals local signs of infection, such as erythema, edema, tenderness, increased warmth and limitation in ROM. Atypical presentation occurs, when there is chronic arthritis, immunocompromised state, extreme age and intravenous drug use or low-grade prosthetic joint infection. Previous use of antibiotics as well as corticosteroids or nonsteroidal anti-inflammatory medication, may mask symptoms.

Laboratory Findings

The white blood cell (WBC) count may be normal to slightly elevated:

- Raised erythrocyte sedimentation rate (ESR)
- *C reactive protein (CRP):* It has been shown to increase more rapidly than the erythrocyte sedimentation rate and may be of great value in the second, third or fourth day of treatment, to evaluate recovery when the sedimentation rate is still increasing
- Blood cultures
- Joint aspiration and culture
- *Synovial fluid analysis:* On gross examination, the fluid is often thick, yellow, and cloudy
- Leukocyte counts greater than 50,000 WBC per cubic millimeter
- *Glucose levels are decreased:* Levels of 20–40 mg/dL below the serum level are consistent with pyoarthrosis.

Imaging Studies

X-ray

X-rays in early stages may show joint subluxation or soft tissue swelling, due to either joint effusion or synovial hypertrophy. Later joint space narrowing and marginal erosions appear radiographically.

MRI

MRI gives excellent resolution of soft tissues and fluid collections with an extremely high sensitivity, demonstrating abnormalities within 24 hours. MRI can clearly demonstrate cartilage destruction and small joint effusions as well as intramedullary bone destruction and marrow edema.

CT Scan

Computed tomography (CT) scan can give better bony resolution than either plain radiographs or MRI, clearly depicting subtle bone destruction.

Bone Scan

Technetium 99m (99mTc) bone scan.

Arthroscopy

Arthroscopy can be a helpful diagnostic as well as therapeutic modality. Arthroscopic examination of a septic joint usually reveals inflamed and friable synovium with fibrinous exudates. Adhesions and loculations of pus may also be present. In addition to visualization of the joint, direct synovial biopsy and culture of multiple sites can be obtained.

Treatment

Prompt recognition, correct diagnosis, joint decompression and an organism specific antibiotic regimen are essential. Initial period of intravenous administration, usually of 3–7 days is followed by oral administration. The total duration of antibiotic regimen varies with the pathogen being isolated, the patient's underlying condition and adjuvant medical or surgical procedures. For gonococcal septic arthritis, 7–10 days are generally recommended. For streptococci or *Haemophilus species,* 2–3 weeks duration is usually adequate. Cases in which more virulent organisms, such as *S. aureus or* gram-negative bacilli are isolated, 4–6 weeks course of appropriate antibiotic is required. Immunocompromised patients or those with a slow clinical response will need the full 6 weeks of treatment.

Antibiotic impregnated polymethylmethacrylate: Antibiotic impregnated, Polymethylmethacrylate (PAMMA) has been used in the treatment of infections of the soft tissue and joint arthroplasty as well as osteomyelitis. The main advantage of this treatment is that it allows for a high concentration of antibiotics to be delivered locally, while minimizing the risk of systemic toxicity.

Evacuation and decompression of the joint: The goals of treatment of septic shoulder include sterilization and decompression of the joint with removal of all inflammatory cells, lysosomal, preoteolytic enzymes and fibrinous materials.

Arthroscopy: The diagnostic advantage of arthroscopy is that it allows for direct visualization of the entire joint. Visualization is essential in determining the extent of the disease and enabling tissue biopsy in atypical or challenging cases. The therapeutic advantage of arthroscopy is that the joint can be adequately drained, thoroughly debrided and copiously irrigated. Prognostically, arthroscopic irrigation and drainage reduces hospital stay and allows for early ROM, which may be helpful in preserving joint function.

TUBERCULOSIS OF THE SHOULDER

This is very rare, constituting nearly 1–2% of skeletal tuberculosis and can start in any of the following sites:
- Glenoid
- Head of humerus
- Synovium (rarely)

Clinical Features

Earlier Stage (Fig. 275)

- Painful limitation of abduction and external rotation occur early
- Marked wasting of the deltoid, supraspinatus other muscles

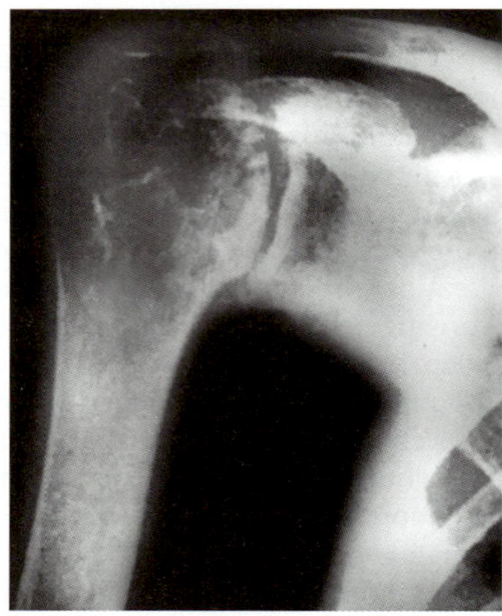

Fig. 275: X-ray shows earlier stage of tuberculosis of the shoulder.

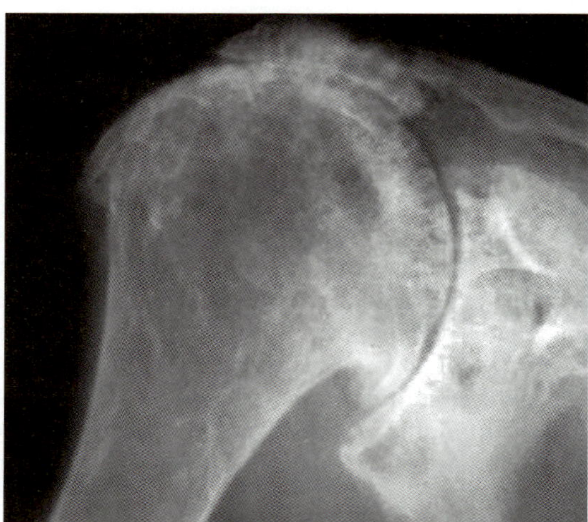

Fig. 276: X-ray shows later stage of tuberculosis of the shoulder.

- Common variety is dry type and is called as caries sicca, since there is no effusion in the joint.
- Cold abscess formed could present at:
  - Supraspinous fossa
  - Deltoid
  - Biceps.

Late Stage (Fig. 276)

- Destruction of the upper end of the humerus and glenoid cavity
- Fibrous ankylosis is the end result.

Radiology

- Generalized rarefaction
- Articular cartilage erosion
- Cavities in the head of humerus
- Periosteal reaction.

Treatment

Chemotherapy is the mainstay of the treatment. Shoulder immobilization by plaster is done, by keeping shoulder spica in 70–90° of abduction, 30° of forward flexion and about 30° of internal rotation, to encourage ankylosis in functional position for 3 months. Also, arthrodesis is the treatment in painful ankylosis, recurrence, etc.

BURSITIS

Subacromial Bursitis (Fig. 277)

The subacromial bursa lies under the upper part of the deltoid and extends upwards underneath the acromion process. This bursa serves to reduce friction and to permit the greater tuberosity of the humerus to rotate inwards under the acromion process in movements of abduction and rotation of shoulder.

The inflammation of bursa occurs mostly as a consequence of a lesion, involving neighboring structures. It is not a structure where disease starts, but it limits disease in the adjacent structures, by temporary adhesions causing fixation of parts. The floor of the bursa is more prone towards pathological changes, owing to relative avascularity and inert supraspinatus tendon, which makes it the most vulnerable part.

Clinical Features

Pain in shoulder is felt on abduction and internal rotation. Pain is usually felt at the insertion of deltoid. Pain is severe at night. Tenderness is present over anterior aspect of humeral head. Usually there is a point of tenderness on the greater tuberosity, which starts disappearing under the acromion on abduction (Dawnbarn's sign). X-ray may show calcareous deposits in the supraspinatus tendon and occasional bony spurs.

Subcoracoid Bursitis

The subcoracoid bursa is situated between the tip of the coracoid process and the capsule of shoulder joint. It extends up to and even over the lesser tuberosity. Strenuous usage of arm causes irritation of bursa from the pressure of the lesser tuberosity against the coracoid. Patients complain of pain in the region of coracoid. Tenderness is present between coracoid and lesser tuberosity.

In late cases, adhesions are present, with marked limitation in lateral rotation and abduction. A diagnostic injection of 5 mL of 1% lignocaine with hydrocortisone into this area produces relief from pain.

Treatment

In acute cases rest of shoulder in sling, together with anti-inflammatory drugs over a course of a week is the treatment. In failed cases injection of 5 mL of 1% lignocaine with hydrocortisone into tender bursa is helpful. However, this is contraindicated in infection.

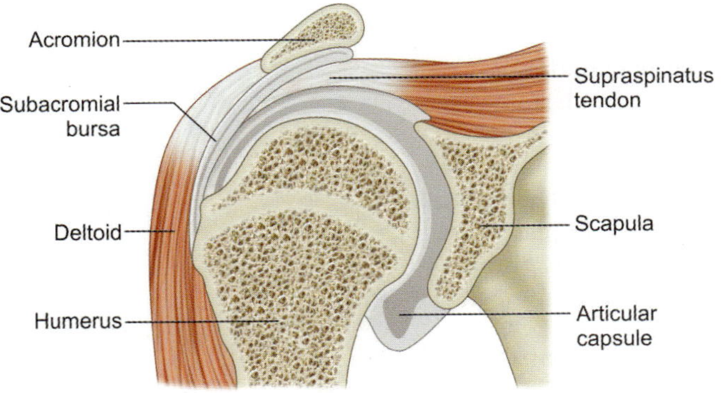

Fig. 277: Anatomical position of subacromial bursa.

In cases of persistent bursitis, exploration and excision of the inflamed bursa together with the removal of calcified deposits in the supraspinatus tendon.

CRYSTALLINE ARTHRITIS

Calcium Pyrophosphate Dihydrate

Calcium pyrophosphate dihydrate (CPPD) deposition disease is a disorder of the articular tissues, resulting from the liberation and deposition of calcium pyrophosphate dihydrate crystals. Clinically, two stages of the disorder have been recognized.

- Occurrence of acute attacks of synovitis precipitated by the liberation, accumulation and reactivity from calcium pyrophosphate crystals within the intra- articular space. These are termed as pseudogout, these attacks clinically resembles gout.
- CPPD arthropathy will evolve from repeated attacks and the accumulation of deposits of pyrophosphate crystals within the articular cartilage. Secondary degenerative arthritis will develop, accompanied by chronic pain. A propensity for elderly women is recognized with this form. X-ray shows crystal deposition in articular cartilage of humeral head and progressive deterioration of GH articulation, as shown in Figure 278.

Laboratory Findings

Synovial fluid analysis: The fluid is often thicker than normal and at times turbid, especially in elderly women.

Characteristic rhomboid-shaped positively birefringent crystals are identified. Some are intracellular, following engulfment by polymorphonuclear cells, as depicted in Figure 279.

Note: Readers are requested to refer Inflammations around Elbow for further reading.

GOUT

Gout is a disease characterized by hyperuricemia and resultant accumulation of sodium urate crystals within tissues and joints. It is the most common inflammatory arthropathy in men older than 40 years of age and its occurrence is at its peak in the fifth decade. It may be the presenting joint in a postoperative flare and in postmenopausal women.

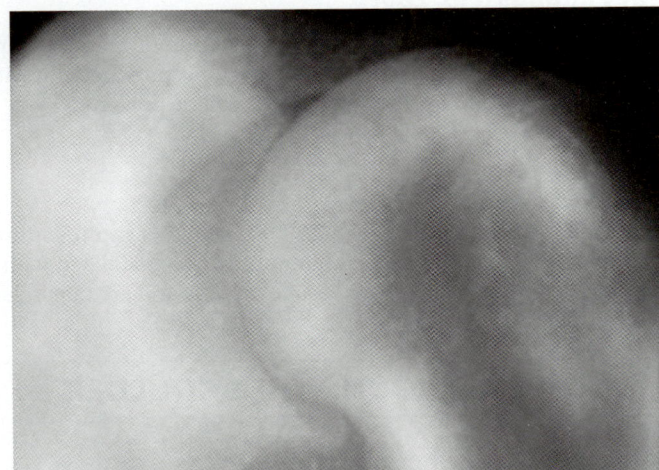

Fig. 278: X-ray shows crystal deposition in articular cartilage of humeral head, resulting in deterioration of glenohumeral articulation.

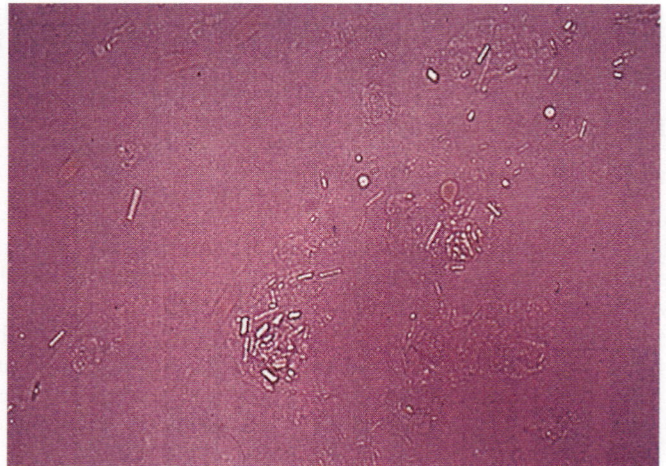

Fig 279: Synovial fluid analysis shows characteristic rhomboid-shaped positively birefringent crystals.

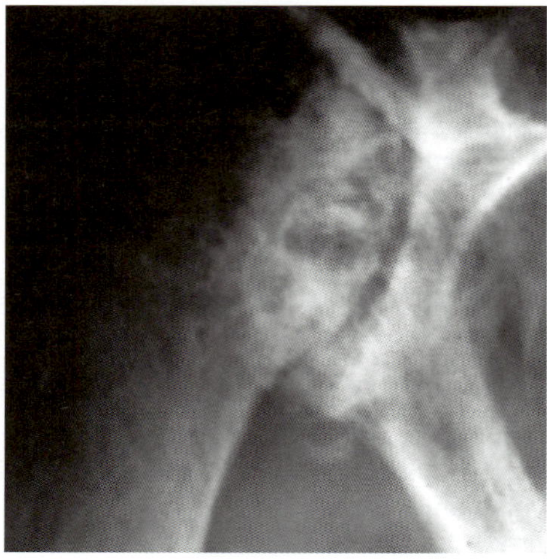

Fig. 280: X-ray shows degenerative manifestations of gout.

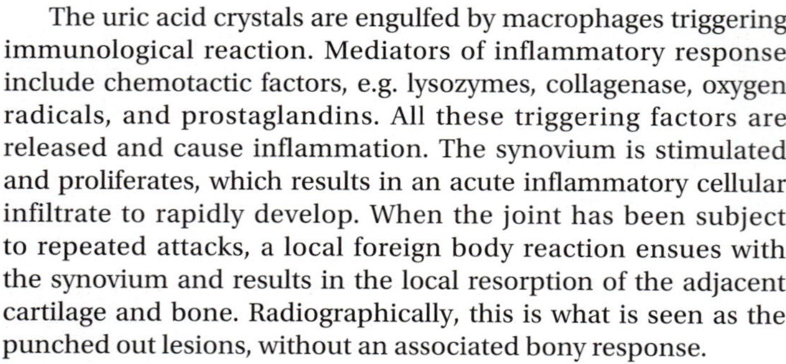

The uric acid crystals are engulfed by macrophages triggering immunological reaction. Mediators of inflammatory response include chemotactic factors, e.g. lysozymes, collagenase, oxygen radicals, and prostaglandins. All these triggering factors are released and cause inflammation. The synovium is stimulated and proliferates, which results in an acute inflammatory cellular infiltrate to rapidly develop. When the joint has been subject to repeated attacks, a local foreign body reaction ensues with the synovium and results in the local resorption of the adjacent cartilage and bone. Radiographically, this is what is seen as the punched out lesions, without an associated bony response.

Clinical Features

- With GH joint involvement, patients will present with an acute onset of shoulder pain.
- These patients are often obese; men are mostly involved and sometimes found to have ingested excessive alcohol.
- Physical findings of an acute gouty arthritis include decreased ROM of the shoulder, overlying warmth, tenderness and perhaps swelling. Occasionally, these patients will have fever.

X-ray Findings (Fig. 280)

Radiographs will show juxta-articular osteopenia and perhaps juxta-articular tophi. Sharply outlined erosions, punched out with sclerotic margins and overhanging edges will be present.

Laboratory Findings

- Elevated serum uric acid levels
- *Synovial fluid analysis (Fig. 281):* Presence of monosodium urate crystals, often intracellular and can be visualized with a polarizing microscope. Needle-like crystals and are negatively birefringent.

TUMORS AROUND THE SHOULDER

Bone Tumors

- Benign
- Malignant.

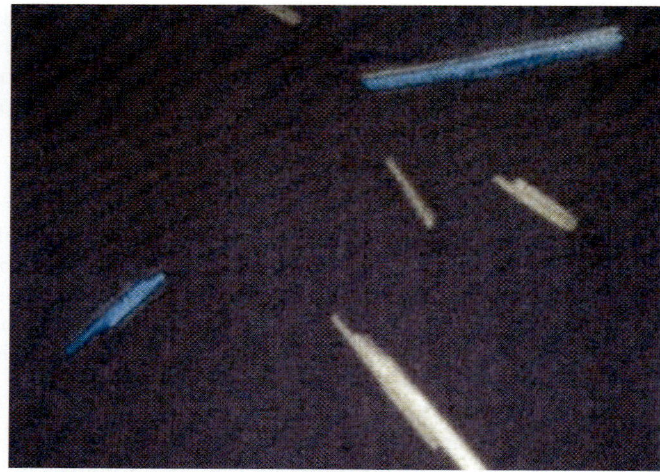

Fig. 281: Synovial fluid analysis shows needle-like crystals of monosodium urate crystals.

Soft Tissue Tumors

- Benign
- Malignant.

BENIGN BONE TUMORS

Benign bone tumors include:
- Osteoid osteoma
- Osteoblastoma
- Osteochondroma
- Chondroblastoma
- Enchondroma
- Unicameral bone cysts
- Aneurysmal bone cyst (ABC)
- Fibrous dysplasia
- Nonossifying fibroma
- Giant cell tumor.

Osteoid Osteoma

This small benign bone tumor occurs in patients of any age, most commonly in children and young adults. It shows predilection for male sex. Only 10–15% of cases of osteoid osteoma occur in the shoulder; main sites are proximal end of the humerus or glenoid.

Symptoms

osteoid osteoma typically displays the classic symptom of night pain, which is relieved by salicylates, e.g. aspirin.

Investigations (Fig. 282)

Radiographically, it is characterized by a large area of reactive bone, surrounding a small, subcentimeter radiolucent nidus. Technetium bone scan, osteoid osteoma has impressive increased activity. The central nidus can be visualized as a distinct cortical hole on computed tomography (CT scanning).

Differential Diagnosis

It consists of osteoblastoma, osteomyelitis (Brodie's abscess) and intraosseous ganglion. Histologically, this lucent nidus is a well demarcated, small area of immature and very active osteoblastic tissue.

Treatment

Preoperative localization is an extremely important strategy, to prevent intraoperative difficulty in locating these lesions and thus minimizing local recurrences.

Operative treatment is curettage, with or without bone grafting, e.g.

- En bloc excision
- CT guided percutaneous radiofrequency ablation. It has been introduced as a successful and minimally invasive method of treating osteoid osteomas.

Osteoblastoma

Osteoblastoma is a larger version of osteoid osteoma (giant osteoid osteoma); it is typified by a large lucent area (greater than 2 cm) of osteoblastic tissue, surrounded by a thin, sclerotic, and reactive rim of bone.

Incidence: About 10% of the total osteoblastoma. It mainly occurs in adults.

Histopathology

- Scattered mitotic figures
- Proliferation of immature plump osteoblasts
- Prominent vascular and stromal tissue component.

Imaging

X-rays (Fig. 283): X-rays show radiolucent lesion, which is surrounded by a thin margin of reactive bone, which may have an expanded aneurysmal appearance.

CT scan and MRI: These confirm preoperative diagnosis and help in determining surgical approach.

Angiography is used for staging aggressive tumors.

Bone scan shows intense radioisotope uptake that helps localize the lesion.

Treatment

En bloc marginal excision is the treatment of choice. Active tumors are more likely to recur, if intracapsular resection is performed. Risk of recurrence after marginal excision of aggressive stage third is 30–50%. Radiation therapy or chemotherapy is not effective.

Osteochondroma

The incidence of cartilaginous tumors in the shoulder is secondary only to those occurring in the pelvis.

Incidence: Solitary osteochondroma or exostosis is the most common benign tumor of the shoulder, fourth of all exostoses occurs in the proximal part of the humerus. It can be found in patients of any age, but it stops growing when skeletal maturity is achieved.

Pathogenesis: It is a developmental abnormality arising from the peripheral growth plate and is typically active and benign lesions during skeletal growth.

Clinical Features

It is usually painless but causes symptoms by pressure on adjacent structures. The cartilaginous cap may impinge adjacent neurovascular structures.

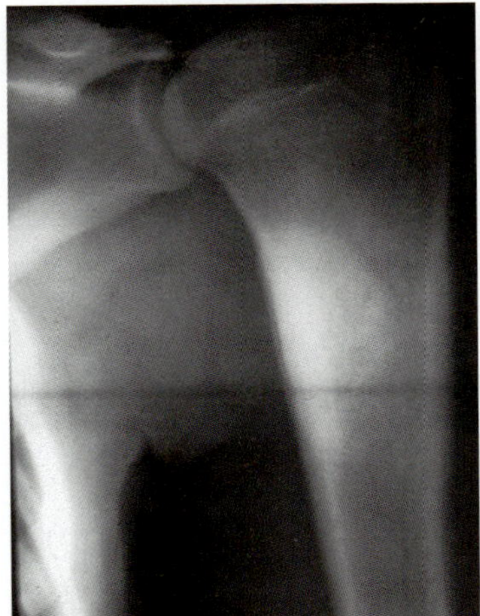

Fig. 282: Osteoid osteoma shows large area of reactive bone surrounding a small, subcentimeter radiolucent nidus.

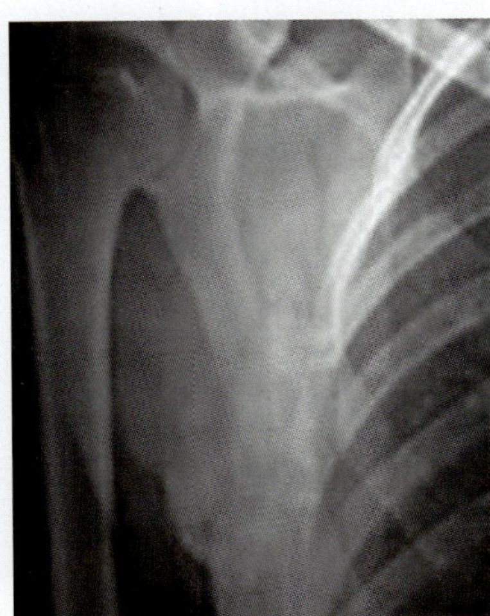

Fig. 283: Osteoblastoma shows radiolucent lesion, surrounded by a thin margin of reactive bone, which have an expanded aneurysmal appearance.

Investigations (Figs. 284A and B)

The plain radiograph is usually diagnostic, a smooth excrescence of metaphyseal cancellous bone that is confluent and continuous with the normal metaphyseal bone.

Histopathology: Exostoses can appear as pedunculated, stalk-like lesions or sessile lesions. The risk of a secondary chondrosarcoma arising out of an exostosis is approximately 1% per lesion, although rates are as high as 10–30% in patients with multiple hereditary exostoses.

Secondary chondrosarcoma can arise in adult patients with pain and an enlarging soft tissue mass or intraosseous bony erosions. Evidence of a thickened cartilaginous cap (1 cm) on CT scan, in association with a soft tissue mass, pain or radiographic evidence of malignant degeneration, suggests a secondary chondrosarcoma.

Treatment

Treatment of a solitary exostosis is done, when it is causing mechanical pressure symptoms or for cosmetic purposes involves excision of the tumor. Excision should be through the base of the lesion and also the cartilaginous cap should be excised to prevent recurrence. In the sessile form, care should be taken to excise the cartilaginous cap, in order to prevent a recurrence.

Chondroblastoma (Fig. 285)

Chondroblastoma is an aggressive benign cartilaginous tumor. Chondroblastoma occur as a round or oval lesion containing fine calcifications, surrounded by a reactive bony margin. It occurs as an active, benign stage II lesion, although it also has a more aggressive stage three form.

Incidence: About 25% of total cases occur in humerus.

Site: Most common site is proximal humerus.

Age: Usually occurs in adolescent or young adult with 2:1 male predominance.

Histologically: It consists of aneurysmal tissue, chicken wire calcifications and immature paving stone chondroblasts.

X-ray: Well-circumscribed lesions, centered in epiphysis, with surrounding rim of reactive bone are seen. 50% of cases will show calcification.

Differential diagnosis: It has to be differentiated from giant cell tumor (GCT). GCT will not have a rim of sclerotic bone and intralesional calcification. It may have soft tissue component.

Treatment

Treatment usually involves extensive intralesional curettage, which results in a large subchondral defect of the humeral head that requiring bone graft, to prevent subchondral and cartilaginous collapse.

An adjuvant agent, such as hydrogen peroxide or cryotherapy can help to decrease local recurrence rates. Patients need to be followed up in every 6 months for 3 years.

Recurrence occurs in 10–20% of cases. Benign pulmonary metastasis occur in 1% of cases should be treated by resection.

Enchondroma

Enchondroma is a benign lesion of hyaline cartilage. They are common and affect all age groups. It is most commonly found in the small tubular bones of the hand, but also occurs in the proximal end of the humerus in 10–15% of cases.

Enchondromas are usually solitary, but multiple, typically unilateral (Ollier's disease) or Maffucci's syndrome (enchondromatosis with multiple hemangiomas of skin or viscera or both). Tumors are located on epiphysis, metaphysis, and even on the shaft.

Clinical Features

Patient can present with deformities, caused by lack of epiphyseal growth and metaphyseal widening.

It is usually painless. Pain may occur when it is associated with some pathological fracture. When an enchondroma occurs adjacent to a joint, which is symptomatic for degenerative reasons, clinical assessment of bone pain related to the enchondroma may be difficult. It makes the initial evaluation of intraosseous cartilage tumors difficult because intrinsic bone pain is an important symptom, suggesting a low grade malignancy. Thus, we have to

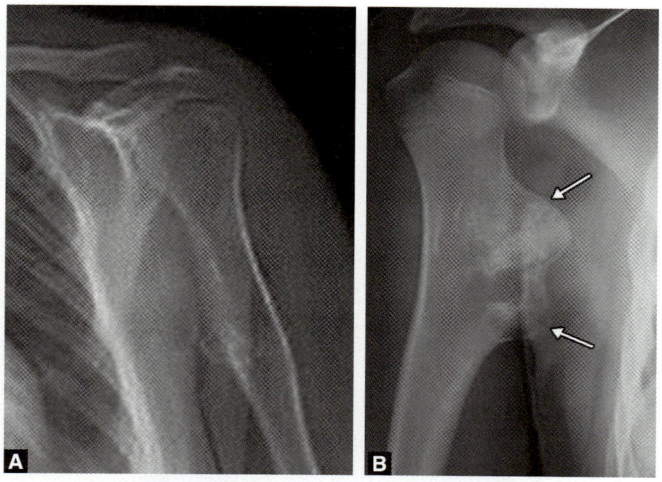

A B

Figs. 284A and B: Osteochondroma, with smooth excrescence of metaphyseal cancellous bone that continue with the normal metaphyseal bone.

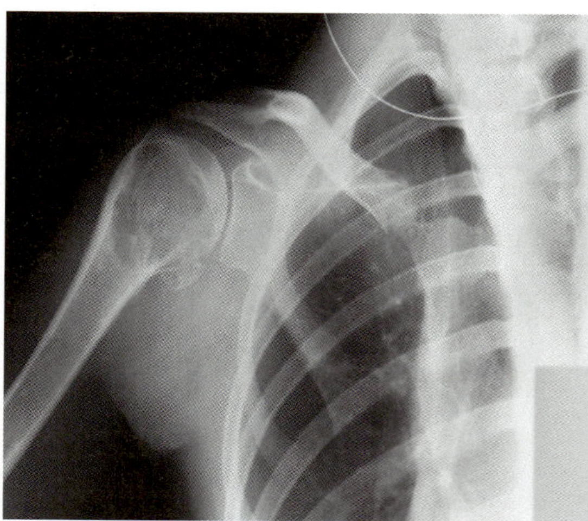

Fig. 285: X-ray shows well circumscribed, chondroblastoma lesion, centered in epiphysis with surrounding rim of reactive bone.

differentiate from the intraosseous symptom with intra-articular symptom.

Investigations

X-ray (Fig. 286): It shows benign appearing lesion, with intralesional calcification. Calcification described as stippled, punctate or popcorn type. Sometimes erosion and cortex expansion is seen. However, if the deep endosteal erosion involves greater than two-thirds of the total cortex thickness, then it suggests a malignancy. If soft tissue mass is present it indicates chondrosarcoma.

Treatment

The risk of malignant transformation of solitary lesions is extremely small. The risk of malignant transformation is 25–30% in Ollier's disease and even higher in Maffucci's syndrome.

Unicameral Bone Cysts (UBC)

They are the common lesions of the childhood more consistent with a developmental or reactive lesion than a true tumor.

Age: Occurs in first to second decade of age.

Sex: Shows 2:1, male predominance.

Site: Most common in proximal humerus. Lesions are active during the skeletal growth and usually heal spontaneously at maturity.

Clinical Features

Usually asymptomatic unless a pathological fracture has occurred. Two-thirds of patients may present with a pathological fracture. Fracture may stimulate a cyst to heal.

Investigation (Fig. 287)

X-ray: Shows centrally located purely lytic lesion well marginated outline.

Cysts may expand concentrically, but it never penetrates the cortex. Occasionally, (20%) thinned cortical fragment fractures and falls into the base of the lesion This fallen fragment sign is pathognomic for unicameral bone cysts with fracture. They are classified as active, when they are within 1 cm of the physis and latent, when they are closer to diaphysis.

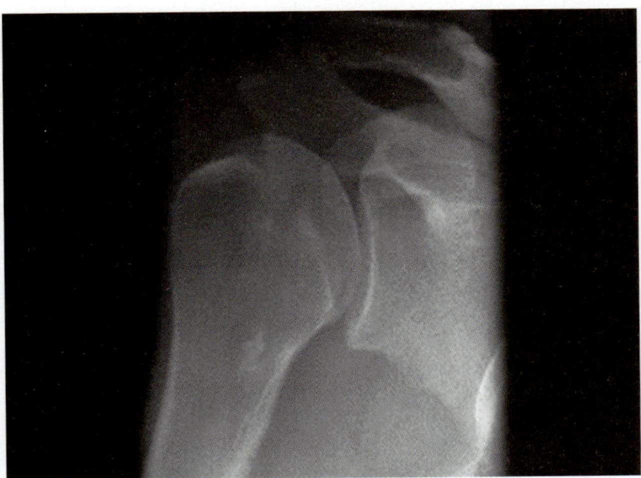

Fig. 286: X-ray shows enchondroma of the shoulder.

Treatment (Figs. 288A and B)

Small asymptomatic cysts can be treated with observation and serial radiographs. Larger lesions are usually treated with curretage with or without bone grafting and internal fixation. Percutaneous aspiration and injection using either:

- Steroid
- Bone marrow aspirate
- Demineralized bone matrix
- Calcium sulfate
- Hydroxy appetite crystals high porosity
- Cancellous allografts.

Aneurysmal Bone Cyst

Aneurysmal bone cyst (ABC) is locally destructive, blood filled reactive lesions of bone, and is not to be considered as true neoplasm.

Site: Most commonly occur at proximal humerus.

Age-sex: Before second decade of life with slight female predominance.

Clinical features: Mild-to-moderate pain present for several weeks to months.

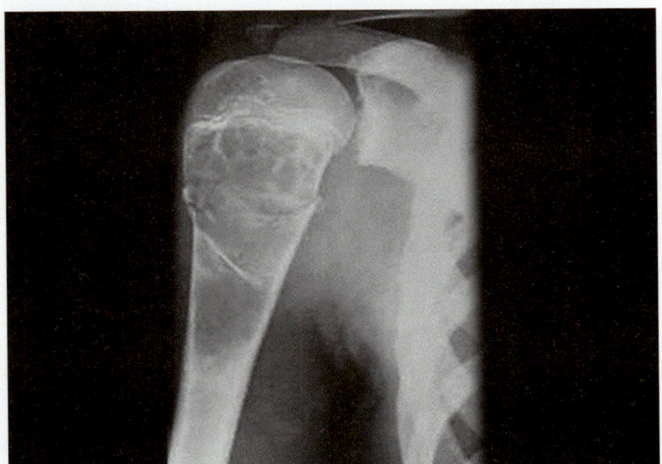

Fig. 287: X-ray shows unicameral bone cysts.

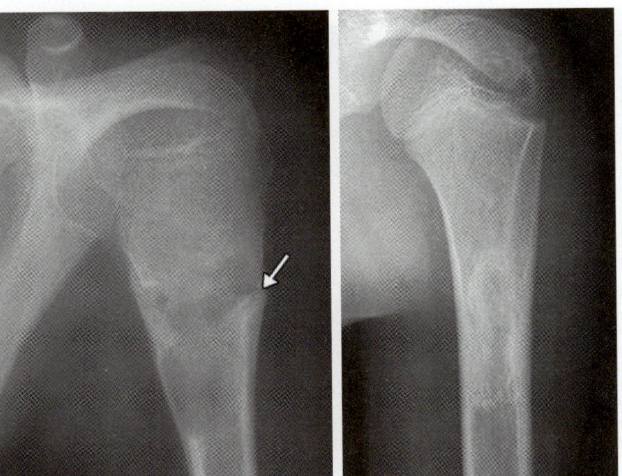

Figs. 288A and B: (A) Unicameral bone cysts, at the upper end of humerus; (B) Follow-up X-ray after one year treated with aspiration and steroid injection.

Radiological Investigations (Fig. 289)

X-ray: Expansile lytic lesion that elevates periosteum, but remained contained by thin shell of the cortical bone. It is most often located in metaphysis.

MRI (Fig. 290): It shows multiloculated cavities and fluid levels when differentiating between a UBC and ABC presence of a double density fluid level and intralesional septations indicates ABC.

Histopathology (Fig. 291)

It shows hemorrhagic tissue, with cavernous spaces, separated by cellular stroma. The lining of cavitary spaces consists of compressed fibroblasts and histiocytes.

Treatment

Extended curettage with a bone graft substitute is usually advised. The recurrence rate after curettage is 10–20%. Recurrence can be treated with the same approach as the primary lesions.

Fibrous Dysplasia

Fibrous dysplasia is a congenital dysplasia of bone, may exist in mono-ostotic or polyostotic form that often presents as a painful lesion secondary to pathologic fracture. The hallmark is replacement of normal bone, by fibrous tissue and small woven spicules of bone.

Site: Epiphysis, metaphysis and diaphysis.

Associated abnormalities: Sexual precocity, abnormal skin pigmentation, intramuscular myxoma and thyroid disease.

Investigations

The typical plain radiograph demonstrates a ground-glass density, with cortical thickening, as shown in the Figures 292A and B. Bone scan also shows increased activity. Histology shows furnace of dysplastic bone activity.

Treatment

When associated with symptoms or pathologic fracture, diaphyseal involvement usually requires intramedullary fixation rather than bone grafting because cancellous bone graft is consistently consumed by the dysplastic process and is ineffective in resolving the weakened dysplastic bone. Deformities are corrected by osteotomy with internal fixation.

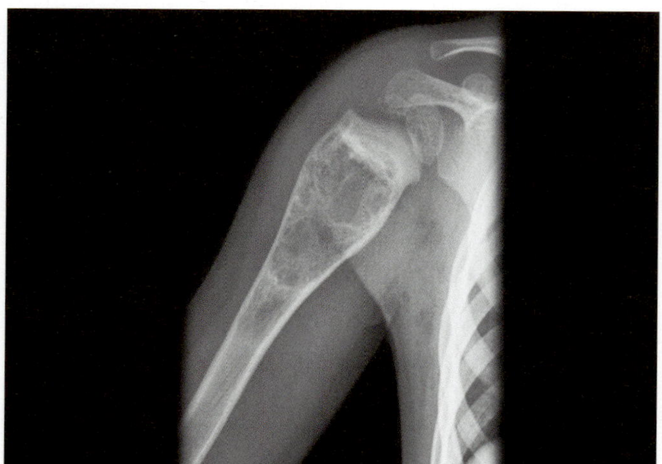

Fig. 289: X-ray shows aneurysmal bone cyst, commonly located in metaphysis.

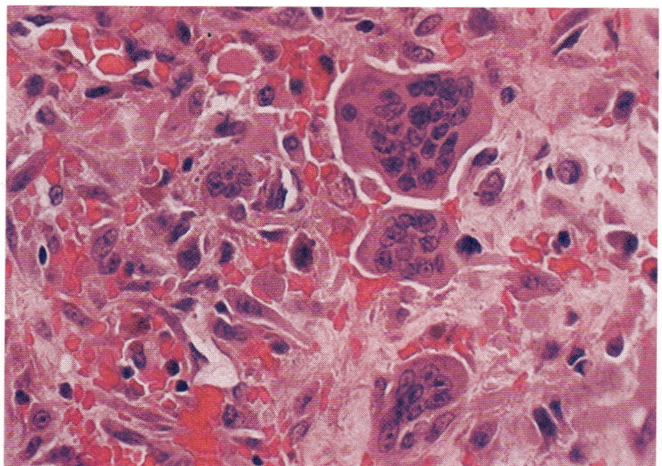

Fig. 291: Hemorrhagic tissue, cavernous spaces, fibroblasts and histiocytes seen in aneurysmal bone cyst.

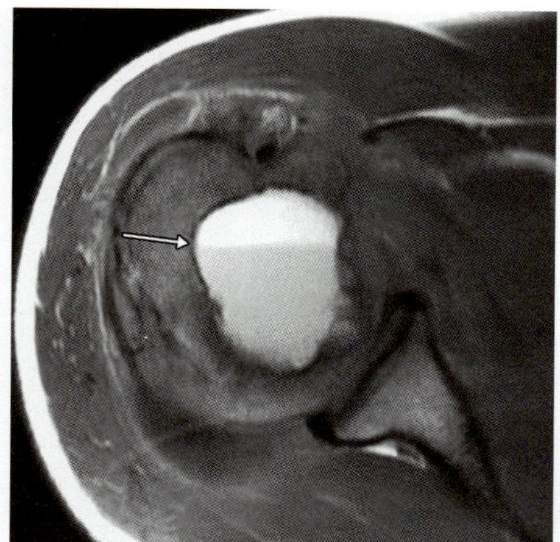

Fig. 290: MRI showing double density fluid level.

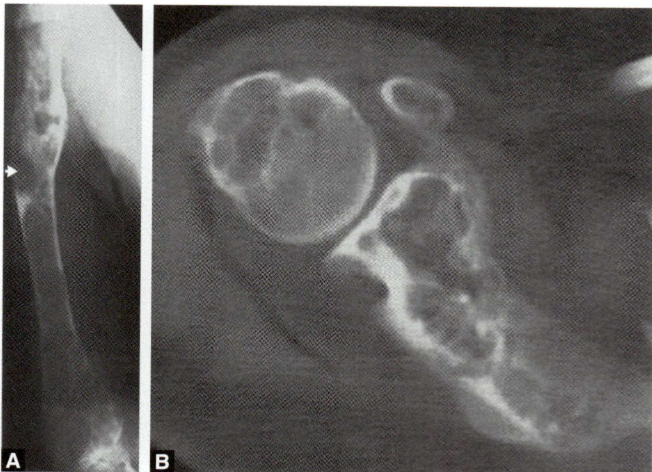

Figs. 292A and B: Radiograph of fibrous dysplasia, demonstrates a ground-glass density with cortical thickening.

Nonossifying Fibroma (Fig. 293)

Nonossifying fibroma is a benign fibrous lesion. Radiographically, it is visible as an eccentric and well defined lucent lesion that has a scalloped border abutting the adjacent cortex.

When the lesion is smaller than 4 cm, it may be referred to as a fibrous cortical defect. When lesions are longer than 5 cm or occupying more than half the transverse diameter of the bone, these lesions are at the risk for pathologic fracture. The majority of nonossifying fibromas heal spontaneously and require no treatment.

Giant Cell Tumor

Giant cell tumor of bone is a benign and locally aggressive lesion.

Site: Uncommon in proximal end of the humerus (5%).

Radiological Findings

Giant cell tumor is a radiolucent, epiphysometaphyseal tumor, which commonly has a distinct bony margin and is associated with extensive subchondral bone erosion. There can be bony expansion, cortical destruction or frank extension of the tumor mass into the soft tissues. Periosteal reaction is uncommon unless there has been a prior pathologic fracture.

Treatment

Treatment alternatives for GCT include:

- Curettage, with or without local adjuvant treatment
- Marginal resection.

Local adjuvant therapy used in conjunction with curettage includes the application of phenol, bone cement (cementation), or liquid nitrogen (cryotherapy). The local recurrence rate after curettage alone is 20–30% for active lesions and 5% after marginal resection.

MALIGNANT BONE TUMORS

Osteosarcoma

Osteosarcoma is the most common malignant primary bone tumor after myeloma. It is the most common primary sarcoma occurring in the shoulder, followed by Ewing's sarcoma and chondrosarcoma. It has typically developed in the adolescent age group, although a significant percentage of patients are the young adults, usually in third decade of their life.

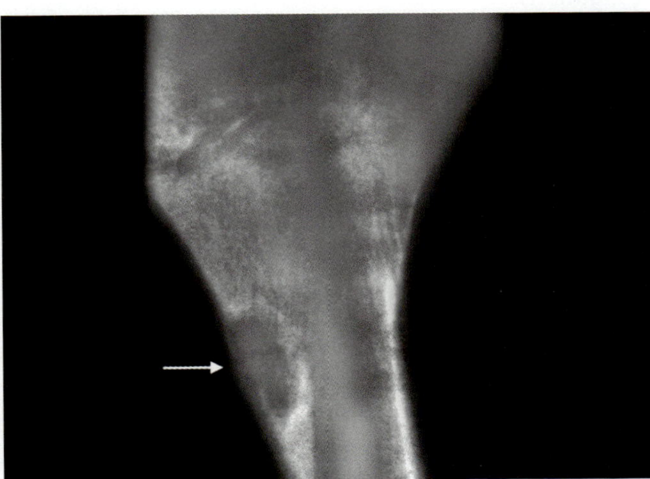

Fig. 293: Nonossifying fibroma.

Clinical Features

- Bone pain
- Night pain
- Pain unrelated to joint motion
- Tender soft tissue mass.

The average duration of symptoms at initial assessment is 3–6 months, which reflects the subtle nature of the preliminary symptoms and the need for early recognition of intraosseous pain and night pain, as a warning symptom.

Approximately 10–15% of all osteosarcomas occur in the proximal part of the humerus, whereas 1–2% developed in the scapula or clavicle.

The typical X-ray for osteosarcoma has a Codman triangle, sunburst or hair on end pattern, with penetration of the adjacent cortex. MRI is gold standard investigation for osteosarcoma; it determines the extent of soft tissue and bony involvement. CT scan determines extent of bony involvement not soft tissue; this is illustrated in Figures 294A to E.

Variants of osteosarcoma include telangiectatic (vascular) osteosarcoma, secondary osteosarcoma (Paget's disease or radiation induced), and various low grade lesions, such as periosteal and parosteal osteosarcoma. The basic histologic criterion for the diagnosis of classic osteosarcoma includes, a malignant stroma producing (spindle cells) tumor or immature neoplastic osteoid.

Classification

Histologically it is classified into three types:

1. Osteoblastic
2. Chondroblastic
3. Fibroblastic.

Treatment

Currently, treatment for high-grade osteosarcoma consists of:

- Neoadjuvant chemotherapy
- Wide or radical surgery (resection or amputation)
- *Adjuvant chemotherapy*: It is a radioresistant malignant bone tumor.

Prognosis

The overall survival rate for patients with osteosarcoma at 5 years of follow-up is approximately 70%, with appropriate chemotherapy and surgery.

Chondrosarcoma

Chondrosarcoma can develop *de novo*, as a primary chondrosarcoma or it can arise out of a pre-existing benign cartilage lesion, known as secondary chondrosarcoma. Primary chondrosarcoma is more commonly seen in the middle decades of life and its incidence in the shoulder is secondary to that in the pelvis or hip joint. It is the most common primary bone malignancy to arise in the coracoid process.

These tumors are typically manifested as intraosseous lesions with poorly defined margins and faint intrinsic calcifications. Secondary chondrosarcoma occurs in young adults and accounts for approximately 25% of all chondrosarcomas.

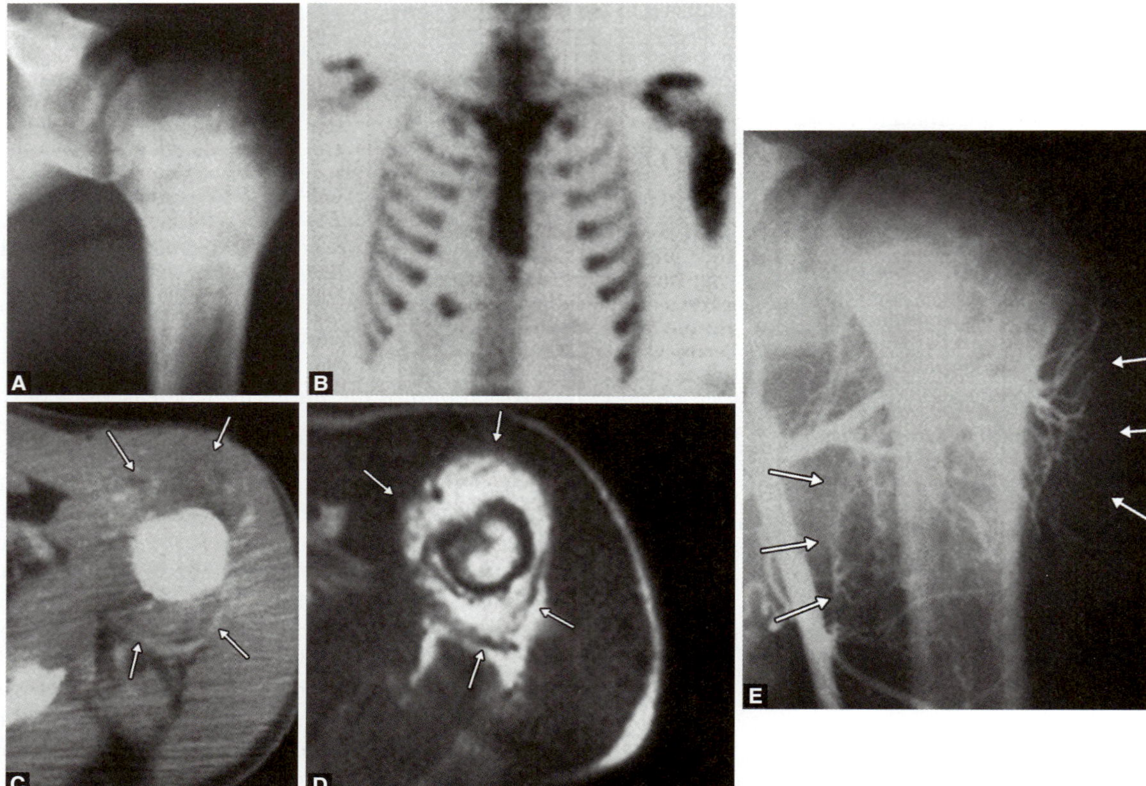

Figs. 294A to E: (A) X-ray shows osteosarcoma of the proximal end of the humerus, suggests soft tissue involvement; (B) Bone scan shows significant extension proximally and distally in the humerus; (C) CT scan of the same patient does not demonstrate the extent of soft tissue extension (arrows); (D and E) MRI through the same area of the humerus, demonstrating circumferential soft tissue involvement (arrows).

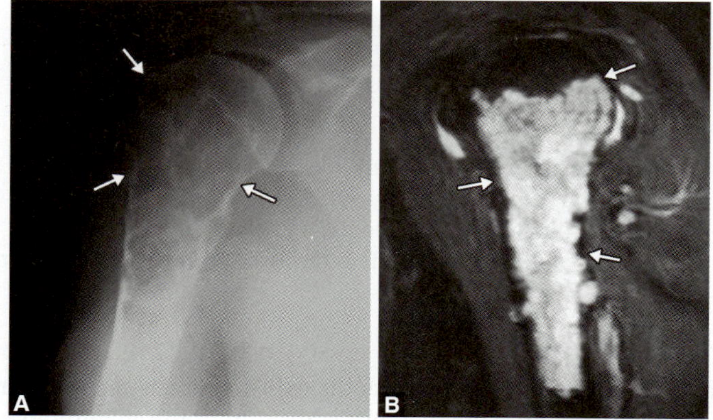

Figs. 295A and B: (A) The distinct endosteal cortical erosions (arrows), suggest a low-grade chondrosarcoma; (B) Sagittal MRI of the proximal end of the humerus, demonstrating high signal intensity the cartilage and the extent of intraosseous involvement (arrows).

Radiological Investigation

X-ray: X-ray finding are enlarging radiolucent areas within the lesion or endosteal cortical erosions along the cortical margins, as shown in Figures 295A and B.

Bone scan: Technetium bone scans are typically moderately hot.

Histopathology

Hypercellularity, pleomorphism, and evidence of mitotic activity, such as double nucleated lacunae and cellular atypia. These findings can also be seen in multiple enchondroma.

Treatment

Low-grade chondrosarcomas may be treated surgically with curettage and bone grafting whereas, high-grade tumors deserve surgical resection and reconstruction of the limb.

Ewing's Sarcoma

It is second most common intraosseous malignancy in adolescence. Children are more commonly affected than adults. It is not a common tumor around shoulder.

Investigations

X-ray: Mottled-moth eaten appearance, destruction of bone, with both lytic and blastic areas. There is periosteal reactive new bone formation, which may form layers, forming classical onion peel appearance.

MRI: It is required to know the extent of bony destruction and soft tissue involvement.

Multiple Myeloma (Figs. 296A to C)

Multiple myeloma is the most common primary malignancy of bone. It occurs in middle decades of life. The shoulder girdle is involved in 5–10% of cases. The most common site of involvement is the axial skeleton.

Prognosis

The overall prognosis is poor, newer treatments involving aggressive chemotherapy and plasma cell antibodies offer hope for the future.

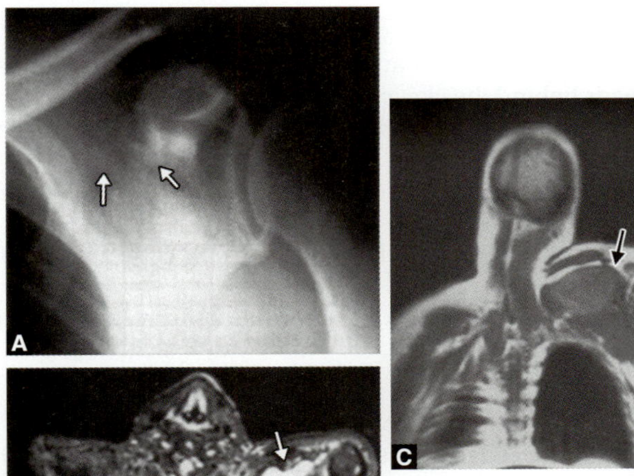

Figs. 296A to C: (A) X-ray of a 42-year-old man, with left shoulder pain and a lytic scapular lesion (arrows); (B) MRI in the same patient, demonstrates a suprascapular soft tissue mass (arrow); (C) MRI view of the same patient, shows a lesion wrapped anteriorly and posteriorly over the scapula (arrows).

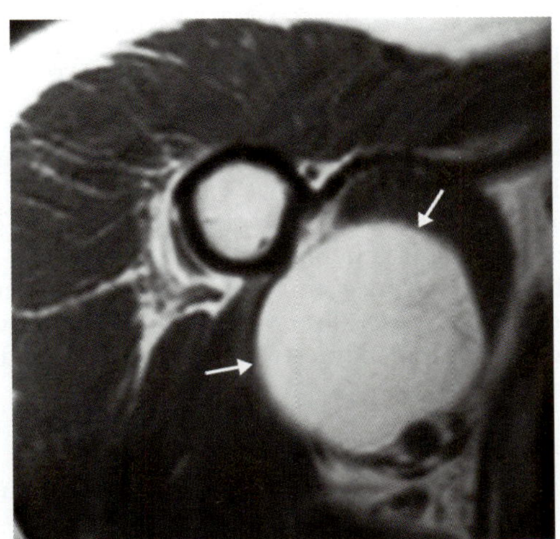

Fig. 297: MRI shows a benign lipoma, usually has a uniform fatty consistency.

BENIGN SOFT TISSUE TUMORS

Ganglion

It is a common soft tissue tumor that is often confused with other cystic lesions. They are filled with a characteristic gelatinous material. In the shoulder, they are often associated with degenerative conditions or a labral tear. When located in the spinoglenoid notch, a ganglion may produce suprascapular nerve palsy secondary to nerve entrapment.

Lipoma (Fig. 297)

Lipomas can occur intramuscularly or within normal fat planes of the axilla or the subscapular planes. They often appear in the anterior part of deltoid as a large, soft, nontender and intramuscular mass. A few lipomas are tender or firm and show history of a change in size.

On MRI or CT scan, a benign lipoma usually has a uniform, fatty consistency.

Hemangioma

Hemangioma typically appears as an enlarging intramuscular lesion in a child or young adult. They are best visualized by MRI and typically have a serpiginous configuration of vessels. If they are intimately involved with a major vessel, they should also be evaluated with an arteriogram. Well localized lesions are more easily resected than the more extensive congenital lesions. Embolization and interferon treatment show mix results in halting the progression of disease.

Fibromatosis

Fibromatosis (desmoid) is a locally aggressive lesion found in young children, teenagers, and young adults. These lesions have a firm consistency on clinical examination and may be associated with osseous erosions or invasion of a neurovascular bundle. Recurrence rate is quite high. Rarely do they have pulmonary metastasis.

MALIGNANT SOFT TISSUE TUMORS

Soft Tissue Sarcoma

Upper extremity is involved in 25% of total cases.

Clinical Features

- Firm mass
- Large (5 cm) or enlarging
- Deep or subfascial
- Non tender.

The most common soft tissue sarcoma in adults is malignant fibrous histiocytoma, which occurs most often in older adults (50–70 years). Liposarcoma typically occurs in the lower extremities in young adults, as a large lesion, with a histology ranging from low-grade to high-grade or pleomorphic. Synovial sarcoma is a less common lesion associated with faint soft tissue calcifications, a juxta-articular location and a high metastatic rate.

Fibrosarcoma, rhabdomyosarcoma, leiomyosarcoma, clear cell sarcoma, and epithelioid lesions are other, less common soft tissue malignancies.

Treatment

Regardless of the tissue type, the grade of the lesion and the anatomic location of the primary tumor are the most significant factors determining prognosis and treatment.

Soft-tissue sarcomas of intermediate grade histology are usually treated with chemotherapy. Synovial sarcoma, epithelioid sarcoma, and rhabdomyosarcoma have high incidence (10–20%) of regional lymph node metastasis and a poor prognosis.

BRACHIAL PLEXUS INJURY AND ITS MANAGEMENT

ANATOMY

The dorsal and ventral rootlets exit the spinal cord and merge to form the spinal nerves, which leave the intervertebral foramina and quickly divide into dorsal and ventral rami, as shown in Figure 298. The origin of brachial plexus is from the ventral rami of C5 through C8 and T1 spinal nerves. Sometimes contributions may originate from, C4 (prefixed) and T2 (postfixed).

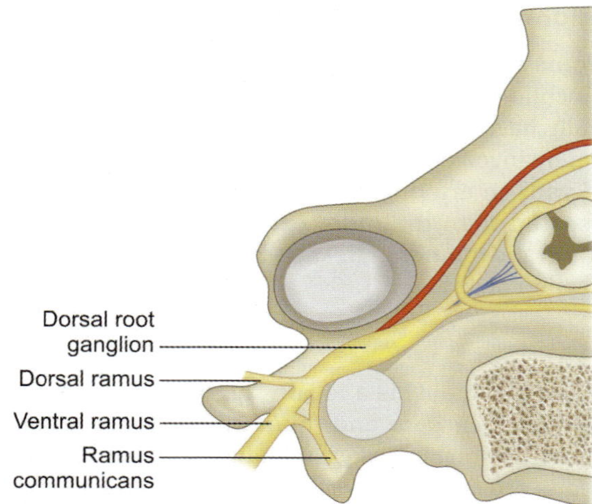

Fig. 298: Origin of spinal nerve from intervertebral foramina forming ventral and dorsal rami.

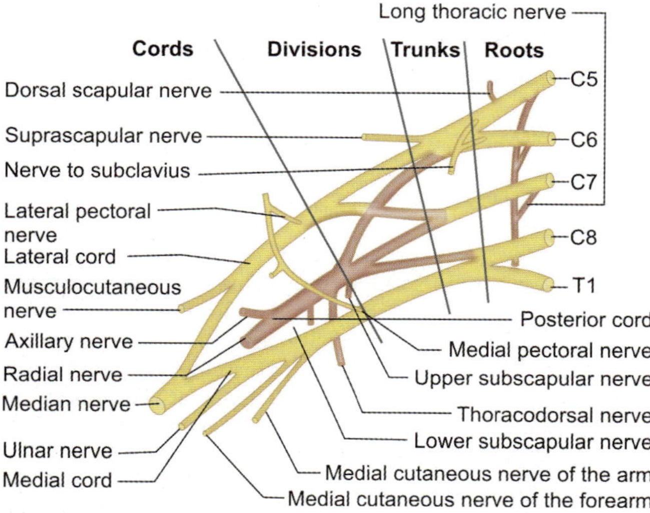

Fig. 299: Brachial plexus and its components.

Roots (Fig. 299)

- The upper roots (C5–C8) descend towards the first rib, whereas the lower T1 root ascend over the first rib to form the brachial plexus.
- Sympathetic fibers join the nerve roots as they traverse between the scalene muscles.
- C5 and C6 receive fibers from the middle sympathetic cervical ganglion and C7–T1, acquire fibers from the cervicothoracic ganglion.
- These sympathetic fibers control blood vessel smooth muscle contraction (vasoconstriction) and sweat gland activity.

Trunks (Fig. 299)

- The ventral rami of C5 and C6 combine to form the upper trunk
- The C7 ramus continued alone as the middle trunk
- C8 and T1 unite to form the lower trunk
- The trunks are located in the posterior triangle of the neck, enclosed by the posterior border of the sternocleidomastoid muscle, anterior border of the upper trapezius, and clavicle.

Divisions and Cords

- Each trunk divides into anterior and posterior divisions and proceeds behind the clavicle
- The divisions then merge into three cords, named in relation to the axillary artery
- The anterior divisions of the upper and middle trunks combine to form the lateral cord
- The anterior division of the inferior trunk continues as the medial cord
- The three posterior divisions converge to form the posterior cord.

Branches

- The cords proceed behind the pectoralis minor muscle into the axilla and divide into two terminal branches
- The lateral cord terminates, as the musculocutaneous nerve and a branch to the median nerve
- The posterior cord divides into the axillary and the radial nerves
- The medial cord continues as the ulnar nerve and a branch to the median nerve
- Several branches arise from the roots, trunks and cords of the brachial plexus.

Branches at the Root Level

- The dorsal scapular nerve arises from C5 and innervates levator scapula and rhomboid muscles.
- The long thoracic nerve arises from C5, C6, and C7 and is supplied to serratus anterior muscle.
- The phrenic nerve arises from C3, C4, and C5 and crosses the anterior scalene muscle to enter the thorax. This nerve may get injured in nerve root injuries, with subsequent hemidiaphragm paralysis.

Branches at the Trunk Level

- The suprascapular nerve arises from the upper trunk and is supplied to supraspinatus and infraspinatus muscles.
- The nerve to the subclavius arises from anterior surface of the upper trunk and innervates subclavius muscle.
- There are no branches from the plexus at the division level.

Branches at the Cord Level

- *From the lateral cord:* The lateral pectoral nerve arises to innervate the clavicular part of the pectoralis major.
- *From the posterior cord*: The upper subscapular, thoracodorsal and lower subscapular nerves:
  - The upper subscapular nerve innervates the upper portion of the subscapularis muscle
  - The lower subscapular nerve innervates the lower portion of the subscapularis muscle and teres major muscle
  - The thoracodorsal nerve originates between the upper and lower subscapular nerves, passes behind the axillary artery and supplies the latissimus dorsi muscle.
- *From the medial cord one motor and two sensory branches arise*:
  - The medial pectoral nerve innervates pectoralis minor muscle and the sternocostal portion of the pectoralis major muscle.

- The medial brachial and medial antebrachial cutaneous nerves are the only sensory branches to arise directly from the brachial plexus and supply the arm and forearm respectively.

ETIOLOGY

Brachial plexus injuries can affect a wide range of individuals from newborns to the elderly. Obstetric brachial plexus palsy can occur during passage through the birth canal, whereas adolescent and adult injury may be secondary to domestic violence, vehicular trauma, athletic endeavors or systemic disease:

- *Trauma*:
  - Nonpenetrating (traction)
  - Penetrating, e.g. knife or gunshot wound (GSW)
- *Nerve entrapment*:
  - Thoracic outlet syndrome
- *Infection*:
  - Viral plexopathy (Parsonage—Turner syndrome)
- *Radiation*:
  - Fibrosis
  - Malignant degeneration after radiation
- *Tumors*:
  - Primary (schwannomas or neurofibromas)
  - Secondary (pulmonary apices)
- Neuropathies
- *Iatrogenic*:
  - Axillary or scalene anesthesia
  - Surgical biopsy
  - Intraoperative positioning
  - Median sternotomy
  - Inadvertent traction.

Nonpenetrating Trauma

- Nonpenetrating trauma is the leading cause of injury to the brachial plexus.
- The mechanism of injury in almost all injuries is traction that produces tension across the brachial plexus.
- The mechanism by which the traction is produced is variable and may be from:
  - Traction to the extremity
  - Forcible head rotation from the shoulder
  - Direct depression of the shoulder girdle
  - Iatrogenic, malpositioning of the patient on the operation theater (OT) table.

Traction Injuries

With traction injuries, there is a stretch of the nerve beyond the physiological limits that nerve can withstand. There is a direct reduction of intraneural blood flow with increasing strain. A 15% elongation will reduce blood flow approximately 80–100%. Continued elongation will cause overt ischemia and disruption of nerve metabolism. Persisted traction will ultimately disrupt nerve continuity. Traction, therefore, can cause nerve injury ranging from a temporary disruption in nerve fiber conduction to functional discontinuity of the nerve fibers and sheath. The upper plexus is taut with the arm dangling at the side and the lower plexus is taut with the arm abducted and elevated.

Traction with the arm forcibly abducted, can causes lower plexus injuries and with the arm adducted and the neck deviated to the opposite side, causes upper plexus injuries. Lateral traction to the arm, causes middle portion (C7) injuries. Disruptive forces (traction) applied in line with the direction of maximal strain can selectively disrupt portions of the brachial plexus or be disseminated throughout the plexus.

Adult traction injuries: Most of the significant adult brachial plexus traction injuries are motor vehicle accidents, especially motorcycle misadventures. The incidence of brachial plexus injury following motorcycle accident has recently increased and is probably related to mandatory helmet regulations and better transportation of trauma patients who previously would have succumbed to their injuries. Associated injuries are common, including head trauma, fractures or dislocations of the cervical spine, shoulder, forearm, and hand.

Minor stretch injuries (burners, stingers) of the plexus are common in contact sports, especially football, because tackling drives the shoulder downward and forcibly flexes the neck toward the contralateral side. The athlete experiences a burning pain and paresthesia that radiates from the supraclavicular area into the arm. Transient weakness and sensory abnormalities are present. The symptoms and signs of these stretch injuries usually resolve spontaneously over a few minutes. However, a cervical spine fracture, dislocation or a severe brachial plexus injury can occur during impact with subsequent quadriplegia or a permanent neurologic deficit. These injuries will have persistent weakness and limited neck motion. Shoulder dislocations are often related to sporting accidents and can produce nerve injuries of the axillary, suprascapular or musculocutaneous nerves. These are usually (80%) temporary lesions that resolve over 4–6 months. However, violent high energy trauma can cause disruption of nerve fiber integrity at the time of dislocation.

Obstetric traction injuries: Traction injuries can occur during birth and are associated with difficult deliveries. Traction to the head with forceful tilting from the fixed shoulder (lateral neck flexion) during delivery can stretch the upper plexus. Instrumentation (forceps, vacuum) to after coming head in postmature delivery, as demonstrated in Figures 300A to D. Injury can also occur during breech presentation as the lower roots are stretched during hyperabduction of the ipsilateral arm during delivery.

Penetrating Trauma

Penetrating trauma to the brachial plexus is often secondary to gunshot wounds or stabbings. Bullet injuries act as projectile missiles that cause neural injury by means of a blast effect or less commonly direct nerve transection. In contrast, stab wounds transect portions of the plexus or cause vascular injury with secondary nerve compression by expanding hematoma. Most commonly, the upper and midplexus are involved, as clavicle protects the lower elements.

Infection

Infection is an uncommon cause of brachial plexopathy and the exact etiology remains obscure. Both viral pathogens and secondary immunologic factors are proposed as the possibilities. This brachial neuritis, also known as Parsonage-Turner syndrome, presents with an acute onset of intense pain about the shoulder girdle without antecedent trauma. Weakness of the muscles innervated by the affected nerves develops after the initial pain

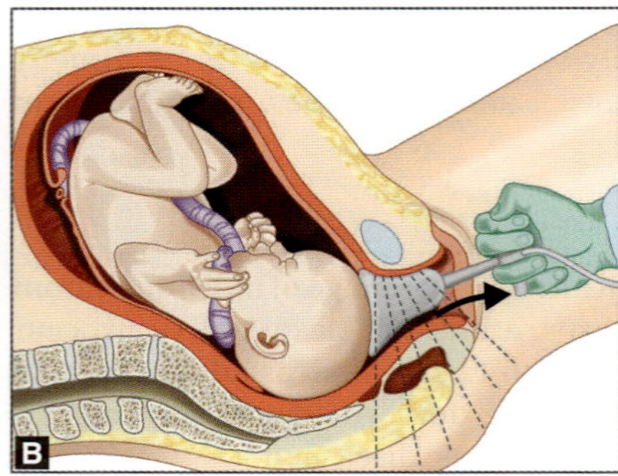

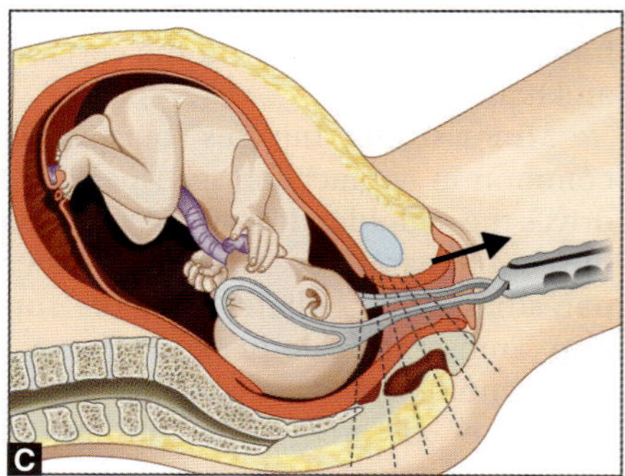

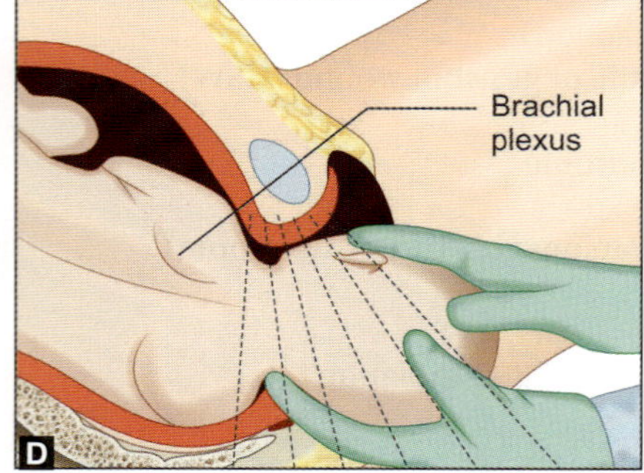

Figs. 300A to D: Use of instruments for delivery can resulted in injuries to brachial plexus.

response. The suprascapular or long thoracic nerve is the most commonly affected. The natural history of brachial neuritis is resolution of the pain followed by improvement in motor function.

Electromyographic abnormalities of the denervated muscles are apparent 3–4 weeks after the initial pain response, with positive sharp waves and fibrillation potentials. The treatment is conservative management with observation and serial examinations. However, prolonged recovery time and persistent weakness is not uncommon even years after the brachial neuritis.

CLASSIFICATION OF BRACHIAL PLEXUS INJURY

The lesion in brachial plexus injury is classified according to the anatomic location and extent of nerve involvement.

Based on Anatomic Location

1. *Supraclavicular lesions:* Affect roots, trunks and divisions.
2. *Infraclavicular lesions:* Affect cords and branches.

Supraclavicular Lesions

Supraclavicular lesions can be due to:
- Avulsion injury or
- Ruptures.

Avulsion Injury

The supraclavicular injury from traction can disrupt the rootlet connection with the spinal cord and is called an avulsion injury. An avulsion separates the motor cell body in the spinal cord from its axons, but the sensory cell body located in the dorsal root ganglion remains connected to its axons. The motor portion of the nerve, therefore, undergoes wallerian degeneration with degradation of the axons and myelin sheaths. The sensory fibers are spared from wallerian degeneration, but have been irrevocably detached from the spinal cord. The injury will cause a clinical motor and sensory loss, whereas electrodiagnostic studies will reveal abnormal motor findings with intact sensory conduction. Rarely, the rupture can affect only the motor or sensory rootlets.

TABLE 7: Various patterns and roots involved in brachial plexus injuries.

Pattern	*Roots involved*
Upper brachial plexus (Erb-Duchenne paralysis)	C5 and C6
Extended upper brachial plexus	C5, C6 and C7
Lower brachial plexus (Dejerine-Klumpke's paralysis)	C8 and T1

Rupture

The injury interrupting nerve continuity at the trunk level is called a rupture. Ruptures of the plexus separate both motor and sensory cell bodies from their axons and wallerian degeneration occurs across all fibers. Discontinuity by rupture can be treated by various surgical techniques to re-establish nerve continuity, whereas avulsion injuries are irreparable. The diagnosis can be difficult, for traction can cause a combination of rupture and avulsion injuries at different levels, which will complicate accurate diagnosis. Supraclavicular lesions account for most brachial plexus injuries (75% approximately) and are also subdivided into groups according to the pattern of involvement.

PATTERNS OF BRACHIAL PLEXUS INJURIES (TABLE 7)

Erb's Palsy (Erb-Duchenne Palsy)

It involves C5 and C6 or the upper trunk. The most common cause of Erb's Palsy is dystocia. Other causes include pressure on the raised arms during a breech delivery, clavicle fracture in neonates, traumatic fall onto the side of the head and shoulder, as shown in Figure 301. The most commonly involved nerves are suprascapular nerve, musculocutaneous nerve and axillary nerve. It is characterized by:

- Loss of elbow flexion
- Weakness of shoulder abduction and external rotation
- Paralysis and atrophy of the deltoid, biceps and brachialis muscles.

The position of the limb in Erb's palsy is characteristic, the arm hangs by the side and is rotated medially and the forearm is extended and pronated, as depicted in Figure 302. Sensory deficit is apparent in the corresponding dermatome, i.e. on radial side of the forearm and thumb.

Extended Upper Brachial Plexus Lesion

A C7 injury can accompany an Erb's palsy. In addition paralysis of elbow extensors, wrist extensors (extensor carpi radialis brevis) and finger extensors (extensor digitorum communis and proprius) are also present.

Klumpke's Paralysis (Dejerine-Klumpke's Palsy)

It involves C8 and T1, or lower trunk. The injury can be resulted from difficulties in proper handling during child birth, e.g. shoulder dystocia or traction on the abducted arm. It could also be the result of, when someone catching himself by a branch as he falls from a tree. Characterized by absent intrinsic hand musculature and finger flexors (flexor digitorum profundus and superficialis) with intact shoulder, elbow and wrist function.

Sensory deficit is situated over the ulnar side of the forearm and hand. Involvement of T1 may result in Horner's syndrome, as shown in Figure 303, with ptosis, miosis and anhydrosis.

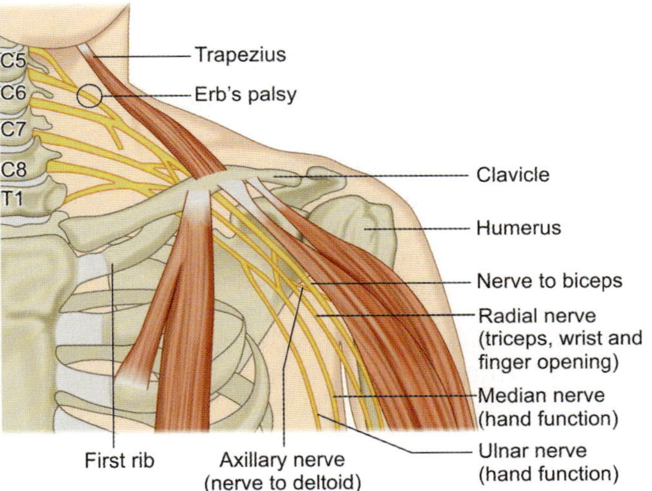

Fig. 301: The roots and trunk involved in Erb's palsy.

Total Brachial Plexus Lesion

The injury can include the entire plexus (C5, C6, C7, C8 and T1), which causes a flail and anesthetic arm. The brachial plexus may be injured by direct violence, gunshot wounds, by violent traction on the arm or by efforts at reducing a dislocation of the shoulder joint. The amount of paralysis will depend on the amount of injury to the constituent nerves. Supraclavicular lesions can also be isolated to peripheral branches, such as the suprascapular or long thoracic nerve. This can be secondary to trauma, infection and surgical positioning (iatrogenic).

Infraclavicular Lesions

They are less common (25% approximately). Usually, these represent stretch injuries from an associated shoulder dislocation or fracture. These injuries represent peripheral nerve lesions of the plexus. The axillary nerve is particularly susceptible to traction because it is securely anchored as it traverses the quadrangular space. However, injury to the musculocutaneous nerve and other elements of the brachial plexus can occur after severe trauma.

BASED ON DEGREE OF INTRANEURAL DAMAGE

- Neuropraxia
- Axonotmesis
- Neurotmesis.

Neuropraxia

It is a segmental demyelination with maintenance of intact nerve fibers and axonal sheath. A temporary conduction block follows, without axonal damage and Wallerian degeneration. Complete recovery occurs over the ensuing days to weeks as remyelinization is completed.

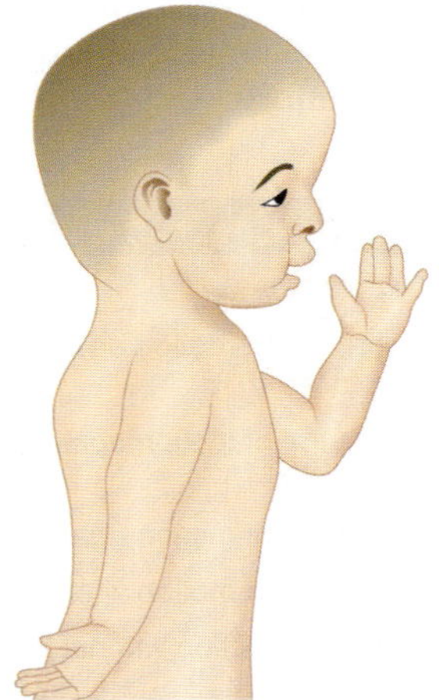

Fig. 302: Typical position of the upper limb in Erb's palsy.

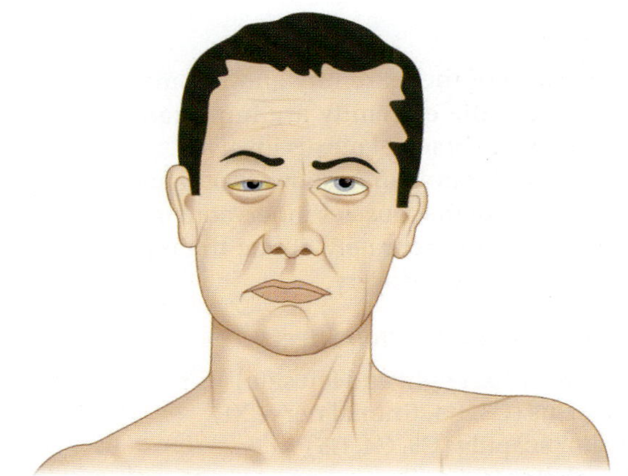

Fig. 303: Horner's syndrome due to the injury involving T1 root.

Axonotmesis

It is disruption of nerve fiber integrity with preservation of the axonal sheath and framework. Wallerian degeneration and nerve fiber regeneration are necessary for recovery. The axons distal to the injury degrade from lack of nutrition and loss of blood supply. The regeneration rate is approximately 1 mm per day or 1 inch per month. The distal nerve injuries have a better prognosis because the extent of Wallerian degeneration is decreased and the proximity to the motor endplates is increased.

Neurotmesis

It is disruption of the nerve fiber and axonal sheath. Transection is the classic example of this injury, but severe traction or contusion can produce a similar injury with irreversible intraneural scarring. The prognosis is bleak without surgical resection of the intervening scar and nerve coaptation by direct repair or graft interposition to allow for nerve regeneration. A severe brachial plexus injury often represents a combined lesion, with elements of neuropraxia, axonotmesis and neurotmesis. This combination injury further complicates accurate diagnosis and predictions for recovery.

EVALUATION OF BRACHIAL PLEXUS INJURY

The clinical evaluation of the patient with a brachial plexus injury begins with a careful history and detailed examination. The examination should include the head, neck, thorax, injured extremity and neurovascular systems. Knowledge of brachial plexus anatomy and concomitant muscle innervation is a prerequisite to accurate diagnosis. Imaging studies and electrodiagnostic tests provide supplemental information to further clarify the extent of injury. The goal of this evaluation is to precisely define the location and extent of nerve injury. This information will direct treatment, which may range from continued observation to prompt surgical intervention.

Adult injury: Usually referred after treatment of any life-threatening injuries.

History taking: Inquiry to the mechanism of injury and degree of energy involved. The force applied (direction, magnitude and duration), position of extremity and concomitant injuries (fractures, dislocations, visceral damage, head trauma and vascular disruptions) are important details. An instantaneous deficit implies nerve laceration, whereas a delayed onset indicates a compressive neuropathy by an expanding hematoma or false aneurysm.

Examination

- The posture of the extremity and the manner by which the patient uses the extremity are important indicators of the segment of the brachial plexus involved.
- Neurological examination shows motor and sensory deficit.
- An inventory of the muscles innervated by the brachial plexus is imperative to accurately define the injury and provides a baseline to assess recovery.

Brachial Plexus Examination Sheet

Muscle tested (both right and left side)

1. Trapezius (C3, C4, Cranial nerve XI)
2. Levator scapula (C3, C4, C5)
3. Rhomboids (C4, C5)
4. Supraspinatus (C5, C6)
5. Infraspinatus (C5, C6)
6. Serratus anterior (C5, C6, C7)
7. Teres major (C5, C6)
8. Subscapularis (C5, C6)
9. Pectoralis major clavicle (C5, C6, C7)
10. Pectoralis major sternocostal (C6, C7, C8, T1)
11. Latissimus dorsi (C6, C7, C8)
12. Biceps and brachialis (C5, C6)
13. Deltoid (C5, C6)
14. Teres minor (C5, C6)
15. Pronator quadratus (C7, C8, T1)
16. Pronator teres (C6, C7)
17. Flexor carpi radialis (C6, C7)
18. Flexor digitorum profundus II, III (C7, C8, T1)
19. Flexor digitorum superficialis (C7, C8, T1)
20. Flexor pollicis longus (C7, C8, T1)
21. Abductor pollicis brevis (C6, C7, C8, T1)
22. Opponens pollicis (C8, T1)
23. Lumbricals (C8, T1)
24. Triceps (C6, C7, C8)
25. Supinator (C5, C6)
26. Brachioradialis (C5, C6)
27. Extensor carpi radialis longus (C6, C7)
28. Extensor carpi radialis brevis (C6, C7, C8)
29. Extensor carpi ulnaris (C7, C8)
30. Extensor digitorum communis (C7, C8)
31. Extensor digiti minimi (C7, C8)
32. Extensor indicis (C7, C8)
33. Extensor pollicis longus (C7, C8)
34. Extensor pollicis brevis (C6, C7)
35. Abductor pollicis longus (C6, C7)
36. Flexor carpi ulnaris (C7, C8, T1)
37. Flexor digitorum profundus IV, V (C7, C8 and T1)
38. Abductor digiti minimi (C8, T1)
39. Abductor pollicis (C8, T1)
40. Opponens digiti (C8, T1)
41. Interossei (C8, T1).

Muscle Grading Chart (Table 8)

Careful examination of the muscles innervated by the proximal branches from the brachial plexus will help define the proximity of the plexus lesion to the spinal cord. Disruption of the dorsal rami (paraspinal muscles), dorsal scapular (rhomboids and levator scapulae) and long thoracic (serratus anterior) nerves are suggestive of an avulsion injury.

TABLE 8: Muscle strength grading chart and its description.

Muscle grade	*Description*
Grade 5 (Normal)	Full range of motion against gravity with full resistance
Grade 4 (Good)	Full range of motion against gravity with some resistance
Grade 3 (Fair)	Full range of motion against gravity
Grade 2 (Poor)	Full range of motion with gravity eliminated
Grade 1 (Trace)	Slight contraction without joint motion
Grade 0 (Zero)	No evidence of contraction

The presence of a Horner's syndrome results in a drooped eyelid, constricted pupil, sunken globe and sweating deficiency that usually implies an avulsion injury at C8 and T1.

Indicators of Avulsion Injuries and Poor Prognosis for Recovery (Table 9)

Percussion of the supra and infraclavicular plexus is performed. A Tinel's sign is indicative of a postganglionic injury, e.g. rupture. This sign will be absent in a preganglionic lesion, e.g. avulsion because the link to the spinal cord and brain has been disrupted. Postganglionic injuries are further localized by examination of the intermediate and terminal branches. The status of the suprascapular (spinati), thoracodorsal (latissimus dorsi), subscapular (subscapularis and teres major), pectoral (pectoralis major and minor) will further define the injury.

Examination of the pectoralis major muscle is particularly helpful because of its dual segmental innervation from the lateral pectoral (C5, C6, and C7) and medial pectoral (C8 and T1) nerves from the lateral and medial cords respectively. Selective atrophy of the clavicular head (lateral pectoral) or sternocostal head (medial pectoral) facilitates diagnosis, whereas complete atrophy implies a global injury.

A peripheral vascular examination is a fundamental component of the evaluation, for damage to the axillary or subclavian vessels can occur. Decreased or absent peripheral pulses, a delayed neurologic deficit (expanding hematoma) and penetrating trauma war rant arteriography.

OBSTETRIC BRACHIAL PLEXUS PALSY

The history is extremely important. Prenatal, postnatal and birth information should be obtained. Risk factors for an obstetric palsy include a difficult or prolonged delivery, large birth weight, shoulder dystocia, breech presentation and forceps or vacuum extraction. A cesarean delivery does not negate the possibility of brachial plexus injury. In fact, bilateral plexus injuries can occur after cesarean section.

Examination

Examination is difficult because of lack of cooperation. Observation of the affected extremity often provides valuable information of the underlying pathology. Upper root or trunk injuries (Erb's palsy) and total plexus palsy are common. Isolated lower root or trunk (Klumpke's palsy) injuries are rare in obstetric injuries.

The presence of a Horner's syndrome (ptosis, miosis, enophthalmos, and ipsilateral facial anhydrosis) is an important observation that implies proximal avulsion injury of the lower trunk, with disruption of the communicating branch supplying sympathetic fibers to the cervicothoracic ganglion.

Palpation of the clavicle and shoulder girdle may reveal crepitation or abundant callus formation. An acute fracture will inhibit voluntary movement and mimic brachial plexus injuries (pseudoparalysis).

Range of motion: A newborn with a brachial plexus injury will have full passive motion, whereas a congenital shoulder dislocation will lack passive motion. Ultrasound may be required to confirm this diagnosis because the newborn humeral head is not calcified.

Assessment of Motor Function

It is a challenging task that requires patience and diligence. The initial goal is to determine the absence or presence of function, as actual grading of muscle strength is impossible.

- *Moro reflex:* The newborn can be aroused by the startle reaction or Moro reflex. This should produce extensor tone in the legs and arms.
- The grasp reaction by palmar stimulation should illicit finger flexion. Absence of these primitive reflexes indicates a neurologic problem.
- In the infant, a collection of toys, rattles and sweets is necessary to incite movement of the injured extremity.
- The effect of gravity can be altered by changing the position of the child to assess weak but functioning muscle.
- Sensory function is also difficult to assess, as the only reaction obtained only to some painful stimuli, which will erase any chance of further cooperation.

Imaging Studies

Radiographic Findings (Table 10)

Angiography: It is indicated if there is any question of the vascular status of the extremity or integrity of the subclavian or axillary vessels.

TABLE 9: Indicators of avulsion injuries and poor prognosis for recovery.

Finding	*Implication*
Denervation of paraspinal muscles	Dorsal rami injury
Denervation of rhomboid muscles	Dorsal scapular (C5) injury
Scapular winging	Long thoracic (C5, C7 and C8) injury
Horner's syndrome	Cervicothoracic sympathetic injury
Absent Tinel's sign	Preganglionic separation from cord
Sensory impairment of neck	Cervical plexus injury
Hemidiaphragm paralysis	Phrenic nerve injury
Cervical transverse process fracture	Avulsion fracture with root injury
Pseudomeningocele	Dura and arachnoid avulsion injury
Anesthesia and intact CV	Dorsal ganglion intact, but avulsion from cord

TABLE 10: Radiographic findings in injuries to the brachial plexus.

Plain X-ray film	*Findings*	*Significance*
Chest	Elevated hemidiaphragm First rib fracture	Phrenic injury, proximal plexus and possible preganglionic avulsion Subclavian or axillary artery injury and lower trunk injury
Cervical spine	Fracture or dislocation	Cervical spine injury
	Transverse process fractured	Preganglionic avulsion injury
Clavicle	Fracture	Possible traction injury to plexus or pseudoparalysis
Shoulder	Glenohumeral dislocation Scapulothoracic dissociation	Infraclavicular injury Severe neurovascular injury

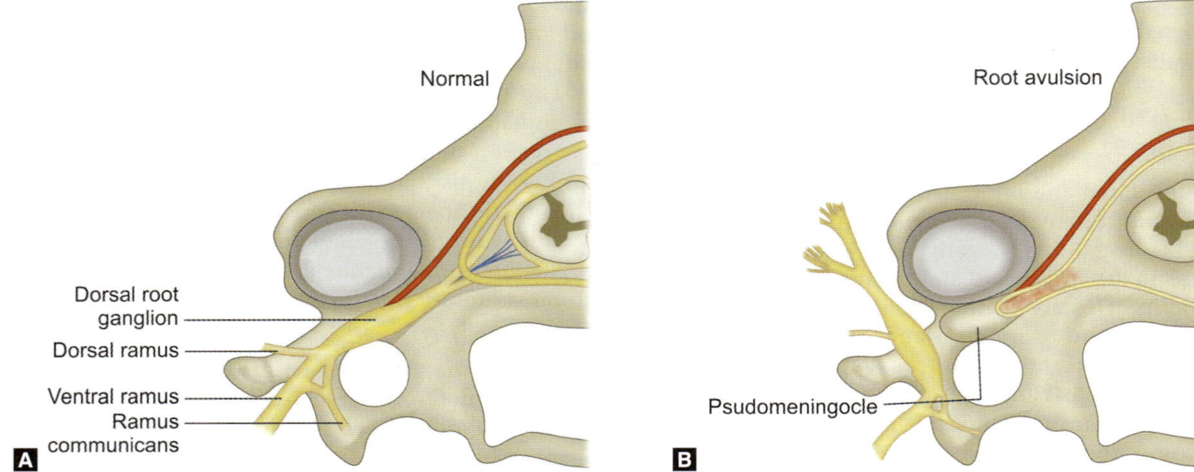

Figs. 304A and B: Formation of pseudomeningocele, due to root avulsion injury: (A) Normal; (B) Pseudomeningocele, extends through the intervertebral foramen into the paraspinal area after root avulsion injury.

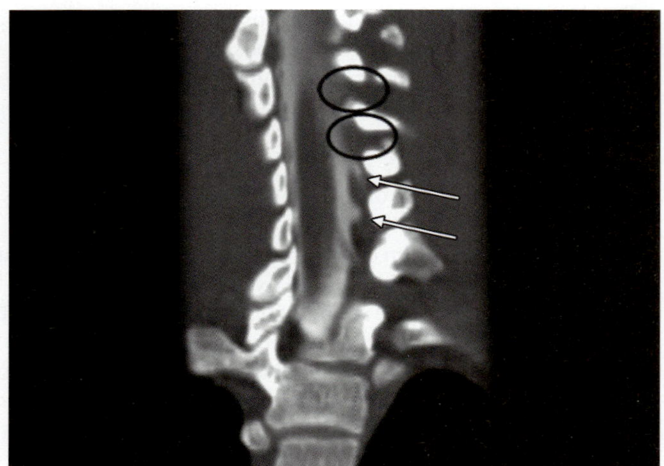

Fig. 305: MRI of spine provides multiplanar imaging to assess the various components of the brachial plexus.

Penetrating trauma or an expanding hematoma also requires angiography.

Myelography (Figs. 304A and B): It is used to define the presence or absence of a pseudomeningocele, a meningeal pouch filled with cerebrospinal fluid that extends through the intervertebral foramen into the paraspinal area. It occurs during root avulsion injury.

Inability to visualize the nerve root on the myelogram further supports the diagnosis of an avulsion injury. However, false-positive pseudomeningocele result has been found in patients in whom the rootlets were intact with isolated dura rupture and false-negative results have been reported during surgical exploration.

Methods recommended to improve the diagnostic accuracy of myelography are to delay the test for 4–6 weeks after injury, to allow for resolution of local swelling and intradural blood clots and also by using computed tomography (CT myelography) to visualize small pseudomeningoceles.

MRI (Fig. 305): Magnetic resonance imaging has become the primary imaging modality. The MRI provides multiplanar imaging to assess the various components of the brachial plexus. Varying the pulse sequence will provide high resolution images that will facilitate identification of plexus pathology.

MRI offers better evaluation of the trunks and cords, with potential verification of a neuroma by an abnormal signal. MRI is the modality of choice to evaluate neoplasms of the brachial plexus. Diagnosis of root avulsion (pseudomeningocele and nonvisualization of a nerve root) is used with MRI.

Electrodiagnostic Studies

Electrodiagnostic testing plays an integral part in the diagnosis and treatment of brachial plexus lesions.

Methods employed are:
- Electromyography
- Nerve conduction velocity measurements
- Somatosensory evoked potentials
- Nerve action potentials.

Electromyography: Electromyography (EMG) records the electrical activity of muscle fibers at rest and during activation. This signal is recorded by the insertion of EMG needles into the muscle. The normal muscle is silent at rest and active during contraction. A denervated muscle will exhibit spontaneous electrical discharge, i.e. fibrillations and positive sharp wave, when the EMG needle is inserted. These findings are not present until 2–4 weeks after denervation. A reinnervated muscle will begin to show reinnervation or nascent potentials (polyphasic low amplitude recordings). EMG examination of the muscles innervated by the brachial plexus can provide valuable information about the degree of injury and early recovery.

An EMG evaluation of the more proximal branches from the brachial plexus can help differentiate an avulsion injury from a rupture. For example, fibrillations and positive sharp waves of the paraspinal muscles (innervated by the dorsal rami from the spinal nerve) imply an avulsion injury, whereas preservation of a normal electrical signal suggests a more distal lesion. The EMG is also useful to differentiate the degree of intraneural injury (neuropraxia, axonotmesis, and neurotmesis) and to follow the progress after injury. A neuropraxia can be differentiated from a more severe nerve injury by the absence of fibrillation potentials and positive sharp waves. These denervation changes will be present in an axonotmesis or neurotmesis. Serial EMG evaluations can distinguish an axonotmetic lesion by the spontaneous return of nascent units or reinnervation potentials that will precede clinical recovery of function. A neurotmetic injury will not exhibit EMG signs of spontaneous recovery.

Conduction velocity: The conduction velocity (CV) is the distance between two sites of stimulation divided by, the time for the nerve action potential to travel from proximal to distal. The integrity of the peripheral nerve is determined by the measurement of the conduction velocity. The motor or sensory latency can be measured depending on the recording of the compound motor action potential (CMAP) or the sensory nerve action potential (SNAP). A severed nerve will lose the capability to conduct an action potential distal to the lesion as the nerve degenerates. However, the distal portion of the nerve may be able to conduct for several days after injury until degeneration occurs. Therefore, testing should be delayed for at least 3 weeks to allow time for loss of conduction and denervation changes in muscle.

The status of the SNAP and corresponding sensory nerve conduction velocity is helpful in differentiating preganglionic avulsion injuries from postganglionic lesions. The presence of an intact sensory CV in an anesthetic part of the arm indicates a preganglionic injury, for the sensory nerve is not separated from its cell body (dorsal root ganglion). The CMAP or motor nerve conduction velocity (NCV) is absent in both preganglionic and postganglionic injuries and is not a distinguishing factor.

Somatosensory evoked potentials (SEP): SEPs are electrical responses of the brain and spinal cord to the stimulation of peripheral sensory fibers. Recordings of the conduction from the stimulating electrode to the central nervous system can be useful for the detection of lesions within the sensory system. This technique can be employed to assess conduction across the brachial plexus and during surgery to define irreparable nerve root avulsions. The absence of SEPs recorded over the spinal cord or contralateral sensorimotor cortex on nerve root stimulation indicates a root avulsion and is a contraindication for nerve grafting.

Nerve action potentials (NAPs): NAPs are used intra-operatively to assess lesions in continuity. Stimulating and recording of a nerve proximal and distal to a neuroma can identify the presence or absence of axonal continuity. The presence of NAPs indicates propagation of an action potential along viable nerve fibers. This can help the surgeon decide between neurolysis or excision and interposition grafting.

Treatment

Conservative Treatment

- *A period of immobilization:* For about 3–4 weeks to allow the fractures and wounds to heal, to prevent further damage. This is achieved by static splints.
- *Physiotherapy:* After 3–4 weeks mobilization of the affected extremity is done in order to prevent contractures.
- *Electrostimulation of paralyzed muscle:* To maintain electrical activity in the paralyzed muscles and also it induces axon regeneration via yet unknown chemotaxis.

Surgical Treatment

Surgical goals: The surgeon should have clear and reasonable surgical goals, which in order of priority are:

- Restoration of elbow flexion
- Restoration of shoulder abduction
- Restoration of sensation to the medial border of the forearm and hand.

Depending on the extent of injury, various surgical techniques may be required, including primary neurorrhaphy, neurolysis, nerve grafting, and neurotization.

Treatment of avulsion injuries: Currently, there is no surgical treatment to restore nerve rootlet connection (avulsion or intraspinal injuries) with the spinal cord. The current treatment options for avulsion injuries are nerve grafting to other viable proximal stumps or a nerve transfer. Neurotization between the intercostal nerves and the musculocutaneous nerve to restore elbow flexion may be considered.

Treatment of lesions in continuity: Neurolysis is performed for lesions in continuity and the extent of neurolysis will vary with the degree of constricting scar. Epineurotomy may be sufficient in instances of external compression from limited fibrosis, whereas epifascicular epineurectomy may be necessary in an advanced interfascicular compression from fibrosis around the fascicles.

Treatment of lesions without continuity: The initial treatment is to resect the neuroma that forms at the proximal and distal nerve stumps until normal nerve consistency and fascicular anatomy is encountered. The distal stumps are now primed for coaptation with a viable inflow for regeneration of axons. Restoration of continuity can be accomplished by nerve grafting or nerve transfer.

Nerve grafting: Nerve grafting is the placement of intercalary nerve grafts that act as scaffolding for regenerating axons. Nerve grafting is the preferred technique for most lesions with loss of continuity. The interposition of nerve segments link the proximal and distal axons and serve as a conduit to channel, the growing axons to the periphery. The donor nerve is usually the sural nerve from the lower extremity, harvested at the time of brachial plexus exploration. Other potential options are the ipsilateral medial antebrachial cutaneous and superficial radial nerves.

Nerve transfer: Nerve transfer is indicated in avulsion injuries and large or extensive defects of the brachial plexus. The indications for nerve transfer increases as the number of avulsed roots multiplies. This technique involves the connection of an expandable donor motor nerve to provide an axonal source for regeneration of the distal stump. The donor neurons will reinnervate the muscle and function will require voluntary control of the transferred nerve. Similar to a tendon transfer, activation of the donor nerve to achieve function will require a period of training. Involuntary muscle activation may occur, until transformation has taken place.

There are numerous donor nerves available for transfer, including the spinal accessory nerve, cervical plexus, phrenic, intercostal nerves, and various portions of the affected plexus (intraplexal transfer).

Oberlin transfer: Transfer of a single fascicle of ulnar nerve to the motor branch of biceps and a fascicle median to the brachialis. Partial transfer of ulnar nerve to the biceps motor branch is made through a longitudinal incision on the anteromedial aspect of the upper arm.

The musculocutaneous nerve is identified after it traverses the coracobrachialis muscle. The biceps motor branch is traced as far proximally as possible and then sectioned. The ulnar nerve is identified at the same level and a longitudinal epineurotomy is done. One ulnar nerve fascicle, carrying motor fibers to the flexor carpi ulnaris (confirmed by electrical stimulation) is minimally dissected, sectioned and coapted to the biceps motor branch with 10-0 nylon sutures. Fascicle of the median nerve that innervated the wrist flexor is identified and coapted with the motor branch to the brachialis, ensuring a tension free nerve anastomosis.

Postoperatively the flexed arm is strapped to the chest for a period of 3 weeks. After that gradually increasing passive exercises are begun. Paralyzed muscles are subjected to electrical stimulation till a grade three power is achieved. After brachial plexus repair and reconstruction, 12–18 months are required to determine the extent of neural regeneration. If recovery is considered inadequate, peripheral reconstruction should be considered.

Tendon transfers, around the shoulder that may be considered include:

- Trapezius to deltoid transfer as described by Saha to improve abduction
- Latissimus dorsi transfer to improve external rotation as described by L'Episcopo.

Shoulder arthrodesis is helpful if active ST motion is preserved and has been shown to improve elbow flexion by preventing uncontrolled internal rotation of the shoulder. Shoulder should be fused in only 20–30° of abduction because most of these patients rely heavily on arm-trunk prehension.

Operations to restore elbow flexion include transfers of:

- Latissimus dorsi
- Pectoralis major
- Triceps
- Sternocleidomastoid
- Flexor pronator mass.

Restoration of elbow flexion is helpful to the patient, even if the hand is functionless.

Amputation: It is performed rarely. If the patient is certain that the dead weight of a functionless upper extremity is disabling, amputation and prosthetic fitting may be helpful. Amputation should never be performed for pain relief.

OBSTETRIC BRACHIAL PLEXUS SURGERY

Surgery for obstetric lesions is usually performed between 6 months and 12 months of age. The obstetric injuries most commonly involve the upper plexus and are usually postganglionic ruptures that can be reconstructed by interposition grafting.

Surgical Methods

Various surgical techniques have been advocated for:

- Root avulsion injuries C5 to T1
- Avulsion of some roots and extraforaminal rupture of other spinal nerves
- Rupture of trunks, cords and individual terminal branches
- Individual nerve injuries.

Root Avulsion of C5 to T1

It can be treated by:

- Conservative treatment
- Nerve transfers

At shoulder: Transfer of 11th cranial nerve (spinal accessory) to suprascapular nerve. Transfer of intercostals nerve to medial pectoral nerve.

At elbow: Transfer of intercostal nerves to musculo-cutaneous nerve.

For sensation: Sensory rami of intercostal nerves are directed preferentially to the median nerve vesicles, to get sensation in the median nerve supplied area.

Avulsion of Roots and Extraforaminal Rupture of other Spinal Nerves

- *Extraforaminal rupture of C5 and root avulsion of C6 to T1:* Neurotization of suprascapular nerve with 11th cranial nerve. C5 extraforaminal root is sutured to the posterior cord and lateral cord origins. Neurotization of intercostals nerves to middle trunk.
- *Extraforaminal rupture C5, C6 and C7 to T1 root avulsions:* Intraplexal neurotization of avulsed C7 to C6. Connecting lateral cord to the stump of C5. Connecting posterior cord to the stump of C6. Repair the suprascapular nerve with 11th nerve.
- *Extraforaminal rupture C5, C6, C7 and C8, T1 avulsions:* C5 and C6 to be sutured (neurorrhaphy). Avulsed C8 division for medial cord is connected to anteroinferior portion of C7. Avulsed C8 division going to the posterior cord is connected to intercostals nerves. Neurotization of 11th nerve to suprascapular nerve.

Rupture of Trunks, Cords, and Individual Terminal Branches

Upper trunk lesions: Connecting posterior part of C5, C6 to posterior cord. Connecting anterior part of C5, C6 to lateral cord. Repair of suprascapular nerve using 11th nerve (Spinal Accessory) transfer.

Lower trunk lesions: Neurotization of medial cord, ulnar nerve and medial origin of median nerve, using intercostals nerves.

Cord lesions: Cord lesions can be repaired by:

- Direct repair
- Nerve grafting.

Deformities in Long Standing Paralyzed Upper Limb in Brachial Plexus Injury

Shoulder: Adduction, internal rotation deformity with inability to abduct and externally rotate.

Elbow: Fixed flexion deformity

Forearm: Supination deformity

Hand: Claw hand.

RECONSTRUCTIVE SURGERIES FOR UPPER LIMB SHOULDER

- *Fairbank's procedure:* Superior portion of tendon of pectoralis major is sectioned at its insertion, entire tendon of subscapularis and anterior capsule of shoulder are divided.
- *Sever's procedure:* Tendons of pectoralis major and subscapularis are completely divided without opening the capsule. When coracobrachialis and short head of biceps are contracted, their tendons at coracoids are released.
- *L'Episcopo and Sever operation:* These constitute the first stage. The teres major is transferred posteriorly over the lateral aspect of humerus, where it acts as an external rotator. The latismus dorsi can be similarly transferred.
- *Green's procedure:* Instead of complete division, the tendons of subscapularis and pectoralis major are lengthened to preserve internal rotation. Both latissimus dorsi and teres major are rerouted to act as external rotators. Overgrowth of coracoids and acromion are excised. Osteotomy of humerus to correct internal rotation also done.
- *Derotation osteotomy of humerus for posterior torsion/ subluxation:* First Sever's operation is done thereby, correcting adduction and internal rotation. This reduces humeral head

back into the glenoid. After sufficient immobilization in the corrected position, the humeral head is held in its normal relationship to glenoid, while surgical neck is osteotomized and distal humerus rotated internally. Immobilization continued until union has occurred.

- *Saha's transfer for supraspinatus and infraspinatus:*
  - *For supraspinatus:* Transfer of sternocleidomastoid, Scalenus anterior and scalenus medius is done.
  - *For infraspinatus:* Transfer of teres major and latissimus dorsi is done.
- *For deltoid paralysis*:
  - *Lange's procedure*: Insertion of trapezius to humerus using silk sutures.
  - *Meyer's procedure:* Used fascia lata instead of silk. But delayed problems of adherence and decreased ROM are seen.
  - *Saha's procedure*: Transfer trapezius along with part of clavicle and spine of scapula to proximal humerus and fixed with screws.

Elbow

Operations to restore active flexor power to elbow include:

- *Steindler's flexorplasty:* Transfer of common flexor origin more proximally.
- *Bunnel's modification of Steindler's flexorplasty:* Common flexor origin transferred proximally and anteriorly.
- Bunnel's anterior transfer of triceps to bicipetal tuberosity. When the pectoralis major and triceps as well as the biceps and brachialis are partially weakened, the further two muscles can be transferred to reinforce the flexor muscle of elbow.
- *Correction of elbow deformity:* Removal of radial head should await skeletal maturity. Arthrodesis of elbow at 90° is an alternative when muscles are unavailable for transfer.

Forearm

Correction of Forearm Deformity

- Fixed pronation deformity, generally left alone.
- *Fixed supination deformity:*
  - Zancolli's transfer for rerouting the biceps.
  - Manual osteoclasis and fixing in needed degree of pronation.

Hand

Correction of claw hand deformity can be done by following procedures:

- Restoration of opposition of thumb
- Restoration of adduction of thumb
- Restoration of abduction of index finger
- Restoration of intrinsic function of fingers.

Restoration of opposition of thumb by:

- Riordans' technique
- Brand technique
- Burkhalter technique
- Groves and Goldner technique
- Litter technique
- Camitz technique.

Restoration of adduction of thumb by:

- Royale-Thompson technique
- Boye's technique
- Smith technique.

Restoration of abduction of index finger: This is done by using palmaris brevis, brachioradialis, and external carpi radialis brevis muscles.

Restoration of intrinsic function of fingers by:

- Bunnel's technique
- Riordan's technique
- Zancollis capsulodesis
- Fowler transfer
- Brand's transfer of extensor carpi radialis Longus (ECRL)
- Brand's transfer of extensor carpi radialis brevis (ECRB)
- Fowler tenodesis.

THORACIC OUTLET SYNDROME

ANATOMY

The thoracic outlet begins just distal to the intervertebral foramina and extends to the coracoid process as depicted in Figure 306. The most common sites of compression in thoracic outlet syndrome (TOS) are:

- Superior thoracic outlet
- Scalene interval or triangle
- Costoclavicular space
- Subcoracoid area.

These sites are enumerated in Table 11. This compression can be static or dynamic with dependence on posture and activity.

Thoracic Outlet Syndrome

The thoracic outlet syndromes comprise three different clinical pathophysiologic entities:

1. Neurologic thoracic outlet syndrome
2. Vascular thoracic outlet syndrome
3. Thoracic outlet syndrome of pain and sensory symptoms.

Neurologic Thoracic Outlet Syndrome (Fig. 307)

Neurologic thoracic outlet syndrome is found mainly in women. It begins to manifest itself as a pain along the medial aspect of the

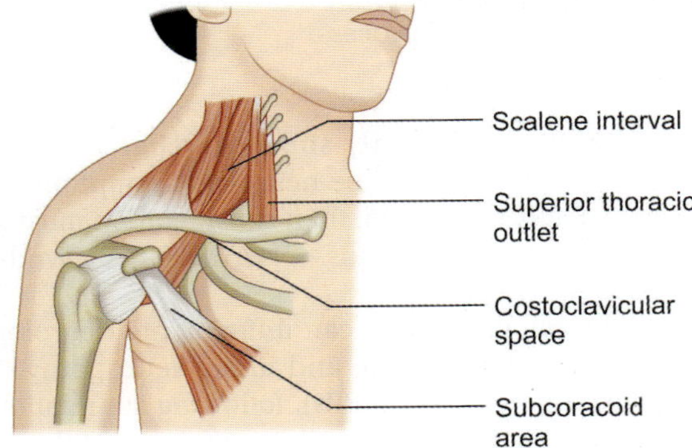

Fig. 306: Extent of the thoracic outlet.

TABLE 11: The most common sites and causes of compression in thoracic outlet syndrome.

Site	*Principal cause*
Superior thoracic outlet	First rib or cervical rib
Scalene interval or triangle	Scalene muscles or fibrous bands
Costoclavicular space	Narrow clavicle—first rib distance
Subcoracoid area	Coracoid process

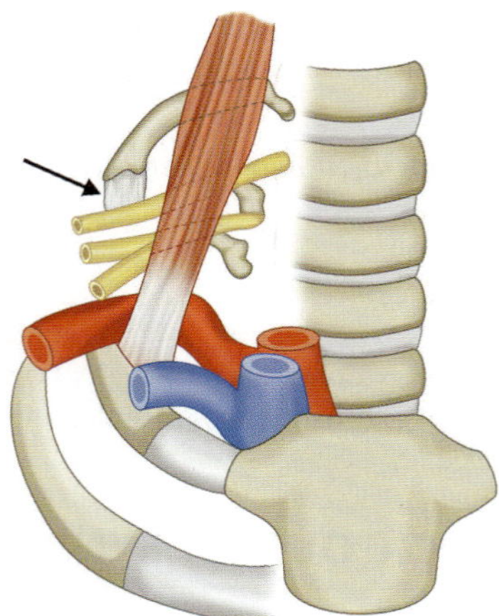

Fig. 307: Rudimentary cervical rib (arrow) with a fibrous band extending to the upper surface of the first rib.

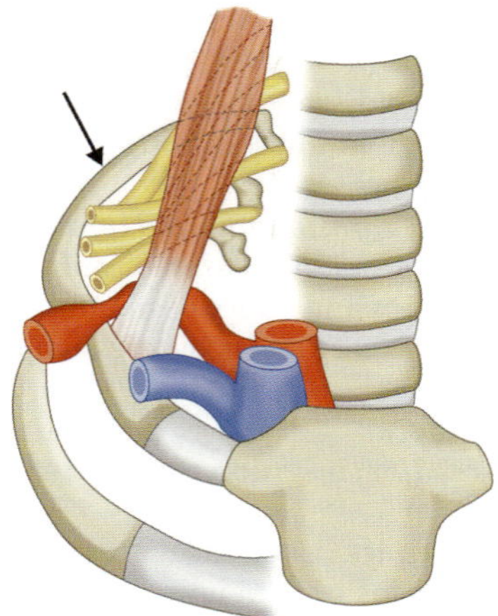

Fig. 308: Vascular thoracic outlet syndrome, subclavian artery wedged between the anterior scalene muscle and the cervical rib that causes its compression.

arm and forearm. Paresthesias are found extending into the ulnar border of the hand. Muscle weakness and atrophy occur later. Muscle atrophy is selective for the abductor pollicis brevis and the opponens muscles of the thenar eminence of hand.

Wasting of all the intrinsic muscles of the hand is possible with the progression of the condition. There are no vascular symptoms. Sensory abnormalities are referrable to the lower trunk of the brachial plexus. A well-developed cervical or rudimentary cervical rib with a fibrous band extending to the upper surface of the first rib may impinge on the lower trunk of the brachial plexus.

Similarly, anatomic abnormalities of the first rib may stretch and angulate the lower trunk of the brachial plexus. The scalenus anticus syndrome involves hypertrophy of the anterior scalene muscle and compression of the brachial plexus as it passes through the interscalene groove between the anterior and middle scalene muscles. Hyperabduction syndrome or subcoracoid-pectoralis minor syndrome involves compression of the brachial plexus with lateral abduction of the arm to an elevated position. In this position, structures, like the brachial plexus and vasculature are compressed by tension of the pectoralis minor muscle and to a lesser extent, the coracoid process.

Investigations

X-rays will almost uniformly show the characteristic bony abnormality, responsible for the neurologic symptomatology. If a bony abnormality is not seen, then consideration must be given to the presence of fibrous bands, scalenus anticus syndrome or hyperabduction syndrome.

Electrophysiologic studies can differentiate neurologic TOS from carpal tunnel syndrome and ulnar neuropathy. Somato sensory evoked potentials (SSEPs), following stimulation of the ulnar nerve at the wrist, may actually be a more useful technique.

Treatment

Supraclavicular exploration with release of the compressive anatomy is the most satisfactory treatment for neurologic thoracic outlet syndrome. Patient experiences immediate relief of pain.

Vascular Thoracic Outlet Syndrome

In patients with a well-developed first rib, the subclavian artery may be angulated over the cervical rib and wedged between the anterior scalene muscle and the cervical rib, as shown in Figure 308. The subclavian artery will become narrowed and will develop an area of poststenotic dilation. Thrombus may accumulate in the poststenotic dilation. Its fragments may embolize to the hand. This produces vascular symptomatology.

Clinical Features

- Intermittent blanching of the hands and fingers.
- Pulses may be diminished or absent.
- A bruit can sometimes be auscultated in the supraclavicular and/or axillary areas.
- The vascular thoracic outlet syndrome consists only of vascular symptomatology without neurologic abnormalities.

Diagnosis

Angiography: Used selectively in suspected cases of vascular thoracic outlet syndrome for visualizing a mural thrombus, stenosis, and aneurysmal dilation.

MRI: Visualize the plexus anatomy and identify areas of compression and anomalous bands.

Treatment

Surgical excision of the cervical rib effectively treats vascular thoracic outlet syndrome.

Thoracic Outlet Syndrome of Pain and Sensory Symptoms

This is more common, but obscure form of thoracic outlet syndrome, where patients present with less clearly defined symptomatology. Such patients will usually present with a diffuse nagging ache and numbness in the arm. The pain in the arm will be made worse by carrying heavy objects or holding the arm in a particular position. Paresthesias may occur concomitantly with the pain or may be temporally distinct. Paresthesias are usually appreciated in the medial aspect of the arm and forearm and sometimes in the hand.

Pathophysiology

The exact pathophysiology is obscure. Various proposed mechanisms include:

- Compression of the subclavian artery and/or brachial plexus between the lower end of the anterior scalene muscle and the first rib
- Vascular factors, i.e. venous rather than arterial compression
- Costoclavicular syndrome.

How to Differentiate Between Cervical Spondylosis and TOS? (Table 12)

Investigations: X-rays, electromyography (EMG), nerve conduction studies, SSEPs, and arteriography are usually normal and of limited value.

Special Tests

Tests for thoracic outlet syndrome indicating compression:

- *Adson or scalene test:* The patient is asked to take and hold a deep breath, extend the neck fully and turn the face into one side. It will tighten the anterior and middle scalene muscles. Diminution or loss of the radial pulse suggests compression.
- *Costoclavicular maneuver or Eden's test (military position):* The back is downward and backward. The costoclavicular space will be narrowed by approximating the first rib and the clavicle. Diminution or loss of the radial pulse suggests compression.
- *Hyperabduction test:* The arm is hyperabducted to 180°. Diminution or loss of the radial pulse suggests compression.
- *Arm claudication test:* The shoulder is drawn backward and upward. The arm is raised horizontally with the elbow flexed to 90°. With exercise of hands, pain and numbness indicates compression.
- *Allen test:* The examiner flexes the patient's elbow to 90° while the shoulder is abducted and extended horizontally and rotated laterally. The patient is asked to turn their head away from the tested arm. The radial pulse is palpated and if it disappears as the patient's head is rotated the test is considered positive.

Hallstead test: This test is like the Adson's maneuver, but here neck is turned to opposite side.

Treatment

- *Physical therapy:* Exercises to counteract and strengthen drooping shoulders have been proposed as a possible treatment.
- First rib resection is often performed in patients with this more obscure but common form of thoracic outlet syndrome.

TABLE 12: Difference between cervical spondylosis and TOS.

Maneuver	*TOS*	*Cervical spondylosis*
Drooping/depression of shoulder	Produces symptoms	Relieves of symptoms
Elevation of shoulder	Relieves symptoms	Produces symptoms

(TOS: thoracic outlet syndrome)

COSTOCLAVICULAR SYNDROME

The costoclavicular syndrome suggests that the subclavian artery and/or the brachial plexus are intermittently compressed between the clavicle and a normal first rib. Patients, who are believed to have costoclavicular syndrome are the women with long necks and drooping shoulders, women with pendulous breasts, patients of new- widow syndrome and women carrying heavy back packs.

Symptomatology has been hypothesized to result from chronic stretching of the brachial plexus. Following symptoms are identified:

- Sense of fullness in the hand and fingers
- Cramping pain in the forearm and hand
- Vague shoulder pain
- Swollen and engorged veins—intermittent
- Shoulder ROM is maintained
- Costoclavicular maneuver and Eden's Test are diagnostic.

CERVICAL RIB SYNDROME

There is a congenital overdevelopment (bony or fibrous) of the C7 costal process. It can be unilateral or bilateral and is usually, asymptomatic. Occurs in 1% of the population and only 10% of those are symptomatic.

Pain and paresthesias in the medial forearm and hand is present, which usually relieved by changing position. Patient can have weakness and difficulty with fine motor control. Prolapse of intervertebral discs (PIVD) of C4, C5, C6 should be considered as a differential diagnosis for the abnormality.

Treatment

Surgical resection of the cervical rib is performed.

REFERENCES

1. Boileau P, Avidor C, Krishnan SG, et al. Cemented polyethylene versus uncemented metal-backed glenoid components in total shoulder arthroplasty: a prospective, double-blind, randomized study. J Shoulder Elbow Surg. 2002;11(4):351-9.
2. Neer CS 2nd. Replacement arthroplasty for glenohumeral osteoarthritis. J Bone Joint Surg Am. 1974;56(1):1-13.
3. Kirkley A, Griffin S, McLintock H. et al. The development and evaluation of a disease-specific quality of like measurement tool for shoulder instability. The WOSI. Am J sports Med. 1998;20:764-72.
4. Bryant D, Litchfield R, Sandow M, et al. A comparison of pain, strength, range of motion, and functional outcomes after hemiarthroplasty and total shoulder arthroplasty in patients with osteoarthritis of the shoulder. A systematic review and meta-analysis. J Bone Joint Surg Am. 2005;87(9):1947-56.
5. Haines JF, Trail IA, Nuttall D, et al. The results of arthroplasty in osteoarthritis of the shoulder. J Bone Joint Surg Br. 2006;88(4):496-501.
6. Frankle M, Siegel S, Pupello D, et al. The Reverse Shoulder Prosthesis for glenohumeral arthritis associated with severe rotator cuff deficiency. A minimum two-year follow-up study of sixty patients. J Bone Joint Surg Am. 2005;87(8):1697-705.
7. Werner CM, Steinmann PA, Glbart M, et al. Treatment of painful pseudoparesis due to irreparable rotator cuff dysfunction with the Delta III reverse-ball-and-socket total shoulder prosthesis. J Bone Joint Surg Am. 2005;87(7):1476-86.

CHAPTER

30 Hip Joint

OBJECTIVES

- Anatomy and Biomechanics of Hip Joint
- Developmental Dysplasia of the Hip
- Congenital Coxa Vara
- Acetabular Fractures
- Fractures of the Femoral Neck
- Intertrochanteric Femoral Fractures
- Subtrochanteric Femoral Fractures
- Traumatic Dislocation of Hip
- Infections of Hip Joint
- Tuberculosis of Hip Joint
- Degenerative Osteoarthritis
- Rheumatoid Arthritis of Hip
- Legg-Calve-Perthes Disease
- Tumors around Hip
- Osteotomies around the Hip
- Surgical Approaches to Hip

ANATOMY AND BIOMECHANICS OF HIP JOINT

Anatomy of Hip Joint (Fig. 1)

Type

Hip joint is ball and socket, variety of synovial joint. The head of femur articulates with the acetabulum of hip bone to form hip joint. It is unique, as it has high degree of stability and mobility.

Articular Surface

Head of the femur

- Directed medially, upward, slightly forward
- Articulates with acetabulum to form hip joint
- Roughened pit situated just below and behind
- The center of the head is called fovea
- Forms more than half-a-sphere and is covered with hyaline cartilage except at the fovea capitis.

Neck shaft angle (Fig. 2)

Neck shaft angle is 120° (115–145°). The axis of the femoral head and neck forms an angle with the axis of the femoral shaft. It is called the angle of inclination/neck shaft angle. It is smaller in women as compared to men, normally, owing to the greater width of female pelvis. With normal angle, the greater trochanter (GT) lies at the level of the center of femoral head.

Angle of anteversion (Fig. 3)

A line parallel to the posterior femoral condyles and line through the head and neck of the femur normally make an angle with each other that average 15–20° in adults without impairment. It is also called as "angle of torsion".

Articular Surface

- *Acetabulum:* It is formed by:
  - *Ilium:* It forms the upper 2/5th region
  - *Pubis:* It forms the anterior 1/5th region
  - *Ischium:* It forms the posterior 2/5th region
- It is a deep, cup-shaped, hemispherical cavity on the lateral aspect of the hip bone

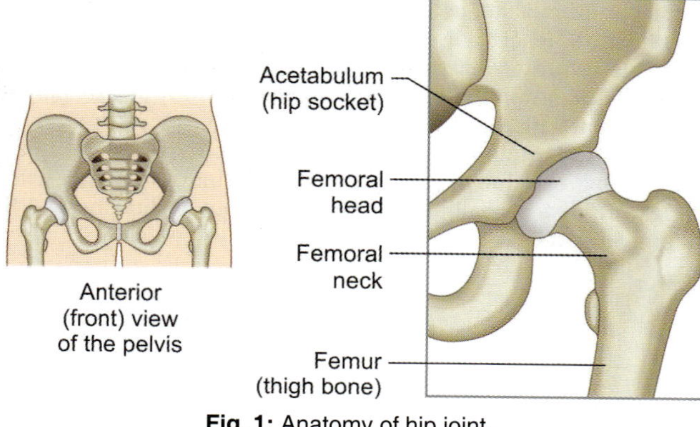

Fig. 1: Anatomy of hip joint.

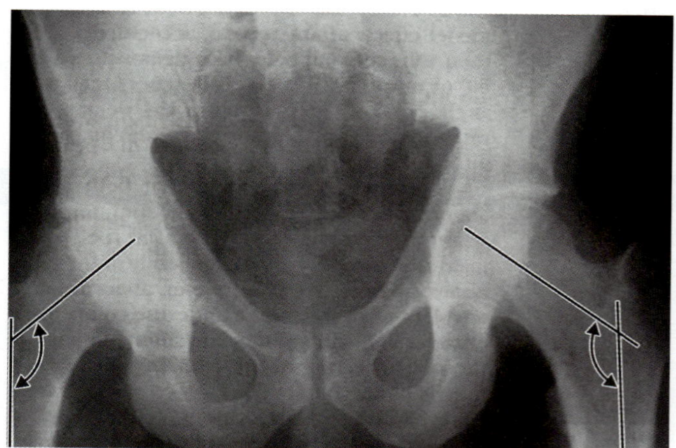

Fig. 2: The axis of the femoral head and neck forms an angle with the axis of the femoral shaft called the angle of inclination. In this adult subject without impairments, the angles are slightly less than 130°, with a couple of degrees of variation from side to side.

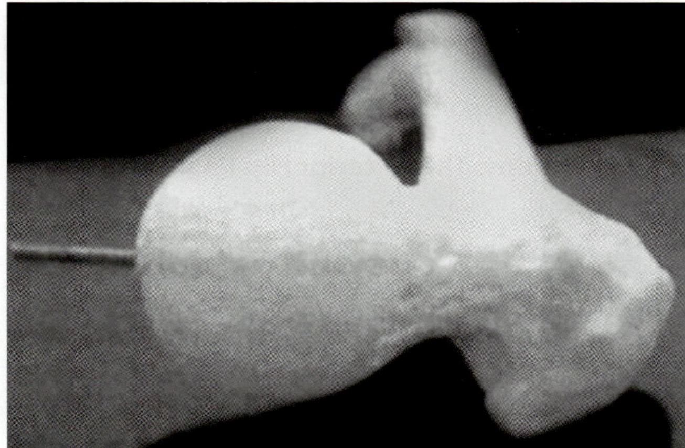

Fig. 3: Angle of anteversion.

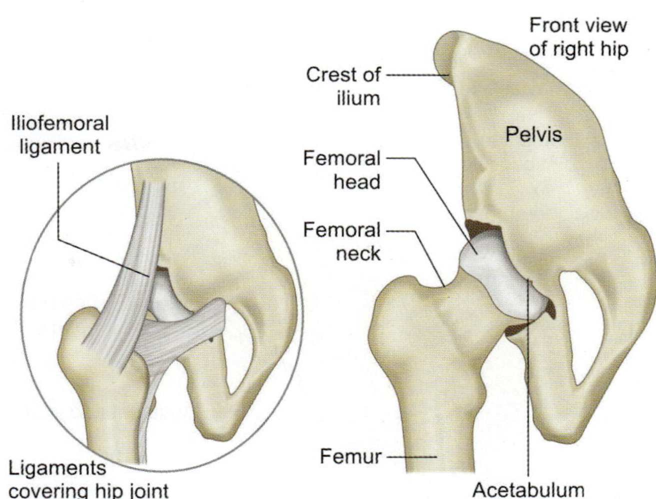

Fig. 4: Different ligaments around hip joint.

- It is directed laterally, downward, and forward
- Margin of the acetabulum is deficient. This deficiency is called "acetabular notch". It is bridged by transverse ligament. Nonarticular roughened floor called acetabular fossa contains mass of fat lined by synovial membrane
- It also has a horseshoe-shaped, lunate articular surface, which is covered by cartilage.

Stability of Hip Joint

Stability of the joint depends on:
- Depth of the acetabulum and narrowing of its mouth by acetabular labrum
- Tension and strength of the ligaments
- Strength of the surrounding muscles
- The length and obliquity of the neck of the femur.

Normal Growth and Development

- Embryologically, the acetabulum and femoral head develop from the same primitive mesenchymal cells.
- Cleft develops in precartilaginous cells on 7th week and this defines both structures.
- At 11 weeks, hip joint is fully formed.
- Acetabular growth continues throughout intrauterine life with development of labrum.
- At birth, femoral head is deeply seated in acetabulum by surface tension of synovial fluid and very difficult to dislocate.
- In developmental dysplasia of hip, this shape and tension is abnormal in addition to capsular laxity.
- The cartilage complex is triradiate, directed medially and cup-shaped laterally.
- Interposed between ilium above and ischium below, and pubis anteriorly.
- Acetabular cartilage forms outer two-thirds cavity and the nonarticular medial wall formed by triradiate cartilage, which is the common physis of these three bones.
- Fibrocartilaginous labrum forms at margin of acetabular cartilage and joint capsule inserts just above its rim.
- Articular cartilage covers the portion articulating with femoral head. On the opposite side is a growth plate with degenerating cells facing towards the pelvic bone it opposes.
- Triradiate cartilage is triphalanged with each side of each limb having a growth plate, which allows interstitial growth within the cartilage causing expansion of hip joint diameter during growth.
- In the infant, the GT, proximal femur, and intertrochanteric portion is cartilage.
- At 4–7 months, proximal ossification center appears, which enlarges along cartilaginous anlage, until adult life when only a thin layer of articular cartilage persists.
- Experimental studies in humans with unreduced hips suggest the main stimulus for concave shape of the acetabulum is the presence of spherical head.
- For normal depth of acetabulum to increase, several factors play a role:
  - Spherical femoral head
  - Normal appositional growth within cartilage
  - Periosteal new bone formation in adjacent pelvic bones
  - Development of three secondary ossification centers
  - Normal growth and development occur through balanced growth of proximal femur, acetabulum, triradiate cartilages, and the adjacent bones.

Ligaments (Fig. 4)

- Fibrous capsule
- Iliofemoral ligament
- Pubofemoral ligament
- Ischiofemoral ligament
- Ligament of the head of the femur
- Acetabular labrum
- Transverse acetabular ligament.

Fibrous capsule (Fig. 5):

The capsule is attached on the hip bone to the acetabular labrum and on the femur to the intertrochanteric line in front. Anterolaterally, the capsule is thick and firmly attached, as this part is subjected to maximum tension in standing posture. The capsule is made of two types of fibers:
1. *Outer fibers:* Longitudinal, forms the retinacula, through which pass the blood vessels supplying the head and neck of femur (NoF).
2. *Inner fibers:* Circular, called as "zona orbicularis".

Iliofemoral ligament:

- Also called as "ligament of Bigelow"

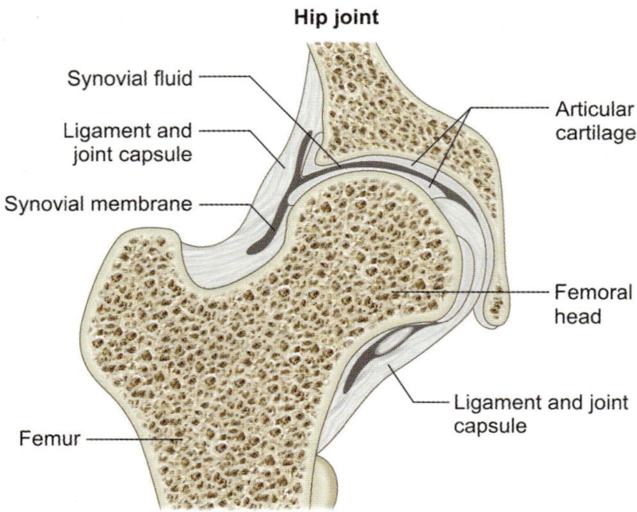

Fig. 5: The fibrous capsule of hip joint.

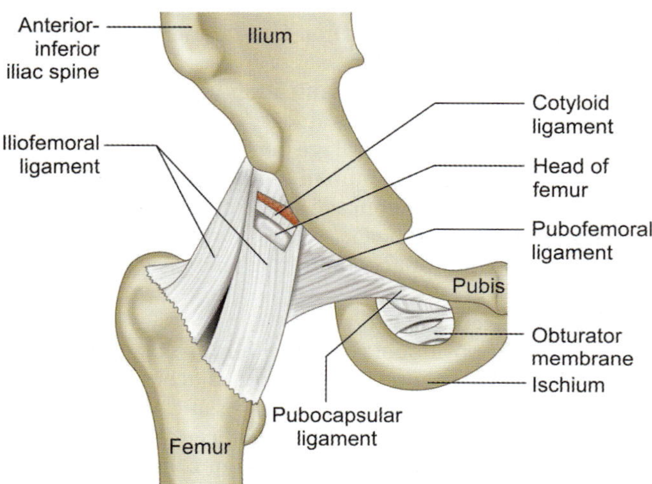

Fig. 6: Different ligaments and their attachments around hip joint.

- It is inverted and Y-shaped. It is one of the strongest ligaments in the body.
- It is the chief stabilizer of the hip in standing position.

Pubofemoral ligament (Fig. 6):
It supports the joint inferomedially.

Ischiofemoral ligament:
- It is comparatively weak
- It covers the joint posteriorly.

Ligament of the head of the femur:
This is also called as "round ligament" or "ligament teres". It is a flat and triangular ligament. The apex is attached to the fovea capitis and the base to the transverse ligament and the margins of the acetabular notch. It transmits arteries to the head of femur from the acetabular branches of the obturator and medial circumflex femoral arteries.

Acetabular labrum:
It is a fibrocartilaginous rim attached to the margins of the acetabulum. It narrows the mouth of acetabulum. This helps in holding the head of femur in position.

Transverse acetabulum ligament:
It is a part of acetabular labrum, which bridges the acetabular notch. Thus, the notch is converted into a foramen, which transmits acetabular vessels and nerve to the joint.

Surface Anatomy: The Anterior Hip Region

Bony Landmarks

- Anterosuperior iliac spine
- Tubercle of the iliac crest at the widest part of the pelvis
- Pubic symphysis in the midline anteriorly
- Pubic tubercle about 1-inch lateral to the symphysis
- The GT
- A line drawn horizontally from the pubic tubercle passes through femoral head.

Superficial Fascia

It is composed of fatty layer and a deep membranous layer. The latter is separated from the deep fascia by loose areolar tissue, but is firmly fused to deep fascia along a horizontal line immediately below the inguinal ligament and to the front of pubis and the pubic arch. Due to this attachment, urinary extravasations from the perineum to the abdomen cannot descend into the thigh.

Fascia Lata

It is thickened deep fascia, covering the thigh. It is attached above at the anterior-superior iliac spine (ASIS), the inguinal ligament, the body of pubic bone, the pubic arch, the ischial tuberosity, the sacrotuberous ligament, and as the gluteal fascia attached to sacrum and the iliac crest. It is extremely strong laterally because in between two layers, there runs a broad band of coarse vertical fibers, the iliotibial band.

Iliotibial Tract/Band

It is a conjoint aponeurosis of tensor fascia latae and the gluteus maximus and runs distally to insert upon the head of fibula and the anterolateral aspect of tibia. The band is often thickened and contracted in poliomyelitis. Shortening of the band produces a flexion and abduction deformity of the hip because the plane of the band lies lateral and anterior to the axis of hip motion.

Long Saphenous Vein

- Superficial epigastric: Superficial circumflex iliac courses along the medial aspect of thigh. It receives three tributaries, which accompany the superficial inguinal branches of femoral artery.
- Superficial external pudendal.
- Long saphenous vein (LSV) then passes through an opening in the fascia lata, the fossa ovalies, to reach the femoral vein. This aperture in deep fascia is located one-and-half inches below and lateral to pubic tubercle, where it is of surgical importance in treating femoral hernia and varicose veins.

Inguinal Lymph Glands

Two groups (superficial and deep). These are shown in Figure 7.

1. *Superficial group:*

- An upper horizontal group, lying below the inguinal ligament and draining the inguinal, lower abdominal, and perineal region.
- The lower group lies about the long saphenous vein and receives superficial lymph vessels from the lower limb.

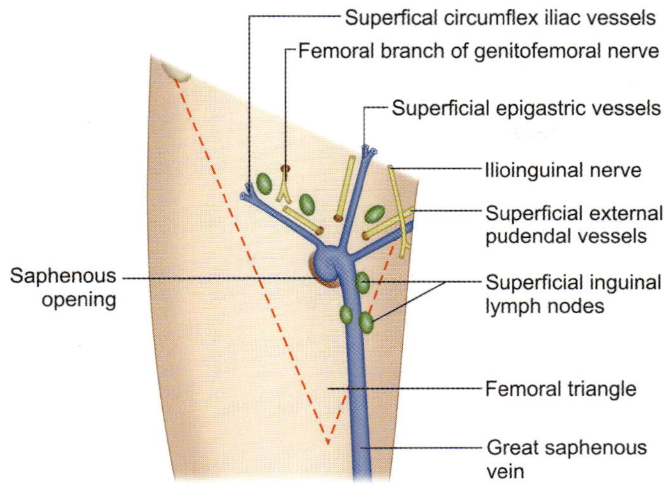

Fig. 7: The anterior hip region, showing inguinal lymph glands.

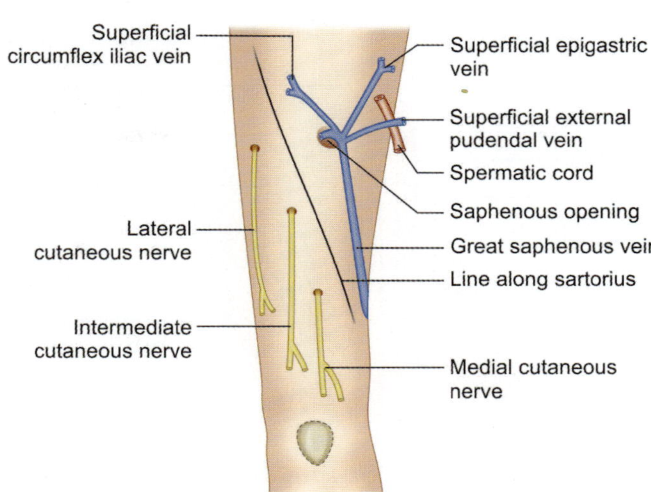

Fig. 8: Cutaneous nerves on anterior thigh/hip region.

2. *The deep group:* One to three in numbers, lies on medial side of the femoral vein in the femoral canal and receives the deep lymph vessels of the lower limb, including those draining the popliteal glands. It also drains the pelvic organs and thus becomes painful and swollen in pelvic inflammatory disease.

Cutaneous Nerves (Fig. 8)

The lateral, intermediate, and the medial cutaneous nerves of thigh (from femoral) supply the lateral, anterior, and medial aspect of the thigh, respectively.

- *The lateral femoral cutaneous nerve:* Often arises from the lumbar plexus and enters the thigh beneath the inguinal ligament close to ASIS. It is involved in meralgia paresthetica, a condition characterized by sensory deficit along the lateral aspect of thigh.
- *Ilioinguinal nerve:* From lumbar plexus L1, emerges superficial inguinal ring and supplies not only the scrotum or labium majus, but also the skin of the adjacent aspect of the thigh.
- *Genitofemoral nerve:* From the lumbar plexus at L1 and L2, sends a femoral branch to supply an area immediately below the inguinal ligament.

Scarpa's or Femoral Triangle

- It is a triangular area, bounded above by the inguinal ligament, laterally by medial border if sartorius and medially by medial border of adductor longus, as shown in Figure 9.
- Floor of the triangle is formed medially by adductor longus and pectineus and laterally by the iliacus and psoas major, as illustrated in Figure 10.
- Roof is formed by—(i) skin, (ii) superficial fascia, containing superior inguinal lymph nodes, femoral branch, or genitofemoral nerve, branches of ilioinguinal nerve, superficial branch of femoral artery and accompanying vein, and (iii) deep fascia, with saphenous opening and cribriform fascia.
- The head of femur can be localized by determining the midinguinal point of crossing of femoral artery, then measuring one inch distally and laterally.

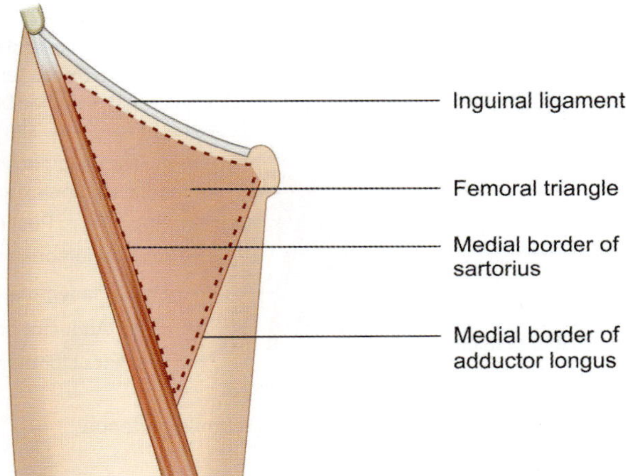

Fig. 9: Boundaries of femoral triangle.

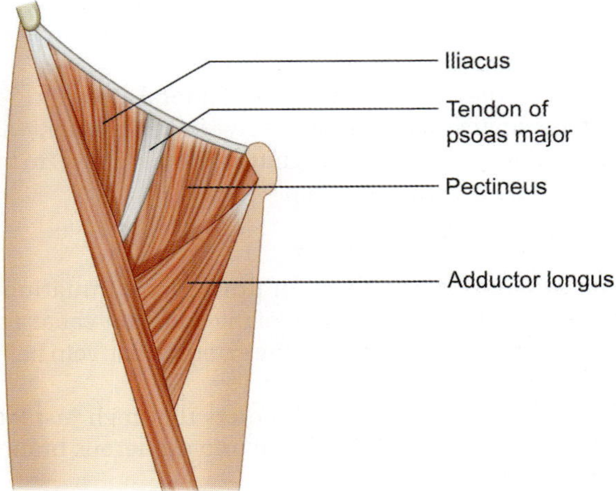

Fig. 10: Structures forming the floor of the femoral triangle.

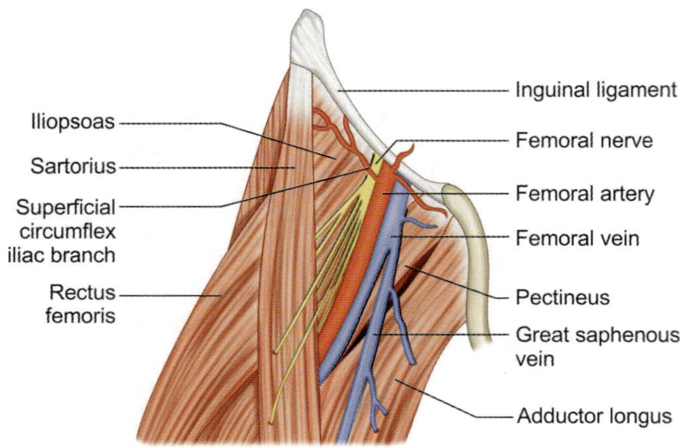

Fig. 11: Course of femoral artery on anterior hip region.

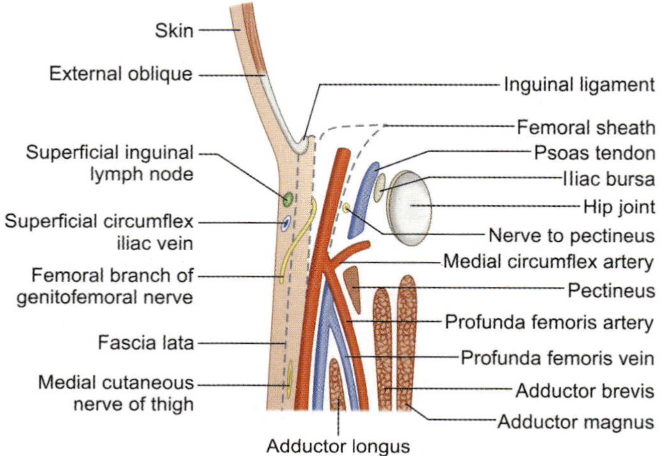

Fig. 12: Course of femoral circumflex arteries.

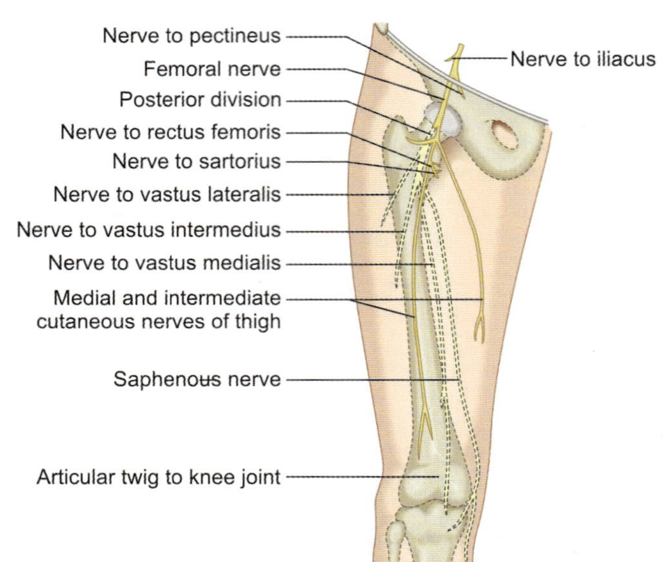

Fig. 13: Nerve supply to the anterior hip/thigh region (Branches of the posterior division are shown in interrupted line).

Blood Supply

- *Femoral artery (Fig. 11):* It runs behind the midinguinal point and enters the femoral triangle.
- *Profunda femoral artery: It* arises from lateral aspect of the femoral artery, at or just below the inguinal ligament.
- *Femoral circumflex artery (Fig. 12):* It has two branches:
  1. The lateral femoral circumflex artery
  2. The medial femoral circumflex femoral artery.

Both these arteries anastomose with each other, with first perforating artery below and the gluteal arteries above, to form the crucial arterial anastomosis of hip.

Femoral Vein and Femoral Nerve

- *Femoral vein:* It begins as an upward continuation of the popliteal vein at the lower end of the adductor canal and ends by becoming continuous with the external iliac vein behind the inguinal ligament.
- *Femoral nerve (L2, L3, L4):* It enters the thigh just lateral to the femoral artery and breaks up into numerous branches, as shown in Figure 13.
  - Its muscular branches include those to pectineus, sartorius, and the quadriceps.
  - Cutaneous branches are the medial and the intermediate femoral cutaneous and the saphenous nerve.

All the adductors are supplied by obturator nerve, except pectineus, which is supplied by femoral nerve. Hence, this explains why some adductor power remains after complete obturator neurectomy.

Muscles of Anterior (Extensor Compartment) of Thigh (Figs. 14A and B)

These are enumerated in Table 1.

- *Sartorius:* Arises by a fibrous origin with inguinal ligament from ASIS.
- *Quadriceps femoris:* This is so called because it is composed of four parts—(1) rectus femoris, (2) vastus lateralies, (3) medialis, and (4) intermedius.
- *Rectus femoris:* Supplied by femoral nerve. It arises by a straight head from the ASIS and by an oblique head from the supra-acetabular rim. It helps in extension of knee and acts as flexors of hip joint.

Muscles of Medial Hip Region (Table 2)

Adductor muscles (Figs. 14A and B): The muscles are disposed in three layers:

1. The anterior layer is composed of pectineus and the adductor longus.
2. The middle layer consists of adductor brevis.
3. The posterior layer is adductor magnus, arises mainly from the side of the pubic arch and is inserted along the back of femur.

Psoas major and iliacus: Both muscles originate intra-abdominally and enter the thigh behind the inguinal ligament. They are inserted by a common tendon into the lesser troch. The united iliopsoas crosses over the capsule of the hip joint, a bursa innervating between the structures. This bursa often communicates with the joint through an aperture in the capsule and is affected by the same disease process that affects the joint. Infection of the upper lumbar spine particularly TB often develops an exudates, which descends downwards beneath the psoas fascia as an abscess at the hip region.

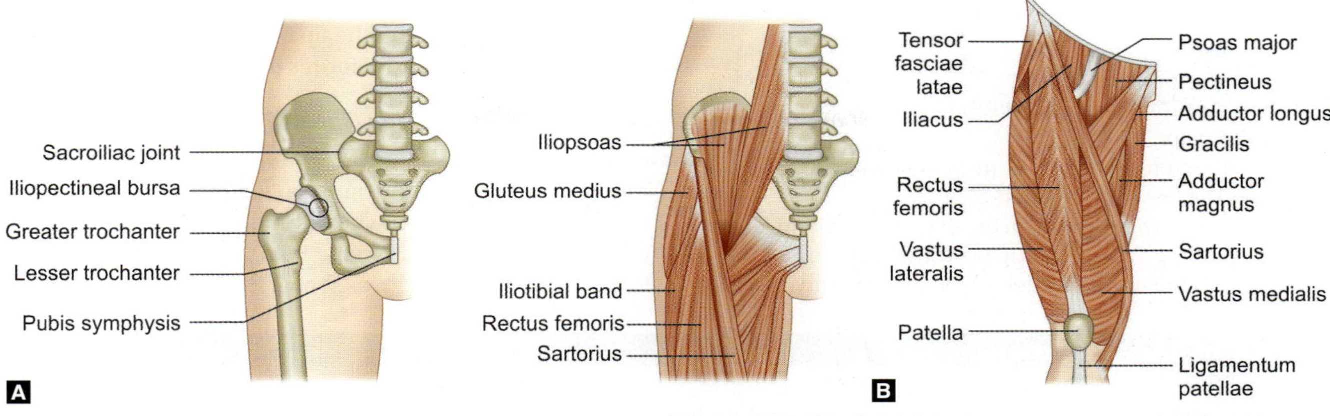

Figs. 14A and B: (A) Muscles in the anterior extensor compartment of hip; (B) Muscles in the medial compartment of thigh or hip.

TABLE 1: Muscles of the anterior or extensor compartment of hip/thigh.

Muscle	*Origin from*	*Insertion into*
Sartorius	• *Anterior*-superior iliac spine Upper half of the notch below the spine	Upper part of the medial surface of the shaft of the tibia in front of the insertions of the gracilis and the semitendinosus
Quadriceps femoris • *Rectus femoris* Fusiform, superficial fibers bipennate, deep fibers straight	• *Straight* head: From the upper half of the anterior-inferior iliac spine • Reflected *head:* From the groove above the margin of the acetabulum and the capsule of the hip joint	Base of patella
• *Vastus lateralis* Forms large part of quadriceps femoris	The origin is linear The line runs along: • Upper part of intertrochanteric line • Anterior and inferior borders of greater trochanter • Lateral lip of gluteal tuberosity • Upper half of lateral lip of linea aspera	• Lateral part of the base of patella • Upper one-third of the lateral border of patella • Expansion to the capsule of knee joint, tibia and iliotibial tract
• *Vastus medialis*	The origin in linear The line runs along: • Lower part of intertrochanteric line • Spiral line • Medial lip of linea aspera • Upper one-fourth of medial supracondylar line	Medial one-third of the base and upper two-thirds of the medial border of the patella
• *Vastus intermedius*	Upper three-fourths of the anterior and lateral surfaces of the shaft of femur	Base of patella *Note:* The patella is a sesamoid bone in the tendon of the quadriceps femoris. The ligamentum patellae is the actual tendon of the quadriceps femoris, which is inserted to the tibial tuberosity

TABLE 2: Muscles of the medial compartment of thigh.

Muscle	*Origin from*	*Insertion into*
• *Adductor longus*		
This is a triangular muscle, forming the medial part of the floor of the femoral triangle. It lies in the plane of the pectineus	It arises by a narrow, flat tendon from the front of the body of the pubis in the angle between the pubic crest and the pubic symphysis	The linea aspera in middle one-third of the shaft of the femur between the vastus medialis and the adductor brevis and magnus
• *Adductor brevis* The muscle lies behind the pectineus and adductor longus	• The *anterior* surface of the body of the pubis • Outer *surface* of the inferior ramus of the pubis between the gracilis and the obturator externus • Outer surface of the ramus of the ischium between the gracilis and the adductor magnus	Line extending from the lesser trochanter to the upper part of the linea aspera, behind the upper part of adductor longus
• *Adductor magnus*		
This is the largest muscles of this compartment. Because of its double nerve supply, it is called a hybrid muscle	• Inferolateral part of the ischial tuberosity • Ramus of the ischium • Lower part of the inferior ramus of the pubis	• Medial margin of gluteal tuberosity • Linea aspera • Medial supracondylar line • Adductor tubercle
• *Gracilis*	• Medial margin of the lower half of the body of the pubis • Inferior ramus of the pubis • The adjoining part of the ramus of the ischium pectin pubis	Upper part of the medial surface of tibia behind the sartorius and in front of the semitendinosus
• *Pectineus*		Line extending from lesser trochanter to the linea aspera
This is flat, quadrilateral muscle	• Upper half of the pectineal surface of the superior ramus of the pubis	
It forms a part of the floor of the femoral triangle	• Fascia covering the pectineus	

Gluteal Region Bony Landmarks

- The iliac crest
- Anterior-superior iliac spine
- Posterior-superior iliac spine (PSIS)
- Ischial tuberosity
  - A line drawn transversely at the level of ischial tuberosity, crosses the lesser trochanter.
  - A line drawn from a point on the iliac crest, a hand-breadth in front of the PSIS. Directly outward to the tip of the GT represents the upper border of gluteus maximus muscle.

By drawing a line from the PSIS to the tip of coccyx, the midpoint of this line extends out to the tip of the GT, which corresponds to the lower border of the pyriformis muscle.

Muscles of Gluteal Region (Table 3)

Gluteus maximus:

The deep fascia over this muscle is thin and transparent. It is a thick fibered rhomboid-shaped muscle innervated by inferior gluteal nerve. It arises from the PSIS, sacrotuberous ligament, the lower sacrum and coccyx, as shown in Figure 15. It passes laterally

TABLE 3: Muscles of the gluteal region.

Muscle	*Origin*	*Insertion into*	*Nerve supply*
• *Gluteus maximus* This is a large, quadrilateral powerful muscle covering mainly the posterior surface of pelvis	• Outer *slope* of the dorsal segment of iliac crest • *Posterior* gluteal line • *Posterior* part of gluteal surface of ilium behind the posterior gluteal line • *Aponeurosis* of erector spinae • Dorsal surface of lower part of sacrum • Side of *coccyx* • *Sacrotuberous* ligament • Fascia *covering* gluteus maximus	• The deep *fibers* of the lower part of the muscle are inserted into the gluteal tuberosity • The greater *part* of the muscle is inserted into the iliotibial tract	Inferior gluteal nerve (L5, S1, S2)
• *Gluteus medius* It is fan-shaped, and covers the lateral surface of the pelvis and hip	Gluteal surface of ilium between the anterior and posterior gluteal lines	The greater trochanter of femur, on oblique ridge on the lateral surface. The ridge runs downwards and forwards	Superior gluteal nerve (L4, L5, S1)
• *Gluteus minimus* It is fan-shaped, and is covered by the gluteus medius	Gluteal surface of ilium between the anterior and inferior gluteal lines	Greater trochanter of femur, on a ridge on the lateral part of the anterior surface	Superior gluteal nerve (L4, L5, S1)
• *Piriformis* Lies below and parallel to the posterior border of the gluteus medius	It arises within the pelvis from: • Pelvic *surface* of the middle three digitations • Upper *margin* of the greater sciatic notch and the adjoining areas of the sacroiliac joint and of the sacrotuberous ligament	The rounded tendon is inserted into the apex of the greater trochanter of the femur	Ventral rami of S1, S2
• *Gemellus superior* Small muscle lying along the upper border of the tendon of the obturator internus	Posterior surface of the ischial spine and upper part of lesser sciatic notch	Blends with tendon of obturator internus, and gets inserted into medial surface of greater trochanter of femur	Nerve to obturator internus (L5, S1, S2)
• *Gemellus inferior* Small muscle lying along the lower border of the tendon of the obturator internus	Upper part of the ischial tuberosity and lower part of lesser sciatic notch	Same as above	Nerve to quadratus femoris (L4, L5, S1)
• *Obturator internus* Fan-shaped, flattened belly lies in pelvis and the tendon in the gluteal region	• Pelvic surface of obturator membrane • Pelvic surface of the body of the ischium, ischial tuberosity, ischiopubic rami, and ilium below the pelvic brim • Obturator fascia	The tendon of the obturator internus leaves the pelvis through the lesser sciatic foramen. Here it bends at a right angle around the lesser sciatic notch and runs laterally to be inserted into the medial surface of the greater trochanter of the femur	Nerve to obturator internus (L5, S1, S2)
• *Quadratus femoris* Quadrilateral muscle lying between interior gemellus and adductor magnus	Upper part of the outer border of ischial tuberosity	Quadrate tubercle and the area below it	Nerve to quadratus femoris (L4, L5, S1)
• *Obturator externus* Triangular in shape, covers the outer surface of the anterior wall of the pelvis	• Outer surface of obturator membrane • Outer surface of the bony margins of obturator foramen	The muscle ends in a tendon which runs upwards and laterally behind the neck of the femur to reach the gluteal region where it is inserted into trochanteric fossa (on medial side of the greater trochanter)	
• *Tensor fasciae latae* Lies between the gluteal region and the front of the thigh	Anterior 5 cm of the outer lip of the iliac crest up to the tubercle	Iliotibial tact 3.5 cm below the level of greater trochanter	Superior gluteal nerve, (L4, L5)

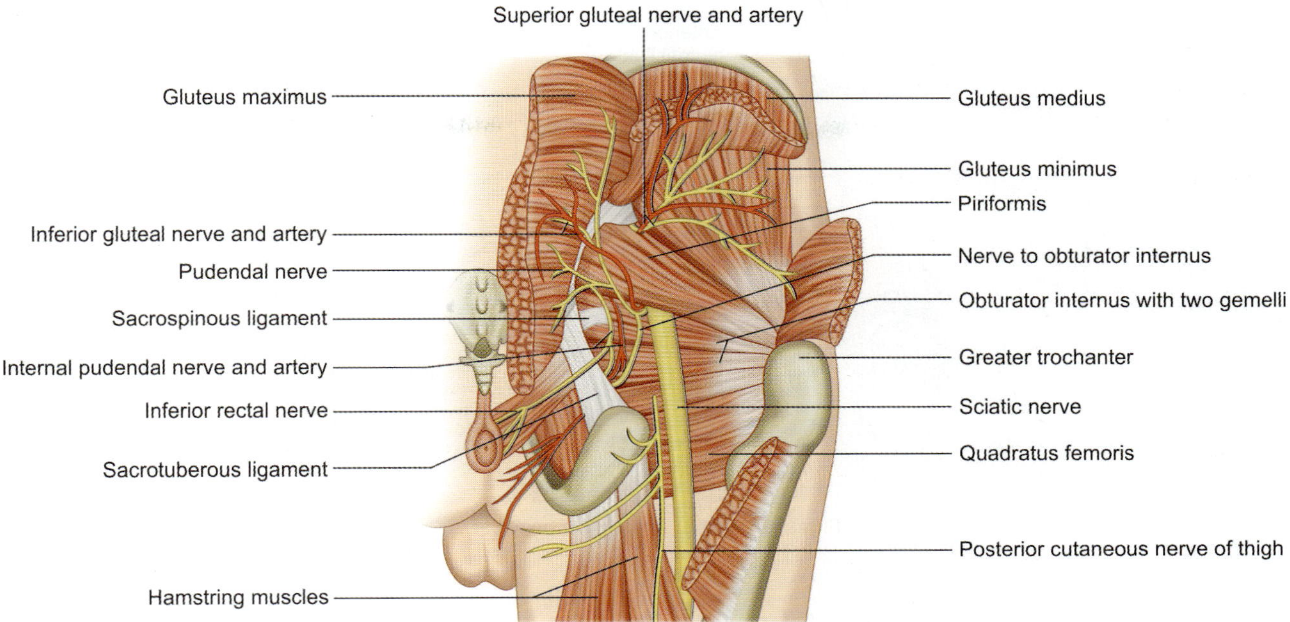

Fig. 15: Gluteus maximus muscle, its origin, blood supply, nerves and surrounding structures.

and distally towards the upper femur, where a portion of its upper fibers insert into the gluteal tuberosity, the remainder ending in a band-like aponeurosis, which joins a similar band-like aponeurosis of the tensor fascia lata, distal to the greater tuberosity to form the iliotibial tract. Its function is to extend the hip joint. Its motion is assisted by hamstrings. Many arteries and veins enter the under surface, in which a muscle splitting incision will cause extensive hemorrhage.

Structures entering at the lower border of pyriformis: This includes:

- Sciatic nerve
- Posterior cutaneous nerve of thigh
- Inferior gluteal nerve and vessels
- Internal pudendal nerve and vessels, which emerge at the lower border of pyriformis.

Structures entering at the upper border of pyriformis: This includes superior gluteal nerves and vessels.

- *Gluteus medius and minimus:* Fan-shaped, arises from most of the lateral surface of the ilium and inserts into the lateral and anterior aspect of GT. It functions as abductors of thigh.
- *Tensor fascia lata:* Arises from ASIS and the outer lip of the iliac crest. It is directed downwards and slightly backwards and is continued as iliotibial tract and innervated by superior gluteal nerve.
- *Quadratus femoris:* It appears to be the proximal portion of the adductor magnus. It arises from lateral border of iliotibial tract (IT) and extends laterally to insert into the quadrate tubercle behind the GT. Nerve to qudratus, lies below sciatic nerve.
- *Obturator internus, superior, and inferior gamellus:* This muscle occupies interval between the pyriformis and the quadratus. Obturator internus arises from the internal aspect of the innominate bone, makes right-angled turn, and goes out through lesser sciatic foramen. Its tendon passes across the posterior surface of ischium and the capsule of hip joint to reach up border of the GT. The superior gamellus arises from ischial spine and the inferior gamellus, from the ischial tuberosity. Both are inserted adjacent to ischial tuberosity. They are the lateral rotators of thigh.

Bony Pelvis (Figs. 16A and B)

It is composed of three main parts:

1. Ilium
2. Ischium
3. Pubis

These three parts meet in a cup-shaped cavity called as acetabulum, which receives the femoral head.

Ilium: It is a large flat fan-shaped bone, lies above the acetabulum. Its crest is subcutaneous and during the growth period is surmounted by an apophysis. Ossification of the apophysis takes place in a line extending along the entire length of the crest. Completion of this line of ossification, coincides with termination of longitudinal growth. This sign is utilized in the management of scoliosis of idiopathic type.

Blood Supply and Nerve Supply of Hip Joint

Blood Supply (Fig. 17)

- The hip is supplied by obturator artery, two circumflex femoral, and two gluteal arteries.
- The median and lateral circumflex femoral arteries form an arterial circle around the capsular attachment on the NoF. Retinacular arteries arise from this circle and supply the intracapsular part of the neck and the greater part of the head of the femur.
- A small part of the head, near the fovea capitis, is supplied by the acetabular branches of the obturator and medial circumflex femoral arteries.

Nerve Supply

- The femoral nerve, through the nerve to rectus femoris
- The anterior division of obturator nerve

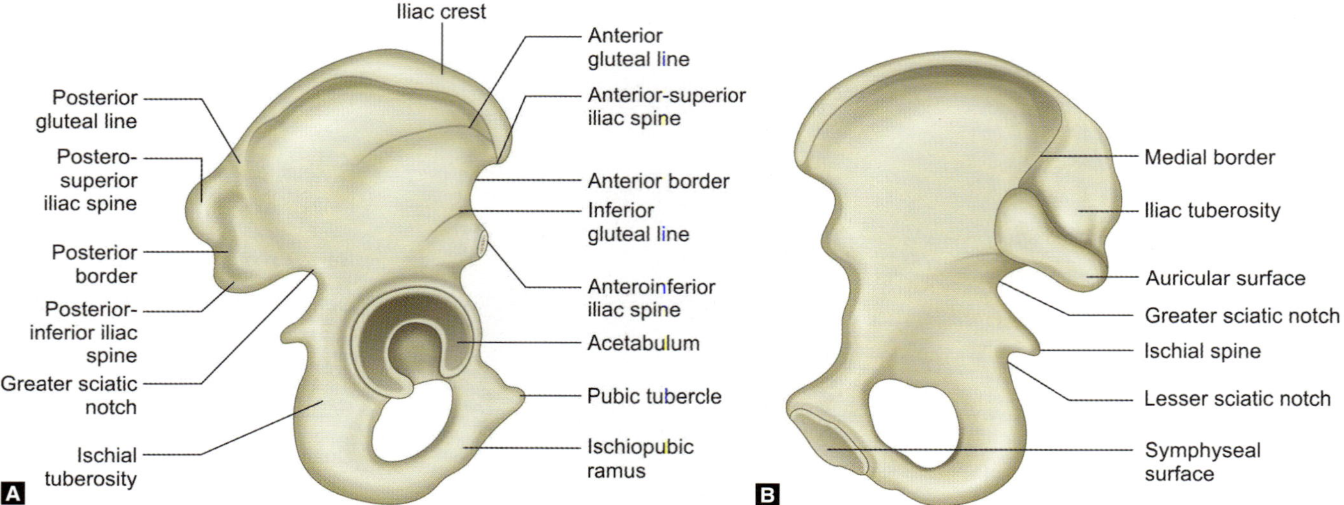

Figs. 16A and B: Anatomy of bony pelvis.

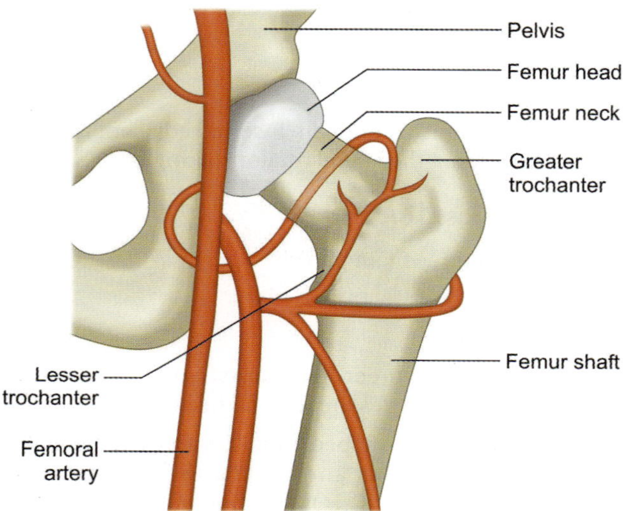

Fig. 17: Course of femoral artery around hip.

- The accessory obturator nerve
- The nerve to quadratus femoris
- The superior gluteal nerve.

Vascular Anatomy of Femoral Head (Figs. 18 and 19)

Growth period: At birth, nutrition of femoral head is derived from three sources.

1. *Lateral epiphyseal (from medial femoral circumflex):* This group of vessels enters the outer part of the femoral head in the region of the trochanteric notch and advances horizontally towards the center of the head.
2. *Metaphyseal, from medial femoral circumflex:* This series of straight vessels ascends vertically through the cartilaginous head.
3. *Ligamentum teres vessels, from acetabular branch of obturator:* These vessels barely supply a superficial portion of the femoral head.

Delay in ossification of the epiphysis commonly observed in congenital diaphragmatic hernia (CDH) could be explained by capsular stretching, obliterating the lateral epiphyseal vessels, while the metaphyseal vessels remain intact. After 4 months of age, the ascending metaphyseal vessels decrease in number. Hence, the main vascular supply at this time is through the lateral epiphyseal arteries. Obstruction of these vessels, theoretically, produces the picture of Legg-Perthes disease.

After 7 years of age, the vessels from ligamentum teres penetrate more deeply and join the lateral epiphyseal vessels in supplying the head. The cartilaginous epiphyseal plate constitutes a barrier to metaphyseal blood flow, until epiphyseal fusion takes place. Vascularity of the metaphysis is profuse during puberty in the period immediately preceding fusion. Hence, when reducing an old slipped epiphysis by open operation, it is advisable to perforate the epiphyseal plate, to allow ready access of metaphyseal vessels into the head.

Adult period: The lateral epiphyseal arteries anastomose with the medial epiphyseal artery, which enters the fovea capitis. These cross the epiphysis horizontally and send branches mainly towards the articular margin. The main source of blood supply to the femoral head is through the lateral epiphyseal arteries, originating from the medial femoral circumflex. It is important to note that the intrinsic vascular tree remains patent with advancing age. Blood supply of femoral head is illustrated in Flowchart 1.

Movements around Hip (Table 4)

- Flexion and extension occur around a transverse axis
- Abduction and adduction occur around AP axis
- Medial and lateral rotation occur around vertical axis
- In general, all axes pass through the head of femur, but none of them is fixed because the head is not quite spherical.
  Hip diseases show an interesting pattern
- Below 5 years of age: CDH and TB
- 5–10 years: Perthes disease
- 10–20 years: Coxa vara
- Above 40 years: Osteoarthritis.

Clinical Anatomy

The region of hip joint is commonly affected by disease or injury. Common hip diseases are:

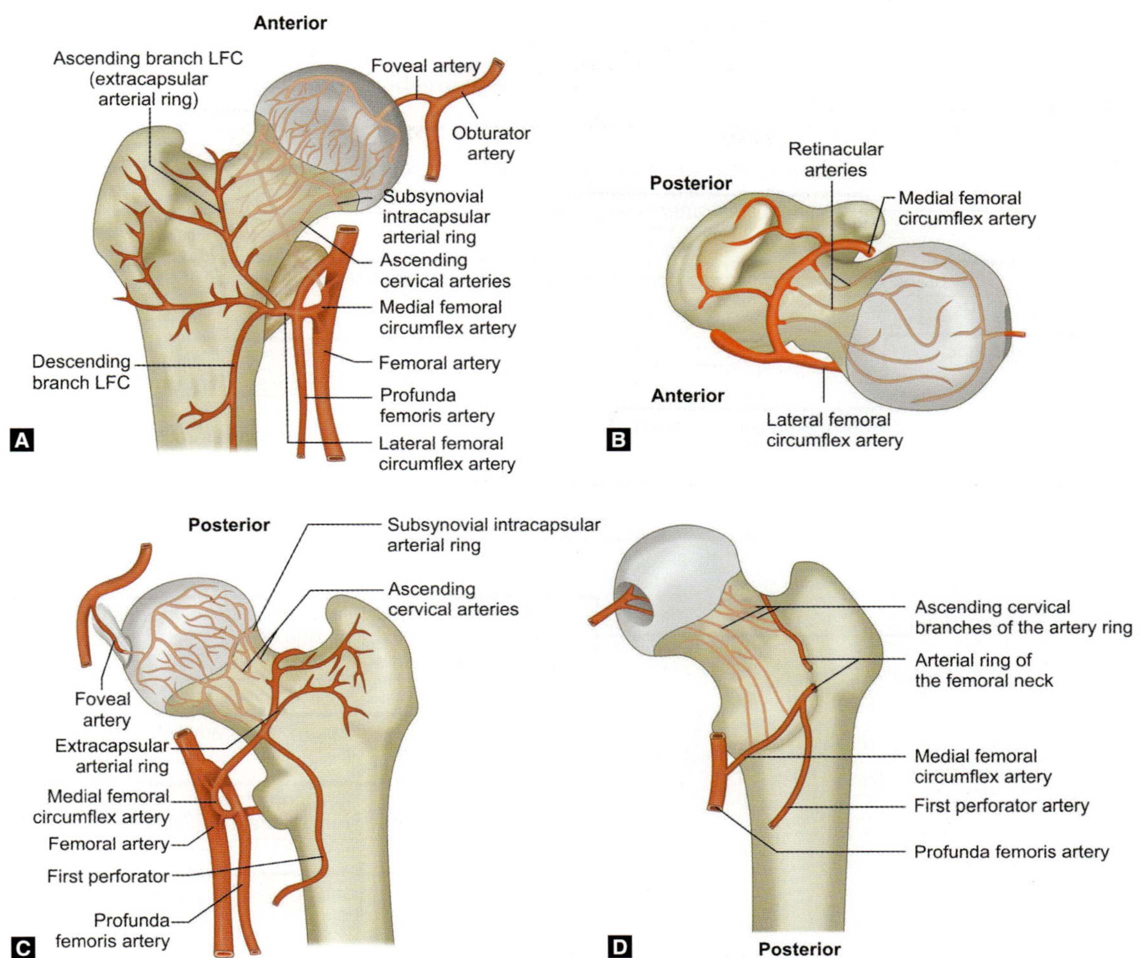

Figs. 18A to D: Blood supply to femoral head.

Congenital dislocation: It is more common in hip joint. Here, the head of femur slips upwards on to the gluteal surface of the ilium because the upper margin of acetabulum is developmentally deficient.

Perthes disease: Characterized by destruction and flattening of the head of femur with increased joint space, seen in X-ray.

Coxa vara: It is a condition, in which the neck shaft angle is reduced from the normal angle of about 150° in a child and 127° in adults.

Injuries: Dislocation of hip may be posterior (more common), anterior (less common), or central (rare).

Various important triangles in hip region are:

- Scarpas as mentioned above
- Babcock's triangle, as seen in TB hip
- Fairbank's triangle seen in coxa vara.

Biomechanics of Hip Joint (Fig. 19)

- The hip joint is a ball-and-socket joint
- In weight-bearing, the pressure forces are transmitted to the head and the neck of the femur at an angle of 165–175° regardless of the position of pelvis.
- The plane of force coincides with the strongly developed trabeculae, which lie in the medial portion of femoral neck and extends upwards through the superomedial aspect of the femoral head.

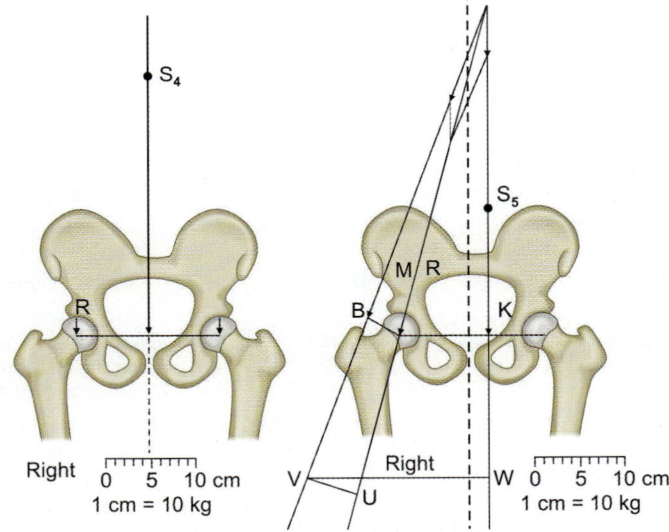

Fig. 19: Biomechanics of hip joint.

- When the weight of the body above the lower extremities rests equally on two normal hip joints, the static force on each hip is one-half of or less than one-third the total body weight.
- The left lower extremity is lifted, as in swing phase of walking. The weight of the left lower extremity is added to that of the

Flowchart 1: Blood supply of femoral head.

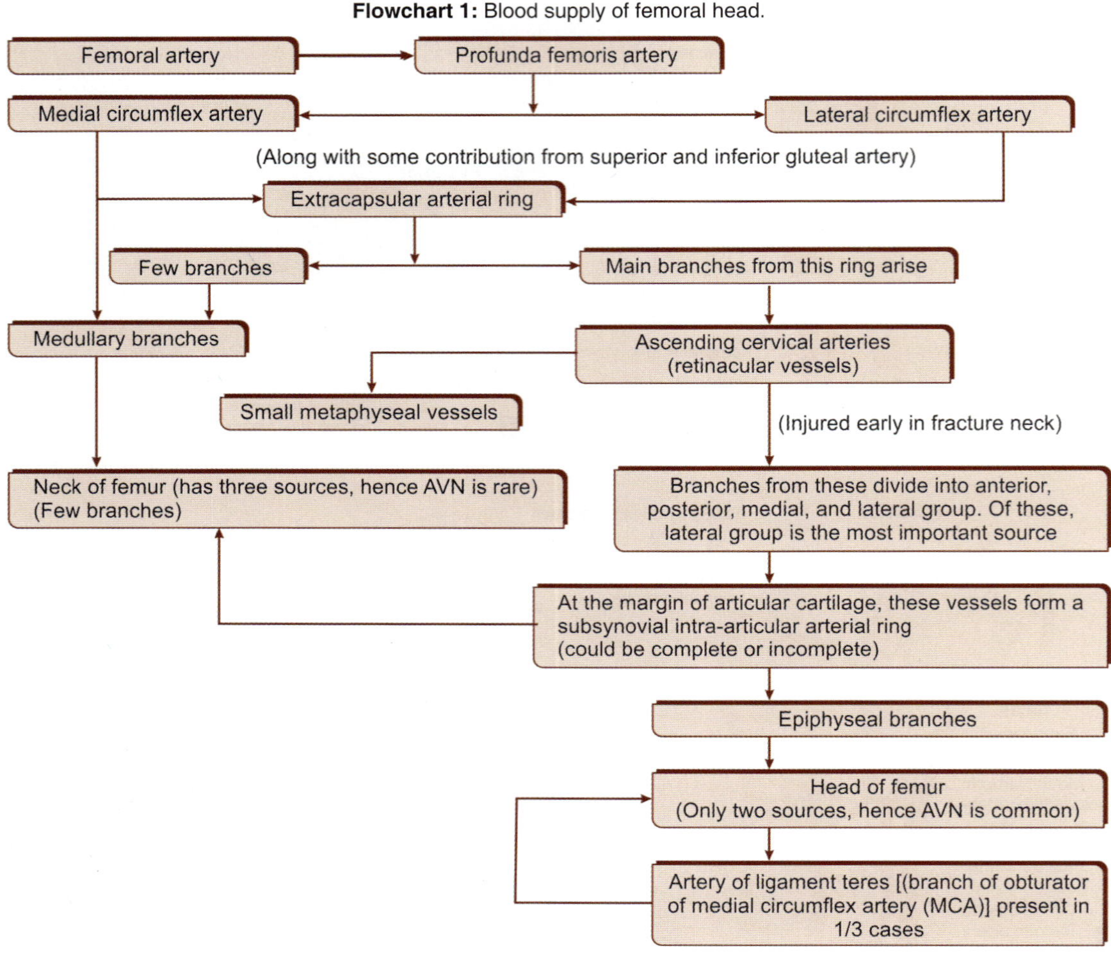

TABLE 4: Movements around hip joint and muscles carrying out those movements and their nerve supply.

Movements	*Axis*	*Range of motion*	*Prime mover*	*Nerve supply*	*Assisted by*
Flexion	Transverse axis	0–120°	Psoas major	L 2-3	Rectus femoris sartorius, pectineus TFL Adductor longus, brevis and magnus
Extension	Transverse axis	0° to 5–20°	Gluteus maximus and hamstrings	Inferior gluteal nerve sciatic nerve	
Abduction	AP axis	0–40°	Gluteus medius	Superior gluteal nerve (L4, 5, S1)	Tensor fascia lata, sartorius, gluteus minimus and maximus
Adduction	AP axis	0–25°	Adductor longus, Magnus brevis	Obturator nerve (L3, 4) and femoral nerve (L2, 3, 4)	Pectineus and gracilis
External rotation	Vertical axis	0–45°	Obturator externus Internus, quadratus femoris, superior and inferior gemelli	S1, 2, 3, 4, L5, S	Sartorius and long head of biceps femoris, pyriformis
Internal rotation	Vertical axis	0° to 35–45°	Gluteus minimus and TFL	Superior gluteal nerve	Gluteus medius

body weight and the center of gravity normally in the median sagittal plane is displaced to the left.

- The abductor muscles exert a counter balancing force to maintain equilibrium. The pressure exerted on the head of the right hip is the sum of these two forces, as shown in Figure 20.
- The pressure exerted on the head of the right femur is the sum of these two forces. Each force is related to the relative length of the levers, as shown in Figure 21.
- If the abductor lever (B to O) is one-third that of the lever arm from the head to the center of gravity (O to C), the downward pull of the abductors must be three times the force of gravity to maintain balance, therefore the total pressure on the head is four times the superimposed weight.
- The longer the abductor lever (i.e. the more laterally placed insertion of the abductors), the less the ratio bet the levers, less the abduction force required to maintain balance and the

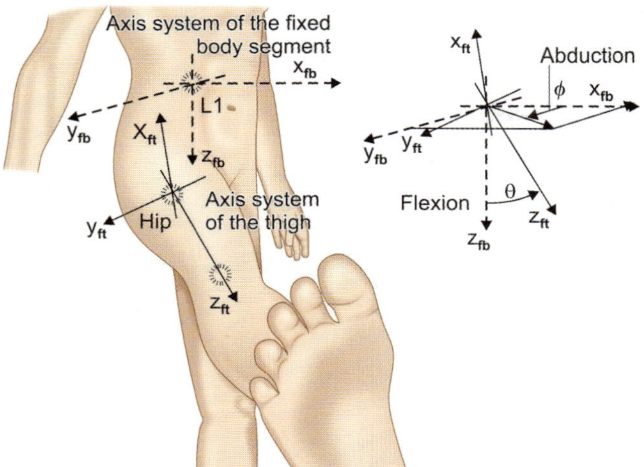

Fig. 20: The abductor muscles acting to counter balance force, exerted on the head of hip to maintain equilibrium.

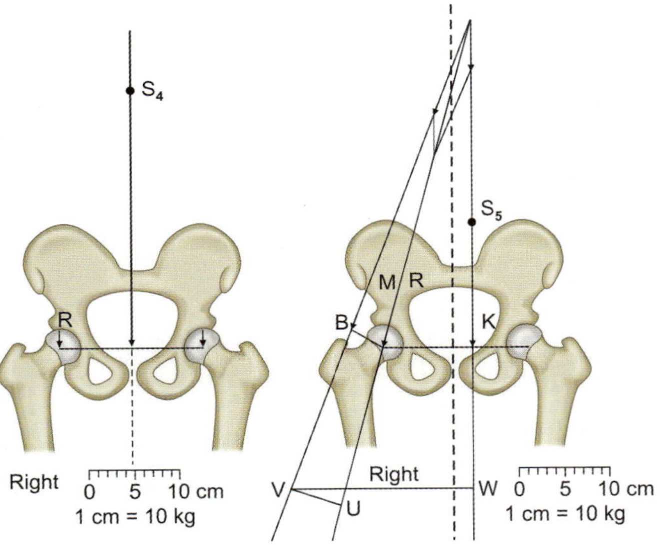

Fig. 21: Forces acting on the head of the femur.

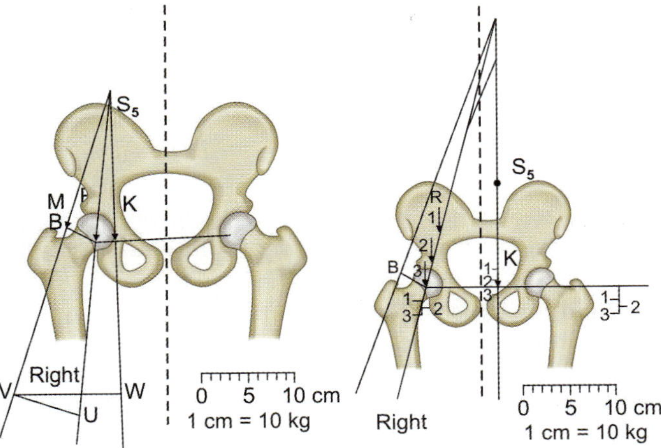

Fig. 22: Abductor lever arm and force ratio required to maintain balance.

less the pressure force upon the femoral head, as illustrated in Figure 22.

Clinical Applications (Figs. 23 and 24)

- When hip is in valgus, the short abductor lever arm requires tremendous abduction pull on the hip and the resultant pressure on the head may be as much as seven or eight times the supported weight.
- To reduce the pressure and pain, the patient lifts the trunk towards the hip and displaces the center of gravity in that direction. Consequently, less pull on the abductors is required and the force on the femoral head is reduced. This is characteristic waddle and limp of coxa valga, a means of relieving stress on the hip.
- The secondary strain on the lumbar spine caused by this lateral lurching produces backache and increased pressure on the femoral head increases degeneration.
- The use of a cane in the opposite hand, by working through the long lever arm can reduce static force on the hip in multiples of pressure force exerted downward on the cane.
- The normal length of femoral neck should be preserved wherever possible, particularly in prosthetic replacement operations. Maintenance of an adequate abductor lever will lessen pressure and enable the prosthesis to withstand stresses for a longer period of time.
- When abductor paralysis exists, equilibrium cannot be attained. The individual shifts laterally and displaces the center of gravity over the affected hip, so that forces are minimal and vertical. During the growth period, the epiphyseal plate tends to remain perpendicular to these forces and consequently shifts to a horizontal position. The result is a coxa valga deformity. A similar mechanism is operative in valgus associated with the congenital dislocation of hip.
- In subluxated hip, the GT is closer to the fulcrum point. The force acts only along the upper border of the acetabulum.
- An adduction osteotomy, to create a varus deformity will produce these effects. The trochanter will be displaced a greater distance from the pelvis, thereby, reducing the load on the femoral head and the line of force will be made to act on the center about a large acetabular area. Relief of pain and fatigue is accomplished.

DEVELOPMENTAL DYSPLASIA OF THE HIP

Introduction

It was previously known as congenital dislocation of the hip, implying a condition that existed at birth. It is a developmental defect and encompasses embryonic, fetal, and infantile periods. It includes congenital dislocation and developmental hip problems, including subluxation, dislocation, and dysplasia. Normal growth and development occurs during this defect. Embryologically, the acetabulum and femoral head develop from the same primitive mesenchymal cells. Cleft develops in precartilaginous cells at 7th week and this defines both structures. On 11th week, hip joint is fully formed and acetabular growth continues throughout intrauterine life with development of labrum. By birth, femoral head is deeply seated in acetabulum by surface tension of synovial fluid and is very difficult to dislocate. In developmental dysplasia of hip, this shape and tension is abnormal in addition to capsular laxity. The cartilage complex is 3D with triradiate shape medially and cup-shape laterally, interposed between ilium above, and ischium below, and pubis anteriorly.

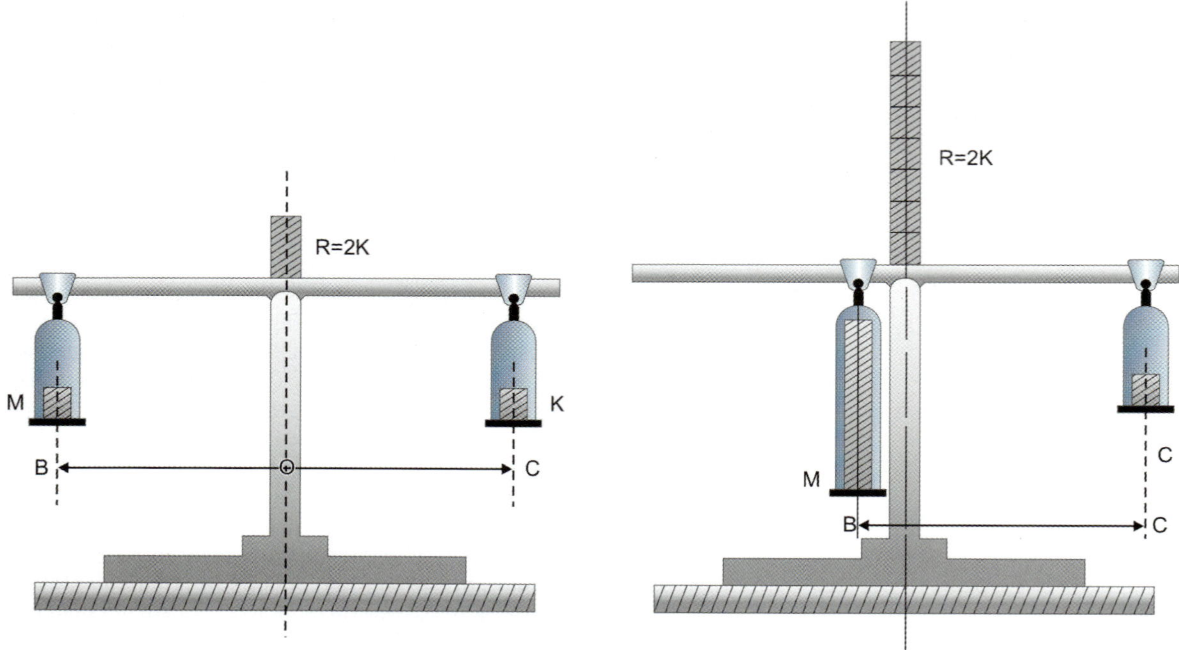

Fig. 23: Illustrating force operating on hip by using simple balance—R. Vector, K. Body weight, M. Muscle force. Superimpose weight R which is equal to 2K is divided equally at M and K, a balancing condition.

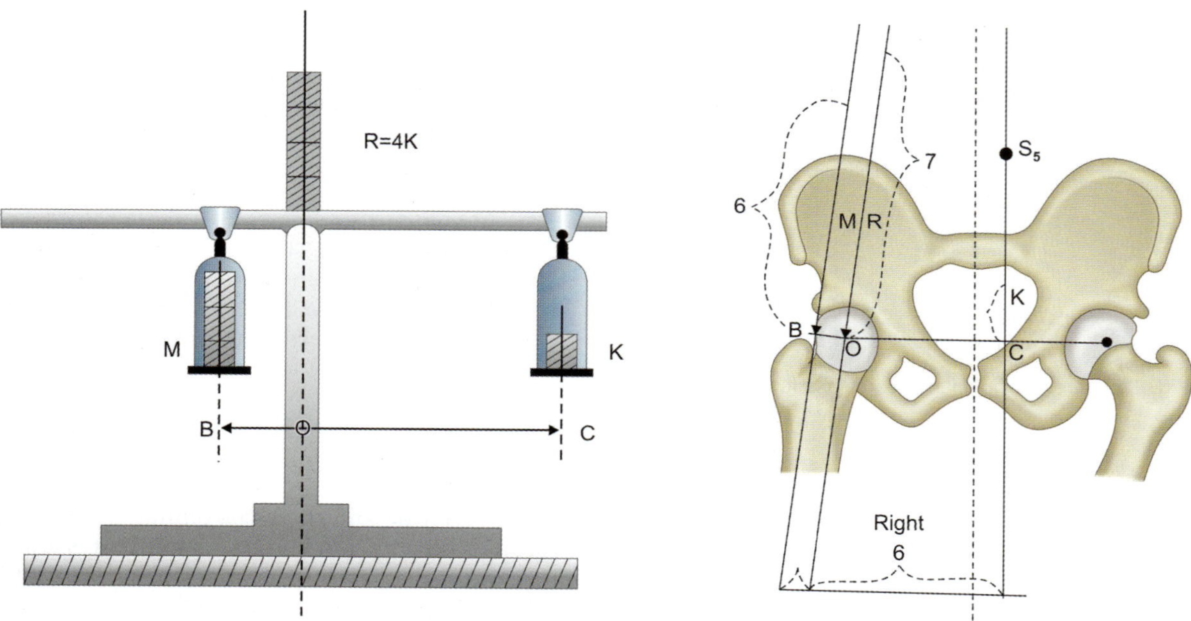

Fig. 24: Forces on valgus hip. The pull of abductor at B is at the end of an abnormally short liver arm, B to O, which is only one sixth of O to C. The pull downward at B must be six times K in order to maintain equilibrium when left foot raised. The total pressure on stationary right hip is seven times K.

Acetabular cartilage forms the outer two-thirds cavity and the nonarticular medial wall is formed by triradiate cartilage, which is the common physis of these three bones. Fibrocartilaginous labrum forms at the margin of acetabular cartilage and joint capsule inserts just above its rim. Articular cartilage covers the portion articulating with femoral head and the opposite side is a growth plate with degenerating cells, facing towards the pelvic bone it opposes. Triradiate cartilage is triphalanged with each side of each limb having a growth plate, which allows interstitial growth within the cartilage causing expansion of hip joint diameter during growth. In the infant, the GT, proximal femur, and intertrochanteric portion are cartilage. Within 5–7 months, proximal ossification center appears, which enlarges along cartilaginous anlage until adult life, when only thin layer of articular cartilage persists. Experimental studies in humans with unreduced hips suggest the main stimulus for the concave shape of the acetabulum is the presence of spherical head. To increase normal depth of acetabulum, several factors play a role. They are as follows:

- Spherical femoral head
- Normal appositional growth within cartilage
- Periosteal new bone formation in adjacent pelvic bones

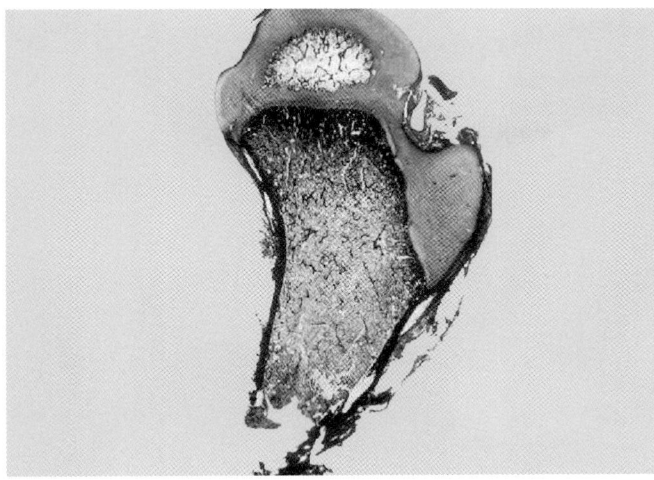

Fig. 25: Normally grown proximal femur.

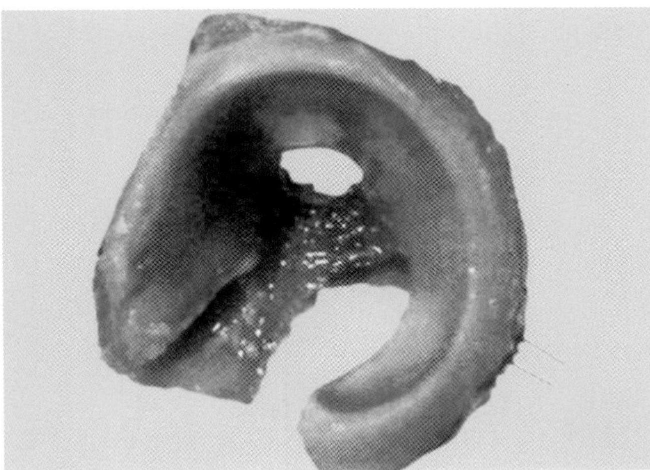

Fig. 26: Normally grown acetabulum, triradiate cartilages and the adjacent bones.

- Development of three secondary ossification centers
- Normal growth and development occur through balanced growth of proximal femur, acetabulum, and triradiate cartilages and the adjacent bones, as shown in Figures 25 and 26.

Developmental dysplasia of the hip is the spectrum of disorders of development of the hip that present in different forms at different ages. The common etiology is excessive laxity of the hip capsule, which fails to maintain the femoral head within the acetabulum, as shown in Figure 27. The syndrome in the newborn consists of instability of the hip, such that the femoral head can be displaced partially (subluxated) or fully (dislocated) from the acetabulum by an examiner.

Epidemiology

- One in 100 newborns examined, have evidence of instability (positive Barlow or Ortolani)
- One in 1,000 live births, true dislocation
- Most detectable at birth in nursery
- Barlow stated that 60% stabilize in the 1st week, and 88% stabilize in the first 2 months without treatment; the remaining 12% are true dislocations.

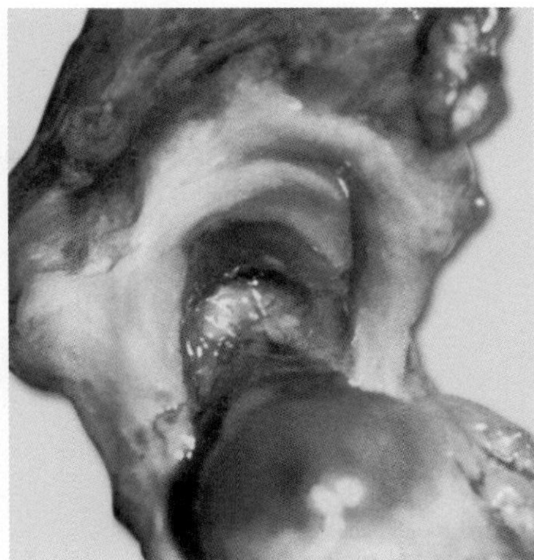

Fig. 27: Due to excessive laxity of hip capsule, it is unable to maintain the femoral head within the acetabulum.

Etiology

- Genetic and ethnic
- Increased in native Americans but very low in southern Chinese and Africans
- Positive family history 12–33%
- Uncommon in India and some Asian countries because of cultural practice
- *Hormonal theory:* It may occur due to maternal relaxin hormone, crossing placental barrier, and leading to joint laxity and dislocation in female fetus.
- *Mechanical theory:* Intrauterine factors that are involved are:
  - Breech position
  - Oligohydramnios
  - Neuromuscular conditions like myelomeningocele.
- *Germ plasma theory:* Teratologic dislocation of the hip are dislocated before birth, having limited range of motion (ROM), and are not reducible on examination associated with myelodysplasias and arthrogryposis.

Pathophysiology

- Shallow acetabulum with steep sloping roof (Fig. 28)
- Hypertrophy of ligamentum teres occurs
- Stretched capsule of hip joint
- Limbus (fibrocartilagenous labrum) folded into the acetabular cavity
- Femoral head is dislocated upwards and laterally
- Epiphysis is small and ossifies late
- Femoral neck is excessively anteverted.

Capsule:
- Capsule could show hourglass constriction, one containing head and the other containing acetabulum.
- Constriction is produced by iliopsoas and the ligamentum teres passes through this constriction and is hypertrophied.

Muscles:
- *Pelvifemoral group:* Adductors, sartorius, gracilis, rectus femoris, hamstrings, and tensor fascia lata are shortened and they prevent the reduction of head.
- *Pelvitrochanteric group:* Obturator, quadrates femoris, and iliopsoas are elongated and the psoas forms an obstacle to reduction.

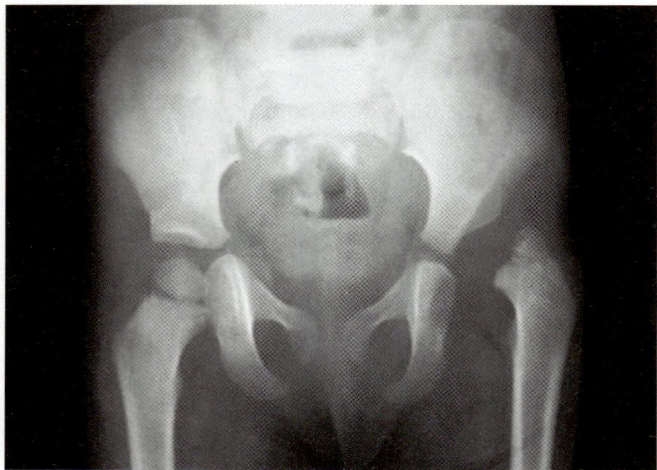

Fig. 28: Shallow acetabulum with steep sloping roof in CDH of hip joint.

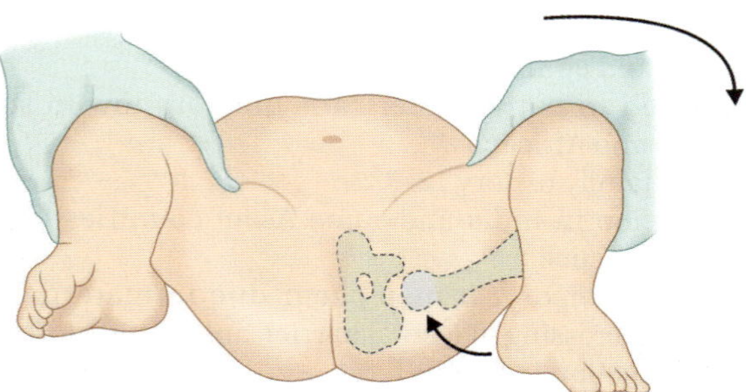

Fig. 29: Ortolani's test.

- *Gluteal muscles:* They show little organic change but power is diminished.

Physical Examination

- *Ortolani test (Fig. 29):* Hip flexion and abduction is done, trochanter is elevated, and femoral head glides into acetabulum.
- *Barlow test (Fig. 30):* It is a provocative test where hip is flexed and adducted, and head is palpated to exit the acetabulum partially or completely over a rim.

Diagnosis

Galeazzi's sign (Fig. 31):

- Flex both hips and one side shows apparent femoral shortening
- Asymmetry gluteal, thigh, or labial folds
- Limb-length inequality
- Waddling gait and hyperlordosis in bilateral cases.

Radiological Diagnosis

X-rays (Figs. 32 to 34):

- Perkins line, vertical line at outer border of acetabulum
- *Hilgenreiner's line* : Horizontal line at triradiate cartilage
- *Shenton's line*: It is a smooth curve between the inferior border of NoF and superior margin of obturator foramen, as shown in Figures 34A and B
- Acetabular index (Fig. 32)
- Center edge (CE) angle of Wiberg (Fig. 33).

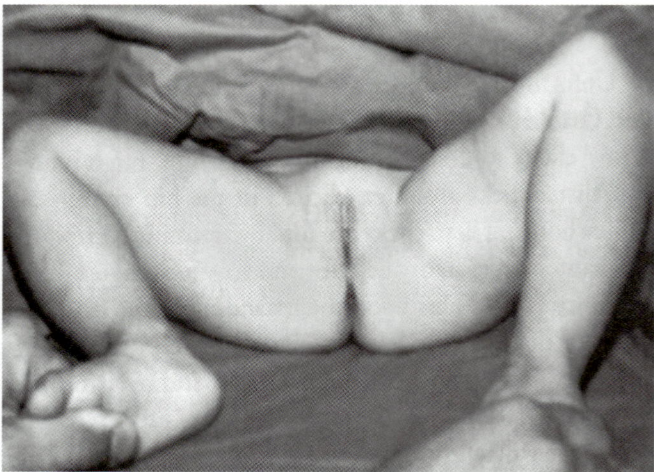

Fig. 30: Barlow's test.

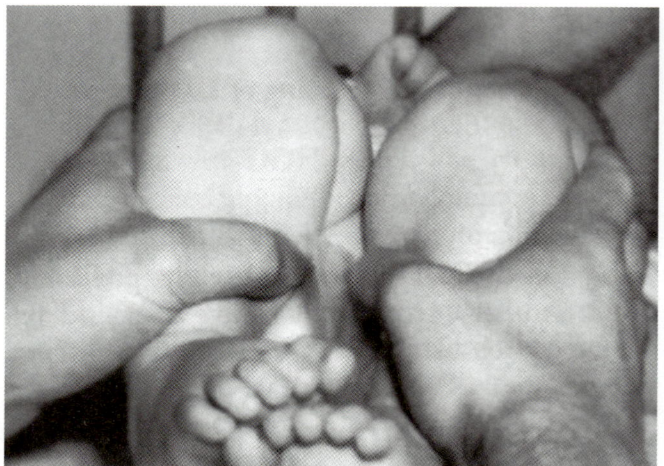

Fig. 31: Galeazzi's sign.

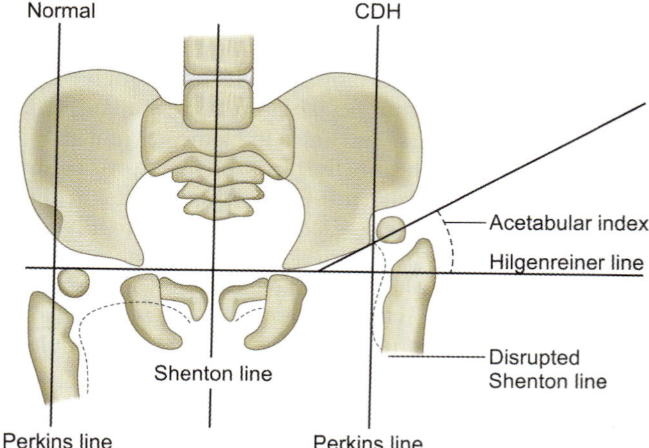

Fig. 32: Acetabular index.

Graff's Ultrasound Classification

- *Type 1:* Normal hip
- *Type 2:* Immature or somewhat abnormal

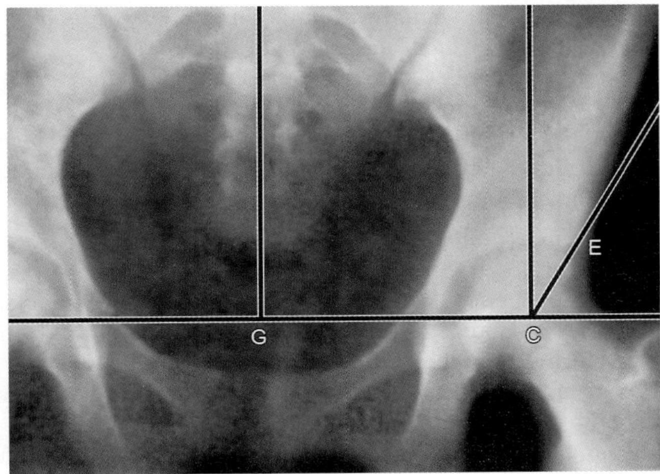

Fig. 33: X-ray showing center edge (CE) angle of Wiberg.

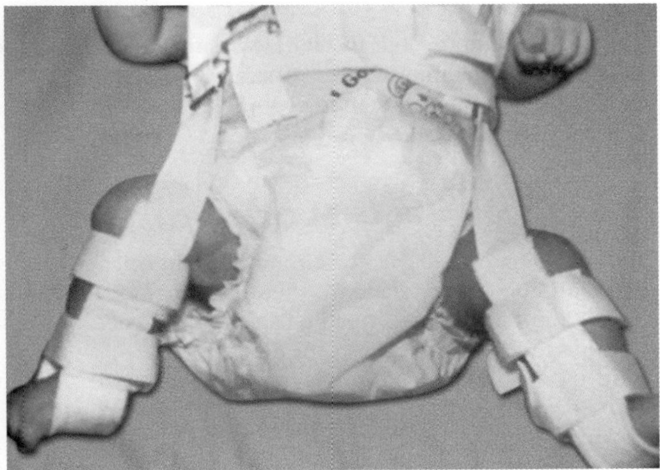

Fig. 35: Newborn with bilateral hip dislocations in a Pavlik harness.

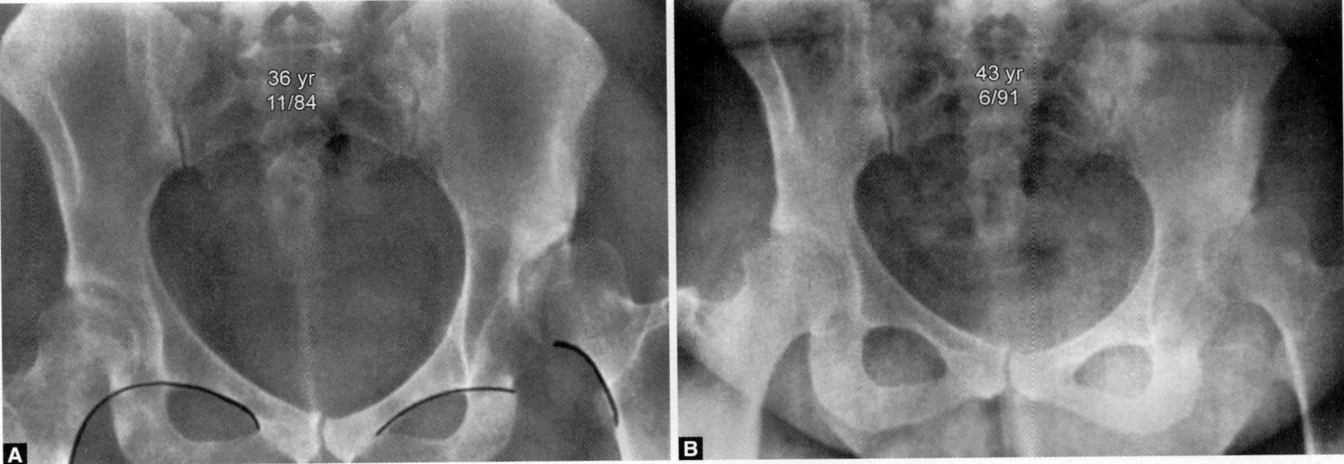

Figs. 34A and B: X-ray showing CDH—(A) Shenton's line, a curve between inferior border of neck of femur and superior margin of obturator foramen; (B) X-ray of pelvis and hip joint.

- *Type 3:* Hips are subluxated
- *Type 4:* Hips are dislocated.

Treatment of Hip Dislocation

0–6 Months:

- Goal is to obtain reduction and maintain reduction, to provide optimal environment for femoral head and acetabular development.
- *Lovell and Winter's:* Treatment is initiated immediately on diagnosis.
- *American Academy of Orthopedic Surgeons (AAOS):* Subluxation often corrects after 3 weeks and may be observed without treatment. If it persists on clinical examination or ultrasonography (USG) beyond 3 weeks, then treatment indicated. If the actual dislocation is diagnosed at birth, treatment should be immediate.
- *Pavlik harness:* The most common device for treatment of developmental dysplasia of the hip (DDH) in a newborn is Pavlik harness, as illustrated in Figure 35. It prevents hip extension and adduction, but allows flexion and abduction, which lead to reduction and stabilization. Success rate is 95%, if maintained full time, 6 weeks. Chest strap at nipple line. Shoulder straps set to hold cross strap at this level. Anterior strap flexes hip 100–110°. Posterior strap prevents adduction and allows comfortable abduction. Safe zone is defined as the arc of abduction and adduction that is between redislocation and comfortable unforced abduction. Indications include, presence of reducible hip and femoral head directed towards triradiate cartilage on X-ray. It is followed by weekly intervals, by clinical examination, and USG for 2 weeks; if it is not reduced, other methods are pursued. Once successfully reduced, harness is continued for children's age at stability for more than 3 months. Worn full time for half interval, if stability continues and then weaned off. End of weaning process, X-ray pelvis is obtained and if normal, harness is discontinued.
- *von Rosen* splint, shown in Figure 36.

Complications:
- *Failure:* Poor compliance, inaccurate position, and persistence of inadequate treatment, greater than 2–3 weeks.
- Femoral nerve compression to hyperflexion.
- Inferior dislocation.
- Skin breakdown.
- Avascular necrosis (AVN).

At 6–18 months:
- Closed reduction and spica cast immobilization recommended.
- Traction is controversial with theoretical benefit of gradual stretching of soft tissues, impeding reduction and neurovascular bundles to decrease AVN.
- Skin traction preferred, however, may vary with surgeon. Usually 1–2 weeks. Scientific evidence supporting this is lacking.
- Traction given may include Bryant's traction. This is shown in Figures 37A and B.
- Reduction maintained in spica cast is well-molded to GT to prevent redislocation. Hip-spica reduction is shown in Figures 38A and B.
- Human position of hyperflexion and limited abduction preferred.

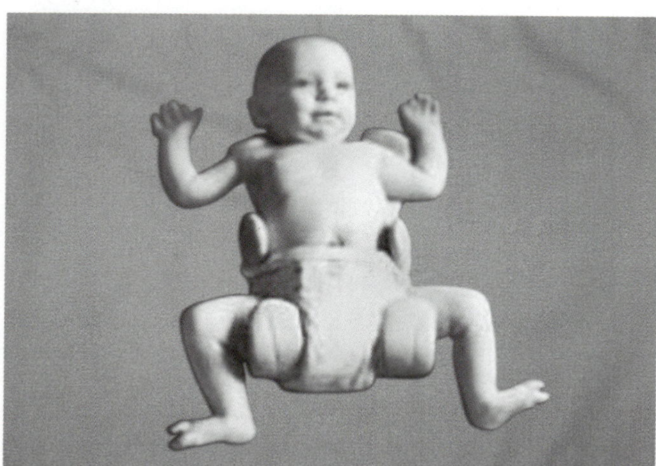

Fig. 36: von Rosen splint.

- Avoid forced abduction with internal rotation, as increased incidence of proximal femoral growth disturbance.
- Cast in place for 6 weeks, then repeat computed tomography (CT) scan, to confirm reduction.
- Casting is continued for 3 months; at which point it is removed and X-ray is done, then placed in abduction orthotic device full time for 2 months, then weaned.

At 18–36 months (Toddlers):
- Failure of closed methods.
- Open reduction indicated. If there is failure of closed reduction, persistent subluxation, reducible but unstable other than extremes of abduction.
- Open reduction is combined with femoral, or pelvic osteotomy, or both and is the treatment of choice.
- Femoral osteotomy is tried first for untreated CDH and is useful in less than 8 years of age.

At 8–18 years (Juvenile and young adults):
- Femoral and pelvic osteotomy should be done. This is shown in Figures 39A and B.
- Total hip replacement (THR) should be thought, when osteoarthritis develops.
- Rarely arthrodesis occurs.

Osteotomies for congenital diaphragmatic hernia:
- Redirectional
  - Salter (hinges on symphysis pubis)
  - Sutherland double innominate osteotomy
  - Steel (triple osteotomy)
  - Ganz (rotational)
- Acetabuloplasties (decrease volume)
  - Hinge on triradiate cartilage (therefore immature patients)
  - Pemberton
  - Dega (posterior coverage in CP patients).
- Salter's osteotomy (Figs. 40A and B)
- Pemberton pericapsular osteotomy (Figs. 41A and B)
- Chiari osteotomy.

At 3–8 years of child:
- Open reduction is treatment of choice
- Usually followed with femoral shortening
- If necessary, pelvic osteotomy may be done.

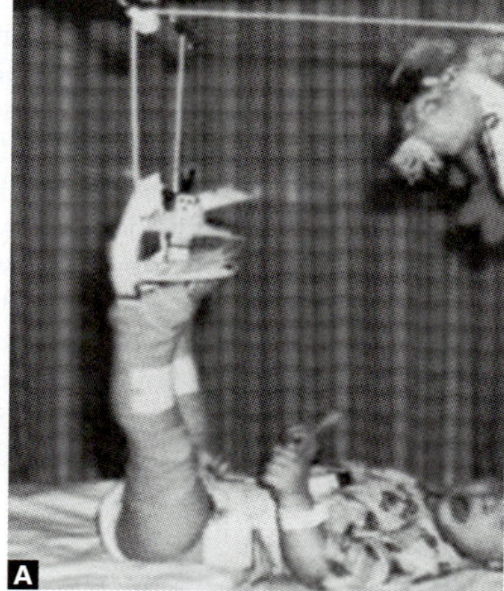

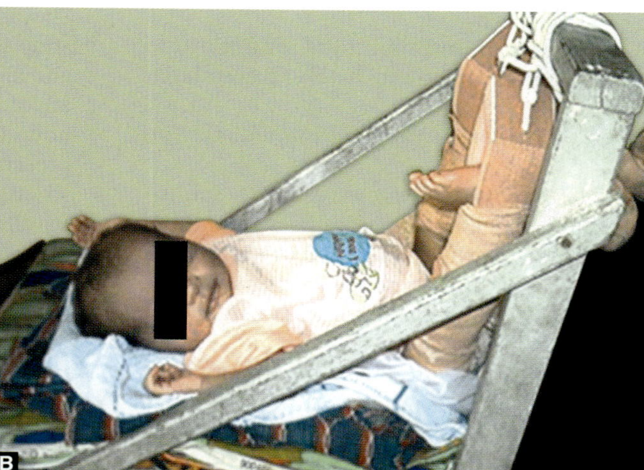

Figs. 37A and B: (A) Position of limb, while giving Bryant's traction; (B) Showing a child with CDH, given Bryant's traction.

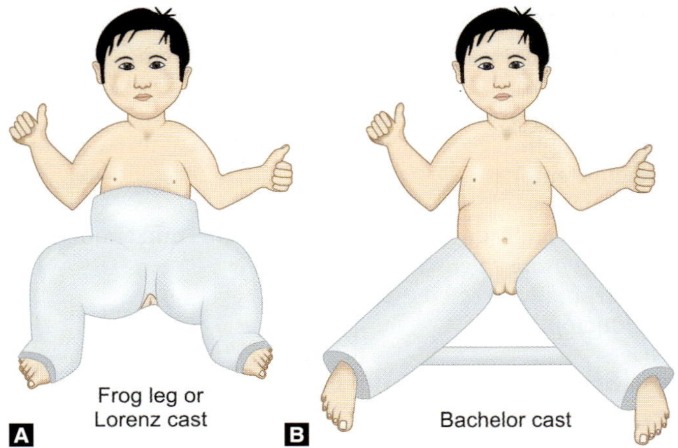

Figs. 38A and B: Reduction maintained in spica cast or hip-spica.

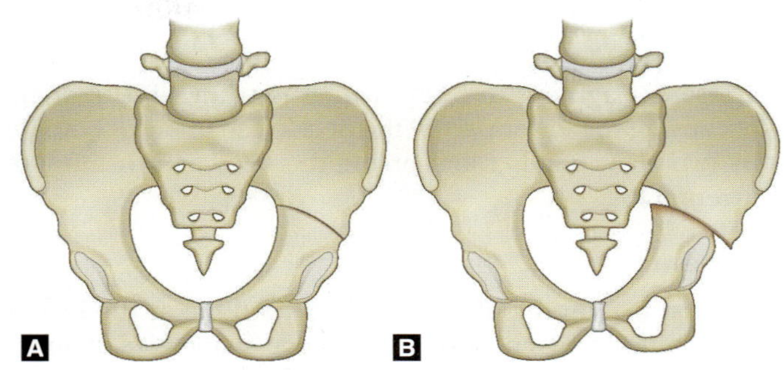

Figs. 39A and B: Femoral and pelvic osteotomy.

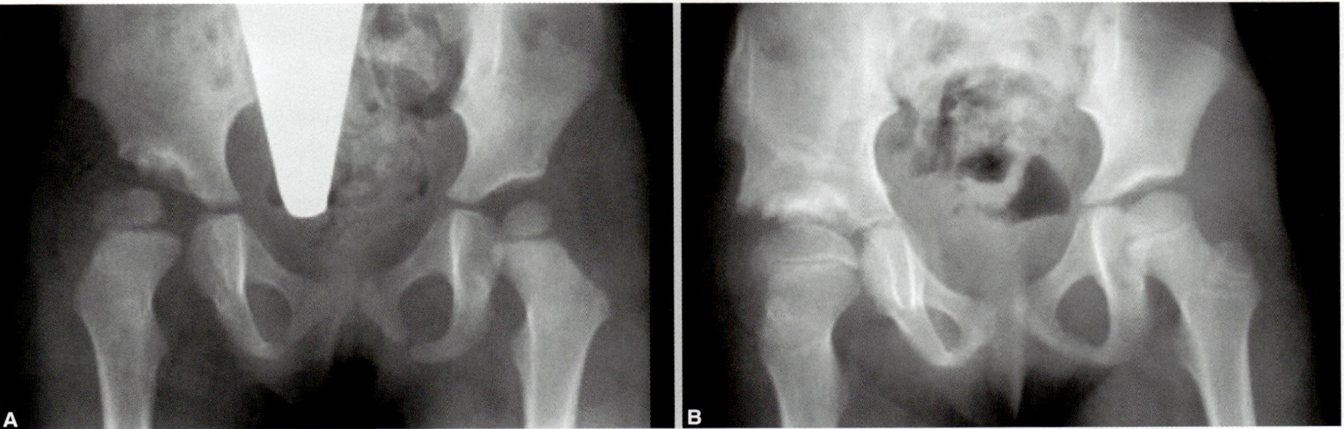

Figs. 40A and B: Salter osteotomy in CDH—(A) Preoperative X-ray; (B) Postoperative X-ray.

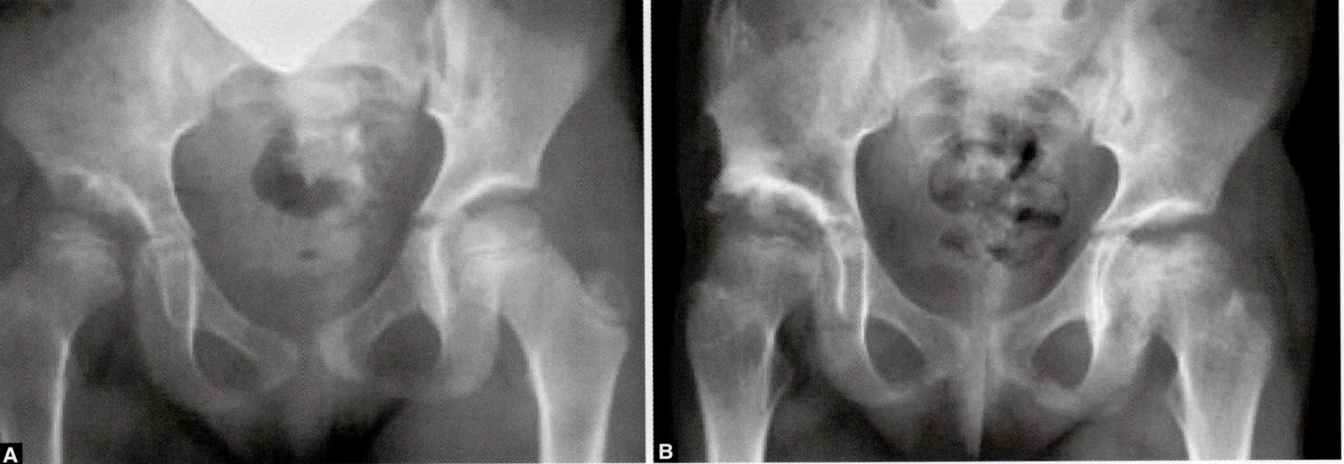

Figs. 41A and B: Pemberton pericapsular osteotomy procedure for carrying out pemberton pericapsular osteotomy; (A and B) X-rays taken before and after performing osteotomy.

CONGENITAL COXA VARA

Introduction

Coxa vara may be a primary congenital deformity occurring alone or in association with other congenital defects, especially defective growth of femur. Congenital coxa vara also sometimes described as "cervical" or "infantile" coxa vara is characterized in radiograph according to Fairbank, by the presence of a triangular piece of neck adjacent to head being separated from the rest of bone. The condition is bilateral. The symptoms appear when the child walks. The patient is small in stature and limps. Often, there is pain and stiffness. On examination, the GT is at higher level, shortening of limb is present, limb is in rotation, and abduction is limited. Flexion contracture may also present.

Radiographic Features

- The angle of neck is reduced to somewhat below right angle.
- Neck varies in length, but is short, and may even become nonexistent, and may be fragmented. Often the neck shows a prolonged lower extremity, which forms down hanging hip.
- Head is translucent and fluffy in appearance.
- There is fragment of bone, which is triangular in shape, occupying the lower part of the neck close to head, bounded by two clear bands transversing the neck and forming the inverted "V".

Treatment

Angulation osteotomy of Dickson type is done at the level of intertrochanteric region. In this, the wedge-shape area of bone is removed and vertical epiphysis becomes horizontal in shape, and relieves the shearing stress, and reduces the varus deformity.

Proximal Femoral Focal Deficiency

In proximal femoral focal deficiency (PFFD), congenital shortening of the femur occurs. Incidence is 1 per 50,000 live births. Dysgenesis of proximal portion of the femur occurs, with partial skeletal defect in the proximal femur, with unstable hip joint and shortening of femur.

Other associated anomalies are:

- Fibular hemimelia
- Agenesis of cruciate ligaments of the knee
- Club foot
- Congenital heart anomalies
- Spinal dysplasia
- Facial dysplasia.

Embryology (Flowchart 2)

Flowchart 2: Schematic representation of embryological development of limbs.

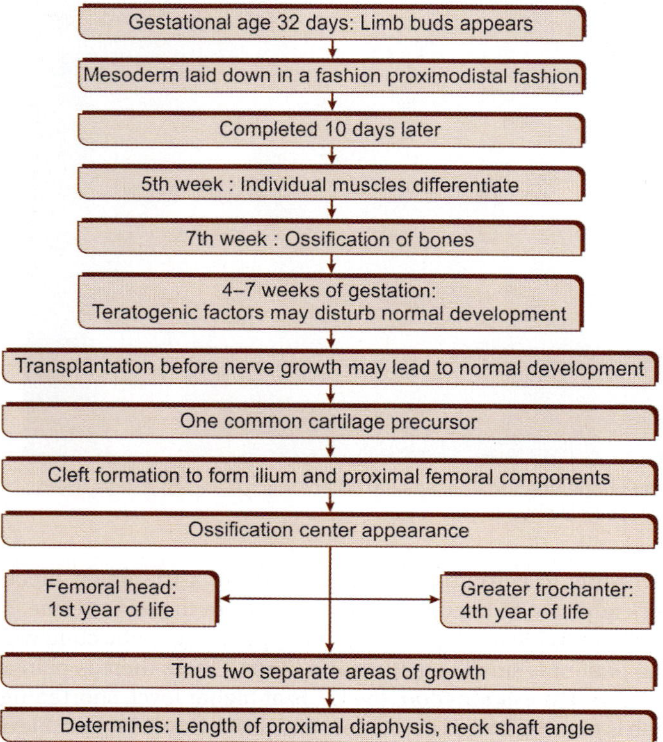

Forces Acting on Femoral Neck

Certain physiological forces tend to force the femoral neck into varus or valgus.

Factors for varus are:

- Body weight
- Rectus femoris
- Hamstrings
- Longitudinally directed fibers of adductors and abductors.

The opposing valgus forces are:

- Horizontally directed external rotators
- Adductors.

Classifications of Proximal Femoral Focal Deficiency

- Aitken's classification
- Pappa's classification
- Kalamchi's classification.

Aitken's Classification (Fig. 42)

Class A:

- Congenital short femur is present with:
  - Bowing
  - Coxa vara
- Normal acetabulum is present along with absence of femoral neck.

Class B:

It contains following features:

- No bony connection between proximal femur and femoral head
- Short femur with sub-trochanteric pseudarthrosis
- Progressive coxa vara and a normal acetabulum.

Class C:

It contains following features:

- Dysplastic acetabulum
- Absent femoral head
- Short femur.

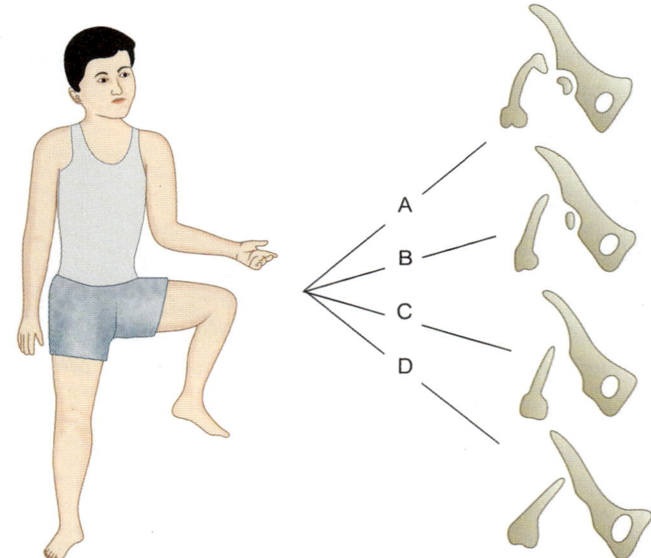

Fig. 42: Schematic representation of the four radiographic subclasses of proximal femoral focal deficiency.

Pappa's classification

Class I

Femoral-pelvic abnormalities	Femur absent ischiopubic bone structures underdeveloped acetabular structure under developed
Associated abnormalities	Fibula absent
Treatment Objectives	Prosthetic management

Tibia

Fig. 43: Class I type of proximal femoral deficiency.

Class D:

It contains following features:

- Acetabulum and femoral head is totally absent
- Proximal femur is extremely short and pointed.

Pappa's Classification

Class I (Fig. 43):

- *Femoral-pelvic abnormalities:*
  - Femur absent, ischiopubic bone structures underdeveloped and deficient
  - Lack of acetabular development.
- *Associated abnormalities*: Fibula absent
- *Treatment objectives*: Prosthetic management.

Class II (Aitken D, Fig. 44):

- *Femoral-pelvic abnormalities:*
  - Femoral shortening (70–90%)
  - Femoral head is absent
  - Ischiopubic bone structures delayed in ossification
- *Associated abnormalities:* Tibia shortened, fibula, foot, knee, and ankle joint abnormal
- *Treatment objectives:* Pelvic femoral stability through prosthetic management.

Class III (Aitken B, Fig. 45):

- *Femoral-pelvic abnormalities:*
  - Femoral shortening (45–80%)
  - No osseus connection between femoral shaft and head
  - Femoral head ossification delayed
  - Acetabulum may be absent
  - Femoral condyles maldeveloped.
- *Associated abnormalities*:
  - Tibia shortened (0–40%)
  - Fibula shortened (5–100%)
  - Patella absent or small and high riding
  - Knee joint instability common
  - Foot malformed
- *Treatment objectives:* Prosthetic management.

Class IV (Aitken A, Fig. 46):

- *Femoral-pelvic abnormalities:*
  - Femoral shortening (40–67%)
  - Femoral head and shaft joined by irregular calcification in fibrocartilaginous matrix.
- *Associated abnormalities*:
  - Tibia shortened (0–20%)
  - Fibula shortened (4–60%)

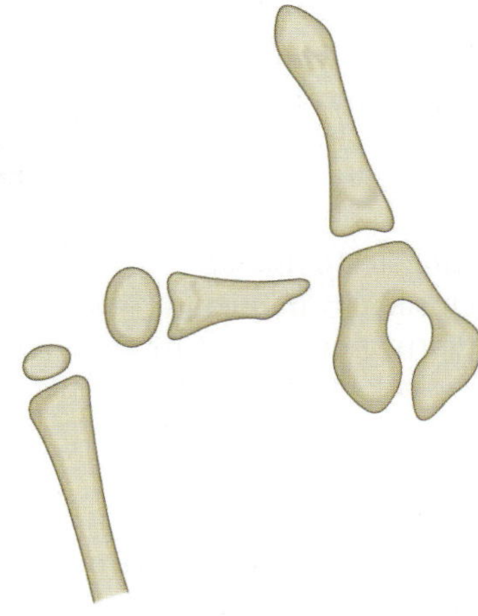

Fig. 44: Class II (Aitken D) type of proximal femoral deficiency.

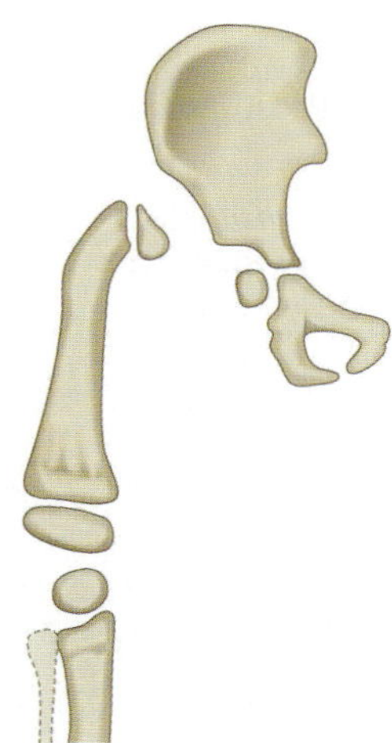

Fig. 45: Class III (Aitken B) type of proximal femoral deficiency.

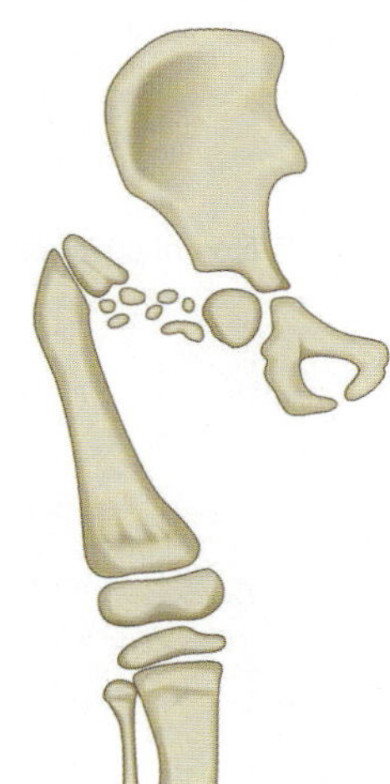

Fig. 46: Class IV (Aitken A) type of proximal femoral deficiency.

  - Knee joint instability frequent
  - Foot malformed with infrequent malformations.
- *Treatment objectives*:
  - Union between femoral head, neck, and shaft
  - Prosthetic management.

Class V (Aitken A, Fig. 47):

- *Femoral-pelvic abnormalities:*
  - Femoral shortening (48–85%)
  - Femur incompletely ossified, hypoplastic, and irregular.
- *Associated abnormalities*:
  - Tibia shortened (4–27%)
  - Fibula shortened (10–100%)
  - Knee joint instability frequent
  - Severe malformations of foot are common.
- *Treatment objectives:* Prosthetic management.

Class VI (Fig. 48):

- *Femoral-pelvic abnormalities:*
  - Femoral shortening (30–60%)
  - Distal femur short, irregular and hypoplastic
  - Irregular distal femoral diaphysis.
- *Associated abnormalities*:
  - Single bone, lower leg
  - Patella absent
  - Foot malformed.
- *Treatment objectives:* Prosthetic management.

Class VII (Fig. 49):

- *Femoral-pelvic abnormalities:*
  - Femoral shortening (10–50%)
  - Coxa vara
  - Hypoplastic femur
  - Proximal femoral diaphysis irregular with thickened cortex
  - Lateral femoral condyle deficiency common
  - Valgus distal femur.
- *Associated abnormalities*:
  - Tibia shortened (<10–24%)
  - Fibula shortened (<10–100%)
  - Lateral high riding patella is common.

Class VIII (Fig. 50):

- *Femoral pelvic abnormalities:*
  - Femoral shortening (10–41%)
  - Femoral-pelvic abnormalities
  - Coxa valga
  - Hypoplastic femur
  - Femoral head and neck smaller
  - Proximal femoral physis horizontal
  - Abnormality of femoral condyled common, with associated boing of shaft and valgus of distal femur.
- *Associated abnormalities*:
  - Tibia shortened (0–36%)
  - Fibula shortened (0–100%)
  - Lateral and high riding patella is common
  - Foot malformed.

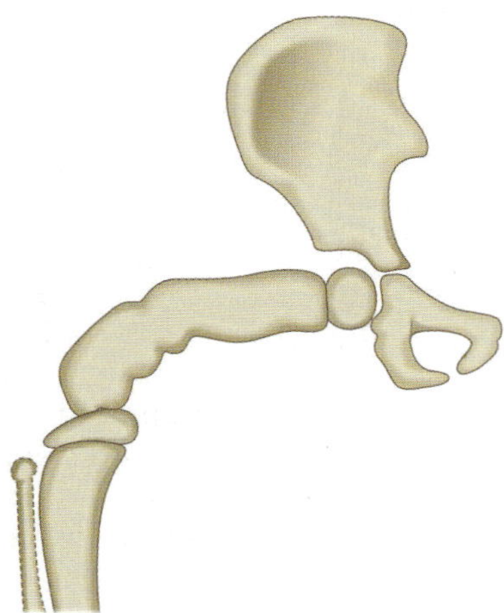

Fig. 47: Class V (Aitken A) type of proximal femoral deficiency.

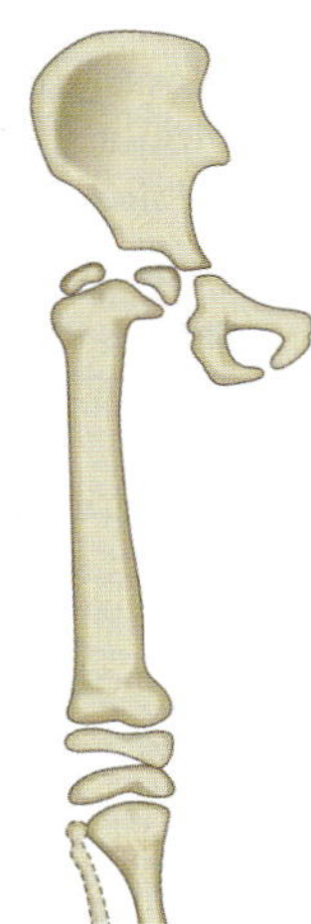

Fig. 49: Class VII type of proximal femoral deficiency.

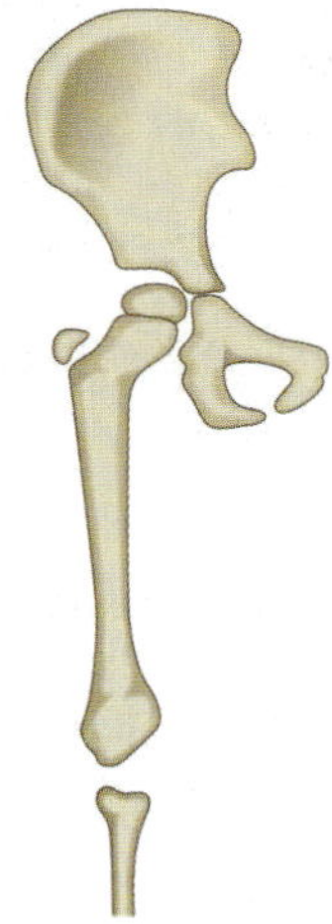

Fig. 48: Class VI type of proximal femoral deficiency.

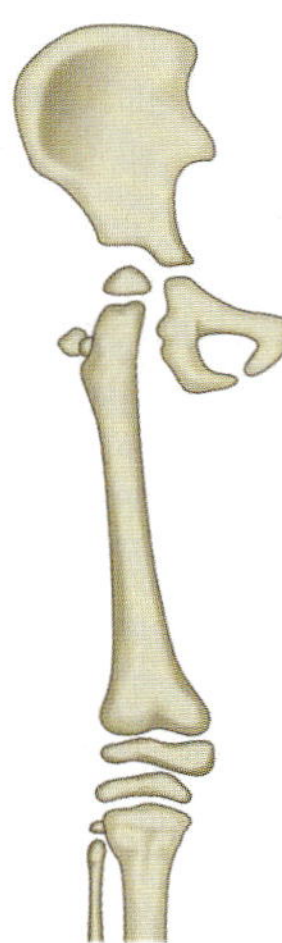

Fig. 50: Class VIII type of proximal femoral deficiency.

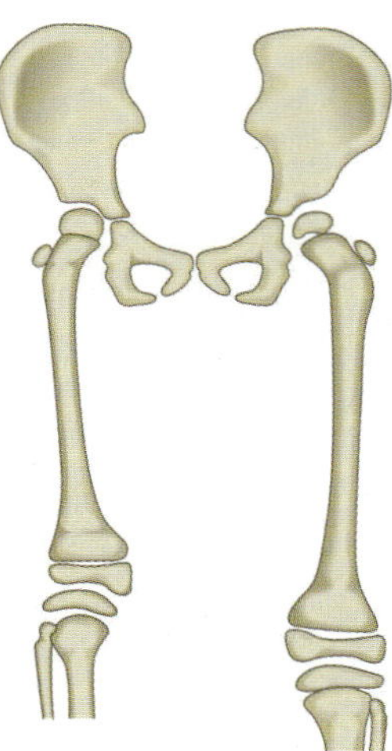

Fig. 51: Class IX type of proximal femoral deficiency.

- *Treatment objectives*:
  - Extremity length equality
  - Improved alignment of
    - Proximal and
    - Distal femur.

Class IX (Fig. 51):

- *Femoral-pelvic abnormalities:*
  - Femoral shortening (6–20%)
  - Hypoplastic femur.
- *Associated abnormalities*:
  - Tibia shortened (0–15%)
  - Fibula shortened (3–30%)
  - Additional ipsilateral and contralateral malformations are common.
- *Treatment objectives:* Extremity length equality.

Kalamchi's Classification

He developed a simple classification scheme, which is as follows:

- *Group I:* Short femur and intact hip joint
- *Group II:* Short femur and coxa vara of hip
- *Group III:* Short femur, well-developed acetabulum, and femoral head
- *Group IV:* Absent hip joint and dysplastic femoral segment
- *Group V:* Total absence of the femur.

Treatment

Proximal femoral focal deficiency presents multiple problems of management, depending upon the degree of various elements of the deformity including:

- Instability of the hip
- Malrotation
- Inadequate proximal musculature
- Inequality of the leg length.

Instability of the Hip

This could be due to iliofemoral maldevelopment and muscle inadequacy. In milder forms, coxa vara leads to proximal displacement of GT, due to abductor insufficiency and lurching gait. In moderate type, pseudarthrosis adds to instability. In severe type, failure of joint formation leads to slip femoral head proximally. When acetabulum can be identified on roentgenogram, cartilaginous head and neck, although not visible, are already present. Allow spontaneous ossification of the head and neck and bony bridging across the pseudarthrosis, to take place. For reducing the degree of coxa vara, bone graft is placed across pseudarthrosis into the femoral head and neck. Before this, presence of proximal element of the femur should be confirmed by arthrography. This surgical procedure is not generally accepted. Moreover, spontaneous ossification, although delayed, generally takes place and the coxa vara deformity can be dealt with later.

In Type 1 or 2 Deformity: Coxa vara is corrected and held with a fixation device. This should be done at an early age.

In Type 3:

- Excise pseudarthrosis
- Correct varus
- Single unit fixation device is inserted alternatively
- Encourage ossification of the proximal femur
- Healing of the pseudarthrosis is done by inserting a bone graft
- Coxa vara can be corrected at second operation.

In Type 4:

- Hypoplastic head widely separated from the tapered
- Sclerotic femoral shaft and it is also associated with muscular hypoplasia
- Results are unrewarding.

In Type 5:

- Acetabulum absent
- Reconstruction is not possible.

Malrotation and Inadequate Proximal Musculature

- Hip usually has a fixed flexion and external rotation contracture.
- Flexion to 90° and abduction to 30° is functionally useful.
- Gluteal muscles are usually good, whereas quadriceps is hypoplastic.
- On active flexion of hip, contraction of sartorius can be demonstrated. Its action is to draw the limb into "sitting tailor" position. Consequently, despite the hip flexion contracture, function is good and treatment for this is not required.

Leg Length Inequality

Generally, femur is 20–40% of normal length. When lower limb inequality is mild, epiphysiodesis or leg lengthening procedure should be done. Usually, the femoral shortening is severe and progressive and may exceed 12 inches at maturity, therefore, foot of the affected leg will come to lie at approximately the same level as the normal knee.

In the following way the progressive deformity should be handled:

- In young child, where the shortening is not yet severe, hence, a shoe elevation is sufficient.
- *Extension prosthesis*: Within the prosthesis, foot is placed on a platform in full equinus.
- *Van Nes rotationplasty (Figs. 52A to E):* Arthrodesis of the knee and rotation of the distal portion of the limb through 180° brings the ankle into a position, where it functions as a knee, with calf muscle acting as a quadriceps. However, gradual derotation takes place with growth and causes difficulty with fitting a functional prosthesis.

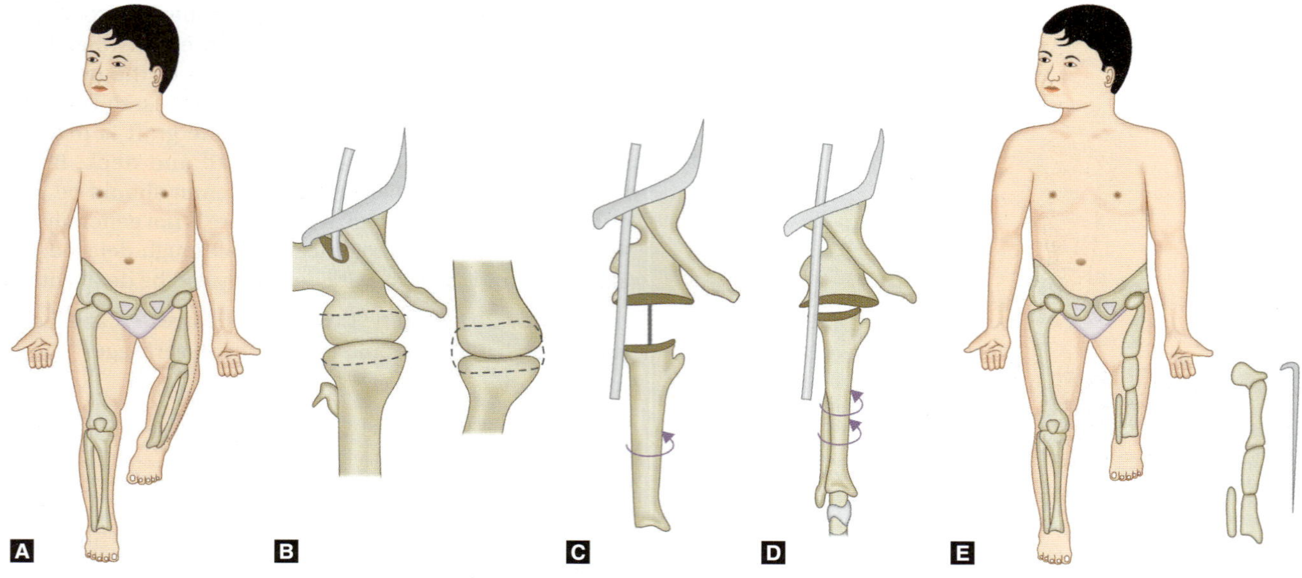

Figs. 52A to E: Van Nes rotationplasty.

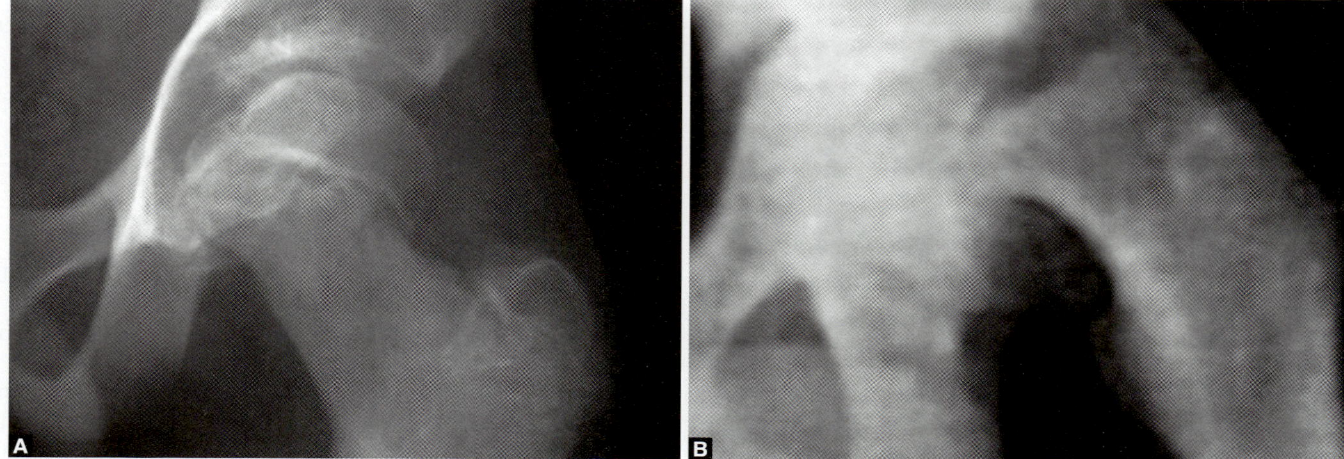

Figs. 53A and B: (A) Slip capital femoral epiphysis; (B) SCFE, where capital femoral epiphysis is displaced from the metaphysis through the physeal plate.

- *Syme's amputation:* This provides an excellent end bearing stump, allowing ready fitting of a prosthesis at an early age, when the child quickly adapts to the prosthesis.
- *Arthrodesis of the knee:* Provides a single skeletal lever so that available muscle can act more efficiently across the hip joint.

The procedure of choice:

- Early Syme's amputation, as soon as walking is established and an end-bearing prosthesis.
- With the growth, thigh-to-leg disproportion increases, hence arthrodesis of the knee is done.

Slipped Capital Femoral Epiphysis

Slip capital femoral epiphysis (SCFE) is a disorder in which capital femoral epiphysis is displaced from the metaphysis through the physeal plate. SCFE is actually a misnomer in that the head is held in the acetabulum by the ligamentum teres and thus, it is actually the neck that comes upward and outwards, while the head remains posterior and downward in the acetabulum. A varus relation exists between the head and neck, but occasionally the slip is into valgus, with head displaced superiorly and posteriorly in relation to the neck, as shown in Figures 53A and B.

Incidence

- Every 2 in 100,000; so, the rate is 0.002%.
- Boys (10–16 years)
- Girls (10–14 years)
- Male to female ratio is 2.5:1
- Blacks are suffering more than white people
- 5% of sufferers having their parents have or had SCFE
- Left hip is twice as often affected as right hip
- Mostly bilateral
- 17–37% in adolescents
- 50% are simultaneous and 50% are sequential
- In younger child (physically or chronologically), the greater risk of subsequent bilateral involvement
- A contralateral slip will usually present within 2 years
- 20% are bilateral at the time of presentation, as shown in Figure 54.

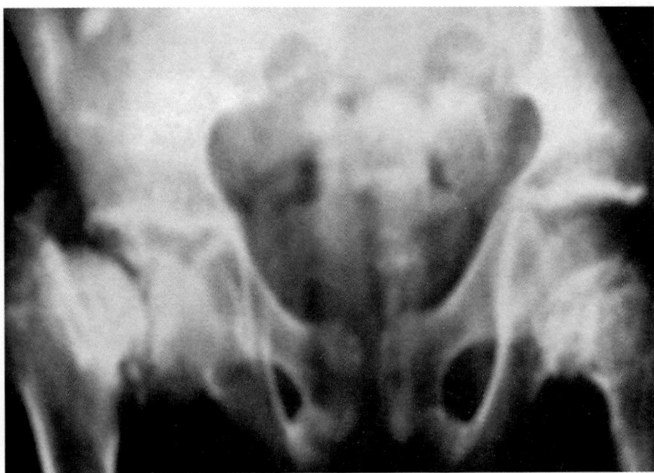

Fig. 54: Slip capital femoral epiphysis, generally have bilateral presentation.

Etiology

- Unknown.
- Hormonal theory.
- Although the softening is due to a failure of maturation of cartilage into bone, analysis of evidence seems to suggest that it is the result of a hormonal imbalance.
- *Siberberg and Sibelberg:* In 1949, Siberberg and Sibelberg have observed with experiments in animals, by administration of hyperestrogen, how to weaken or change in epiphyseal plate.
- Duthie and Barker, in 1955 by cortisone.
- *Harris:* In 1950, Harris showed GH increased thickness of epiphyseal plates, which required less force to slip and estrogen led to thinner, required more force with experiments in rats.
- Unfortunately, there are no human studies to support any theory for hormonal basis for slipping.
- *Burrows:* In his careful survey of 100 cases, Burrows found that a quarter of boys and two-thirds of girls showed evidence of some endocrine defect, quite apart from those who are unusually fat.
- Moreover, although line of separation is at the usual level at the junction is at the metaphysis with epiphyseal cartilage, epiphysis in its backward and downward displacement does not carry with it a triangular fragment from the margin of the diaphysis, over which it is displaced as it does in other epiphyseal injuries.

Traumatic theory:

- There is no doubt that trauma and static influences are both important factors in the development of SCFE.
- *Key:* In 1930, Key pointed out pathological conditions may be neither in the bone nor in the epiphyseal cartilage, but in the periosteum of femoral neck. In childhood, periosteum is thick and thrown into ridges or folds known as "retinacula of Weitbrecht", which is the chief factor in holding the head in place. In adolescence, this periosteum begins to atrophy and to approach the adult type, thus producing weakness at epiphyseal line. Moreover, coxa vara gives a history of rapid growth prior to epiphyseal displacement and during this period, the periosteum crossing the epiphyseal line is stretched, thinned, and consequently weakened, thus permitting the epiphysis to be easily separated.
- *Fairbank:* Fairbank pointed out that the epiphysis is set obliquely on the neck and faces upwards and medially. This setting, somewhat insecure as a means of supporting the body weight is strengthened by a spur projecting from the lower half of the metaphysis.
- *Haas:* In 1948 Haas showed, once the periosteum has been stripped off the humeral epiphysis of rats, the middle zone of epiphyseal plate will slip when a shearing stress is applied.
- *Walmsley:* In 1938, Walmsley showed that the spur provides a natural ledge, on which the epiphysis rests. Occasionally the spur ossifies from a separate secondary center, which may remain isolated from the rest of metaphysis by a strip of cartilage till puberty. This increase in amount of cartilage weakens the neck in proportion to the body weight, while the inadequacy of the spur, increased occasionally by fragmentation of its center, allows the epiphysis to slide downward.

Proven associations:

- Hypothyroidism
- Renal disease (renal osteodystrophy)
- Hypogonadism or hypopituitarism
- Secondary to mechanical disturbances
- Increased retroversion, increase force on epiphysis
- Obesity
- Secondary to biochemical abnormality in cartilage collagen
- Sometimes, adults men suffering from Simmond's disease
- Hypopituitarism resulting from intracranial tumor
- Affected boys may have excessive fat with hypopituitarism of French type, i.e. undeveloped testis and absence of pubic hair and axillary hair.

Pathology

Synovium shows:

- Synovitis with hypertrophy
- Hyperplasia of synovial cells
- Villus formation
- Increased vascularity
- Round cell infiltration
- Light microscopic studies reveal that physis is widened and irregular, sometimes reaching 12 mm in width. In SCFE hypertrophic zone may constitute up to 80% of the physis width
- Slip occurs through the zone of cell hypertrophy, with occasional extension into the calcifying cartilage.

Symptomatology

Idiopathic:

- Onset is gradual
- Patient gets tired easily after walking or standing
- Pain is confined to hip, but usually radiates down to lower thigh and knee, relieved by rest in early stage. It is also accompanied by limping
- Limitation of abduction
- Affected leg gradually becomes shorter and smaller. Movements are restricted and leg may be in full external rotation.

Traumatic:

- History of trauma (fall or blow on hip) and is very trivial
- Dull ache associated with little disability in the hip. Although occasionally, pain is severe and it prevents from being able to walk.

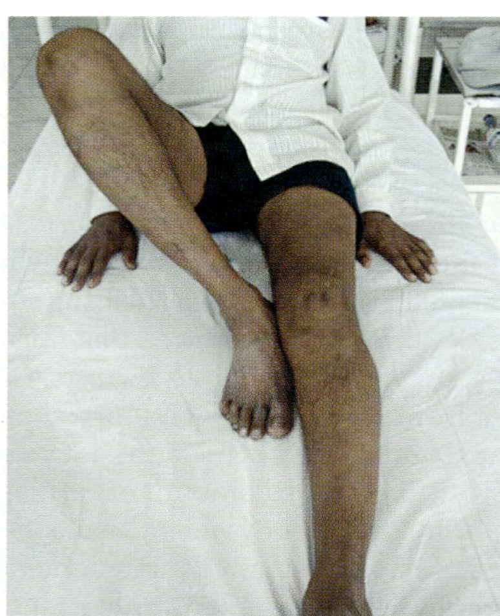

Fig. 55: Position of the leg in recumbent position.

Physical Signs

At early stage:
- Pain
- Waddling gait
- Body sways over affected side
- Pelvis on sound side tends to drop when weight borne on affected extremity.

On standing:
- Leg rotated laterally, abducted, and pelvis tilted on affected side
- Slight scoliosis towards affected side is present lumbar and in sound side thoracic buttock atrophied and gluteal fold lower than normal side.

On recumbent position (Fig. 55):
- *Position of leg:* Lateral rotation and slight abduction. Flexion is limited up to 80–90° and as thigh is flexed, it rotates laterally.
- *Axis deviation:* Adduction and lateral rotation are free, but abduction, medial rotation, and extension are greatly restricted.

Radiological Findings (Figs. 56A to C)

X-rays:
- AP view
- True lateral view
- Frog leg lateral view–Lauenstein view (Fig. 56C)

Preslipping stage:
- Minimal slipping, indicated by the absence of normal shoulder on the upper aspect of neck and head, i.e. Trethowan's sign, as shown in Figures 57A and B. A line drawn from superior surface of the neck will pass above the femoral head rather than it passing through 20% of the head normally.
- Lateral view shows slightest backward displacement.
- *Billing's lateral view of hip (Fig. 58):* An accurate measurement of epiphyseal slip can be obtained, with patient lying in supine on X-ray table and the knee in 90° of flexion. The hip is allowed to fall into a position of external rotation and abduction. The knee is supported to bring the shaft of the femur to a position of 25° of elevation, while the height of malleolus is adjusted.
- *Interpretation:* The neck axis is indicated by relatively straight anterior border of distal half of femoral neck, and shaft axis by anterior border of upper third of femoral shaft line, connecting anterior and posterior margins of epiphysis define epiphyseal plane.

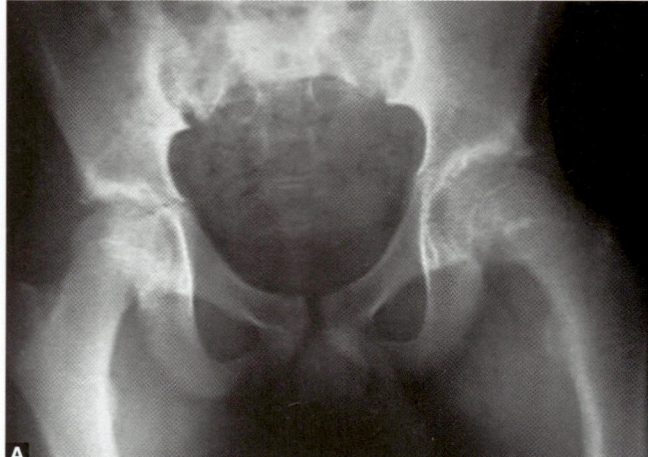

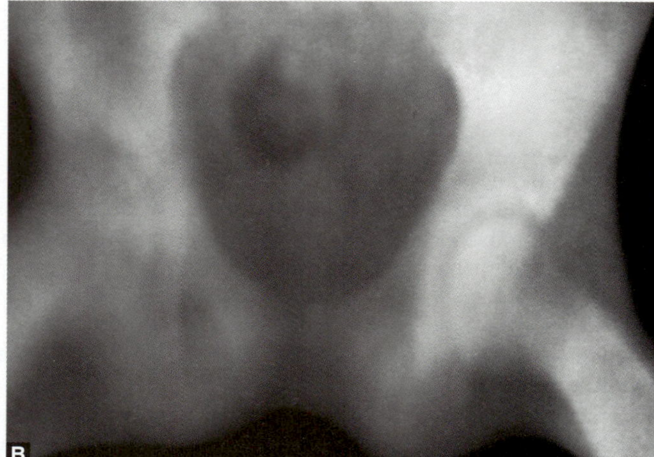

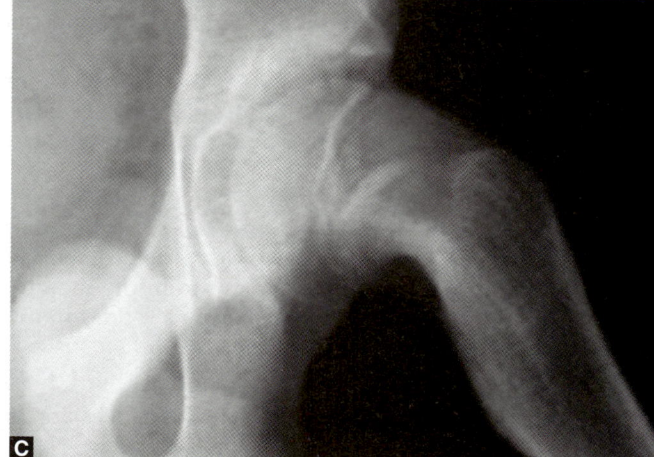

Figs. 56A to C: Lateral view showing slipped capital femoral epiphysis.

Early Radiographic Sign

- *Lateral view:* Cup-shaped epiphysis. No longer fitting into cup surface of metaphysic.
- *AP view:* Decrease in depth.

Late Radiographic Sign

AP view: Epiphysis lies well below its normal level with backwards rotation.

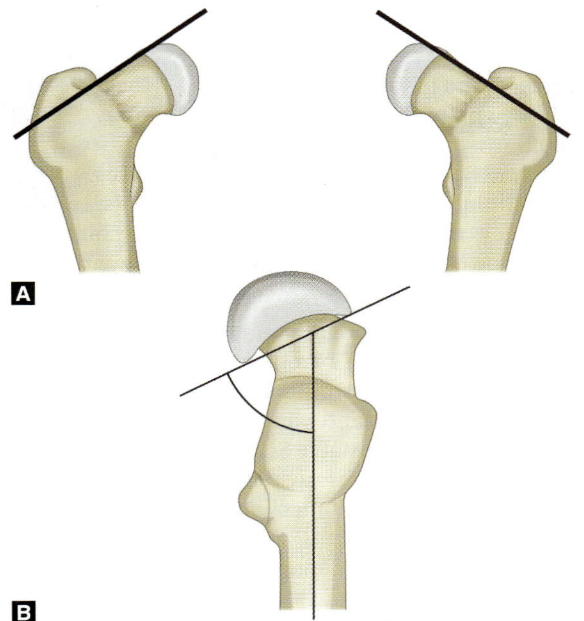

Figs. 57A and B: Trethowan's sign. (A) Lateral view; (B) A view from above.

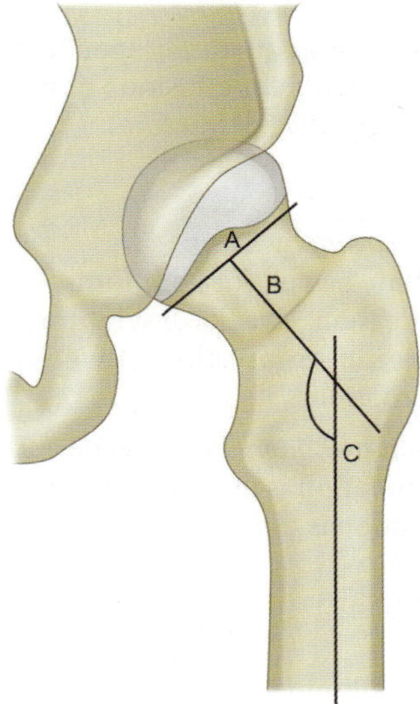

Fig. 59: The angle form between this two line is anteroposterior head shaft angle (normal 145°)—(A) Line drawn across the base of epiphysis connecting both superior and inferior margins of epiphysis; (B) Another line drawn perpendicular to it; (C) A straight line drawn over shaft of femur joining the perpendicular line.

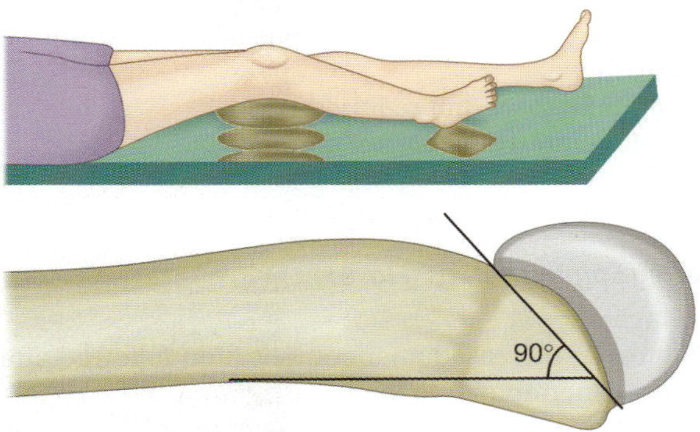

Fig. 58: Billing's lateral view of hip.

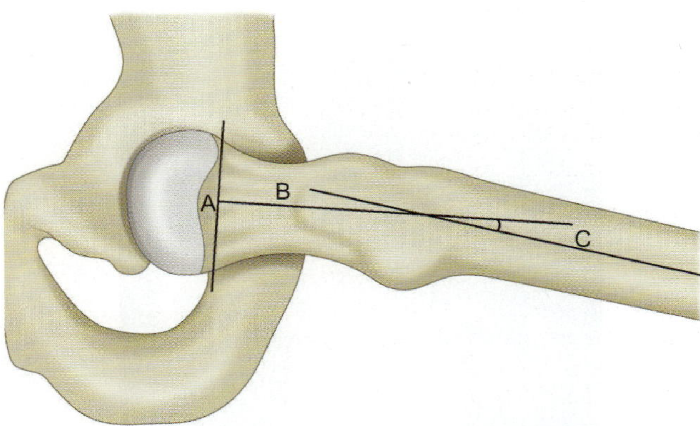

Fig. 60: Frog leg lateral head shaft angle—(A) Line drawn across the base of epiphysis connecting both superior and inferior margins of epiphysis; (B) Another line drawn perpendicular to it; (C) A straight line drawn over shaft of femur joining the perpendicular line.

Anteroposterior head shaft angle:

- Line drawn across the base of epiphysis connecting both superior and inferior margins of epiphysis.
- Another line drawn perpendicular to it.
- A straight line drawn over shaft of femur joining the perpendicular line.
- The angle form between these two lines is AP head shaft angle (normal 145°), as shown in Figure 59.
- This angle difference between the two sides represents the amount of correction needed on the anterior surface of femur.
- Frog leg lateral head shaft angle, as shown in Figure 60.
- Lines are drawn in the same fashion. In both normal and affected sides angle is determined (normal range 0–25°).
- The difference of retroversion between affected and normal sides determines the lateral wedge to be removed, to correct the posterior angulation.

Severity

It can be seen in radiograph and classified by maximal anatomic displacement, either on AP or lateral view.

- *Minimal slip:* Maximal displacement is less than one-third the diameter of the neck.
- *Moderate slip:* Greater than 1 cm of displacement, but less than half the diameter of the neck.
- *Severe slip:* Displacement more than 50% diameter of the neck.

Other Investigations

Computed tomography scan:

Findings: CT is a sensitive method for measuring the degree of tilt and detecting disease, it can help in defining whether growth plate is open.

Magnetic resonance imaging:

Findings: The earliest way to detect SCFE is by using magnetic resonance tomography. With MRI, early marrow edema and slippage can be demonstrated. MRI can be considered in patients for whom the clinical suspicion of SCFE is high and in whom the radiographs appear normal. MRI can be considered for follow-up imaging of the contralateral hip.

Ultrasound:

Ultrasonographic findings are rarely specific and the sensitivity of sonography is unknown. Hip effusions of blood often have been reported and are suggestive of fracture.

Classification (Fig. 61)

Traditional classification by Dunn

- Acute—less than 3 weeks of symptoms
- Chronic—more than 3 weeks of symptoms
- Acute on chronic—more than 3 weeks of symptoms and sudden exacerbation.

Newer classification by Loder (Figs. 62A and B):

- *Unstable:* Ambulation is impossible, with or without crutches
- *Stable:* Ambulation is possible with or without crutches.

Surgical Treatment

Goals:

- Prevent further slipping
- Close the growth plate
- Safely restore normal anatomy
- Reduction or osteotomy.

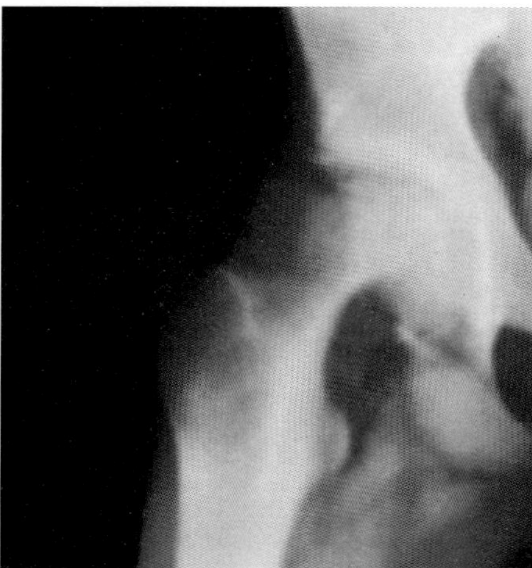

Fig. 61: Acute SCFE.

Treatment Options

- Pin in situ
- Reduction and pinning
- Bone peg epiphysiodesis
- Osteotomy
- Reconstruction by arthroplasty and arthrodesis
- Each technique has proponents and opponents, and the choice of treatment must be individualized for each child, depending on age, type of slip, and severity of displacement.

Pinning in situ (Figs. 63 and 64):

- Internal fixation with single cannulated screws or pins (Moore or Knowles). Screws are extremely effective for stable SCFE.
- There is decreased complications compared to multiple pins (pin protrusion and chondrolysis), however, its use is controversial in the unstable SCFE.
- Some advocate two screws, while others have excellent results with single screw. No biomechanical benefit found with two screws.
- The fixation device must enter the epiphysis perpendicular to physeal plate of femoral head and must cross it, but well short of subchondral cortex.

Reduction:

- It is very controversial, becoming timely
- Reduction gives poor results especially in a chronic SCFE
- Necessity
  - In mild cases, not required
  - Moderate, probably not required
  - Unstable, severe slips.
- Can make pinning technically easier.

Bone Peg Epiphysiodesis (Fig. 65)

Advantages:

- Popularity increased after complication followed after pin or screw penetration into joint.
- Rapid physeal closure and low incidence of complication.
- Useful in moderate or severe slips.

Disadvantages:

- Need longer operating time, increased blood loss, longer hospitalization, and rehabilitation.
- Bad results in mild, acute, and chronic slips.

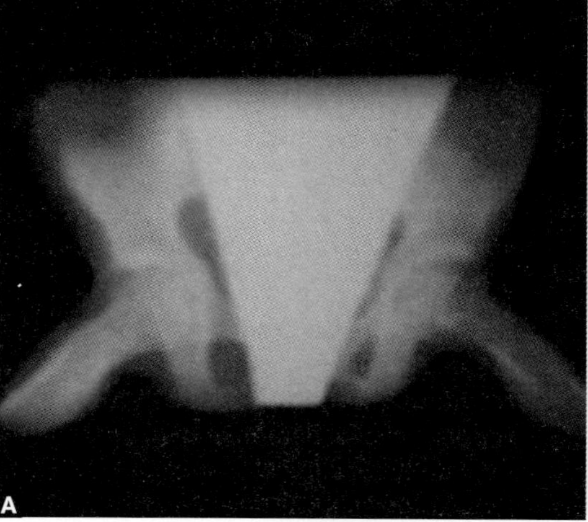

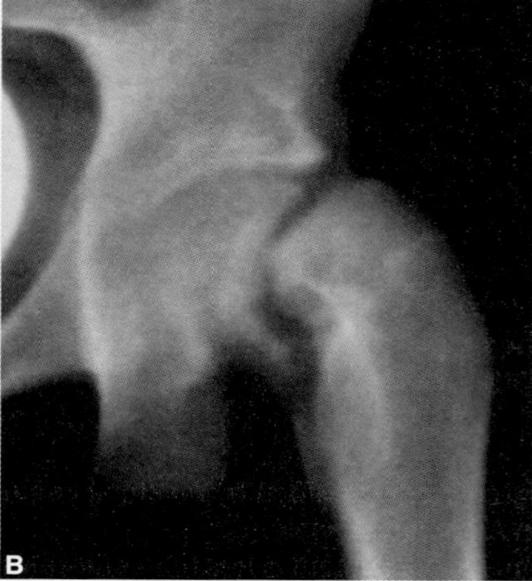

Figs. 62A and B: (A) Frog leg view; (B) AP view showing SCFE.

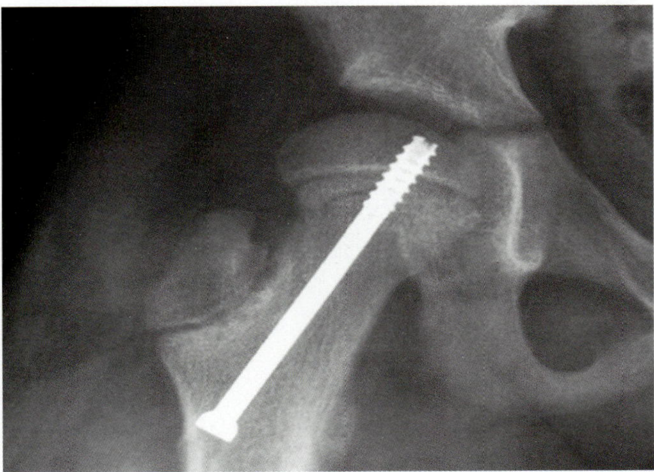

Fig. 63: Internal fixation, with single cannulated screws in SCFE.

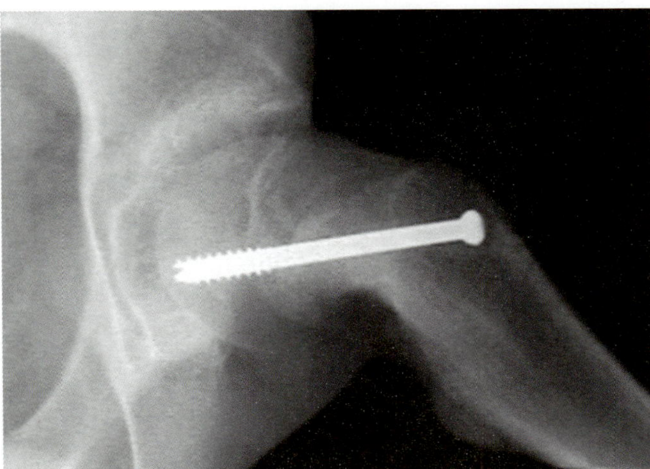

Fig. 64: Screw fixation in case of stable SCFC.

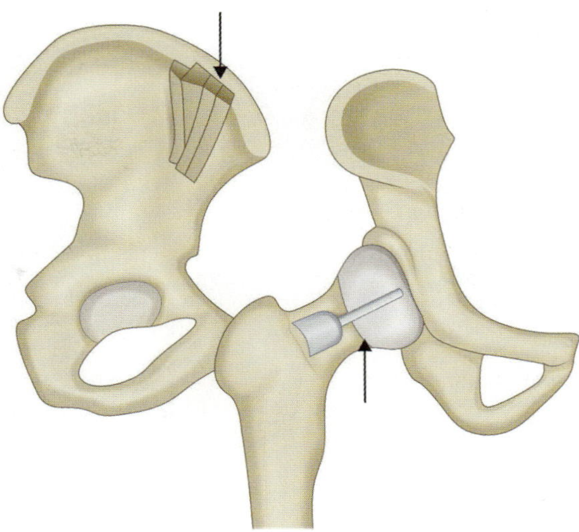

Fig. 65: Bone peg epiphysiodesis.

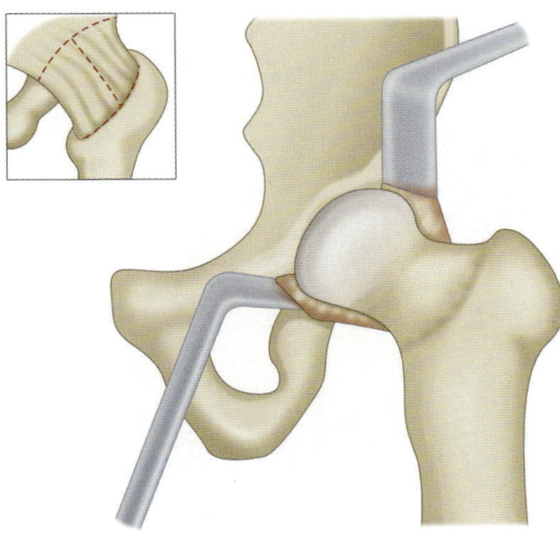

Fig. 66: Cuneiform osteotomy of femoral neck, joint capsule incised longitudinally.

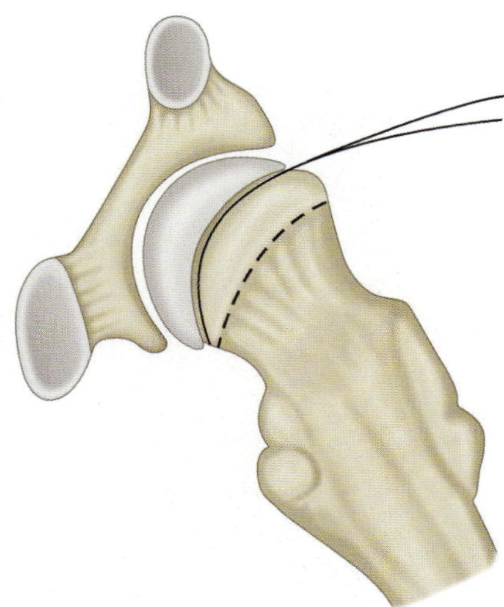

Fig. 67: Osteotomy made distal to physis.

Osteotomy (Fig. 66)

Indications:

- Moderately or severely displaced chronic slips
- Malunion of a chronic slip in poor position
- Femoral neck osteotomies.

Cuneiform osteotomy of femoral neck by Fish is shown in Figures 66 to 71.

Cuneiform osteotomy of femoral neck by Duun is shown in Figures 72 to 76.

Compensatory basilar osteotomy of femoral neck by Kramer is shown in Figures 77 to 79.

Cross osteotomy of head is shown in Figure 80.

Extracapsular base of neck osteotomy by Abraham is shown in Figures 81 to 84.

Intertrochanteric osteotomy (Figs. 85 and 86):
Slip capital femoral epiphysis, when chronically slipped and united in poor position, a trochanteric osteotomy to produce an opposite deformity may be indicated.

Biplane wedge osteotomy by Southwick:

- Transverse line drawn on anterior and lateral surface of bone.
- At level of lesser trochanter, junction of lateral and anterior surface identified.

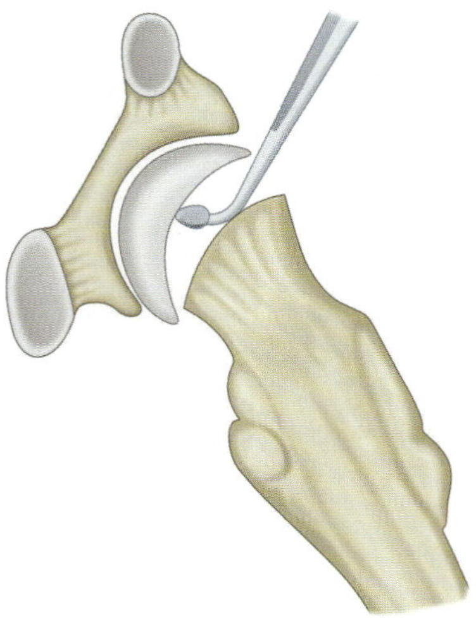

Fig. 68: Wedge of bone removed.

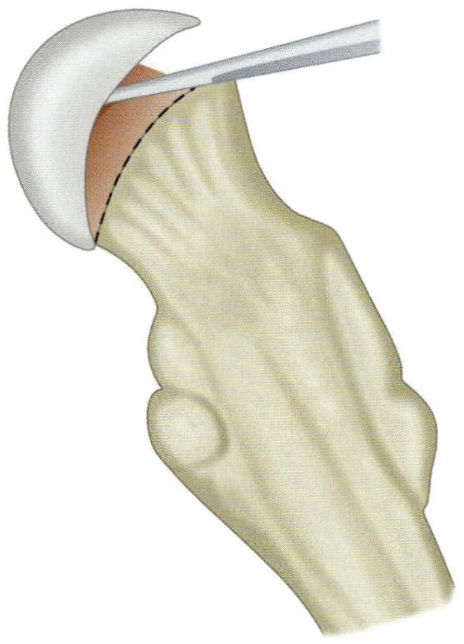

Fig. 69: More bone removed.

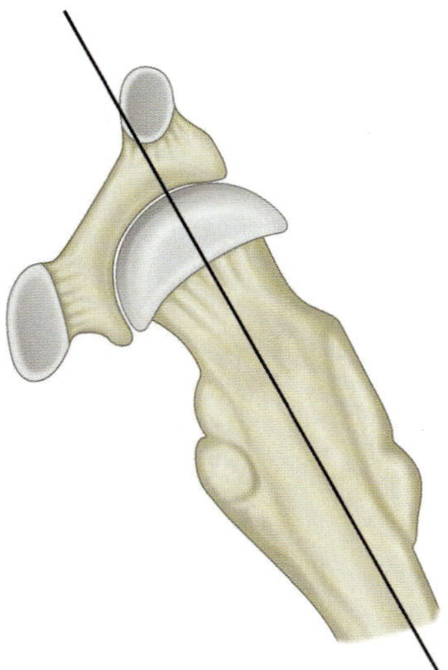

Fig. 70: Alignment obtained.

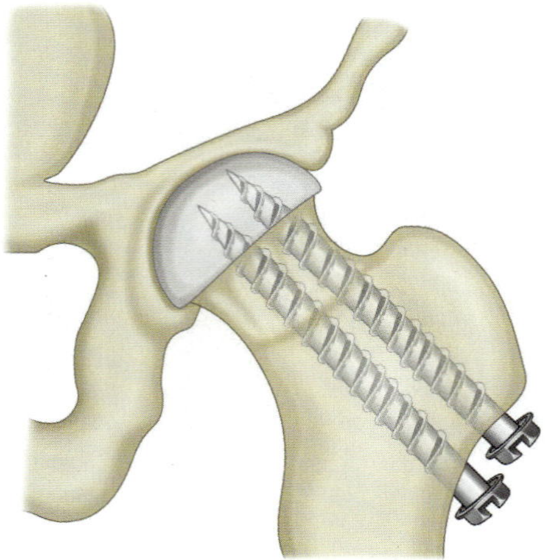

Fig. 71: Epiphysis fixed with pins.

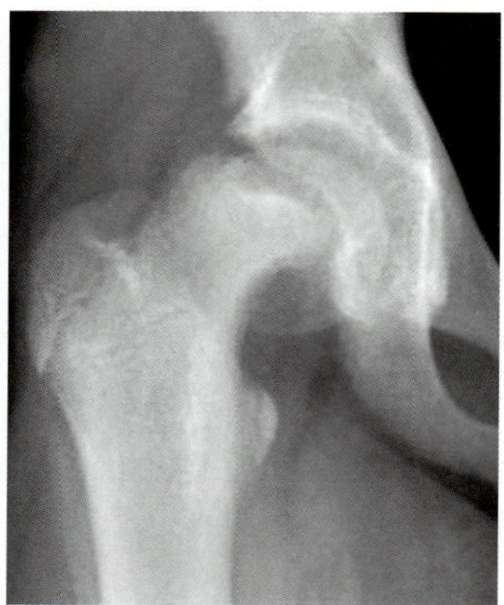

Fig. 72: Beak of new bone.

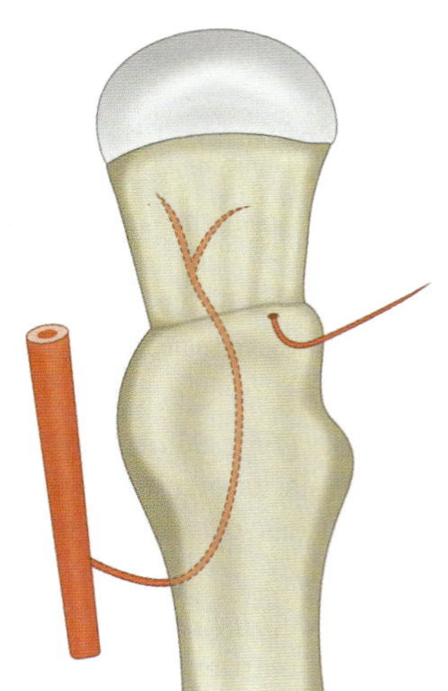

Fig. 73: Vascular synovium on back of neck.

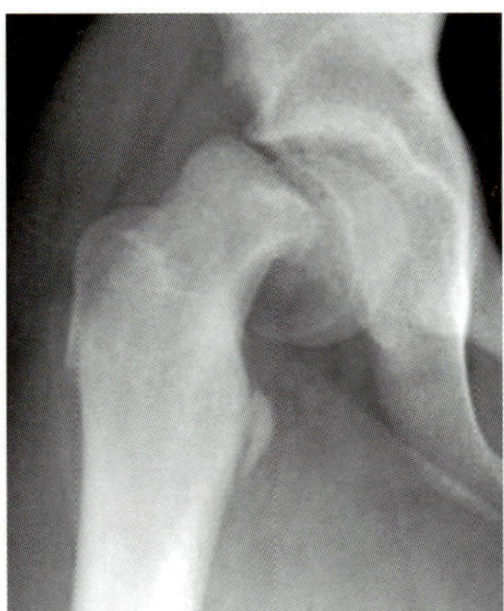

Fig. 74: Incision in synovium and head detached, preserve blood supply and exposing beak of new bone.

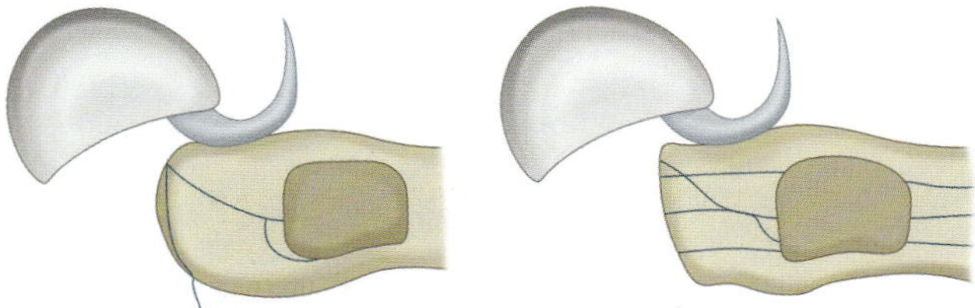

Fig. 75: Beak removed and threaded pins inserted.

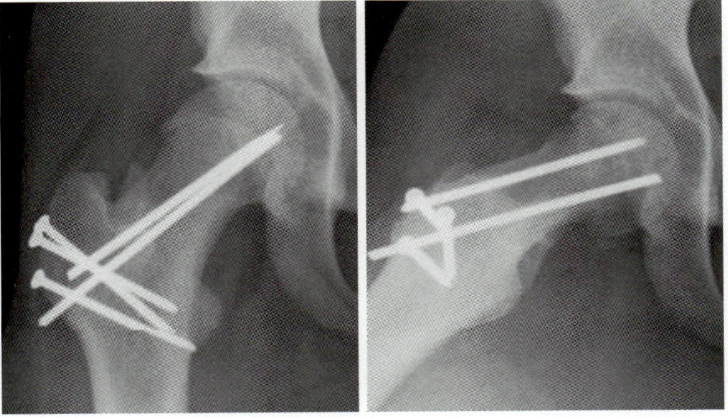

Fig. 76: Head square on neck and deformity is reduced.

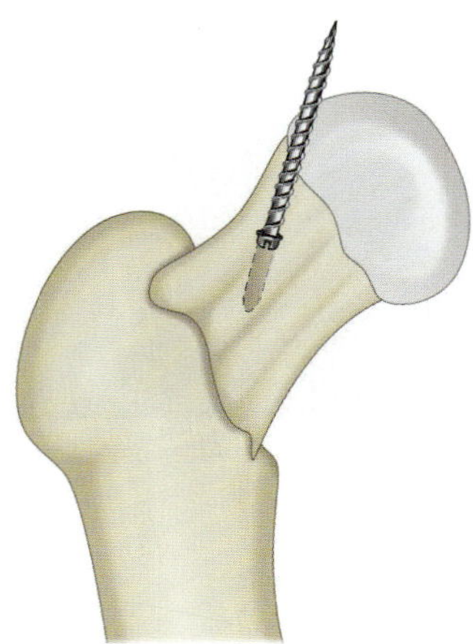

Fig. 77: Widest part of wedge in line with widest part of slip.

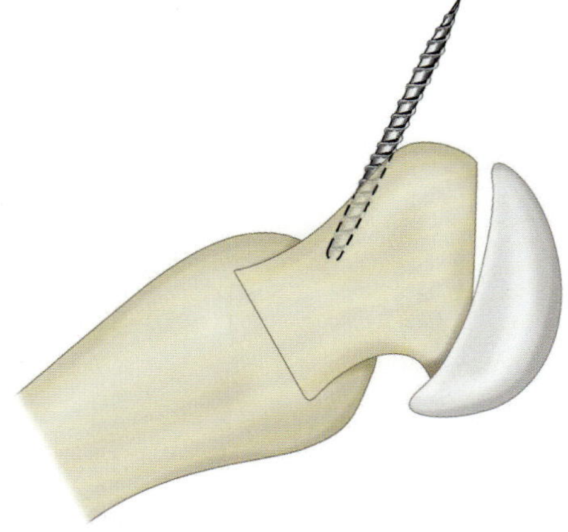

Fig. 78: Steinmann pin inserted into femoral neck.

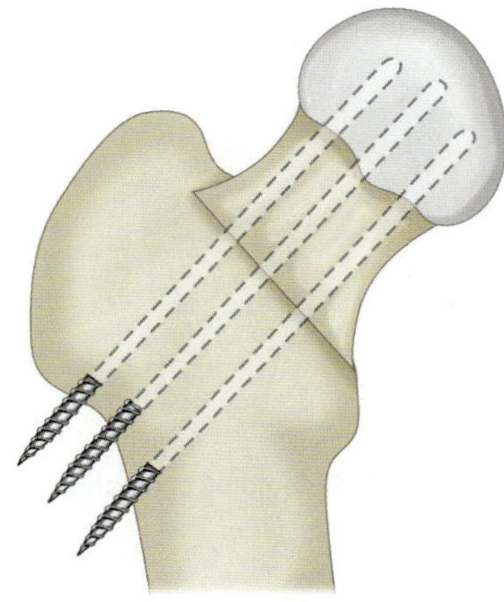

Fig. 79: Osteotomy closed and pins inserted from outer cortex of shaft through neck.

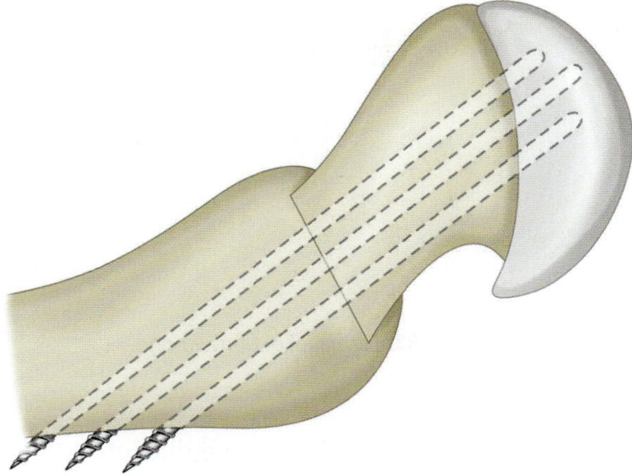

Fig. 80: Pins fix osteotomy and cross physis, prevent further slip.

Complications

Avascular Necrosis

Etiology:

- Single most repeatable finding is reduction.
- *Stable SCFE:* Iatrogenic with reduction

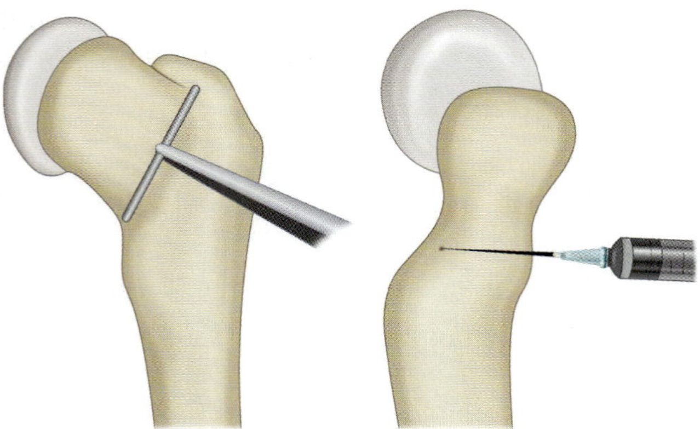
Fig. 81: Determination of proximal osteotomy cut.

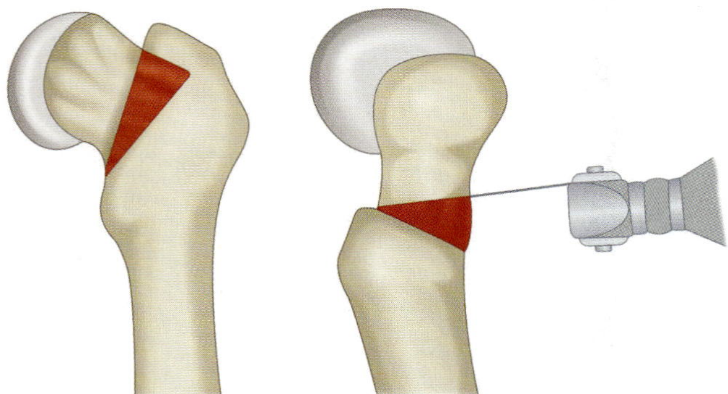
Fig. 82: Osteotomy cut made.

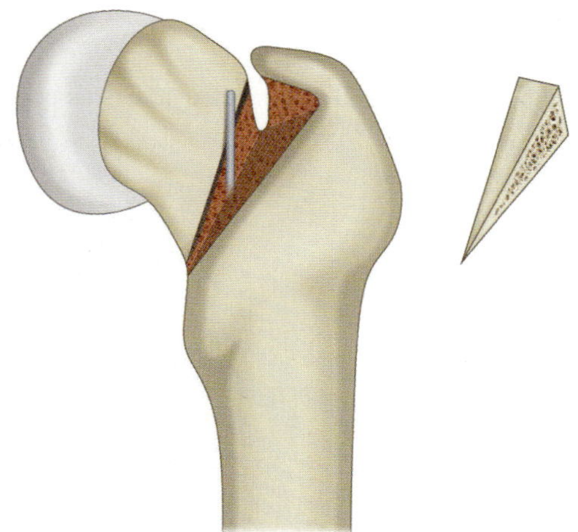
Fig. 83: Removal of bony wedge.

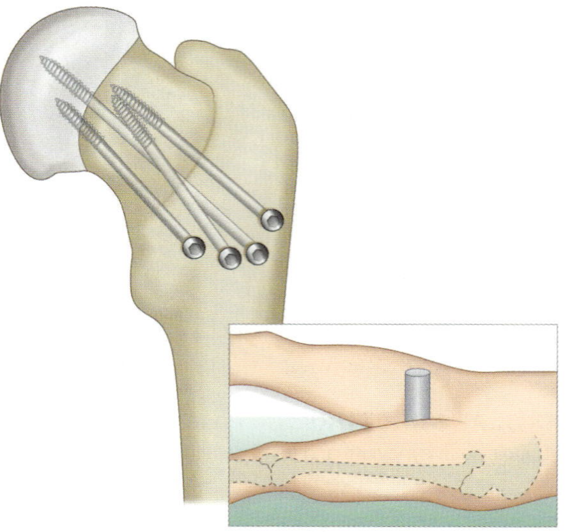
Fig. 84: Fixation with cannulated screw.

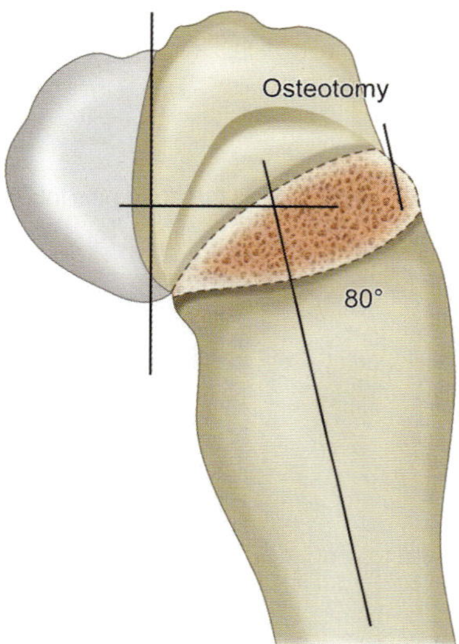

Fig. 85: Intertrochanteric osteotomy.

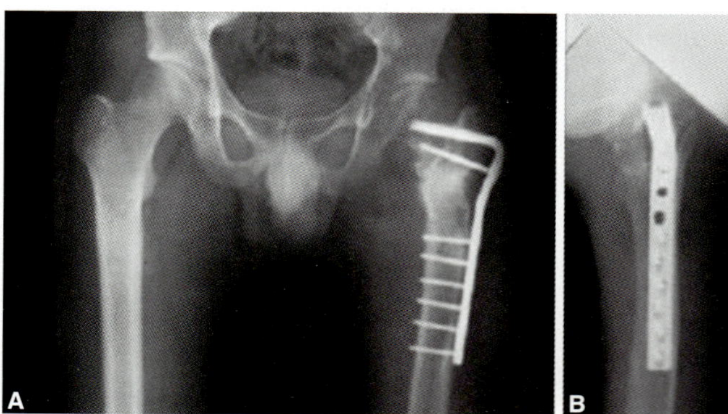

Figs. 86A and B: After osteotomy.

- *Unstable SCFE*:
  - More likely the result of slip, not reduction
  - Immediate reduction and fixation vs. traction prior to fixation to reduce AVN
  - One screw vs. two
  - Role of pretreatment bone scan
- *Chondrolysis associations*:
  - 5–7% of SCFE
  - Increased incidence in more severe slips
  - Increased with spica casts
  - Pin penetration.

Chondrolysis

Diagnosis:
- *Clinical:* Pain out of proportion to SCFE severity
- *Radiographic:*
  - Increased joint space narrowing 50%
  - Persistent juxta-articular osteoporosis
  - Subchondral erosion of femoral head/acetabulum
- *Bone scan:* Marked periarticular uptake.

Treatment:
- Remove protruding pins
- Rest and nonweight-bearing (NWB)
- Nonsteroidal anti-inflammatory drug (NSAID).

ACETABULAR FRACTURES

Acetabular fractures are generally caused by high-energy trauma, and associated injuries are common. Treatment should follow advanced trauma life support (ALTS) protocol with management of acetabular fractures appropriately integrated. The patient is placed in skeletal traction to maintain reduction, while the other acute injuries are treated. In general, operative treatment should not be considered emergency, except, in open fracture management and fracture associated with irreducible dislocation of hip to prevent AVN.

Anatomy

Letournel and Judet described the acetabulum as being composed of two columns in the shape of an inverted Y. These columns support the articular surface of the acetabulum. The columns are connected to the sacroiliac joint by a thick strut of bone, the sciatic buttress, as shown in Figures 87A and B.

Anterior column: It is formed by:
- Bone of the iliac crest
- Iliac spines
- Anterior half of the acetabulum
- Pubis (Fig. 88).

Posterior column: It is composed of:
- Ischium
- Ischial spine
- Posterior half of the acetabulum
- Dense bone forming the sciatic notch, as shown in Figure 88

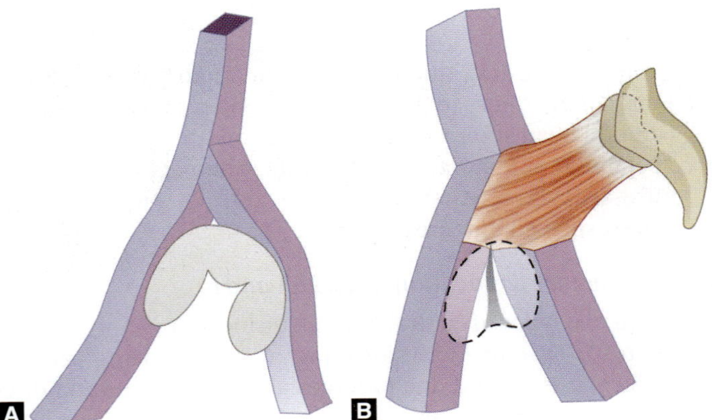

Figs. 87A and B: Acetabular columns supporting articular surfaces of the acetabulum, with sciatic buttress.

- *Dome of the acetabulum:* It is the weight-bearing portion of the articular surface that supports the femoral head, as shown in Figure 89.

The column concept is used in:
- Classification of these fractures
- Fracture patterns
- Operative approaches
- Internal fixation
- Anatomical restoration of the dome with concentric reduction of the femoral head is the goal in both nonoperative and operative management.

Classification (Flowchart 3)

Simple fracture types (Figs. 90A to E):
- Posterior wall fractures
- Posterior column fractures
- Anterior wall fractures
- Anterior column fractures
- Transverse fractures.

Associated fracture types (Figs. 91A to E):
- Posterior column and posterior wall fracture
- Transverse and posterior wall fracture
- T-shaped fracture
- Anterior column and posterior hemitransverse fracture
- Complete both column fractures.

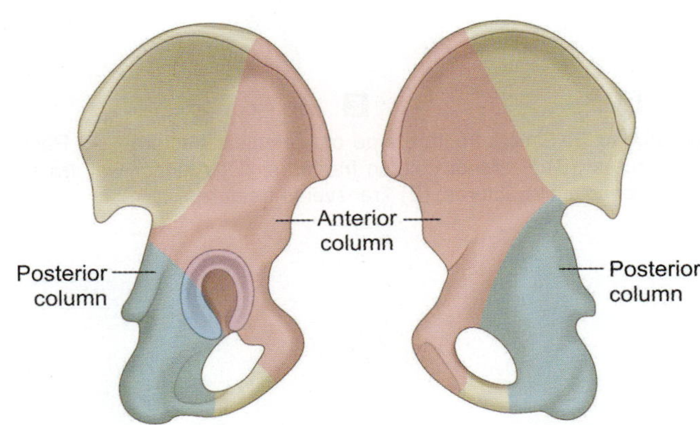

Fig. 88: Anterior and posterior columns around acetabulum.

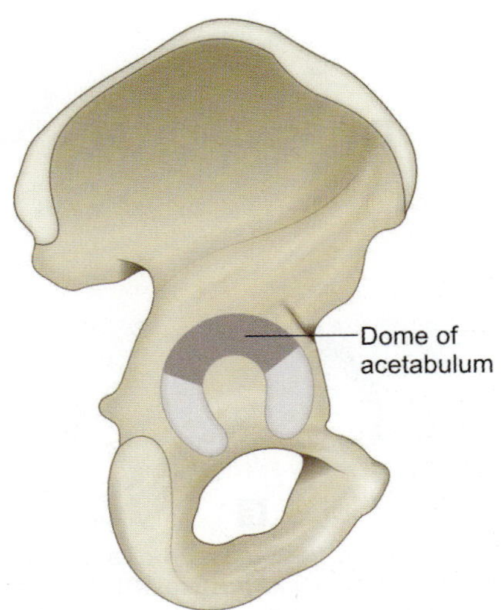

Fig. 89: Dome of the acetabulum (gray surface).

Flowchart 3: Letournel and Judet classification of acetabular fracture.

- Letournel and Judet
  - Simple fracture types
  - Associated fracture types

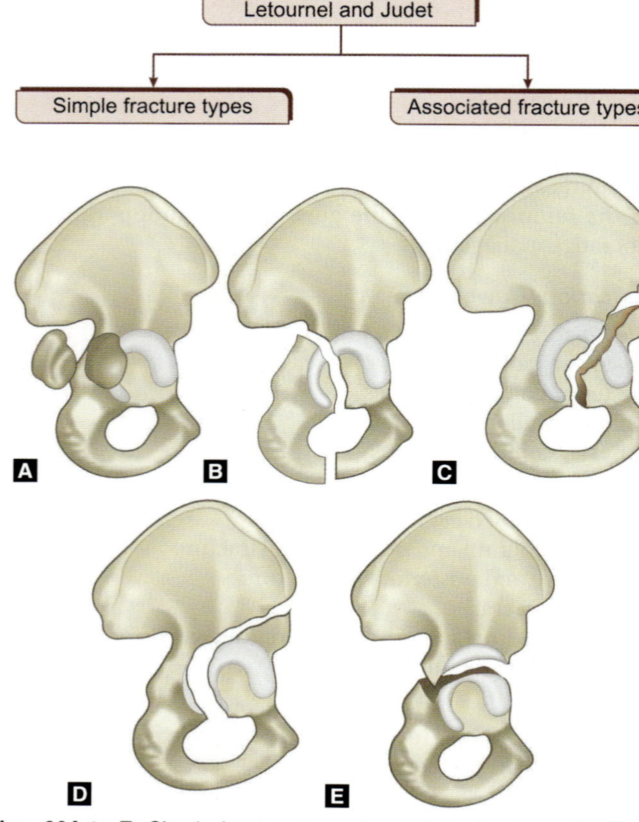

Figs. 90A to E: Simple fracture type of acetabular fracture—(A) Posterior wall fractures; (B) Posterior column fractures; (C) Anterior wall fractures; (D) Anterior column fractures; (E) Transverse fractures.

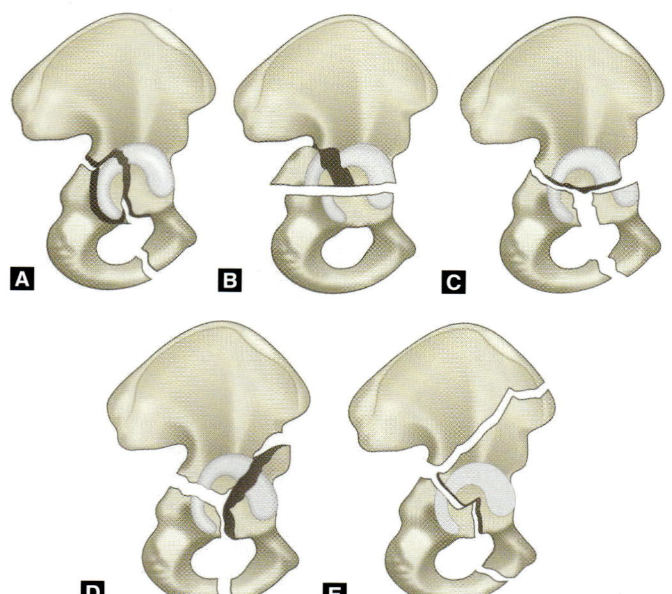

Figs. 91A to E: Associated fracture types of acetabular fracture—(A) Posterior column and posterior wall fracture; (B) Transverse and posterior wall fracture; (C) T-shaped fracture; (D) Anterior column and posterior hemitransverse fracture; (E) Complete both column fracture.

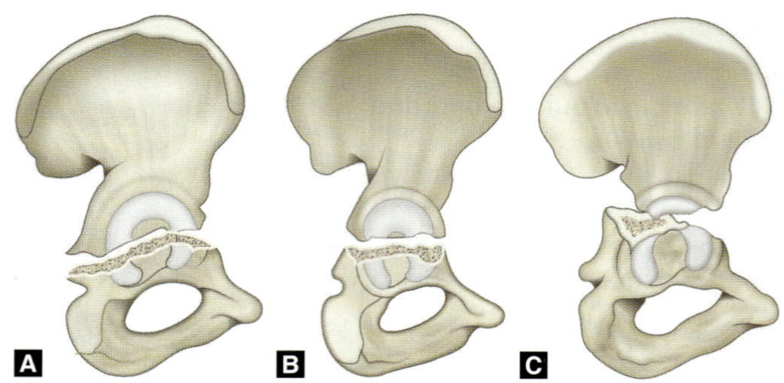

Figs. 92A to C: Transverse fracture types—(A) Infratectal fracture below cotyloid fossa; (B) Juxtatectal fracture through cotyloid fossa; (C) Transtectal fracture. Above the condyloid fossa.

Transverse fracture types (Figs. 92A to C):
- Infratectal fracture below cotyloid fossa
- Juxtatectal fracture through cotyloid fossa
- Transtectal fracture.

AO Classification

It is based on the severity of the fracture:
- *Type A:* Fractures of a single wall or column
- *Type B:* Fractures of both anterior and posterior columns
- *Type C:* Fractures of both columns, but all articular segments are detached from the remaining segment of intact ilium
- Each type has subtypes 1, 2, and 3 depending on the characteristics of the fracture.

Type A fractures (Figs. 93A to D):
- Posterior wall fracture
- Posterior column fracture
- Anterior wall fracture
- Anterior column fracture.

Type B fractures (Figs. 94A to D):
- Transverse fracture
- Transverse and posterior wall fracture
- T-shaped fracture.

Type C fractures (Figs. 95A to C):
- Anterior wall/column and posterior hemitransverse fracture
- Aberrant crypt foci (ACF) extending of iliac crest
- ACF extending to anterior border ilium
- Fractures enter sacroiliac joint.

Tiles Classification

Tile proposed adding qualifiers, i.e. the factors that affect the prognosis of the injury to the AO classification. These include:
- Femoral head subluxation or dislocation
- Acetabular or femoral articular surface damage
- Intra-articular fragments
- Non-displaced fractures.

Central Fracture Dislocation (Figs. 96A and B)

There are two types of central fracture dislocation:
1. *Group I:* Fracture with an intact weight-bearing articular surface. It is caused due to forces along the femur and direct forces to the trochanter.
2. *Group II:* Acetabulum is reduced to bag-of-bones. It is caused by direct injury to the trochanter or pelvis.

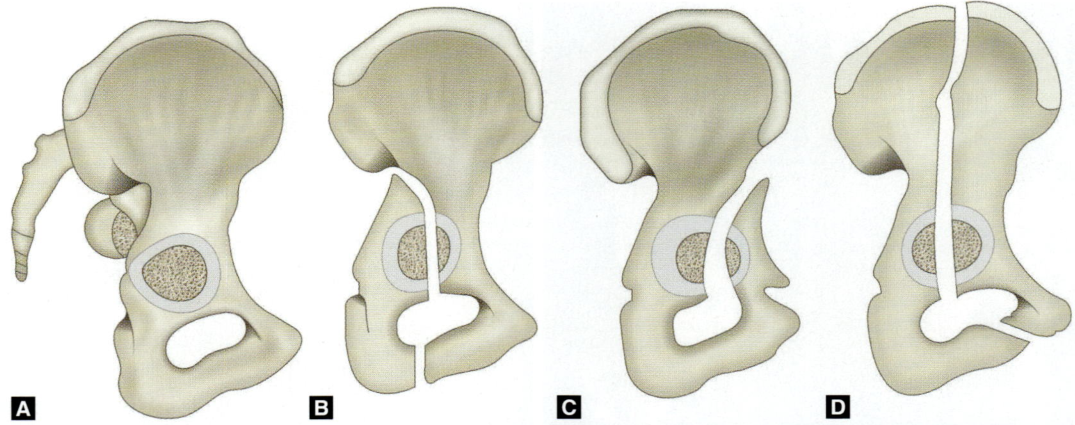

Figs. 93A to D: Type A fractures—(A) Posterior wall fracture; (B) Posterior column fracture; (C) Anterior wall fracture; (D) Anterior column fracture.

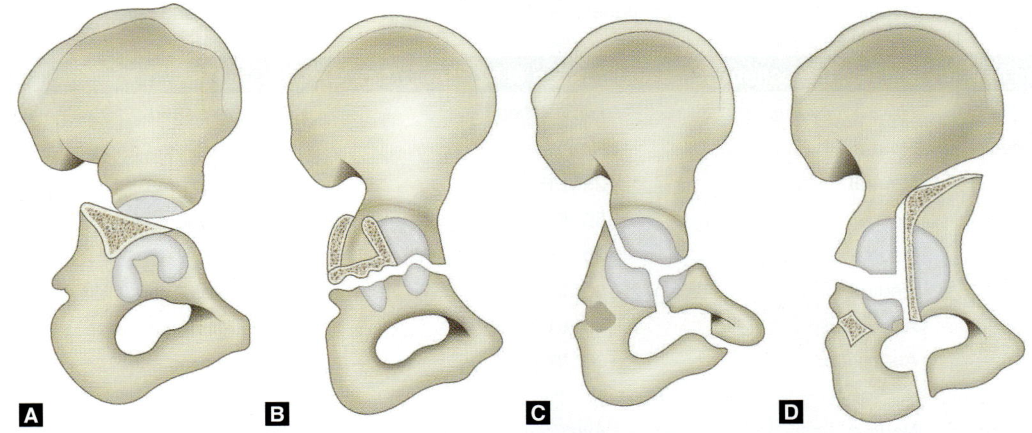

Figs. 94A to D: Type B fractures—(A) Transverse fracture; (B) Transverse and posterior wall fracture; (C) T-shaped fracture; (D) Anterior wall/ column and posterior hemitransverse fracture.

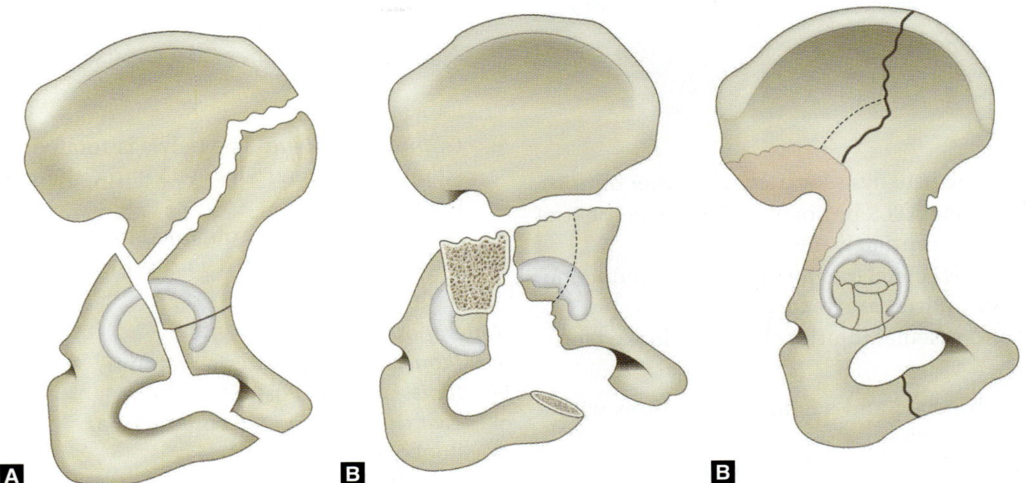

Figs. 95A to C: Type C fractures—(A) ACF extending to iliac crest; (B) ACF extending to anterior border of ilium; (C) Fractures enter sacroiliac joint.

Mechanism of Injury (Table 5)

Acetabular fractures are generally caused by high-energy trauma. These fractures occur as force is transmitted from the femur to the pelvis via femoral head. The fracture pattern depends on:

- Position of the hip at the time of injury
- Direction of the impact
- Magnitude of the impact
- Strength of the bone, as in osteoporotic bones, there may be low energy trauma.

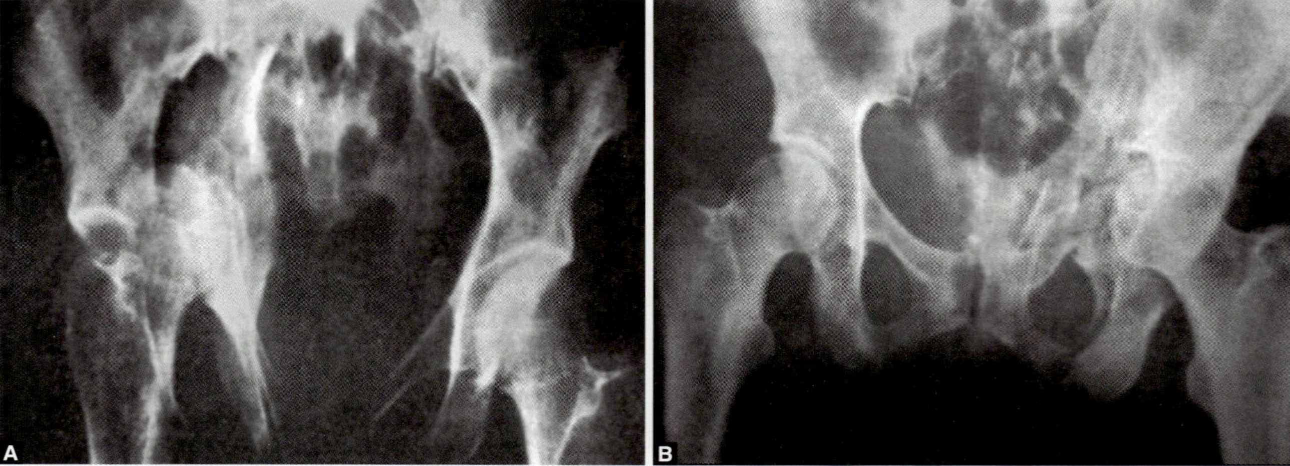

Figs. 96A and B: Central fracture dislocation of acetabulum— (A) Group I fracture, with an intact weight-bearing articular surface; (B) Group II, acetabulum is reduced to bag of bones, caused by direct injury to the trochanter and pelvis.

TABLE 5: Mechanism of injury and fracture pattern, force and position of hip during injury.

Force	*Hip abduction*	*Hip rotation*	*Fracture pattern*
Along axis of femoral neck	Neutral	Neutral	Anterior column and posterior hemitransverse
	Neutral	25° ER	Anterior column
	Neutral	50° ER	Anterior wall
	Neutral	20° IR	T-shaped
	Neutral	50° IR	Posterior column
	Adduction	20° IR	Transtectal transverse
	Abduction	20° IR	Juxta/infratectal
			transverse
Along axis of femoral shaft (hip flexed 90°)	Neutral Abduction Adduction	Any Any Any	Posterior wall Transverse and posterior wall Posterior hip dislocation
Along axis of femoral shaft (hip extended)	Neutral Abduction	Any Any	Posterosuperior fracture of posterior wall Transtectal transverse

Clinical Picture

- Acetabular fractures are usually associated with other injuries.
- Treatment should follow ATLS protocol with management of acetabular fractures appropriately integrated.
- The patient is placed in skeletal traction to maintain reduction, while the other acute injuries are treated.
- Any neurological and vascular injuries should be looked for.

Morel-Lavallee lesion:
- It may occur in both pelvic and acetabular fractures with a shear component to the injury.
- It occurs when the skin is separated from the fascia.
- This creates a pocket where bleeding can occur.
- A large hematoma can threaten the viability of the above skin.
- Treatment includes wound drainage or radical incision.

Radiological Evaluation

The views to be taken are:
- AP view
- Judet views
- *Iliac oblique*: The pelvis is rotated 45° with unaffected side up
- *Obturator oblique*: The pelvis is rotated 45°, with the injured side up. A proper view will show the coccyx centered over femoral head
- *Pelvic inlet view*: It is obtained by 40° caudocranial projection
- *Pelvic outlet view*: It is obtained by 40° craniocephalic projection.

Anteroposterior view (Fig. 97):
- *Iliopectinal line:* Anterior column
- *Ilioischial line:* Posterior column
- *Tear drop:* Relation of columns tear
- Roof of acetabulum
- Anterior column/wall
- Posterior column/wall.

Iliac oblique view:
Figure 98 shows iliac oblique view.

Obturator oblique view (Fig. 99):
- Roof arc measurements (Matta). It is done to quantify acetabular dome after fracture, as shown in Figures 100A to C.
  - Medial roof arc measured on AP view
  - Anterior roof arc measured on obturator oblique view

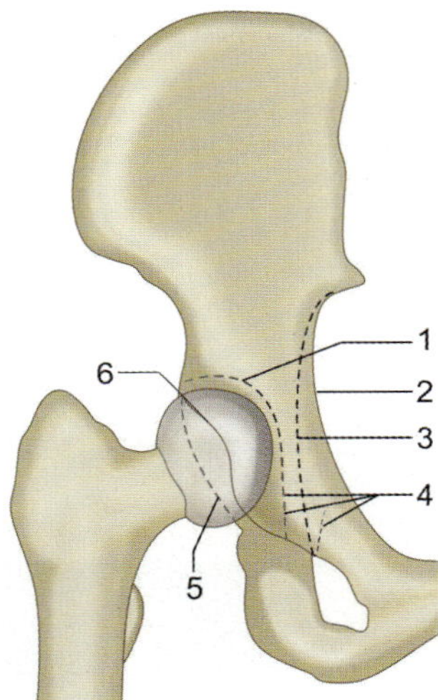

Fig. 97: AP view of hip joint—1. Roof of acetabulum; 2. Iliopectoreal line; 3. Ilioischial line; 4. Teardrop; 5. Posterior column/wall; 6. Anterior column/wall.

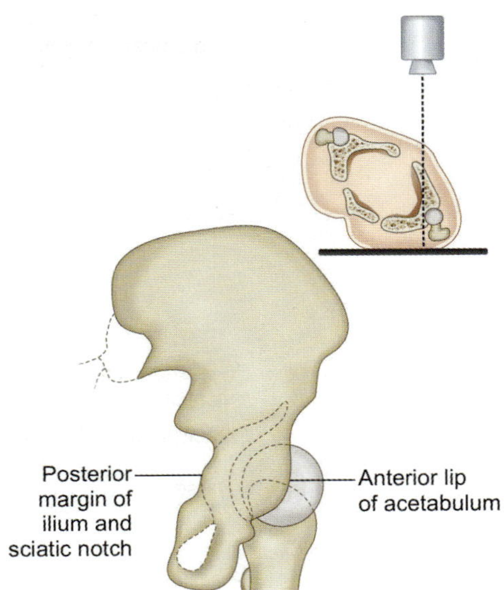

Fig. 98: Iliac oblique view.

- *Posterior roof arc measurement on iliac oblique view:* It is measured by drawing a vertical line through the center of femoral head and second line through center of the head to the location of fracture at the articular surface. If the measurements in a displaced fracture is less than 45°, operative treatment is indicated.

Spur sign (Figs. 101A and B):
- It is demonstrated on obturator iliac view
- Pathognomonic of both column fracture
- It represents the remaining portion of ilium still attached to sacrum and is seen projected lateral to medially displaced acetabulum.

Inlet and outlet views (Figs. 102 and 103):
- These views are not mandatory for acetabular fractures.
- These can be done to diagnose and characterize concurrent injuries to the pelvic ring.

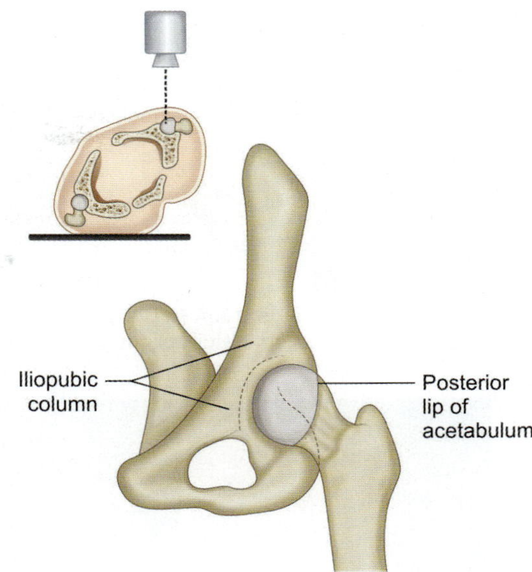

Fig. 99: Obturator oblique view.

Computed Tomography Scan

- CT scan is helpful in detecting
  - Rotational displacements
  - Marginal articular impactions
  - Intra-articular fragments
  - Associated femoral head injuries
  - Accurate assessment of size of a posterior wall fragment.
- 3D CT is helpful for understanding the relationship between multiple sites of injury, but is not a replacement for plain X-ray.

Treatment

Conservative

Criteria for conservative management are:
- Nondisplaced and minimally displaced fractures
- Roof arc measurements are more than 45°
- No femoral head subluxation on three X-rays, taken without traction
- Fractures with displacement, but the region of the joint involved is unimportant prognostically
- Secondary congruence in both column fractures
- No fracture involvement in cranial 10 mm of joint on CT (CT subchondral arc)
- For posterior wall fractures, more than 40% of width of wall on CT
- Medical contraindication to surgery
- Local soft tissue problems.

Operative

Criteria for operative treatment are:
- Roof arc measurements are more than 45°
- Subluxation of femoral head from a displaced acetabular fracture noted on any of three standard views
- More than 50% involvement of the articular surface of posterior wall or clinical instability with hip flexion to 90° in posterior wall fractures
- Incarcerated fragments in acetabulum after closed reduction of a hip dislocation

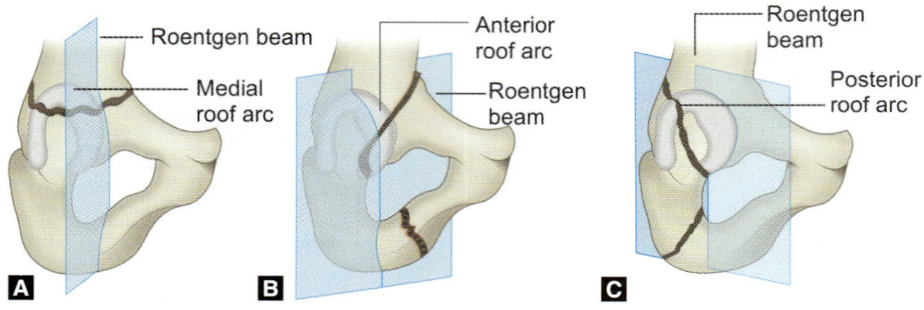

Figs. 100A to C: (A) Medial roof arc measurement on AP; (B) Anterior roof arc on obturator oblique view; (C) Posterior roof arc measurement on iliac oblique view.

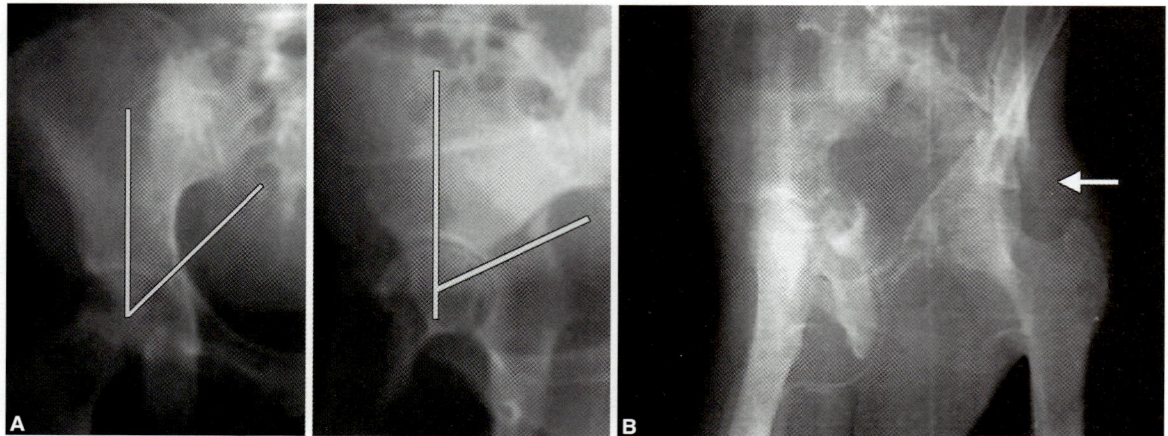

Figs. 101A and B: Spur sign.

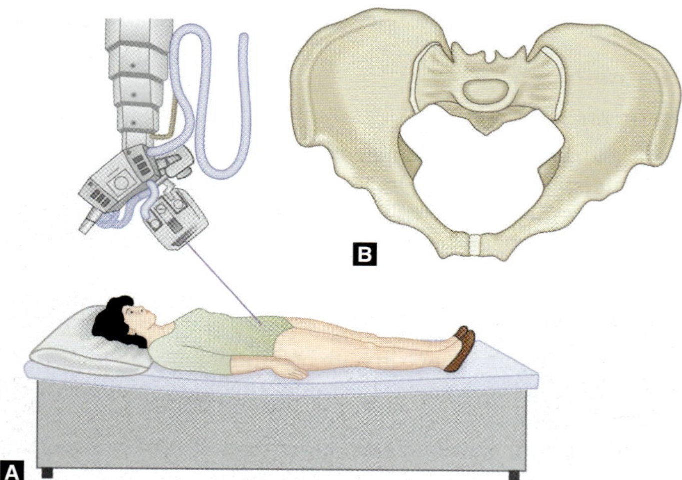

Figs. 102A and B: Pelvic inlet view.

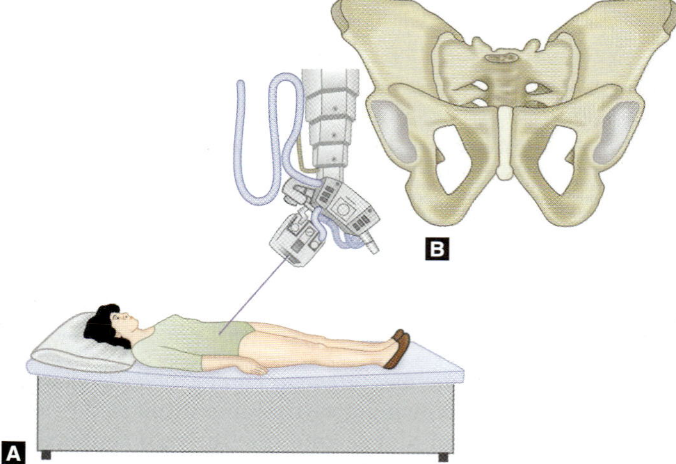

Figs. 103A and B: Pelvic outlet view.

- Prevention of nonunion and retention of sufficient bone stock for later reconstructive surgery.

Surgical Approaches

The various approaches used are:

- Kocher-Langenbeck
- Ilioinguinal
- Extended iliofemoral
- Combined approaches.

Treatment of Specific Fractures

For accurate reduction and fixation:

- Thorough understanding of anatomy of normal and injured innominate bone.
- Preoperative X-rays must be evaluated and the fracture pattern classified correctly.
- The presence and number of free articular fragments and areas of marginal impaction must be identified.

Posterior wall fractures (Fig. 104):

- Most common of the acetabular fractures
- Treated through Kocher-Langenbeck approach
- Patient is positioned in either prone or lateral position
- Fixation is done by using lag screws and reconstruction plate placed from the ischium over the retroacetabular surface onto the lateral ilium.

Posterior column fracture:

- Relatively uncommon fractures
- Kocher-Langenbeck is used
- Rotational deformity is corrected with a Schanz in ischium to control rotation
- Fixation is done with lag screw combined with a contoured reconstruction plate along the posterior column, as shown in Figure 105.

Anterior wall fracture:

- Isolated anterior wall fractures are uncommon.
- They are sometimes associated with anterior hip dislocation.
- Ilioinguinal or iliofemoral approaches are used for its reduction.
- Fractures are fixed with a buttress plate from iliac fossa to superior ramus, as shown in Figure 106.
- Interfragmentary screws are also used.

Anterior column fractures:

- These fractures are approached through ilioinguinal or iliofemoral approach.
- They are fixed with a contoured plate along the pelvic brim and several lag screws are placed between inner and outer tables of innominate bone, as illustrated in Figure 107.

Transverse fractures:

- Posterior, ilioinguinal, or combined approach.
- Posterior fixation, by buttress plate along posterior column with anterior fixation with 3.5 mm lag screw from above the acetabulum.
- Anterior fixation, by contoured plate along the pelvic brim with lag screw directed down the posterior column, as shown in Figures 108 and 109.

Posterior column and posterior wall:

- Kocher-Langenbeck approach with or without trochanteric osteotomy.
- Column fracture is reduced first and a short reconstruction plate is placed posteriorly along posterior edge of column.
- A separate plate is used for wall fragment and screws through this plate, secure rotational reduction of posterior column, as shown in Figure 110.

Transverse fracture and posterior wall:

Combined approach is necessary, as the posterior wall fragment requires a posterior exposure, but anterior part of the transverse fracture is difficult to reduce through this approach. Fixation is variable depending on the specific fractures, as shown in Figure 111.

T-type and anterior column posterior hemitransverse fractures:

These two patterns can be treated by ilioinguinal approach. If both the anterior and posterior components of the fracture are significantly displaced, then a combined approach is required. Fixation is done with a contoured plate placed along the pelvic brim with lag screws extending into either posterior/anterior column, as shown in Figure 112.

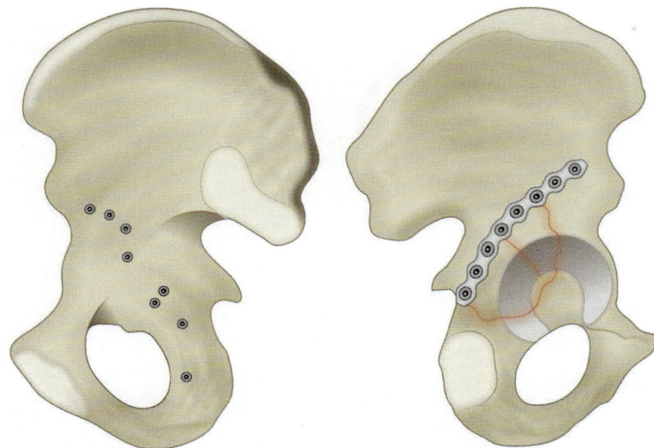

Fig. 104: Fixation of posterior wall fracture, using lag screws and reconstruction plate.

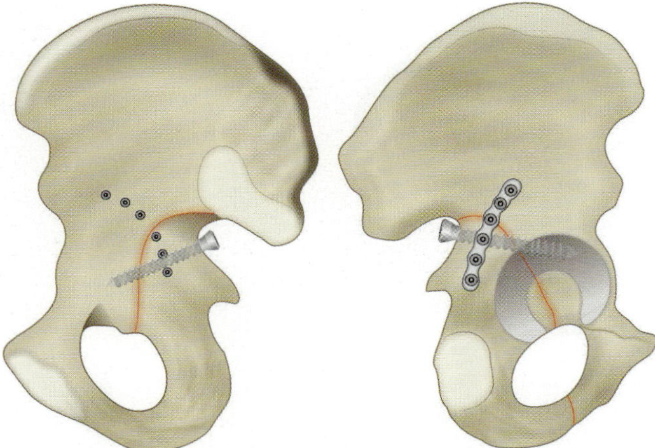

Fig. 105: Posterior column fracture repair, with lag screw combined with a contoured reconstruction plate.

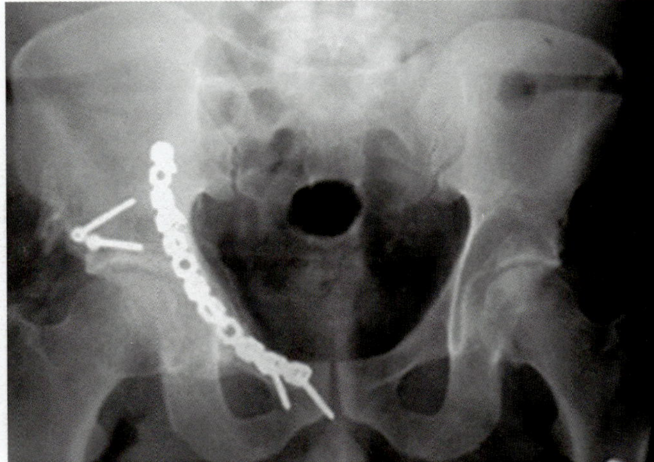

Fig. 106: Anterior wall fracture fixation with a buttress plate from iliac fossa to superior ramus.

Both column fractures:

These fractures can be treated through an anterior ilioinguinal approach, but a posterior approach is required for sacroiliac joint involvement, a significant posterior wall fracture or intra-articular

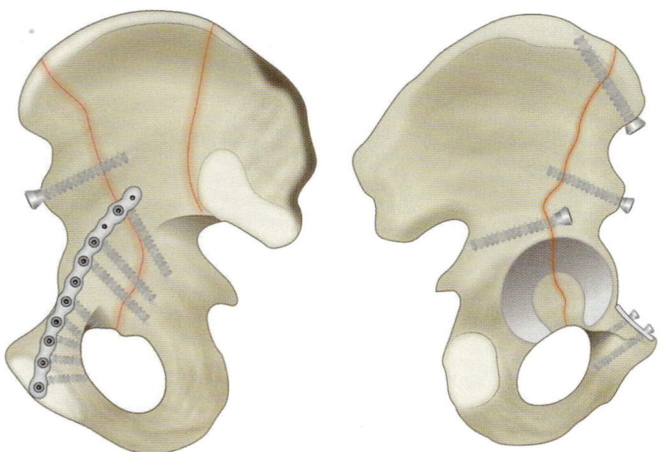

Fig. 107: Anterior column fracture, fixed with a contoured plate along the pelvic brim and several lag screws.

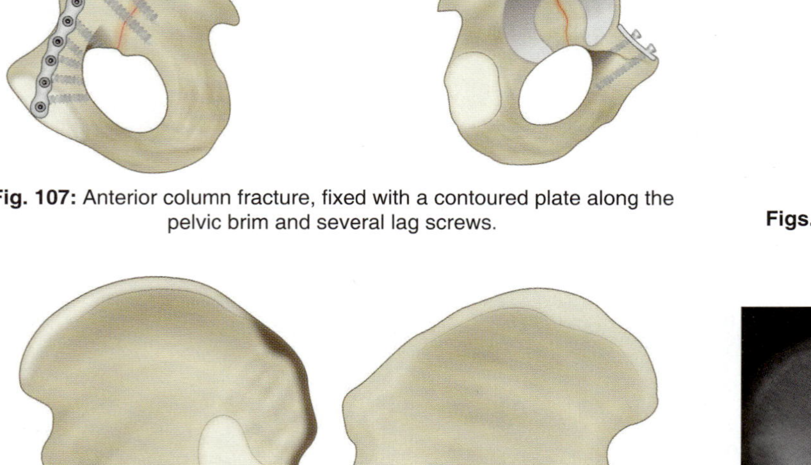

Fig. 108: Anterior fixation, by contoured plate along the pelvic brim with lag screw directed down the posterior column.

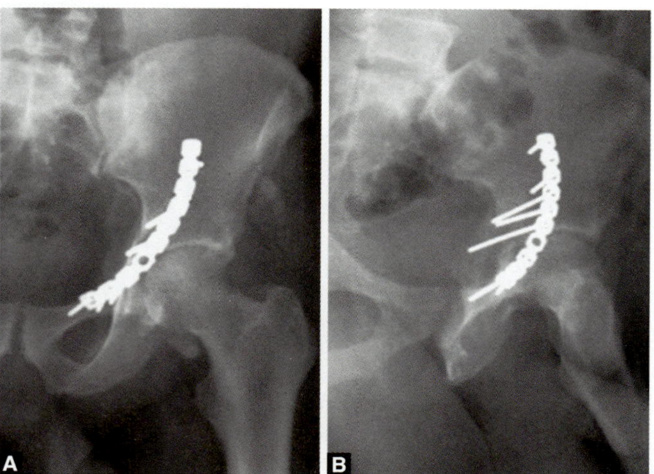

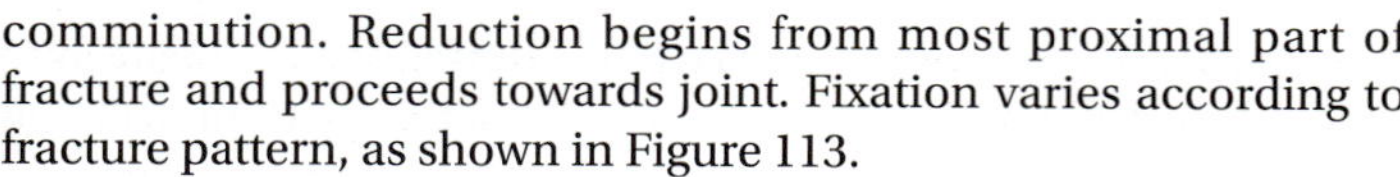

Fig. 109: A separate plate is used for fixing posterior wall and column fragment.

comminution. Reduction begins from most proximal part of fracture and proceeds towards joint. Fixation varies according to fracture pattern, as shown in Figure 113.

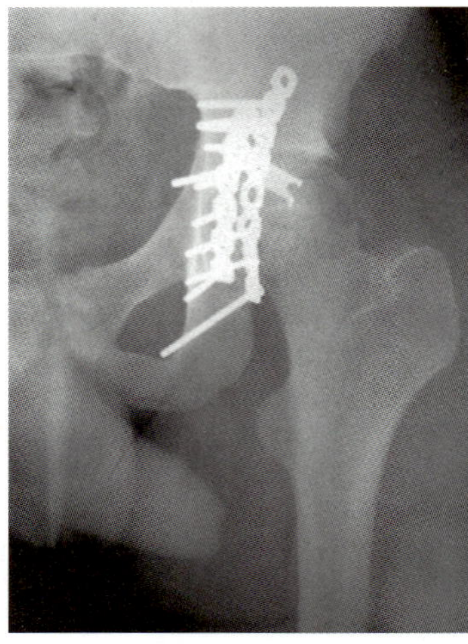

Figs. 110A and B: X-ray showing the transverse fracture fixation.

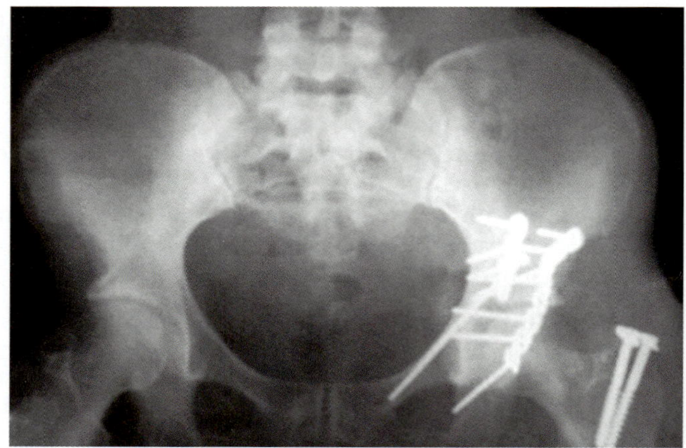

Fig. 111: Combined approach used for fixing transverse and posterior wall fracture.

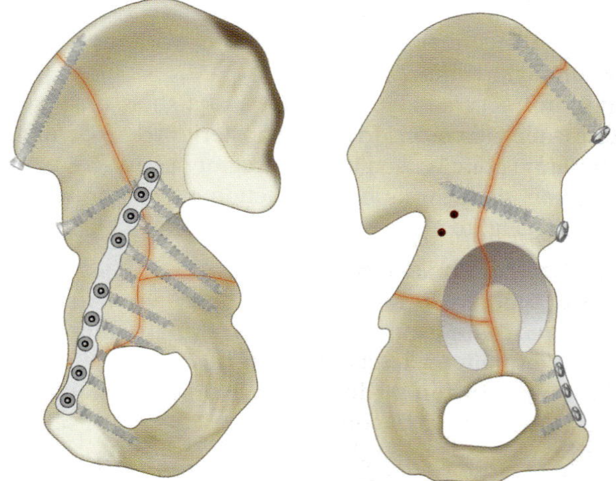

Fig. 112: T-type and anterior column posterior hemitransverse fractures reduction by ilioinguinal approach.

Central fracture dislocation:

Group I: Conservative treatment includes traction applied in two planes: (1) Longitudinal traction to leg by Hamilton Russell, using

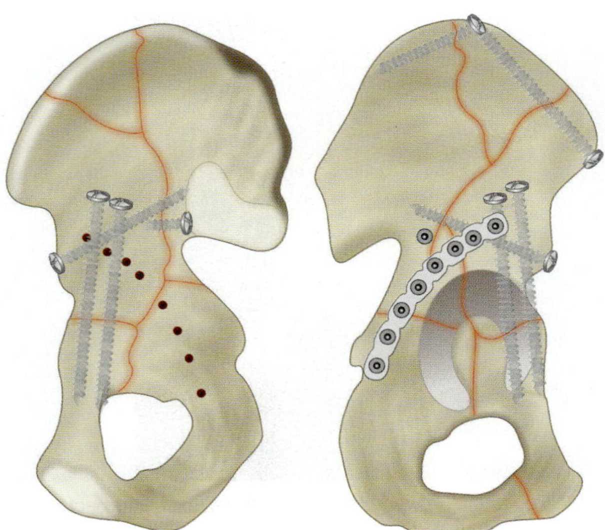

Fig. 113: Both column fracture reduction by ilioinguinal approach.

a tibial Steinmann's pin and (2) Lateral traction, to correct central displacement of femoral head.

Operative treatment: Posterior approach is taken. Reduction is maintained, by a small four hole plate screwed into adjacent parts of iliac and ischial components.

Group II: Conservative: These fractures are better left in displaced portion or pulled out as far as longitudinal traction permits.

Postoperative Management

- Closed suction drain for 2 days
- Antibiotics for 5 days
- Passive motion of hip on 2nd day
- Touch down ambulation with crutches on 4th day and progression depending on other injuries
- Minimal weight-bearing for 8 weeks, for simple fractures and 12 weeks in others.

Complications

- Post-traumatic arthritis
- AVN of femoral head
- Infection
- Sciatic nerve palsies
- Heterotopic ossification
- Deep vein thrombosis.

Post-traumatic arthritis:
The incidence is about 17%. Imperfect reduction increases the chances of arthritis. Both column and transverse-posterior wall fractures have worse results than associated types, due to imperfect reduction. Even after perfect reduction, the rate of arthritis is about 10%. Primary THR can be done for a comminuted, incongruous, both column fracture. Secondary THR has been done for post-traumatic arthritis, though loosening and revision rates for cemented acetabular sockets are a common problem.

Avascular necrosis:
More frequent in fractures associated with posterior dislocation. The rate after dislocation is about 7.5%. It is roentographically apparent within 2 years in most patients. AVN of posterior wall can be caused by the injury or by excessive exposure, as the only blood supply is the injured posterior capsule of the hip.

Infection:
It occurs in 1–5% of cases. Factors which increase the risk of infection are:

- Suprapubic catheter in ilioinguinal approach
- Morel-Lavalle lesion.

Sciatic nerve palsies:
Due to initial injury, incidence is 10–15%. Due to surgery, incidence is 2–6%. It is more often associated with:

- Posterior fracture pattern
- Kocher-Langenbeck approach
- Extensile exposures.

Heterotopic ossification:
It occurs in about 14–50% patients. It is more common after extensile or Kocher-Langenbeck approaches.

Prophylaxis:

- *Indomethacin:* 25 mg TDS for 4–6 weeks.
- *Radiation:* One time dose of 700 cGy in patients, in whom indomethacin is contraindicated.

Deep vein thrombosis:
It can occur in 8–61% and the reported risk of pulmonary embolism range from 2% to 6%.

Prophylaxis:

- Subcutaneous enoxaparin and intermittent compression boots preoperatively.
- Anticoagulation, with enoxaparin followed by warfarin for 6 weeks, unless medically contraindicated.

FRACTURES OF THE FEMORAL NECK

Fractures of the neck of the femur have always presented great challenges to orthopedic surgeons and remain in many ways today the unsolved fracture as far as treatment and results are concerned. With life-expectancy increasing with each decade, our society is becoming increasingly an active geriatric society, with significant numbers of hospitalized and nursing home patients with femoral neck fractures and their sequel.

Fracture Fixation

Femoral neck fractures in young patients usually are caused by high-energy trauma and often are associated with multiple injuries and high rates of osteonecrosis and nonunion. Results after this injury apparently depend on:

- The extent of the injury, such as the amount of displacement, the amount of comminution and whether the circulation has been disturbed
- The adequacy of the reduction
- The adequacy of fixation.

Even when nondisplaced, there is no assurance that a fracture of the femoral neck will attain an excellent result. Early anatomical reduction, compression of the fracture and rigid internal fixation are used to promote union, but the surgeon probably has less control over osteonecrosis because the blood supply to the femoral head after femoral neck fracture is quite precarious. Crock described the blood supply to the proximal end of the femur, dividing it into three major groups:

1. An extracapsular arterial ring located at the base of the femoral neck
2. Ascending cervical branches of the arterial ring on the surface of the femoral neck
3. Arteries of the ligamentum teres, as shown in Figure 114.

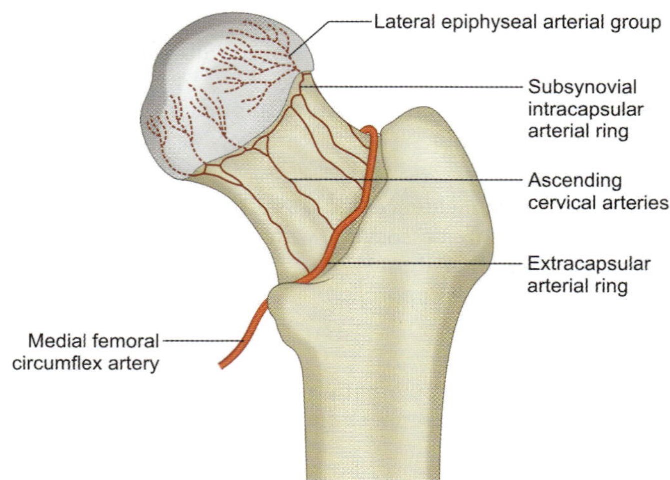

Fig. 114: Arteries of the ligamentum teres.

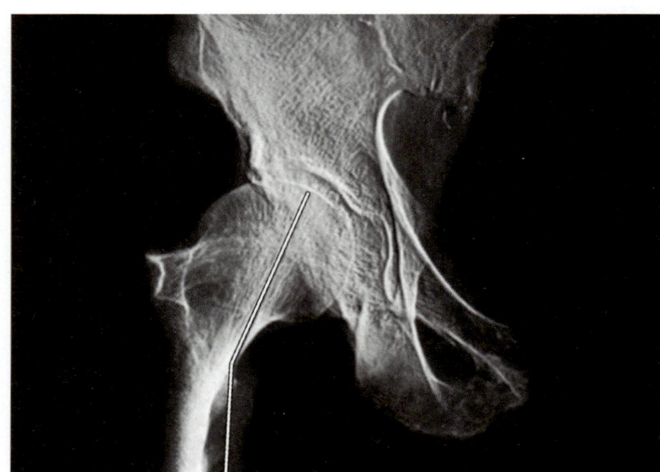

Fig. 115: The angle between the central compressive trabeculae, within the femoral head and the medial cortex of the femur is measured.

The extracapsular arterial ring is formed posteriorly, by a large branch of the medial femoral circumflex artery and anteriorly by a branch from the lateral femoral circumflex artery. The ascending cervical branches or retinacular vessels ascend on the surface of the femoral neck in anterior, posterior, medial, and lateral groups. The lateral vessels are the most important. Their proximity to the surface of the femoral neck makes them vulnerable to injury in femoral neck fractures. As the articular margin of the femoral head is approached by the ascending cervical vessels, a second less distinct ring of vessels is formed, referred by Chung as the subsynovial intra-articular arterial ring. It is from this ring of vessels that vessels penetrate the head and are referred to as the epiphyseal arteries, the most important being the lateral epiphyseal arterial group supplying the lateral weight-bearing portion of the femoral head. These epiphyseal vessels are joined by inferior metaphyseal vessels and vessels from the ligamentum teres.

Nonunion

Femoral neck fractures are usually entirely intracapsular and common to all intracapsular fractures, the synovial fluid bathing. The fracture may interfere with the healing process because the femoral neck essentially has no periosteal layer. All healing must be endosteal. Angiogenic-inhibiting factors in synovial fluid can also inhibit fracture repair. These factors along with the precarious blood supply to the femoral head make healing unpredictable and nonunions fairly frequent. With anatomical reduction and stable fixation, the incidence of nonunion should be acceptably low.

Osteonecrosis

As with nonunion, the development of osteonecrosis correlates with the extent of initial trauma and the displacement of the fracture, with some questions concerning the tamponading effect of the intracapsular hematoma. Urgent gentle reduction and fixation of these fractures should be done, especially in younger patients. They suggested that prompt reduction of the displacement possibly may open some of the retinacular vessels that are temporarily closed by kinking or stretching and rigid fixation may permit re-establishment of some vascular continuity that otherwise might not be preserved, if reduction and fixation are delayed. In the meta-analysis of Damany et al. however, there was no statistically significant difference in osteonecrosis rates in fractures treated early (<12 hours) compared with fractures treated late (>12 hours), or in fractures treated with open reduction compared with closed reduction. Radiographic evidence of osteonecrosis does not always indicate a poor functional result and the late effects of osteonecrosis may take many years to develop. Some scientists showed that intracapsular pressures after femoral neck fractures are higher in nondisplaced fractures than in displaced fractures and Harper, Barnes, and Gregg showed increased intraosseous pressure within the femoral head after intracapsular femoral neck fractures. Joint aspiration lowered the intraosseous pressure and increased the pulse pressure within the femoral head. They and others recommended routine aspiration or capsulotomy, to decompress this increased intracapsular pressure. No study to date has conclusively shown a decreased rate of osteonecrosis with routine capsulotomy or hip aspiration. We do not routinely decompress the hip joint by aspiration or capsulotomy in geriatric patients, but we may decompress the hip capsule in younger patients.

The method of fracture fixation can have an effect on the rate of osteonecrosis and nonunion with femoral neck fractures. The use of a single large compression hip screw for fixation of femoral neck fractures was shown by Madsen et al. and Christie et al. to result in lower rates of union for intracapsular fractures. In some intracapsular femoral neck fractures at the base of the femoral neck and in severely comminuted femoral neck fractures, however, multiple pin fixations is not ideal because of the lack of an adequate posteromedial buttress. For these fractures, the use of a hip compression screw with side plate is indicated, usually with the addition of a supplemental antirotation screw, a short barrel, and possibly a lateral buttress plate, if the fracture extends into lateral cortex. The adequacy of reduction attained with displaced femoral neck fractures has been shown to affect the rates of nonunion and osteonecrosis. Garden originally described his alignment index, as a guide to adequacy of a given reduction. On the AP view, the angle between the central compressive trabeculae within the femoral head and the medial cortex of the femur is measured. According to Garden, this angle is normally 160°, as shown in Figure 115. On the lateral view, the major trabeculae are in the same axis as the axis of the femoral neck or lie at an angle of 180°. Garden showed higher rates of union and lower rates of osteonecrosis, if the compressive trabeculae of the femoral head were aligned with the medial cortex

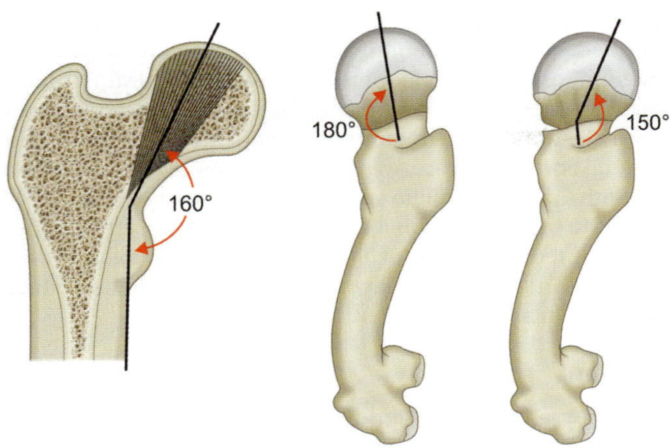

Fig. 116: On the lateral view, an acceptable reduction to be within the same range of 155–180°.

of the femur on the AP view between an angle of 155° and 180°. On the lateral view, he described an acceptable reduction to be within the same range of 155–180°, although he strived to correct the entire anterior angulation. This is illustrated in Figure 116. He found that osteonecrosis was universal, when in the AP view, fractures were reduced with an alignment index of less than 150° or more than 185°, implicating angular and rotational malunion in the incidence of osteonecrosis. Other authors, such as Smyth and Shah, reported similar findings.

Multiple methods have been used to determine preoperatively the vascularity of the femoral head in femoral neck fractures. To date, bone scans have failed to show adequate sensitivity or specificity to have useful predictive value. Speer et al. found no evidence of osteonecrosis within the first 48 hours after displaced fracture on standard T1 and T2 weighted MRI. They hypothesized that the fatty marrow within the femoral head was relatively resistant to the anoxic insult, with fat cell death occurring over 2–5 days and that this fatty marrow was responsible for the normal signal seen within the femoral head on MRI. A postoperative bone scan has been shown to correlate with eventual rates of nonunion and osteonecrosis in femoral neck fractures. Scientists showed that bone scans performed within 2 weeks of operative treatment were able to determine the healing course in 306 fractures (uneventful healing, hardware failure, nonunion, and osteonecrosis) with a prognostic accuracy. The patients were followed, until fracture union, until conversion to hip arthroplasty, or for 2 years. Of these patients, some healed and had no evidence of osteonecrosis. Thirteen patients eventually had arthroplasty for osteonecrosis, nonunion, or both.

Classification

Various classifications have been described for fractures of the femoral neck. Structurally, there are:

- Impacted fractures
- Nondisplaced fractures
- Displaced fractures.

Causatively, in addition to fractures resulting from trauma without other complicating conditions, there are:

- Stress fractures
- Pathological fractures
- Postirradiation fractures.

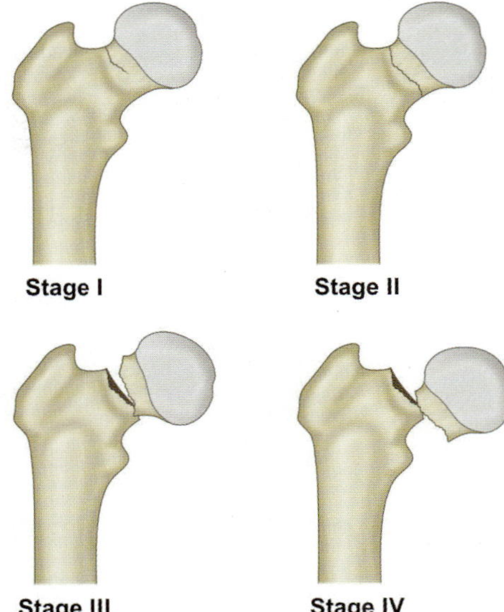

Fig. 117: Common classification of displaced femoral neck fractures, by Garden.

The latter three are discussed separately in this chapter. The most common classification of displaced femoral neck fractures is that of Garden, which is based on the degrees of displacement, as shown in Figure 117. He believed that the various types of femoral neck fractures represent different stages of the same displacing movement. In his classification, the direction of the medial or compression trabeculae coming from the calcar and rising superiorly into the weight-bearing dome of the femoral head is used to indicate the degree of rotation of the fracture in the AP radiograph. These trabeculae normally lie in alignment with their projections in the pelvis and form an angle of 160–170° with the medial cortex of the femoral shaft. They also align with similarly oriented trabeculae in the acetabulum. On the lateral projection, the trabecular alignment from the head fragment to the neck fragment normally should be 180°. Angulation of the head fragment into more anteversion or retroversion would affect the alignment of these trabeculae.

- *Stage I:* In Garden stage I fractures, the fracture is incomplete, with the head tilted in a posterolateral direction. Practically speaking, this is an impacted fracture.
- *Stage II:* Garden stage II fractures are complete, but undisplaced.
- *Stage III:* Garden stage III fractures are complete and partially displaced, as judged by the direction of the trabecular stream in the head fragment, but the two fragments remain in contact with each other.
- *Stage IV:* In Garden stage IV fractures, the fragments are completely displaced and the trabeculae of the femoral head realign themselves with the trabeculae within the acetabulum.

Although Garden's classification system is the most commonly used, it has been difficult to apply without significant interobserver variability. The distinction between displaced and nondisplaced fractures (stages I and II compared with stages III and IV) was much more consistent and was thought by many to be the only reliable distinction.

In the AO classification system, as shown in Figure 118, fractures of the femoral neck are classified as subcapital with no or minimal displacement (type B1), transcervical (type B2) or

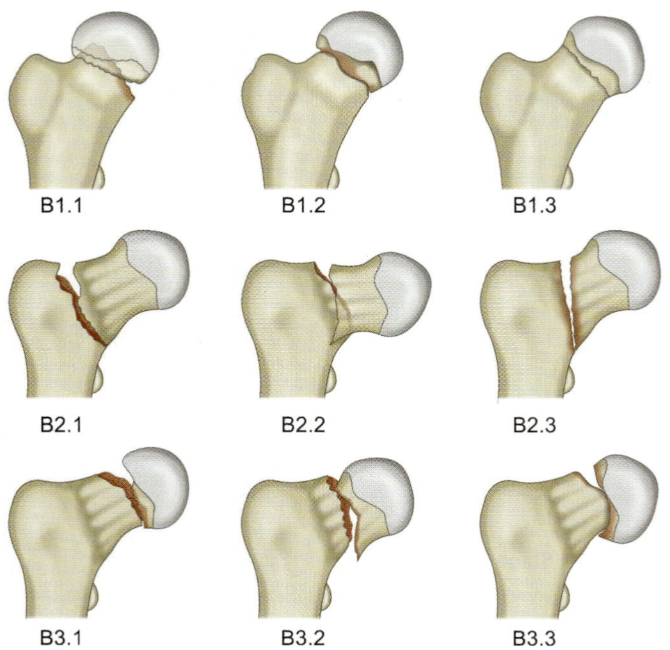

Fig. 118: AO classification of femoral neck fracture.

displaced subcapital fractures (type B3). Each of these types is identified further. Type B1 fractures may be impacted in valgus of 15° or more (type B1.1), impacted in valgus of less than 15° (type B1.2) or nonimpacted (type B1.3). Transcervical (type B2) fractures may be basicervical (type B2.1), midcervical with adduction (type B2.2) or midcervical with shear (type B2.3). Displaced subcapital fractures (type B3) may be moderately displaced in varus and external rotation (type B3.1), moderately displaced with vertical translation and external rotation (type B3.2) or markedly displaced (type B3.3). Type B3 fractures have the worst prognosis.

Whichever classification system is used, impacted fractures must be distinguished from nondisplaced fractures of the neck of the femur. Impacted fracture surfaces are crushed together or invaginated, so that the trabeculae and usually the cortex of the neck are pushed into the soft trabecular bone of the head. This impaction imparts a significant amount of stability at the fracture site and suggests a conservative or nonoperative approach. In nondisplaced fractures of the femoral neck (Garden stage II), there is no impaction and no inherent stability and almost all subsequently displace, if not internally fixed. Rates of nonunion and osteonecrosis for nondisplaced fractures are low, when these fractures are treated with multiple screw fixation. Many different devices have been devised for internal fixation of femoral neck fractures, but currently two are commonly used:

1. Multiple cannulated screws and
2. Collapsible compression screw and side plate combinations that are typically used with an additional antirotation screw.

The following principles of preoperative preparation, reduction of the fracture, fluoroscopic control, surgical exposure, and insertion of internal fixation are common to many of the techniques. Fixation with cannulated screws usually is adequate for most femoral neck fractures. In a review of femoral neck fractures in young patients, Kyle determined that the most consistently good results were obtained with anatomical reduction and fixation with some form of multiple screw fixations. Scientists have found a distinct correlation between fixation with screws and the strength of the lateral cortex. Based on their studies, they concluded that if the lateral cortex does not provide sufficient stability to prevent toggling of the screws and reduction of torsional forces, complications and nonunions occur more frequently. We most often use cannulated screws for fixation of femoral neck fractures. If osteopenia or comminution of the lateral cortex is severe, we infrequently use a compression hip screw with a small side plate and accessory screws, as advocated by scientists to control rotational forces around the lag screw further. If satisfactory reduction cannot be obtained by closed methods, open reduction is indicated. Satisfactory reduction should be evaluated by the Garden alignment index.

Treatment

We prefer manipulation and closed reduction of femoral neck fractures and perform open reduction, only when anatomical closed reduction is not attainable and the patient is not a good candidate for a hemiarthroplasty with a femoral head prosthesis.

Closed Reduction

Whitman described a method that involves traction on the limb in extension, internal rotation in extension and abduction, and abduction and internal rotation. We usually have success with this method. With the patient supine on the fracture table, the normal extremity is tied to the footplate.

The fractured extremity is tied to the other footplate in an externally rotated position. With the extremity externally rotated, it is abducted approximately 20° and enough traction is applied to regain slightly more than normal length. The extremity is internally rotated, until the patella is internally rotated 20–30°. Scientists described a technique of manipulation with the hip in flexion that we have found satisfactory, when the Whitman technique is unsuccessful. In his technique, the affected limb is flexed at the hip to 90° and the thigh is slightly internally rotated, traction is applied in line with the femur. The limb is circumducted into abduction, maintaining the internal rotation and is brought down to table level in extension. Scientists evaluated the reduction with a "heel-palm" test, in which the patient's heel is placed in the palm of the surgeon's outstretched hand. If reduction is complete, the limb does not externally rotate spontaneously. The foot is tied to the footplate with the extremity in only 15–20° of abduction, neutral flexion and extension, and firm internal rotation of approximately 20°. This position usually places the head, neck, and trochanter on a horizontal plane. The position is verified, by image intensification in the AP and lateral planes.

Evaluation of Reduction (Fig. 119)

On the lateral fluoroscopic view, only the slightest variation from the anatomical position is permissible. On the AP view, anatomical position or a slight valgus relationship of the head and neck is acceptable. Garden proposed an index for acceptable reduction, using the trabecular pattern alignment, as viewed in the AP and lateral radiographic planes. On the AP view, the angle formed by the central axis of the medial trabecular system in the head fragment and the medial cortex of the femoral shaft should measure no less than 160° and no more than 180°. An angle less than 160° denotes an unacceptable varus reduction and an angle more than 180° indicates severe valgus, which has been shown to increase the risk of osteonecrosis and degenerative changes within the joint caused by hip joint incongruity. On the lateral view, Garden's alignment index should be within 20° of the normal 180° straight line along the

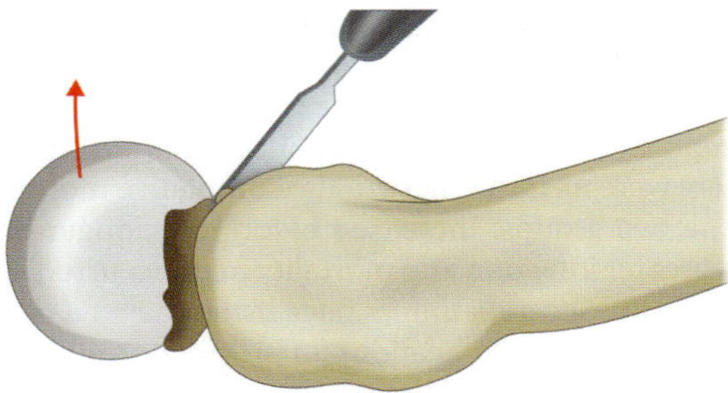

Fig. 119: An osteotome or elevator inserted into the anterior aspect of the fracture can be used to manipulate the femoral head fragment.

neck. If the femoral head is anteverted or retroverted and this angle is less than 150°, an unstable, nonanatomical reduction is present and remanipulation should be considered. Any variation from these rigid requirements demands that the hip be remanipulated. If remanipulation is necessary, the limb first must be brought into full external rotation because the internally rotated position locks the fragments and prevents successful manipulation.

If the position is unsatisfactory after a second or third attempt, either the fracture must be reduced under direct vision by open reduction or a femoral head prosthesis must be inserted. If the patient is younger than 70 years old and a satisfactory reduction has not been obtained, open reduction through a Watson-Jones approach is preferred. If the patient is older than 70 years, a femoral head prosthesis is usually inserted. Variations from these age-related guidelines should be based on the patient's associated medical conditions and are discussed in detail in the following section. Reduction can be difficult, when comminution is extensive, especially along the posterior part of the neck; large comminuted posterior fragments may make the fracture unstable. The inability to reduce by manipulation a wedge-shaped or a serrated margin of the fracture into its corresponding defect may be caused by a pedunculated flap of capsule or other soft tissue or a sharp edge of the anterior or posterior margin of the neck may have become caught in the intact capsule. During manipulation, the capsule may become more tightly impaled between the fracture surfaces, making proper apposition impossible. As already stated, an accurate reduction is an absolute requirement for internal fixation, if it is not obtained, internal fixation should not proceed further.

Open Reduction and Internal Fixation (Figs. 120A to F)

Patient positioning and draping after fracture reduction are performed in a similar manner to that described for internal fixation of intertrochanteric fracture. If open reduction is performed, the usual lateral incision is extended proximally and anteriorly, as in a Watson-Jones approach. The capsule is opened and the fracture is reduced under direct vision. Open reduction in this manner is not an easy surgical exercise. If the extremity is kept in the extended position in traction, the exposure to the femoral neck through the anterior capsule can be extremely difficult because of the tightness of the anterior and anterolateral thigh and hip muscles in this position. The femoral head is largely covered and within the acetabulum, it is difficult to manipulate and the fracture is not easily aligned, even with it exposed and visible. Flexing the hip 20° or 30° greatly aids in the exposure and reduction. An osteotome or elevator inserted into the anterior aspect of the fracture can be used to manipulate the femoral head fragment, as shown in Figure 119. When the fracture has been satisfactorily reduced, guide pins are inserted for provisional fixation, and views with the image intensifier are obtained to check their position. The fracture can be fixed definitively with three screws.

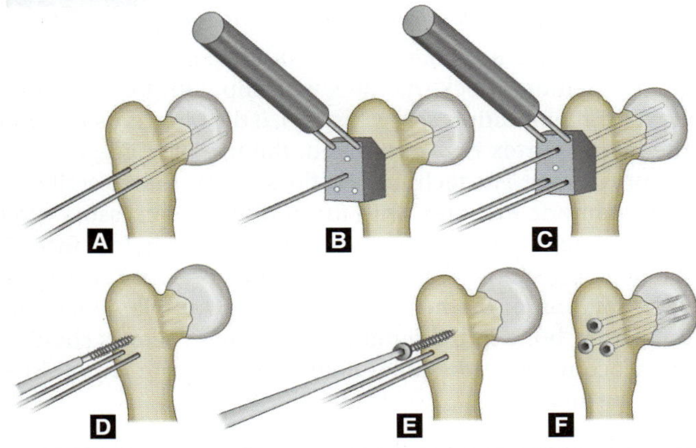

Figs. 120A to F: Open reduction and internal fixation after reduction guide pins are inserted for provisional fixation. The fracture can then be fixed definitively with three screws.

Some surgeons have suggested open reduction through a posterior approach, but we have had no experience with this approach. The reason for nonanatomical reduction often involves comminution of the posterior femoral neck and advocates of the posterior approach have suggested that this is the most direct route to obtain anatomical reduction. If a posterior approach is used for open reduction, further damage to the most important vascular supply to the femoral head, traversing the posterior femoral neck through its retinaculum and the lateral epiphyseal arterial group is a distinct risk. Many authors have evaluated the number of screws and the configuration in the neck for the greatest degree of stability. The usual number of screws recommended is three to four and the location and arrangement of the screws in the neck should be as recommended by Booth et al. in the calcar and more peripheral positions. Screws positioned along the posterior femoral neck may resist retroversion forces, as screws along the calcar resist varus forces.

After Treatment

The patient is allowed to sit on the day after surgery. Ambulation with a walker is allowed as soon as possible. Weight-bearing varies depending on the stability of the fracture construct (quality of the bone, reduction, and screw fixation), but there is evidence that with adequately fixed fractures, at least partial weight-bearing can be allowed immediately in most patients with no increased incidence of hardware failure. Scientists analyzed weight bearing after femoral neck intertrochanteric hip fractures and found that patients allowed to bear weight, as tolerated voluntarily, which will limit the amount of weight they apply to their fractured hip and increase the weight gradually as the fracture heals. We encourage our patients to ambulate with "protected" weight bearing and try to not let a strict NWB status restrict the patient's rehabilitation. Many of these patients become unable to ambulate at all, if weight bearing is restricted, so we usually err on the side of allowing weight to be applied to the hip, rather than have the patient be in bed or a chair for a prolonged time. The patient is encouraged to bear full weight by 6–8 weeks.

Fixation with a Compression Hip Screw and Plate

Although current literature reviews indicate poorer results after fixation of femoral neck fractures with hip compression screws alone than after multiple screw fixation, if the bone is osteoporotic or the lateral cortex is comminuted, the use of a side plate and accessory screws. The technique is the same as that described for intertrochanteric fractures, with the addition of accessory screws inserted through the femoral neck into the head before insertion of the large lag screw. The function of the accessory screws is to prevent rotation of the neck, while inserting the large lag screw into the hard bone in the femoral head. These screws should be left in place to resist torsional deformation of the femoral neck fracture further.

Prosthetic Replacement for Recent Femoral Neck Fractures

For displaced fractures of the femoral neck, reduction, compression, and rigid internal fixation are required, if union is to be predictable because nonunion and osteonecrosis develop frequently after internal fixation of displaced femoral neck fractures, many surgeons recommend primary prosthetic replacement, as an alternative in elderly ambulatory patients. Although, the use of a prosthesis avoids nonunion and osteonecrosis, it also may be followed by complications. Their study showed a higher rate of revision in patients older than 80 years treated with internal fixation of a displaced femoral neck fracture compared with patients, who were treated with hemiarthroplasty. There was no difference, however, in the revision rates of nondisplaced fractures treated by internal fixation or hemiarthroplasty in this age group. In patients 65 to 80 years old, regardless of the amount of displacement, no difference was noted in revision rates after hemiarthroplasty or internal fixation. These authors noted a significantly higher mortality rate associated with internal fixation than with hemiarthroplasty for patients in this age group.

Complications, revision rates, and other outcomes were the same regardless of whether a unipolar or bipolar prosthesis was used and whether an anterior or posterior approach for hemiarthroplasty was used in patients 65–80 years old. After the first month, there were no differences in the cumulative mortality rates between the two groups. Increased blood loss, longer operative times, and greater infection and mortality rates occurred, however with arthroplasty. Several authors have listed the advantages and disadvantages of and the indications for prosthetic replacement for recent displaced fractures of the femoral neck and no two totally agree. The advantages and disadvantages can be summarized as in Boxes 1 and 2.

Based on the relative advantages and disadvantages, various authors have proposed indications for prosthetic replacement and internal fixation for displaced intracapsular fractures. Many indications for the use of a prosthesis are controversial; some of the indications are enumerated in Boxes 3 and 4. A treatment algorithm based on our treatment preferences—closed reduction and internal fixation (CRIF); not applicable (NA) then open reduction and internal fixation (ORIF).

Selection of a Prosthesis

With the development of bipolar endoprostheses, the use of fixed head endoprostheses has declined. Although, the Austin-Moore prosthesis has produced excellent results, thigh pain, and protrusio acetabuli in younger patients have been associated with this device. Revision to a total hip arthroplasty is also difficult and the complication rate is much higher when an Austin-Moore prosthesis has been used. We still use the Austin-Moore prosthesis on rare occasions, but only in patients with extremely limited ambulation and short life-expectancy. Modern low cost femoral stems, with modular unipolar or bipolar femoral heads are currently in use that allows revision to a total hip arthroplasty, often without revision of

Box 1: Advantages of prosthetic replacement.

- Prosthetic replacement allows immediate weight bearing to return elderly patients to activity and help avoid complications of recumbency and inactivity.
    - When the concept of prosthetic replacement was first introduced, this perhaps was the most important advantage.
    - As patients with internal fixation devices are more aggressively mobilized than in the past, and most are allowed at least partial immediate weight bearing, this advantage is less distinct than previously thought.
- As a primary procedure, prosthetic replacement eliminates osteonecrosis and nonunion as complications of femoral neck fractures.
    - There still is no completely reliable way of identifying femoral heads with a significantly damaged blood supply before definitive surgery.
    - Developing technology may allow definitive preoperative identification of these avascular femoral heads and provide useful information in making the decision between prosthetic replacement and internal fixation.
- Prosthetic replacement of displaced femoral neck fractures reduces the incidence of reoperation compared with internal fixation.

This argument applies only to elderly individuals with a limited life expectancy because the cumulative rate of reoperation for prosthetic replacement increases with time.

Box 2: The recognized disadvantages of using a prosthesis in a fresh femoral neck fracture.

- After the femoral head and neck have been discarded in favor of a metal implant, salvage procedures become complicated if there is mechanical failure or infection.
    - The use of a prosthesis for most fractures of the femoral neck ignores the fact that at least two-thirds of patients treated by internal fixation have functional hips that last the remainder of their lifetimes.
    - *It is appropriate to remember Boyd and Salvatore's comment:* "The sacrifice of the head and neck and replacement by a metallic foreign substance is not the answer for the majority of patients; in over half, the best available material is in the acetabulum, and its indiscriminate removal should be avoided."
- The operation for inserting a prosthesis generally is considered to be more extensive than that required for an uncomplicated internal fixation procedure.
    - Larger exposure is required, and blood loss is greater. Many authors have reported slightly higher perioperative mortality rates for patients treated with prosthetic replacement than for patients treated with internal fixation. This finding has a definite selection bias, however, because patients undergoing hemiarthroplasty tend to be more elderly and have more medical comorbidities.

Box 3: Relative indications for hemiarthroplasty.

- *Advanced physiological age:* Advanced age alone is not a true indication for a prosthesis, although some local and systemic diseases that occur in older patients, especially if they occur in combination, might be. Prosthetic replacement probably should be reserved for patients 70 years old or older with a life expectancy of no more than 10–15 years. Some definite exceptions to this statement are mentioned later.
- *Fracture-dislocation of the hip in an older patient:* If the fracture involves the superior weight-bearing surface of the head (Pipkin type II; the Pipkin classification system is discussed in the section on dislocation and fracture-dislocation of the hip), the insertion of a prosthesis is preferable to closed treatment or open reduction of the fragment. If a substantial fragment of the inferior part of the head is fractured (Pipkin type I), the dislocation should be reduced promptly and, if the head fragment is not caught in the joint, treated closed;
  - If necessary, open reduction of the hip can be performed, and the fragment can be removed. Such treatment results in a good hip if the superior weight- bearing surface of the head is intact.

Box 4: Stronger indications for hemiarthroplasty.

- A fracture that cannot be satisfactorily reduced or fixed with stability, especially with posterior comminution.
- Femoral neck fractures that lose fixation several weeks after operation.
- *Some preexisting lesions of the hip:* In patients with preexisting lesions, an arthroplasty already may have been indicated and the fracture merely makes the decision immediate
  - Patients with osteonecrosis of the head of the femur from unknown causes, from irradiation, or from a previous dislocation and patients with severe rheumatoid or degenerative arthritis of the hip probably would have a better hip after insertion of a prosthesis than before the fracture.
  - In one study of rheumatoid patients, Strömqvist, Kelly, and Lidgren reported a 95% rate of loss of reduction or superior segmental collapse compared with 50% in a matched non-rheumatoid group most of these patients are candidates for total hip arthroplasty rather than femoral head replacement.
- *Malignancy:* A malignancy may be an indication for the insertion of a prosthesis. A patient with a short life expectancy, whether the fracture is pathological or primarily the result of trauma, is best treated with a prosthesis.
  - If the fracture is pathological, the insertion of a prosthesis offers not only a good solution, but also an opportunity to perform an open biopsy and to establish a definite diagnosis.
  - In pathological fractures, supplementing the fixation with methyl methacrylate usually provides sufficient ability.
- *Neurological disorders:* Patients subject to uncontrolled epileptic seizures and patients with severe uncontrolled Parkinson is mare treated better with a primary prosthesis. Many of these disorders are controllable, however, and the indication may not always be absolute.
- Old, undiagnosed fractures of the femoral neck. Occasionally, a fracture of the femoral neck goes undiscovered for several weeks. Sometimes multiple injuries may delay treatment of a fractured femoral neck even after its diagnosis.
  - An untreated, unreduced, and unimpacted fracture of the femoral neck that is more than 3 weeks old should have a primary prosthesis, other things being equal.
  - Before the use of prostheses, we saw many patients with fractures of the femoral neck 3 weeks old that healed satisfactorily with nothing more than reduction and rigid internal fixation.
  - The odds for favorable results decline, however, with the passage of time after a displaced fracture.
- Fracture of the neck of the femur with complete dislocation of the femoral head. This lesion is rare and is best treated by primary prosthetic replacement because osteonecrosis of the head is certain under these circumstances.
- A patient who probably cannot withstand two operations. If a patient's general condition prohibits a second operation, a primary prosthesis is justified. In patients who have unstable multiple medical problems, we occasionally perform a closed reduction with percutaneous multiple screw fixation using intravenous sedation and generous amounts of local lidocaine infiltration anesthesia.
- Patients with psychoses or mental deterioration. Elderly patients with fractures of the femoral neck often already have Alzheimer disease, and protected weight bearing in such patients may be unreliable, with immediate unprotected weight bearing resulting in possible loss of fixation, especially in severely comminuted fractures. A primary prosthesis may be justified in these circumstances.

the femoral component. They also allow some adjustment of the prosthetic femoral neck length for stability and offset considerations. For active patients in whom a prosthesis is indicated, we prefer a cemented or cementless total hip femoral component with a bipolar or unipolar head attachment.

Bipolar versus Unipolar

- The complications of persistent pain and protrusio acetabuli with unipolar hemiarthroplasties have led many surgeons to choose a bipolar system.
- Studies suggest that the current generation of bipolar hemiarthroplasties have a lower incidence of protrusio acetabuli than do earlier designs. Some authors have found, however, that the motion of the inner bearing surface may not last and that all bipolar hips functionally become unipolar implants.

Cemented versus Cementless

- Emery et al. found significantly better pain relief after cemented Thompson hemiarthroplasties than after the use of uncemented Austin-Moore prostheses.
- This has also been our experience and we cement many endoprostheses used for femoral neck fractures.
- We use contemporary cement techniques that include distal femoral canal occlusion, pulsatile lavage of the canal, and meticulous drying of the canal before cement insertion with a cement gun, avoiding significant cement pressurization.
- As many patients have compromised cardiopulmonary reserve and a recent long bone fracture, we avoid further metabolic insult of cement pressurization.
- If uncemented hemiarthroplasty is done for femoral neck fracture, we prefer to use a proximally porous textured total hip style stem, rather than a nonporous "press-fit" type stem.
- The lack of biological fixation of the nontextured stem inserted without cement may cause long-term thigh pain.

Total Hip Arthroplasty

Primary total hip arthroplasty is indicated in patients with significant preexisting joint destruction caused by rheumatoid disease, osteonecrosis, or osteoarthritis. The clinical results and survivorship of primary hip arthroplasty in this setting have varied from excellent to poor. There seems to be a definite increased risk of dislocation in this population compared with the risk after purely elective total hip arthroplasty. Scientists, reported their results after total hip arthroplasty for femoral neck fractures and noted that although results were good, the complication rate was higher than those reported in other studies of hemiarthroplasties. We rarely perform total hip arthroplasty for a femoral neck fracture.

Surgical Approaches

We most frequently use a posterior approach for the insertion of femoral head prostheses after acute fractures of the neck of the femur. Numerous authors recommend a more anterior approach, such as a Hardinge approach because complications, especially infection and prosthetic dislocation occur more frequently, when a posterior approach is used. Advocates of an anterior approach state that infection and dislocation are infrequent with that approach because of the greater distance of the anterior incision from the perineum and the absence of an incision through the strong posterior capsule. Unquestionably, getting these elderly patients out of bed to a sitting position places considerable stress on the posterior capsule and posterior approaches can make the hip more vulnerable to dislocation. We occasionally use an anterior approach in patients with bowel incontinence, in unreliable patients, who are likely to violate the standard total hip range-of-motion precautions and in patients, who are spastic and tend to flex and adduct their hips in household ambulation. An adductor tenotomy may be indicated in this last group of patients. Patients with Parkinson's disease have been identified, as being at risk for posterior dislocation. Failures after internal fixation of fractures of the hip can be caused by:

- Infection
- Loss of fixation
- Nonunion
- Osteonecrosis.

Infection after internal fixation of intertrochanteric fractures or fractures of the femoral neck is serious and usually leads to significant compromise of hip function. Many patients have diseases, such as diabetes or infections of other organ systems, which have been shown to retard fracture repair. Incisions for hip surgery are near the perineum and are easily contaminated. Intraoperative wound contamination from wide exposure and prolonged operating time and postoperative hematomas are other factors. Disoriented patients sometimes remove the postoperative dressing and directly contaminate the wound. Adding to the problem is the fact that many infections are not evident, until after the patient has been discharged and the patient may not exhibit the classic signs and symptoms of an infection. Even when none of the cardinal signs and symptoms of infection, such as fever, chills, redness, or drainage are present, an infection should be suspected, if a patient complains of persistent pain, especially if motion is painful, if the sedimentation rate is elevated, if the joint space is progressively becoming more narrow on radiographs, if there is progressive loss of bone density around the head, neck, or acetabulum, or if there is any sign of loosening of the internal fixation appliance. Aspiration of the hip joint may allow early diagnosis. Organisms normally considered to be contaminants or nonpathogens may produce infections that appear late. Superficial infections usually appear within the first 1–2 weeks after surgery and usually respond to drainage and antibiotics. Early deep infections generally produce all the cardinal signs and symptoms of an acute infection and demand aggressive early treatment with wide drainage and appropriate antibiotics. If the infection involves the hip joint in a patient with a femoral neck fracture, the internal fixation usually should be removed, only if it is unstable, however, control of the infection takes precedence over further efforts to obtain union of the fracture.

In many patients, femoral head resection is required because the head becomes a sequestrum. If an intertrochanteric or subtrochanteric fracture becomes infected, it should be widely drained. The internal fixation device is left in place, however, if it is still providing rigid fixation of the fracture and the joint is not involved. The infection may continue in a subacute or chronic form, as long as the device remains in place, but union of the fracture can occur despite this. The fixation device can be removed after union and the infection can usually be cleared. Late deep infections without joint involvement should be managed in a similar manner with drainage and appropriate antibiotics, leaving the fixation device in place, if fracture healing is incomplete or removing it, if the fracture has united.

Stress Fractures of the Femoral Neck

Stress fractures of the femoral neck can occur in young, vigorous individuals with unaccustomed strenuous activity, such as athletics, running, or marching long distances. In elderly individuals, they can occur because of one of the metabolic disorders of bone. Frequently, routine AP and lateral radiographs initially are normal with the diagnosis confirmed by bone scan or MRI.

Femoral neck stress fractures have been classified according to the location of the fracture in the femoral neck.

- *Type I:* Lateral fractures, often referred to as "tension fractures", are more unstable and prone to displacement. We recommend internal fixation with multiple screws for this fracture.
- *Type II:* Medial compression fractures can be treated nonoperatively with rest followed by a period of protected weight bearing. Radiographs should be made at multiple intervals to confirm progression toward union without displacement. If a patient cannot comply with activity restriction, internal fixation is recommended.
- *Type III:* Fractures, are displaced and require closed or open reduction with screw fixation or hemiarthroplasty, depending on the patient's age and medical circumstances.

Pathological fractures of the femoral neck:
The proximal end of the femur is a common location for the spread of metastatic disease. Pathological fracture in this area is commonly the presenting symptom that leads to and establishes the diagnosis of malignancy. Pathological fractures or impending pathological fractures in the subtrochanteric and intertrochanteric region should be fixed internally, using techniques and devices discussed in the previous sections. In addition to internal fixation, the bulk of the tumor at the pathological site can be removed and fixation supplemented with polymethylmethacrylate (PMMA). We prefer to use a cephalomedullary reconstruction nail for pathological fractures of the intertrochanteric and subtrochanteric regions and to stabilize the entire femur prophylactically, with or without PMMA. Depending on the aggressiveness of the tumor, fractures so treated may heal. Pathological fractures arising from metastatic disease in the femoral head and neck usually are best treated by removal of the head and neck and replacement with a femoral head prosthesis. The prosthesis should be secured in the medullary canal with PMMA.

Box 5: Indications for inserting prosthesis instead of using internal fixation for pathological fractures.

- If the fracture is the result of irradiation and has been present for some time, efforts to correct the deformity and preserve the head usually fail. Fractures with minimal deformity and of recent onset should be fixed internally
- If the patient's life expectancy is uncertain because of an aggressive malignancy, this fact favors a method that would provide early function and ambulation.

The stages of the primary malignancy must be considered; the presence of multiple metastatic lesions or a life expectancy of only a few weeks or months would favor the use of a prosthesis.

Postirradiation fractures of the femoral neck:
If a patient has received radiation therapy for pelvic malignancy months or years before sustaining a fracture of the femoral neck, the surgeon should try to determine whether the fracture is pathological and the result of irradiation, whether it is a pathological fracture arising from a metastatic lesion or an extension of the primary tumor or whether it is a simple fracture totally attributable to trauma. Clinical signs and symptoms suggesting irradiation, as the cause of fracture are prodromal pain localized to the hip or radiating to the knee, followed by a gradually increasing limp and disability, as might occur with a slipped femoral epiphysis. Although, the patient is able to walk, coxa vara deformity may have already occurred. Some scientists described the radiographic characteristics as:

- The fracture is subcapital or high in the neck
- Before the fracture occurs, an irregular transverse line of increased density is the only evidence that fracture is impending
- Scattered areas of increased translucency sometimes may be seen in the femoral neck
- Characteristically, there is a coxa vara deformity, as in an adduction fracture
- Rotation or angulation of the head is slight on the AP and lateral view
- After the fracture heals, considerable sclerosis can be seen at the fracture and in the adjacent bone.

The fracture is preceded by a loss of trabecular bulk and the blood supply is not obliterated and is not responsible for the bony changes; the meager blood supply of the femoral head can be increased by radiation therapy, unless intensive direct irradiation has produced complete cellular destruction. They recommended early internal fixation, without manipulation of the fragments. They found that these fractures heal well, often with "skillful neglect" as the treatment that many heal in less time than average and that the usual complications of nonunion and osteonecrosis of the femoral head probably are less common than after fractures that occur purely from trauma. Internal fixation was used when the fracture continued to displace or when separation of the fragments already existed. Only in the old and markedly displaced fractures was a major reconstructive procedure necessary in deciding whether to insert a prosthesis instead of using internal fixation for a pathological fracture of the femoral neck. This is illustrated in Box 5.

Fractures of the Femoral Neck with Ipsilateral Femoral Shaft Fractures

Fracture of the femoral neck with ipsilateral femoral shaft fracture is an unusual segmental fracture of the femur that initially was reported by Delaney and Street, as an incidental finding during intramedullary nailing of a femoral fracture. Approximately 19% of ipsilateral femoral neck fractures are discovered late or during treatment of femoral shaft fractures. Fractures of the femoral shaft can occur in combination with subtrochanteric fractures, intertrochanteric fractures, nondisplaced femoral neck fractures or displaced femoral neck fractures. Shaft fractures with displaced femoral neck fractures, as expected have the worst prognosis. More than 60 different methods have been advocated in the literature for treatment of this rare injury. This is a better prognosis than is usually seen for femoral neck fractures, and it is attributed to the fact that most of the energy, causing the fractures is dissipated to the femoral shaft, with less resultant displacement of the femoral neck fracture. Any patient sustaining high-energy trauma should be thoroughly examined with a radiographic survey of the femoral neck area, to rule out this combination of injuries. We routinely re-examine the femoral neck under fluoroscopy after all intramedullary nailings of the femur. The best treatment of these fractures is controversial.

Considering the greater significance of failure of femoral neck fractures in young patients, most authors emphasize making the fracture of the femoral neck a greater priority. Some authors now recommend femoral neck fixation with screws and an intercondylar retrograde femoral nail. The use of a hip compression screw and long side plate has also been reported. The Russell-Taylor reconstruction nail was designed specifically for this injury. It allows fixation by two self-compressing lag screws in the femoral head, for control of torsional forces around the femoral neck, in conjunction with a cephalomedullary nail. In a series of 30 consecutive femoral neck and shaft fractures treated with Russell-Taylor reconstruction nails, Azar and Russell reported one femoral neck nonunion and one patient who developed osteonecrosis. We advocate anatomical reduction of femoral neck fractures before stabilization with the implant.

Many new cephalomedullary implants with a reconstruction mode are now available. We currently use the Trigen nail in the Recon mode or a retrograde intramedullary nail with cannulated screws placed into the femoral neck proximal to the nail to treat these injuries. Although, we have had good results with closed reduction of the shaft after preliminary neck fixation and insertion of a reconstruction nail, the technique requires careful and constant imaging of the femoral neck fracture, to ensure no displacement occurs during nailing. Two screws must be used for femoral head fixation, and the threads must be placed well into the head for adequate stability of the femoral neck portion. When an undetected femoral neck fracture is found after conventional intramedullary nailing of a femoral shaft fracture, the nail should be left in place and cannulated screws should be inserted from the lateral shaft of the femur, anterior to the femoral nail, into the middle of the femoral head to fix the femoral neck fracture.

INTERTROCHANTERIC FEMORAL FRACTURES

Most intertrochanteric femoral fractures occur in patients older than 70 years old. It includes fractures from the extracapsular part of the neck to a point 5 cm distal to the lesser trochanter.

Classification

Boyd and Griffin classified fractures in the peritrochanteric area of the femur into four types. Their classification, which included fractures from the extracapsular part of the neck to a point

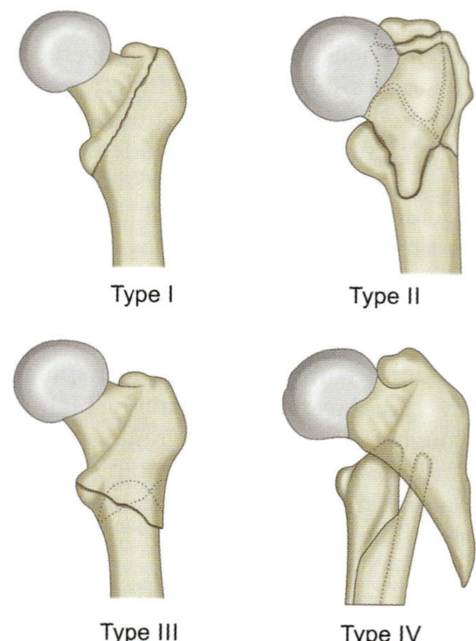

Fig. 121: Classification of intertrochanteric femoral fractures.

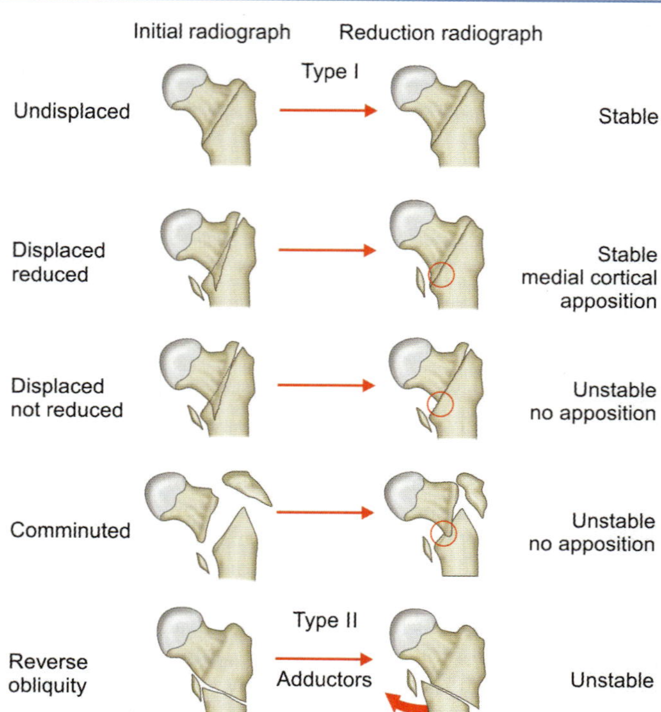

Fig. 122: Evans classification system based on the division of fractures into stable and unstable groups.

5 cm distal to the lesser trochanter, follows. These are shown in Figure 121.

1 *Type I:* Fractures that extend along the intertrochanteric line from the greater to the lesser trochanter. Reduction usually is simple and is maintained with little difficulty. Results generally are satisfactory.
2 *Type II:* Comminuted fractures, the main fracture being along the intertrochanteric line, but with multiple fractures in the cortex. Reduction of these fractures is more difficult because the comminution can vary from slight to extreme. A particularly deceptive form is the fracture, in which an AP linear intertrochanteric fracture occurs, as in type 1, but with an additional fracture in the coronal plane, which can be seen on the lateral radiograph.
3 *Type III:* Fractures that are basically subtrochanteric with at least one fracture passing across the proximal end of the shaft just distal to or at the lesser trochanter. Varying degrees of comminution are associated. These fractures usually are more difficult to reduce and result in more complications at operation and during convalescence.
4 *Type IV:* Fractures of the trochanteric region and the proximal shaft, with fracture in at least two planes, one of which usually is the sagittal plane and may be difficult to see on routine AP radiographs. If open reduction and internal fixation are used, two-plane fixation is required because of the spiral, oblique or butterfly fracture of the shaft.

The most difficult types to manage are types III and IV, which are accounted for only about one-third of the trochanteric fractures in Boyd and Griffin's series. Evans devised a widely used classification system based on the division of fractures into stable and unstable groups, as shown in Figure 122. He divided unstable fractures further into those, in which stability could be restored by anatomical or near-anatomical reduction and those in which anatomical reduction would not create stability. In an Evans type I fracture, the fracture line extends upward and outward from the lesser trochanter. In type II, reverse obliquity fracture, the major fracture line extends outward and downward from the lesser trochanter. Type II fractures have a tendency toward medial displacement of the femoral shaft because of the pull of the adductor muscles.

The AO group classified trochanteric fractures as described in Figure 123. A1 fractures are uncomminuted, A2 fractures have increasing comminution and A3 fractures have subtrochanteric extensions or reverse obliquity. AO fractures A1.1 through A2.1 are commonly described as stable and fractures A2.2 through A3.3, usually are unstable. The orientation of the trabeculae is along the lines of stress, with thicker trabeculae coming from the calcar and passing superiorly into the weight-bearing dome of the femoral head, as shown in Figure 123.

Nonoperative Treatment

Closed methods of treatment of intertrochanteric fractures have largely been abandoned.

Rigid internal fixation of intertrochanteric fractures with early mobilization of the patient should be considered standard treatment. Medical complications after internal fixation are fewer and less serious than complications after nonoperative treatment. Only comfortable nonambulatory patients or patients with brief life expectancies should be treated nonoperatively.

Operative Treatment

One goal of operative treatment is strong, stable fixation of the fracture fragments. Scientists listed the following variables, as those that determine the strength of the fracture fragment-implant assembly:

- Bone quality
- Fragment geometry
- Reduction
- Implant design
- Implant placement.

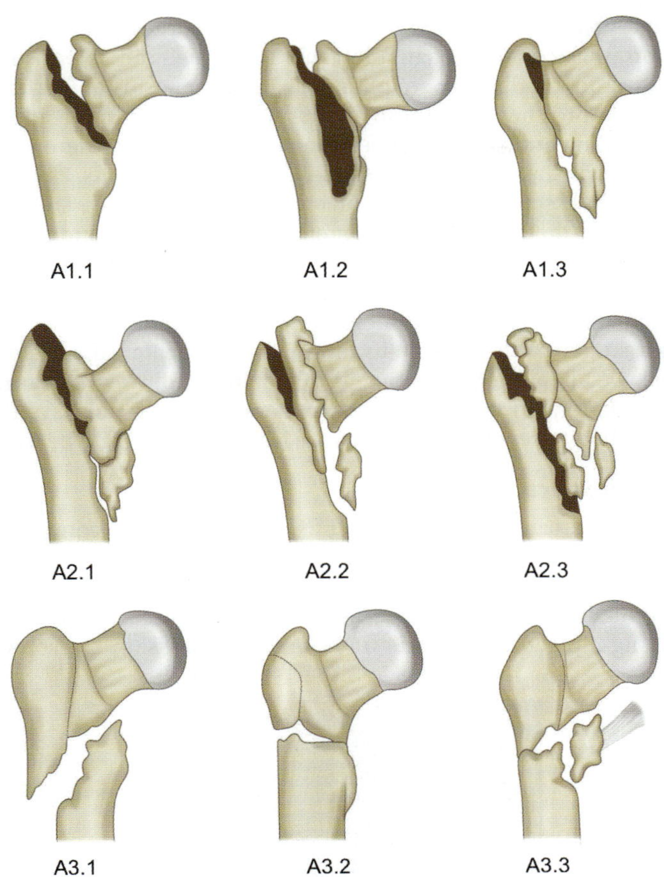

Fig. 123: AO classification of trochanteric fractures.

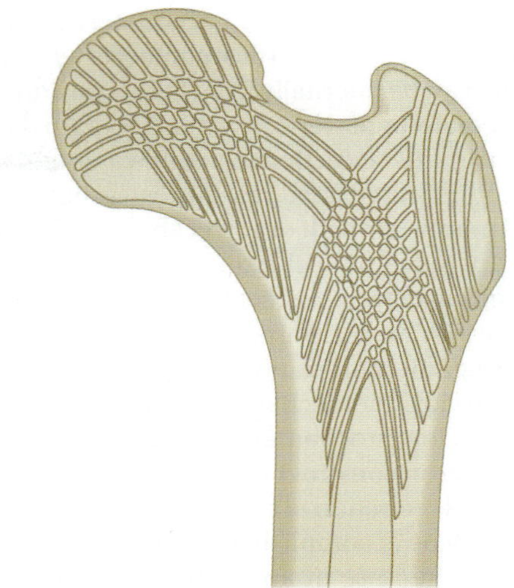

Fig. 124: Internal trabecular system of femoral head.

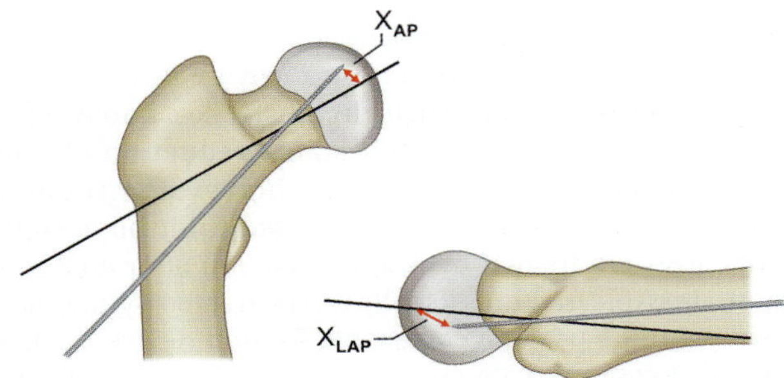

Fig. 125: The tip-apex distance, as the sum of the distances from the apex of the femoral head to the tip of the lag screw on anteroposterior and lateral radiographs, correcting for magnification.

Of these five elements of stable fixation, the surgeon can control only the quality of the reduction and the choice of implant and its placement. As most patients with intertrochanteric fractures have considerable osteopenia, with the quality of bone for the purchase of fixation within the femoral head and neck less than desirable, it is important that the internal fixation device be placed in that part of the head and neck where the quality of bone is best. A scientist described the internal trabecular system of the femoral head, as illustrated in Figure 124. The orientation of the trabeculae is along the lines of stress, with thicker trabeculae coming from the calcar and passing superiorly into the weight-bearing dome of the femoral head. Smaller trabeculae extend from the inferior region of the foveal area across the head and the superior portion of the femoral neck and into the trochanter and to the lateral cortex. The calcar is a dense, vertical plate of bone extending from the posteromedial portion of the femoral shaft under the lesser trochanter and radiating laterally to the GT, reinforcing the femoral neck posteroinferiorly. The calcar is thickest medially and gradually thins, as it passes laterally. The quality of bone for purchase within the head and neck varies from one quadrant to another. Although, the optimal position of a compression screw within the head and neck is controversial, all agree that it should be central or slightly inferior and posterior.

The bone of poorest quality is in the anterosuperior aspect of the head and neck. Optimal positioning of the device is controlled by the surgeon. A scientist described the tip-apex distance, as the sum of the distances from the apex of the femoral head to the tip of the lag screw on AP and lateral radiographs, correcting for magnification. Scientists have found that, if this sum was less than 25 mm, there were no failures caused by cutting out of the lag screw, as depicted in Figure 125. Scientists showed that the tip-apex distance also is crucial, when using intramedullary nails and compression hip screws to prevent cutout and loss of reduction.

It is important before treatment to distinguish by radiographs, whether the intertrochanteric fracture is stable or unstable based on fracture geometry and whether reduction can restore cortical contact medially and posteriorly. The status of the lesser trochanter is important in evaluating the stability of the reduction. If the lesser trochanter is displaced with a large fragment, a significant cortical defect is present posteromedially, and the fracture geometry indicates a potentially unstable reduction. The surgeon should carefully inspect the radiographs for this defect or palpate this region to feel for a defect. If the defect is seen on preoperative radiographs, the decision may be made to change internal fixation devices from a plate to an intramedullary device. Reduction can be done by open or closed means, with either method, the objective is a stable reduction, whether anatomical or nonanatomical.

Usually, closed reduction by manipulation should be attempted initially. In most fractures, an anatomical reduction with posteromedial apposition is possible. Fluoroscopy, with good-quality AP and lateral views, is used to evaluate the quality of the reduction, with special attention paid to the cortical contact medially and posteriorly. If good medial cortical contact is seen on the AP view and good posterior cortical contact is seen on the lateral view, the fracture can be internally fixed in this position. If a gap or overlap exists medially or posteriorly, adjustments in the traction or rotation may correct the reduction to a stable anatomical position. Frequently, in comminuted fractures, the distal shaft fragment sags posteriorly and may be difficult to correct by closed manipulation. In such cases, open anatomical reduction should be considered and the posterior sag may be corrected by lifting up with a hip skid under the fracture by an assistant. This position may need to be maintained during internal fixation to prevent recurrence of the deformity. In an in vitro, biomechanical study of posterior sag of 30° or more in two-part intertrochanteric fractures, scientists found no significant difference in construct strength or stability. If necessary, an open anatomical reduction of the medial and posterior cortical support can usually be accomplished by applying a bone-holding forceps across the fracture in an AP plane while adjusting the traction and rotation.

When an anatomically stable reduction has been achieved, a compression hip screw or other device can be used to secure the reduction. In rare cases, if the fracture is severely comminuted, anatomical reduction even by open means is difficult, if not impossible. In such circumstances, it may be wise to accept the nonanatomical, but stable reduction obtained by medial displacement techniques; however, a reduction that is nonanatomical and unstable should not be accepted. Stable fractures are treated by internal fixation after anatomical reduction. Unstable fractures usually can be treated by anatomical reduction, with the use of a collapsible fixation device, such as a hip compression screw or cephalomedullary nail. Such collapsible internal fixation devices permit the proximal fragment, to collapse or settle onto the fixation device, seeking its own position of stability, with the shaft usually displacing medially, as shown in Figures 126A to C. Enlarged width to improve purchase in soft bone. We routinely use prophylactic antibiotics in the perioperative. Some authors have suggested that unstable trochanteric fractures in patients with severely osteoporotic bone are best thought of as pathological fractures and that the use of PMMA, to augment the fixation can improve stability in these patients. They recommended PMMA augmentation for unstable trochanteric fractures in elderly patients with severe osteoporosis, for whom no better form of fixation is available and the bone is too porotic to hold a screw. Some orthopedic manufacturers have introduced "super lag" screws that have screw threads of a period. Generally, a first generation cephalosporin is administered immediately before surgery and is continued for 24 hours after surgery. Some form of prophylactic anticoagulation therapy is also indicated, such as ultra-low-molecular-weight heparin (enoxaparin) or warfarin (Coumadin), however these are associated with complications of bleeding and postoperative hematomas. As of yet, there is no ideal prophylaxis for thromboembolism in these patients. Physical therapy is essential for successful restoration of mobility. The goal of physical therapy is a return to prefracture ambulation and overall function. Age younger than 85 years and the absence of multiple comorbid conditions correlated with the resumption of prefracture ambulatory status. We routinely have patients ambulating the day after surgery. When stable fixation has been achieved, as is our goal, we allow weight bearing as tolerated or full weight bearing immediately. In this population, patients often do not have the upper body strength or balance to be less than full weight bearing.

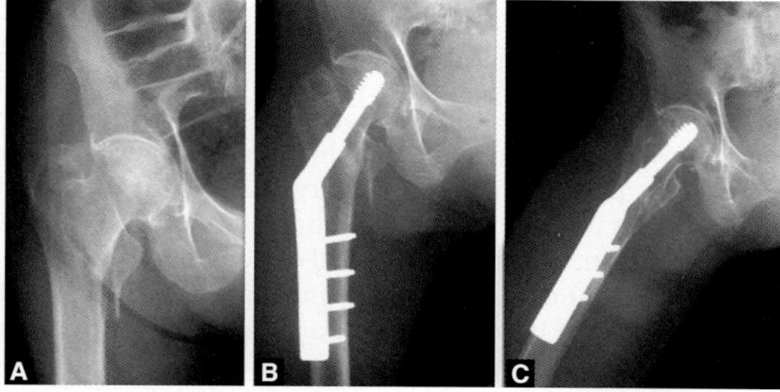

Figs. 126A to C: Unstable fractures treated by anatomical reduction, with the use of a collapsible fixation device, such as a hip compression screw or cephalomedullary nail.

Implant Selection

Two broad categories of internal fixation devices are commonly used for intertrochanteric femoral fractures, sliding compression hip screws with side plate assemblies, as shown in Figure 127 and intramedullary fixation devices, shown in Figures 128A and B. Sliding hip screws, include traditional compression hip screws

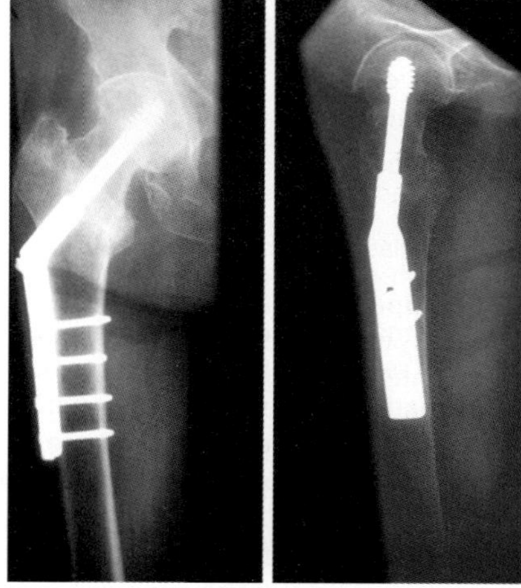

Fig. 127: Intertrochanteric femoral fractures treatment, using sliding compression hip screws with side plate assemblies.

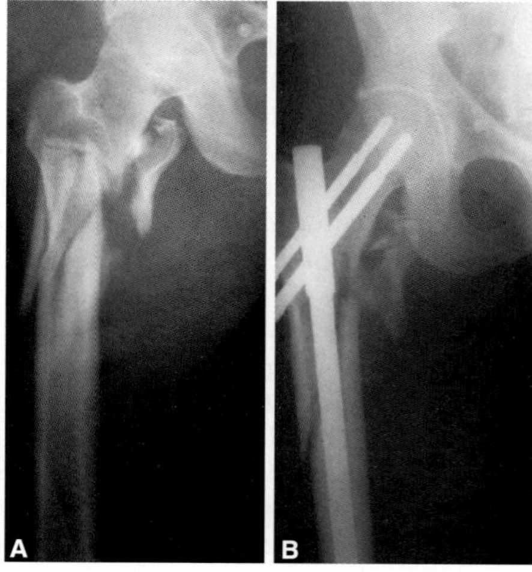

Figs. 128A and B: Intertrochanteric femoral fractures treatment, using intramedullary fixation devices.

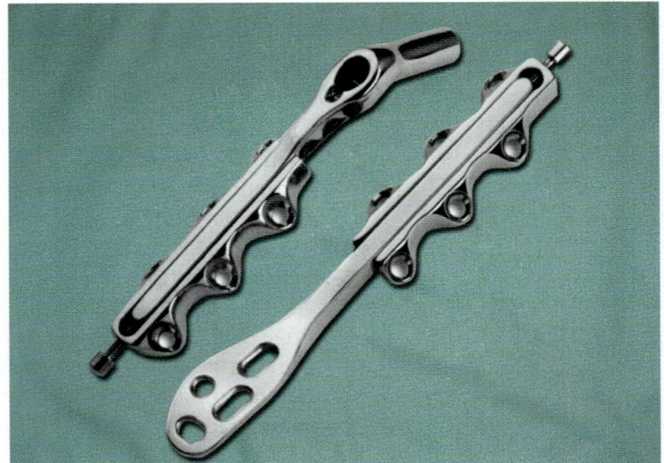

Fig. 129: Sliding hip screws, include traditional compression hip screws that provide compression in the intertrochanteric plane and compression plates that provide additional compression axially.

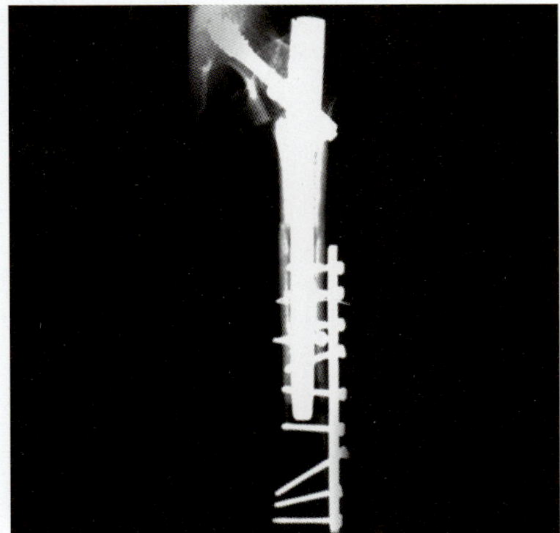

Fig. 130: Intramedullary nails.

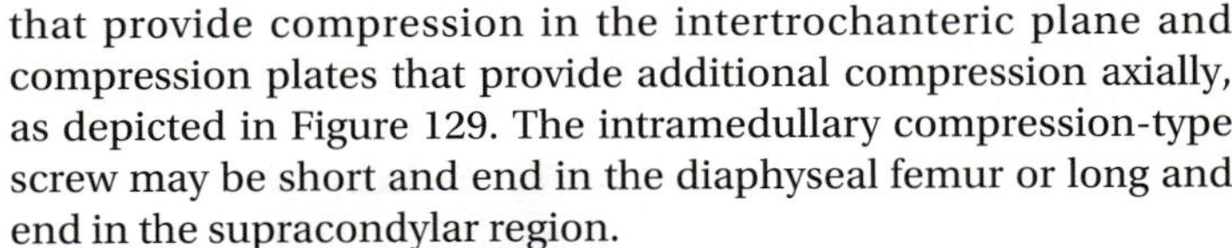

that provide compression in the intertrochanteric plane and compression plates that provide additional compression axially, as depicted in Figure 129. The intramedullary compression-type screw may be short and end in the diaphyseal femur or long and end in the supracondylar region.

The preferred type of device is controversial. Intramedullary nails have a biomechanical and biological advantage over standard compression hip screws. Intramedullary nails can be inserted with less exposure of the fracture and less blood loss, although they require more fluoroscopic exposure and have been associated with fracture comminution. Biomechanically, nails allow for stable anatomical fixation of more comminuted fractures, without shortening the abductor moment arm or changing the proximal femoral anatomy. These devices provide fracture stability by virtue of allowing the lateral aspect of the head and neck, to come to rest against the nail in the medullary canal. Due to complication, we prefer the longer version of these implants, which extends to the supracondylar region of the femur, as shown in Figure 130. Intramedullary nails seem to have some advantage in unstable fractures, especially fractures with reverse obliquity and subtrochanteric extension that cannot be treated easily with standard hip compression screws institution. Stable fractures (AO A1.1 through A2.1) may be treated by either devices, but the literature does not support the routine use of intramedullary nails in stable fractures because of concerns over the added complexity of the procedure and added expense of the intramedullary implants.

Fixation with Sliding Compression Hip Screw Devices

Sliding compression screw assemblies were introduced, to allow compression of some intertrochanteric fractures. The depth to which the lag screw fixation is inserted into the head is crucial for maximal purchase on the proximal fragment; the screw should be inserted to within 1 cm of the subchondral bone. The optimal angle between the barrel and the side plate of a hip compression screw is controversial. Many authors have argued that 150° plates are preferable because the angle of the lag screw more closely parallels the compressive forces within the femoral neck. Theoretically, this should lead to less binding of the screw within the barrel of the side plate and less chance of failure of the implant from bending. In clinical studies, however no difference has been found in the compression ability of 135° hip compression screws and 150° devices. Plate fracture secondary to failure in a bending mode has been reported only rarely in true intertrochanteric fractures. More problematic is the placement of 150° lag screws in the center of the femoral head because they tend toward superior placement within the head, leading to a higher chance of screw cutout. Due to the 135° devices are easily placed and because their clinical results are similar to those for the 150° plates, the higher angle plates are only rarely indicated for extremely valgus femoral necks and more distal fractures.

In the past, with fixation devices that did not allow collapse, medial displacement osteotomy was performed more frequently. They found that in four-part intertrochanteric fractures, anatomical reduction with the sliding hip screw, regardless of the presence of a posteromedial fragment, provided significantly higher compression across the calcar region and significantly lower tensile strain on the side plate than did medial displacement osteotomy. Scientists compared unstable intertrochanteric fractures treated with anatomical reduction and a hip compression screw with fractures treated with medial displacement osteotomy and found no significant differences in eventual healing or walking ability, although surgery time and blood loss were higher in the osteotomy group. These researchers concluded that there was no advantage to medial displacement osteotomy in these fractures. A short-barrel side plate is often needed with this technique, to prevent impingement of the compression screw against the barrel in the neck of the femur with this configuration. Disadvantages include a larger plate profile and the possibility of mechanical failure of the angle-locking mechanism. This aids in resisting lateral sliding of the proximal fragment and maintaining an anatomical reduction, as illustrated in Figure 131. The current version of this device, allows for sliding of the screw in the barrel and is applied on top of a compression hip screw. This technique adds to surgical time, blood loss, and amount of dissection needed to apply the device. The two barrels and screws are inserted in the head of the femur and all screws are inserted percutaneously. We have limited experience with these devices and the literature has not supported their widespread use.

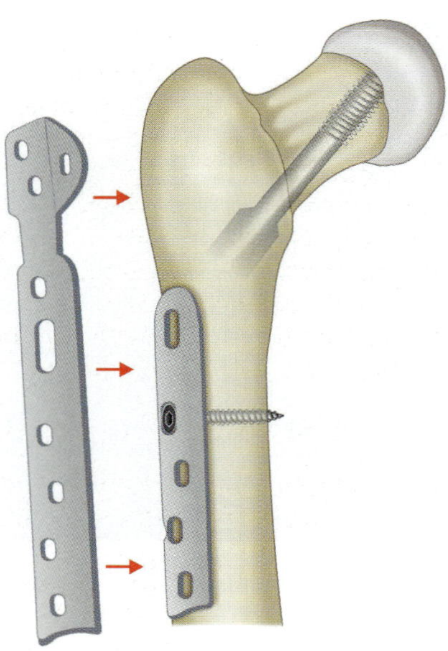

Fig. 131: Reduction with a hip compression screw and medial displacement osteotomy. A short-barrel side plate often is needed with this technique, to prevent impingement of the compression screw against the barrel in the neck of the femur with this configuration.

Compression Hip Screw Fixation of an Intertrochanteric Hip Fracture

The techniques for hip screw insertion are similar for all devices. The technique described next is for the Richards classic compression screw.

After treatment:
The patient is mobilized the day after surgery and active exercises of the upper and lower extremities are begun. Depending on the patient's condition and the stability of the internal fixation, weight-bearing to tolerance is begun using a walker.

Biaxial Compression Plate Fixation

Medoff modified the standard compression hip screw, recognizing the need for axial compression until stability is obtained, especially in intertrochanteric fractures with a significant subtrochanteric component. His modification includes the traditional proximal screw in a barrel, a two-part sliding plate, and a distally positioned compression screw, to compress the proximal femoral fracture fragment to the shaft in the subtrochanteric region.

The plate that is applied to the lateral part of the femur is in two parts, with the barrel and proximal part sliding into a slot on the distal part that is fixed to the femur with oblique screws. It is usually recommended for unstable intertrochanteric fractures and subtrochanteric fractures. The Medoff plate comes in two versions—six-hole and four-hole plates. The six-hole plate has an axial compression screw at the end of the plate and a proximal blocking screw, to prevent barrel back-out in highly comminuted fractures and to provide for more axial and anatomical compression.

Intertrochanteric Osteotomy

Emphasizing that restoration of medial continuity is essential to successful internal fixation of three-part and four-part intertrochanteric fractures, as shown in Figure 132. More recent studies have indicated, however, that anatomical reduction allows greater load sharing, by the bone than does medial displacement osteotomy and that with sliding hip compression screw devices, stability is not improved by osteotomy. Knowledge of these techniques is still occasionally useful in some extremely comminuted fractures, in which anatomical reduction is not feasible.

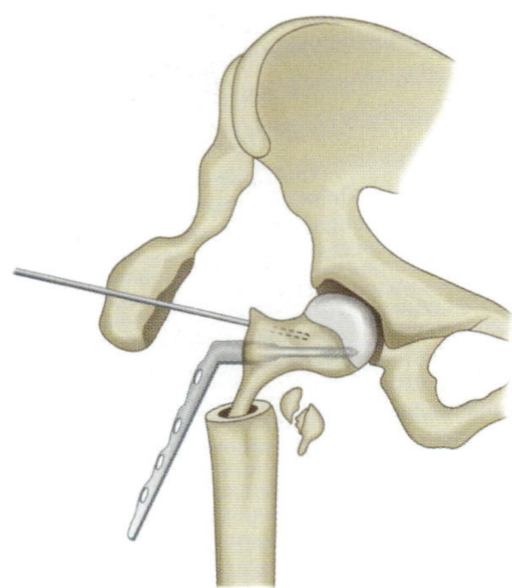

Fig. 132: Intertrochanteric osteotomy.

Fixation with Intramedullary Devices

Intramedullary devices have at least theoretical advantages over open reduction procedures in that the surgical procedure for insertion is much less extensive, the fracture is not opened, and the operating time and blood loss may be lessened. With the fixation device within the medullary canal, the bending moment on it is considerably less than on standard compression screw and side plate devices. Cephalomedullary nails, such as the Gamma nail, the intramedullary hip screw, and interlocking intramedullary nails inserted in the Recon mode, have been used for fixation of unstable intertrochanteric fractures. These devices are centromedullary nails with proximal fixation into the femoral head by nails, screws, or blades.

The Gamma nail and intramedullary hip screw began, as shorter nails than reconstruction nails, with the device ending within the diaphysis of the femur. This allows relatively reliable targeting of the distal interlocking screws through a proximally attached insertion guide.

Changes in the angle of the nail and a smaller diameter have decreased the incidence of this complication, but because there is still a risk of late fracture and because this patient population is at risk for further falls, we advocate the use of long intramedullary nails that end at the supracondylar region of the femur. Unless, there is extensive comminution that increases the risk for shortening, or unless the medullary canal is unusually large increasing the risk for late malrotation, we usually do not lock the distal ends of these long nails when used for intertrochanteric fractures.

The literature on these devices and our experience are limited. These devices seem to have some benefit in reverse obliquity intertrochanteric fractures and in fractures with subtrochanteric extension, but not for routine, stable intertrochanteric hip fractures. The technique for intramedullary hip screw placement is similar to the Gamma nail technique and is useful in the treatment of unstable peritrochanteric fractures, reverse obliquity fractures, and subtrochanteric fractures. The intramedullary hip screw nail is cannulated with a 4° mediolateral bend, to allow for insertion through the GT. It is used with a standard Richards AMBI/Classic lag screw (½-inch thread diameter) and compression screw. A sleeve over the lag screw is used to prevent rotation, while allowing the lag screw to slide. The long nail is designed for subtrochanteric fractures, femoral reconstruction after tumor resection, prophylactic nailing of impending pathological fractures, and leg-length discrepancies after femoral fracture. The nail has a distal diameter of 10 mm and is available in lengths of 34 cm, 38 cm, and 42 cm and angles of 130° and 135°. A slight bend in the nail conforms to the natural bow of the femoral shaft and the 10° of anteversion, matches the angle of the femoral head in relation to the shaft of the femur. Distal locking is accomplished with 4.5 mm locking screws. The long nail has a proximal diameter of 17.5 mm. The operation is performed on a standard fracture table and requires the use of an image intensifier, which produces images in two planes. AP and lateral views of the proximal one-half of the femur should be obtained preoperatively or fluoroscopically, at the time of surgery. Severe deformities of the femoral canal or excessive anterior bowing may preclude the use of an intramedullary device.

After treatment:

In peritrochanteric fractures, with a stable configuration (i.e. where the medial cortical buttress and lesser trochanter remain intact), early full weight-bearing is permitted. The patients are mobilized the first day after surgery and full weight bearing is allowed as tolerated.

Prosthetic Arthroplasty

In patients with severe osteoporosis with significant comminution, prosthetic replacement may be considered; however, the extensive surgery necessary may be unjustified in elderly patients with low activity demands and limited life expectancies.

Prosthetic replacement is a useful technique for the occasional patient with an intertrochanteric nonunion and failure of fixation, when the head is damaged or the bone is poor, as shown in Figures 133A and B. In calcar replacement, femoral components usually are needed because of loss of most of the femoral neck and possibly the lesser trochanter.

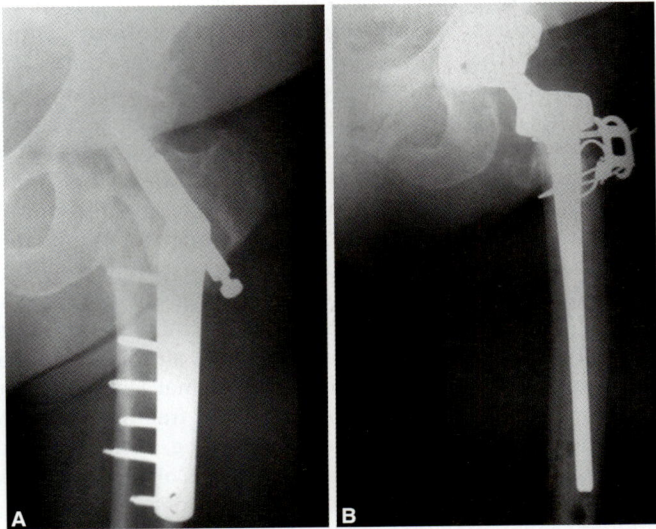

Figs. 133A and B: Prosthetic replacement for intertrochanteric nonunion and failure of fixation.

Salvage Procedures

If there is a nonunion or loss of fixation of an inter-trochanteric fracture and the articular cartilage of the head has not been damaged by the implant, the hip may be saved by revising the internal fixation and bone grafting the fracture. In a series of 20 patients (mean age 58 years) by Haidukewych and Berry, 11 patients had secondary hip fixation with an angled blade plate, five had a dynamic hip screw, three had a condylar screw, and one had a cephalomedullary nail. Bone grafting was used in all patients and 19 of the 20 healed. We usually change from intramedullary to extramedullary forms of fixation (or vice versa).

SUBTROCHANTERIC FEMORAL FRACTURES

Some scientists called attention to subtrochanteric fractures, as a variant of peritrochanteric fractures and noted their higher incidence of unsatisfactory results after operative treatment. Since that time, subtrochanteric fractures have been variously defined, but most authors limit the term to fractures between the lesser trochanter and the isthmus of the diaphysis. They have a bimodal age distribution and different mechanisms of injury. Older patients typically sustain low-velocity trauma, whereas in younger patients, these fractures commonly result from high-energy trauma and often are associated with other fractures and injuries. Restoration of femoral length and rotation and correction of femoral head, and neck angulation to restore adequate abductor tension and strength are essential, to restoring maximal ambulatory capacity.

Classification

The introduction of various classification systems gives some insight into the evolution of treatment options and indicates the uncertainty regarding the treatment and prognosis of this complex fracture. Boyd and Griffin in their classification of trochanteric fractures, included subtrochanteric elements in types III and IV. According to Fielding's classification of subtrochanteric fractures, a type I fracture is at the level of the lesser trochanter, a type II fracture is 2.5–5 cm below the lesser trochanter and a type III fracture is 5–7.5 cm below the lesser trochanter. Transverse fractures fit this classification well, but oblique and comminuted fractures may involve more than one of the levels described and should be classified according to, where the major portion of the fracture occurs. Traditionally, fractures at the upper level have a better prognosis for union than fractures at the lower level. Seinsheimer developed the following classification system based on the number of fragments, and the location and configuration of the fracture lines, as shown in Figure 134 and Table 6.

With the development of modern reconstruction nails, also known as second-generation intramedullary nails, the classification schemes of Fielding and Seinsheimer have become less useful because they do not separate fractures according to the different treatment methods. At this institution, Russell and Taylor devised a classification scheme based on lesser trochanteric continuity and fracture extension posteriorly on the GT involving the piriformis fossa, the major two variables influencing treatment, as shown in Figure 135.

Type I fractures do not extend into the piriformis fossa, whereas type II fractures do involve the piriformis fossa, in the past, the most commonly used nail entry portal. In type IA fractures, the lesser trochanter is intact and in type IB fractures, the lesser trochanter is fractured. In type IA fractures, comminution and fracture lines

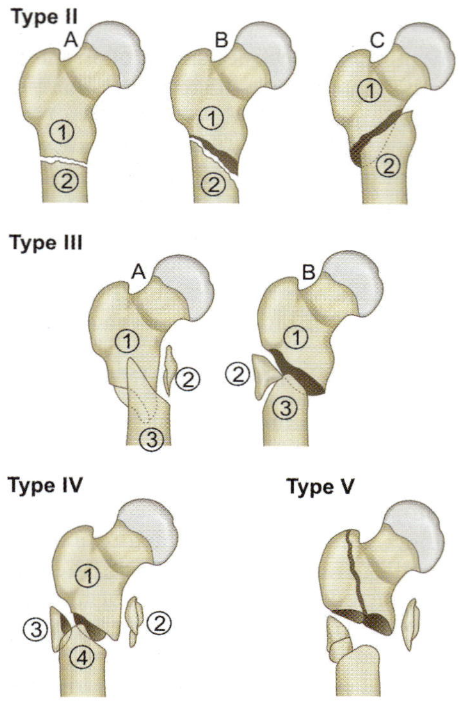

Fig. 134: Seinsheimer, classification of femoral subchondral fractures.

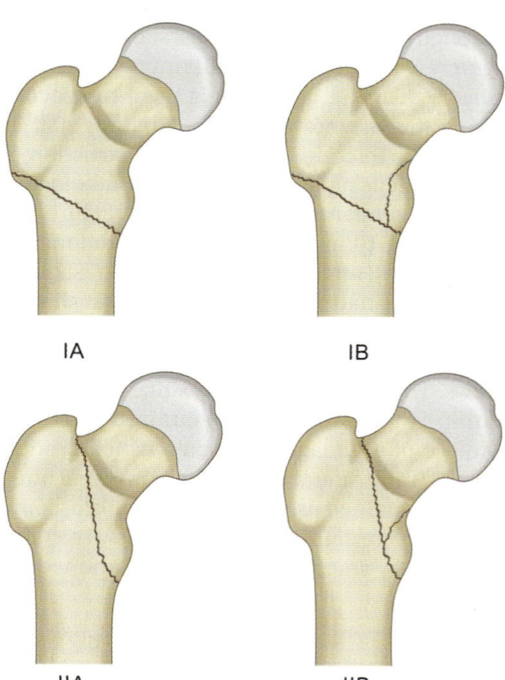

Fig. 135: Russell and Taylor classification of femoral subchondral fractures.

TABLE 6: Seinsheimer, classification system for femoral subchondral fractures.

Type I:	Nondisplaced fracture or one with less than 2 mm of displacement
Type II:	Two-part fracture
Type IIA:	Transverse fracture
Type IIB:	Spiral configuration with the lesser trochanter attached to proximal fragment
Type IIC:	Spiral configuration with the lesser trochanter attached to distal fragment
Type III:	Three-part fracture
Type IIIA:	Three-part spiral configuration with the lesser trochanter a part of the third fragment
Type IIIB:	Three-part spiral configuration with the third part a butterfly fragment
Type IV:	Comminuted fracture with four or more fragments
Type V:	Subtrochanteric-intertrochanteric configuration

extend from below the lesser trochanter to the femoral isthmus, any degree of comminution may be present in this area, including bicortical comminution. Type IB fractures have fracture lines and comminution, involving the area of the lesser trochanter to the isthmus (see Figure Type IIA fractures extend from the lesser trochanter to the isthmus, with extension into the piriformis fossa, as detected on lateral radiographs, but significant comminution or major fracture of the lesser trochanter is not present). In type IIB fractures, the fracture extends into the piriformis fossa with significant comminution of the medial femoral cortex and loss of continuity of the lesser trochanter. In type I fractures, closed intramedullary nailing has the advantage of minimizing vascular compromise of the fracture fragments. In type II fractures, the extension into the piriformis fossa complicates closed nailing techniques. In type IA and IIA fractures, the lesser trochanter is intact, making medial stability more likely. Plate fixation may be the device of choice. With the development of nails that are placed through a trochanteric portal, it is even more likely that the nail's entry portal will be fractured. For this reason, careful attention to surgical technique is necessary, to avoid further comminution of the fracture or inadvertently displacing the fracture during nail insertion.

Treatment

Treatment methods for subtrochanteric fractures have included nonoperative methods, such as traction techniques, which yielded variable results. Plate and screw fixation of subtrochanteric fractures is still advocated by many authors, especially for fractures with intertrochanteric extension, such as Russell-Taylor types IIA and IIB fractures. In this group, all fractures united and there were no deep infections. Compression hip screws have been a popular method of internal fixation for subtrochanteric fractures. They credit at least a portion of their good results to the approach that preserves the fracture's vascularity. Advantages of intramedullary devices also include retained blood supply to bone fragments, less operative blood loss, and less disruption of the fracture environment. Modern reconstruction nails have greatly improved the outcome and ease of treatment of subtrochanteric fractures. The first modern cephalomedullary reconstruction nail, the Russell-Taylor reconstruction nail is a closed-section, stainless steel nail with proximal interlocking screws that extend into the femoral head and distal interlocking screws similar to standard first-generation interlocking nails. In the original series of patients treated with this device, 59 subtrochanteric fractures all healed uneventfully without the need for bone grafting, auxiliary fixation, immobilization, or nail dynamization (removal of the distal locking screws to allow fracture impaction in cases of delayed union).

Short cephalomedullary nails, principally the Gamma nail and similar devices, including the intramedullary hip screw have been used for high subtrochanteric fractures and for intertrochanteric fractures with subtrochanteric extension. A potential complication of these devices is late femoral fracture at the tip of the device, this does not occur with nails that extend well into the distal metaphysis of the femur. For this reason, we usually do not use short intramedullary devices. Before the development of closed-section interlocking reconstruction nails, complex subtrochanteric fractures were treated at our institution with compression hip screws and side plates with bone grafting, if the medial cortex was comminuted. Difficulty often was encountered, when comminution was extensive. Cephalomedullary interlocking nailing allows length and rotational control, even when the lesser trochanter is not intact. Involvement of the piriformis fossa, the entry portal for the device, does not contraindicate its use, but does increase the technical difficulty of placement. The choice of treatment of subtrochanteric fractures depends on several factors.

- When the greater and lesser trochanters are intact, conventional interlocking intramedullary nailing may be indicated.
- In fractures with extension into the lesser trochanter, the Russell-Taylor reconstruction nail, inserted with closed techniques is our treatment of choice.
- Plate and screw fixation probably is best used for fractures in patients with preexisting deformities of the proximal femur, previous implants or Russell-Taylor type IIA fractures.
- Pathological fractures of the subtrochanteric area are best treated with reconstruction nails, which allow stabilization of the entire femur.
- In general, our treatment recommendations are based on the involvement of the piriformis fossa or GT, as the usual entry portals for nails.
- Regular interlocking intramedullary nails can be used for fixation of most femoral fractures between the distal fifth of the femur and a point just distal to the lesser trochanter.
- We prefer a cephalomedullary reconstruction nail, for fractures with extension into the lesser trochanter (Russell-Taylor type IB), as shown in Figures 136A and B.

Russell-Taylor types IIA and IIB fractures can be treated with reconstruction nails, although the technique becomes more demanding, as shown in Figures 137A to C. Closed techniques, with image intensifier guidance can be used. Determination of the proper entry portal is more difficult, improper positioning of the nail can occur, if the guidewire or nail, itself slips posteriorly in the comminution around the trochanteric or piriformis fossa entry portal, stabilization of the posterior fragment may be inadequate and nail placement lateral to the correct portal predisposes to varus deformity at the fracture. In a series of 61 unstable subtrochanteric fractures treated at this clinic with Russell-Taylor reconstruction nails, 12 displayed extension of the fracture into the piriformis fossa (Russell-Taylor types IIA and IIB). Careful attention to proper guidewire positioning, allowed successful nail placement in all 12 fractures. Type II fractures, with involvement of the piriformis fossa, can also be fixed with a hip compression screw or Medoff plate and an indirect reduction technique. For type IIB fractures, autogenous bone grafting should be considered at the time of fixation of the fracture if the fracture is opened.

Fixation with an Interlocking Reconstruction Nail

Care must be taken, however, to avoid the same complications that occur with nailing of any fracture, in which the entry portal is involved in the fracture site, displacement of the fracture and the nail not being contained within the bone. In subtrochanteric fractures, there is a tendency for the nail to fall posteriorly out of the femur proximally, if the GT is comminuted and a portal is placed there. The TriGen nail has replaced the Russell-Taylor nail at our

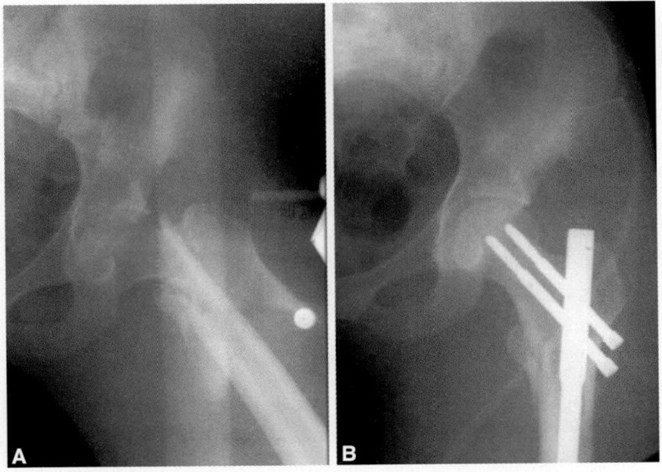

Figs. 136A and B: Intramedullary nailing: Cephalomedullary reconstruction nail for fractures with extension into the lesser trochanter.

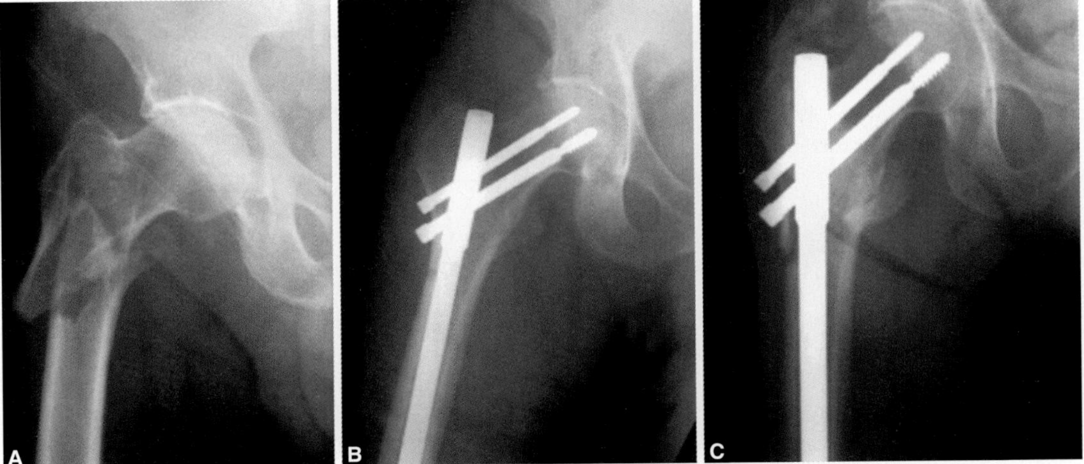

Figs. 137A to C: Reconstruction nailing in Russell-Taylor types IIA and IIB fractures.

clinic, as the cephalomedullary nail of choice in subtrochanteric fractures. It is a titanium closed-section nail that has a 5° lateral proximal bow, to make use of a trochanteric entry portal. Two holes in the nail allow two 6.4 mm, titanium, and partially threaded locking screws, to be inserted into the femoral head. The angle between the shaft of the nail and the proximal locking screws is 135°. Lengths range from 30–50 cm and the nail comes in 10 mm, 11.5 mm, and 13 mm diameters.

After treatment:
The patient is allowed to ambulate partial weight bearing, with crutches the day after surgery. Progressive weight bearing is based on radiographic evidence of callus formation.

Fixation with Hip Compression Screw and Side Plate

Biomechanical and clinical studies have indicated that Russell-Taylor type II subtrochanteric fractures can be fixed adequately with a hip compression screw and side plate combination.

Newer systems have improved fatigue characteristics and loss of fixation usually occurs from cutout of the screw from the femoral head, rather than from fracture of the plate, as occurred with older designs. For subtrochanteric fractures, detailed preoperative planning is essential. Lag screw fixation of major fragments should be planned carefully, to avoid placing the screws in areas that would be compromised by plate application. We use an AO femoral distractor and the indirect reduction technique described by Kinast et al. After provisional reduction has been obtained and is held with Kirschner wires, the hip compression screw is inserted in the standard manner. At least four screws should engage both cortices in the distal fragment. Lag screws can be used through the plate, but screw fixation in the proximal fragment, prevents the compression screw from obtaining some dynamization. The hip compression screw device used should prevent rotation of the lag screw in the barrel. If medial dissection is necessary, autogenous iliac bone grafting should be used. In a similar way, the Medoff plate can be used, especially if the comminution does not extend distally down the shaft of the femur.

Indirect Reduction and Fixation with a 95° Condylar Plate

Some scientists compared their results of open reduction and blade plate fixation of subtrochanteric fractures with indirect reduction and fixation.

After treatment:
After treatment is similar to that for hip compression screw fixation of intertrochanteric fractures. Generally, the medial buttress is not completely restored and only touch-down weight bearing is allowed, until signs of early fracture healing are present at 6–8 weeks. Full weight bearing, is usually delayed for up to 3 months after surgery.

TRAUMATIC DISLOCATION OF HIP

Introduction

Hip dislocations were once a rarity and have become increasingly common due to increased number of automobile accidents and high speed transportation.

Traumatic dislocation of hip joint includes pure hip dislocation, dislocation with fracture femoral neck and dislocations with fracture of acetabulum.

Joint Contact Area (Fig. 138)

Throughout ROM:
- 40% of femoral head is in contact with acetabular articular cartilage.
- 10% of femoral head is in contact with labrum.

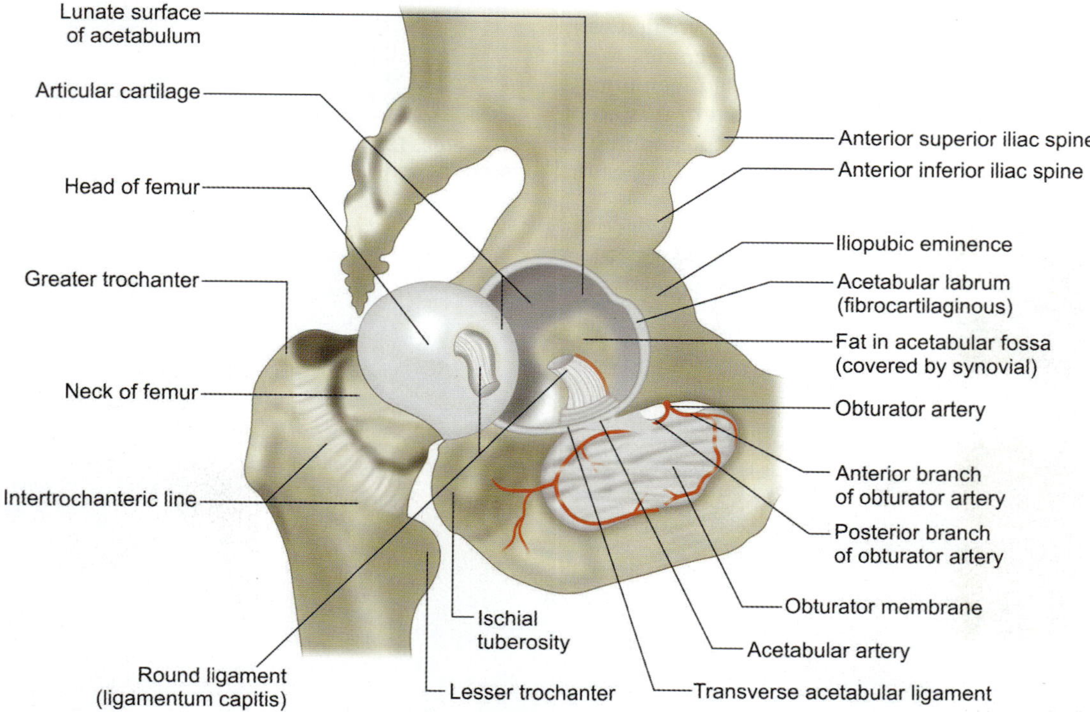

Fig. 138: Hip joint opened lateral view, showing joint contact areas.

Hip Joint Capsule (Fig. 139)

Extends from intertrochanteric ridge of proximal femur to bony perimeter of acetabulum. It has several thick bands of fibrous tissue.

Iliofemoral ligament:

- Upside-down "Y"
- Blocks hip extension
- Allows muscle relaxation with standing.

Acetabular labrum (Fig. 140):

- Strong fibrous ring
- Increases femoral head coverage
- Contributes to hip joint stability.

Blood Supply to Femoral Head (See Figs. 18A to C)

Artery of ligamentum teres

- Most important in children
- Its contribution decreases with age and is probably insignificant in elderly patients
- *Ascending cervical branches (Fig. 141):* Arise from ring at base of neck. Ring is formed by branches of medial and lateral circumflex femoral arteries. Penetrate capsule near its femoral attachment and ascend along neck. Perforate bone just distal to articular cartilage. It is highly susceptible to injury with hip dislocation.

Sciatic Nerve (Fig. 142)

- It is formed from roots of L4 to S3.
- Peroneal and tibial components differentiate early, sometimes as proximal as in pelvis.
- Passes posterior to posterior wall of acetabulum.
- Generally, passes inferior to piriformis muscle, but occasionally the piriformis will split the peroneal and tibial components.

Classification of Hip Dislocation

- Congenital
- Acquired
  - Traumatic

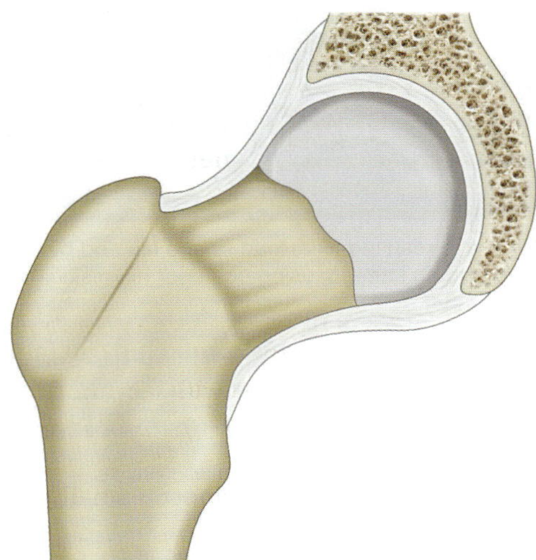

Fig. 139: Hip joint capsule.

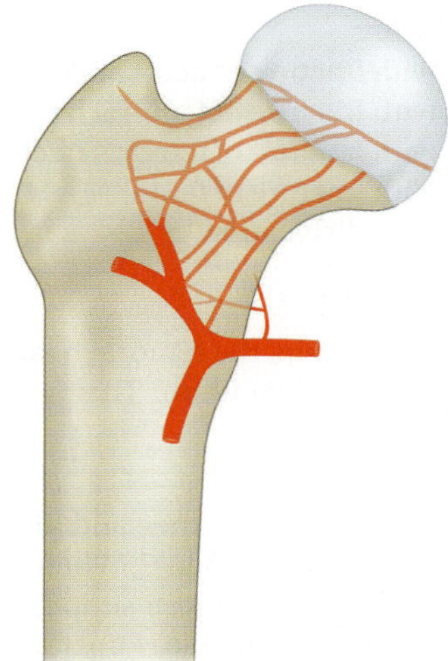

Fig. 141: Arteries of ligamentum teres, showing ascending cervical branches.

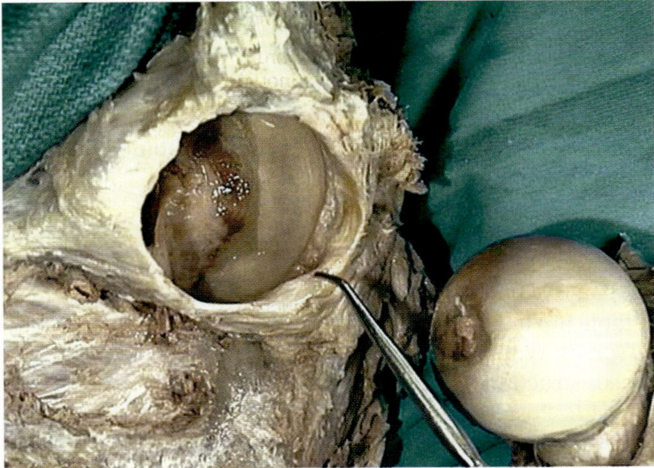

Fig. 140: Opened hip joint with acetabular labrum.

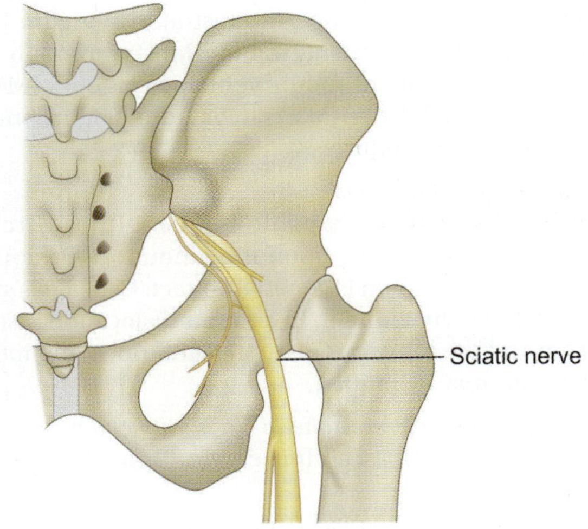

Fig. 142: Sciatic nerve origin and course, as it passes posterior to posterior wall of acetabulum.

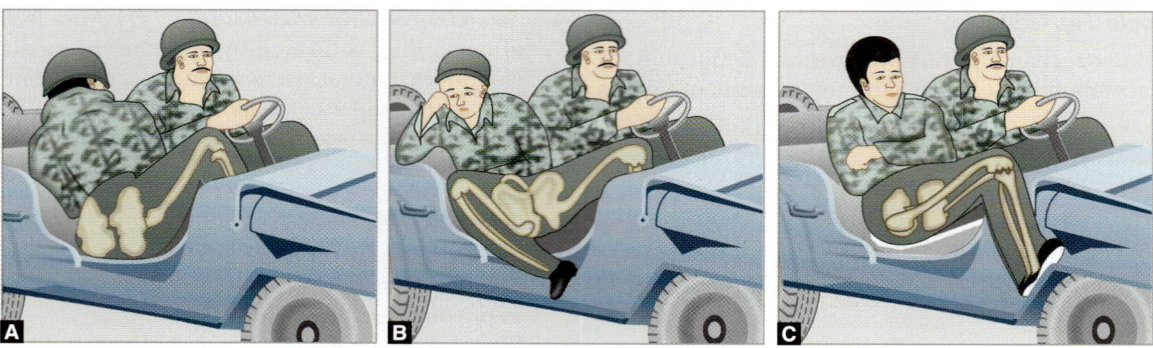

Figs. 143A to C: Different mechanisms of posterior hip dislocation.

- Pathological, e.g. tubercular arthritis and pyogenic arthritis
- Paralytic, e.g. poliomyelitis and cerebral palsy.

Classification of traumatic dislocation hip:

- Simple dislocations
  - Posterior dislocation
  - Anterior dislocation
- Fracture dislocations
  - Associated with fracture of acetabular rim
  - Associated with fracture of femoral head
  - Associated with fracture of femoral neck
  - Associated with fracture of femur
  - Central fracture dislocation.

Posterior Dislocation of Hip

In posterior dislocation of hip, the femoral head rests posterior to the coronal plane of the acetabulum. This is the most common type of dislocation.

Mechanism of injuries:

It is due to the force applied to the knee and hip in varying degree of flexion, as shown in Figures 143A to C. When femur is flexed and adducted, the femoral head is not well supported by acetabulum and more dependent on the capsule. Funsten called them dash board injuries, as they occurred in the motor vehicle accidents. If the limb is in slight abduction, fracture of rim of acetabulum and femoral head also takes place. Generally, results from axial load applied to femur, while hip is flexed. Most commonly caused by impact of dashboard on knee, as illustrated in Figure 144. It is almost always due to high-energy trauma. Most commonly involve unrestrained occupants in motor vehicle accidents (MVAs). It can also occur in pedestrian-MVAs, falls from heights, industrial accidents, and sporting injuries.

Pathoanatomy of dislocations:

In posterior dislocation, capsule is torn either directly or inferoposteriorly depending upon the amount of flexion at the time of injury. "Y" ligament is generally intact. Capsule is stripped from its acetabular attachment. In anterior dislocation, psoas acts as a fulcrum and the capsule is disrupted anteriorly and inferiorly. Femoral vessels may be injured.

Effect of dislocation on femoral head circulation:

- When capsule tears, ascending cervical branches are torn or stretched.
- Artery of ligamentum teres is torn.
- Some ascending cervical branches may remain kinked or compressed, until the hip is reduced.

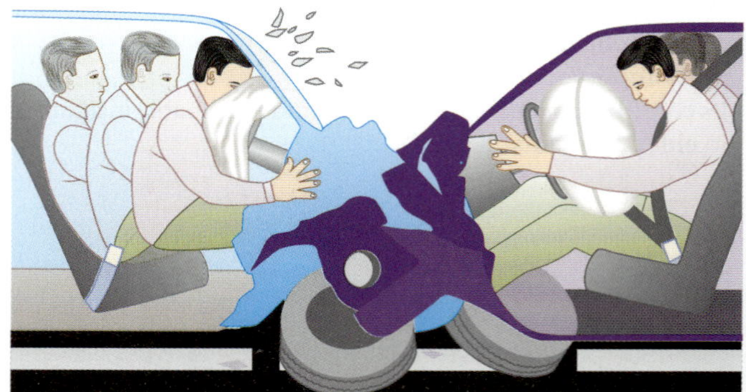

Fig. 144: MVA with resulted axial load on the hip and by the impact of dashboard on knee, causing posterior hip dislocation.

- Thus, early reduction of the dislocated hip can improve blood flow to femoral head.

Thomas and Epstein classification of hip dislocations (most well-known):

- *Type I:* Pure dislocation with at most a small posterior wall fragment.
- *Type II:* Dislocation with large posterior wall fragment.
- *Type III:* Dislocation with comminuted posterior wall.
- *Type IV:* Dislocation with "acetabular floor" fracture (probably transverse and posterior wall acetabulum fracture-dislocation).
- *Type V:* Dislocation with femoral head fracture.

Pipkin Classification (Fig. 145)

- *Type I:* Fracture inferior to fovea
- *Type II:* Fracture superior to fovea
- *Type III:* Fracture of femoral head, with fracture of femoral neck
- *Type IV:* Fracture of femoral head with acetabulum fracture.

Brumback Classification (Figs. 146 and 147)

- *Type I:* Posterior hip dislocation with fracture of the involving inferomedial portion of femoral head.
- *Type IA:* With minimum or no fracture of the acetabular rim and stable hip joint after reduction.
- *Type IB:* With significant acetabular rim and stable joint after reconstruction.
- *Type II:* Posterior hip dislocation with fracture of the femoral head involving the supermedial portion of the femoral head.
- *Type IIA:* With minimum or no fracture of the acetabular rim and stable joint after reduction.

- *Type IIB:* With significant acetabular fracture and hip joint instability.
- *Type III:* Dislocation of the hip with femoral neck fracture.
- *Type IIIA:* Without fracture of femoral head.
- *Type IIIB:* With fracture of femoral head.
- *Type IV:* Anterior dislocation of femoral head.
  - *Type IVA: Indentation type:* Depression of the superolateral surface of the femoral head.
  - *Type IVB: Transchondral type:* Osteocartilaginous fracture of the weight-bearing surface of the femoral head.
- *Type V:* Central fracture dislocation of the hip with femoral head fracture.

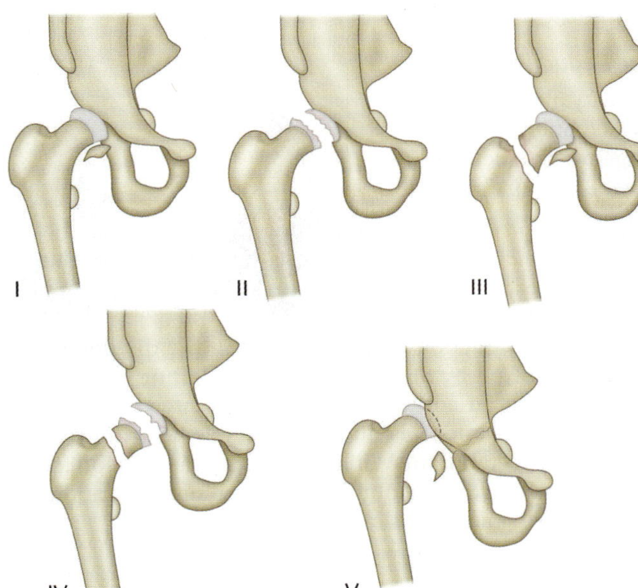

Fig. 145: Pipkin classification of hip dislocation.

Stewart and Milford Classification

- *Type I:* Simple dislocation without fracture
- *Type II:* Dislocation with one or more rim fragments, but with sufficient socket to ensure stability after reduction
- *Type III:* Dislocation with fracture of the rim producing gross instability
- *Type IV:* Dislocation with fracture of the head and NoF.

Evaluation

History:
- Significant trauma, usually MVA.
- Awake, alert patients have severe pain in hip region.

Physical examination:
Classical appearance of posterior dislocation of hip, as shown in Figure 148.

Unclassical presentation (posture) if:
- Femoral head or neck fracture
- Femoral shaft fracture
- Obtunded patient.

Signs and symptoms:
- Pain on palpation of hip
- Pain with attempted motion of hip
- Possible neurological impairment
- Vascular sign of Narath positive
- Femoral head can be palpated in the gluteal region
- Associated ligamentous injury to the ipsilateral knee
- Fracture of the head of femur, femora shaft, and acetabulum
- Sciatic nerve injury
- Patient might be in shock.

Investigations:
X-rays: These include:
- AP X-ray
- Oblique lateral view of pelvis
- Posterior oblique view
- Full length femur.

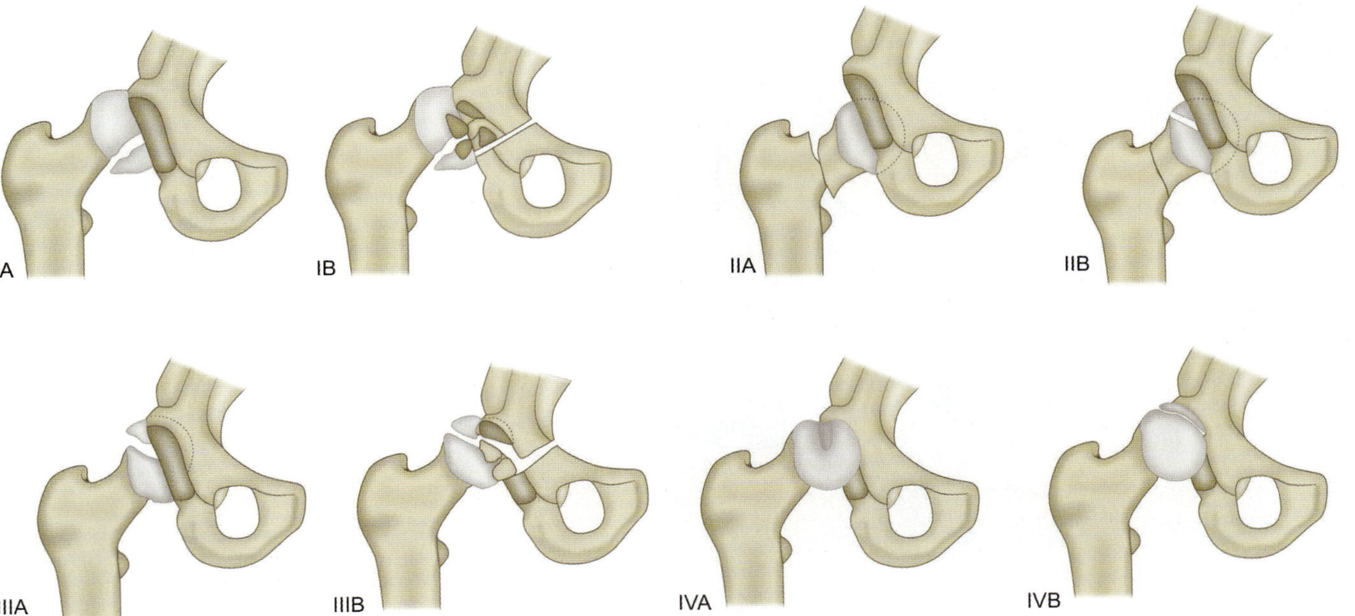

Fig. 146: Brumback classification of hip dislocation.

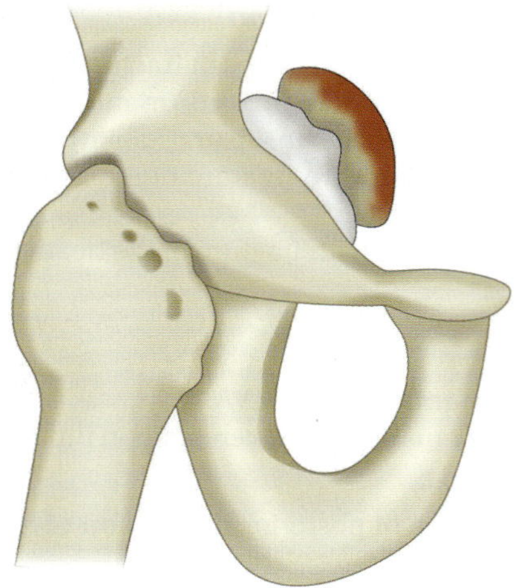

Fig. 147: Brumback classification of hip dislocation—Type V central fracture dislocation of hip.

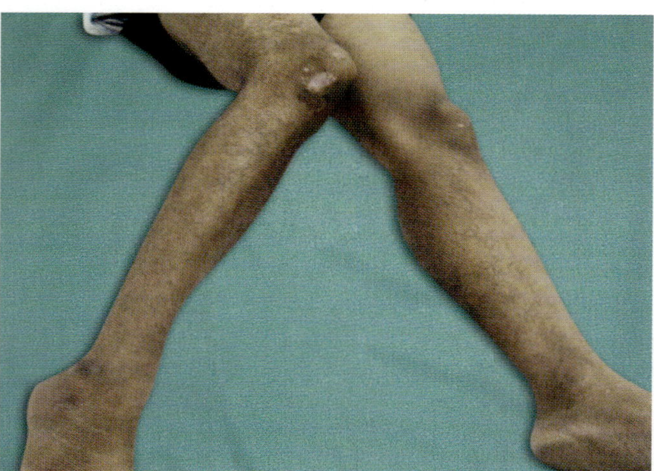

Fig. 148: Posterior dislocation—Hip flexed, internally rotated and adducted.

X-ray findings:

- Loss of congruence of femoral head with roof of acetabulum
- Head will appear smaller than the contralateral head
- Overlapping of the head with the acetabulum
- Lesser trochanter lies apparent and neck seen due to internal rotation
- Break in Shenton's line.

CT scan to delineate fracture fragments size and location.
Routine laboratory investigations.

Management

- Supportive treatment, e.g. treat shock
- Definitive treatment
- Closed reduction
- Open reduction.

Closed Reduction

- Gravity method of Stimson
- Allis maneuver
- Bigelow's maneuver
- East Baltimore method.

Bigelow's maneuver (Figs. 149A to D):

Patient is supine: Assistant applies pressure to the ASIS. Surgeon then grasps the affected limb by the ankle and places his opposite forearm behind the patient's flexed knee.

Longitudinal traction is then applied in the direction of the deformity, followed by the flexion of hip to 90° or greater, while maintaining it in an adduction internally rotated position. This relaxes the "Y" ligament. Femur head comes near the posterior inferior rim of acetabulum. While continuing the traction femoral head is relocated in the acetabulum, by combination of abduction, external rotation and extension of hip.

Gravity method of Stimson (Fig. 150):

Associated injuries prevented, using method. Patient is positioned in prone. Assistant stabilizes pelvis. Involved hip and knee flexed 90°. Grasp knee, just distal to flexed knee. Apply longitudinal force and gentle internal and external rotation.

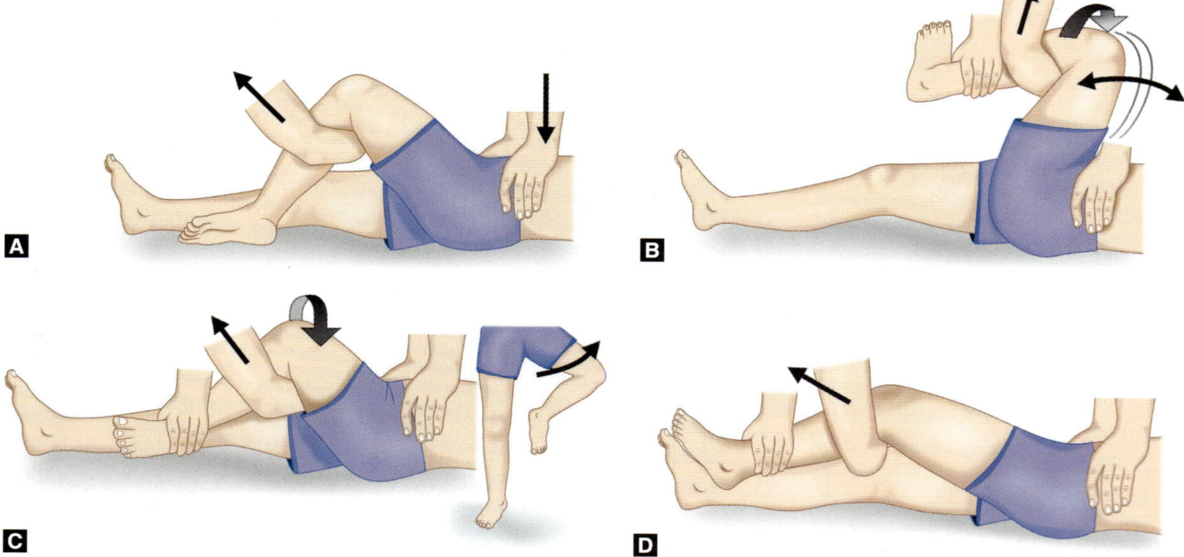

Figs. 149A to D: Different steps of Bigelow's maneuver of closed reduction.

Allis maneuver (Figs. 151A to D):
Patient is supine. Pelvis is stabilized, by assistant applying pressure to ASIS. Surgeon applies longitudinal traction in line of deformity, followed by flexion of the hip to 90°, while continuing traction. Internal and external rotation of hip is then performed until reduction is achieved. Limb is then brought to neutral position.

East Baltimore lift:
Patient is placed supine. Patient's leg is flexed so that the hip and the knee are in 90°. Surgeon places his arm, which is closest to the patient's head under the proximal calf of the patient. Cradling the leg in his elbow, with his hand resting on the shoulder of his assistant. His other hand grasps the patient's ankle. The assistant's arm passes under the proximal calf of the patient and rests on the surgeon's shoulder. Surgeon and assistant squat slightly with knees bend. Then they straighten up together to apply traction to the hip without straining their backs. The surgeon rotates the leg and the ankle and the second assistant stabilizes the pelvis.

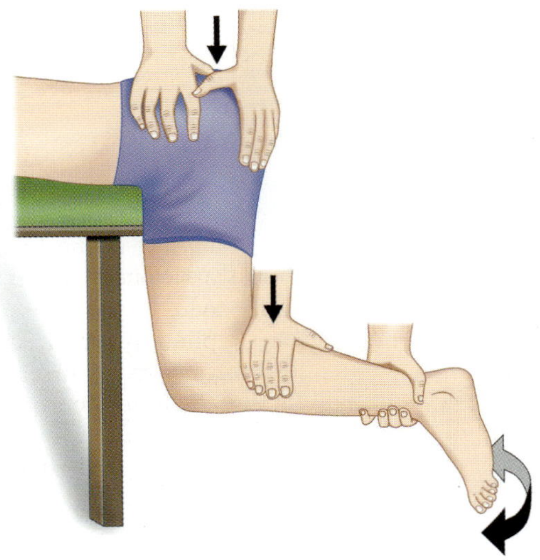

Fig. 150: Gravity method of Stimson for reduction.

Management after closed reduction:
After closed reduction, light skin or skeletal traction is recommended to provide comfort and allow capsular healing. Traction prevents recurrent dislocation, by keeping it in extension, abduction, and external rotation. Traction is maintained until hip is pain free and good ROM achieved. Time of weight bearing is controversial. Stuck and Valerian recommended NWB for 6–12 weeks. Stewart recommended weight bearing 2–4 weeks after reduction.

Open Reduction

Indications of open reduction:
- If closed reduction is not possible after one or two attempts
- Button holing of the femoral head through capsule
- Displacement of piriformis muscle across the acetabulum
- Concentric reduction is prevented by invested acetabular labrum
- Presence of osteochondral loose bodies within the acetabulum.

Three approaches have been described:
1. Anterior approach (Smith Petersons anterior iliofemoral approach)
2. Posterior approach (Osborne)
3. Posterolateral approach (Kocher-Langenback).

Posterior approach is superior to anterior approach because most offending structure are more easily reached through the posterior approach. Anterior approach has more chances of AVN, as posterior retinacular vessels are damaged during dislocation and this approach damages the remaining anterior vascular supply.

After treatment:
Thomas or Buck's traction is given, to immobilize the hip when reduction is stable. Active exercises and physical therapy advocated by 3–10 days. Weight bearing is gradually resumed after 3–4 weeks.

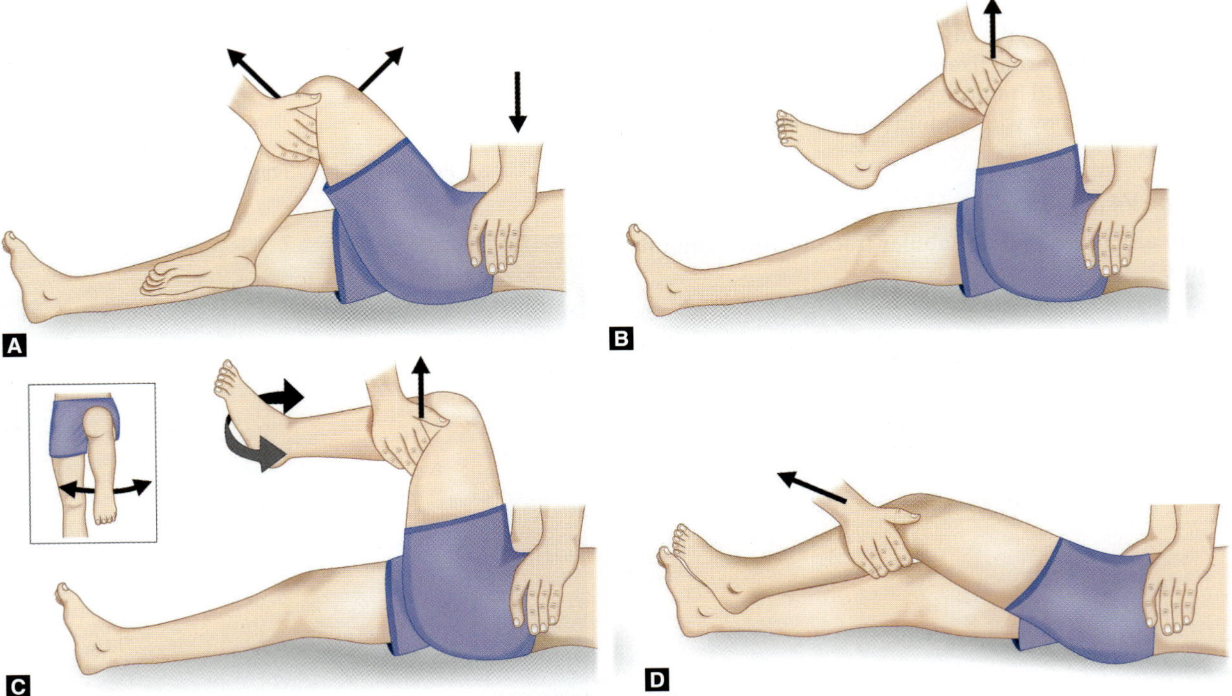

Figs. 151A to D: Allis maneuver of reduction.

Treatment of Type II, III and IV Dislocation

Primary closed reduction, dislocation with acetabular fracture should be reduced, as quickly as possible. If fails, open reduction is done to prevent further damage to femoral head.

Primary Open Reduction

Indications of primary open reduction:
- Large posterior hip fragment that did not get reduced on closed method
- Presence of fracture bone fragments in the acetabulum
- Fracture of the femoral head prevented reduction
- Displaced posterior rim fracture associated with sciatic nerve palsy
- Comminuted fracture of acetabulum
- Unstable joint after closed reduction.

Unstable hip: After closed reduction, stability of the joint should be evaluated by carrying the hip through a range of flexion to 90° with adduction to 20° and posterior pressure on the hip. If hip dislocates, it is unstable.

Treatment of Type V1 Pipkin (Fig. 152)

- Closed reduction should be tried.
- If reduced, 6 weeks traction followed by protective weight-bearing walking is recommended.
- Surgical excision of fragments is done, only if closed reduction is unsuccessful.

Treatment of Type V2 (Fig. 153)

- Closed reduction tried and anatomical reduction achieved
- If fails, open reduction
- CT scan should be taken, to locate the fragments before opening
- Internal fixation of fragments, by Hebert screw.

Treatment of Type V3 (Fig. 154)

- This is associated with femoral neck fracture
- Usually occurs, while closed manipulation of V1 and V2
- Open reduction and internal fixation of femoral neck fracture followed by femoral head fracture done
- Alternatively arthroplasty with endoprosthesis can be done in elderly patients.

Treatment of Type V4 (Fig. 155)

- In this, there are associated acetabular fracture with femoral head fracture

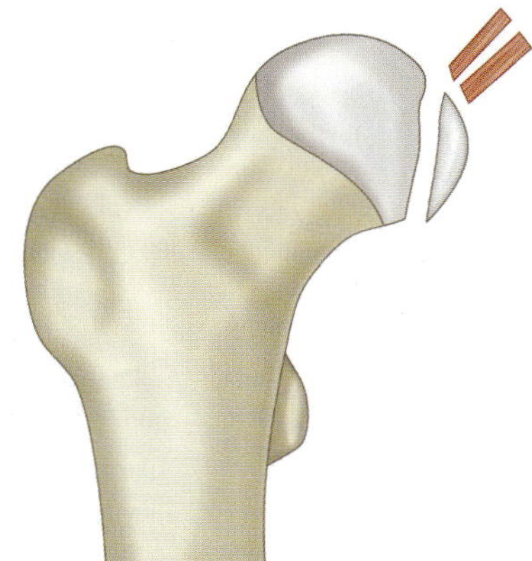

Fig. 152: Type V1 hip dislocation-fracture.

- Acetabular fractures are fixed first followed by femoral head fractures.

Complications

Early complications:
- Sciatic nerve peresis
- Irreducile posterior dislocation
- Missed knee ligamentous injury.

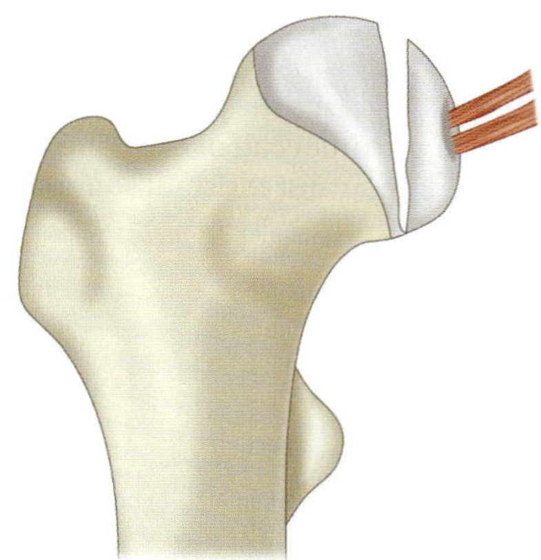

Fig. 153: Type V2 hip dislocation-fracture.

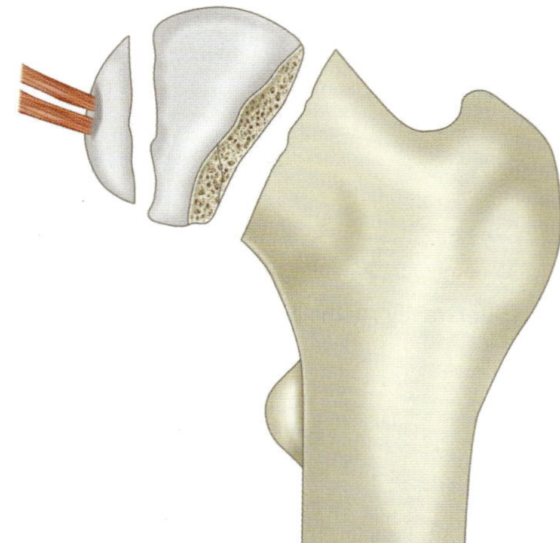

Fig. 154: Type V3 hip dislocation-fracture.

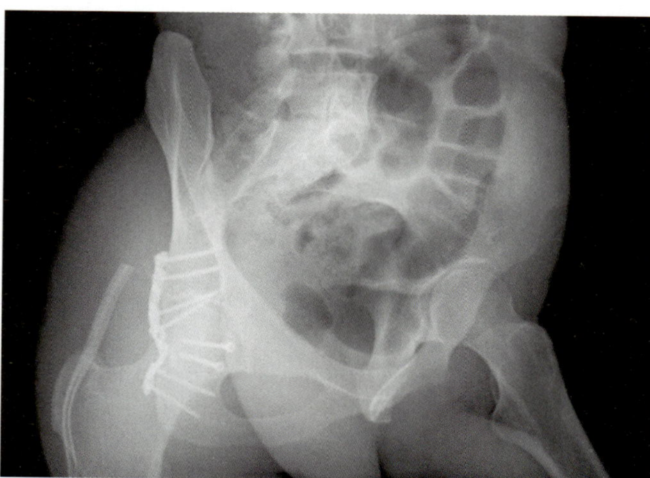

Fig. 155: Acetabular reconstruction with head fixation.

Late complications:
- Recurrent posterior dislocation
- Myositis ossificans
- AVN
- Post-traumatic arthritis
- Unreduced posterior fracture
- Heterotrophic calcification
- Malunion.

Sciatic Nerve Paresis

Sciatic nerve paresis is of two types:
1. *Prereduction paresis:* Commonly peroneal component is involved. 8–19% patients present with these complications. There is a direct contusion and ischemia of sciatic nerve takes place. 60–70% recover partially or completely. Management, include patients with simple dislocation, reduction of the dislocation. In patients, with associated fracture of posterior lip decompression is corrected with ORIF.
2. *Postreduction paresis:* Surgical exploration is indicated, to check if the nerve has been trapped in the joint. Thomas splint should not be used because the ring of the splint draws the nerve tighter. If complaints of pain and paresthesia present, the hip should be extended and the knee flexed, in order to reduce the nerve stress.

Rehabilitation, after sciatic nerve injury include:
- A well-padded short leg plaster cast with tibial pin, maintains the foot in position and prevents pressure ulcers.
- After open reduction, to relieve pressure on nerve is done. Care should be taken to avoid fixed flexion deformity.
- Periodic electromyograms and physical examination after every 3 weeks should be done.
- If permanent sciatic paralysis foot-drop splint and walking calipers for good function should be given.
- If common peroneal is paralyzed, transfer of tibialis posterior tendon through interosseus membrane with triple arthrodesis can be done.

Recurrent posterior dislocations: It occurs in 0.3–1.2% of all dislocated hips. Two theories have been given:
1. Buildup of the hydrostatic pressure in the joint cavity, owing to a one way valve in the posterior capsule forced the head of femur across the acetabular rim.
2. Repeated injury and a chronically intoxicated state a shallow acetabulum, deficient posterior rim, and a massive soft tissue injury.

Causes:
- Acetabular or femoral dysplasia
- Acetabular fracture
- Joint infection
- Paralysis
- Generalized ligamentous relaxation
- Massive soft tissue damage
- Delayed reduction of hip
- Inadequate reduction of the previously dislocated hip.

Management:
- Combined CT with arthrography should be done, to locate the tear in the capsule
- Tear are usually anterior with anterior dislocation and posterior with posterior dislocation.

Various procedures:
- Posterior bone block and innominate osteotomy
- Plication of the enlarged capsule and posterior muscles including quadratus femoris and gemelli
- Transfer of the piriformis tendon over the posterior capsule for posterior dislocation
- Transfer of iliopsoas for anterior dislocation
- Modified Bankarts type repair through the posterolateral approach for post-traumatic posterior recurrent dislocation of hip.

Anterior Dislocation

It consists of 10–15% of traumatic dislocations of hip. In anterior dislocation of hip, the femoral head rests anterior to the coronal plane of the acetabulum.

Classification

Modified Epstein classification
- *Type I:* Superior pubic/subspinous
  - *Type IA:* No associated fractures
  - *Type IB:* Associated fractures of head and NoF
  - *Type IC:* Associated fracture of acetabulum
- *Type II* **:** Inferior obturator/perineal dislocation
  - *Type IIA:* No associated fracture
  - *Type IIB:* Associated fracture of head and neck femur
  - *Type IIC:* Associated fracture of acetabulum.

Mechanism of Injury

It occurs mainly in automobile accidents, when knee strikes the dashboard with the thigh abducted. In fall from a height, or secondary to a blow to the back of the patient, while in squatted position. The neck of the femur or the GT impinges on the rim of the acetabulum and thereby levers the head of the femur, out of the acetabulum through a tear in the anterior hip capsule. The degree of flexion determines, whether a superior or inferior type of dislocation.

Clinical Diagnosis

- Attitude of limb is flexion or extension, abduction and external rotation.
- Extremity is slightly short in superior type and long in inferior type.
- In superior dislocations, the femoral head is palpable in the vicinity of ASIS and is palpable in the groin in the pubic type.
- In inferior type, fullness in palpable in the region of the obturator foramen.
- Extreme abduction with external rotation of hip.
- Anterior hip capsule is torn or avulsed.
- Femoral head is levered out anteriorly.
- Inferior type of dislocation, results from simultaneous hip abduction and external rotation, whereas superior type dislocation results from hip abduction, external rotation, and hip extension.
- The mechanism of bilateral anterior dislocation is with the pelvis fixed both the legs are forced into flexion, abduction, and external rotation.
- Anterior dislocation is usually associated with femoral head fractures.
- Anterior dislocation with femoral neck fracture is rare.

Investigations

X-rays:

- AP X-ray
- Oblique lateral view of pelvis
- Posterior oblique view
- Full length femur.

CT scan, to delineate fracture fragments size and location.
Routine laboratory investigations.

Management

Early diagnosis and prompt closed reduction under general anesthesia (GA) are the treatment of choice, however, certain dislocations require open reduction, if hip cannot be reduced in GA. Gravity method of Stimson, is primarily used for posterior dislocation of hip. In inferior obturator type of dislocation, reduction can be achieved by this method, whereas superior dislocation of the pubic type, in which the hip presents in extension are not amenable to the procedures.

Reverse Bigelow's Maneuver

The position of the patient is partial flexion and abduction. Two methods of reduction are indicated:

1. First is the lifting method, in which a firm jerk is applied to the flexed thigh. This method often results in reduction except in pubic dislocations.
2. If the lifting method fails, the second method is used, in which the hip is adducted sharply, internally rotated, and extended. Complication of this method is fracture of the femoral neck.

Allis's Maneuver

Assistant stabilizes the pelvis, by holding at the ASIS. Longitudinal traction is applied in the line with the axis of the femur and the hip is slightly flexed. Then, gently adduct and internally rotate the femur, to achieve the reduction.

Open Reduction

If a large area of weight-bearing surface of the femoral head is fractured, from the superior and the anterolateral aspects, then open reduction and internal fixation is done, using Watson Jone approach and Smith Petersons technique.

Postreduction management

It includes traction angles from 8 days to 4–6 weeks. Controlled ROM is instituted during this time, to aid nutrition of articular cartilage. Avoid extremes of abductions and external rotation, to avoid redislocation.

Complications:

- *Neurovascular compromise:* Direct pressure on the femoral artery, vein, or nerve resulting in distal neurovascular compromise in pubic or subspinous dislocation.
- *Irreducibility:* Obstruction to the closed reduction, include bone locking in the obturator foramen and interposition of the tissues, including the rectus femoris, iliopsoas muscle, and anterior hip capsule.
- *Recurrent dislocation:* Inadequate immobilization during the postoperative reduction.

Chronic Unreduced Hip Dislocations

Dislocation more than 3 months is considered to be chronic. They can be either:

- Anterior dislocation
- Posterior dislocation.

Chronic Anterior Hip Dislocation

- It is rare
- Surgical treatment is done, by intertrochanteric osteotomy. It is done to correct the deformity and improve body mechanics and balance. Two methods are used to perform intertrochanteric osteotomy:
  1. Aggarwal and Singh method
  2. Modified girdlestone arthroplasty by Nagi.

Aggarwal and Singh method:

This is usually followed, in which Gibson's approach is taken. Femur is divided along the line joining the GT and the lesser trochanter. Limb is then adducted, extended, and internally rotated. Patient is given skin traction for 6 weeks to prevent rotational deformity. Crutch walking at 6 weeks and full weight-bearing walking at 3–4 months.

Nagi method:

In this method, the femoral neck is exposed by the Smith Petersons or the Watson and Jones approach. Subcapital osteotomy is performed, attempting to leave as much neck as possible without disturbing the femoral head. By manipulating the leg, the cut femoral neck is displaced into the acetabulum. Postoperatively, 5 kg traction is maintained for 6 weeks. NWB walking by 6 weeks and gradual weight-bearing started at 3 months.

Comparison:

Nagi method is easier to do. THR after this operation as the anatomy of the proximal femur is undisturbed, while Aggarwal and Singh method is more stable, where a fixed hip can be achieved.

Chronic Posterior Hip Dislocation

- More common
- Two main causes are:
  1. Fracture of the femoral head or acetabular rim and
  2. AVN.

Treatment of Type I:

Gupta method: Tibial pin traction is given for 18 kg weight. Patient is kept in sedation and muscle relaxation during traction. By fifth day, usually femoral head is at or below the level of acetabulum. Limb is then abducted every 4th day and weight reduced by 3.6 kg. After head is reduced in acetabulum, 7 kg weight traction maintained for next 2 weeks. NWB at 4 weeks and weight bearing at 3 months.

Treatment of Type II, III, IV:

- Skeletal traction
- Open reduction and fixation of the fracture fragments
- In young patients arthrodesis, if come with complications as AVN.

Central acetabular fracture dislocation:

In this type of fracture dislocation, involving the medial acetabular wall or the superior weight-bearing dome of the acetabulum is present, with or without associated control displacement of the head of the femur. It occurs in all adult age groups. It is now considered as fracture of the acetabulum.

INFECTIONS OF HIP JOINT

Pyogenic Arthritis

It is a purulent infection of the joint cavity, due to pyogenic organisms and productive of purulent exudates. It is also known as septic arthritis and suppurative arthritis. It is more common

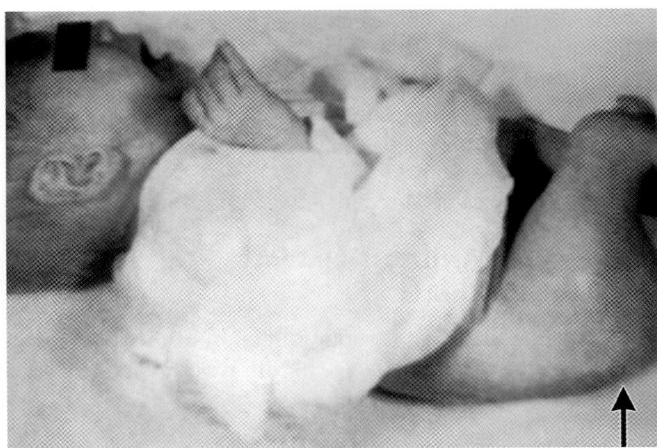

Fig. 156: Pyogenic arthritis of hip in an infant.

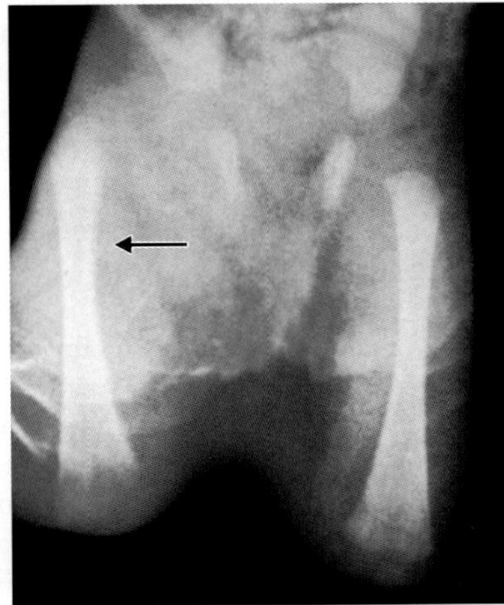

Fig. 157: X-ray showing pyogenic hip arthritis in infant.

in childhood and the ratio of the pyogenic arthritis in adult, as compared to the children's is 1:1.5. Infant and young children's hip are more commonly involved. Multiple joint involvement occur in 5% of cases and 75% of the cases occur in children under 5 years of age, as shown in Figures 156 and 157.

Etiology

Common organisms: These include, *Staphylococcus aureus*; most common, pneumococci, gonococci, *E. coli* and *H. influenzae* (account for the most of the cases between 6 months and 2 years of age).

Susceptible group:

- Infants and neonates
- Elderly patients with pre-existing joint diseases
- Immunocompromised patients.

Route of infections: Route of infection is divided into three types:

1. *Hematogenous spread:* Infection is usually in gastrointestinal tract (GIT), urinary tract, teeth, tonsil, pneumonia
2. *Direct extension:* Spread from local abscess, osteomyelitis or infected compound fracture
3. Direct implantation of bacteria through puncture wound.

Pathology

The reaction of the joint is determined by the virulence of the organisms and the resistance of the individuals, in any case there is exudation of the fluid in the joint cavity. It will be serous, seropurulent, or may frankly purulent.

- *Serous type:* Joint is distended with clear serous fluid, with dilatation of vessels of synovial membrane and capsule. The effusion may subside or may recur or it may become seropurulent or actually purulent.
- *Serofibrinous arthritis:* In this, the synovial membrane is not only hyperemic, but inflamed so the joint is covered with serofibrinous exudate and cavity filled with cloudy fluid with large number of polymorphs and large mononuclear cell. Organisms present in the joint fluid.
- *Purulent arthritis:* Most severe type of arthritis. In this, most of the joint and surrounding structure are quickly involved, considerable exudate in the joint cavity containing polymorph, bacteria, red blood count (RBC) and fibrin. Capsule and synovium are engorged edematous. There is a destruction of the articular cartilage. Mechanism, causing destruction: enzymes, like plasmin, kinase, collagenase, protease, cathepsins B and D and prostaglandin raised. Encroaching granulation from synovia, synovium completely detached to lie free in the joint cavity in the pool of pus. Thus, bone are exposed, infection may spread and causes osteomyelitis, which lead to sequestration, suppuration, and necrosis. Intra-articular ligaments may be destroyed and finally capsule is perforated and pus escaping from the joint, to form an extra-articular or periarticular abscess and at the end results complete resolution, dislocation, absorption of head, and ankylosis.

Clinical Features

Serous type (acute synovitis):

- Tense painful swelling of the joint
- Local rise of temperature
- Severe tenderness in the joint
- Muscle spasm present.

Serofibrinous type:

- Joint is exquisitely tender and swollen
- High fever and night pain occur
- Movement are severely restricted
- Muscle spasm.

Suppurative type:

- It is most severe form of disease
- In the early stages, symptoms are those of the acute synovitis
- In this, the patient feels extremely ill and joint is more painful and limb wastes rapidly.

Investigations

- Total count is raise, with polymorphonuclear leukocyte
- Erythrocyte sedimentation rate (ESR) raised
- C-reactive protein (CRP) elevated
- Blood culture may be positive
- Joint aspirate examine for the culture and sensitivity, gram stain-cocci or bacilli, glucose is low, but protein are high and its turbid appearance
- *Radiograph:* In the early stage shows increase joint space and the soft tissue shadow

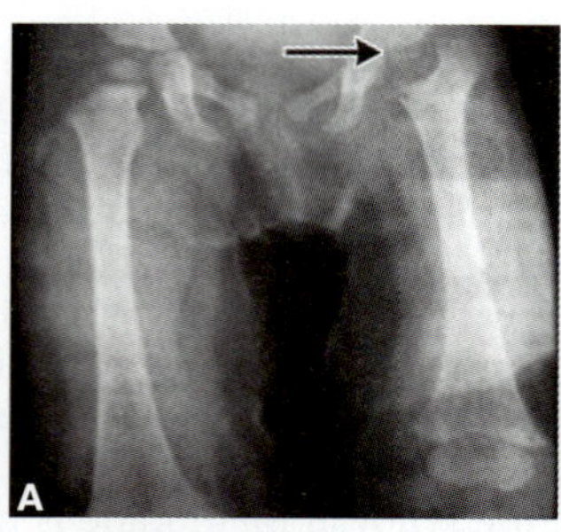

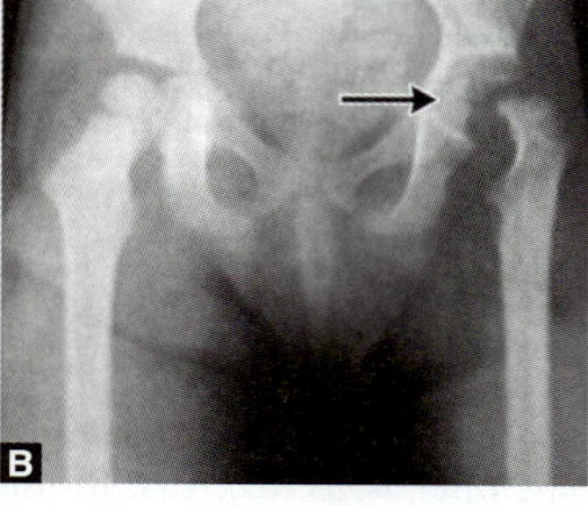

Figs. 158A and B: Later stage of pyogenic arthritis, show osteoporosis, cartilage destruction, decreased joint space, bone necrosis, epiphyseal premature closure and fibrous or bony ankylosis is present—(A) Arrow showing destruction of femoral head; (B) Arrow showing involvement of acetabulum.

- In the later stage, shows osteoporosis, cartilage destruction, decreased joint space, bone necrosis, epiphyseal premature closure and fibrous or bony ankylosis is present, as shown in Figures 158A and B
- Ultrasound, it detect joint effusion
- Isotope bone scan are performed, to distinguish cellulitis, septic arthritis, and osteomyelitis.

Differential Diagnosis

- Acute rheumatism and rheumatoid arthritis (RA)
- Acute osteomyelitis
- Acute (nonsuppurative) arthritis.

Complications

- Joint stiffness
- Joint instability-subluxation dislocation
- Arthritis
- Epiphyseal growth disturbance
- Ankylosis-cartilagenous, fibrous and bony
- Amyloidosis
- Pelvic abscess
- Chronic osteomyelitis.

Treatment

Principles of treatment are:
- Early diagnosis
- Antibiotics required for 4–6 weeks and used higher antibiotics
- Immobilized and give rest to joint by splintage or light traction and hip should be in abduction to prevent dislocation
- Removal of pus and decompression to prevent cartilage destruction.

Treatment consists of bed rest:
- *Antibiotic:* Intravenous cloxacillin and ampicillin is given as soon as sample of blood and synovial fluid collected for culture and antibiotic must be given for 3–6 weeks.
- *Immobilization:* Relieved the pain and spread of the infection and it is achieved by light skin traction CR splintage with compression bandage, with hip in abduction and is to continue till patient is pain-free.
- *Joint decompression:* It reduces the intra-articular tension, and also prevents AVN of femoral head, and subluxation or dislocation of hip.
- *Aspiration of hip joint:* In the children, anterior aspiration technique is used and in adult posterior aspiration technique used.
- *Posterior drainage:* Ober technique is used and done by taking the Moore's approach.
- *Anterior drainage:* It is done, by taking the Smith Peterson approach.
- Lateral drainage.
- Medial drainage.
- *Arthroscopic lavage:* A recent advance technique.

Acute Infective Arthritis of Infants (Tom Smith's Arthritis)

It is a pyogenic arthritis or septic infection of the joint in small infants below one year of the age. Smith was the first to describe septic arthritis in neonate and infants.

Etiology

Secondary to neighboring bone lesion, i.e. from metaphysis to epiphysis because vessels from metaphysis penetrate the growth plate, up to the age of one and half year. Joint may be infected through the bloodstream, usually from the infected umbilicus, oronasal infection, respiratory tract infection, etc. Proteolytic enzymes derived from leukocytes and bacteria cause cartilage destruction. The most common organism is *S. aureus* followed by *Streptococcus influenzae, Pneumococcus, E. coli,* etc.

Pathology

Infection starts in synovial membrane lining the joint. This rapidly inflamed and edematous, and from its surface, it poured out synovial fluid, plasma, and leukocyte. Filling the joint with turbid exudates, containing a large number of polymorphonuclear leukocyte and fibrin. If the infection is severe, mesothelium lining of the synovial membrane is destroyed and its place is taken by mass of the granulation tissue. Articular cartilage is also involved and lead to impairment of joint function.

Clinical Features

- Child is very ill, toxic, high grade fever, and irritable
- Joint is swollen, painful, and hot
- Movement of the limb are painful
- Hip may be flexed, abducted, and slightly externally rotated
- Sometimes extensive fluctuant abscess may be present in the thigh or buttocks
- Sometimes, when child may be brought, a month later, the limb is shortened and the child has an unstable hip gait. The joint is hypermobile.

Differential Diagnosis

- Acute rheumatic fever
- Tuberculous arthritis
- Traumatic synovitis
- Hemophilic arthritis.

Investigation

- Total count is raised and polymorphonuclear leukocyte is present
- Blood for culture demonstrates septicemia
- Aspiration of the joint fluid, establishes diagnosis
- *X-rays:* First sign is swelling due to joint effusion and edema of soft tissue.

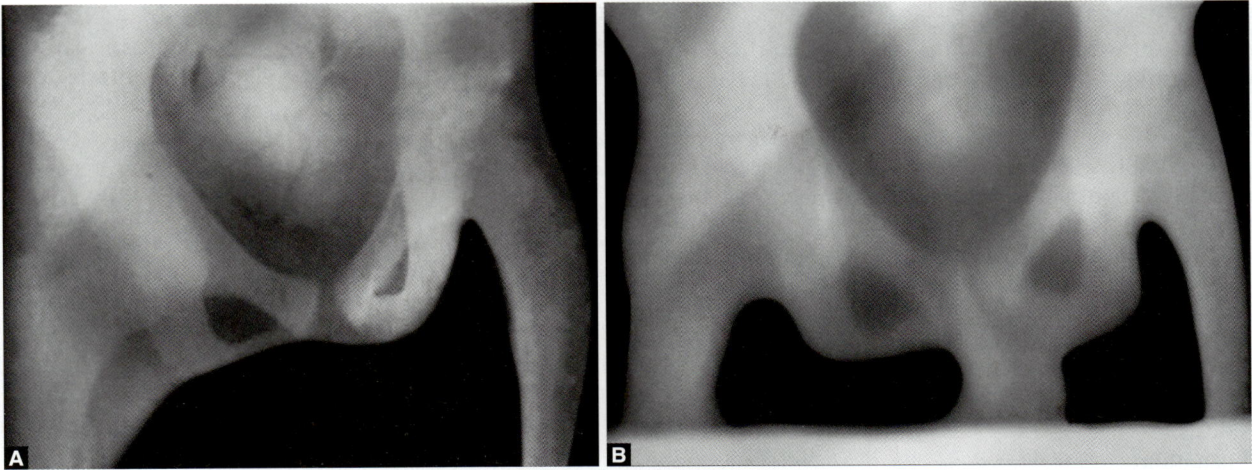

Figs. 159A and B: Sequelae of Tom Smith arthritis.

TABLE 7: Johari's classification of Tom Smith arthritis.

Group I:	Loss of CFE/neck, metaphyseal spike present—sable Group II: Loss of CEF and neck—unstable
Group IIIA:	Dislocation, CFE present—unstable Group IIIB: Subluxation, CFE present—unstable
Group IV:	Articular incongruity, AVN, coxa magna, breva, trochanteric overgrowth—stable
Group V:	Pseudarthrosis of neck of femur—stable/unstable

Radiographs (Figs. 159A and B)

Classification:

- *Eyre-Brook classification:*
  - *Type 1:* Recovery occurs with coxa magna.
  - *Type 2:* Destruction or severe damage to the capital epiphysis with the femoral neck remaining in the acetabulum or a deformed femoral head in valgus or varus.
  - *Type 3:* Destruction or severe damage to the growth plate.
  - *Type 4:* Destruction of the capital epiphysis with dislocation or severe subluxation of hip.
- *Choi's classification:*
  - *Type 1:* Deformity involved transient ischemia of the epiphysis, with or without mild coxa magna, and these hips did not need reconstruction.
  - *Type 2:* Deformity included deformity of the epiphysis, physis, and metaphysis and these hips needed an operation to prevent subluxation; the goal of operation included improvement in acetabular coverage.
  - *Type 3:* Deformity involved malalignment of femoral neck with extreme anteversion or retroversion or with a pseudarthrosis of femoral neck that needs realignment osteotomy of proximal part of femur or bone grafting for pseudarthrosis.
  - *Type 4:* Deformity, which included severe limb length discrepancy and incompetent articulation of hip needs operation such as Pemberton osteotomy, trochantric arthroplasty, arthrodesis, and lengthening of ipsilateral tibia.
- *Johari's classification (Table 7)*
  This is also shown in Figures 160A to F.

Radiology and Diagnosis of Sequelae

- Ossification of the head and neck is delayed and translucency persists

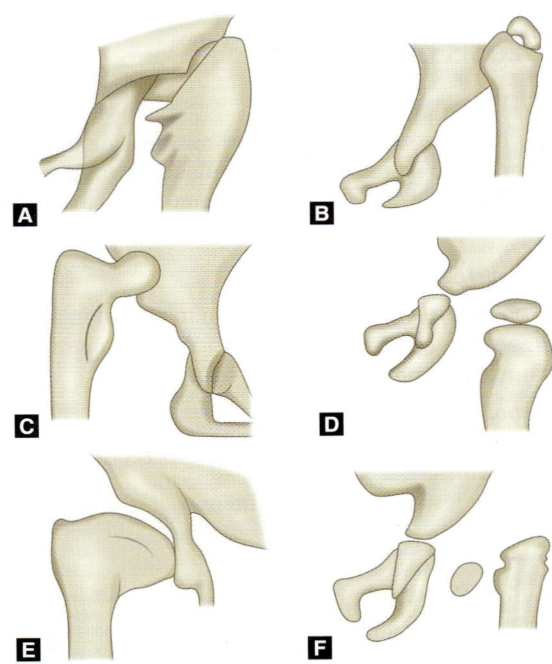

Figs. 160A to F: Johari's classification of Tom Smith arthritis. (A) Group I arthritis; (B) Group II; (C) Group IIIA; (D) Group IIIB; (E) Group IV; (F) Group V arthritis.

- On X-ray, telescopic sign is positive.
- Differential diagnosis, with positive telescopic sign:
  - Dislocation of hip
  - Pseudarthrosis of the NoF
  - Complete destruction of the head and neck
  - On X-ray telescopic sign is negative, then head may be osteoporotic, AVN and may be partially destroyed.

Treatment

- *Type I:* Lesion, with no instability or significant deformity should be simply kept under observation, with the use of the abduction plaster cast or brace.
- *Type II:* Sequelae, with a deformed coxa vara or valga may need treatment initially with the orthosis. If there is dislocation or severe coxa valga or vara, then femoral or pelvis osteotomy needed.
- *Type III:* Sequelae, the pseudarthrosis, and nonunion may be treated with subtrochantric osteotomy, with bone grafting and internal fixation with lag screw.
- *Type IV:* Lesion, reconstructive surgeries done.

Operation to Stabilize the Hip

- Arthrodesis
- Pelvic osteotomy
- High femoral osteotomy
- Trochanteric arthroplasty combined with proximal femoral osteotomy
- Harmon or L-Episcopo reconstruction
- *To correct deformities:* Flexion and adduction contracture is treated, by an adductor tenotomy and hip is ankylosed in flexion and adduction, then it is treated by intertrochanteric osteotomy
- Operation to equalized leg length, which is done only after all reconstructive operation are done.

TUBERCULOSIS OF HIP JOINT

Introduction

Tuberculous disease of the hip is very common. The frequency of the involvement is next to spinal tuberculosis. In long series, it is 15% of total skeletal TB and age group affected is first three decades of life.

Pathology (Fig. 161)

The initial focus of the tuberculosis lesion may start in acetabular roof, epiphyses, metaphyseal region (Babcock's triangle), GT, and rarely in synovial membrane.

Acetabular roof:

- The joint involvement is late
- Mild symptoms are seen
- No extensive destruction of acetabular roof is seen.

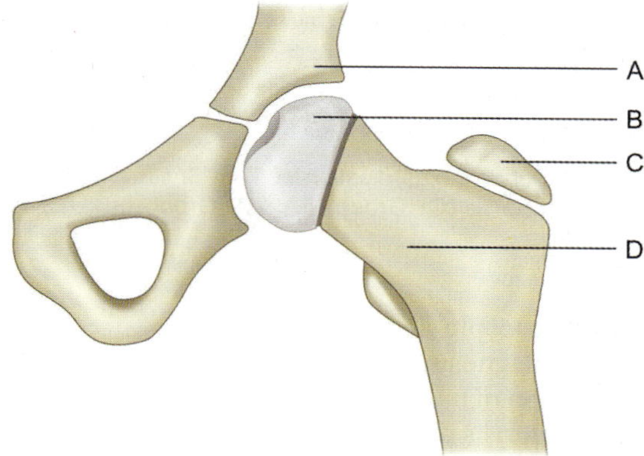

Fig. 161: Main foci of tuberculosis lesions—(A) Roof of acetabulum; (B) Epiphysis; (C) Greater trochanter; (D) Babcock's triangle.

Greater trochanter:

- Overlying bursa is involved
- Joint involvement is late.

Epiphyses and metaphyseal region:

- As intracapsular early involvement of joint
- Both are rapidly destructive.

Synovium:

- Involvement of the synovium is very rare
- Early joint involvement seen.

It may form cold abscesses, which may penetrate the joint and inferior weak part of capsule or rarely on the acetabular floor and from this it is perforated and present in femoral triangle, inguinal region, medial, lateral, or posterior aspect of thigh, ischiorectal fossa or pelvis and lower part of thigh knee because of spread along neurovascular bundle.

In the acetabular roof, psoas abscess and pelvic abscess are there. If it is above urogenital diaphragm then, it will track above inguinal ligament. If it is below urogenital diaphragm, then will track into ischiorectal fossa.

Clinical Features

- *Night cries:* Patient wakes up from sleep during night because of pain. Pain is because of the relaxation of protective muscle spasm there is irritation of eroded cartilage gives rise to pain
- *Pain:* Pain is more towards the end of the day and it is referred to the medial aspect of the thigh and knee
- *Limping:* It is most common symptom seen in the TB hip. Patient is with the typical antalgic gait (this is early stage), short limb gait is seen
- *Cold abscesses:* Present in the 8% of total patients. Cold abscess is palpable with or without sinuses
- *Tenderness:* Felt by direct pressure on the hip in the femoral triangle or medial to the GT posteriorly
- Fullness is present around the hip
- Stiffness and restriction of movement
- Muscle spasm, seen in the lower abdominal muscle and the adductor of thigh
- Pathological subluxation and the dislocation hip
- Constitutional symptoms, loss of weight, loss of appetite, low grade fever, and cough.

Stage I (Tuberculous Synovitis)

- In the early disease of the hip joint due to the juxta articular osseous lesion, causing the irritable hip
- Joint held in position of maximum capacity, i.e. flexion, abduction, and external rotation leading to apparent shortening
- No true shortening
- Only the movement are painful and limited.

Stage II (Early Arthritis) (Fig. 162)

- Actual destruction or damage to articular cartilage
- Local signs become more prominent because of spasm of adductor and flexors
- Assume deformity of flexion, adduction and internal rotation
- True shortening of less than 1 cm
- Appreciable muscle wasting
- Restriction of movement in all direction due to pain and muscle spasm.

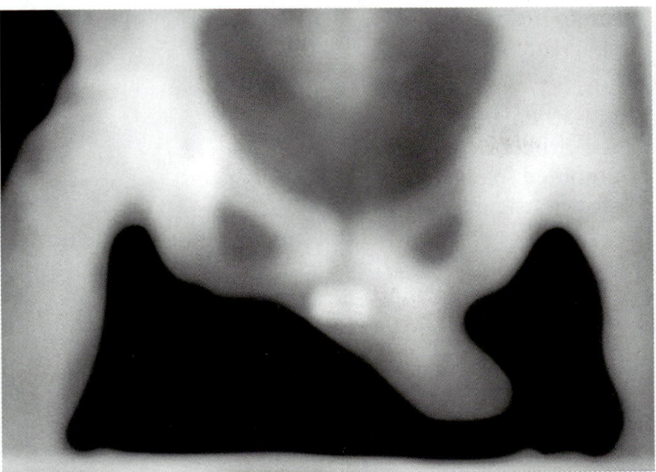

Fig. 162: Stage II early tubercular arthritis.

- *X-ray shows*
  - Osteoporosis of bone
  - Slight diminution of joint space
  - Erosions of articular cartilage margins.

Stage III (Advanced Arthritis)

- Further advancement of destruction
- Flexion, adduction, and internal rotation deformities will pronounced
- Restriction of movement
- Apparent as well as true shortening
- Gross restriction of femoral head and acetabulum
- Muscle wasting
- Capsule is further destroyed and thickened and contracted.

Stage IV (Advanced Arthritis with Subluxation/Dislocation)

- Further destruction of femoral head, acetabulum, capsule, and upper end of femur is displaced upwards and dorsally, in wondering or migrating acetabulum
- Shenton's arc is broken
- Destruction of capsule may lead to frank pathological posterior dislocation of femoral head
- Movements are increased as compared to previous stages
- X-ray showing wandering acetabulum, as shown in Figure 163.
- Other X-ray findings (Fig. 164):
  - Gross osteoporosis of bone
  - Destroyed head and acetabulum
  - Mostly posterior dislocation, rarely protrusio acetabuli can occur
  - Shenton's line broken
  - Morter and Pestle appearance.

In certain cases of tuberculous arthritis (stages 2, 3, and 4), the hip may not assume the classical triple deformity of flexion, adduction, and internal rotation, instead the deformity may be that of flexion, abduction, and external rotation with the lateral aspect of thigh of the diseased hip resting on bed. This is due to adaptation of latter posture for relief of pain or due to destruction in iliofemoral " Y" ligament by tuberculous process.

Radiological Classification

Shanmugasundaram (1980), C for child and A for adult

- Normal appearance (C)

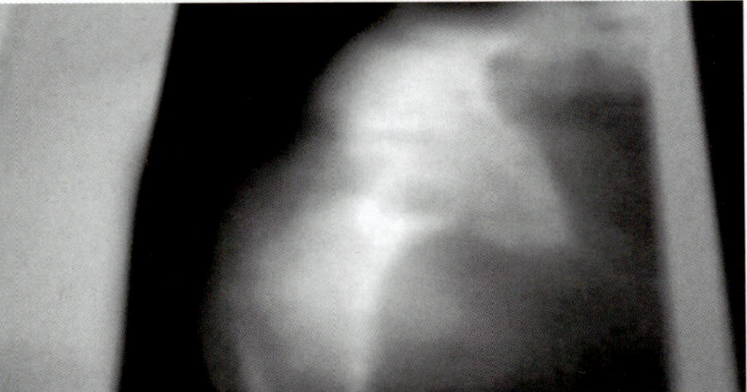

Fig. 163: X-ray showing wandering acetabulum in advanced tubercular arthritis.

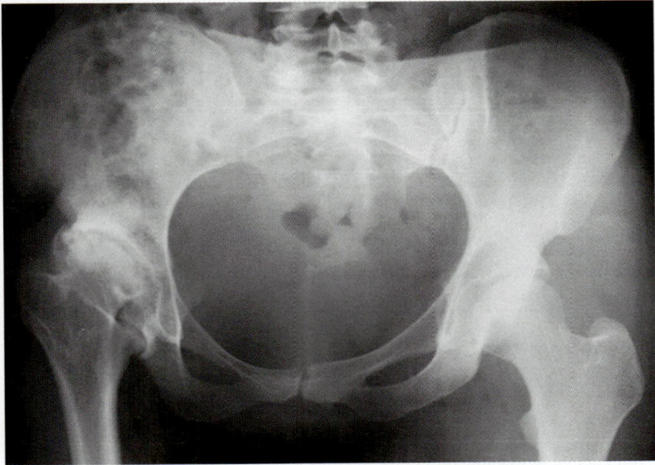

Fig. 164: Stage IV (advanced arthritis with subluxation/dislocation).

- Traveling acetabulum (C, A)
- Perthes type (C)
- Dislocated hip (C)
- Protrusion acetabuli (C, A)
- Atrophic type (A)
- Morter and Pestle type (C, A).

Investigation

- Hemoglobin (Hb percent)
- ESR, raised in active stage
- Mantoux test (in children), indicates an active infection and sensitization of child to *Mycobacterium* infection
- TB Enzyme-linked immunosorbent assay (ELISA) (usually in gram titer, is active)
- X-ray hip AP and lateral and X-ray chest PA view
- Biopsy and histopathological examination.

Treatment

General

- Good nutrition diet
- Fresh air
- Rest
- Analgesics
- Proper positioning of limb
- Maintenance of good hygiene
- Traction.

Advantages of traction
- Gives rest to the part
- Relieves muscle spasm and pain
- Prevents subluxation and dislocation, by keeping leg in abduction
- Maintains joint space and keep the articular surface away.

Chemotherapy—Antitubercular Treatment (ATT)

For first 4 months
- Isoniazid 300 mg/kg body weight
- Rifampicin 450 mg/kg body weight
- Ethambutol 1200 mg/kg body weight

For second 4 months
- Isoniazid 300 mg/kg body weight
- Pyrazinamide 1500 mg/kg body weight

For third 4 months
- Isoniazid 300 mg/kg body weight
- Rifampicin 450 mg/kg body weight

For fourth 4 months
- Isoniazid 300 mg/kg body weight
- These are the triple regime.

Management of cold abscess: Any palpable cold abscess may be aspirated with instillation of streptomycin with or without isoniazid.

Surgical Treatment

Indications for surgery are:
- If response to the conservative treatment is not favorable
- Patient presenting with sound ankylosis in bad position
- Mobility at hip joint.

Synovectomy and debridement:
Indications:
- Synovitis
- Early arthritis
- In addition to synovectomy; removal of loose bodies/rice body, debris, pannus covering articular cartilage, loose articular cartilage and careful curettage of osseous juxta-articular foci can be performed.

Complications
- AVN
- SCFE in children
- Fracture of femoral neck and acetabulum
- Secondary infections.

Osteotomy:
Indications:
- Sound ankylosis in bad position, require upper femoral corrective osteotomy.
- Unsound ankylosis in bad position becomes an osseous fusion, by a high femoral corrective osteotomy.
- Can be done at any age.
- Ideal site is as near as possible to the deformed joint.

Arthrodesis:
- Done in adult patients
- Can be done in active as well as healed stage
- Failure of conservative treatment
- Recurrence of pain and deformity
- Certain destructive lesion, e.g. the formation of the sequestra in head or NoF or in acetabulum.

Methods:
- Intra-articular
- Extra-articular
- Combined (panarticular)
- In extra-articular methods
  - Iliofemoral arthrodesis (Hibb's) in abduction deformity
  - Ischiofemoral arthrodesis (Britain's technique) in adduction deformity.

Disadvantages of arthrodesis: Activities not possible after arthrodesis are:
- Bending
- Sitting cross leg
- Squatting
- Sports and running
- Bicycling.

Complications of arthrodesis:
- Early development of degenerative arthritis of
  - Lumbosacral spine
  - Ipsilateral knee
  - Contralateral hip.
- Increased energy expenditure of ambulation.

Girdlestone's excision arthroplasty:
- Girdlestone's excision arthroplasty can safely be carried out in healed or active disease after completion of growth potential of hip.
- This procedure provides mobile and painless hip joint, with control of infection and correction of deformity.
- Excision of:
  - Femoral head and neck
  - Proximal part of trochanter
  - Acetabular rim.
- Safely done in healed/active disease after completion of growth potential.
- Procedure provides painless, mobile hip joint with control of infection and correction deformity.
- Postoperative skeletal traction in abduction for minimum 3 months minimizes shortening and gross instability. Instability will be minimized due to maturation and contractures of soft tissues around hip.

Disadvantages:
- Relative unstable joint, when disease heals without much fibrosis and scarring.
- Stabilization can be done by:
  - Pelvic support osteotomies
  - Acetabular shelf procedure.

Replacement arthroplasty:
- Most debated and can be done in highly selected cases
- At least 10 years, after last evidence of active infections
- Antitubercular treatment (ATT) is must
- Reactivation of infection is noted in about 10–30% of cases.

Amniotic arthroplasty:
- In the treatment of tuberculous arthritis of hip, multilayered cap of amniotic membrane was used.
- Vishwakarma (1986) stated that of the out 28 patients, 25 showed good range of painless movement and stable joint.

Recent Advance Techniques in Management of Tuberculosis of Hip Joint

- Amniotic arthroplasty for tuberculosis of hip
- Charnley low friction arthroplasty in tuberculosis of hip
- Gene therapy in tuberculosis of hip
- Interpositional arthroplasties
- THR.

Gene therapy in tuberculosis of hip: Impressive advances, in our knowledge of the molecular genetic basis of skeletal disorders and fracture healing, have led to the development of novel therapeutics based on ectopic expression of one or more genes in patient cells that can influence repair or regenerative processes in bone. Gene therapy is an attractive new approach to the treatment of bone disorders. Orthopedics has become one of the most promising areas of research into gene therapy. This is because many potential orthopedic targets for gene therapy, unlike traditional targets, such as cancer and severe genetic disorders, neither present difficult delivery problems nor require prolonged periods of gene expression. Gene therapy offers new possibilities for the clinical management of orthopedic conditions that are difficult to treat by traditional surgical or medical means. Impaired bone healing, need for extensive bone formation, cartilage repair, and metabolic bone diseases are all conditions, where alterations of the signaling peptides involved may provide cure or improvement. Several preclinical studies have shown that gene transfer technology has the ability to deliver osteogenic molecules, to precise anatomical locations at therapeutic levels for sustained periods of time. Both in vivo and ex vivo transduction of cells, can induce bone formation at ectopic and orthotopic sites. Genetic engineering of adult stem cells from various sources with osteogenic genes has led to enhanced fracture repair, spinal fusion, and rapid healing of bone defects in animal models. Although, still a relatively immature field, proof-of-principle for enhanced bone formation through skeletal gene therapy has already been established. The challenge now is to more precisely define optimal cellular targets and therapeutic genes and to develop safe and efficient ways to deliver therapeutic genes to target cells. Skeletal gene therapy can have an enormous impact on patient care. The next 5 years will present us with unparalleled opportunities to develop more effective therapeutic strategies and overcome obstacles, presented by current gene transfer technologies.

Obesity: Twice as prevalent in obese.

Occupation: With physical activities involving repetitive use of particular joints over period of time.

Mechanical factors: Mechanical stress, gross anatomical damage, subtle mechanical derangement (IDK-long standing), joint hypermobility and direct articular cartilage damage.

DEGENERATIVE OSTEOARTHRITIS

Introduction

It is characterized by degenerative changes in articular cartilage of diarthrodial joints and subsequent new bone formation at the articular margins. The term osteoarthritis was coined by John Spendon. However, it is a misnomer and the right term is osteoarthrosis or degenerative joint disease. Pathologically, it may be defined as a condition of synovial joints characterized by:

- Focal loss of articular hyaline cartilage, as shown in Figure 165.

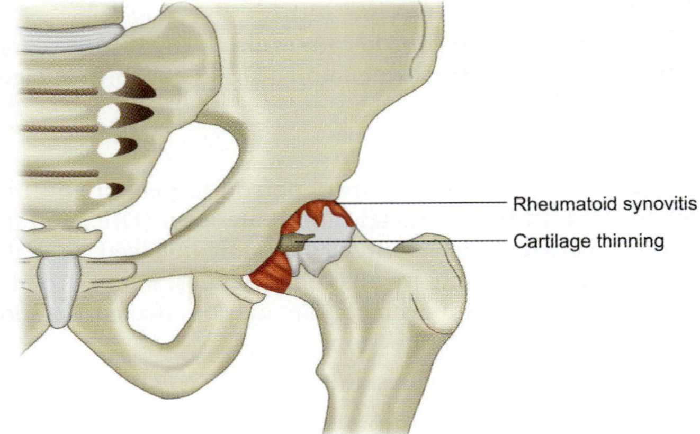

Fig. 165: Degenerative changes in articular cartilage, with focal loss of articular hyaline cartilage.

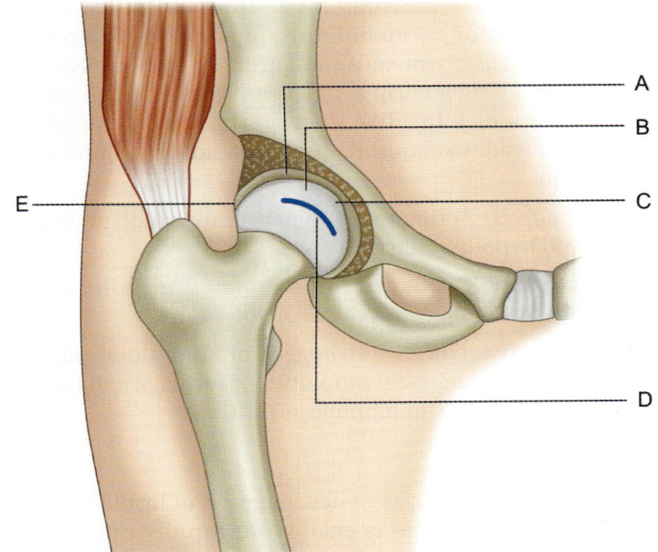

Fig. 166: Proliferation of new bone and remodeling of joint contour, with focal degenerative changes—(A) Proliferation of new bone; (B) Remodeling of joint contour; (C) Head of femur; (D) Articular surface of femur; (E) Defect in articular surface.

- Simultaneous proliferation of new bone, with remodeling of joint contour. This is illustrated in Figure 166.

Incidence: By the age of 40 years, about 40% of population has radiological sign of osteoarthrosis of major weight-bearing joints (knee, hip). 50% of these will be symptomatic.

Risk Factors

- Age
- Female sex
- Race
- Genetic factors
- Major joint trauma
- Repetitive stress
- Obesity
- Congenital development defects
- Metabolic endocrine disorders.

Etiology

Age: Process begins in second decade of life and by 50 to 65 years of age 80% have radiological evidence of disease, as shown in Figure 167.

Sex: Female > male

Areas of involvement: Varies from person to person and from joint to joint. In female distal interphalangeal (DIP) and first carpometacarpal (CMC) is most commonly involved. In males, hip are most commonly involved. In females, knees are most commonly involved. Any synovial joint may be affected, but those under compression are more prone.

Inflammatory process: like RA destroys articular cartilage.

Traumatic cause: Acute or chronic (occupational, sports).

Metabolic disorders, like hemochromatosis, Wilson's disease, Gaucher's disease, gouty deposits of urates and alkaptonuric ochronosis deposits, make cartilage susceptible to destruction.

Biomechanical factors: Structural abnormalities like articular fracture, dislocation, acetabular dysplasia, slipped epiphysis, and Perthes disease will cause abnormally high pressure over articular surface, and predispose it for early degeneration. Similarly misalignments of joint, like genu varum and genu valgum, meniscal tear leads to abnormal stresses, leading the joint to early degeneration.

Hormonal effects: Acromegaly, hyperparathyroidism, diabetes mellitus, and hypothyroidism.

Chemical injury: Corticosteroids injected in joint or given systemically, tends to destroy joints on long-term.

Repeated intrasynovial hemorrhage: Iron and blood pigments, alters physical and chemical properties of cartilage and causes its early degeneration, e.g. hemophilic arthritis.

Pathophysiology

The primary lesion consists of degeneration of hyaline cartilage. As a result, the cartilage is easily and rapidly eroded, until ultimately the bone matrix is exposed. The erosion of the cartilage is not uniform, so relatively at first area of bone are exposed in a patchy fashion and there are intervening islands of relatively normal cartilage. The perichondrium and the cartilage round the periphery of the joint are stimulated into activity and as a result, the nonarticular areas of the bones are elevated above the remainder of the surface and project circumferentially, to give the appearance known as "lipping".

Formation of osteophytes: These cartilaginous outgrowth ossifies to form osteophyte. Local periosteal new bone formation, particularly around capsular attachment also leads to osteophyte formation.

Synovitis and capsulitis: Detached cartilaginous flakes, which lie freely in the joint cavity are readily absorbed by synovial membrane and leads to synovitis followed by fibrosis. Proteoglycans leaks from damaged articular cartilage, produces irritation to synovial membrane and capsule, which undergoes hyperplasia.

Subchondral sclerosis: Proliferation of blood vessels along the subchondral bone leads to osteoporosis initially, followed by invasion of larger blood vessels, leading to subchondral sclerosis, as shown in Figure 168.

Formation of subchondral cyst: Edema of subchondral bone marrow, followed by formation of mucinous fatty marrow with dilatation of surrounding sinusoids, leads to cyst formation. There is mucoid secretion within the center of this area and the expansion of the cyst cavities, by osteoclastic resorption of bony trabeculae. Surrounding this, there is some osteoblastic response and a sclerotic wall is formed. Other theories are that these cysts arise from herniation of synovial fluid through cracks within the denuded subchondral bone plate, as shown in Figures 169A and B.

Formation of loose bodies: The synovial membrane and capsule are involved in the late stages and are the site of inflammation and adhesions. The synovial tags or polypi are insinuated into the joint and when very exuberant the process is referred to as "lipoma arborescens". Occasionally, cartilage formation occurs in these tags and they are liable to be broken off into the joint, when they form loose bodies.

Eburnation: The exposed bone ends of the articular surface are subjected to considerable friction, in consequence the bone trabeculae in the immediate neighborhood fracture and repair and the marrow space are obliterated. The change involves only a thin layer abutting on the joint and when the surface of this layer gradually becomes more and more smooth and polished, as a result of the continual rubbing, the process is known as eburnation. An osteoarthritic joint rarely, if ever, becomes completely ankylosed,

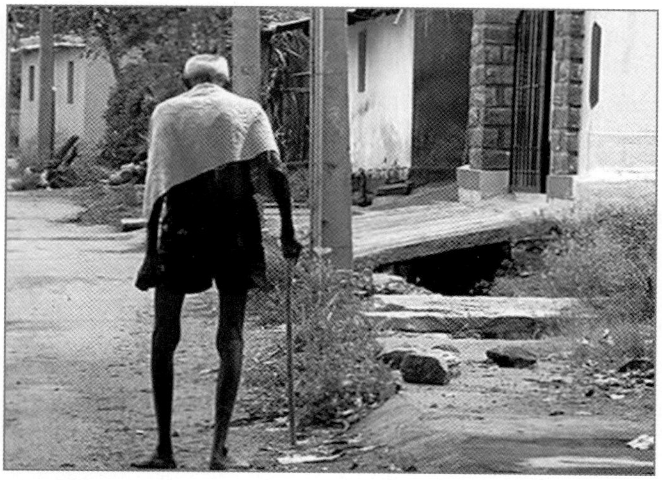

Fig. 167: Degenerative changes of joints are common in old age group.

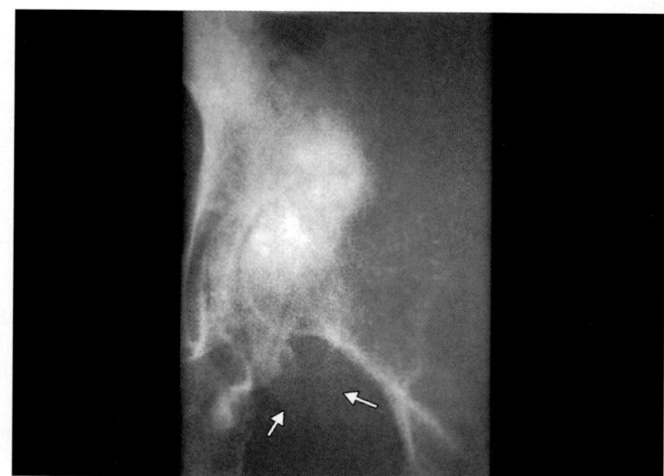

Fig. 168: X-ray showing subchondral sclerosis of hip joint. Arrows showing osteophytes.

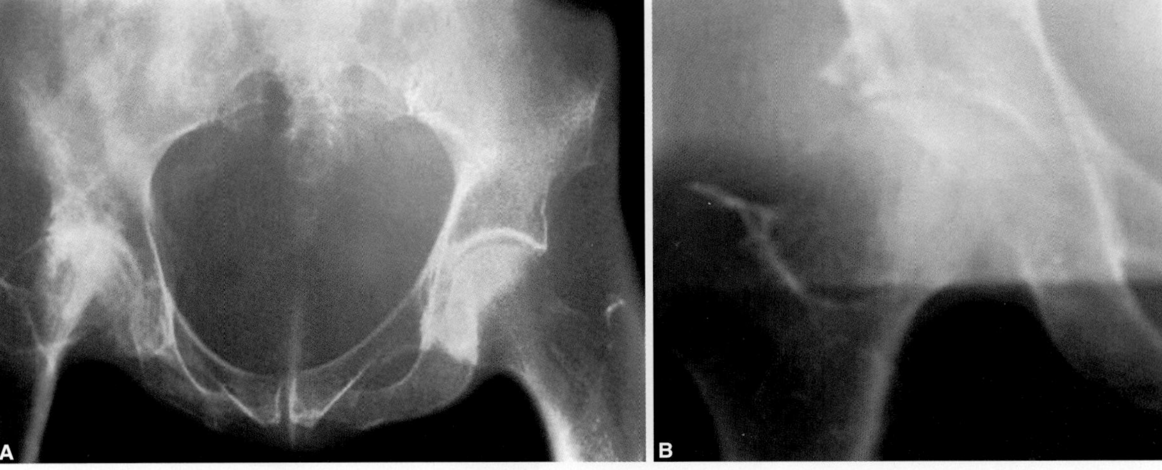

Figs. 169A and B: Progression of osteoarthritis of the hip over period of time. There is narrowing of joint space, early cyst formation and early thickening of the both femoral head and acetabulum.

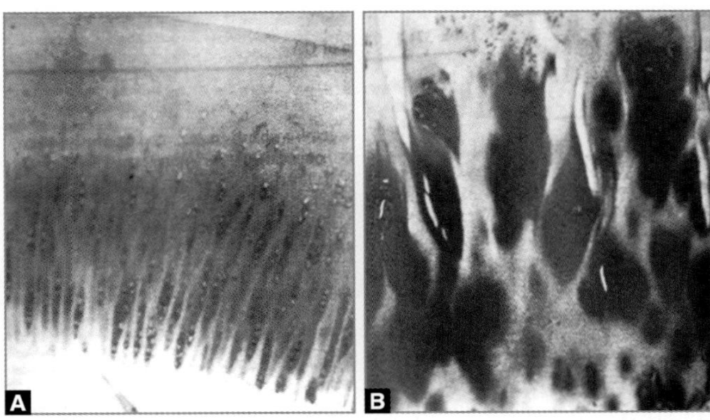

Figs. 170A and B: Early changes in osteoarthritis (as seen under light microscope).

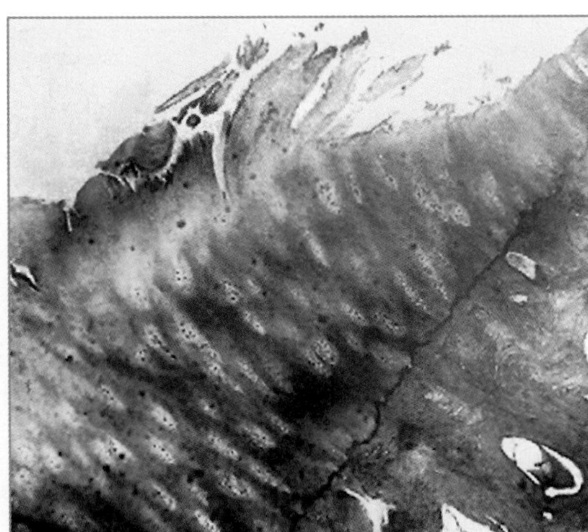

Fig. 171: Moderately advanced changes in osteoarthritis (as seen under light microscope).

in contrast to the rheumatoid form, in which ankylosis is frequent. Nevertheless, the gross peripheral proliferation and the presence of osteophytic outgrowths and dense capsular fibrosis may impede the free movements of the joint and even simulate a degree of fusion, which does not, in fact, exist.

Stages of Osteoarthritis as Seen under Light Microscopy

Early (Figs. 170A and B):

- Surface irregularities or fibrillation with small clefts not extending beyond superficial zone
- Slight hypercellularity
- Minimal loss of mucopolysaccharides.

Moderately advanced (Fig. 171):

- More extensive loss of surface
- Clefts extending into middle zone and occasionally into calcified zone
- Loss of mucopolysaccharides, extend into middle zone
- Hypercellularity in clusters of cells or chondrocyte clones.

Advanced changes (Fig. 172):

- Thickness of cartilage reduced
- Clefts may extend down to subchondral bone
- Mucopolysaccharides markedly reduced through entire thickness of cartilage

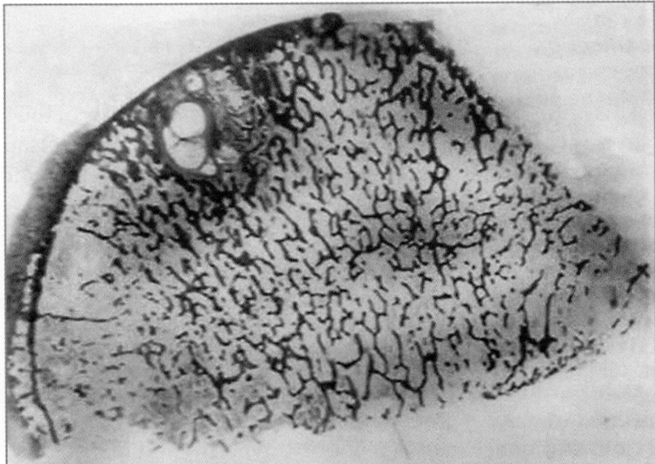

Fig. 172: Advanced changes in osteoarthritis (as seen under light microscope).

- In some areas, complete loss of cartilage with exposure of thick and eburnated subchondral bone.

Sites of osteoarthritis:

Figure 173 shows different sites of osteoarthritis.

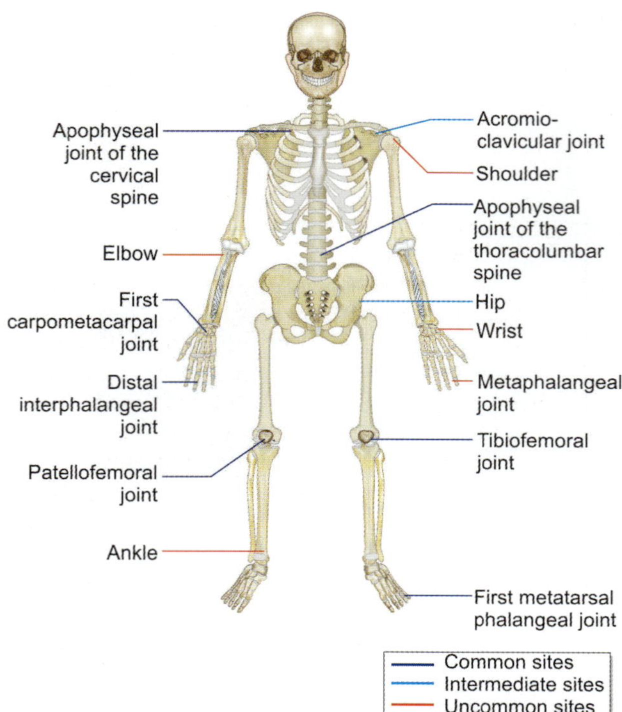

Fig. 173: Different sites of osteoarthritis.

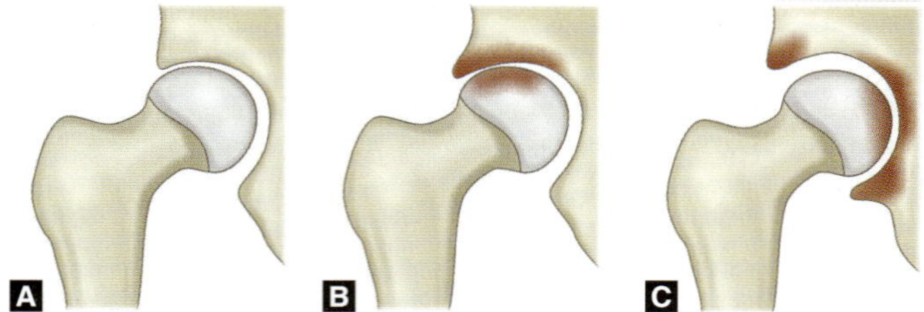

Figs. 174A to C: Osteoarthritis of hip, often unilateral at presentation and progresses with superolateral migration of the femoral head.

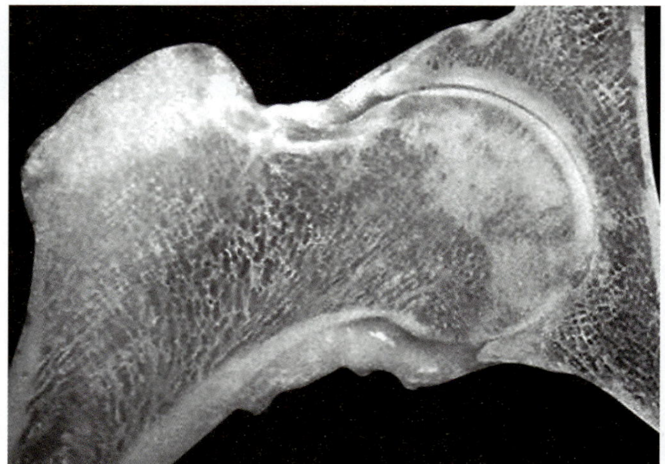

Fig. 175: Pathological changes in OA of hip.

Osteoarthritis of Hip (Figs. 174A to C)

- Familiarly called as malum coxa senilis.
- Most commonly targets the superior aspects of the joint.
- Often unilateral at presentation, often progresses with superolateral migration of the femoral head and has a poor prognosis.
- The less common central (medial) OA, shows more central cartilage loss and is largely confined to women.
- It is often bilateral at presentation, may associate with nodal generalized OA, uncommonly progresses with axial femoral migration and has a better prognosis.

Classification

Primary OA of hip:

- This is idiopathic and forms 50% of the osteoarthritis of the hip
- In this variety, the exact cause is not known and the causative factors suspected are increased anteversion and the trabecular microfracture, causing stiffening of the subchondral bone.

Secondary OA of hip:

Following factors are responsible:

- Incongruity of the articular surface, e.g. trauma, perthes, CDH, slipped epiphysis, etc.
- Instability of the hip, e.g. subluxation.
- Concentration of pressure load, e.g. coxa vara, anteversion.
- Direct injury, e.g. infection, trauma, etc.
- Constitutional cause, e.g. obesity, hyperthyroidism, etc.
- Bone diseases, like AVN, RA, etc.

Pathology (Fig. 175)

The earliest change in OA begins in the hyaline cartilage. Harrison believed that this is not at the summit of the femoral head of the femur (i.e. at the main pressure area), but at the nonpressure area of the lower part of the head, which is opposite to the acetabulum without an articular lining. He said that use and compression are necessary, to maintain the nutrition of the articular cartilage. The intermittent pumping action of alternate pressure and rest forces the synovial fluid into the cartilage. Hence, where pressure is absent, nutrition is likely to be absent and degeneration occurs more readily. The immediate reaction of the cartilage is proliferation of the subchondral blood vessels, which is interpreted as an attempt to bring about repair. Calcification and ossification take place in the deeper layers of the cartilage, then the blood vessels enter this calcified cartilage and further calcification takes place ahead of them. In nonpressure areas, this process continues indefinitely, the vessels spread outwards, preceded by a vanguard of calcification capped with a layer of fibrocartilage, this gradually increasing the size of the bone to form osteophytes. In vascular zone, beneath the pressure area cysts are formed and these cysts always communicate with the joint through small openings. The cyst increases in size from the intermittent pressure of the synovial fluid. At the late stage the hyperemic bone, no longer protected by its coverings of articular cartilage, decreases in height as a result of successive trabecular fractures. Areas of hyperemia, as well as venous stasis are seen and cause the severe, constant night pain in late disease. In response to the progressive breakdown of articular cartilage with loss of matrix proteoglycan and collagen and death of chondrocytes, there is response in the residual tissue of cellular division and increased glycosaminoglycan synthesis. In any event, the repair response of the cartilage is never sufficient to effect repair. Thus, inevitable gradual progression of the disease occurs.

Synovial Membrane and Capsule (Figs. 176A and B)

As matrix proteoglycan begins to leak out of the damaged articular cartilage, it produces direct irritation and inflammation of the synovial membrane, which undergoes hyperplasia of the lining layer and hyperemia. With the progressive accumulation of more cartilage and late bone debris, the inflammation persists and inflammatory cells are seen in the subsynovial tissue. With the hyperplasia, the synovium is thrown into folds and villi though these are never so profuse, as in RA. Fragments of cartilage and bone are engulfed by the synovial membrane and are seen in the subintima. Metaplasia of the synovium may occur with the point of attachment to the articular margins. These pedunculated masses may break off into the joint to form loose bodies or "joint mice". Loose fragments of cartilage and bone from the degenerating articular surface or from osteophytes may also remain free in the joint, giving rise to symptoms of "locking". The underlying capsule also becomes involved by the inflammatory process. As fibrosis commences in the synovium and capsule, the latter becomes thickened and shortened with resultant reduction in joint movements.

Clinical Features

- *Pain:* Often described as a deep ache and is localized to the involved joint. Typically, the pain of OA is aggravated by joint use and relieved by rest, but as disease progresses, it may become persistent
- Stiffness of the hip joint
- Muscle spasm
- Restriction of terminal movements
- Deformity-thigh is flexed, adducted, and externally rotated
- Shortening leading to limp, while walking
- Disturbed sleep.

Physical Examination

- Localized tenderness and bony or soft tissue swelling
- Bony crepitus are palpable, sometimes audible, coarse crepitus (rough articular surface)
- Joint line tenderness or periarticular tenderness
- Synovial effusions, if present are usually not large
- Palpation may reveal some warmth over the joint
- Periarticular muscle atrophy may be due to disuse or to reflex inhibition of muscle contraction
- In advanced stages of OA, there may be gross deformity, bony hypertrophy, subluxation, and marked loss of joint motion.

Deformity in OA Hip

In 80%, there is adduction, external rotation, and flexion deformity with joint space narrowing, cysts, and sclerosis in the superior segment of the femoral head and acetabulum. There is a somewhat valgus position of the femoral neck and a bony buttress develops on the inferior aspects of the neck. In 10%, there is external rotation of the femur but the leg is in neutral of slightly abducted. The radiological changes are seen mostly in the medial segment of the joint and there is a varus deformity of the femoral neck. In further 10%, there is concentric loss of cartilage space on the radiographs and the deformity is of flexion and slight abduction. The appearance may be similar to those of RA, except that there is hypertrophy of bone rather than atrophy of subchondral bone.

Investigations

- Routine investigations in primary OA are usually in normal limits
- Analysis of synovial fluid reveals mild leukocytosis, with a predominance of mononuclear cells
- Other investigations are depending upon the predisposing factors, if present
- Radiographs of both the hips
- Ultrasound, arthroscopy, and MRI have limited role.

Radiology (Fig. 177)

- *Stage I:* Hyperemia with periarticular osteoporosis.
- *Stage II:* Reduction in joint space.
- *Stage III:* Osteophytes formation, with subchondral sclerocystic changes.
- *Stage IV:* Complete loss of joint space with or without subluxation.

Differential Diagnosis

The diagnosis of chronic arthritis is seldom difficult, unless pain and swelling are limited to one joint. When the onset is acute, gout, pseudogout, rheumatic fever, and infective arthritis have

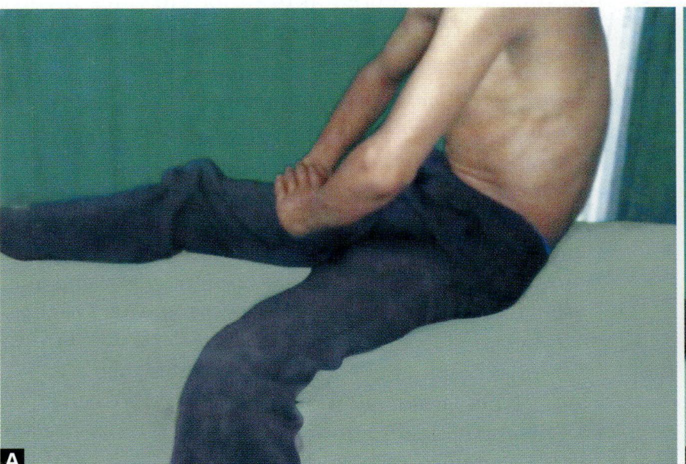

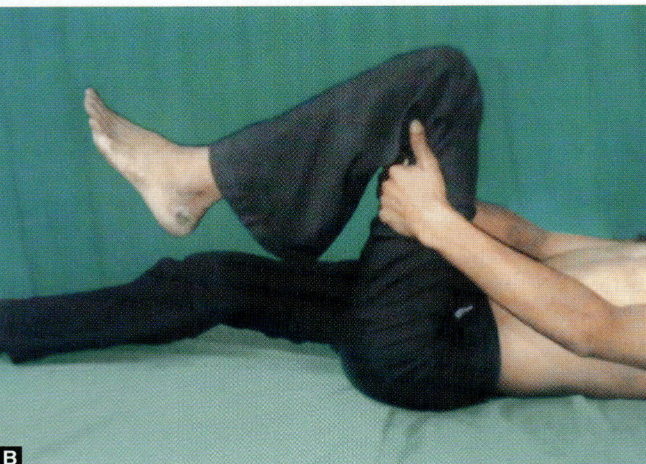

Figs. 176A and B: Effect of inflammatory changes on synovial membrane and joint capsule.

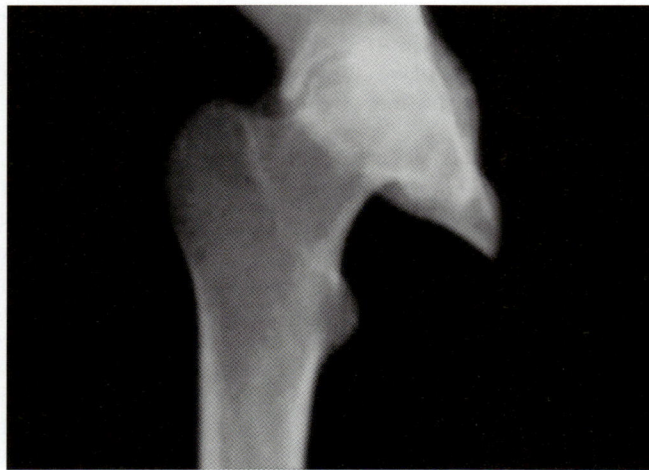

Fig. 177: Radiograph showing OA of hip.

TABLE 8: Laboratory differentiation in rheumatoid arthritis and osteoarthritis.

	Rheumatoid arthritis	*Osteoarthritis*
Agglutination reactions Sedimentation rate	Positive in over 50% of typical cases Usually greatly increased; tends to return to normal as patient improves	Never definitely positive Normal or only slightly increased
Roentgenographic appearances	*Early:* Osteoporosis, periarticular swelling, and joint effusion *Late:* Narrowing of joint space, bone destruction, ankylosis, and deformities	*Early:* No osteoporosis; slight lipping at joint margins *Late:* Marked lipping, osteophytes narrowing of joint space deformation of articular bone ends

first to be considered. In the younger people, it may be necessary to distinguish between RA, gouty diasthesis, gonococcal arthritis, and tuberculosis.

Laboratory and radiological differentiation in RA and OA illustrated in Table 8.

Treatment Options

- Medications
- Injections
- Physical therapy
- Weight loss
- Nutrition consult
- Surgery.

Conservative

- Rest
- Active and passive ROM
- Abstinence from weight bearing
- Vertical load reduction
- Traction
- Physical therapy
- Orthotics
- Heat therapy
- Graduated exercise
- Drug therapy.

Drug Therapy

- NSAIDs
- Chondrosynthesis drugs
- Chondroprotective and disease modifying drugs
- Antioxidants vitamins
- Antioxidants minerals
- Semi-invasive treatment.

NSAIDs

Diclofenac and aceclofenac: These drugs produce their anti-inflammatory and analgesic effect, by inhibiting cyclo-oxygenase and thus, preventing production of prostaglandins from arachidonic acid. In addition, aceclofenac has shown some stimulatory effects on cartilage matrix synthesis that may be linked to ability of drug to inhibit IL-1 activity.

Chondrosynthetic drugs:

Glucosamine: Rejoint is the sulfate derivative of amino monosaccharide glucosamine, a normal constituent glucosaminoglycan in the cartilage. Given orally in the dose of 1500 mg daily in divided doses for long periods, it is claimed to slow down the progression of OA.

Chondroitin:

- Nonspecific slow acting chondroprotective, but helps in chondrosynthesis.
- Supplement action of glucosamine.
- Inhibits proinflammatory prostaglandin/leukotrienes.
- Inhibit hyaluronidase enzyme, e.g. breakdown hyaluronic acid (HA) molecule and viscosity of synovial fluid.

Chondroprotective and disease modifying drugs:

- Inhibit pain by inhibiting synthesis of cytokines.
- Improves mobility, by stimulating the production of collagen II and proteoglycan.
- Reduces stiffness, by stimulating the production of hyalurons.

Others:

- Antioxidant vitamins, e.g. vitamin C, E, beta-carotene.
- Antioxidant minerals, e.g. selenium, Mn, Zn.

Newer drugs:

- Diacerein
- Dosage 50 mg twice daily
- Inhibits the production of IL-1
- Also inhibits the secretion of other enzymes involved in cartilage destruction, like myeloperoxidase, glucuronidase, and elastase.

Semi-invasive treatment corticosteroids:

- *Intra-articular cortisone:*
  - Temporary relief.
  - Satisfying and lasting in mild and moderate cases.
  - When there is no response to conservative treatment in acute inflammatory phase.
  - In case of severe OA, there is pain in pericapsular site (outside joint)—Pes anserinus and biceps. Local steroid, shows good result:
    - Risk of joint infection
    - Hypopigmentation
    - Subcutaneous atrophy
    - Osteonecrosis.
- Repeated—Long-acting depot preparation.

- *Intra-articular injection of hyaluronic acid*: It includes viscosupplementation therapy:
  - Safe and effective
  - Pain, improves joints function for months
  - Five injections, weekly.

Physical Therapy

- Flexibility
- Strength
- Walking pattern
- Leg length
- Shoes
- Weight
- Lifestyle
- Goals
- *Flexibility (Figs. 178 and 179)*
- *Strength (Figs. 180A to C)*
  - Slow
  - Rhythmic
  - Light resistance
  - 30 min/day
  - 6 days/week
- *Walking pattern and shoes (Figs. 181A and B)*
- *Leg length (Figs. 182A and B)*
- *Body weight and lifestyle*
  - For every 1 pound of body weight you lose, it takes 3 pounds of pressure off your hips
  - Losing 10 pounds, takes 30 pounds of pressure off your hips
  - Create a manageable schedule
  - Alternate heavy tasks with light tasks
  - Change positions frequently
  - Plan rest breaks during your activities
  - Apply heat and/or cold
  - Heat, increases blood circulation

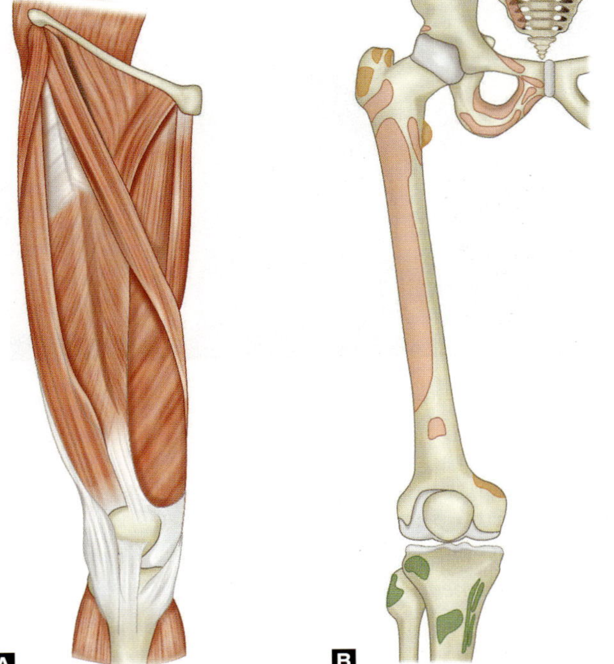

Figs. 178A and B: Musculature around hip joint.

  - Cold, decreases inflammation and pain
  - 15 minutes maximum.

Operative Treatment

Indications:
- Pain unrelieved by conservative treatment
- Limitation of movements
- Flexion adduction deformity, with pelvic tilt and distortion of the lumbar spine.

Surgical options:
- Synovectomy
- Arthroscopic lavage with debridement
- Osteotomies
- Arthrodesis
- Arthroplasties.

Arthroscopy:
- Joint clean-up
- Symptom relief
- 50–90% for cartilage tears of socket
- Limited benefit for arthritis.

Arthrodesis (Figs. 183 and 184):
- Usually Watson Jones arthrodesis is performed
- Hip is exposed through a Smith Petersen approach
- The head and the acetabulum are thoroughly denuded
- The nail is inserted through the neck and the head, so that 1 inch of the nail engages in the pelvis
- A bone graft removed from the ilium is inserted through a slot in the superior acetabular rim and fixed by a screw to the neck, as shown in Figure 182.

Osteotomies:
- Correction of mechanical malalignment
- Brings into contact nondamaged articular surface, hence, reducing friction and pain
- Alters weight-bearing and joint reaction forces
- Decongests venous stasis and venous hypertension in metaphyseal trabecular bone.

Intertrochanteric osteotomy (Fig. 185): Intertrochanteric osteotomy for the relief of pain in an OA hip was introduced by McMurray, which is based on principle of providing pelvic support through the shaft of femur. Pain was relieved because of the altered thrust of weight bearing and rotation of the femoral head, which brought an unaffected portion of the femoral articular cartilage in contact with the acetabulum. It requires displacement of the distal femoral fragments beneath the inferior acetabular rim.

Pauwel's varus osteotomy (Figs. 186 and 187): The clinical indications for varus osteotomy, according to Blount, are hips with painless, adequate abduction, and limited painful adduction, an antalgic gait and apparent lengthening. Varus osteotomy consists of resecting a segment of bone from the intertrochanteric area, with its base directed medially. The wedge must be removed from the proximal fragment, so that the level of transection of the distal shaft fragment lies transverse and therefore, will not interfere with rotation. External rotation and flexion deformity are corrected, by rotating the extremity inward, with the base of the wedge extended towards the posterior aspect to permit anterior angulation.

Valgus osteotomy (Figs. 188 and 189): An abduction (valgus) osteotomy is indicated for the OA hip in patient who walks with a

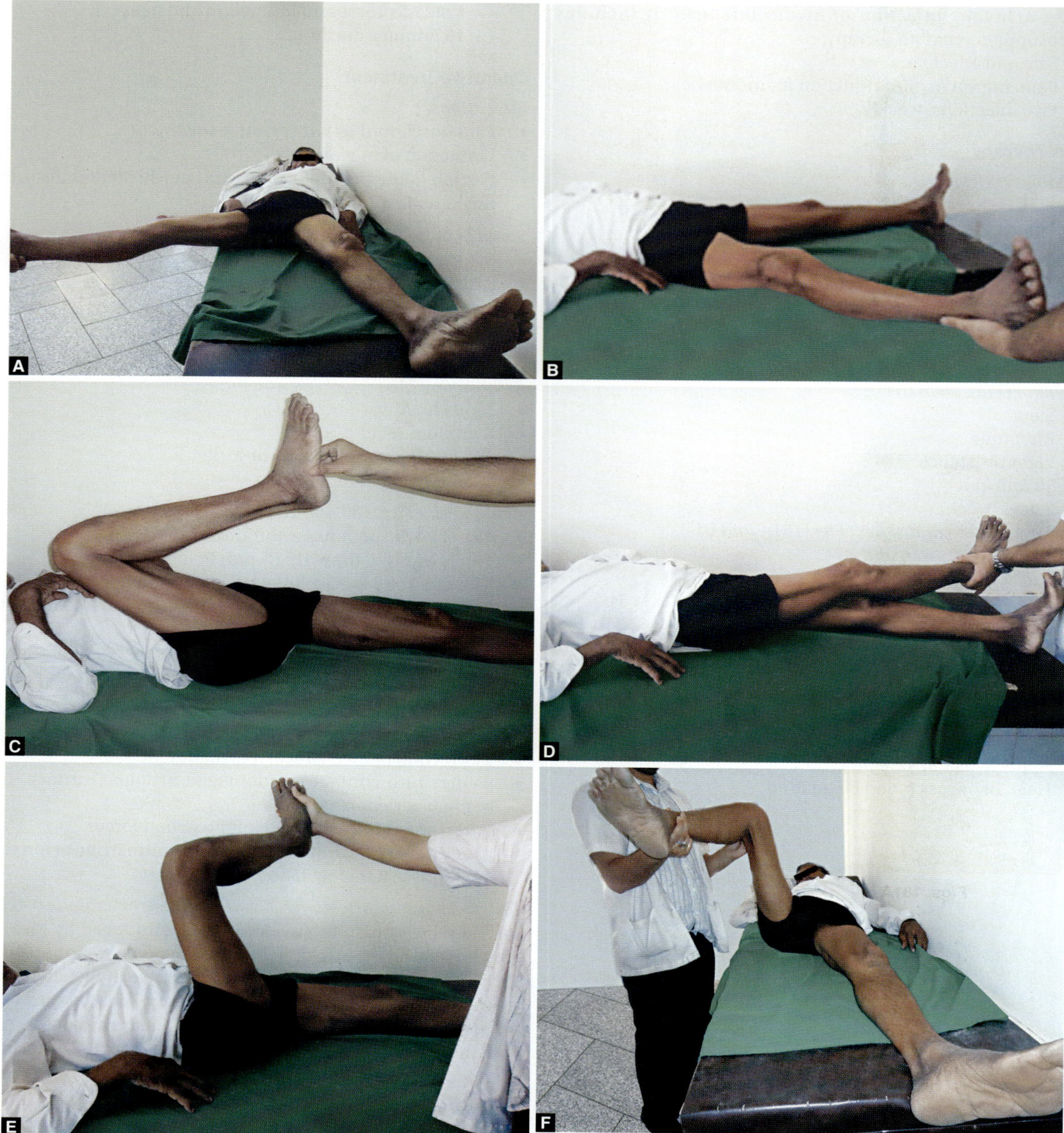

Figs. 179A to F: Lower limb flexibility exercises.

Trendelenburg Lurch and has an adduction deformity and in whom further abduction is not possible, adduction is limited and painful and repositioning of the femoral head within the acetabulum is demonstrable on the roentgenogram, when the hip is adducted. Wedge of bone is resected laterally. Insertion of nail plate forms an angle with outer aspect of shaft. Shaft has been abducted, fragment ends were approximated and compression device is in place. Compression is applied and first screws are inserted.

Arthroplasty

- Interposition (cup) arthroplasty
- Excision arthroplasty
- Total replacement arthroplasty.

Total hip replacement (Figs. 190 and 191):

- Uncemented THR
- Cemented THR
- Surface replacement.

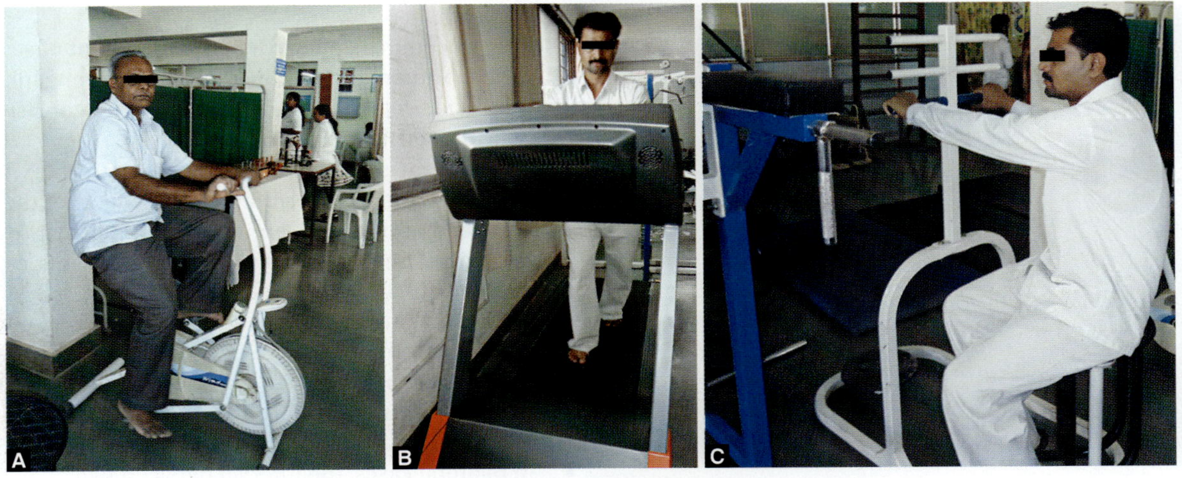

Figs. 180A to C: Strength building exercises of lower limb.

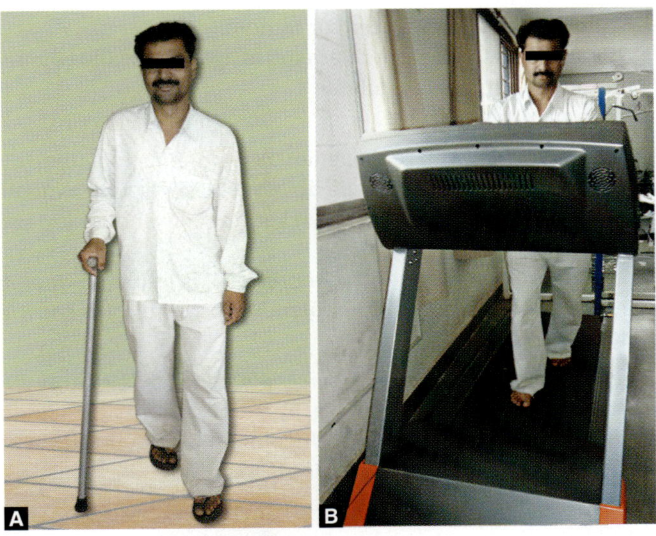

Figs. 181A and B: Walking pattern.

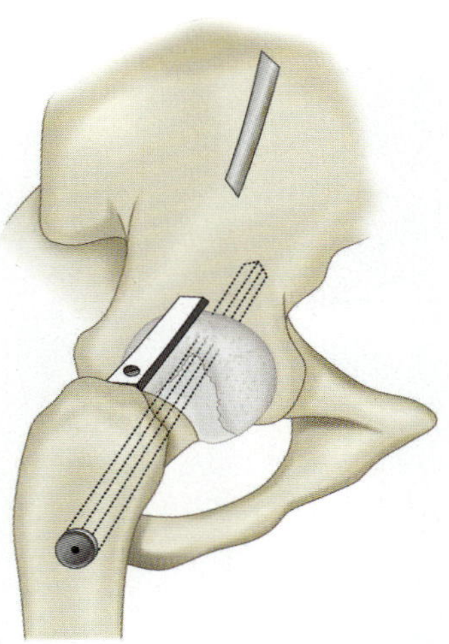

Fig. 183: Hip arthrodesis: A bone graft removed from the ilium is inserted through a slot in the superior acetabular rim and fixed by a screw to the neck.

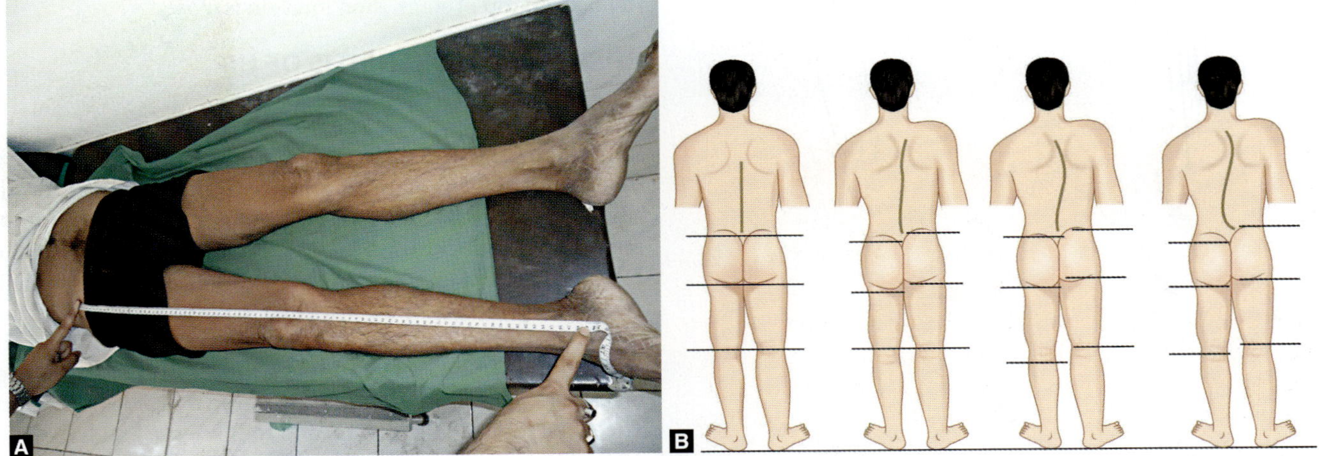

Figs. 182A and B: Limb length measurement.

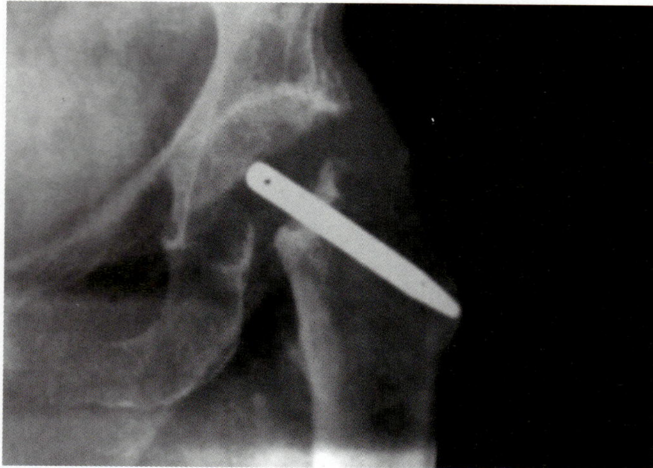

Fig. 184: Hip prosthesis, Judet type. Roentgenographic appearance. This was the forerunner of the modern hip prosthesis. The head was composed of acrylic. Breakage and loosening were frequent.

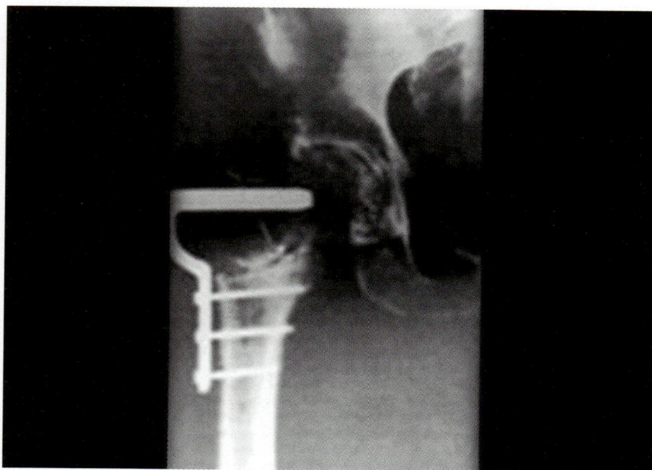

Fig. 185: Intertrochanteric osteotomy for pain relief.

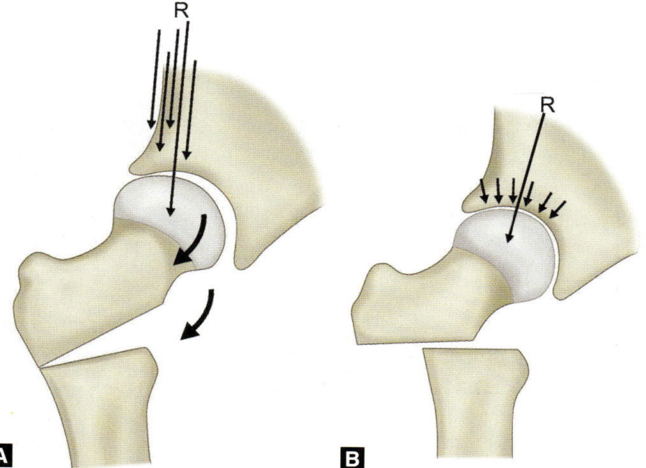

Figs. 186A and B: Pauwel's varus osteotomy. Arrow forces directed acetabulum to head of femur.

Indications:
- The procedure is effective in the treatment of severe osteoarthritis, primary or secondary to trauma, congenital dysplasia, protrusio acetabulae, AVN, local benign neoplasm, and metabolic disease.
- The patient should be over 60 years of age, because the durability and long-term biological effects of the component and cement materials are not yet established (exceptionally, the procedure may be done in younger patients, especially with bilateral hip disease).
- If the previous operations (e.g. prosthesis, cup arthroplasty, and osteotomy) were unsuccessful, infection as a cause of failure must be ruled out, prior to THR. In doubtful cases, the hardware must be removed and cultures obtained before THR at a later date.
- In bilateral cases, the interval between two operations should be less than 3 months.

Contraindications:
- When the infection is recent or remote
- When the person is under 60 years of age, especially when the alternative surgery is available
- When pain is not severe.

Charnley principles: Hip replacement components include:
- Acetabular component made up of metal shell, with a medical grade plastic or metal inner socket liner, as shown in Figure 192A.
- The femoral component (stem portion), is made up of metal. Femoral head is made, either of metal or ceramic, as shown in Figure 192B.

Hip replacement: cemented or uncemented (Figs. 193 and 194): Cemented implant is held in place, by a type of epoxy cement that attaches the metal to the bone. Uncemented implant has a fine surface (mesh of holes) allowing tissue to grow.

Surgical procedure (Figs. 195 and 196): Incision made on the side of the thigh. Socket is reshaped, to fit new cup implant that replaces the diseased socket. New cup is placed in the socket. Femur is prepared for the stem and hip stem is implanted and the ball is put in place on top of stem, then incision is closed.

RHEUMATOID ARTHRITIS OF HIP

Introduction

Rheumatoid arthritis (RA) is a chronic inflammatory systemic disease of young or middle-aged adults, characterized by destructive and proliferative changes in synovial membrane, periarticular structures, skeletal muscle, and perineural sheaths. Eventually, joints are destroyed, ankylosed, and deformed. RA is a systemic inflammatory disorder that mainly affects the diarthrodial joint. The clinical course of the disorder is extremely variable, ranging from mild, self-limiting arthritis to rapidly progressive multisystem inflammation with profound morbidity and mortality. The small joints of the fingers and toes are the first to be affected. As the disease progresses, it tends to spread to involve the wrists, elbows, shoulders, knees, ankles, subtalar, and midtarsal joints.

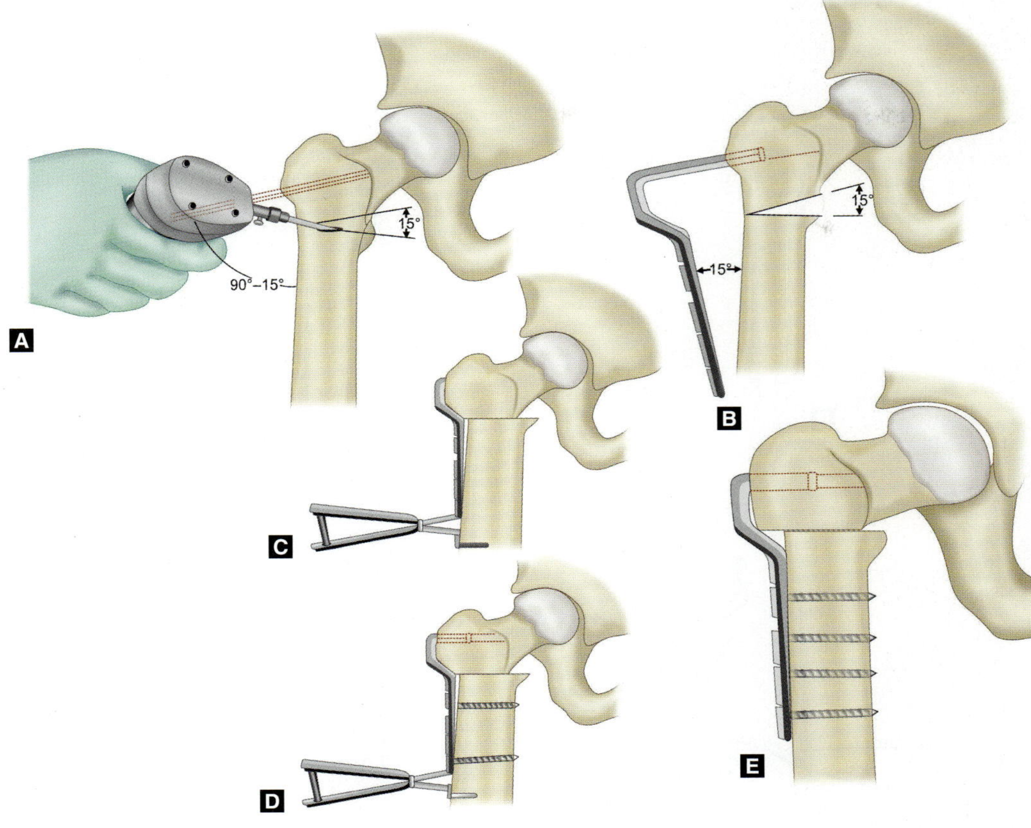

Figs. 187A to E: Different steps in performing varus osteotomy—(A to C) Resecting a segment of bone from the intertrochanteric area, with its base directed medially. The wedge must be removed from the proximal fragment, so that the level of transection of the distal shaft fragment lies transverse and therefore, will not interfere with rotation; (D and E) External rotation and flexion deformity are corrected by rotating the extremity inward, with the base of the wedge extended towards the posterior aspect to permit anterior angulation.

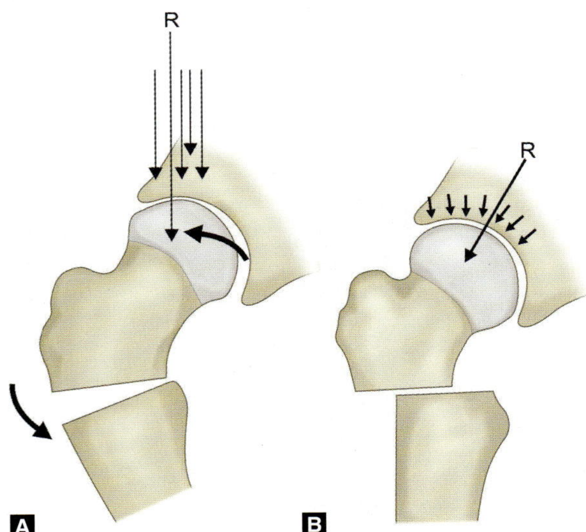

Figs. 188A and B: An abduction (valgus) osteotomy.

Etiology

- Cause remains unknown
- Might be manifestation of the response to an infectious agent in a genetically susceptible host. Possible causative agents are: *Mycoplasma, Epstein-Barr virus* (EBV), *Cytomegalovirus, Parvovirus* and *Rubella virus*
- Environmental trigger, e.g. smoking
- Genetic traits, e.g. HLA-DR4 and DR1.

Epidemiology

- RA has a high prevalence in the Indian population (around 0.75%)
- Thus, projected population of at least 7 million patients
- Male : female ratio is 1:3
- The peak age of onset is in the fourth decade in females and slightly later in males
- 40–60% with advance RA will
  - Survive 5 years or less following diagnosis
  - Die 10–15 years earlier than expected.

Pathogenesis (Fig. 197)

In RA, the immune system loses its ability to recognize synovial tissue, as self-tissue and thus, attacks the synovial tissue and causes inflammation and destruction. The macrophages or antigen presenting cells (APCs) are responsible for recognizing the antigen and presenting them to the T cells, which in turn leads to activation of T cells. Activated T cells recruit more T cells and B cells. Release of cytokines, lead to proliferation of rheumatoid synovial tissue and destruction of bone, as shown in Figure 198. B cells produce antibodies, which attract polymorphonuclear leukocytes, which in turn release more cytotoxins and free oxygen radicals. The resultant production of immunoglobulin and rheumatoid factor can lead to immune complex formation with consequent complement activation and exacerbation of the inflammatory process.

Pannus (Fig. 199):

Rheumatoid nodules (Fig. 200): Rheumatoid nodules are made up of central necrotic area, palisade formation by mononuclear cells, round cell infiltration, and fibrous capsule.

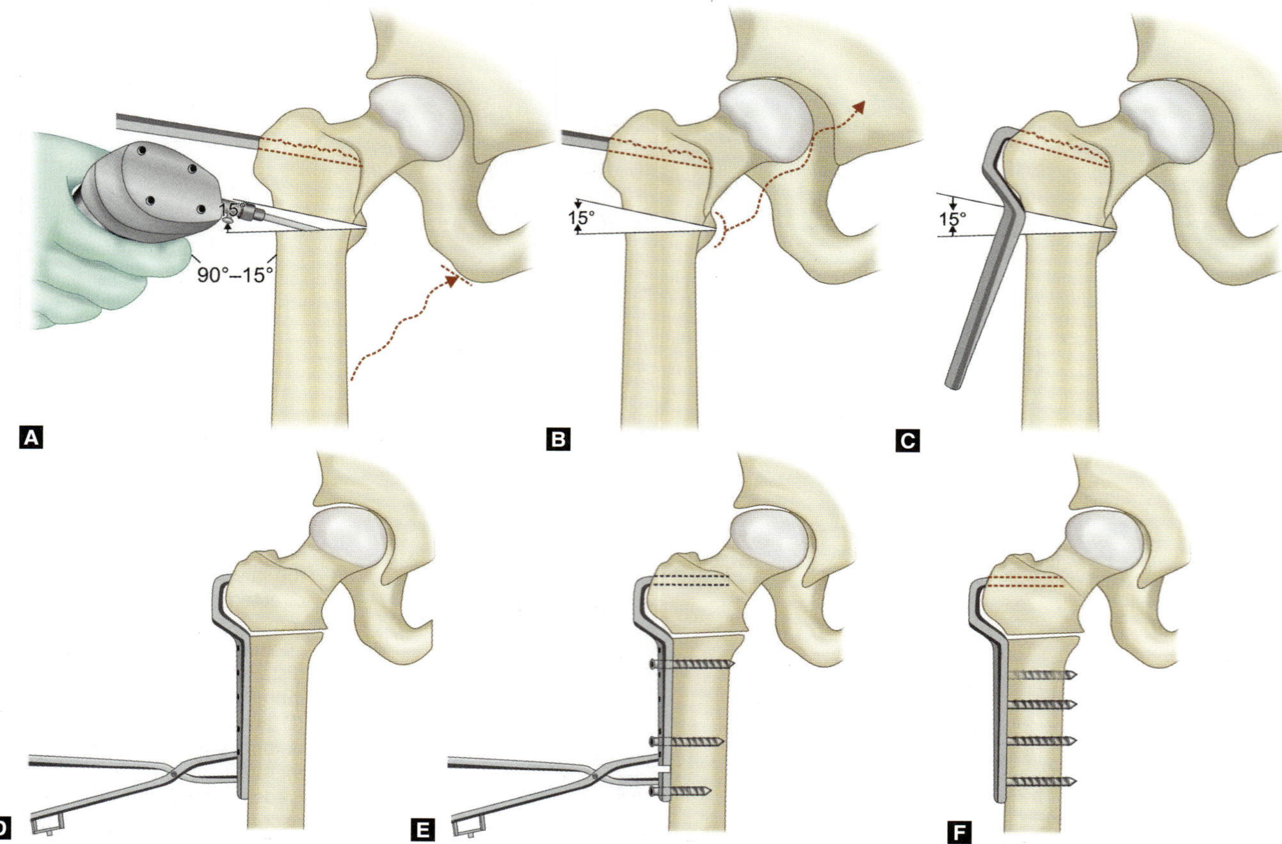

Figs. 189A to F: (A to C) Wedge of bone is resected laterally. Insertion of nail plate forms an angle with outer aspect of shaft; (D to F) Shaft has been abducted, fragment ends were approximated and compression device is in place. Compression is applied and first screws are inserted.

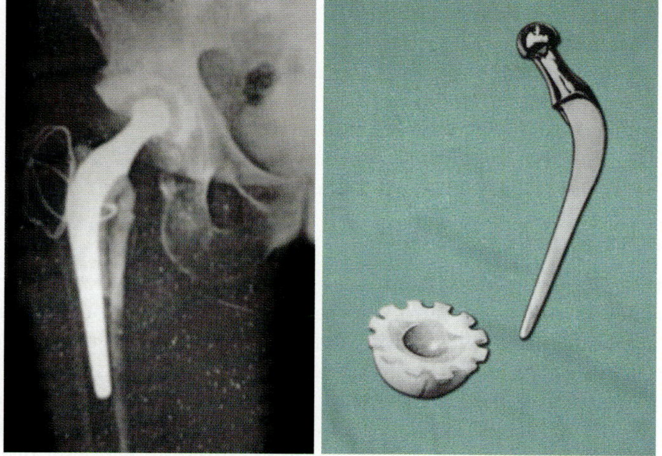

Fig. 190: Cemented THR with hip prosthesis.

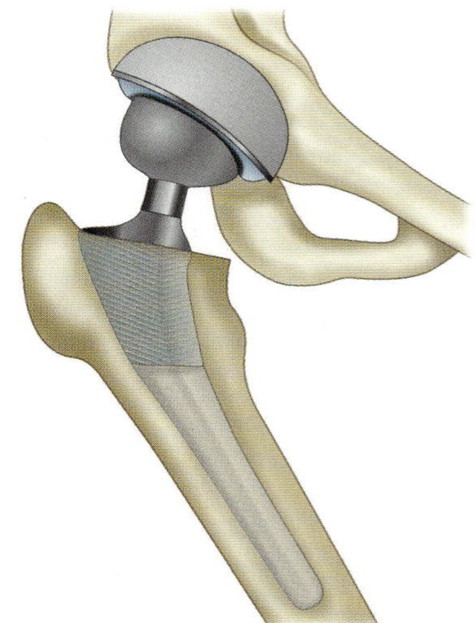

Fig. 191: Uncemented total hip replacement.

Clinical Features

- Joint swelling
- Pain/stiffness (commonly in morning and lasting for more than 1 hour) and pain on motion
- Tenderness
- Weakness
- Deformity
- Fatigue
- Malaise
- Fever
- Weight loss
- Depression.

Extra-articular manifestations: The extra-articular manifestation of RA is listed in Table 9.

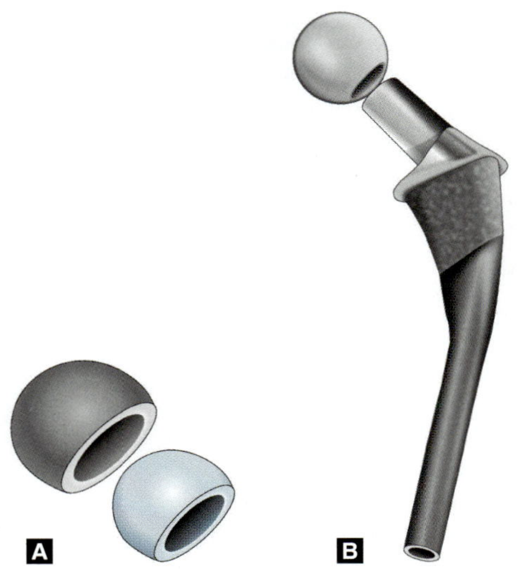

Figs. 192A and B: (A) Acetabular component; (B) Femoral component.

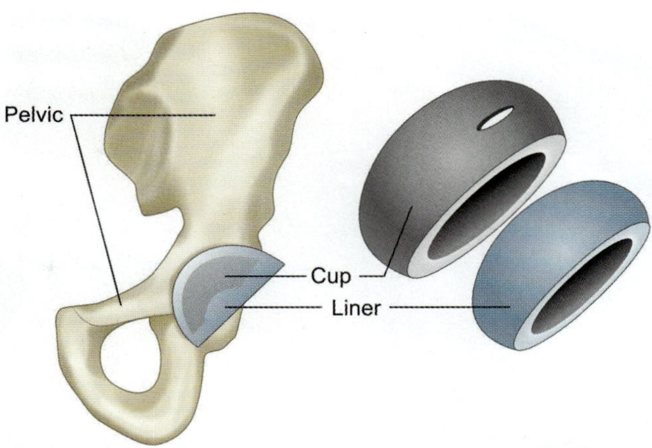

Fig. 195: Incision made on the side of the thigh. Socket is reshaped, to fit new cup implant that replaces the diseased socket.

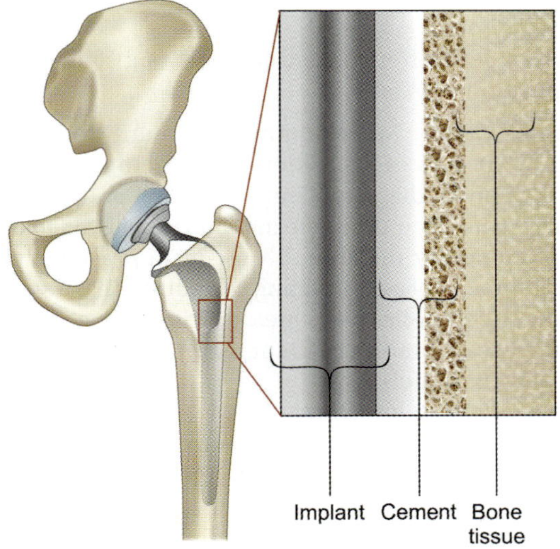

Fig. 193: Cemented hip replacement.

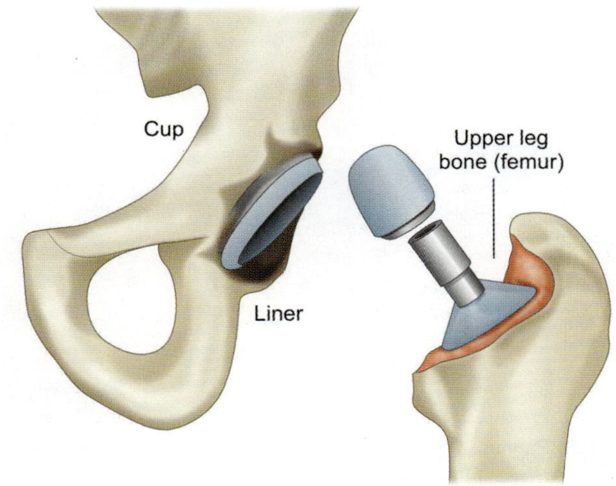

Fig. 196: New cup is placed in the socket. Femur is prepared for the stem and hip stem is implanted and the ball is put in place on top of stem, then incision is closed.

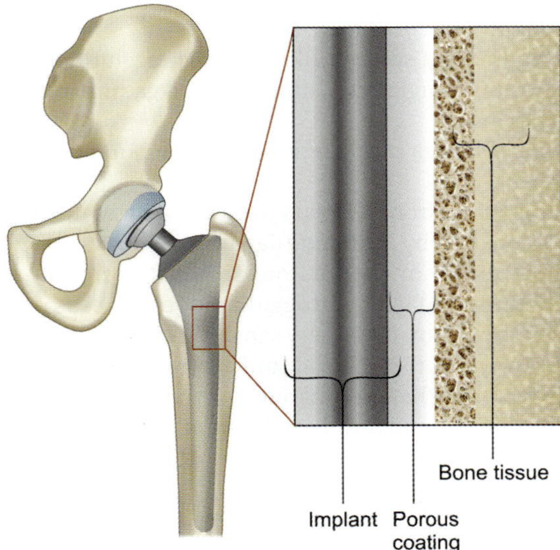

Fig. 194: Uncemented THR.

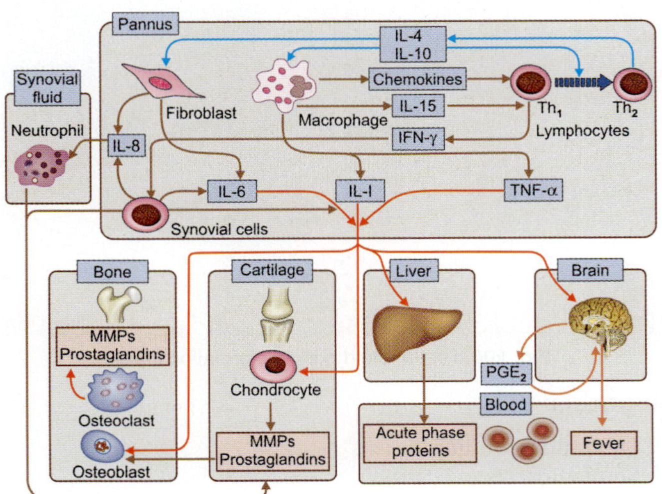

Fig. 197: Pathogenesis of RA of hip.

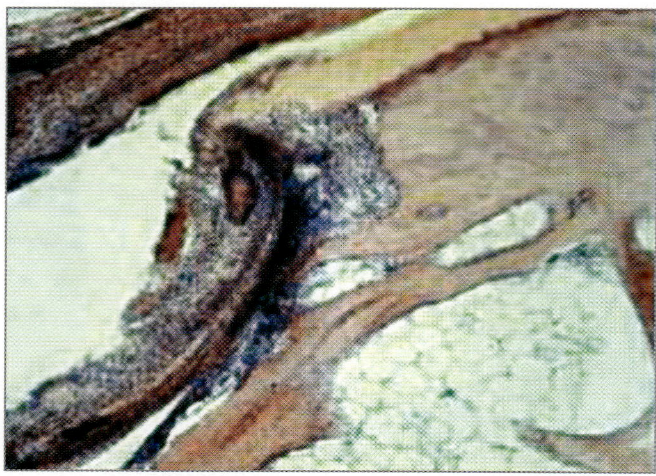

Fig. 198: Rheumatoid synovial tissue.

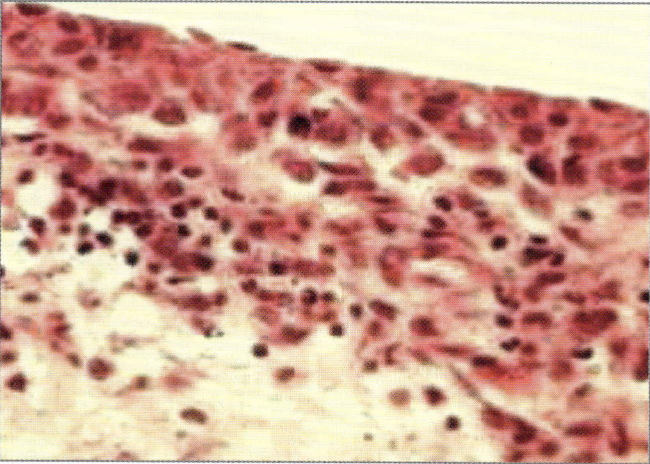

Fig. 199: Pannus: Thickened synovium with lymphocytic infiltrate and neovascularization.

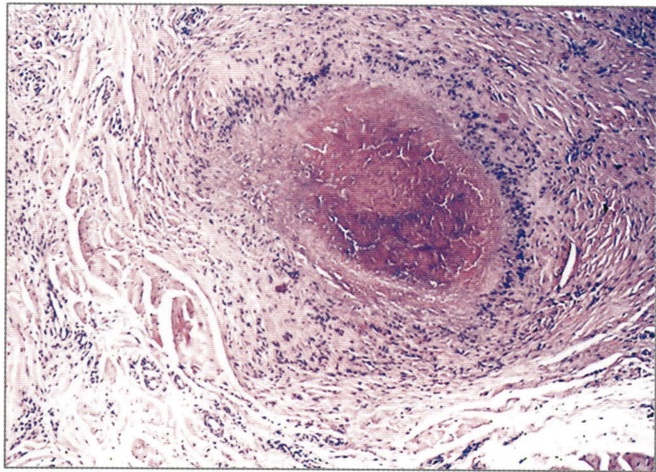

Fig. 200: Rheumatoid nodules formation in RA.

Diagnosis

- Laboratory findings
- Serologic tests
- Roentgenographic findings.

TABLE 9: Extra-articular manifestation of RA.

Organ system	*Involvement*
Skin	Rheumatoid nodules
Ocular	Episcleritis and scleritis
Cardiac	Pericarditis and myocarditis
Pulmonary	Nodules and pleural effusion
Neurological	Neuropathy and cervical cord compression
Lymphatic	Splenomegaly
Musculoskeletal	Muscle wasting and tenosynovitis
Hematologic	Anemia and thrombocytosis
Vascular	Vasculitis

Laboratory findings:
- ESR is elevated particularly during active stage
- During periods of remission ESR continues to increase, but to a lesser extent
- Hypochromic normocytic anemia is frequently associated.

Serologic tests:
- *RA factor:* Serum from patient contains a substance of unknown composition—RA factor.

Rheumatoid factor: Most common autoantibody in RA and detected in 70–80% of RA patients. RA factor does not have a predictive value for diagnosis, but has a good predictive value for poorer outcome. Their presence in joints is believed to contribute to the inflammatory reaction. RA factor in presence of gamma globulin is capable of agglutinating certain strains of streptococci, sensitized sheep cells, and latex particles. A convenient lab procedure uses a standard suspension of latex particles in a solution of gamma globulins.
- *Latex fixation test on serum:*
  - *Latex suspension:* Unknown serum and gamma globulin.
  - *Agglutination occurs:* Serum contains, adequate amount of RA factor.
  - *No agglutination:* Serum contains inadequate amount of RA factor.
  - If there is no agglutination, then second more sensitive test must be performed.
- *The inhibition test:*
  - Rheumatoid serum of known high agglutinating activity, unknown euglobulin, and standard gamma globulin latex suspension
  - This test uses characteristics of euglobulin from unknown serum
  - Euglobulin from normal serum neutralizes the rheumatoid factor, thereby inhibiting agglutination
  - Euglobulin of rheumatoid serum has no effect on the rheumatoid factor and agglutination proceeds unhindered
  - The inhibition test is very sensitive. It is likely to be positive, even when the rheumatoid factor is present in minute amounts. When an unknown serum shows negative latex fixation test and positive inhibition test, the arthritis may be a part of rheumatoid spondylitis or a lupus erythematosus.

Roentgenographic findings (Fig. 201):

Early changes: Osteoporosis, periarticular swelling, and joint effusion.

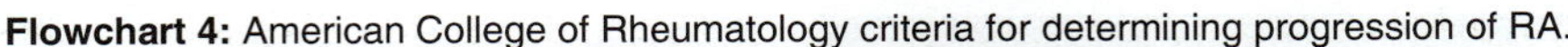

Flowchart 4: American College of Rheumatology criteria for determining progression of RA.

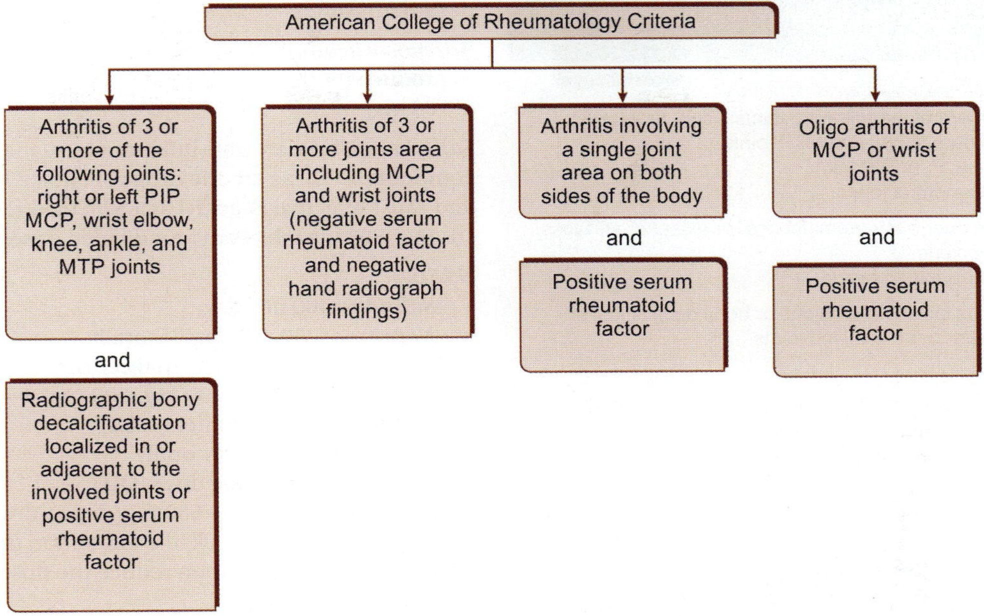

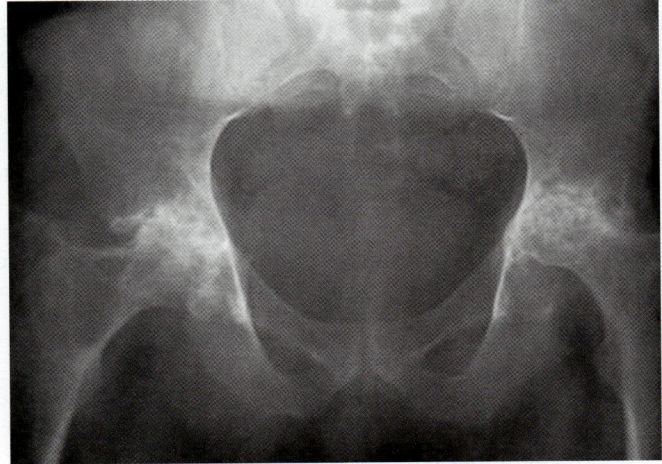

Fig. 201: X-ray showing pathological changes in hip due to RA.

Late changes: Narrowing of joint space, bone destruction, ankylosis, and deformities.

Criteria for Diagnosis

- Morning stiffness
- Pain on motion or tenderness in at least one joint
- Swelling (soft tissue thickening or fluid; not bony outgrowth alone) in at least one joint continuously for not less than 6 weeks
- Swelling of at least one other joint
- Symmetrical joint swelling
- Subcutaneous nodules
- X-ray changes typical of RA
- Positive latex fixation test
- Poor mucin clot
- Characteristic histologic changes in synovial membrane
- Characteristic histologic changes in nodules. *Classic:* Any seven criteria for at least 6 weeks. *Definite:* Any five criteria for at least 6 weeks. *Probable:* Any three criteria for at least 4 weeks.

American College of Rheumatology Clinical Classification Criteria for Rheumatoid Arthritis

This is based on history, physical examination, laboratory, and radiographic findings, as shown in Table 10.

American College of Rheumatology (ACR) Classification Criteria for Determining Progression of RA is shown in Flowchart 4.

American College of Rheumatology Classification Criteria for Determining Clinical Remission in Rheumatoid Arthritis

Five or more of the following are present in at least two consecutive months:

1. Morning stiffness less than 15 minutes
2. No fatigue
3. No joint pain
4. No joint tenderness or pain on motion
5. No soft tissue swelling in joints or tendon sheaths
6. ESR (Westergren method) less than 30 mm/hour for a female or 20 mm/hour for a male.
7. Maintenance of function. This is illustrated in Flowchart 5.

American College of Rheumatology Classification Criteria of Functional Status in Rheumatoid Arthritis

- *Class I:* Completely able to perform usual activities of daily living (self-care, vocational, and avocational).
- *Class II:* Able to perform usual self-care and vocational activities, but limited in avocational activities.
- *Class III:* Able to perform usual self-care activities, but limited in vocational and avocational activities.
- *Class IV*: Limited ability to perform usual self-care, vocational, and avocational activities.

Treatment

The goals of the therapy of RA are:

- Relief of pain
- Reduction of inflammation

TABLE 10: American College of Rheumatology (ACR) clinical classification criteria for RA of the following must be present with 1 through 4 present a minimum of 6 weeks.

Morning stiffness > 1 hour
• Arthritis of three or more of the following joints: Right or left PIP, MCP, wrist, elbow, knee, ankle, and MTP joints – Arthritis of wrist, MCP, or PIP joint – Symmetric involvement of joints
• Rheumatoid nodules over bony prominences, or extensor surfaces, or in juxta-articular regions – Positive serum rheumatoid factor
• Radiographic changes including erosions or bony decalcification localized in or adjacent to the involved joints

Flowchart 5: Treatment goals in RA pyramid of therapeutic options in rheumatoid arthritis.

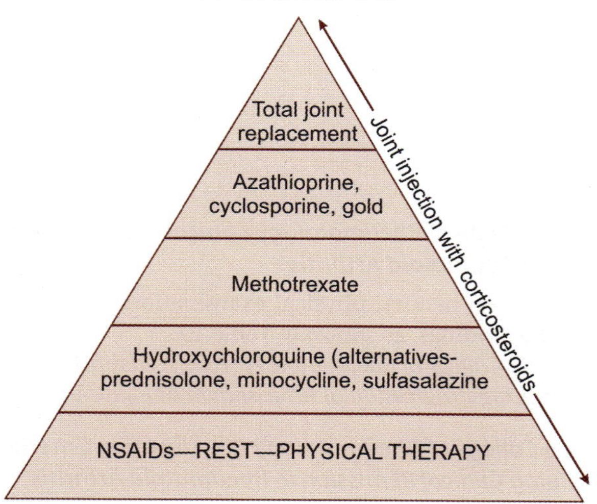

Treatment of RA can be divided into three modes:

1. Conservative
2. Surgical
3. Rehabilitation.

Conservative Treatment

Rest: Complete bed rest.

Removal of foci of infection: Teeth, tonsils, sinuses, and pelvic organs are investigated and infections are eliminated.

Nutritious diet: A diet high in calories and high in vitamins is essential.

Transfusions and hematinics: These are continually necessary during entire course of disease.

Hormones: Combination of estrogen and androgen are given for their anabolic effect, to bone structure.

Dilute HCl: It is given to combat achlorhydria that leads to anemia.

Splinting: Inflamed joint is immobilized in plaster splint, to relieve pain and reduce inflammation and the position of function is desirable in event that ankylosis occurs.

Position of rest for inflamed hip:

- 5° of flexion, 5° of abduction, and neutral rotation.
- *Cortisone:* 17-hydroxy-11-dehydrocorticosterone.

Synthetic steroids: Prednisone, prednisolone, triamcinolone, and dexamethasone.

Adrenocorticotropic hormone (ACTH): Stimulates adrenal cortex to produce more of compound E and F. It is injected in daily dose of 100 mg.

Salicylates: These are anti-inflammatory, analgesic, and antipyretic compounds. These are the drugs of choice for RA. Most common and most effective is acetyl salicylic acid (aspirin, ASA). Around 10–15 g, 300 mg tablets in four divided doses are given.

NSAIDs

- *Sulindac:* 400 mg/day
- *Naproxen:* 250–500 mg BD orally
- *Tolmetin:* 1,200 mg/day in three divided doses
- *Ibuprofen:* 300 mg, 400 mg, 600 mg, 3–4 times/day half hour before or 2–3 hours after meals
- *Piroxicam:* 20 mg/day orally
- *Indomethacin:* 25 mg doses QID
- *Phenylbutazone:* 300–600 mg/day in divided doses, if there is no response for 1 week, then abandon the drug, and if there is adequate response then reduce the dose to less than 400 mg/day.
- *Gold salts:* Gold sodium thiomalate (myochrysine)
  - *Procedure:* It is given deep intramuscular.
  - *Dosage:* First injection of 10 mg dose is given for the first week followed by 25 mg dose, second week is followed by 50 mg dose and third week 50 mg dose is repeated weekly for 4–5 months, until total of 1 g of dose is given. With each dose 10 mL of 10% calcium is given, to decrease the possibility of reaction. Another course, given after 6–12 months or after remission
  - Change of symptoms is expected after 6–15 weeks. If there is no improvement after 5 months, then abandon the drug
  - Sensitivity test to be done. Toxic reactions that can occur are:
    - Pruritus
    - Stomatitis
    - Diarrhea
    - Microscopic hematuria
    - Albuminuria
    - Granulocytopenia
    - Thrombocytopenia
    - Every 2 weeks a complete blood count and platelet count is done
    - The reduction of hemoglobin, leukocytes, platelets and tendency to eosinophilia are danger signals
    - In case of toxic reactions British-Anti-Lewisite (BAL), dimercaprol is given
  - *Contraindications:* Hepatic or renal damage and blood dyscrasias.
- *Combined cortisone and gold therapy:* Has a little advantage over gold therapy alone.
- *Manipulation:* Gentle prolonged traction and gradual spontaneous correction by active motion.
- *X-ray treatment:* More useful in RA of spine.
- *Relief of muscle spasm:* Drugs most commonly used for this are:
  - Myanesin
  - Carisoprodol
  - Diazepam.

- *Aspiration:* It is done, when there is recurrent effusion that causes pain.
- *Hydrocortisone injections*
  - When only one or two large joints involved.
  - Compound injected intra-articularly.
  - Reduces inflammation and eliminates pain.
  - Constitutional effects are avoided.
  - *Dose:* 1 mL of suspension.
- *Intra-articular irradiation:*
  Radioactive colloidal gold injected into the joint.
- *Special drugs:*
  - *Antimalarial compounds:*
    - Chloroquine
    - Hydroxychloroquine.
  - *Immunosuppressive agents:*
    - Azathioprine
    - Penicillamine
    - Cyclophosphamide.
  - *Protozoacides:*
    - Clotrimazole
    - Copper sulfate.

Surgical Treatment

- Hip is generally involved at a late stage of severe generalized disease
- Multiple joint involvement of both lower extremities is the rule
- Flexion contractures of hips and knees are common
- The objectives are relief of pain, provision of increased motion, and maintenance of stability.

Surgical options
- Synovectomy
- THR
- Arthroplasty of Smith Peterson
- Arthrodesis
- Pseudarthrosis.

Synovectomy: Role of synovectomy is to remove large bulk of diseased tissue, so that drugs can have an effect on the joint.

THR: Complete prosthetic replacement, using both acetabular and femoral components is the ideal procedure. Procedure is generally reserved for adults in middle age and beyond. Done preferably before the advanced destructive stage of disease.

Arthroplasty of Smith Peterson: A vitallium mold (65% cobalt, 30% chromium, and 5% molybdenum) is interposed, the articular surfaces become lined with smooth glistening fibrocartilage and the underlining bone becomes more firm.

Reankylosis is less likely than when other interposing material, such as fascia lata is used. Recurrence of stiffness and deformity is greater in RA than in degenerative, but some useful motion is gained, permitting ambulation with canes and sitting on high chairs. Rarely the femoral head and neck within the cup may undergo resorption, subluxation, or dislocation.

Technical principles for arthroplasty: Enlarge the acetabulum, consistent with stability of mold and neck. Excise the entire capsule and diseased synovial tissue. Replace the blood lost. Coagulate raw bone surfaces after reshaping, to prevent new bone formation. Adapt modifications to RA, to gain more mobility in spite of marked ankylosis.

a. *Whiteman reconstruction:* Remove head, reshape neck, and displace GT downward, before interposing cup.
b. *Colonna:* Remove head and neck, reshape trochanter, which forms new articulating surface, detach and reattach trochanteric muscles at lower level.

Arthrodesis: Bilateral arthrodesis is not advisable. With one freely movable hip joint, the other can be fused, providing stability and freedom from pain.

Pseudarthrosis: The procedures of Girdlestone and Batchlor restore movement and correct deformity. Instability is unlikely or minimal because of surrounding soft tissue fibrosis.

Rehabilitation

- Positive mental attitude
- Regular medication
- Use of joints and regular exercises (physiotherapy)
- Energy conservation
- Assisted devices like stick, walker, splints, braces
- Adequate sleep
- Massage: Myofacial and centrifugal
- Relaxation techniques
- Modification in daily activities, like use of western toilets, bath aids, railings, long handle broomsticks, and mop to clean the floors.

LEGG-CALVE-PERTHES DISEASE

Introduction

Legg-Calve-Perthes disease (also known as Perthes, osteochondritis deformans juvenilis and coxa plana) is a self-limiting, affection of the hip occurring in children characterized by aseptic necrosis of the whole or part of the femoral head produced by interruption of its blood supply, followed by subchondral fracture, revascularization, and repair of dead bone.

History

- *1909* Waldenstrom, was the first to describe the condition and mistakenly ascribed it as tuberculosis of hip.
- *1910* Legg and Calve and Perthes, described the condition independently.
- *1913* Perthes gave a precise description of the disease and recognized its ischemic nature.
- *1922* Waldenstrom correctly interpreted and described the stages of the disease.

Incidence

- Disorder of the hip in young children
- Usually ages 4–8 years
- As early as 2 years, as late as teens
- Boys: girls ratio is 4 to 5:1
- Bilateral 10–12%
- No evidence of inheritance
- It is rare in blacks, Indians and Polynesians, with higher incidence seen in whites and Eskimos.

Predisposing Factors

- *Age:* Predominately affected are children between the ages of 3 and 12 with its peak at 6 years of age.
- *Sex:* Males have more predilection with ratio of 4:1.
- Either hip may be affected. Bilateral cases are rare with about 15% of incidence.

- *Genetic factor:* The disease is found to be familial in 6–4% of cases. It occurred more often in later-born children, particularly the third to sixth child.
- A higher than normal incidence of minor congenital genitourinary anomalies, such as renal abnormalities, inguinal hernia, or undescended testicles is seen in children with Perthes disease.
- *Abnormal growth and development:* The bone age of children with Perthes disease is typically lower than their chronological age by 1–3 years. The affected child are smaller in all dimensions (except head circumference), with disproportionately smaller distal segment of the extremities.
- *Environmental factors:* Although, the effect of environment on the incidence of the disorder is unclear, a high percentage of involved children come from low socioeconomic groups, whether this reflects dietary or environmental influence, or a combination thereof is certain.
- *Regional factor:* The disease occurs predominately in Eskimos and whites, have a higher incidence of the disease, whereas Australians, American, Indians and blacks have a lower incidence.

Etiology

- Perthes disease is produced by impairment of the blood supply to the femoral head
- Multiple episodes of infarction are required to produce the pathological defect of Perthes disease.
- The exact cause of interruption of blood supply remains obscure.
- Numerous theories/hypothesis speculating on the pathogenesis of the disease have been proposed.

Trueta hypothesis: This hypothesis is based on the variation of vascular pattern of femoral capital epiphysis with advancing growth. After 8 years, the foveolar arteries of the ligamentum teres contribute blood supply to femoral head and with lateral epiphyseal again provide a double source of blood and the incidence of disease begins to decline at this age. Thus, Trueta postulated that the solitary blood supply between the age 4 and 8 years, makes this group vulnerable to ischemic necrosis.

Caffey's hypothesis: According to Caffey, the radiological features of perthes are more consistent with an AVN, resulting from intraepiphyseal compression of blood supply to ossification center. The increased density of the necrotic bone is at first, a result of compression of femoral head by the acetabular roof and later by newly formed bone superimposed on yet unresorbed old necrotic bone.

Other theories: Increased intra-articular pressure and tamponade compression of the retinacular vessels around the femoral neck and a casual relationship between acute transient synovitis and Perthes have been postulated. Kleinman and Black reported increased blood viscosity in Perthes patients. The venous drainage have been disturbed in Perthes, due to increased intravenous pressure. Patients with Perthes disease have low levels of somatomedin C.

Pathogenesis

Loss of blood supply produces AVN of the epiphyseal ossification center, followed by resorption of dead bone and replacement with newly formed immature bone. The process is described in stages.

Incipient or synovitis stage (Fig. 202):

- Lasts 1–3 weeks
- Synovium is swollen, hyperemic, and edematous.
- Joint fluid is increased and absence of inflammatory cells.

Stage of avascular necrosis (Fig. 203):

- AVN involves portion of ossific nucleus situated anteriorly
- Amorphous debris fills the marrow spaces
- Trabeculae are crushed into minute fragments and compressed into a compact bone accounting for increased density on radiograph
- The increased opacity is contrasted
- Marked demineralization of adjacent metaphysic, as a result of hypervascularity, constitutes preparation for invasion of vascular connective tissue towards necrotic bone
- The cartilage is viable, nutrition is derived from synovial fluid
- Stage lasts 6 months to 1 year.

Stage of fragmentation or regeneration:

- Necrotic bone resorbed and replaced by viable bone
- Radiographic fragmented appearance results many tonge-like roads of vessels, which appear to come from ligamentum teres periosteum and metaphysis
- Subchondral fractures of necrotic bone, multiple minute trabecular fragments compressed together
- Cartilage remains normal

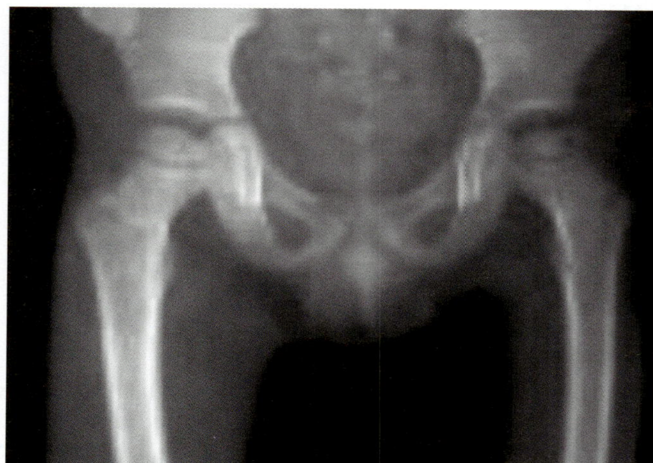

Fig. 202: Incipient or synovitis stage.

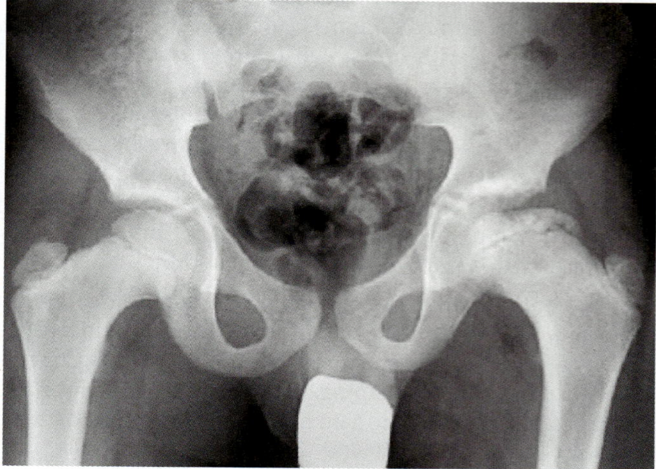

Fig. 203: Stage of AVN.

- The contour of the newly formed soft bone develops in response to the external forces
- Stage extents over 2–3 years.

Healed or residual stage:
- Formation of normal bone, alongside replacing slowly resorbing bone
- Newly formed bone is immature, formed of slender trabeculae, and easily compressed together with necrotic fragments
- The compression is limited to anterior portion of head, creating a cup-shaped defect seen on frog leg view
- Defect appears cystic
- The ossific nucleus assumes a mushroom-shaped contour
- *Appearance of GT:* It becomes strikingly large in some cases. Since longitudinal growth of the femoral neck may cease completely at 12–14 years of age, whereas growth of the GT continues until 17–18 years, a discrepancy in growth and the GT may result. The elevation impairs the power of pelvitrochanteric abductor muscles, manifested by positive Trendelenburg sign, as shown in Figure 204.

Clinical Features

Symptoms
- Most children present with mild and intermittent pain in the thigh, or a limb, or both
- The onset of pain may be acute or insidious
- The classical presentation is described as a "painless limb"; the child limps, but does not complain of discomfort
- Pain is aggravated by movement of hip and relieved by rest
- History of trauma, usually mild, is present.

Examination
- Antalgic gait
- Proximal thigh atrophy
- Muscle spasm, secondary to irritable hip
- Limitation of abduction and internal rotation
- Focal-film distance (FFD) is present
- Axis deviation is present due to central collapse

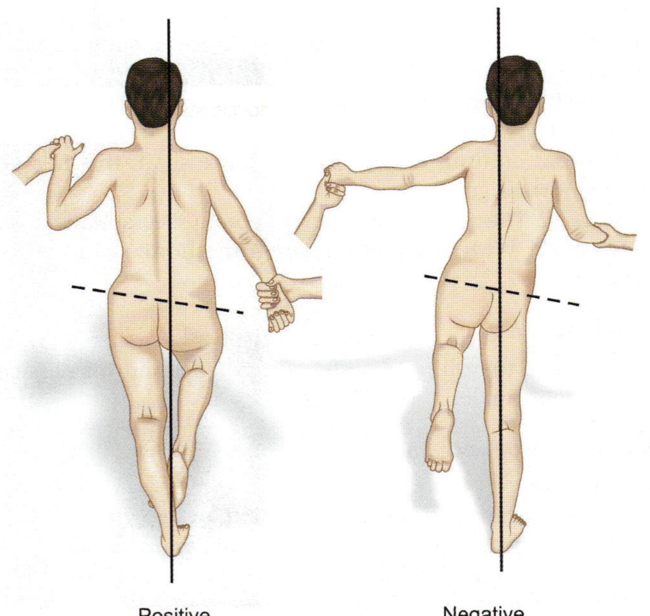

Fig. 204: Trendelenburg sign.

- Differential rotation
- Trendelenburg test positive with free abduction and adduction range.

Imaging
- AP pelvis
- Frog leg lateral
- USG
- Bone scan
- Arthrography
- MRI role is undefined.

Radiographic Studies (Fig. 205)
- Increased head socket distance (Waldenstrom's sign)
- Bulging of the joint capsule
- Rarefaction or rounding of the lateral margin of metaphysis (Gage' sign)
- A strip, shaped subcortical area ventrolaterally in the epiphysis
- Rarefaction in the lateral outline of the epiphysis close to the epiphyseal plate
- Band shaped osteoporosis in the metaphysis close to epiphyseal plate
- Translucent area in the medial metaphyseal zone
- Changes in roof on the acetabulum
- The capital epiphysis smaller than in the unaffected hip but shape and structure of the epiphysis normal
- Enlargement of NoF
- The tear-shaped phenomenon, widening of Kohler's tear-shaped figure
- Thickening of epiphyseal plate.

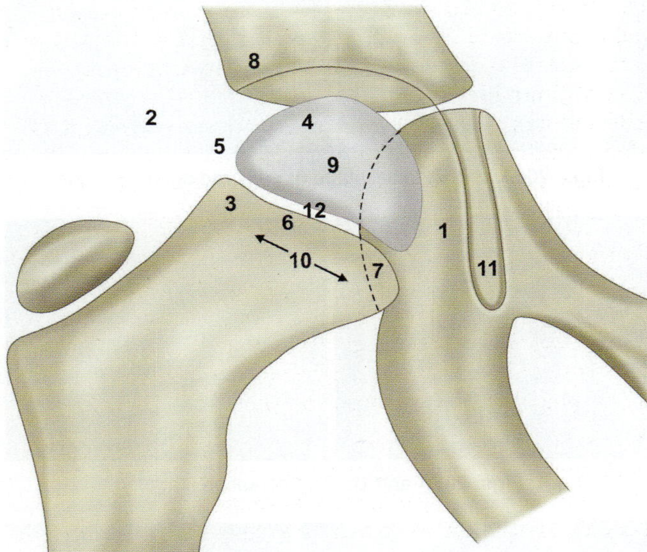

Fig. 205: 1. Increased head socket distance (Waldenstrom's sign); 2. Bulging of the joint capsule; 3. Rarefaction or rounding of the lateral margin of metaphysis (Gage' sign); 4. A strip, shaped subcortical area ventrolaterally in the epiphysis; 5. Rarefaction in the lateral outline of the epiphysis close to the epiphyseal plate; 6. Band shaped osteoporosis in the metaphysis close to epiphyseal plate; 7. Translucent area in the medial metaphyseal zone; 8. Changes in roof on the acetabulum; 9. The capital epiphysis smaller than in the unaffected hip but shape and structure of the epiphysis normal; 10. Enlargement of neck of femur; 11. The tear shaped phenomenon, widening of Kohler'stear-shaped figure; 12. Thickening of epiphyseal plate.

Radiographic Stages

Four Waldenstrom stages have identified:
1. Initial stage
2. Fragmentation stage
3. Reossification stage
4. Healed stage

Initial stage (Figs. 206A and B)

Early radiographic signs are:
- Failure of femoral ossification to grow
- Widening of medial joint space
- "Crescent sign"
- Irregular physeal plate
- Blurry/radiolucent metaphysis.

Fragmentation stage (Figs. 207A and B)
- Bony epiphysis begins to fragment
- Areas of increased lucency and density
- Evidence of repair aspects of disease.

Reossification stage (Figs. 208A and B)
- Normal bone density returns
- Alterations in shape of femoral head and neck evident.

Healed stage
- Left with residual deformity from disease and repair process
- Differs from AVN following fracture or dislocation.
- "Head at risk sign"
  - A transradiant "V" on the lateral side of epiphysis, formed by small osteoporotic segment, which is seen on the AP X-ray
  - Calcification lateral to epiphysis
  - Lateral subluxation of the femoral head, measured as an increase in the width of the inferomedial joint space
  - A horizontal epiphyseal line seen in AP view
  - Diffuse metaphyseal changes.
- Extensive involvement of elective orthopedic center (EOC)
- Child over 6 years of age
- Early closure of the epiphyseal plate
- Stage of disease advanced, when first seen
- Female patient invariably has group 3 or 4
- When any two of the first five signs listed above are found, a head at risk is said to exist. Catteralls head at risk signs (poor prognosis)
  - Clinically
    - Progressive loss of movement
    - Adduction contracture
    - Heavy child.
  - Radiological
    - Lateral subluxation of head (head partially uncovered) most important
    - Whole of head involved
    - Calcification lateral to epiphysis
    - Metaphyseal cysts
    - Gage sign
    - Horizontal physis.

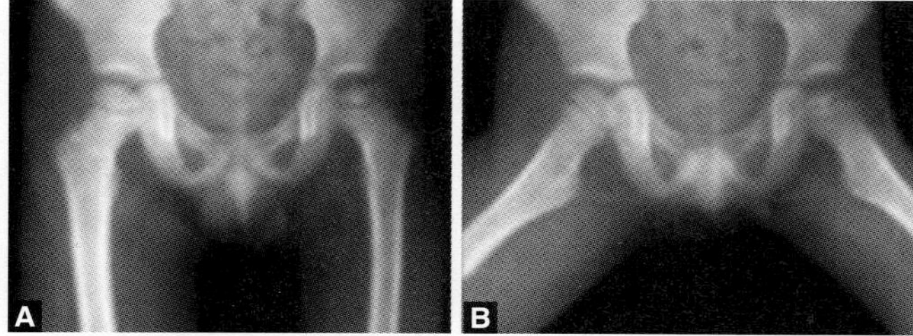

Figs. 206A and B: Initial stage or early radiographic signs.

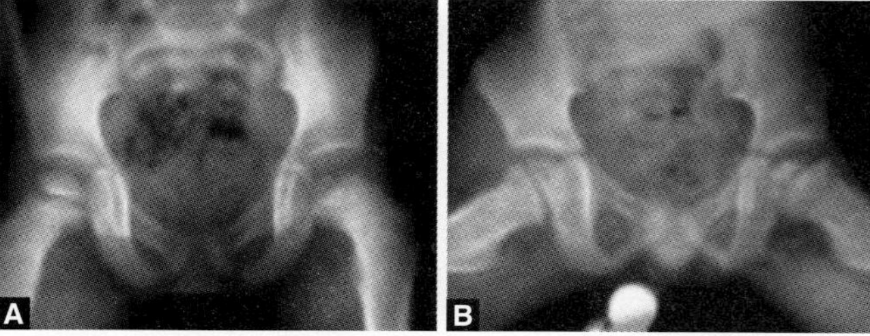

Figs. 207A and B: Fragmentation stage.

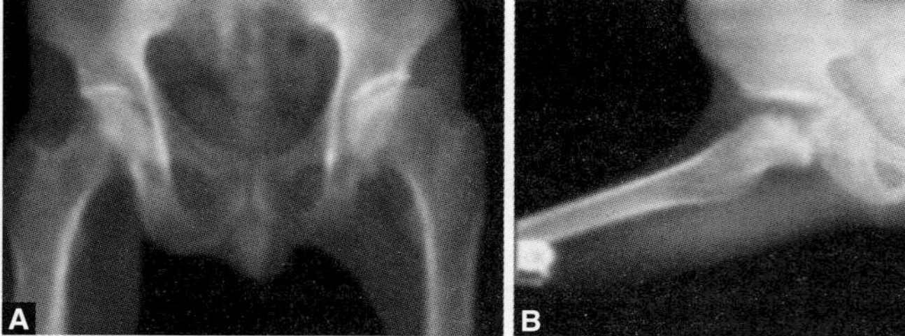

Figs. 208A and B: Radiographical findings in reossification stage of RA.

Ultrasonography

- Effusion of hip (which when persistent should make one suspicion of Perthes).
- Thickening and enlargement of articular cartilage of the epiphysis.
- Lateral and anterior uncoverage of head and flattening of femoral head.
- Irregularity and deformation of bony epiphysis.

Bone Scan

During the course of Perthes disease bone scan shows following stages:
- *Stage I:* The whole ossific nucleus appears avascular.
- *Stage II:* When revascularization takes place by recanalization, a lateral column is seen on the bone scan, this is a good prognostic sign.
- *Stage III:* The anterolateral part of epiphysis gradually fills.
- *Stage IV:* With complete healing, the bone scan comes to normal.

Arthrography

It is indicated to in-hinged abduction, osteochondritis dessicans, or a torn labrum.

Magnetic Resonance Imaging

Demonstrates:
- Contour of femoral head
- Degree of extrusion and uncoverage of femoral head
- Degree of superolateral subluxation of femoral head
- Extent of necrosis.

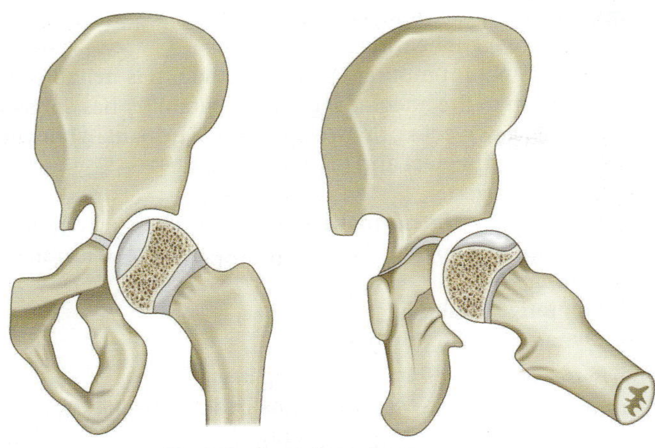

Fig. 209: Stage I of Catteralls classification.

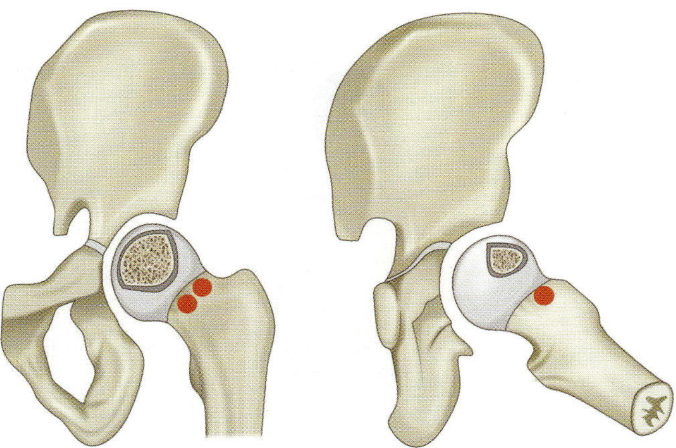

Fig. 210: Stage II of Catteralls classification.

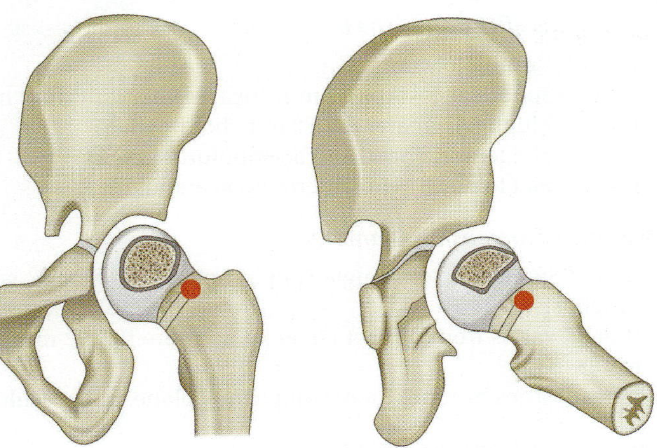

Fig. 211: Stage III of Catteralls classification.

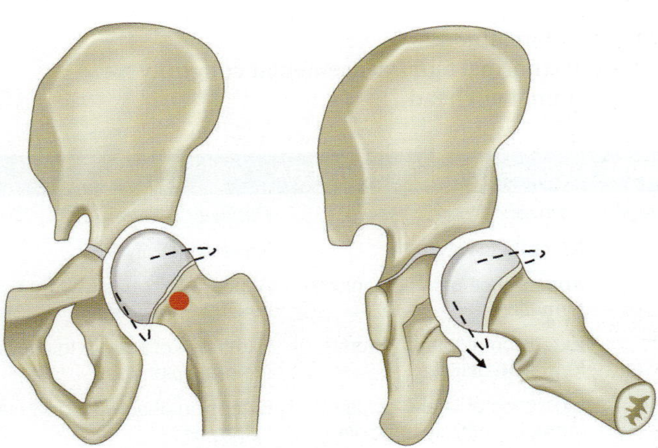

Fig. 212: Stage IV of Catteralls classification.

Classification

Catteralls Classification

- *Stage I:* Anteromedial portion head involved and no collapse, metaphyseal changes do not occur and the epiphyseal plate is not involved. Heal without sequelae. This is shown in Figure 209.
- *Stage II:* There is a fragmentation of involved segment. The involved segment shows increased density and uninvolved pillars of normal bone prevent significant collapse. Regeneration without much loss of height and the end result is good. Metaphyseal reaction localized, as shown in Figure 210.
- *Stage III:* More of the head involved. Shows head within head. The metaphysis is diffusely involved. Broad neck and the epiphyseal plate is unprotected. Results are poor. This is illustrated in Figure 211.
- *Stage IV:* Whole is involved and sever collapse occurs early. Metaphyseal changes are extensive. Epiphyseal plate involved, abnormal growth present, like coxa magna, coxa breva, coxa vara, and coxa valga, as shown in Figure 212.

Herrings Classification (Lateral Pillar Classification)

- *Group A:* There is no collapse of the lateral pillar.
- *Group B:* Lateral pillar margins, has more than 50% of original height.
- *Group C:* Collapse of lateral pillar more than 50%.

Salter-Thompson

- *Stage A:* Lateral portion of femoral epiphysis present, same as Catterall 1st and 2nd stages (less than 50% head involved).
- *Stage B:* Lateral portion of femoral capital epiphysis absent, same as Catterall 3rd and 4th stages (more than 50% head involved, lateral margin of epiphysis protects from stress).

Ponsetti Classification

- Those with 50% less involved head
- Those with more than 50% of involved head.
- *Deformities at maturity:*
  - Coxa magna—enlarged head
  - Hanging rope sign, characteristic of old Perthes
  - Coxa brevis, short neck, and overgrowth of trochanter, as a result of premature femoral neck physeal growth arrest.
  - *Coxa irregularis:* Collapse and lateral extrusion of the femoral head, forming a groove under the lateral edge of acetabulum
    - Osteochondritis dessicans.

Stulberg Classification of the End Result

- *Class 1:* Completely normal
- *Class 2:* Spherical, less than 2 mm coxa magna, with short neck
- *Class 3:* Elliptical, greater than 2 mm, but not flat
- *Class 4:* Flat femoral head and acetabulum
- *Class 5:* Flat femoral head and round acetabulum.

Mose-ring of Increasing Diameter

- If head conforms to a single ring in both X-ray planes, good prognosis.
- If head varies from perfect circle by no more than 2 mm, fair result.
- If head varies by more than 2 mm in any plane, poor result.

Conway Classification (Table 11)

It is based on nuclear scanning (Scintigraphy). This is illustrated in Figure 213.

Treatment

Principles of treatment:
- Preserve normal femoral acetabular congruity
- Containment of head

TABLE 11: Conway classification of RA.

Stage	*Pathway A*	*Pathway B*
I	No radioactivity	No radioactivity
II	Appearance of lateral column formation	Appearance of activity from base of epiphysis
III	Extension of lateral column formation activity	Extension of activity to capital femoral epiphysis
IV	Extension of lateral column formation activity to whole epiphysis	Extension of activity to whole epiphysis

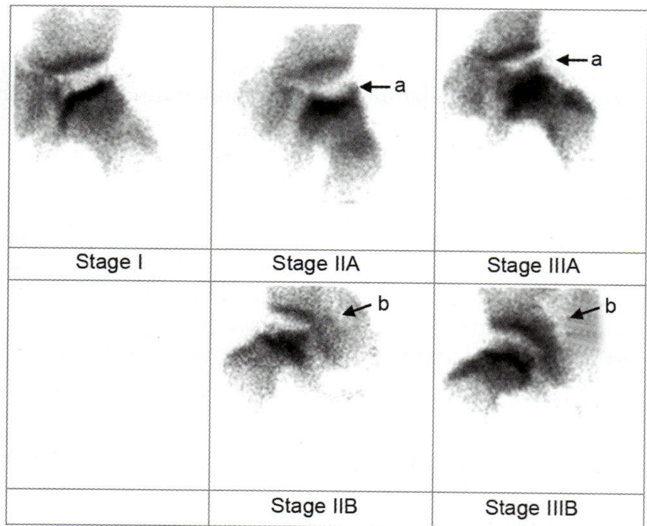

Fig. 213: Scintigraphic stages of Conway classification of LCP. Stage I (total avascularity of proximal femoral epiphysis) is observed at initial stage of disease. Appearance of lateral column formation, a. characterizes a pathway (stages IIA and IIIA). In b pathway, as neovascularization progresses, extension of activity from metaphysis is observed (stages IIB and IIIB), without lateral column formation b.

- Eliminate or reduce load bearing
- Encourage weight bearing in abduction
- Continue hip joint motion. As long as the hip is irritable, give skin traction to the affected leg. Once irritability has subsided (usually takes 3 weeks), there is a choice of treatment between: (1) supervised neglect and (2) containment.
- *Supervised neglect:*
  - Child attains the normal activity and is checked regularly.
  - If symptoms appear, then containment of head is done.
- *Containment:*
  - Operative methods
  - Dynamic abduction braces.

Conservative treatment:
- Broomstick plaster or Scottish rite abduction brace (Figs. 214)
- Newington children's ambulatory brace (Fig. 215).

Nonoperative Treatment

- *Check serial radiographs:*
  Q3 and 4 mostly with ROM testing.

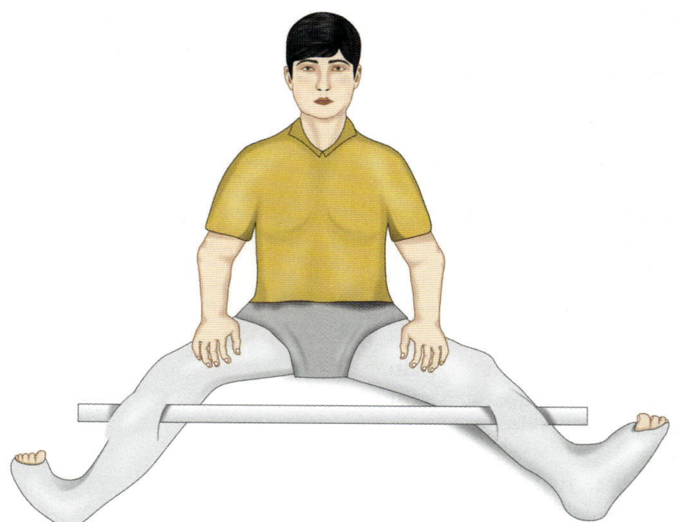

Fig. 214: Broomstick plaster or Scottish rite abduction brace.

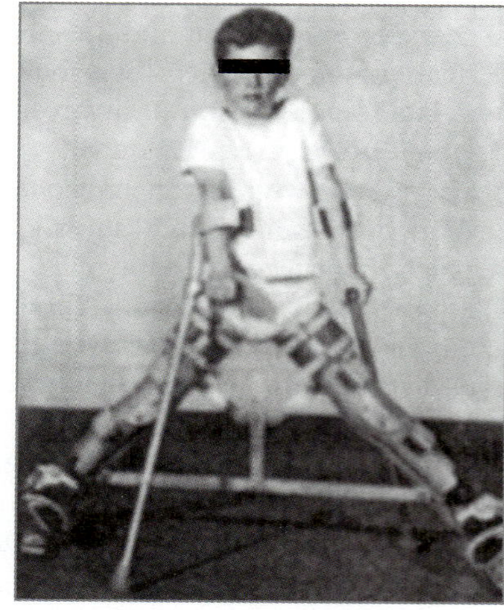

Fig. 215: Newingtons children's ambulatory brace.

- *Continue bracing until:*
  - Lateral column ossifies
  - Sclerotic areas in epiphysis gone.
- Cast/brace uninvolved side.

Operative Treatment

- If nonoperative treatment cannot maintain containment
- Surgically, ideal patient:
  - 6–9 years
  - Catterall II-III
  - Good ROM
  - Less than 12 months surgery
  - In collapsing phase.

Benjamin Joseph's criteria for containment surgery in late onset Perthes disease (in children of age 7–12 years)

- *Stage I:* Containment surgery indicated
- *Stage II:* Containment surgery indicated
- *Stage III:* Containment surgery not indicated
- *Stage IV:* Containment surgery not indicated.

The concept of containment with weight bearing: Although, others had previously recommended immobilization of the hip in wide abduction combined with complete bed rest, Petrie and Bitenc were the first to propose the position of wide abduction for the purpose of diminishing abduction forces on the femoral head, while permitting full weight bearing. The efficacy of the concept of containment of the femoral head was demonstrated in experimental investigation of AVN of the femoral head in young pigs by Salter et al. Subsequently, Lloyd-Roberts et al. concluded that methods of early treatment, either surgical or nonsurgical that do not include the concept of containment, seem to be of little value in Legg-Perthes disease.

Basic premises concerning treatment: Children, who acquire Legg-Perthes disease are not systemically ill. They have only a local disease. From humanitarian point of view, treatment should interfere, as little as possible with the child's normal psychological and physical development. Legg-Perthes disease is a self-healing process. Therefore, the only justification for treatment is the prevention of femoral head deformity and secondary degenerative arthritis. The decision concerning the need for the treatment of a given child, should be based on a knowledge of the prognosis for that particular child. Lloyd-Roberts, et al. made an important contribution, in emphasizing that no children with Group-I involvement and relatively few with Group-II involvement, require any treatment whatsoever. All forms of the treatment should be based on a sound understanding of the underlying pathogenesis of the disease.

Basic principles of all forms of treatment: Obtain and maintain a full or almost full ROM of the hip joint. Obtain and maintain containment of the femoral head in the position of weight bearing, by preventing or correcting subluxation of the hip. Provided these two principles have been achieved, then and only then encourage full weight bearing, on the involved hip (a turnabout from the principle of NWB that prevailed during the first five decades, following the original description of the disease).

Classification of currently acceptable forms of management:

- Observation only
- Intermittent symptomatic treatment (temporary), brief periods of traction, slings and springs, or crutches (with or without a Snyder sling or Salter stirrup)
- Definitive early treatment (to prevent deformity)
  - Non-surgical
    - Abduction casts (Petrie and Bitenc)
    - Abduction orthoses (Toronto, Newington, New Orleans, Atlanta, and others)
  - Surgical
    - Femoral osteotomy
      Varus (Soeur and de Racker)
      Rotation (Axer)
      Combined varus and rotation (Somerville, Lloyd-Roberts et al. and Catterall)
    - Innominate osteotomy (Salter et al.) combined with adductor tenotomy and iliopsoas release.
  - Late surgical treatment (to correct existing deformity)
    - Muscle release and arthrotomy, followed by abduction casts
    - Partial excision of the femoral head
      Peripheral cheilectomy (Garceau et al.)
      Central (loose fragment of osteochondritis dissecans)
    - Abduction (valgus) osteotomy of the femur (Salter et al. and Catterall)
    - Distal and lateral transfer of the GT
  - Late surgical treatment (for secondary degenerative arthritis)
    - Femoral osteotomy
    - Arthrodesis
    - Arthroplasties including prosthetic joint replacement.

Definitive early surgical treatment (to prevent deformity).

Indications

- Involvement of more than half of the femoral head (Catterall groups III and IV or Salter group B)
- Age at onset for more than 6 years (possibly more than 5 years in girls)
- Loss of containment of femoral head, i.e. subluxation of femoral head in the position of weight bearing.

Prerequisites

- A full or almost full ROM at hip joint (which may necessitate traction or slings and springs, to overcome irritability of the hip or even surgical release of the adductor muscles, to overcome contractures, followed by abductor casts for a few weeks or longer)
- A round or almost round femoral head and hence, reasonable congruity of the hip joint in abduction (which may have to be established by an arthrogram, if there has been significant resorption of the femoral head).

Contraindications

- Lack of a good indication (because the child does not need surgical treatment)
- Lack of the prerequisites (because the child cannot be helped by such surgical treatment).

Surgical options:

- Pelvic osteotomies, like Salter, Chiari, and Shelf
- Varus derotation osteotomy
- Late stages, valgus extension osteotomy, and cheilectomy
- Arthrodesis should be preserved for patient, with severe deformity and done after skeletal maturity.

Prognosis
- 60% of children do well without treatment.
- Age is key prognostic factor:
  - Less than 6 years, shows good outcome regardless of treatment
  - Six to eight years, not always good results, with just containment
  - More than 9 years, containment option is questionable, poorer prognosis and significant residual defect.
- Flat femoral head incongruent with acetabulum, have worst prognosis.
- Do not treat in reossification stage (> 15 months).

Differential diagnosis:
- Important to rule out infectious etiology (septic arthritis and toxic synovitis).
- *Others:*
  - Chondrolysis
  - Neoplasm
  - Juvenile RA
  - Sickle cell anemia
  - Osteomyelitis
  - Traumatic AVN
  - Lymphoma
  - Medication.

Late effects or sequelae of Legg-Calves-Perthes
- Coxa magna
- Coxa irregularis, irregular head formation
- Physeal arrest patterns
- Osteochondritis dessicans
- Coxa breva, due to relative overgrowth of GT and short femoral head
- Hinged abduction of the hip
- Osteoarthritis.

TUMORS AROUND HIP

Tumors around hip can be:
- Benign
- Malignant.

Benign Tumors around Hip

- Bone forming tumors:
  - Osteoid osteoma
  - Osteoblastoma.
- Cartilaginous tumors:
  - Osteochondroma
  - Chondroma (enchondroma and periosteal chondroma)
  - Multiple enchondromatosis (Ollier disease) III. Fibrous lesions
  - Fibrous cortical defect
  - Benign fibrous histiocytoma
  - Fibrous dysplasia
  - Desmoplastic fibroma
  - Giant cell reaction (giant cell reparative granuloma).
- Cystic lesions:
  - Unicameral cyst
  - Aneurysmal bone cyst (ABC).
- Miscellaneous:
  - Neural tumors
  - Osteochondromatosis
  - Synovioma
  - Pigmented villonodular synovitis (PVNS).

Malignant Tumors around Hip

- Chondrosarcomas
- Osteosarcomas
- Chordomas
- Metastatic tumors.
  Multiple myeloma:
- Lymphoma.

Commonly found tumors around hip are:
- Osteochondroma
- Osteosarcoma
- Chondrosarcoma
- Multiple enchondromatosis (Ollier's disease)
- Aneurysmal bone cyst
- Unicameral bone cyst (UBC)
- Fibrous dysplasia
- Chondroma.

Osteochondroma

It is the most common benign bone tumor. It accounts for 20–50% of benign bone tumors and 10–15% of all bone tumors. Approximately, 15% of patients with osteochondromas have multiple lesions. It is an offshoot from the spongy bone tissue covered with a cartilaginous cap, as shown in Figure 216.

Classification of Osteochondroma

WHO classification:
- Lichtenstein classification of primary bone tumors
- Classification of bone tumors (Briston University)
- ABC classification by Charles Price
- Enneking's system of staging.

Enneking's system of staging (Table 12):
- Based on degree of anaplasia, it is divided into two types:
  - G1-low grade
  - G2-high grade.
- Based on the tumor location:
  - Intracompartmental (T1)
  - Extracompartmental (T2).

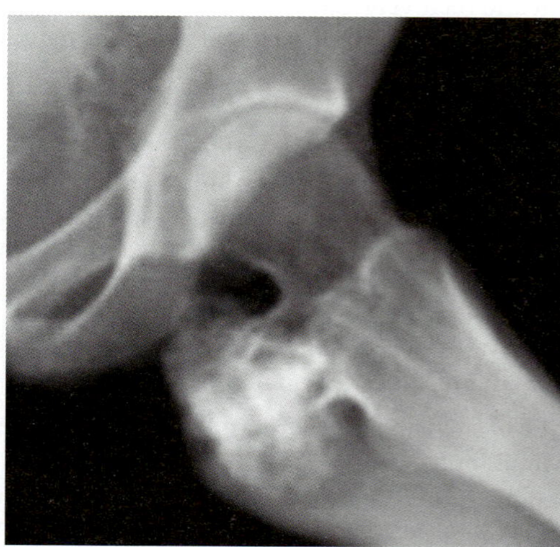

Fig. 216: Osteochondroma of hip.

TABLE 12: Enneking's system of staging.

I-A	G1, T1, M0	Low grade, intracompartmental, no metastasis
I-B	G1, T2, M0	Low grade, extracompartmental, no metastasis
II-A	G2, T1, M0	High grade, intracompartmental, no metastasis
II-B	G2, T2, M0	High grade, extracompartmental, no metastasis
III-A	G1 or G2, T1, M1	Any grade, intracompartmental, metastasis
III-B	G1 or G2, T2, M1	Any grade, c metastasis

- Based on metastasis:
  - Absent (M0)
  - Present (M1).

Age: Common during the growth period.

Sex: Male preponderance (male/female ratio 1.5:1).

Area: Sites of tendinous attachments and metaphysis of femur around hip.

Theory of Histogenesis

Exact cause is not known. Cambium layer of periosteum retains throughout life its ability to form cartilage and bone, due to perverted activity of periosteum that it reverts to its role as "perichondrium". At point of tendinous insertion, there are focal accumulation of embryonic connective tissue.

Clinical Features

Symptoms: Usually symptomless. Patient may complain of pain, swelling, bursitis, malignant change, fracture, neuropathies, etc.

Signs:
- Firm nontender swelling fixed to bone around the joints
- An inflamed bursa causes tenderness and local warmth
- Decreased joint movements and tumor causing mechanical block.

Roentgenographic Findings (Figs. 217 and 218)

Osteochondromas are of two types:
1. Stalked
2. Broad based or sessile.
   Sessile lesions cover a wide area and as a result cause metaphyseal widening or a "trumpet shaped deformity" on X-ray.

Treatment

Usually it requires no treatment. Surgical treatment excision should consist of an en bloc resection. It is indicated when:
- Joint interference
- Painful bursitis
- Fracture of the bony stalk
- Malignant change
- Pressure on the neighboring vessels/nerves.

Prognosis

The risk of malignant transformation to chondrosarcoma in hereditary multiple osteochondromatosis is unknown, but may be 25–30% compared to approximately 1% for a solitary osteochondromas.

Osteosarcoma

It is a malign and primary bone tumor, arising from multipotent mesenchymal tissue of bone. It is characterized by direct formation of bone or osteoid, by proliferating tumor cells, as shown in Figures 219A to H.

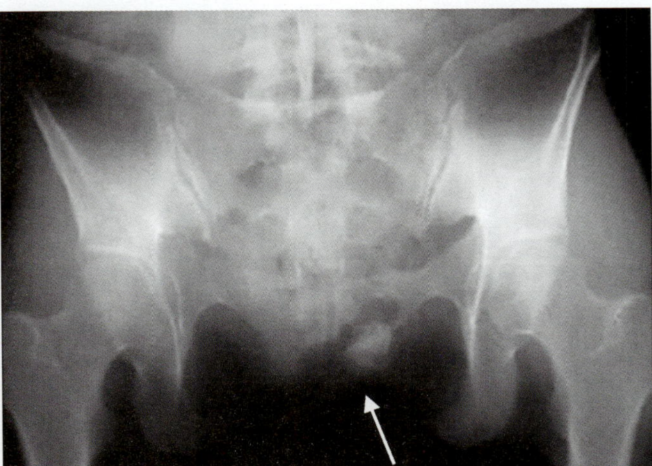

Fig. 217: X-ray PBH-AP showing osteochondroma of pelvis. Arrow showing osteosarcoma of pelvis.

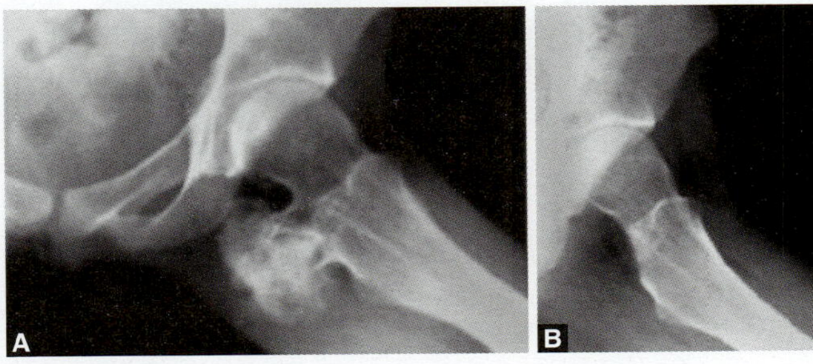

Figs. 218A and B: Osteochondroma of hip: Sessile lesions cover a wide area and as a result cause metaphyseal widening or a "trumpet shaped deformity"—(A) Preoperative roentgenogram; (B) After excision of lesion.

Incidence

- Common malignant tumor
- Occurs in young, between 10 and 20 years of age.

Sites (Fig. 220):
- Metaphysis of long bones
- Proximal one-third of femur.

Exciting Factors

The predisposing factors of the tumors are:

Virus:
- *DNA virus:* Polyoma and SV-40 virus
- *RNA virus:* Harvey and Moloney sarcoma virus. These are known to produce tumors in animals and not in humans.

Radiation:
A dose of 2000 rads, can set malignancy in the bone.

Chemicals:
Beryllium compounds and methylcholanthrene.

Clinical Features

- Pain is the initial and dominating symptom
- Bony swelling appears after some weeks
- Swelling progressively increases in size.

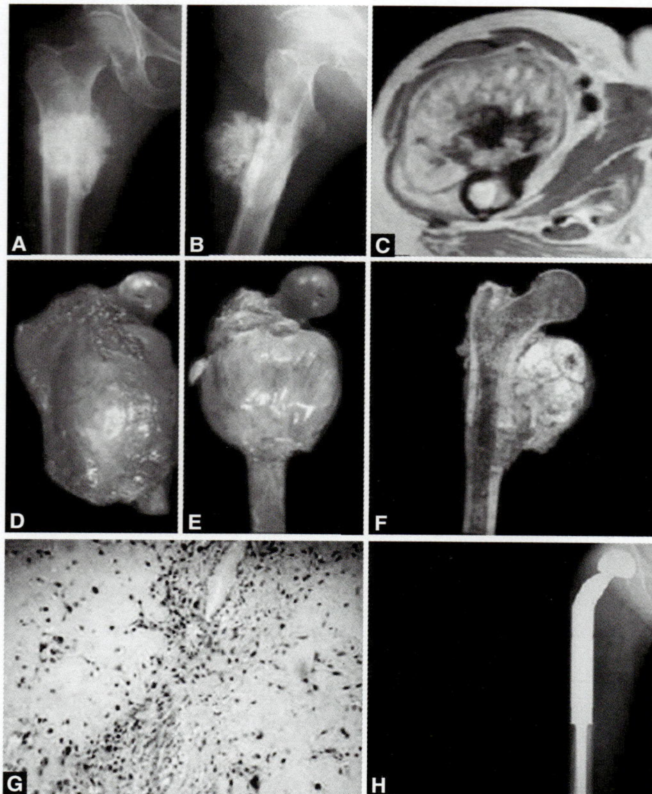

Figs. 219A to H: (A) to (F) Different stages of osteosarcoma of hip; (G) Histological findings; (H) Prosthetic replacement of the hip.

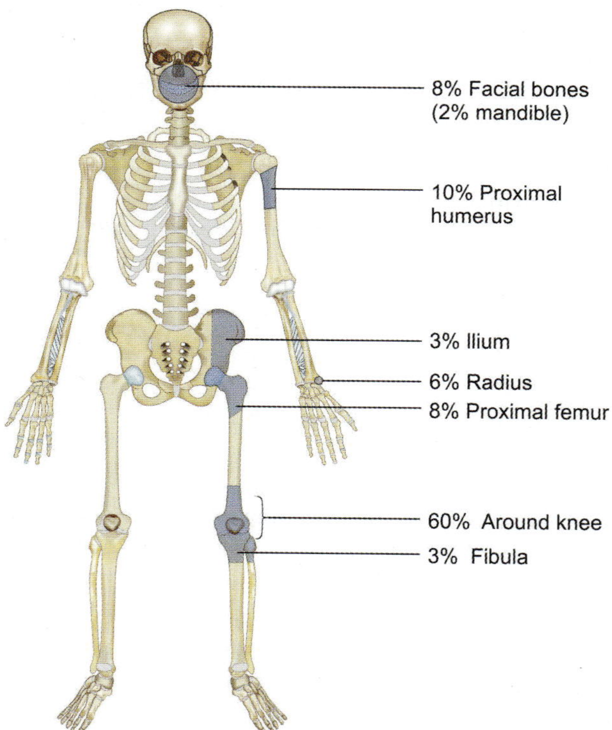

Fig. 220: Distribution of osteosarcoma in body.

General Examination

- General health deteriorates with anemia, loss of weight, and cachexia
- Patient develops pulmonary symptoms due to secondaries.

On examination

- Swelling is fusiform
- Skin is stretched, shiny and vascular, with prominent veins
- Swelling is warm to touch and show pulsation, if tumor is highly vascular
- It is firm to hard in consistency
- In late stages, tumor fungates.

Classification of Osteosarcoma

Primary osteosarcomas:

- Conventional:
  - Osteoblastic
  - Chondroblastic
  - Fibroblastic
  - Small cell
  - Telangiectatic.
- Surface (juxtacortical) osteosarcoma
  - Parosteal osteosarcoma
  - Periosteal osteosarcoma
  - High grade surface osteosarcoma.

Secondary osteosarcoma:

- Post-irradiation
- Paget's sarcoma
- Solitary/multiple osteochondromatosis
- Bone infarction
- Chronic osteomyelitis
- *Miscellaneous:* Gaint cell tumor (GCT), fibrous dysplasia, chondroblastoma and osteoblastoma.

Rare osteosarcoma:

- Li Fraumeni syndrome
- Osteosarcoma of the jaw
- Multicentric osteosarcoma.

Pathology

Grossly: It is a large tumor with areas of destruction gives an appearance of leg of mutton. Consistency ranges from hard to soft. Color of tumor could be white, if fibroblastic; yellowish white, if osteoblastic and bluish, if cartilaginous. At the areas of rapid growth, there are areas of cavitation, necrotic foci, and hemorrhages. Sun-ray appearance seen is due to the bone disposition along the vessels. Codman's triangle is the reactive bone formation parallel to the bone.

Histology

- Small spindle cells with hyperchromatic nuclei
- Shape may be round, cuboidal, and columnar
- Cells are pleomorphic in nature
- Giant cells are often present
- Matrix may be myxomatous, cartilaginous, or osseous
- Areas of hemorrhages may be present.

Radiological Features

Tumor arises from metaphyseal region of the bone either centrally or from cortex. Mottled area of rarefaction, with areas of osteosclerosis. When it extends beyond the cortex, the periosteum is raised and there is new bone formation in lines at right angle to the cortex. This causes sun-ray appearance on X-ray. Codman's triangle is seen at the junction of normal bone and tumor area it is a reactive new bone formation subperiosteally, ghost shadow, and chest X-ray (CXR) may show secondaries in chest.

Treatment

The aim of treatment is to confirm the diagnosis and to evaluate the spread and to execute adequate treatment. Confirmation of diagnosis is done clinically, histologically, radiologically, and laboratory findings. Evaluation of the spread of the tumors is done. Lung is common area of metastasis CXR should be done. CT and MRI will detect the extent of tumor and soft tissue involvement. Bone scan will detect skip lesions.

Surgery:
- Early and radical ablation is the surgery of choice.
- Limb salvage, if no joint involved
- En block resection of proximal femur
- Reconstruction-bipolar with long stem, combined with allograft
- Amputation remains the mainstay. Level of amputation is upper end femur-hind quarter amputation and hip disarticulation.

Newer techniques:
- Limb salvage, with tumor endoprosthesis.
- Juxta-articular-intraepiphyseal resection and biological reconstruction.
- *Megavoltage radiotherapy:* Radiation is given preoperatively, to decrease the viable cells that get disseminated into bloodstream. It is a useful adjuvant in the treatment of resectable tumors. Radiation destroys tumor cells, with minimal effect on uninvolved parts. Total dose is 6,000–8,000 rads or 230 rads/day or 1,000 rads/week.
- *Chemotherapy:* It is given pre- and postoperatively, to control the micrometastasis. Drugs are methotrexate, citrovorum factor, endoxan, and cisplatinum.
- *Immunotherapy:* New concept. The sensitized lymphocytes from the survivors are infused in the patient. Follow-up, every 6–8 weeks for recurrence and metastasis.

Prognosis

Without therapy, death occurs in 2 years to 6 months and with surgery and chemotherapy. Five years of disease free life, seen in 70% of patients.

Chondrosarcoma (Figs. 221 and 222)

It is malignant slow growing tumor. It arises from cartilage cell. It ranges from being locally aggressive to high grade malignancy.

Incidence: Second in frequency to osteosarcoma.

Site: Common are proximal femur.

Sex: Males commonly affect then females (male/female ratio 1.5:1).

Location: Long bone from diaphyseal-metaphyseal region.

Age: Twenty to sixty years of age.

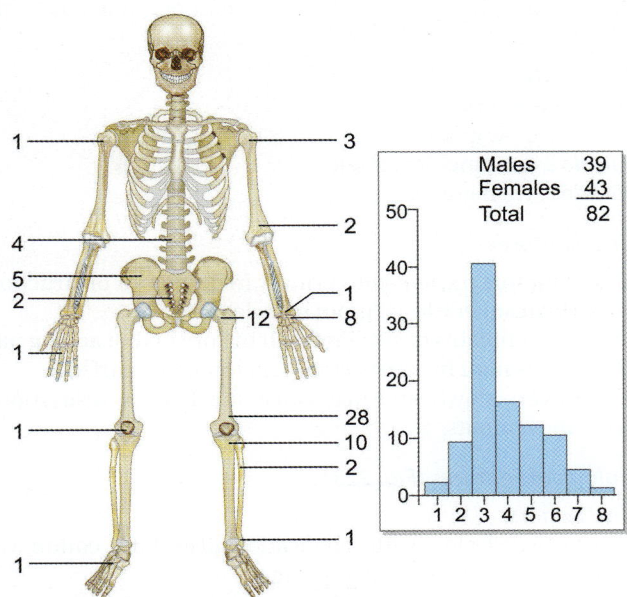

Fig. 221: Distribution of skeletal chondrosarcoma.

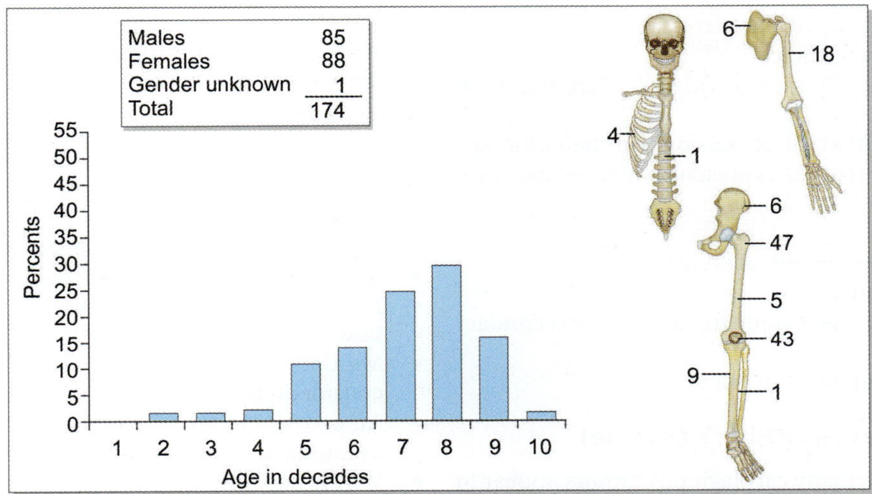

Fig. 222: Distribution of dedifferentiated chondrosarcoma.

Classification

Primary:
- Central (medullary) type
- Juxta-cortical (peri/parosteal)
- Clear cell chondrosarcoma
- Mesenchymal chondrosarcoma
- Dedifferentiated chondrosarcoma.

Secondary:
Arising from pre-existing benign condition, like exostosis or multiple enchondroma.

Pathology

Microscopically:
- Tumor is lobulated appears as white or bluish mass
- Firm in consistency
- Areas of myxomatous degeneration and softening
- Irregular patchy areas of calcification seen microscopically
- Masses of cartilage cell with more than one nucleus, hyperchromatic.

Histologically:
Tumor is graded as:
- *Grade 1:* Low grade
- *Grade 2:* Intermediate grade
- *Grade 3:* High grade.

Clinical Features

- Pelvic tumors present with urinary frequency or obstruction or may masquerade as "groin muscle pulls".
- Patient complains of swelling with history of dull aching pain.
- Swelling is hard in consistency with lobulated surface.
- Grows very slowly and may cause mechanical restriction of joint movements.

Radiological Features (Fig. 223)

Central tumors:
- Central lytic lesion, with calcification gives fluffy, cotton wool, popcorn, or breadcrumb appearance.
- It invades the soft tissue little or no periosteal reaction.

Peripheral tumors (Fig. 224):
Very large tumors and central part is calcified.

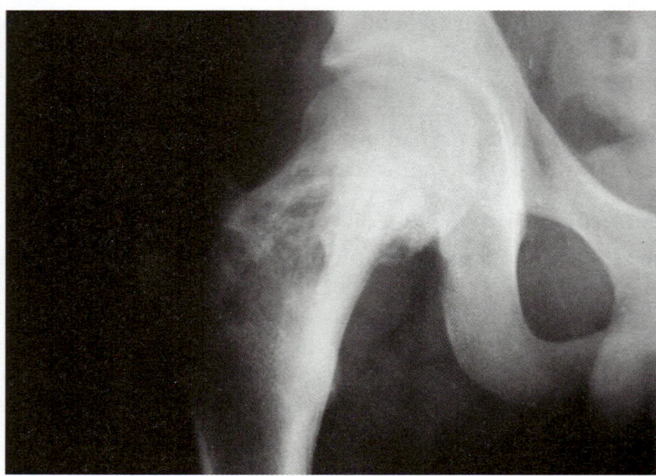

Fig. 223: Radiograph showing chondrosarcoma.

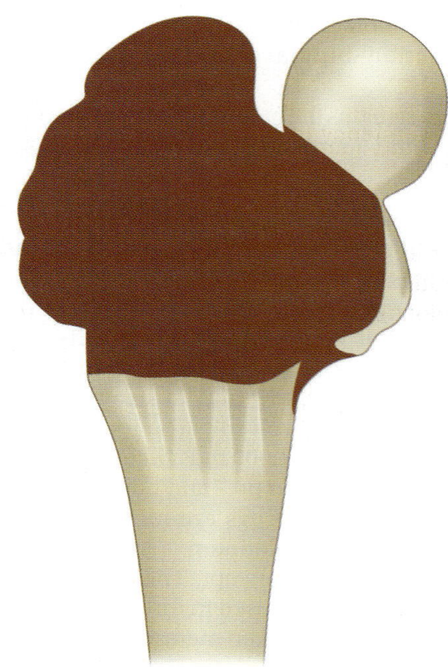

Fig. 224: Chondrosarcoma of hip.

Treatment

- Surgery is the treatment of choice
- Low and medium grade, requires wide excision, e.g. hind quarter for pelvic girdle
- High grade lesion, requires radical excision and chemotherapy
- *Palliative radiotherapy:* If tumor is present in inaccessible area.

Prognosis

- Poor in axial skeleton and proximal bone tumors
- Childhood and young adults
- Cytologically, suggesting high grade malignancy or secondary chondrosarcoma
- Survival time after treatment is 10 years.

Multiple Enchondromatosis (Ollier's Disease)

It is a rare disease, in which many cartilaginous tumors appear in both the large and small tubular bones and in the flat bones. It is caused by failure of normal endochondral ossification, as shown in Figure 225.

Age: 25–40 years.

Site: Located in the epiphysis and the adjacent parts of the metaphysis and shaft and many bones, or only a few may be affected.

Deformities resulting from the tumors include:
- Shortening caused by lack of epiphyseal growth
- Broadening of the metaphysis
- Bowing of the long bones
- Multiple lesions of the small bones of the hand may cause considerable disability
- An occasional lesion has the characteristics of both fibrous dysplasia and enchondromatosis
- When associated with hemangiomas of the overlying soft tissues, the disease is known as Maffucci syndrome.

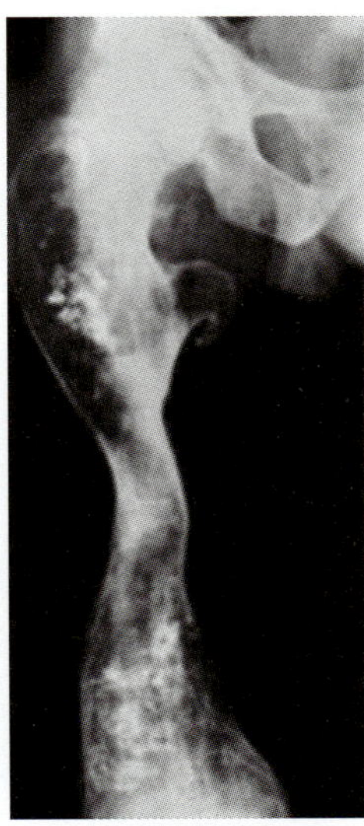

Fig. 225: Multiple enchondromatosis (Ollier's disease).

The individual lesions are quite similar to solitary enchondromas, but often the cellular changes are more bizarre, they have a definite tendency to become malignant. The diagnosis of enchondroma is made on roentgenogram.

Treatment

If malignant transformation is suspected, open surgical biopsy is mandatory. Although, the individual lesions are usually not treated, the more obvious deformities can be corrected by osteotomy.

Aneurysmal Bone Cyst

Aneurysmal bone cysts is benign cystic lesion of bone, composed of blood filled spaces separated by connective tissue septa containing fibroblast, osteoclast-type giant cells, and reactive woven bone. Benign solitary and expansible, an erosive lesion of bone. ABC can be a tumor of undefined neoplastic nature.

Incidence: 1% of benign bone lesion.

Age: Most frequent in children (85% cases < 20 years old).

Sex: Female to male ratio is 2:1.

Radiological Classification of Juxtaphyseal Aneurysmal Bone Cyst (Campanacci's Classification)

- *Type I:* Cyst in middle with little or no expansion.
- *Type II:* Lesion substitutes the whole bone segment.
- *Type III:* Eccentric interosseous lesion with little or no expansion.
- *Type IV:* Subperiosteal cyst and superficial erosion of cortex.
- *Type V:* Periosteum eroded and expansion into soft tissue.
- Primary lesion (de novo)
  - *Incidence:* 70% of ABCs
  - *Cause:* Trauma or vascular disturbances.
- Secondary with precursor lesion
  - *Incidence:* 30%
  - *Cause:* Common precursor lesion is GCT 19–39%
  - *Other precursor lesion:* Osteoblastoma, fibroma, chondroblastoma, osteosarcoma, and UBC.

Treatment

Recommended surgeries:
- Curettage with bone grafting
- Curettage with cementing
- Cryosurgery
- En bloc excision, with or without reconstruction of skeletal defect.

Local recurrence: Young age and open growth plates are associated with an increased risk of local recurrence.

Unicameral Cyst

This is thin walled cavity in metaphysis of long bone closely adjacent to the growth plate and migrates away from it, as it matures. Pathological fractures are common. This rarely affects epiphyseal growth plate.

Etiology

- Unknown
- Popular theory—local trauma
- Local venous congestion
- Increase in intraosseous pressure
- Reactive bone resorption
- Cyst fluid—prostaglandin IL and IB
- Bone resorption.

Types

- Active cyst:
  - Under 10 years
  - Fills most of the metaphysis
  - Thin bony wall
  - Continue to enlarge
  - Pathological fractures.
- Passive cyst:
  - Over 12 years
  - Separated from growth plate
  - Thick bony wall
  - Cease to expand
  - *Age:* 50% lesion in less than 10 years, 40% in 10–20 years. At proximal end femur in adolescent and adult, with mean age of 20
  - *Sex:* Male to female ratio is 2:1
  - *Location:* Always in metaphysis of upper end femur (40% cases) and less common site is ilium.

Pathology

Gross area of fusiform expansion and periosteum lifts away.

Underlying tissue: Egg-shell thin, semitranslucent, bluish, and easily penetrated.

Cavity: Single chamber containing yellow fluid. Following a healed fracture cavity, divided by fibro-osseous septe.

Microscopic: The connective tissue composed of fibroblasts lying on vascular collagenous tissue containing multinucleated giant cells, foam cells containing hemosiderin, lipids, and cholesterol crystals.

Clinical Features

- Asymptomatic, until trivial trauma
- Local aching pain, due to fracture through cyst wall
- Local swelling and tenderness
- Intermittent limp in weight-bearing bones
- Pathological fractures (50% cases)
- Infarction of the thinned cortex (25% cases)
- Displacement of the cyst down the shaft
- Growth disturbances
- Coxa vara deformity in proximal femoral region
- Shortening and overgrowth.

Diagnosis (Figs. 226A to F)

- X-ray
  - Large, well-localized, radiolucent, expansile defect in metaphysis. Regional cortex attenuated.
  - Pseudoloculated form, following a fracture healing
  - Fallen leaf sign, fragment of cortex in the cyst
  - In proximal femur, cyst in subcapital area of neck, calcar is preserved.
- *CT scan:* Only useful if lesion in pelvis.
- *MRI:* Not useful, as it demonstrates only fluid signals.
- *Bone scan:* Light peripheral uptake with cold center.
- *Fluid aspiration:* Aspiration of fluid and injection of radio-opaque substance. Aspirated fluid shows increased level of PG E2.
- Open biopsy and cytology.

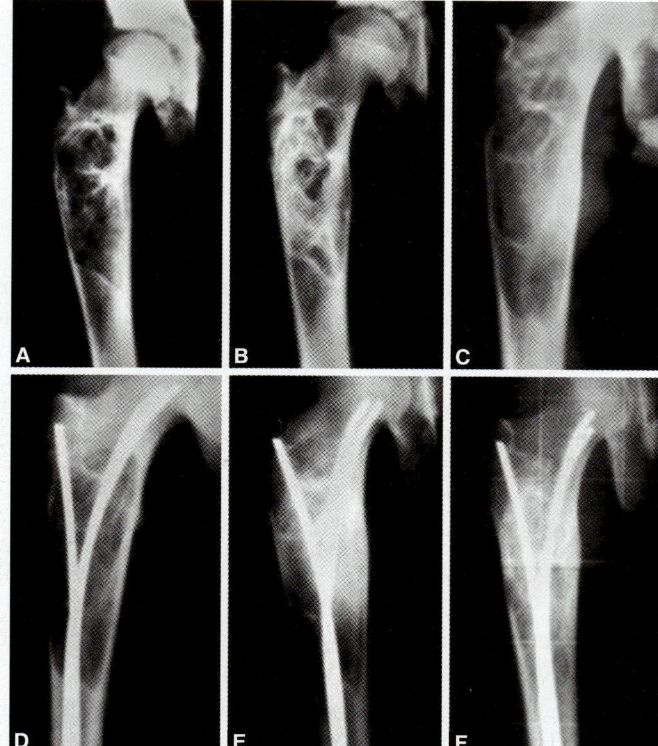

Figs. 226A to F: (A) Solitary bone cyst in femur of 7-year-old child; (B) After three infiltrations of methylprednisolone; (C) Recurrence of cyst after five infiltrations; (D) After nailing with three ender nails because of large size of cyst; (E) One month after operation; (F) Eight months after operation, remodeling of bone tissue is evident.

Differential Diagnosis

- Eosinophilic granuloma
- Enchondroma
- Fibrous dysplasia
- Giant cell tumor
- Aneurysmal bone cyst.

Simple Bone Cyst

- Minimal pain unless fracture
- Fluid filled cavity
- Slightly expansile
- X-ray shows few loculations
- MRI shows prominent fluid-fluid levels
- It has membranous lining.

Aneurysmal Bone Cyst

- Aching pain without fracture
- Blood filled cavity
- Very expansile
- X-ray shows many loculations
- In MRI, no fluid-fluid levels
- Mesenchymal tissue lining.

Treatment

Goal: Prevention of pathological fracture.

Modalities:

- Curettage and bone grafting:
  - High recurrence rate
  - For active cyst (50%)
  - For passive cyst (10%).
- Steroids:
  - *Methyl-prednisolone:* 80–200 mg infused in cavity
  - Unpredictable response
  - Failure in weight-bearing bones
  - *Autologous bone marrow injection:* Unsatisfactory response (F Lokeiec et al.)
  - *Multiple drill holes:* Unpredictable response (T Shinozaki et al.)

Fibrous Dysplasia

It is a skeletal developmental anomaly of the bone forming mesenchyme that manifests as a defect in osteoblastic differentiation and maturation. Thus, leading to replacement of normal marrow and cancellous bone, by immature bone and fibrous stroma. It is an uncommon benign disorder characterized by a tumor, like proliferation of fibro-osseous tissue. Etiology is unknown.

Types

- Monostotic—confined to one bone
- Polyostotic—multiple bone involvement.

Age: Disease of childhood may progress beyond puberty and through adulthood.

Sex: Equal distribution.

Location

- Monostotic form (70–80%)—Femur (23%)
- Polyostotic form (20–30%)—Femur (91%), pelvis (78%), then long bones of lower limb and metaphyseal.

Pathology

Gross appearance: Bony structure is replaced by avascular fibrous tissues, in which thin trabaculae are formed. Gross appearance shows bony irregularity and bent appearance. Cortex is thin and bulged outward. Tissues are reddish-gray and tough fibrous. Pathological fractures are undisplaced, usually heal readily with deformity. Shepherd Crook deformity is present, as shown in Figure 227.

Microscopic appearance: Dense, mature, collagenase tissues with fibrous bone trabaculae. Fibroblast are elongated and placed in linear or whorled intersecting bundles. Trabaculae appear as Chinese letter or alphabet soup fashion. Classic lesion, in which bone develops by metaplasia, absence of osteoblast and giant cells are sparse.

Clinical Features

- Early childhood
- Mild and asymptomatic
- Onset of symptoms > 10 years
- Limp, pain in leg, and fracture
- Females show abnormal vaginal bleeding
- Bending deformity in weight-bearing bones
- Shepherd Crook deformity
- Skull show hyperostosis at the base and is asymmetrical
- Café-eu-late spots in polyostotic
- Sexual precocity in females
- *McCune-Albright syndrome*
  - Polyostotic fibrous dysplasia
  - Pigmentation
  - Sexual precocity in female.

Diagnosis

Laboratory findings: Normal
- Serum calcium
- Serum phosphorus
- Serum alkaline phosphatase raised in severe conditions.

Radiological Findings

- *X-ray:*
  - Localized, well-circumscribed lesion in shaft
  - Ground glass appearance

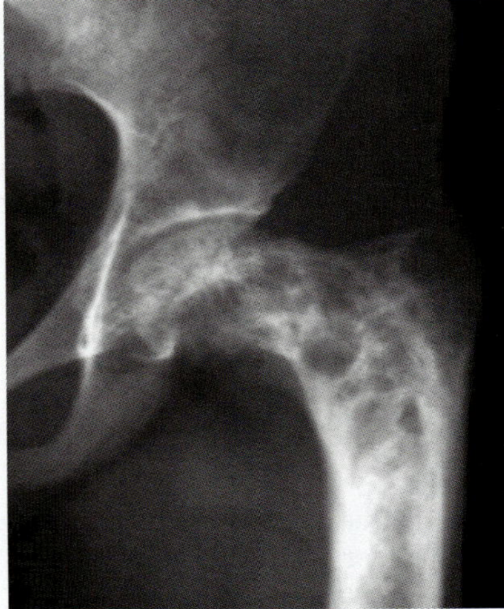

Fig. 227: Gross pathological appearance in fibrous dysplasia, with Shepherd Crook deformity.

  - Cystic or multilocular
  - Cortex—thinned and expanded
  - Skull—hyperostotic formation at base
- *Bone scan:*
  - Active lesion—increased uptake
  - Inactive lesion—decreased uptake
- *CT scan:* To evaluate extent of bone involvement
- *MRI:* To find sarcomatous changes
- *Biopsy:* Is confirmatory.

Differential Diagnosis

- Hyperparathyroidism
- Osteogenesis imperfecta
- Neurofibromatosis
- Paget's disease.

Management

Medical: Biphosphonate (Fosamax)
- 35 mg weekly for children
- 70 mg weekly for adults
- Long-term therapy for symptomatic and large lesions.

Postoperative

- IV bisphosphonate including zoledronic acid, symptomatic or critical lesions, monthly for 3–6 months.

Surgical (Figs. 228A to C):
- Curettage–high rate of local recurrence
- Curettage and bone grafting, preferably in NWB bones
- Curettage with cortical bone grafting and implant fixation in weight-bearing bones
- In proximal femur, rigid intramedullary fixation, with strongest possible device.

Radiotherapy:
Contraindicated: Increased risk of sarcomatous changes.

Prognosis

- *Mono-ostotic:* Excellent, if the bone can be strengthened
- *Polyostotic:* Several operative procedures, to achieve bone strength and correct deformity
- *Malignant degeneration:* Extremely rare.

Chondroma

Including enchondroma and periosteal chondromas. It is a benign tumor of mature hyaline cartilage (chondromas), are usually located centrally in bone, and are known as enchondromas. Less frequently, they are located sub-periosteally and are known as juxtacortical or sub-periosteal chondromas.

Age: Occur during the second, third, and fourth decades of life.

Site: Most common sites of manifestations include:
- Metaphysis is usually involved.
- Enchondroma, the most frequent tumor of bone in the hand, rarely exhibits aggressive behavior and is sometimes referred to as cartilaginous hamartoma.
- The long bones of the extremities are involved less frequently, but enchondromas of the humerus and femur are not rare.
- Vertebral involvement has been reported.

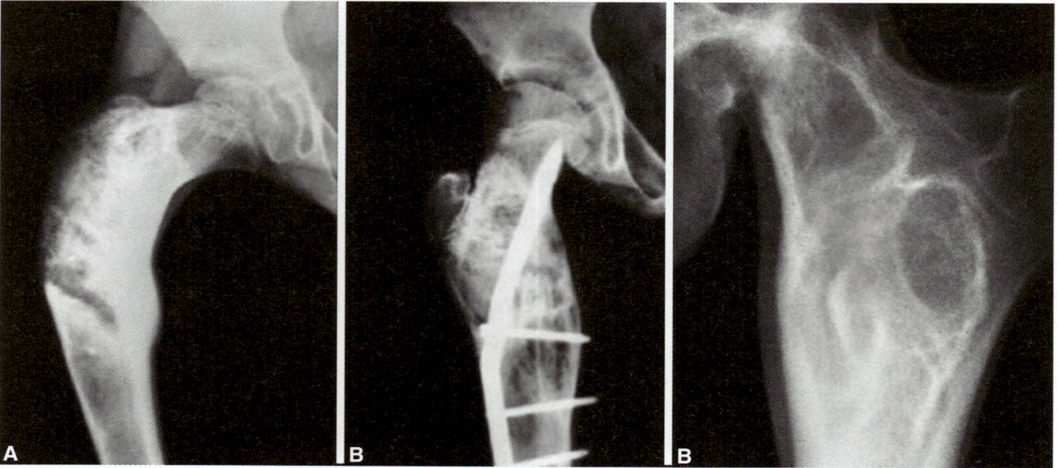

Figs. 228A to C: Fibrous dysplasia—(A and B) Shepherds Crook deformity; (C) Deformity has been corrected by osteotomy and cystic lesion has been filled with grafts.

Symptoms

- Often are nonspecific and some lesions being discovered incidentally, during an unrelated roentgenographic examination.
- Usually the tumor is found after a pathological fracture.
- Pain is an ominous symptom and suggests that the tumor is growing and may be malignant.

Roentgenographic Findings (Figs. 229A to C)

- It depends on the location and extent of calcification of the tumor.
- A central lesion in a small tubular bone of the hand or foot, usually appears as a well-circumscribed area of rarefaction, most frequently diaphyseal. Cortex around it may be expanded.
- A juxtacortical lesion is eccentric and is located beneath the periosteum in a well-defined cortical defect.
- Small flocculent foci of calcification are often seen within the tumor and in a long bone, the tumor may be highly calcified and radiopaque.

Pathology

The differentiation of benign from malignant cartilaginous tumors is one of the most difficult problems in bone pathology. All available tissues must be examined and even then the diagnosis may depend more on the clinical and roentgenographic features, than on the microscopic changes. Juxtacortical chondromas and enchondromas of the hands may be quite cellular and contain many atypical cells and still be benign. Conversely, enchondromas of long bones often appear benign microscopically, but tend to recur after removal. Some uncalcified enchondromas, may mimic a variety of lytic lesions, both clinically and on roentgenograms and the heavily calcified enchondromas of long bones may resemble bone infarcts or so-called bone islands.

Treatment

- Curettage is done and the wall is cauterized if the tumor is small
- Surgery done in cases of large tumors, excision and removal of capsule is to prevent recurrence
- Radical resection done for tumors of long bones and pelvis.

Less commonly tumors found around hip are:

- Osteoid osteoma

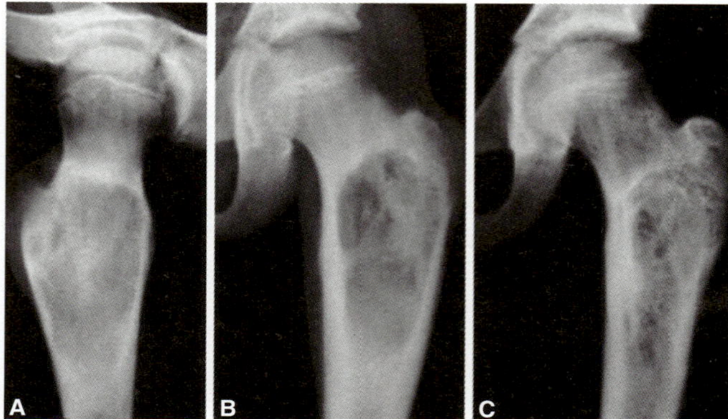

Figs. 229A to C: X-rays showing enchondroma in proximal femur of a boy of 11 years of age. Patient was followed up for 15 years, after curettage of enchondroma and there was no evidence of recurrence found.

- Giant cell tumor
- Chordoma
- Metastatic tumors
- Multiple myeloma
- Osteochondromatosis
- Synovioma
- Pigmented villonodular synovitis
- Lymphoma
- Fibrous cortical defect
- Benign fibrous histiocytoma
- Neural tumors
- Desmoplastic fibroma.

Osteoid Osteoma

Osteoid osteoma is a benign osteoblastic tumor.

Sex: Young adults between 10 and 25 years of age. Male to female ratio is 2:1.

Age: Found in the first three decades of life, but an occasional lesion has been reported in older patients.

Location: The proximal femur is the most common location. Osteoid osteoma is found in the diaphysis or the metaphysis of the proximal end of the bone more often than the distal end.

Incidence: Approximately, 10% of benign bone tumors. 5% are subperiosteal, and 5% of sciatica are due to osteoid osteoma.

Pathology

Vascular mesenchymal type of connective tissue stroma, with proliferating fibroblasts and osteoblasts surrounds abundant pink staining osteoid tissue. Osteoid forms irregular branching network, surrounding the poorly formed tissue at the center of lesion is marked bony proliferation. Marrow is fibrous, cartilage is never found.

Clinical Features

- The typical patient has pain that is worse at night and relieved by aspirin (aspirin tumor)
- The person may limp
- When the lesion is near a joint, swelling, stiffness, and contracture may occur
- When in a vertebra, scoliosis may occur. Occasionally, osteoid osteoma occurs with minimal pain
- In children, overgrowth and angular deformities may occur
- Systemic symptoms are absent.

Radiographic Findings (Fig. 230)

- Small rarefied lesions less than 2 cm in diameter in cortex, subcortical, or subperiosteal regions
- Surrounded by thick sclerotic bone
- Small dense center of ossification—Nidus
- CT/MRI useful to identify and localize the lesion
- A bone scan is helpful in detecting small lesions that may be overlooked on roentgenograms
- The "double-density sign", which is a focal area of increased activity with a second smaller area of increased uptake superimposed on it is said to be diagnostic of osteoid osteoma.

Treatment

Conservative: Rest to the part and analgesics (aspirin).

Surgical

- To affect a cure, the entire nidus must be removed.
- Block resection of the nidus; however, if the lesion is in cortical bone, this method increases the risk of subsequent fractures (Figs. 231A and B).

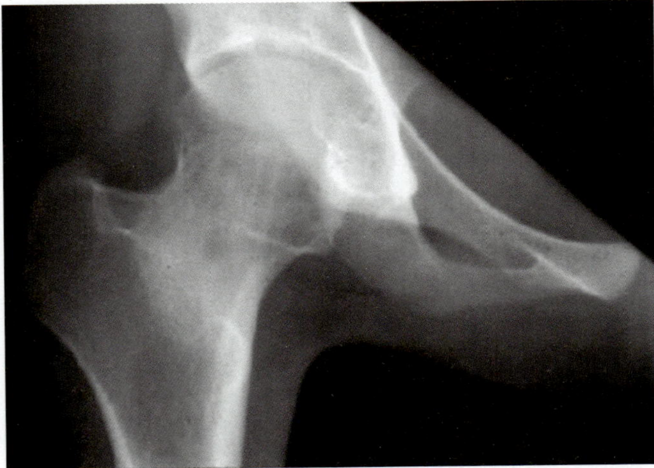

Fig. 230: Osteoid osteoma of hip.

- An alternative method suggested by Johnston, is to shave the reactive bone with a sharp osteotome, until the nidus is encountered then curet the exposed nidus.
- CT-guided percutaneous resection allows precise localization and removal of the nidus through a small access without the need for removal of an excessive amount of bone.
- Percutaneous radiofrequency ablation of osteoid osteomas and believe their results are equivalent to operative excision.
- For rare intra-articular situations, arthroscopically assisted excision.
- MRI guided cryotreatment.

Recurrence and malignancy:

- After complete removal of tumor along with nidus recurrence is very rare.
- No malignant change has ever been documented.

Giant Cell Tumor

Benign giant cell tumor is an osteolytic tumor, arising from the epiphysis and is common in young adults. Though, it is benign it is locally malignant.

Sex: The male to female ratio is 1.5:1.

Age: It is common between 15 and 35 years of age (80% occur in more than 20 years of age and the average age group is 35 years).

Sites: It is shown in Figure 232:

- Giant cell tumor may occur in the sacrum
- Upper end of femur.

Pathology

Grossly, the tumor consist of ragged, friable, and bleeding tissue filled with old or fresh blood clot, with various sized cysts and cavities. Color varies from red and brown. Epiphyseal end of the bone is distorted. Tumor extension in the joint cavity is usually not seen and there is no evidence of periosteal reaction.

Microscopically, the tumor is encompassed, by a fibrous capsule at the periphery. Presence of abundant tumor giant cells, are quiet characteristic. These cells are characterized by their larger size, multiple nuclei more than 150 in number, which are distributed throughout the cell. Appearance of spindle cell, indicate malignant potential.

Histological Grading (Jaffe's Criterion)

- *Grade I:* Presence of characteristic stromal cell, little intercellular collagen and spindle are adjacent to the necrotic tissue.
- *Grade II:* Random distribution of giant cell are seen among the stromal cells.
- *Grade III:* Nuclei of giant cell are identical to those of the stromal cells.

Clinical Features

- The course of the tumor is chronic.
- Unlike osteogenic sarcoma, pain is not the presenting feature but trauma is the patient complains of swelling, which is situated on one side of the bone.
- Skin over the tumor is stretched, but there are no dilated vein.
- Tenderness is moderate or absent egg-shell crackling sensation may be present or absent.
- Invasion in the joint is rare and joint effusion is rare.
- Pathological fracture is a late feature.

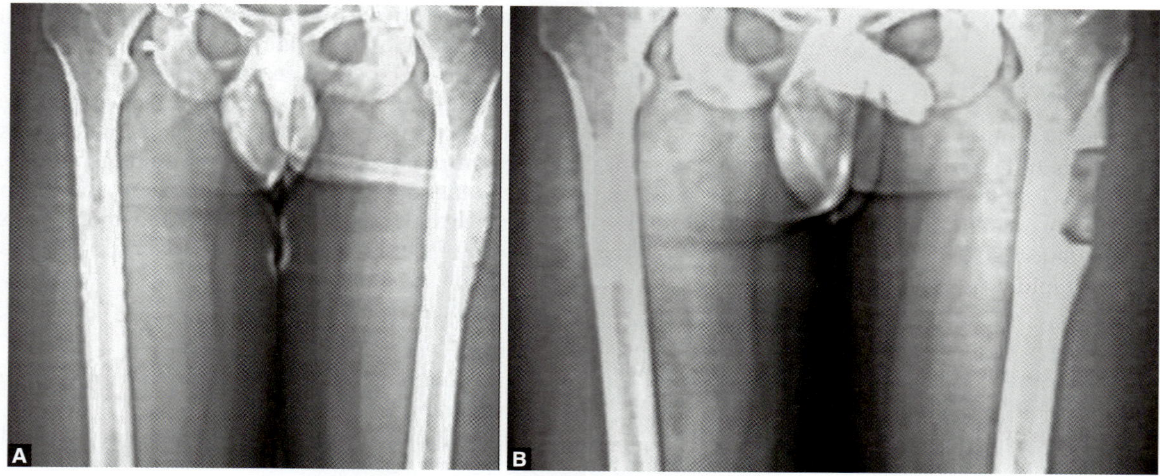

Figs. 231A and B: Osteoid osteoma (preoperative and postoperative).

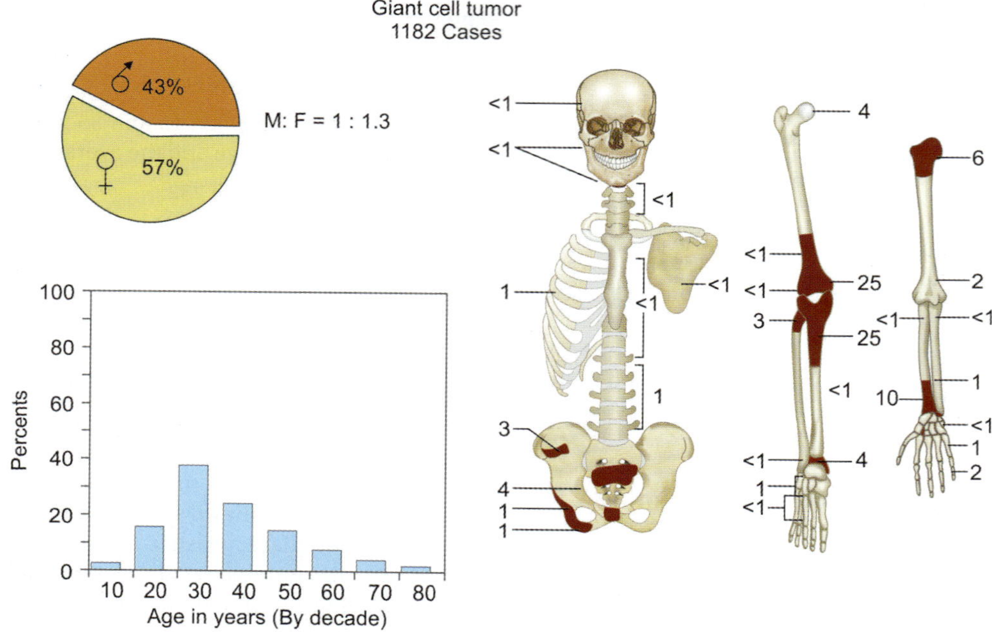

Fig. 232: Common site of occurrence of GCT.

Radiology (Fig. 233)

- An osteolytic area is seen near the epiphysis
- The cortex is thin and expanded
- There is no periosteal new bone formation
- Thin septa of bone transverse the interior of bone and gives it soap-bubble appearance
- The cortex may be disrupted in late stages
- Joint extension is rare.

Companacci's radiographic grading:

- *Grade 1:* Cystic lesion
- *Grade 2:* Cortex is thin, but not perforated
- *Grade 3:* Cortex is perforated, with extension in the soft tissue.

Enneking's staging of benign GCT:

- Stage 1 (Latent):
  - Incidence is 10– 15%
  - Discovered accidentally

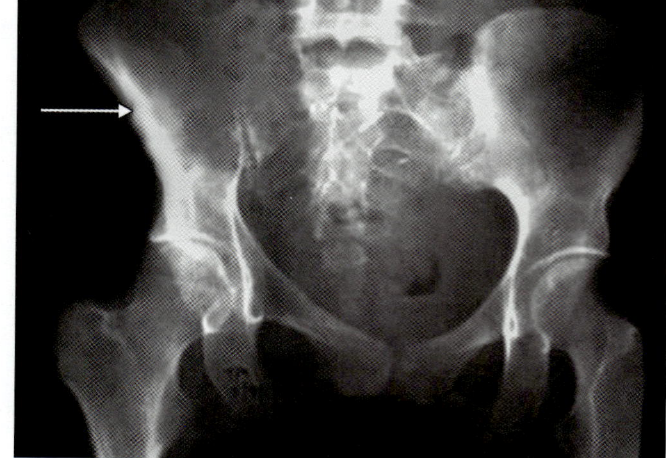

Fig. 233: X-ray showing GCT of hip, arrow showing GCT.

- No symptoms
- Pathological fractures may be present.

- Stage 2 (Active):
  - Incidence is 70%
  - Symptomatic
  - Pathological fracture may be present
  - Benign.
- Stage 3 (Aggressive):
  - Incidence is 10–15%
  - Symptomatic rapidly growing
  - Benign
  - Cortex is perforated.

Treatment

- Intralesional excision by "extended" curettage is the treatment of choice
- Curettage and bone grafting
- En bloc resection
- Curettage and acrylic bone cementation
- Curettage and cryosurgery
- Arthrodesis
- Arthroplasty
- Radiotherapy.

Chordoma

Chordoma is a rare malignant neoplasm that arises from notochord remnants, as shown in Figure 234. Chordomas account for 1–4% of all bone tumors. The ratio of male to female is 2:1. Chordoma is the most common primary malignancy of the sacrum. Over 50% of chordomas arise in the sacrococcygeal area. Peak incidence for sacrococcygeal chordomas occurs in the fifth through seventh decades. Most series demonstrate a marked male predominance (as high as 3:1), especially for sacrococcygeal tumors.

Clinical Features

- Sacrococcygeal tumors often present as low back pain, with no characteristic pattern or time course.
- Bowel and bladder dysfunction.
- Presacral tumors can sometimes be palpated on rectal examination.
- Sacral tumors are often large at presentation, as a large volume of tumor can be accommodated within the pelvis.

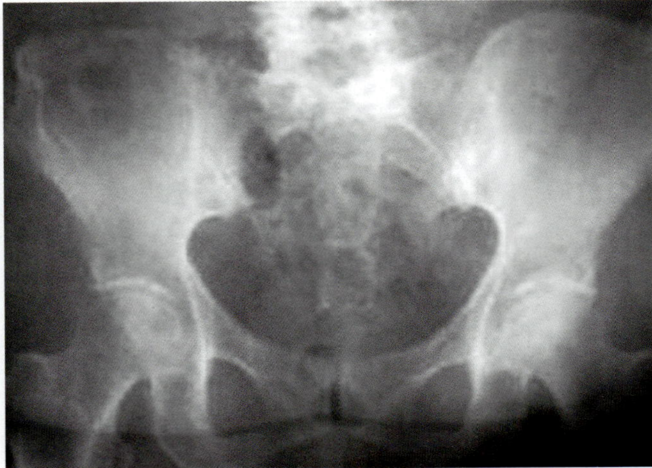

Fig. 234: Chordoma of hip.

X-rays: On plain X-ray, chordomas appear as a solitary mid-line lesion with bony destruction. There is often an accompanying soft tissue mass. Approximately, half of the time focal calcifications are present.

CT and MRI scans help demonstrate the soft tissue component, calcifications, and epidural extension. MRI is helpful in identifying local recurrences.

Bone scan: Chordomas have reduced uptake on bone scan.

Examination (Figs. 235A to D)

On gross examination chordomas are soft, blue-gray, lobulated tumors.

There are gelatinous translucent areas and often a capsule is present.

The lesion often tracks along nerve roots in the sacral plexus or out the sciatic notch in planes of least resistance.

Under the microscope:

The chordomas are characterized by lobules and fibrous septa. The malignant cell has eosinophilic cytoplasm. Prominent vacuoles of mucus push the nuclei to the side, resulting in "physaliferous" cells from the Greek word for bubble or drop.

Treatment

The treatment of chordomas is difficult. Wide surgical excision is desirable, but rarely feasible based on the anatomic location of the tumor. With sacrococcygeal tumors, sexual function, and sphincter control may be compromised after surgery. Radiation is used, if complete resection is impossible. Chordomas metastasize to lymph nodes, lungs, liver, and bone. Chemotherapy can be used for late stage disease.

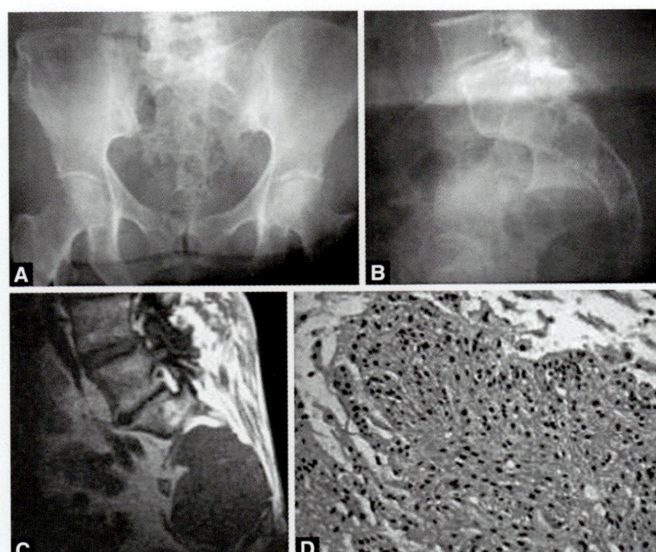

Figs. 235A to D: Anteroposterior (A) and lateral; (B) views of sacrum of patient with sacrococcygeal chordoma. This lesion could easily be missed because of overlying bowel gas; (C) MRI clearly demonstrates lesion; (D) Typical microscopic appearance of chordoma. Cells with abundant vacuolated cytoplasm (physaliferous cells) are arranged in cords with mucinous background.

Metastatic Tumors of Bones

These are cancerous tumors originating in the other organs and involving the skeletal structures of the body. Bones may be involved by:

- Direct invasion,
- Blood-borne metastasis, and
- Very rarely, through the lymphatics.

Incidence: 27–70%

Tendency percentage wise:

- Carcinoma breast (73%)
- Lung (32%)
- Kidney (24%)
- Rectum (13%)
- Stomach (11%).

Sites: Sites of frequent metastasis to the skeleton are shown in Figure 236.

Clinical Features

- Adult and middle age patient
- Pain, pathological fracture or anemia. Pathological fractures are frequent in femur.

Diagnosis

- Blood picture show anemia, thrombocytopenia, leukocytosis or leukopenia, eosinophilia, etc.
- Alkaline phosphatase has increased
- Acid phosphatase increased in cancer of prostate.

Investigation

- Radiology (Fig. 237)
- Osteolytic and osteoblastic variety
- Periosteal reaction and mottled or marble appearance
- Bone scan
- Fine needle biopsy.

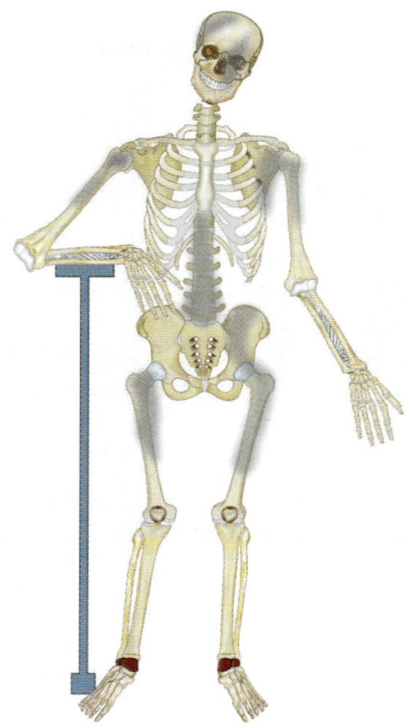

Fig. 236: Sites of frequent metastasis to the skeleton (gray highlighted area) commonly involves pelvis and proximal end of femur.

Treatment (Figs. 238 to 241)

- Radiotherapy 3000–4000 rads for 3–4 weeks
- *Surgery:* Internal fixation with acrylic cement for pathological fractures
- Hormone therapy
- Radioisotope therapy

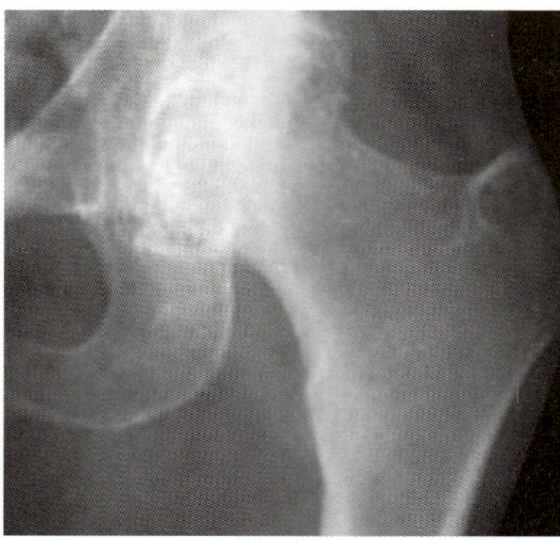

Fig. 237: X-ray showing malignant osteoblastic and osteolytic tumors of hip.

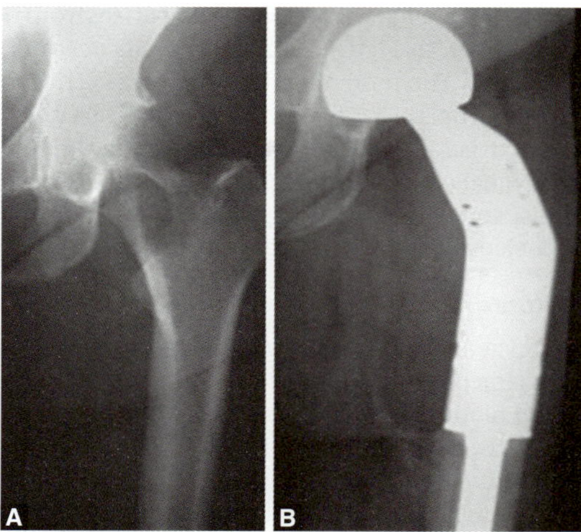

Figs. 238A and B: (A) X-ray showing malignant tumor of hip; (B) Tumor excision followed by prosthesis implantation.

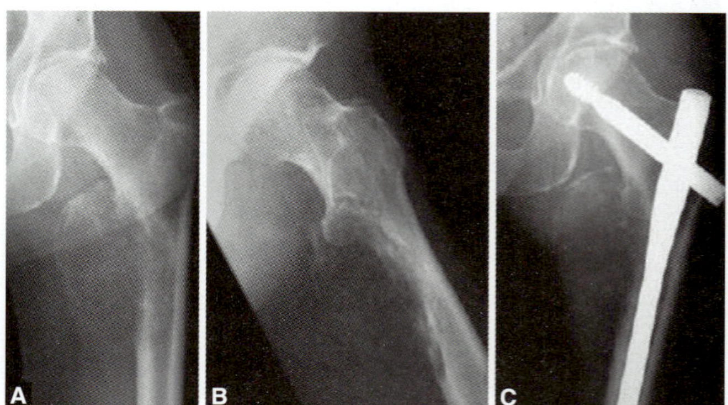

Figs. 239A to C: Anteroposterior (A) and lateral (B) Roentgenograms of left hip of a 44-year-old man, with metastatic bladder cancer; (C) Anteroposterior view after prophylactic fixation with long gamma nail.

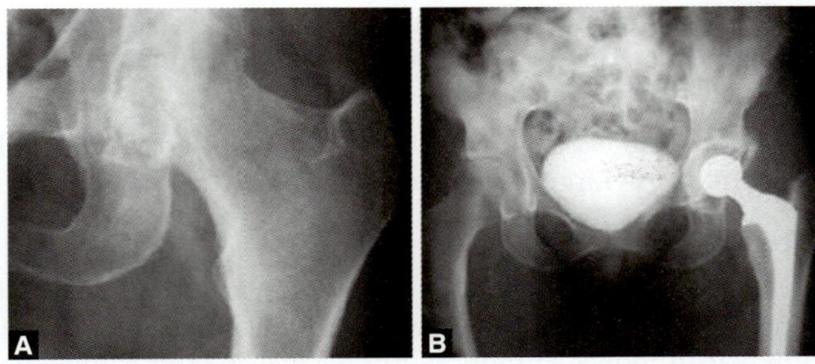

Figs. 240A and B: (A) Anteroposterior view of left hip of patient treated with radiation for metastatic breast cancer. She subsequently, developed avascular necrosis of femoral head; (B) Anteroposterior view of pelvis after treatment with cemented total hip arthroplasty. As the bone had been irradiated, both femoral and acetabular components were cemented.

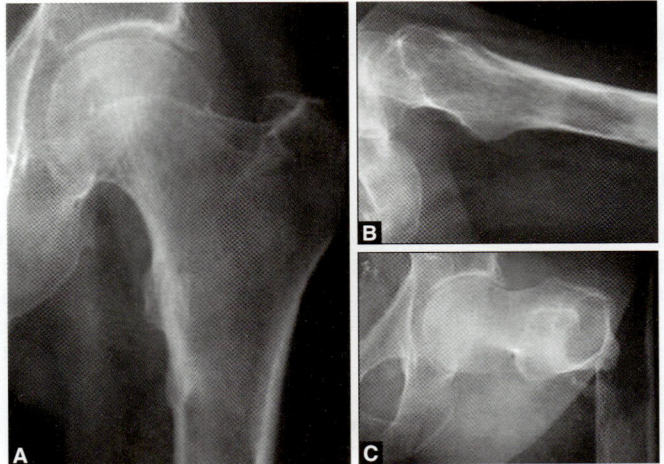

Figs. 241A to C: Anteroposterior (A) and lateral (B) roentgenograms of proximal femur of an 82-year-old man, with metastatic kidney cancer reveal multiple lytic lesions. Patient failed to respond to radiation treatment. Prophylactic internal fixation was scheduled, however operation was cancelled because patient was considered medically unstable for surgery; (C) Anteroposterior view of left hip of same patient several weeks later after sustaining pathological fracture. Surgery is now more difficult and patient has experienced greater morbidity.

- Chemotherapy
- Radiofrequency ablation.

Multiple Myeloma

Malignant tumor arising from plasma cell of reticuloendothelial cell of bone marrow. It can occur as a solitary plasmocytoma, multiple myeloma or generalized myelomatosis. This is shown in Figures 242A to D.

Incidence: Accounts for 45% of total malignant tumors.

Age: Fifty to eighty years of age. Males are commonly affected (male to female ratio is 2:1).

Site: Proximal femur and pelvis.

Pathology

Grossly:

- Tumor is dark red in color
- Soft in consistency and lies within medulla
- The cortex is thin and broken.

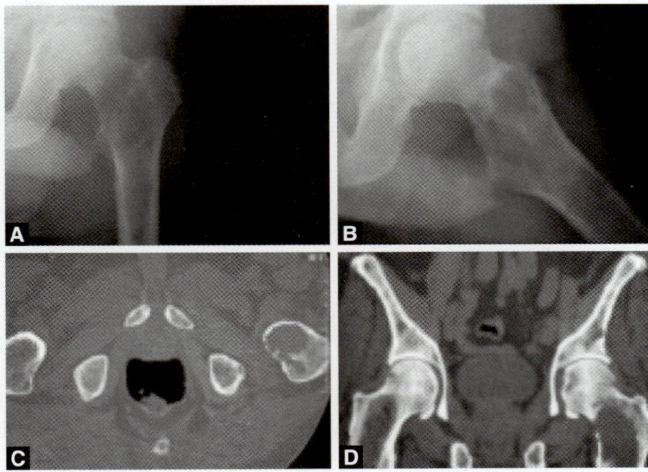

Figs. 242A to D: Anteroposterior (A) and lateral (B) roentgenograms of proximal femur of 61-year-old man with multiple myeloma demonstrate multiple lytic lesions; (C and D) CT better demonstrates extent of lesions and need for prophylactic fixation.

Microscopically:

- Consist of round cells with eccentrically placed nucleus with nucleolus.
- Chromatin is sparsed and is arranged in spokes of wheel fashion.
- Perinuclear halo typical of plasma cell not seen in multiple myeloma.

Associated pathology:

- Interstitial fibrosis in the kidney
- Nodules in the lungs
- Amylodosis may occur.

Clinical Features

General examination:

Patient becomes severely anemic, loses weight, and becomes cachetic. In the late stage, patient develops hyperazotemia, uremic syndrome, hypercalcemia, hyperuremic syndrome, and hemorrhagic diasthesis.

Sign and Symptoms

- Generalized bone pain and pain in back.
- Pain may be intermittent, but later become intense.
- In the early stages, there are hardly any clinical symptoms.
- Late stages, patient complains of soft tissue swelling and sign of pathological fracture.
- Tumor is chronic and tubular block due to protein cast may be seen causing renal failure (myeloma kidney).

Investigation:

- Radiological features
  - Affected bone shows diffuse osteoporosis or lytic lesion.
  - Punched out lesion in the pelvis; skull bones; ribs.
- Laboratory findings
  - Low Hb%
  - High ESR
  - Increased total protein A/G ratio reversed
  - Increased serum calcium
  - Low to normal alkaline phosphatase

- Urine Bence-Jones protein are found in 30% of patients
- *Serum electrophoresis:* Abnormal spike of gamma globulin in 90% of cases
- *Sternal puncture:* Myeloma cell may be seen
- Bone biopsy
- Bone scan
- Open biopsy
- Alpha-2 microglobulin tumor marker.

Treatment

- Chemotherapy is the mainstay of the treatment.
- Drugs used are melphalan, cyclophosphamide, vincristine, and steroids.
- High dose of vincristine, doxorubicin, and dexamethasone (VDD) is the new and better alternative. Tumor is radiosensitive and localized lesions are treated with radiation for pain relief.

Surgery:
- In case of pathological fractures
- Decompression of cords in neurological involvement.

Prognosis:
- Disease is widespread and fatal
- Death in 3- 5 years.

Complications:
- Pathological fractures of rib
- Spinal cord or nerve root compression
- Renal failure
- Severe infection
- Amylodosis.

Osteochondromatosis (Fig. 243)

Osteochondromatosis can be (1) Hereditary multiple osteocartilagenous exostoses (H MOCE) and (2) Hereditary multiple exostoses (HME). HMOCE is a rare, autosomal dominant condition, where a genetic error of bone growth results in the formation of multiple osteochondromas. The condition can range from a mild nuisance to a very severe, disabling, and even potentially deadly problem, depending on the number and location of the lesions. HMOCE is an autosomal dominant condition. The condition is genetically heterogeneous and it has been linked to three loci including 8 *q*24.1 (EXT1), 11*p*11-12 (EXT2) and 19 *p* (EXT3). EXT1 and EXT2

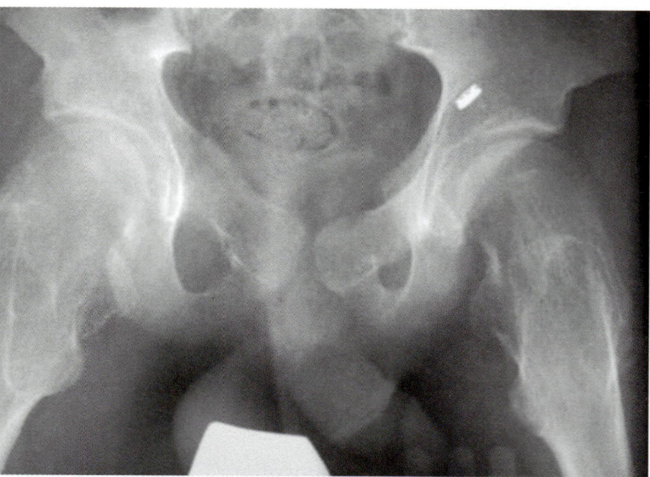

Fig. 243: Osteochondromatosis of hip.

are proposed tumor supressor genes, which may be lost in HMOCE, resulting in the growth of the lesions. The condition can lead to both sessile and pedunculated lesions.

Occurrence: The lesions may occur on different bones or on the same bone and symptoms present in the first decade of life.

Clinical Features

Patients may have short stature. Limb-length discrepancies. The lesions cluster at the metaphyseal ends of the bones near the joint and may lead to loss of motion, hip dysplasia, joint subluxation, nerve compression, vascular pseudoaneurysm, cord compression, and pain. The risk of malignant transformation to chondrosarcoma in hereditary multiple osteochondromatosis is unknown, but may be 25–30% compared to approximately 1% for a solitary osteochondromas. The risk of malignant degeneration increases as the number and size of the osteochondromas increases. Large deep osteochondromas, often located on the pelvis or the spine, where malignant transformation, may be more likely and much more difficult to treat.

Treatment

Surgical removal of troublesome lesions or lesions, which appear to possess malignant potential is associated with a good outcome. Significant angular deformities of the lower limb can be reduced or eliminated with realignment procedures, which should improve function and reduce pain. Early surgical corrections of deformities have been advocated to improve function. Indications for surgical removal include persistent pain, functional impairment, joint subluxation, neuropraxia, and others.

Synovioma

The synovioma (synovial sarcoma, synovial sarcomesothelioma, cancerous synovial tumor) is a slow growing malignant tumor occurring in juxtaposition to and often attached to synovial tissue, but almost invariably lies outside the joint.

Pathology

Grossly, the tumor is sharply circumscribed, rounded, and lobulated. As it grows, it compresses the surrounding tissue, which becomes attenuated to form a pseudocapsule.

Microscopically: Three basic patterns, indicating a synovial origin are formation of tissue spaces, formation of cell tufts. Epithelia, like cells on a supporting stroma of tissue.

Clinical Features

Age: Young adults 25- 40 years.

Site: Lower extremity.

Position: In soft tissue, outside the joint.

Symptoms:
- Painful swelling begins in periarticular or peritendinous site
- Increases slowly, large swelling with severe pain
- Swelling is firm or soft, moderately tender.

Course: Very slow, metastasizes eventually to lungs.

Roentgenographic Findings

- Soft tissue technique reveals a rounded and lobulated shadow
- Stippling is observed, if tumor contains small areas of calcification.

Prognosis and Treatment

- Tumor is slow-growing and metastasizes late
- Local excision is inadequate
- Radical amputation is indicated.

Pigmented Villonodular Synovitis

Pigmented villonodular synovitis (PVNS) is a locally aggressive synovial tumor. There are two forms of PVNS—(1) diffuse and (2) nodular. PVNS occurs in the hips.

Incidence: PVNS has the highest prevalence during the third and fourth decades and it affects males and females equally.

Signs/symptoms: It presents as a painless or mildly painful joint with swelling. Mechanical interference causes stiffness, locking, limitation of motion, and snapping sensations at times.

Lymphoma

Lymphoma may involve bone primarily or secondarily.

Occurrence: Lymphoma can occur at any age, but becomes more common in the sixth and seventh decades of life.

Sex: The male to female ratio is approximately 1.5:1.

Location: The femur is the most common bone involved, followed by the pelvis.

Signs/Symptoms: Most patients complain of localized pain or swelling.

Roentgenographically: Lymphoma usually appears as an ill-defined area of bone destruction, frequently diaphyseal and often has a permeative appearance. The cortex may be thickened, but a periosteal reaction rarely is seen.

Microscopically, osseous lymphomas are composed of a mixture of both large and small lymphoid cells with both cleaved and noncleaved nuclei. A discussion on the classification of lymphomas is beyond the scope of this text.

Prognosis: Patients with primary lymphoma of bone have a better prognosis (approximately 55%, 5 years survival) than those with systemic disease (less than 25% and 5 years survival).

Treatment: The primary treatment of lymphoma is chemotherapy. Local control usually is attained with radiation treatment. Surgical intervention is therefore rarely needed, but may be indicated for treatment of impending or actual pathological fractures.

On aspiration: Thick orange brown fluid containing cholesterol in large amounts is pathognomonic. Hemosiderin is also present.

Radiological appearance of PVNS depends on the location. Bone erosion or cysts will be present in tighter joints, like the hip. The joint space is usually preserved and there may be an effusion.

CT scan is able to pick up the hemosiderin and demonstrates the extent of the synovial involvement as well as bone erosion and cysts. Hemosiderin appears as low or absent signal on both T1 and T2 weighted images.

Pathology: On gross examination, the diffuse form of PVNS is a tanned mass of villi and folds of synovium. The lesion may be sessile or have several pedunculated nodules. Bony invasion through the joint capsule is possible. The local form of PVNS is a pedunculated firm nodule.

Treatment: Treatment of PVNS is surgical excision. Recurrences are common due to the difficulty of complete surgical excision. Hence, radiotherapy has been recommended.

Benign Fibrous Histiocytoma

Fibrous histiocytoma was first described by Dahlin in 1978. This lesion occurs most frequently in the soft tissues and is less common in bone. Although, it is histologically similar to that of nonossifying fibroma, it is a much more aggressive tumor in its biological behavior and roentgenographic characteristics. Unlike, nonossifying fibroma, which usually is an eccentric metaphyseal lesion, benign fibrous histiocytoma may occur in the diaphysis or epiphysis of long bones, or in the pelvis. It is further distinguished by its occurrence in older patients between the ages of 30 and 40 years. Roentgenographically, benign fibrous histiocytoma is a well-defined, lytic, expanding lesion with little periosteal reaction. Bone scans usually are mildly positive. Unlike, nonossifying fibroma, this lesion is considered a true neoplasm.

Treatment: Due to its tendency for local recurrence (persistence), aggressive curettage or when feasible, wide excision is necessary.

Fibrous Cortical Defect

Fibrous cortical defects, although classified as bone tumors are probably developmental abnormalities and are believed to occur in as many as 35% of children. Generally, these lesions occur in the metaphyseal region of long bones in individuals between the ages of 2 and 20 years and occur predominantly in males. Approximately, 40% are found in the femur, although some occur in the ilium.

On plain roentgenograms, a fibrous cortical defect appears as a circular or oval, eccentrically located radiolucent area, near the physis of a long bone. The margins of the defect are smooth or lobulated with a well-defined thin rim of sclerosis. CT may be useful, especially if the diagnosis is uncertain.

Histologically, the defect is filled with spindle-shaped cells distributed in a whorled or storiform pattern. There is fibroblastic proliferation with high cellularity. Multiple fibrous cortical defects occur in approximately 50% of patients. Usually, they are bilateral and symmetrical. 5% of patients with multiple fibrous cortical defects also have neurofibromatosis. Several authors have suggested stress or trauma as a cause. Regardless, the defects resolve without treatment, the disappearance perhaps being the result of physiological remodeling of bone.

Neural Tumors

Neurogenous tumors of bone are quite rare, but definite neurilemomas have been described. On roentgenograms, they are seen as discrete lytic lesions. Their microscopic appearance is similar to that of neurilemomas of soft tissue. Neurofibromas also develop in bone, especially in von Recklinghausen disease. A variety of other musculoskeletal abnormalities not necessarily related to the presence of discrete neurofibromas may be found, such as hypertrophy of parts, kyphoscoliosis, congenital bowing of bones, and congenital pseudarthrosis of bones.

Desmoplastic Fibroma

Desmoplastic fibroma is a rare, densely collagenized tumor of fibrous tissue histologically similar to the soft tissue desmoid tumors.

Sex: Males and females are affected with nearly equal frequency.

Age: The lesion has been seen in patients as young as 8 years of age and as old as 80.

Location: The long tubular bones are involved most often, but involvement of the pelvis has been reported.

Clinical findings: Include pain late in the clinical course and swelling. It may present as an effusion if near a joint. The roentgenograms reveal a lytic defect centrally located and usually well-circumscribed. Plain X-ray shows an osteolytic, expansile, medullary lesion with well-defined sclerotic margins. The oval tumor is often found in the metaphysic, aligned with the long axis of the bone. There is usually thinned cortex and the fine intralesional trabeculae give a lobulated appearance that is described as "soap-bubbly". Microscopically, it is hypocellular and fibroblastic, and contains much collagen and few mitoses.

Treatment: This tumor does not metastasize, but local recurrence or persistence is common. Wide local resection is the preferred surgical treatment, since persistence after curettage occurs in 40–66% of patients. One study has recommended "aggressive curettage" as a surgical option. Radiotherapy is not recommended because of the increased risk of sarcomatous change. Tamoxifen and indomethacin have been reported to reduce the size of soft tissue desmoid tumors and may be useful as adjuvants in the bony counterpart.

OSTEOTOMIES AROUND THE HIP

Introduction

With the advent of arthroplasty, numbers of osteotomies around hip have decreased, but they can still be used in pediatric and healthy young patients, who have a longer life expectancy.

Indications

Children

- DDH
- Slipped capital femoral epiphysis
- Legg-Calve-Perthes disease.

Adults

- Osteoarthritis
- Nonunion fracture neck femur
- Osteonecrosis.

Developmental Dysplasia of Hip

These can be divided according to the age group of the child.
- *Toddler:* 18–36 months of age
- *Juvenile*: 3–8 years
- *Adult:* More than 8 years.

Toddler (18–36 Months)

Femoral derotation osteotomy:
Proximal femoral derotation or varus osteotomy is indicated in subluxation or dysplasia of the hip, when reorientation can stabilize a reduction, resolve mild subluxation, or stimulate remodeling of the joint. Often, it is used to achieve a congruent joint in the weight-bearing position after closed or open reduction, to allow a child of walking age to ambulate with less risk of subluxation. When acetabular dysplasia persists after reduction, femoral osteotomy can stimulate remodeling of the acetabulum, if done by 5 years of age. The usual deformity of the femur in congenital hip dysplasia is excessive anteversion. This contributes to anterolateral subluxation in the weight-bearing position and encourages superolateral subluxation in the sitting position. Femoral derotation alone is generally sufficient to correct the deformity. Internal fixation is necessary for femoral osteotomy. Rigid fixation with a small plate (for derotation alone) or a pediatric blade plate (for a varus osteotomy in an older child) is advocated. The perineum will appear wide, until the child grows and that a limp may persist for 2–3 months, but will eventually disappear. The osteotomy is done at the intertrochanteric or subtrochanteric region and a medial wedge removed for varus positioning, followed by derotation of the distal fragment and application of the plate.

Juvenile (3–8 Years)

Treatment osteotomies can be divided into: (1) pelvic osteotomies and (2) femoral osteotomies. The pelvic osteotomies include:
- Osteotomy of the innominate bone–Salter's
- Acetabuloplasty–Pemberton
- Osteotomies that free the acetabulum
- Steel, Dega, Tonnis, Tachdjian
- Periacetabular osteotomy–Ganz (bernese)
- Shelf operation–Staheli
- Innominate osteotomy with medial displacement of the acetabulum–Chiari.
  - *Salter's osteotomy (Figs. 244A and B):* It is designed to limit anterolateral subluxation, by improving coverage in this area. The Salter osteotomy, as it goes completely through the pelvis, allows anterior and lateral rotation of the acetabulum through an axis, formed by the sciatic notch and the pubic symphysis, as illustrated in Figure 244A. The osteotomy is held open anterolaterally, by a wedge of bone and thus the roof of the acetabulum is shifted more anteriorly and laterally, as shown in Figure 244B. It is contraindicated in patients with nonconcentric hips or severe dysplasia.

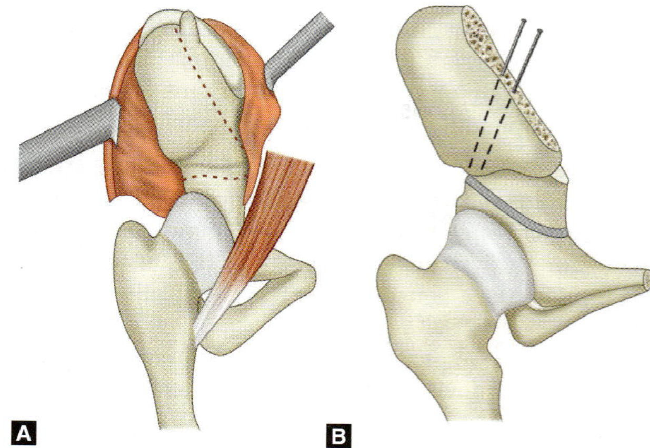

Figs. 244A and B: Salter's osteotomy—(A) In the pelvis, it allows anterior and lateral rotation of the acetabulum through an axis, formed by the sciatic notch and the pubic symphysis; (B) The osteotomy is held open anterolaterally, by a wedge of bone and thus the roof of the acetabulum is shifted more anteriorly and laterally.

- *Pemberton osteotomy (Fig. 245):* It is an incomplete pericapsular osteotomy of the ilium that hinges the anterolateral acetabular roof on the flexible triradiate cartilage for correction. This actually changes the configuration of the acetabulum and introduces joint incongruence that must be corrected by remodeling during growth. It is indicated, when there is an elongated, dysplastic acetabulum, but it is most effectively done in children younger than 8 years, as there is still flexibility in the triradiate cartilage and growth remains for remodeling of the joint surfaces. Wedge of bone is impacted into the open osteotomy site.
- *Osteotomies that free the acetabulum (Fig. 246):* These osteotomies free part of the pelvis, creating a movable segment of bone that includes the acetabulum. They are indicated in patients with residual dysplasia and subluxation, in whom remodeling of the acetabulum is not possible. These surgeries place the articular cartilage over the femoral head.
  - *Steel (triple innominate) osteotomy:* In this, the ischium, the superior pubic ramus and the ilium, superior to the acetabulum are all divided and the acetabulum is repositioned and stabilized by a bone graft and metal pins.
  - *Eppright (dial) osteotomy:* The entire acetabulum superiorly, posteriorly, inferiorly, and anteriorly is freed and a single segment of bone is redirected to cover the femoral head.

Steel makes the pubic cut through an inguinal incision and the ischial cut through the buttock. Tönnis uses a posterior gluteal approach for the ischial cut. He felt that redirection should emphasize more lateral and less anterior coverage of the hip than advocated by Salter or Steel. Tachdjian performs the ischial cut anteromedially through a subinguinal incision between the adductor magnus and obturator externus, as shown in Figures 247A to C.

- *Dega osteotomy (Figs. 248A to D):* It is a transiliacosteotomy for treatment of residual acetabular dysplasia. It involves osteotomy of the anterior and middle portions of the inner cortex of the ilium, leaving an intact hinge posteriorly, consisting of the intact posteromedial iliac cortex and sciatic notch.
- *Periacetabular osteotomies-Ganz (bernese) osteotomy (Figs. 249 and 250):* It is a triplanar periacetabular osteotomy for adults, with dysplastic hips that require correction of congruency and containment to the femoral head. It redirects the position of the acetabulum, to reduce sheer forces and decrease compressive forces on the articular

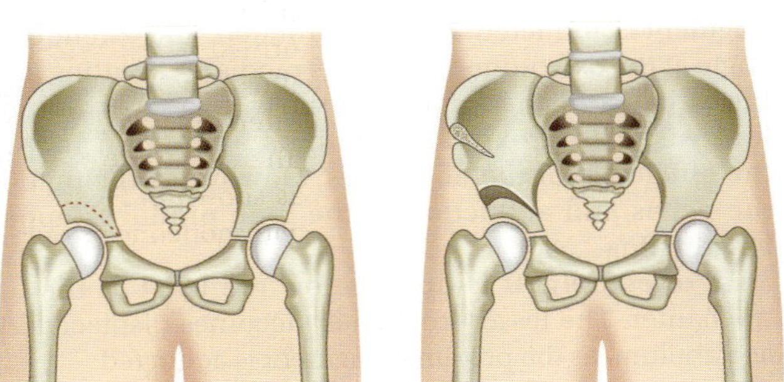

Fig. 245: Pemberton osteotomy.

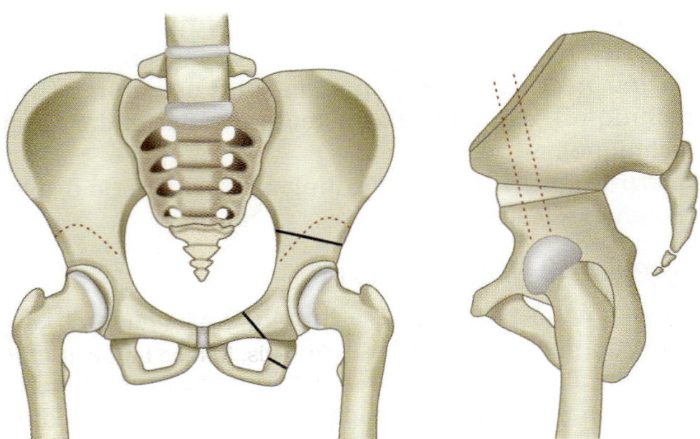

Fig. 246: Osteotomies that free the acetabulum.

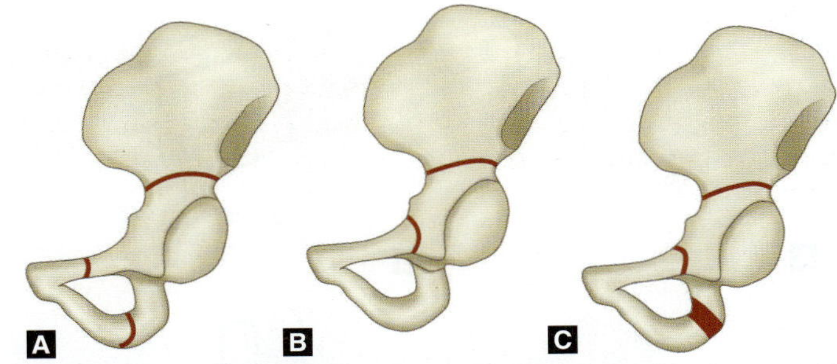

Figs. 247A to C: Tachdjian osteotomy, where the ischial cut is made anteromedially, through a subinguinal incision between the adductor magnus and obturator externus.

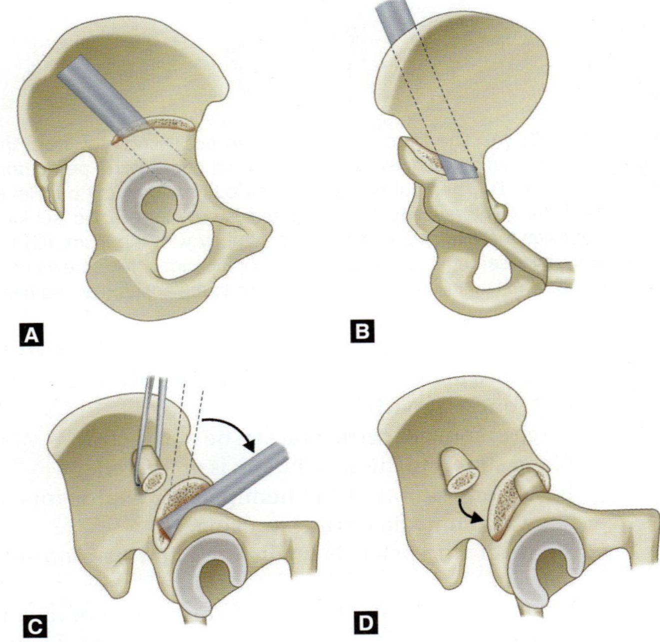

Figs. 248A to D: Dega osteotomy—(A and B) Osteotomy of the anterior and middle portions of the inner cortex of the ilium, leaving an intact hinge posteriorly; (C) Osteotomy site is leaving open to accept bone graft; (D) Second graft inserted more posteriorly.

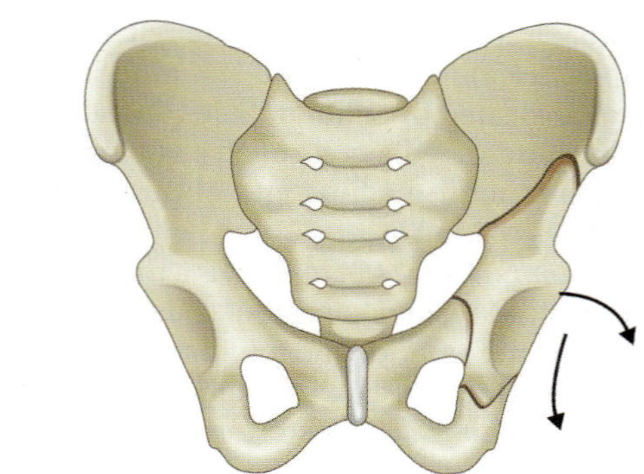

Fig. 249: Ganz (bernese) osteotomy.

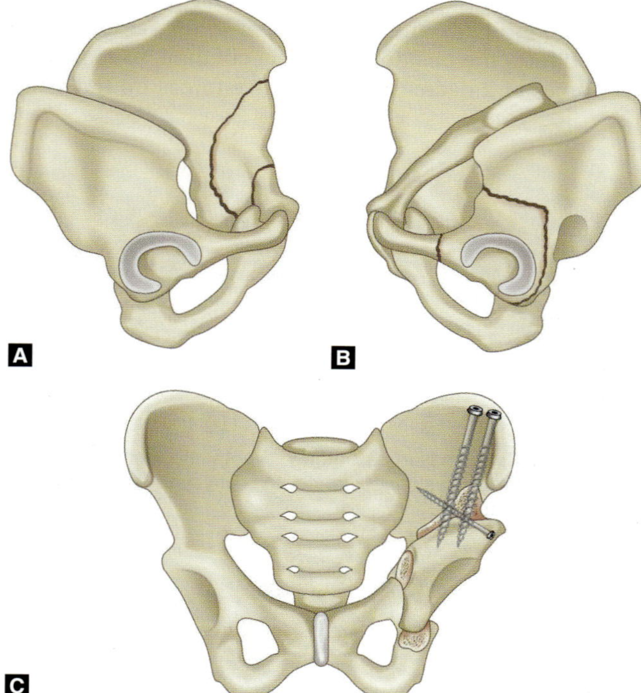

Figs. 250A to C: (A) The ilium is cut, using an oscillating saw from the ASIS toward the sciatic notch, stopping 10–15 mm short of the pelvic brim (iliopectinate line); (B) Then cut across the pelvic brim. Next cut parallel to the posterior column intersecting with the previous cut made in the ischium. The final cut frees the acetabulum from its continuity with the ilium; (C) Fix the osteotomy, by inserting three or four AO 4.5 or 3.5 mm pelvic screws from the superior iliac crest in an inferomedial direction into the acetabular segment.

cartilage. The quantity of cartilage that already exists is rotated into a more favorable position. The advantages are:
- Only one approach is used
- Large amount of correction can be obtained
- Blood supply to the acetabulum is preserved
- Posterior column of the hemipelvis remains intact, allowing immediate crutch walking
- Shape of true pelvis is unaltered, allowing a normal delivery
- It can be combined with trochanteric osteotomy, if needed.

The ilium is cut, using an oscillating saw from the ASIS toward the sciatic notch, stopping 10–15 mm short of the pelvic brim (iliopectinate line). Then cut across the pelvic brim. Next, cut parallel to the posterior column intersecting with the previous cut made in the ischium. The final cut frees the acetabulum from its continuity with the ilium. Insert the angled osteotome into the medial osteotomy of the quadrilateral surface and transect the ilium from medial to lateral, carefully avoiding the hip joint. Reorient the acetabulum fragment, to improve both lateral and anterior coverage of the femoral head. Fix the osteotomy by inserting three or four AO 4.5 or 3.5 mm pelvic screws from the superior iliac crest in an inferomedial direction into the acetabular segment.
- *Staheli osteotomy (Figs. 251A to C):* It is a shelf procedure. It establishes a congruous joint with apposition of the articular cartilage of the acetabulum to the femoral head. The acetabular roof is extended laterally, posteriorly, or anteriorly, by a graft or by turning the acetabular roof and part of the lateral cortex of the ilium over the femoral head.
- *Chiari osteotomy (Figs. 252A and B):* It is an innominate osteotomy, with medial displacement of the acetabulum. It is a modified shelf operation that places the femoral head beneath a surface of bone and joint capsule and corrects pathological lateral displacement of the femur. The osteotomy is made at the level of the acetabulum and femur are displaced medially. The inferior surface of the proximal fragment forms a roof over the femoral head.

Adults (More than 8 Years)

- *Lorenz bifurcation osteotomy (Figs. 253A to C):* It is an oblique osteotomy below the level of lesser trochanter. The proximal end of the distal fragment is displaced into the acetabulum. The distal end of the proximal fragment abuts against the side of the shaft.
- *Schanz low-subtrochanteric osteotomy:* The osteotomy of the femur is done at the level of the tuber ischii. The distal fragment is abducted, internally rotated, and extended. The angle at the osteotomy site points medially, abutting against the pelvis and the angle anteriorly corrects the lumbar lordosis. The proximal fragments adduction increases the efficiency of the abductors. Downward inclination of the pelvis and abduction of the limb produces apparent lengthening.
- *Hass osteotomy:* It is done below the level of the lesser trochanter. The lesser trochanter becomes displaced in the acetabulum, as the proximal fragment is adducted.

Slipped Capital Femoral Epiphysis

- *Proximal femoral osteotomy:*
  - *Physeal osteotomy:* Dunn procedure and cuneiform osteotomy (fish procedure).
- *Basilar neck osteotomy:* Intracapsular osteotomy (Kramer technique), extracapsular osteotomy (Barmada/Abraham technique).
- *Intertrochanteric osteotomy:* Biplane trochanteric osteotomy (Southwick technique).

Dunn's Procedure (Figs. 254A to C)

Indication for this procedure is a chronic SCFE of more than one-third the diameter of the physis or an acute-on-chronic SCFE, radiographically demonstrated by the presence of new bone along the posterior aspect of the metaphysis. After achieving reduction, two osteotomies are done. The first is in the long axis of the neck to remove the bony beak. The second is to shorten the neck a few millimeters.

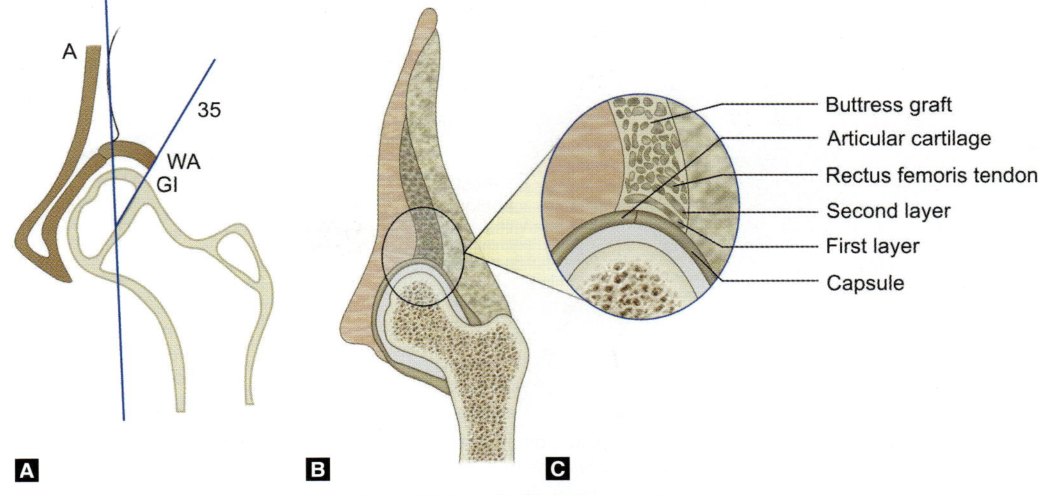

Figs. 251A to C: Staheli osteotomy.

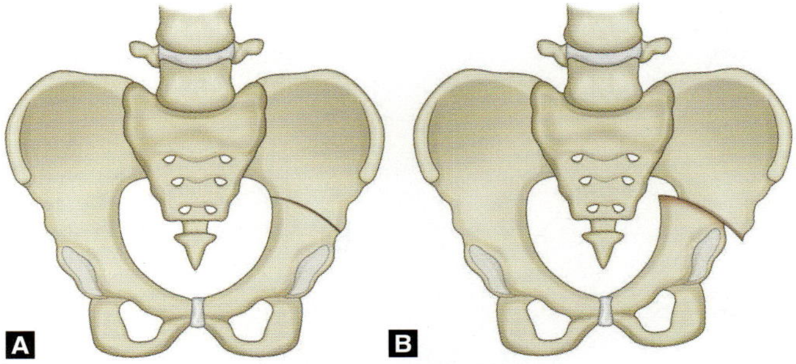

Figs. 252A and B: Chiari osteotomy.

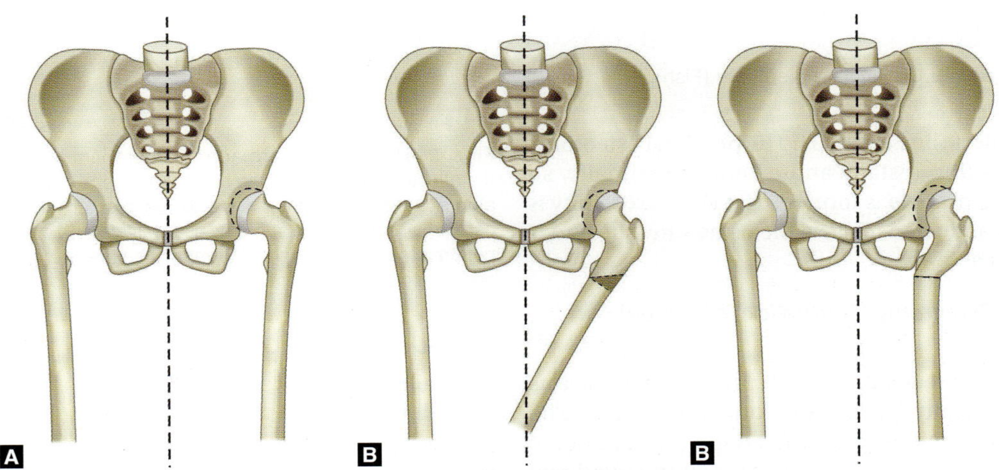

Figs. 253A to C: Lorenz bifurcation osteotomy.

Cuneiform Osteotomy (Fish) (Figs. 255A and B)

The indication is an SCFE greater than 30° with an open physis. The osteotomy is made at the metaphyseal region, by removing small pieces of bone with a sharp osteotome and mallet. Further removal of the physeal cartilage with a curet and then reduction of the epiphysis on the metaphysis is carried out. After reduction of the epiphysis, it is fixed with three or four threaded pins.

Kramer's Technique

Indications are an SCFE greater than 40°, on either the AP or the lateral radiographic view. The widest part of the wedge is removed in line with the widest portion of the slipped epiphysis, in the anterior and superior aspects of the neck. The distal osteotomy is made first, perpendicular to the femoral neck and following the anterior intertrochanteric line from proximal to distal. The second osteotomy is done obliquely, so that the cutting edge of the osteotome remains distal to the posterior retinacular blood supply. It is fixed with Steinmann pins.

Barmada and Abraham (Extracapsular) (Figs. 256A to C)

The indication is an SCFE greater than 50°. The distal osteotomy starts at the base of the neck inferiorly and extends obliquely

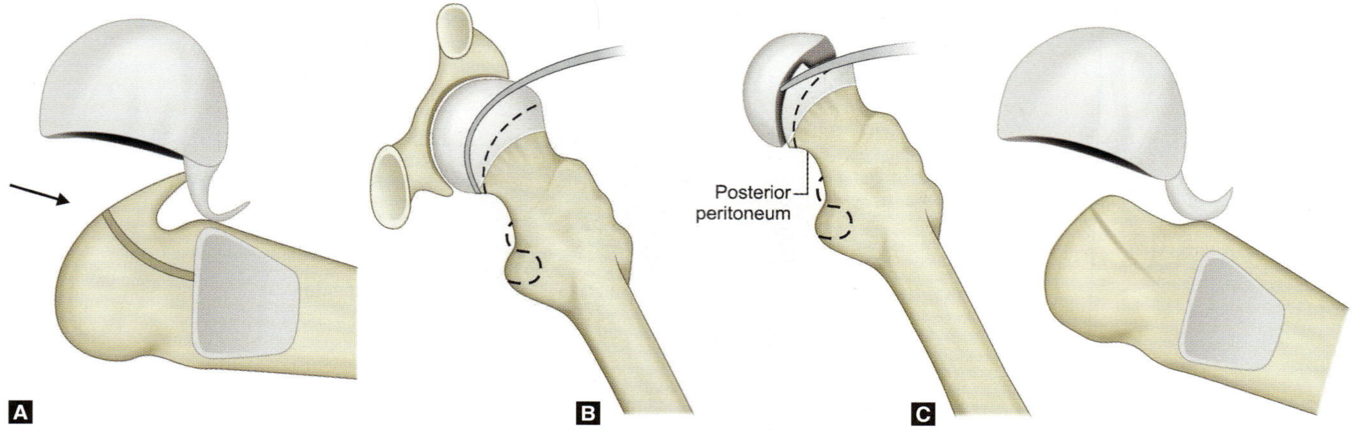

Figs. 254A to C: Dunn's procedure—(A) After achieving reduction, osteotomy is done in the long axis of the neck to remove the bony beak; (B) and (C) Second osteotomy is done to shorten the neck a few millimeters.

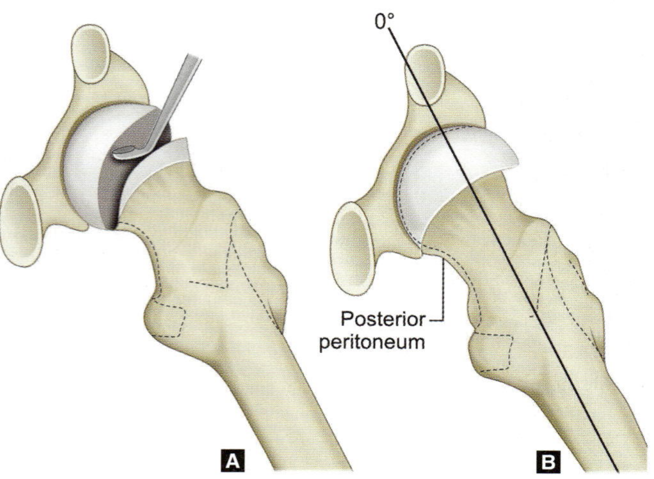

Figs. 255A and B: Cuneiform osteotomy (Fish).

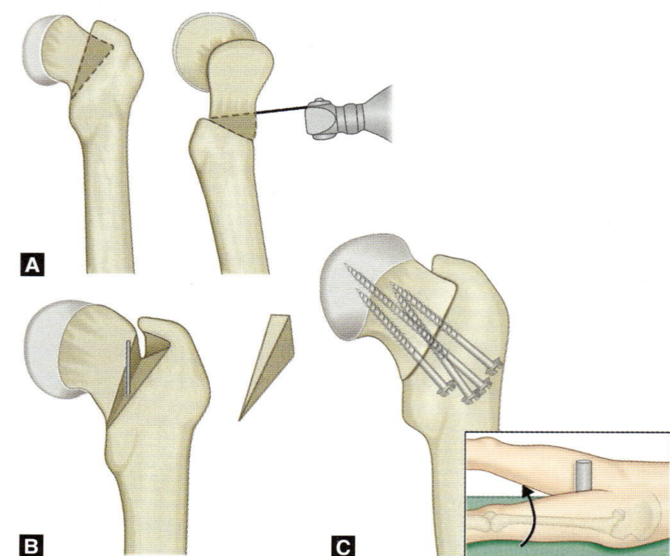

Figs. 256A to C: (A) Barmada and Abraham (extracapsular)—and (B) The distal osteotomy starts at the base of the neck inferiorly and extends obliquely along the intertrochanteric line to the greater trochanter; (C) The proximal osteotomy starts at the same position distally and extends proximally, so that a proximally based triangle is formed. The lower extremity is internally rotated and abducted to close the osteotomy site and is fixed with three to four screws.

along the intertrochanteric line to the GT. The proximal osteotomy starts at the same position distally and extends proximally, so that a proximally based triangle is formed. The lower extremity is internally rotated and abducted to close the osteotomy site and is fixed with three to four screws.

Biplane Trochanteric Osteotomy (Southwick Technique) (Figs. 257A to C)

The indication is an SCFE greater than 30°. This osteotomy corrects all three planes of deformity (varus, rotation, and flexion). The biplane osteotomy, corrects the varus and adduction-rotation of the distal fragment, relative to the proximal corrects the rotational deformity. The osteotomy is made and the bone wedge removed. The remainder of the medial and posterior transverse cut is made and while controlling the proximal fragment, the distal fragment is abducted and flexed, bringing the osteotomy surfaces together.

Legg-Calvé-Perthes Disease

- *Femoral osteotomy:*
  - Varus derotational osteotomy
  - Valgus derotational osteotomy
- *Pelvic osteotomy:*
  - Salter innominate osteotomy.

Varus Derotational Osteotomy

The child should have at least 30° of hip abduction to perform this procedure. If the femoral head levers out of the joint with abduction (hinge abduction), this osteotomy is contraindicated. The osteotomy is usually performed at the subtrochanteric level. The amount of varus is based on the amount of abduction required to cover the lateral portion of the femoral head under the acetabulum. Fixation is done with one of the blade plates or screw plate devices specifically designed for children, as shown in Figures 258A and B. If the femoral head levers out of the joint with abduction (hinge abduction), a varus osteotomy is contraindicated.

Reverse wedge technique:

Removal of wedge one-half of calculated height medially and inserting laterally and fixation with prebend plate. Advantages are—(1) shortening minimized and (2) minimum wedge. POP (hip spica) applied for 6–8 weeks.

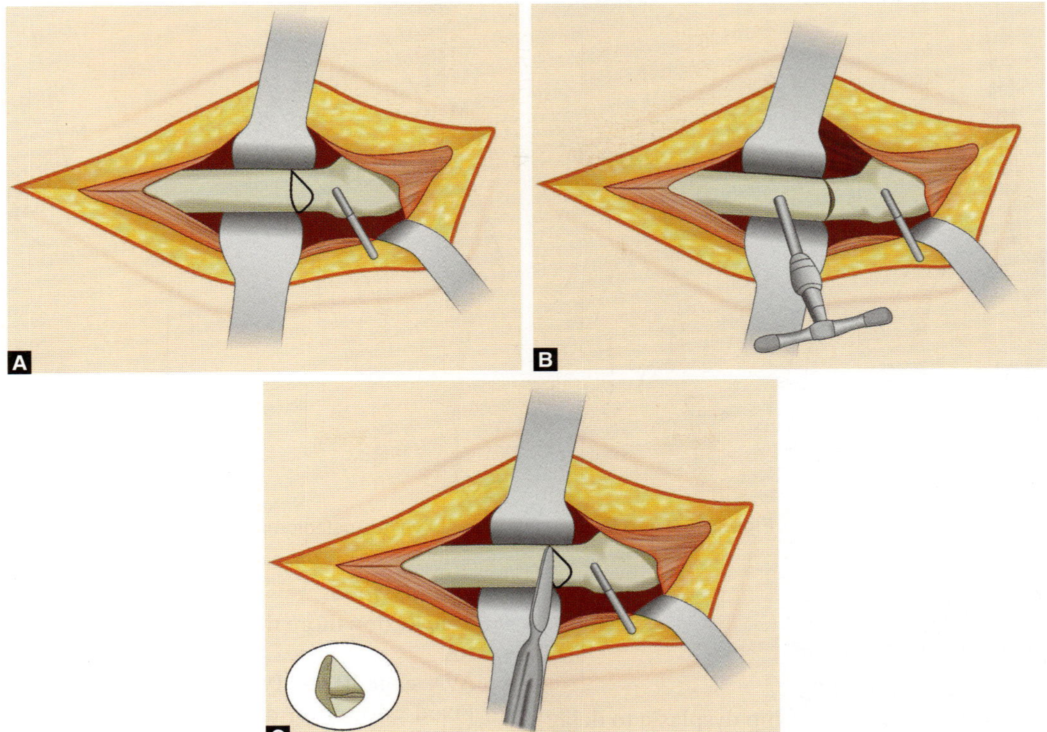

Figs. 257A to C: Biplane trochanteric osteotomy (Southwick technique)—(A) The osteotomy is made and the bone wedge removed; (B and C) The remainder of the medial and posterior transverse cut is made and while controlling the proximal fragment, the distal fragment is abducted and flexed, bringing the osteotomy surfaces together.

Osteotomies in Adults

Indications

- Osteoarthritis
- AVN
- Nonunion neck femur
- Ankylosis after septic arthritis
- Osteoarthritis hip.

Aims

- To relieve pain
- Restoration of motion
- Correction of deformity
- Restoration of stability
- Reversal of degenerative process.

Theories of Pain Relief

- Hemodynamic—decreases venous hypertension
- Biomechanical
- Reducing muscle force
- Displacing fulcrum
- Relaxing capsule
- Restoring acetabulofemoral congruency.

Preoperative Planning

Detailed physical examination:

- Preoperative X-rays—standing AP and lateral
- Hip in maximum abduction and adduction.
  - If adduction is restricted—adductor tenotomy
  - If head fixed in abduction—varus osteotomy
  - If head fixed in adduction—valgus osteotomy
  - At least 70° free flexion must be there.

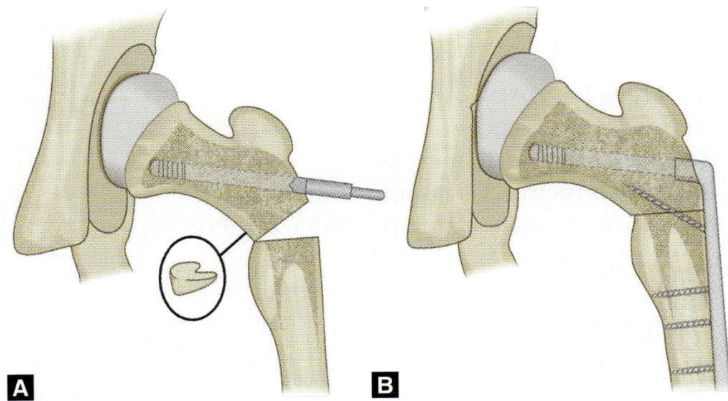

Figs. 258A and B: Varus derotational osteotomy—(A) The osteotomy performed at the subtrochanteric level; (B) Fixation is done with one of the blade plates or screw plate devices.

Blount's Indications

Valgus osteotomy:

- Trendelenburg limp
- Adduction deformity
- Adduction beyond add deformity
- Painful abduction.

Varus osteotomy:

- Antalgic gait
- Abduction deformity
- Abduction beyond abduction deformity
- Painful adduction.

Varus osteotomy alone done for (See Figs. 187A to E):

- Steps involved in performing varus osteotomy
- Spherical head

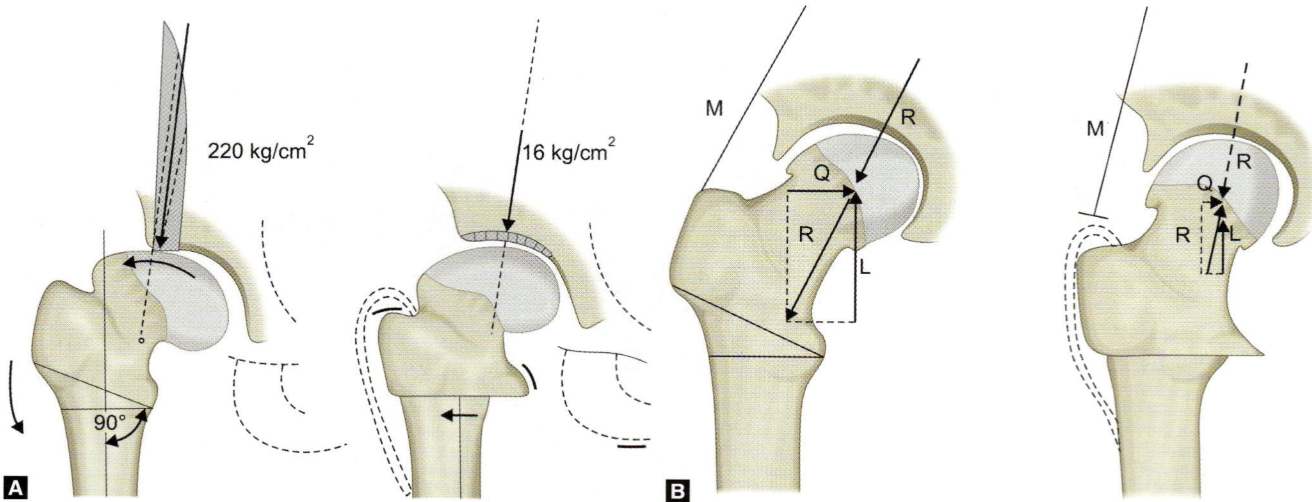

Figs. 259A and B: Steps involved in valgus osteotomy.

- Little or no acetabular dysplasia
- Sign of lateral overloading
- Valgus neck shaft angle more than 135°.

Valgus osteotomy alone (Figs. 259A and B):
- In patients older than 50 years with OA hip dysplasia to delay THR
- Patient in sixth decade with medial head osteophyte and subchondral sclerosis in lateral roof
- Seventh decade with OA for pain relief, whom THR is contraindicated
- Protrusive OA.

Pauwel's type 1 varus:
- Medially based wedge
- Abduction lever arm increased
- Relaxes abductors, psoas and adductors
- Extension obtained by taking wedge posteriorly.

Disadvantages:
- Shortening
- Trendelenburg gait
- Prominence of GT.

Pauwel's type 2 valgus (See Figs. 189A to F):
- Steps involved in the correction of Pauwel's type 2 valgus
- Acetabular dysplasia, with femoral head uncovered antero-laterally
- Extension added by taking wedge posteriorly
- Increase weight-bearing area of femoral head, but no muscle relaxation.

Complications:
- Nonunion
- Unpredictable results.

Müller Technique (Figs. 260A to D)

- Lateral approach
- Medially based wedge taken from proximal fragment
- Fixed with compression blade plate
- Müller's modification—short wedge taken medially and placed laterally.

Contraindications:
- Free flexion more than 50
- RA
- AVN stage III and IV
- Fixed adduction deformity for varus and fixed abduction deformity for valgus
- Fixed external rotation deformity more than 25°
- Knock knee for valgus.

Blount's Displacement Osteotomy (Figs. 261A to D)

- Just proximal to lesser trochanter
- Oblique direction
- Angle of osteotomy decided from preoperative X-ray
- Lateral approach, distal fragment displaced medially
- Blade plate
- Postoperative crutch walking after few days
- Weight bearing after solid union.

McMurray Osteotomy

- Severe OA with large hypertrophic loose spurs on head preventing rotation into valgus/varus, so that adduction or abduction gets fixed
- Nonunion fracture of NoF
- Neither increase nor decrease weight-bearing surface of femur
- Done to relieve pain in patient who are not suitable for THR
- *Principle:* Preliminary traction and adductor tenotomy. Oblique osteotomy from lower border of lateral aspect of shaft below lesser trochanter to a level above lesser trochanter medially, as shown in Figure 262. Shaft displaced medially, in nonunion completely displaced distal fragment is under head, in OA only 20° displaced. POP–spica applied for 2 weeks
- *Disadvantage:* Instability and shortening.

Milch-Batchelor Osteotomy (Fig. 263)

It is a salvage osteotomy. Indications are:
- OA for pain relief
- Old unreduced dislocation with pain and instability
- Combination of Girdlestone and Schanz.

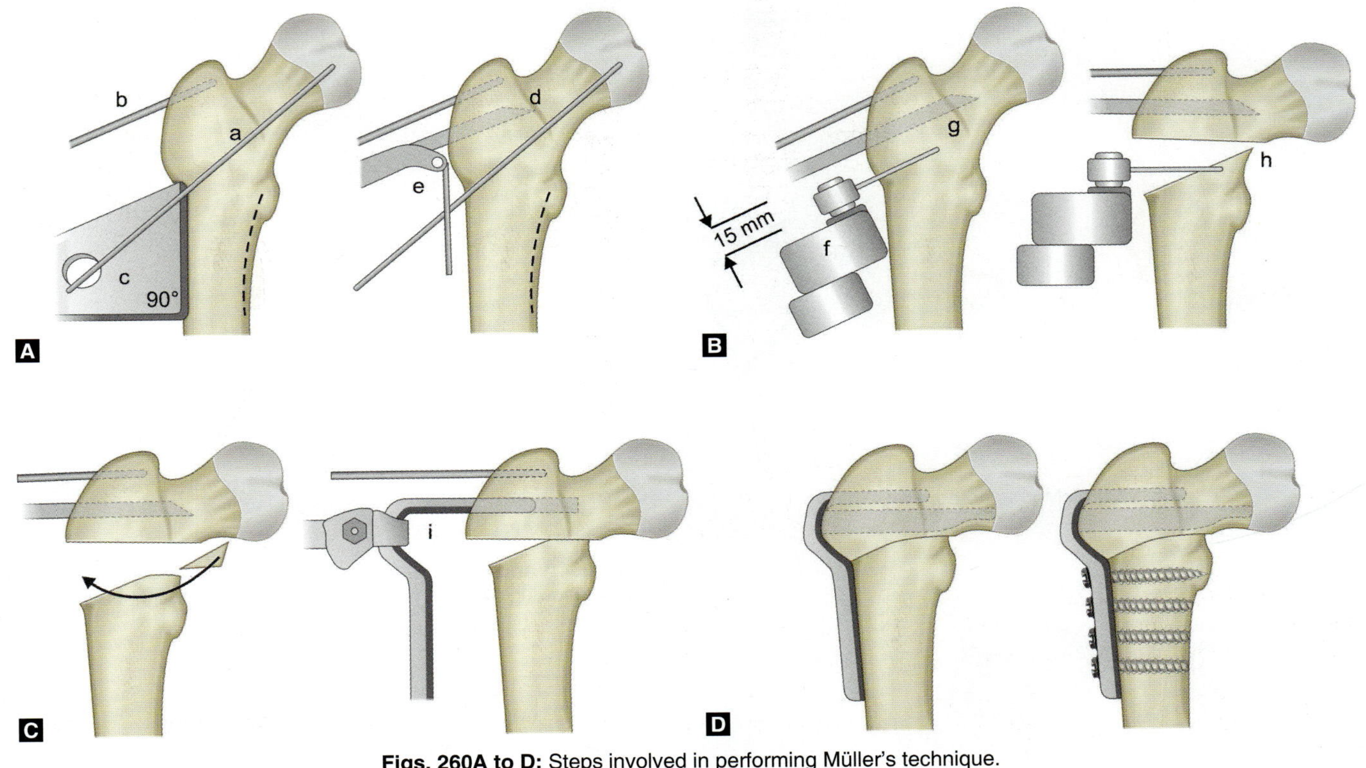

Figs. 260A to D: Steps involved in performing Müller's technique.

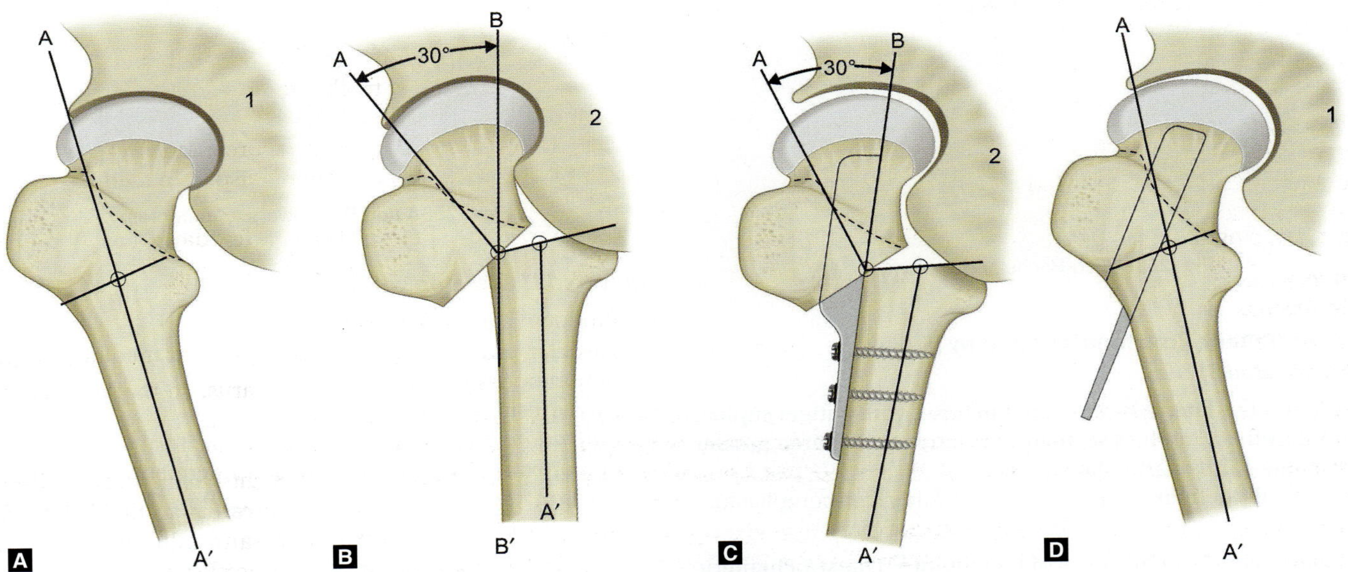

Figs. 261A to D: Blount's displacement osteotomy.

Disadvantage: Instability, weak muscular control, prolonged period of traction, and bed rest.

Advantage: Lengthening, bony support, lever arm more, correct lordosis, and rotation deformity.

Smith Peterson approach:

- Level at tuber ischii
- Ci-opposite hip ankylosed in abduction.

Avascular Necrosis Femoral Head

Aims

- Reposition of necrotic anterosuperior part of femoral head into NWB portion
- Femoral head and neck segment rotated anteriorly, so weight bearing on posterior articular surface, which is not involved
- Useful in stage I and II
- Postoperative degenerative change in stage III.

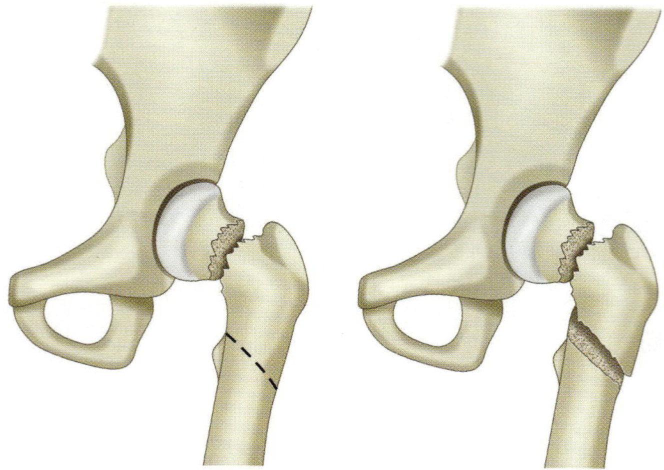

Fig. 262: McMurray osteotomy.

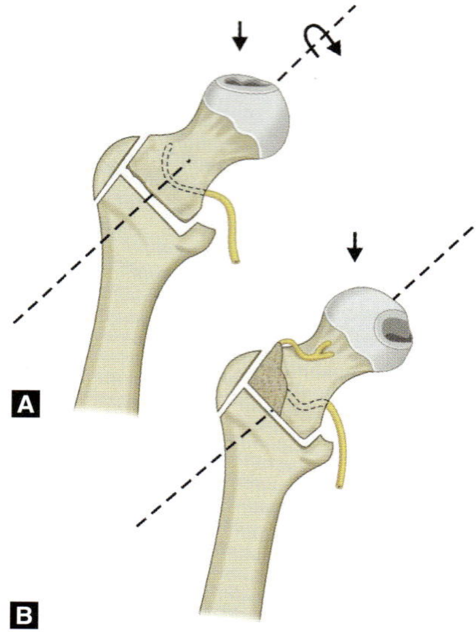

Figs. 264A and B: Transtrochanteric rotational osteotomy (Sujioka), arrow showing direction of rotation to change the weight-bearing area.

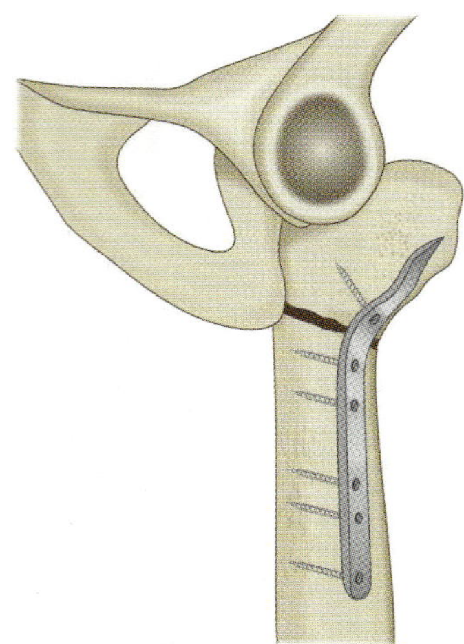

Fig. 263: Milch-Bachelor osteotomy.

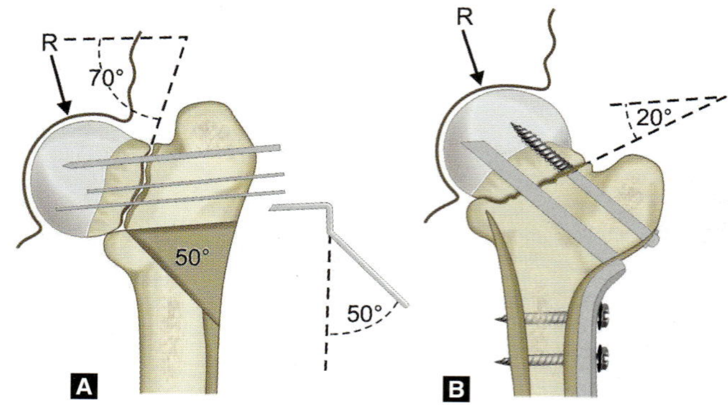

Figs. 265A and B: Pauwel's "y" osteotomy.

Transtrochanteric Rotational Osteotomy (Sujioka) (Figs. 264A and B)

- Preoperative lateral view of femoral head, with patient supine, hip flexed 90°, abducted, neutral rotation intact area greater than one-third of articular surface.
- Technically demanding procedure with fairly high complication rates.

Technique: Capsule cut near rim of acetabulum. Transtrochanteric osteotomy is done 10 mm distal to intertrochanteric line. Leave lesser trochanter with distal fragment and head rotated 45–90°. Postoperative skin traction given for 3 weeks, weight bearing for 8 weeks and crutches for a year.

Nonunion Fracture of Neck of Femur

- Children, adults less than 60 years with viable neck
- *Principle:* Weight bearing shifted medially and shearing force at fracture site becomes horizontal.
- *Disadvantage*: Excessive valgus, short abductor lever arm, shortening and instability.

Pauwel's "Y" Osteotomy (Figs. 265A and B)

- Produce valgus neck shaft angle
- Vascular proximal end of shaft displaced medially to bridge nonunion site
- Prerequisite—viable head
- *Indication:* Nonunion fracture of NoF with absorption of neck and proximal displacement of distal fragment
- *Dickson high geometric:* Osteotomy below GT, distal fragment is abducted to 60° and fixed with blade plate
- *Puttis osteotomy:* Nonunion transcervical fracture
- Displacement osteotomy with horizontal section of femur in intertrochanteric region and distal fragment displaced beneath fracture line, as shown in Figures 266A and B.

Septic Arthritis Ankylosed Hip

Ankylosis in unsound position treated by intertrochanteric osteotomy, as illustrated in Figures 267A to C.

- *Transverse opening wedge (Gant):* Level of osteotomy is proximal to lesser trochanter. It is a very simple procedure, causes limb lengthening. Nonunion in adults are common and is usually unstable initially.

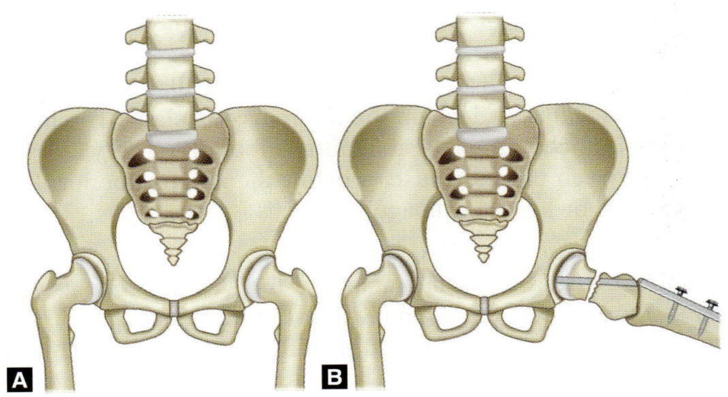

Figs. 266A and B: Displacement osteotomy with horizontal section of femur in intertrochanteric region and distal fragment displaced beneath fracture line.

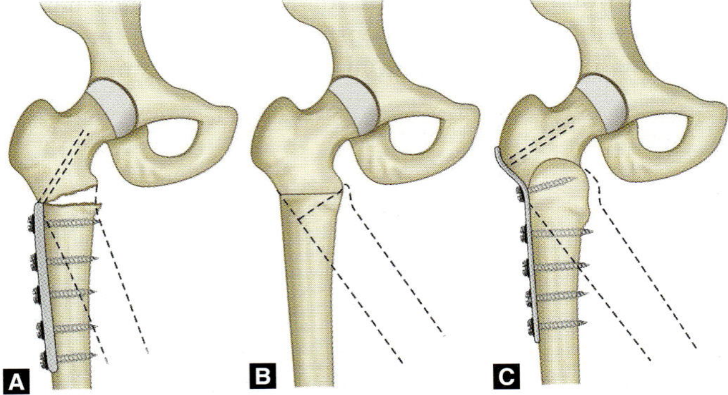

Figs. 267A to C: (A) Transverse opening wedge (Gant); (B) Whitman closing wedge; (C) Brackett ball and socket technique.

- *Whitman closing wedge:* It is a stable, shortening osteotomy. Lateral based wedge osteotomy procedure.
- Brackett ball and socket.
- Stability without shortening.
- Extensive dissection.
- In biplane deformities difficult to perform.

SURGICAL APPROACHES TO HIP

Surgical approaches to the hip may be classified as:
- Anterior
- Anterolateral
- Posterolateral
- Lateral
- Posterior
- Medial.

Anterior Approach (Figs. 268 to 273)

Smith Peterson approach improved and revived interest in the anterior iliofemoral approach and now it used often and gives safe access to the hip joint and ilium. It exploits the internervous plane between the sartorius (femoral nerve) and tensor fasciae latae (superior gluteal nerve) to penetrate the outer layer of the joint musculature.

Anterior approach by two techniques:
1. Smith Peterson
2. Somerville.

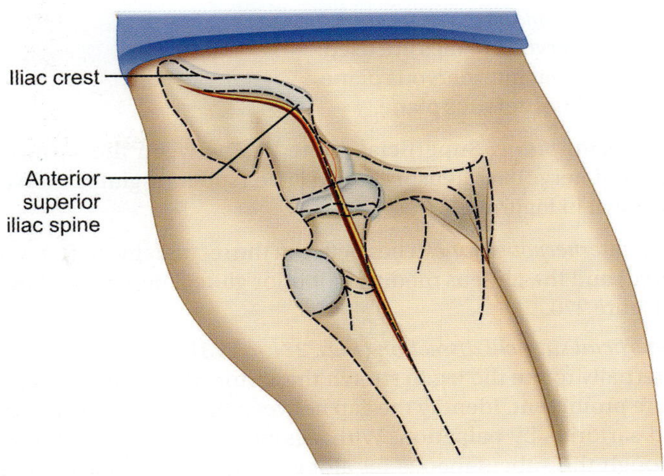

Fig. 268: Make a long incision at the middle of the iliac crest. Carry it anteriorly to the anterosuperior iliac spine and then distally and slightly laterally 10–12 cm.

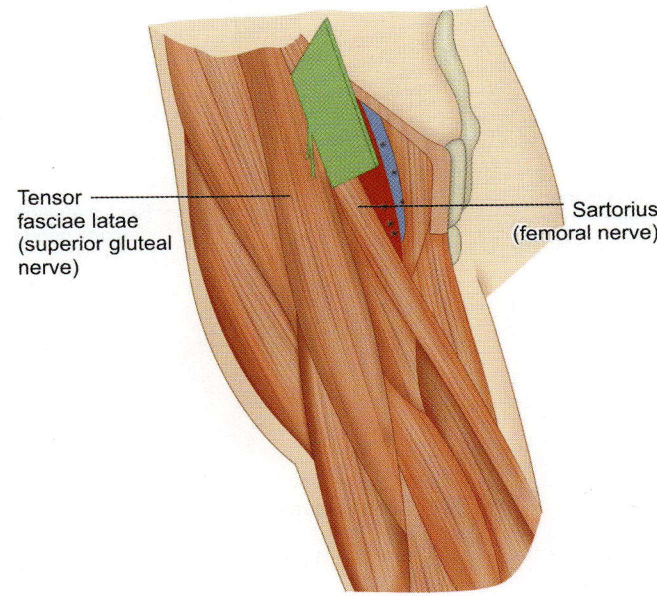

Fig. 269: Superficial plane of incision.

Smith Peterson Approach

Position of patient: Place the patient supine on operating table. If the approach is to be used for pelvic osteotomy then place sandbag under the affected buttocks, to push the hemipelvis forward.

Landmarks and incision:

Landmarks: The anterosuperior iliac spine is subcutaneous and easily palpable in thin patients. In obese patients it is covered by adipose tissue and is more difficult to find. You can locate it most easily, if you bring your thumbs up from beneath the bony protuberance.

Incision: Make a long incision at the middle of the iliac crest or for a larger exposure, as far posteriorly on the crest as desired. Carry it anteriorly to the anterosuperior iliac spine and then distally and slightly laterally 10–12 cm, as shown in Figure 268.

Internervous planes

Two internervous planes are used:

1. Superficial internervous plane
2. Deep internervous plane.

Superficial plane: Superficial plane lies between the sartorius (femoral nerve) and tensor fasciae latae (superior gluteal nerve), as shown in Figure 269.

Deep internervous plane: It lies between the rectus femoris (femoral nerve) and the gluteus medius (superior gluteal nerve), as shown in Figure 270.

Superficial surgical dissection (Figs. 271 to 273):

Externally rotate the leg to stretch the sartorius muscle, making it more prominent. Identify the gap between the tensor fasciae latae and sartorius by palpation. With scissors carefully dissect down through the subcutaneous fat along the intermuscular interval. Avoid cutting the lateral femoral cutaneous nerve, which pierces the deep fascia of the thigh close to the intermuscular interval. Incise the deep fasciae on the medial side of the tensor fascia latae. Retract the sartorius upward and medially and the tensor fasciae latae downward and laterally. Detach the iliac origin of the tensor fasciae latae to develop the internervous plane. The large ascending branch of the lateral femoral circumflex artery crosses the gap between the two muscles below the anterosuperior iliac spine. It must be ligated or coagulated.

Deep surgical dissection (Figs. 274 to 276):

Retracting the tensor fasciae latae and the sartorius brings you onto two muscles of the deep layer of the hip musculature, the rectus femoris (femoral nerve) and gluteal medius (superior gluteal nerve), as shown in Figure 274. The rectus femoris originate from two heads, the direct head from the anteroinferior iliac spine and the reflected head from the superior lip of the acetabulum. The reflected head also takes origin from the anterior capsule of the hip joint. If you have difficulty in identifying the plane between the rectus femoris and the gluteus medius, palpate the femoral artery. The femoral pulse is well medial to the intermuscular

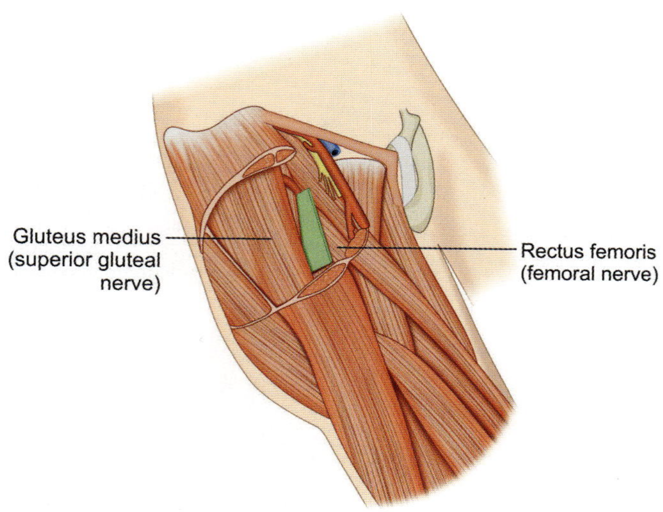

Fig. 270: Deep intravenous plane.

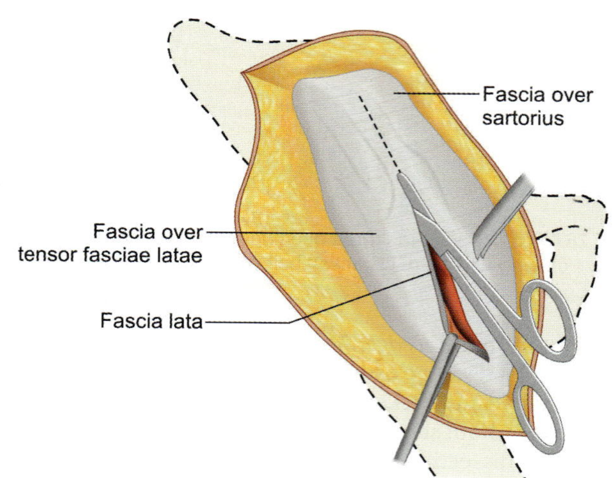

Fig. 272: Incise the deep fascia on the medial side of the tensor fasciae latae.

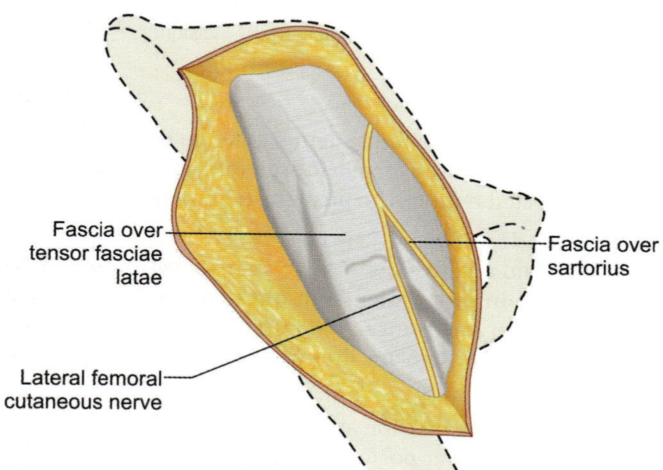

Fig. 271: With scissors carefully dissect down through the subcutaneous fat along the intermuscular interval in the gap between the tensor fasciae latae and sartorius.

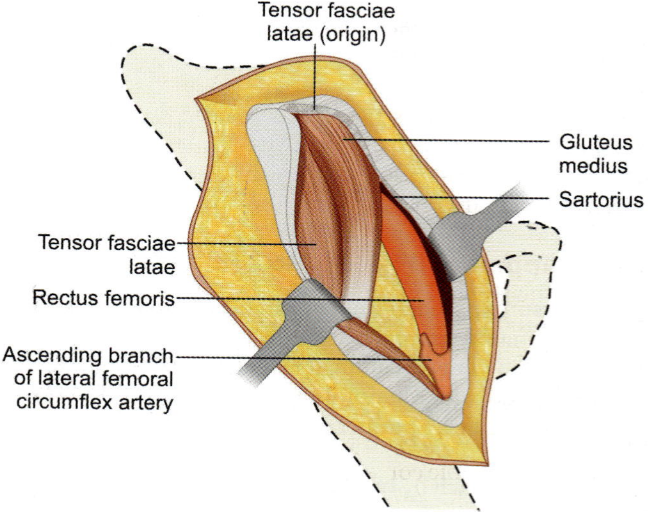

Fig. 273: Retract the sartorius upward and medially and the tensor fascia latae downward and laterally. Detach the iliac origin of the tensor fascia latae to develop the internervous plane.

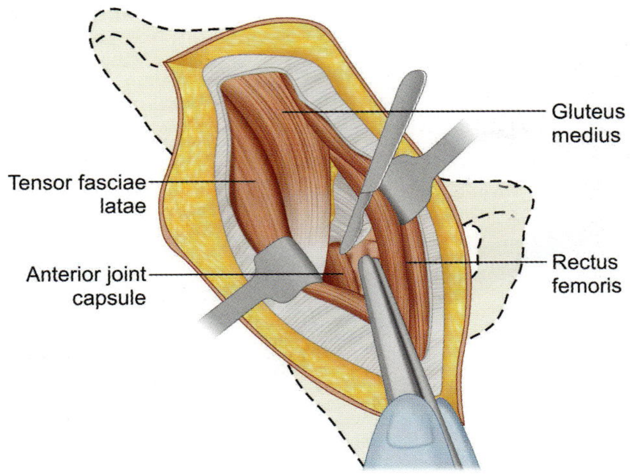

Fig. 274: Retracting the tensor fasciae latae and the sartorius brings you onto two muscles of the deep layer of the hip musculature, the rectus femoris (femoral nerve) and gluteal medius (superior gluteal nerve).

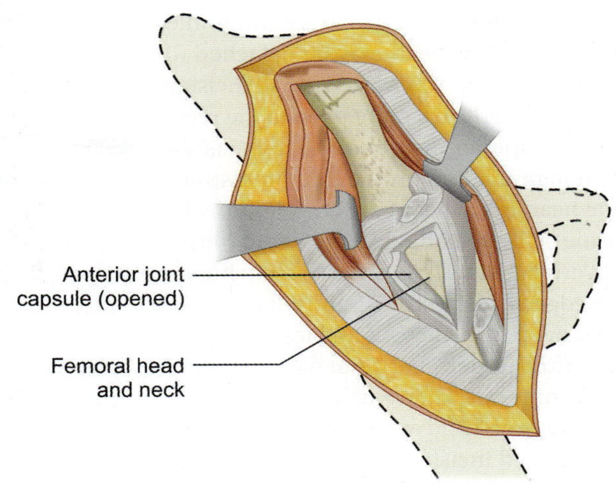

Fig. 276: Incise the hip joint capsule as surgery requires, with either a longitudinal or T-shaped capsular incision. Dislocate the hip by external rotation after the capsulotomy.

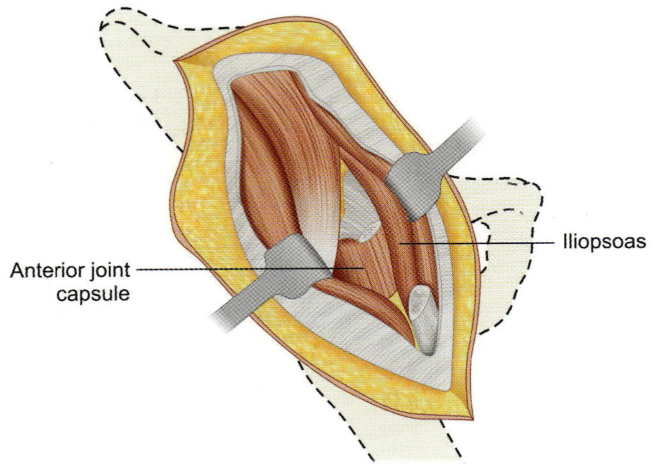

Fig. 275: Detach the rectus femoris from both its origin and retract it medially. Retract gluteus medius laterally.

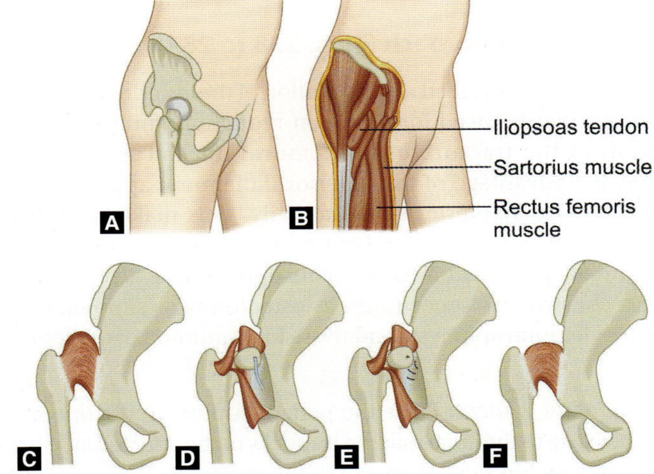

Figs. 277A to F: Somerville anterior approach—(A) A transverse bikini incision made; (B) Expose the reflected head of the rectus femoris and separate it from the acetabulum and capsule, leaving straight head attached to the anteroinferior spine; (C) Near the acetabular rim make a small incision in the capsule and extend it anteriorly to a point deep to the rectus and posteriorly to the posterosuperior margin of the joint; (D) Exert enough traction on the limb to distract the cartilage of the femoral head from that of the acetabulum about 0.7 cm and examine the inside of the acetabulum visually; (E) Radial incision in acetabular labrum and removal of all tissue of all tissue from depth of true acetabulum; (F) Capsulorrhaphy after excision of redundant capsule.

interval, if you dissect near it, you are out of plane. Detach the rectus femoris from both its origin and retract it medially. Retract gluteus medius laterally. Capsule of the hip joint is now exposed. Inferomedially, you can see the iliopsoas, as it approaches the lesser trochanter, retract it medially. Iliopsoas is often partly attached to the inferior aspect of the hip joint capsule and must be release from it. Inferolaterally, the shaft of the femur lies under cover of the vastus lateralis. Adduct and fully externally rotate the leg, to put the capsule on stretch, define the capsule with blunt dissection. Incise the hip joint capsule as surgery requires, with either a longitudinal or T-shaped capsular incision. Dislocate the hip by external rotation after the capsulotomy.

Somerville Approach (Figs. 277A to F)

Somerville described anterior approach using the transverse bikini incision, for irreducible congenital dislocation of the hip in a young child. This approach allows sufficient exposure of the ilium. For dislocated hip, the following sequential steps must be performed, psoas tenotomy, complete medial capsulotomy, including transverse acetabular ligament, excision of hypertrophied ligamentum teres, and reduction of femoral head into the true acetabulum. Place the sandbag beneath the affected hip. Make the straight skin incision, beginning anteriorly inferior and medial to the anterosuperior iliac spine and coursing obliquely superiorly and posteriorly to the middle of iliac crest.

Deepen the incision and expose crest. Then reflect the abductor muscle subperiosteally from the iliac wing distally to the capsule of the joint. Increase the exposure of the capsule by separating tensor fasciae latae from the sartorius for about 2.5 cm inferior to the anterosuperior spine. Next expose the reflected head of the rectus femoris and separate it from the acetabulum and capsule, leaving straight head attached to the anteroinferior spine, as shown in Figure 277B. The head may be detached to increase exposure. Near the acetabular rim make a small incision in the capsule and extend it anteriorly to a point deep to the rectus and posteriorly to the posterosuperior margin of the joint, as shown in Figure 277C. Exert enough traction on the limb to distract the cartilage of the femoral head from that of the acetabulum about 0.7 cm. Examine the inside of the acetabulum visually, as illustrated in Figure 277D. If no inverted limbus seen, insert a blunt hook and palpate the joint for free edge of an inverted limbus. If one is found, place the tip of the hook deep to the limbus and force it through its base and then separate from its periphery that part of the limbus lying anterior to the hook come out. Then with Kocher forceps, grasp the limbus by the end thus freed and excise it with strong curved scissor or make radial T-shaped incision to evert the limb and allow reduction of femoral head as illustrated in Figure 277E. Reduce the head into the acetabulum by abducting the thigh 30° and internally rotating it. Hold the joint in this position and close the capsule, as depicted in Figure 277F. Reattach the muscle to the iliac crest, close the skin, and apply the spica cast.

Anterolateral Approach (Figs. 278 to 281)

Smith Petersen described a modification of the anterior iliofemoral approach that he used for the open reduction and the internal fixation of the fracture of the femoral neck. This approach retains the advantage of the anterior iliofemoral approach, but expose the trochanteric region laterally. This makes aligning a fracture or osteotomy of the femoral neck and inserting pins or nail under direct vision easier. This approach is also useful in such reconstructive procedures, as osteotomy for slipping of the proximal femoral epiphysis and those for nonunion of the femoral neck.

Position of the patient: Place the patient supine on the operating table, so close to the edge that the buttocks of the affected side hang over. Tilt the table away from you as the patient lie flat.

Landmarks and Incision

Landmarks: The anterosuperior iliac spine is subcutaneous. It is easy to palpate in all, but difficult to palpate in the obese patient, who have the thick layer of the adipose tissue covering it. To palpate it, bring your thumbs up from beneath the bony protuberance. The GT is a large mass of the bone that projects up and back from the junction of the shaft of the femur and its neck.

Incision: Make the skin incision along the anterior third of the iliac crest and then along the anterior border of the tensor fascia latae muscle, curve it posteriorly across the insertion of this muscle into the iliotibial band in the subtrochanteric region (usually at a point 8–10 cm below the base of the GT) and end it there.

Anterolateral Surgical Approach

- Incise the fascia along the anterior border of the tensor fascia latae muscle. Identify and protect the lateral femoral cutaneous nerve, as illustrated in Figure 279.
- Next cleanly incise the muscle attachment to the lateral aspect of the ilium, along the iliac crest to make the periosteum elevation easier. Reflect it as continuous structure, without fraying distally to the superior margin of the acetabulum, as shown in Figure 280.
- Then divide the muscle attachment between the anterosuperior iliac spine and the acetabular labrum. The flap thus, reflected consists of the tensor fascia latae, the gluteal minimus, and the anterior part of the gluteus medius. This is illustrated in Figure 281.
- Inferiorly carry the fascial incision across the insertion of the tensor fascia latae into the iliotibial band and expose the lateral part of the rectus femoris and anterior part of the vastus lateralis muscle.
- Begin the capsular incision on the inferior aspect of the capsule just lateral to the acetabular labrum from this point extend it proximally, parallel with the acetabular labrum to the superior aspect of the capsule and then curved it laterally continuing on beyond the capsule to the base of the GT.
- This incision divides that part of the reflected head of the rectus femoris that blend into capsule inferior to its insertion into the

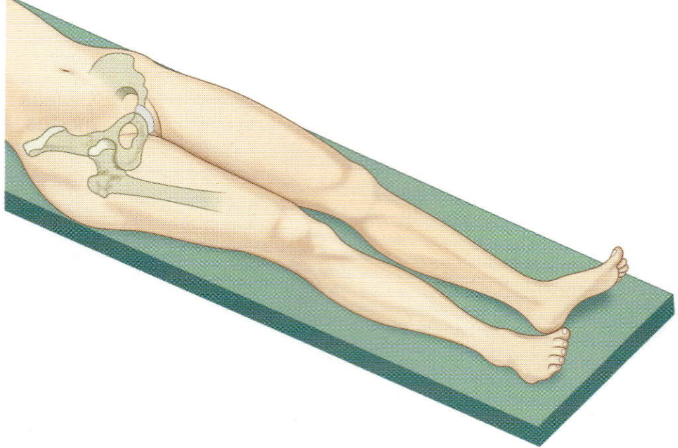

Fig. 278: Anterolateral surgical approach.

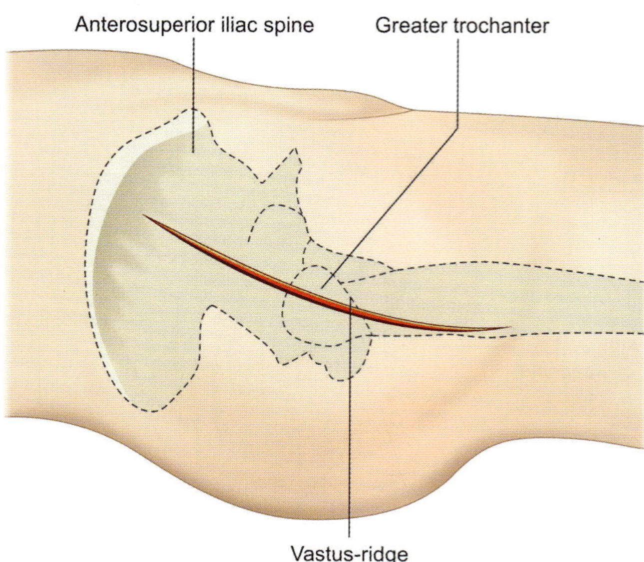

Fig. 279: Incise the fascia along the anterior border of the tensor fascia latae muscle.

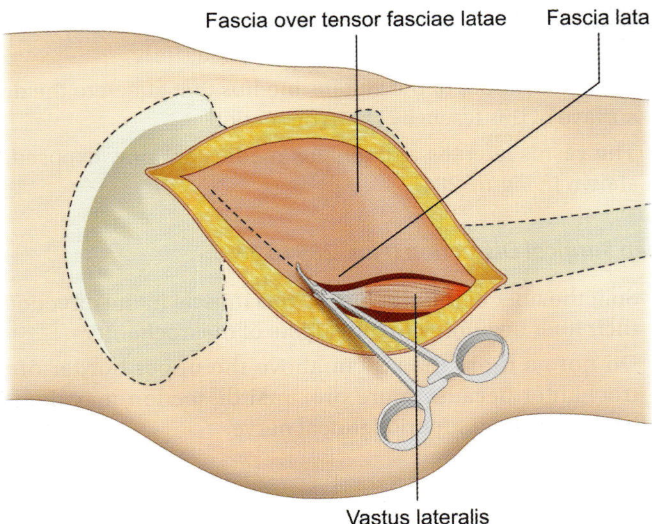

Fig. 280: Next cleanly incise the muscle attachment to the lateral aspect of the ilium along the iliac crest to make the periosteum easier.

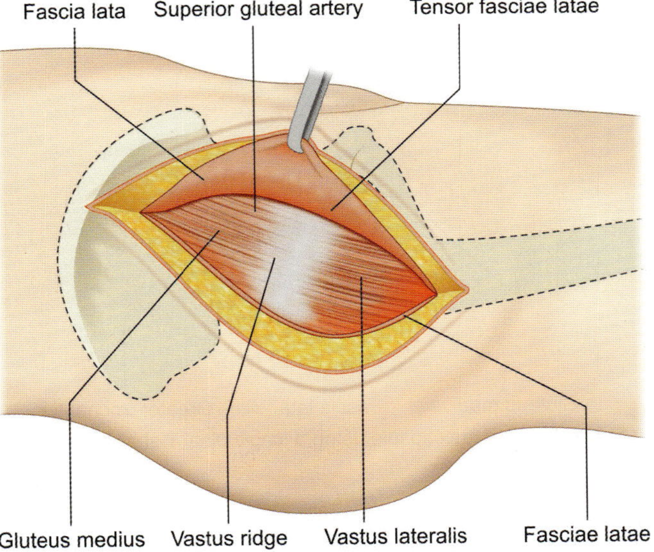

Fig. 281: Divide the muscle attachment between the anterosuperior iliac spine and the acetabular labrum. The flap thus, reflected consist of the tensor fasciae latae, the gluteal minimus and the anterior part of the gluteus medius.

superior margin of the acetabulum. By reflecting it with the capsule, flap is inforced and repair is thus made easier.

Lateral Approach (Figs. 282 to 284)

Lateral approach or transgluteal approach is described by Watson Jones, Harris, MacFarland and Osborne, Hardinge, McLauchlan, and Hay.

Position of the patient: Place the patient supine on the operating table, with the GT at the edge of the table. This allows the buttocks muscle and gluteal fat to fall posteriorly away from the operating table.

Landmarks and Incision

Landmarks: Palpate the anterosuperior iliac spine upward from below. Palpate the lateral aspect of the GT and below that the line

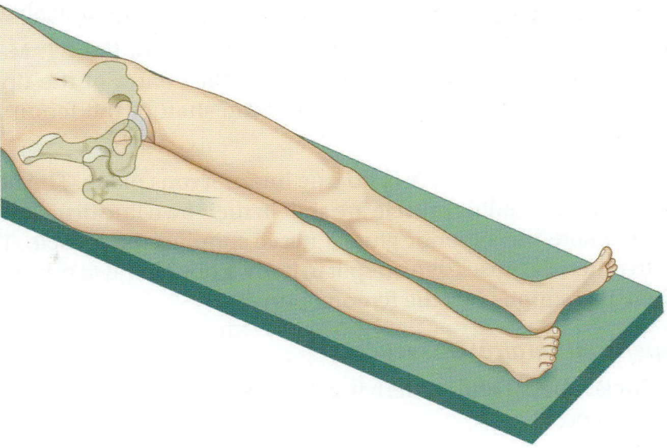

Fig. 282: Position of the patient for lateral surgical approach.

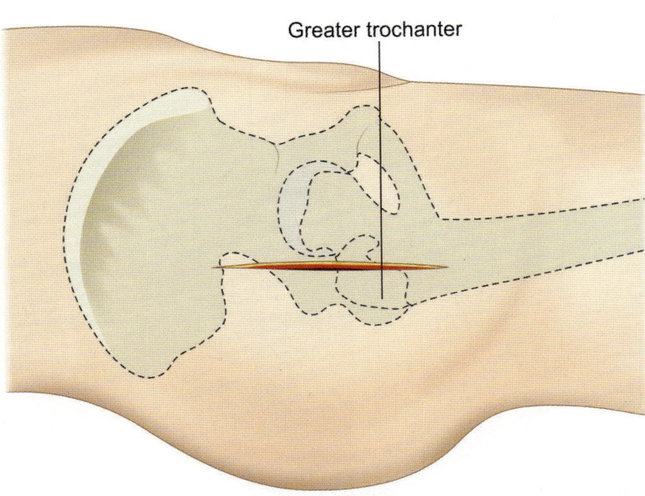

Fig. 283: Incision line for lateral approach, a longitudinal incision is made that passes over the center of the tip of the greater trochanter and extends down the line of the shaft of the femur for approximately 8 cm.

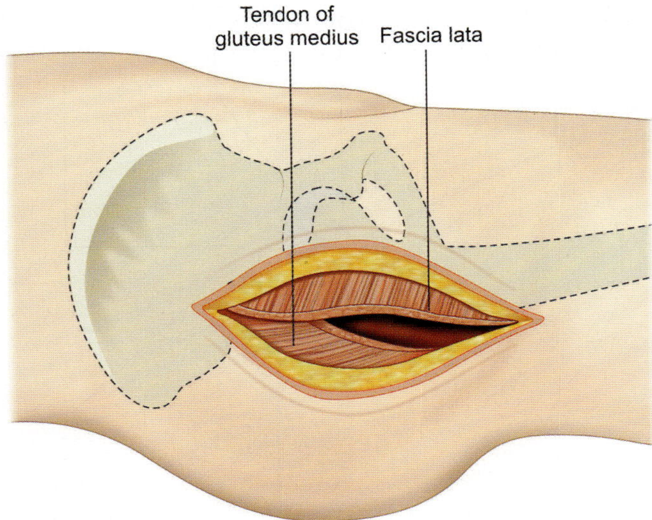

Fig. 284: Superficial surgical dissection in lateral approach, vastus lateralis and gluteus medius are now exposed.

of the femur that feel like a resistance against the examining hand.

Incision: Begin the incision 5 cm above the tip of the GT. Make a longitudinal incision that passes over the center of the tip of the GT and extends down the line of the shaft of the femur for approximately 8 cm.

Internervous plane: There is no true internervous plane. The fiber of the gluteus medius muscle are split in their own line distal to the point, where the superior gluteal nerve supplies the muscle. The vastus lateralis muscle is also split in its own line lateral to the point, where it is supplied by the femoral nerve.

Superficial Surgical Dissection

- Incise the fat and underlying deep fascia in line with the skin incision
- Retract the cut edge of the fascia to pull the tensor fascia latae anteriorly and the gluteus maximus posteriorly
- Detach any fiber of the gluteus medius that attach to the deep surface of this fascia by sharp dissection
- The vastus lateralis and gluteus medius are now exposed, as shown in Figure 284.

Deep Surgical Dissection (Figs. 285 to 289)

- Split the fiber of the gluteus medius muscle in the direction of their fiber beginning in the middle of the trochanter.
- Do not go more than 3 cm above the upper border of the trochanter because more proximal dissection may damage branches of the superior gluteal nerve.

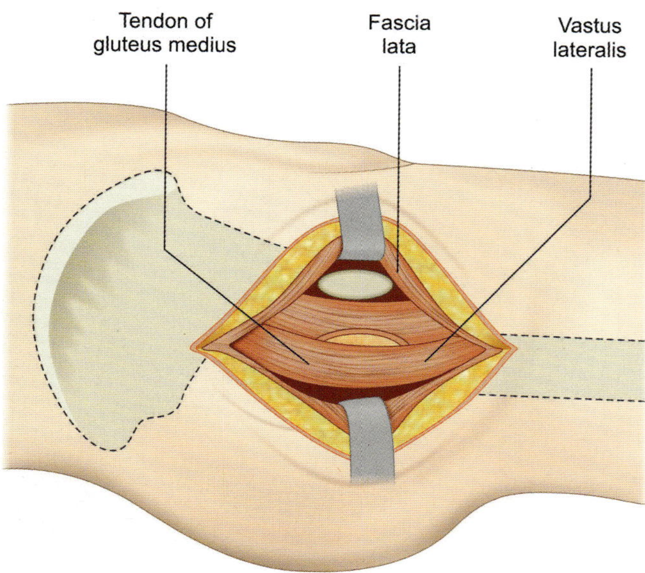

Fig. 285: Deep surgical dissection detaches the muscle from greater trochanter, either by sharp dissection or by lifting off a small flake of bone.

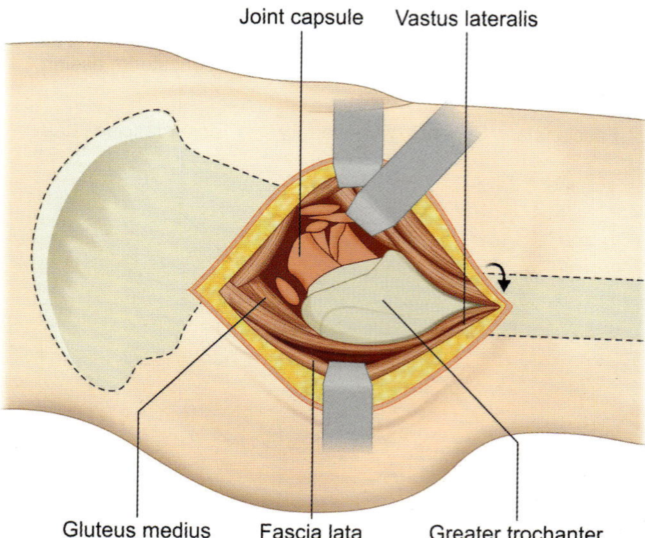

Fig. 287: Enter the capsule using a longitudinal T-shaped incision.

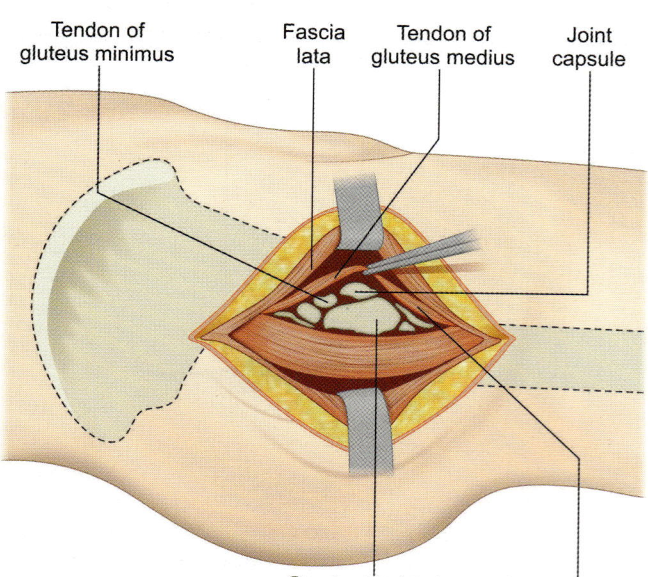

Fig. 286: Detach the insertion of the gluteus minimus tendon to the anterior part of the greater trochanter.

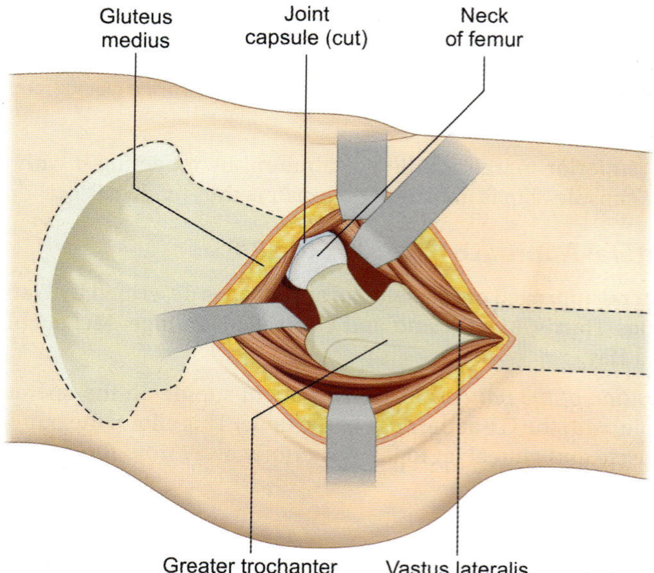

Fig. 288: Osteotomize the femoral neck.

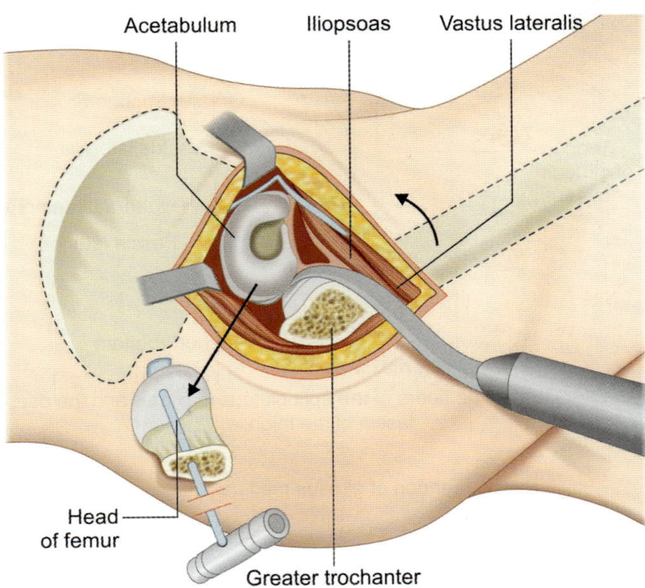

Fig. 289: Complete the exposure of the acetabulum, by inserting appropriate retractors around the acetabulum.

- Split the fiber of the vastus lateralis muscle overlying the lateral aspect of the base of the GT.
- Next, develop an anterior flap that consists of the anterior part of the gluteus medius muscle with the underlying gluteus minimus and anterior part of the vastus lateralis.
- You will need to detach the muscles from GT, either by sharp dissection or by lifting off a small flake of bone, as illustrated in Figure 285.
- Continue developing this anterior flap, following the contour of the bone onto the femoral neck, until the anterior hip joint capsule is fully exposed.
- You need to detach the insertion of the gluteus minimus tendon to the anterior part of the GT.
- Enter the capsule using a longitudinal T-shaped incision.
- Osteotomize the femoral neck.
- Extract the femoral head using a cork screw.
- Complete the exposure of the acetabulum, by inserting appropriate retractors around the acetabulum.

Dangers

Nerves: The superior gluteal nerve runs between the gluteal medius and minimus muscle approximately 3-5 cm above the upper border of the GT. More proximal dissection may cut this nerve or may produce the traction injury. The femoral nerve, the most lateral structure in the anterior neurovascular bundle of the thigh, is vulnerable to inappropriately placed retractor. Anterior retractor should be placed strictly on the bone of the anterior aspect of the acetabulum.

Vessels: The femoral artery and nerve are also vulnerable to inappropriately placed anterior retractor. The transverse branch of the lateral circumflex artery of the thigh is cut as the vastus lateralis is mobilized and it must be cauterized during the approach.

Posterior Approach (Figs. 290 to 292)

Posterior approach is the most common and practical of those used to expose the hip joint and popularized by Moore. It is also called the "southern approach". The uses of the posterior approach are as follows:

- Hemiarthroplasty
- THR
- Open reduction and internal fixation of posterior acetabular fracture
- Dependent drainage of hip sepsis
- Removal of loose bodies from the hip joint
- Pedicle bone grafting
- Open reduction of the posterior hip dislocation.

Position of the patient: Place the patient in the true lateral position, with the affected limb uppermost. As most of the patients requiring surgery are elderly and have delicate skin, it is important to protect the bony prominences of the leg and pelvis with pads placed under the lateral malleolus and knee of the bottom leg and pillow between the knees. Drape the limb free to leave room for movement during the procedure, as shown in Figure 290.

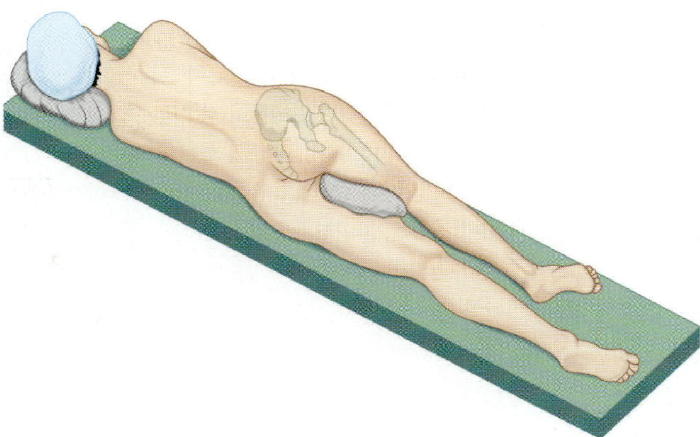

Fig. 290: Position of the patient for posterior surgical approach.

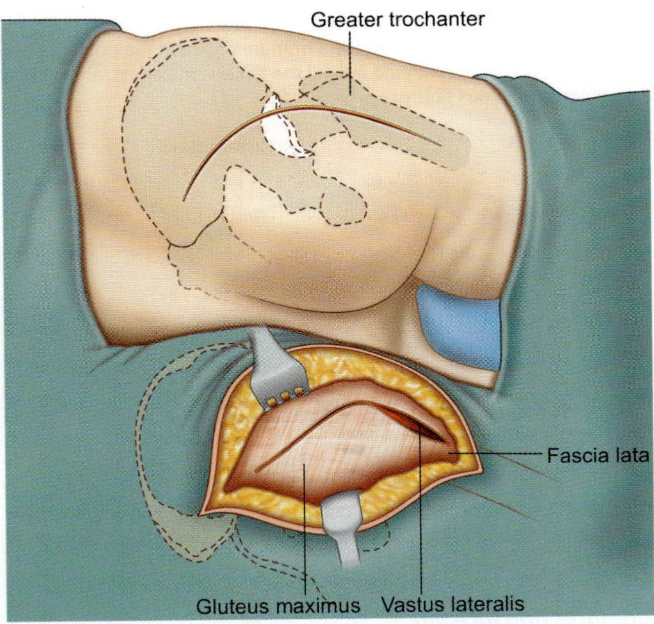

Fig. 291: Incision for posterior surgical approach begins some 6–8 cm above and posterior to the posterior aspect of the greater trochanter.

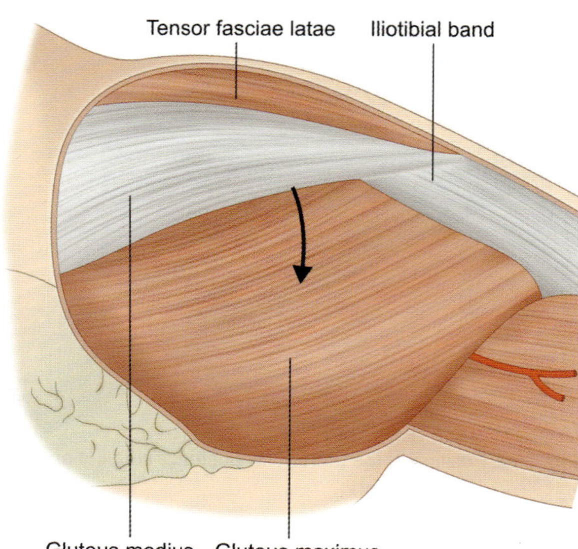

Fig. 292: The part of the incision runs from this point to the posterior aspect of the trochanter is in line with the fiber of the gluteus maximus, arrow showing line of gluteus maximus fibers.

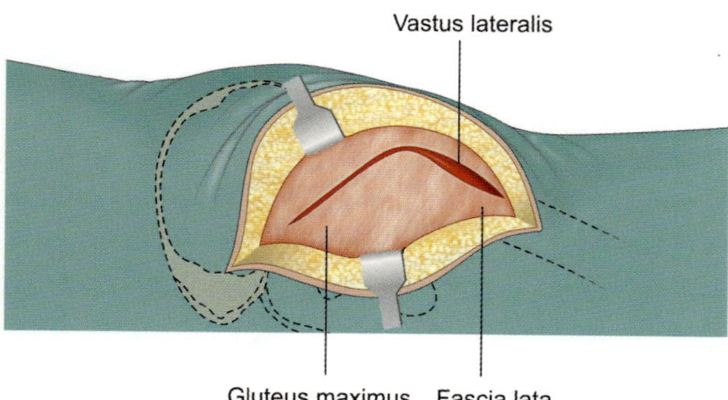

Fig. 293: Lengthen the fascial incision superiorly in line with the skin incision and split the fibers of the gluteus maximus by blunt dissection.

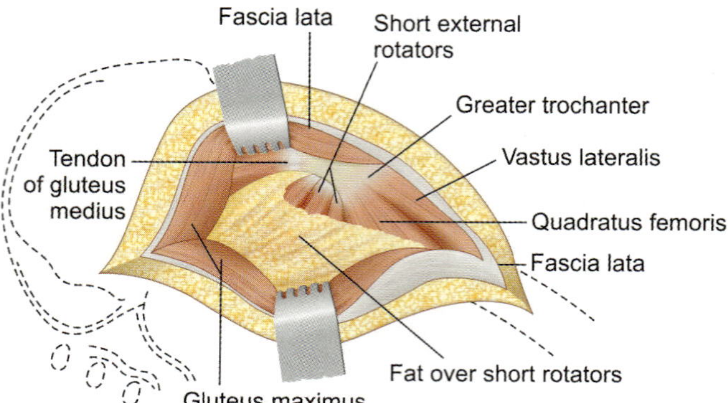

Fig. 294: Retract the fibers of the split gluteus maximus and the deep fascia of the thigh.

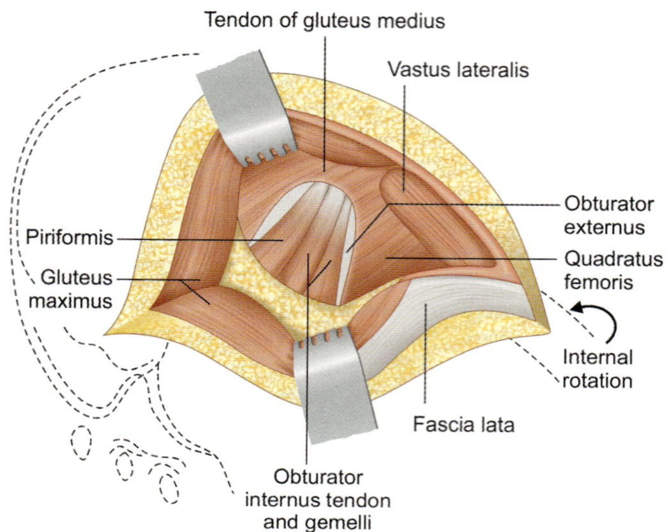

Fig. 295: Underneath is the posterolateral aspect of the hip joint, still covered by short external rotators muscles, which attach to the upper part of the posterolateral aspect of the femur.

Landmarks and Incision

Landmarks: Palpate in detail the grater trochanter on the outer aspect of the thigh. The posterior edge of the trochanter is more superficial than the anterior and lateral portions and as such it is easier to palpate.

Incision: Make a 10–15 cm curved incision centered on the posterior aspect of the GT. Begin your incision some 6–8 cm above and to the posterior aspect of the GT. The part of the incision that runs from this point to the posterior aspect of the trochanter is in line with the fiber of the gluteus maximus, as illustrated in Figures 291 and 292.

Internervous plane: There is no true internervous plane in this approach. However, gluteus maximus, which is split in the line of its fibers, is not significantly denervated because it receives its nerve supply well medial to the split.

Superficial Surgical Dissection

- Incise the fascia lata on the lateral aspect of the femur to uncover the vastus lateralis
- Lengthen the fascial incision superiorly in line with the skin incision and split the fibers of the gluteus maximus by blunt dissection, as shown in Figure 293
- The gluteus maximus received its blood supply from the superior and inferior gluteal arteries, which enter the deep surface of the muscle
- In addition to the arterial bleeding venous bleeding must be anticipated
- If you split the muscle gently, you may be able to pick up, coagulate, and cut the crossing vessels before they are stretched and avulsed by blunt dissection of the split.

Deep Surgical Dissection (Figs. 294 to 297)

- Retract the fibers of the split gluteus maximus and the deep fascia of the thigh
- Underneath is the posterolateral aspect of the hip joint, still covered by short external rotators muscles, which attach to the upper part of the posterolateral aspect of the femur
- Remember that the sciatic nerve leave the pelvis through the greater sciatic notch and runs down the back of the thigh on the short external rotator muscle

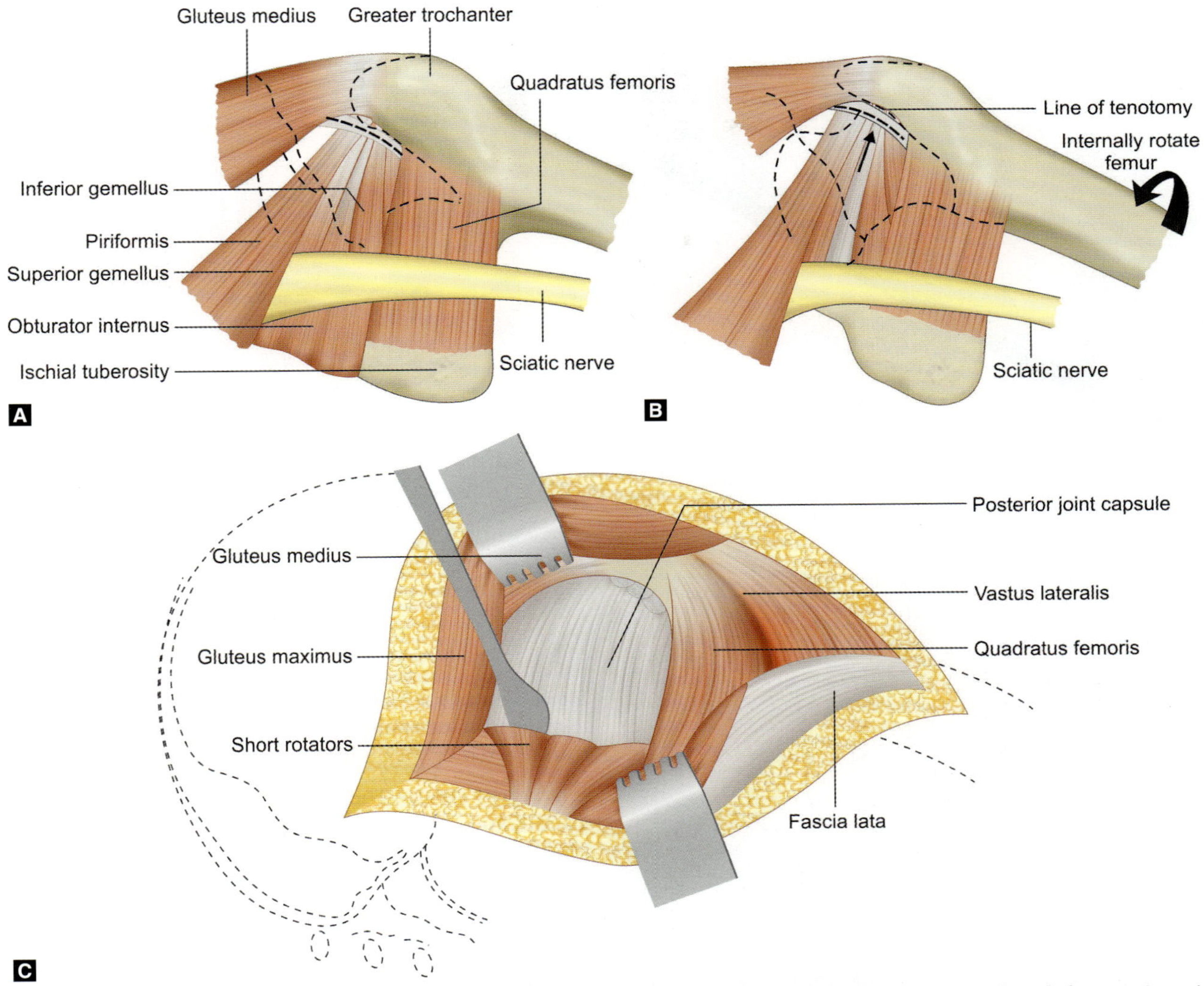

Figs. 296A to C: Detach the muscle close to their femoral insertion and reflect them backward, laying them over the sciatic nerve to protect it during the rest of the procedure.

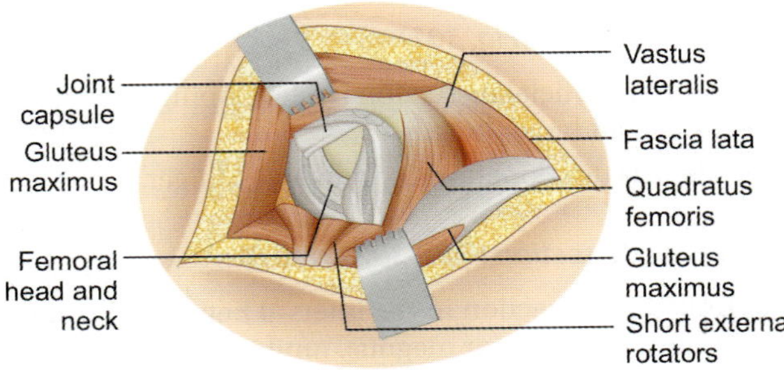

Fig. 297: Posterior joint capsulotomy exposed the femoral head and neck.

- The nerve crosses obturator internus, two gemelli, and the quadratus femoris before disappearing beneath the femoral attachment of the gluteus maximus muscle
- You can find the nerve lying on the short external rotators and it can be easily palpated
- Internally rotate the hip to put the short external rotators muscle on the stretch (making them more prominent)
- Insert stay suture into the piriformis and obturator internus tendon just before they insert into the GT
- Detach the muscle close to their femoral insertion and reflect them backward, laying them over the sciatic nerve to protect it during the rest of the procedure, as shown in Figures 296A to C
- The posterior aspect of the hip joint capsule is now fully exposed
- The joint capsule can be incised with a longitudinal or T-shaped incision
- Dislocation of the hip is achieved by internal rotation after capsulotomy
- Posterior joint capsulotomy will have exposed the femoral head and neck.

Medial Approach (Figs. 298 to 300)

The medial approach attributed to Ludloff was originally designed for surgery on flexed, abducted, and externally rotated hips. The uses of the medial approach in open reduction of congenital dislocation of the hip, include biopsy and treatment of the tumors

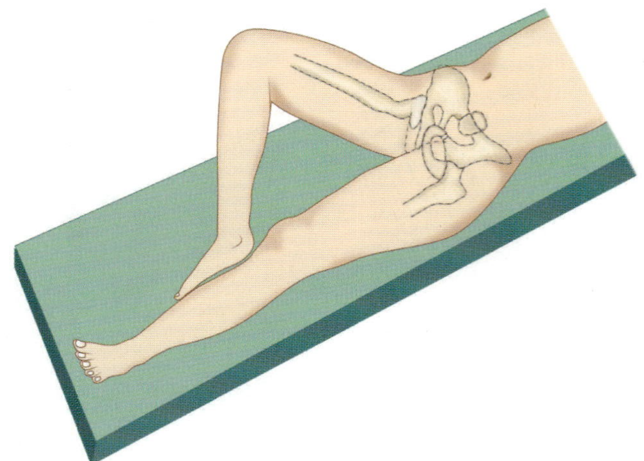

Fig. 298: Patient's position in medial surgical approach.

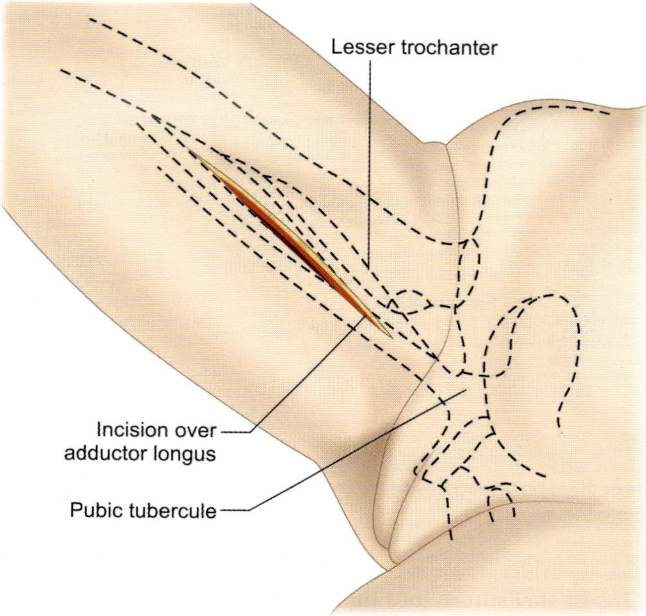

Fig. 299: A longitudinal incision is made on the medial side of the thigh, starting at a point 3 cm below the pubic tubercle. The incision runs down over the adductor longus.

of the inferior portion of the femoral neck, in release of the psoas muscle and obturator neurectomy.

Position of the patient (Fig. 298): Place the patient supine on the operating table with affected hip flexed, abducted, and externally rotated.

Landmarks and Incision

Landmarks: Palpate the adductor longus from the medial side of the thigh and follow it up to its origin at the pelvis in the angle between the pubic crest and symphysis. With your finger anchored on the GT, move your thumb along the inguinal creases medially and obliquely downward until you can feel the pubic tubercle.

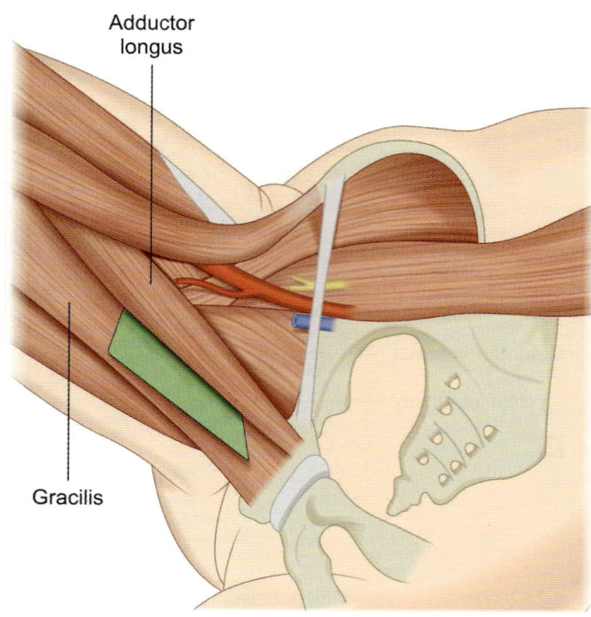

Fig. 300: The plane of the dissection lies between the adductor brevis and adductor magnus.

Incision: Make a longitudinal incision on the medial side of the thigh, starting at a point 3 cm below the pubic tubercle. The incision runs down over the adductor longus, as shown in Figure 299.

Internervous plane: The superficial dissection does not exploit an internervous plane, since both the adductor longus and gracilis are innervated by the anterior division of the obturator nerve. The plane nevertheless safe for the dissection, both muscles receive their nerve supplies proximal to the dissection. More deeply, the plane of the dissection lies between the adductor brevis and adductor magnus. The adductor brevis is supplied by the anterior branch of the obturator nerve. The adductor magnus has two nerve supplies—its adductor portion is supplied by the posterior division of the obturator nerve and its ischial portion is supplied by the tibial part of sciatic nerve.

Superficial Dissection (Fig. 301)

- Begin the superficial dissection by developing plane between gracilis and adductor longus
- This plane is developed with your gloved finger.

Deep Surgical Dissection (Figs. 302A and B)

- Continue the dissection in the interval between the adductor brevis and the adductor magnus, until you feel the trochanter on the floor of the wound
- Try to protect the posterior division of the obturator nerve
- Place the narrow retractor (such as bone spike) above and below the lesser trochanter to isolate the psoas tendon.

Dangers

Nerves: The anterior division of the obturator nerve lies on the top of the obturator externus and run down the medial side of

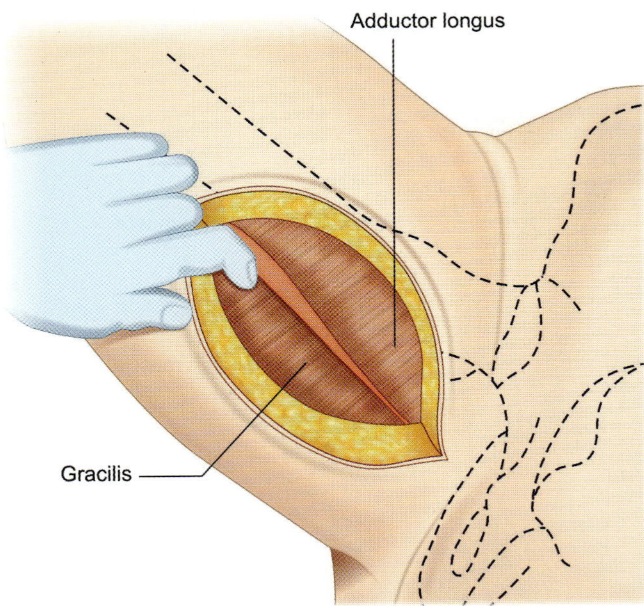

Fig. 301: Superficial dissection approach.

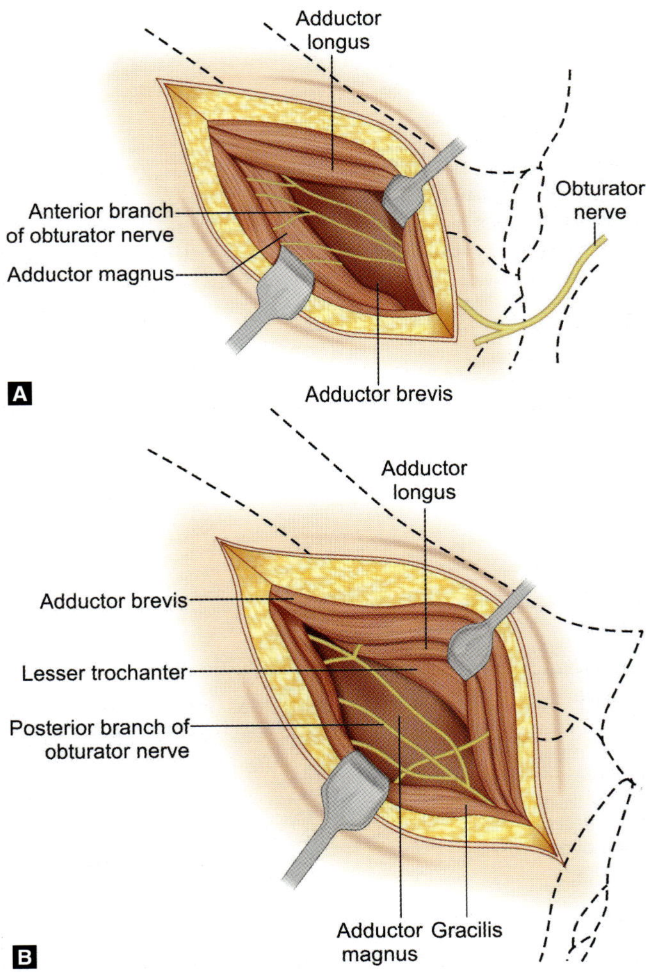

Figs. 302A and B: Deep surgical dissection approach.

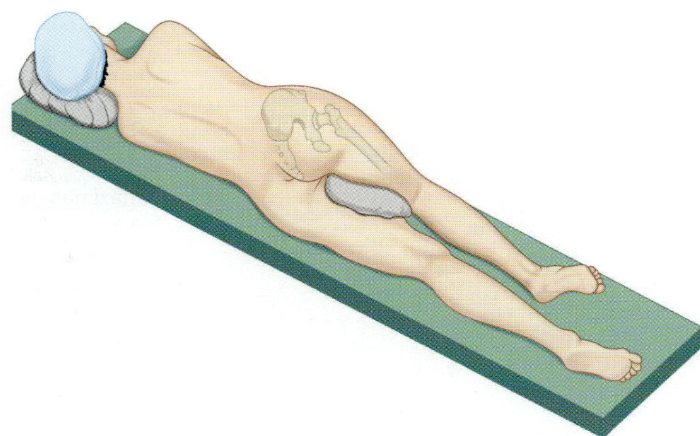

Fig. 303: Position of the patient in posterolateral surgical approach.

the thigh between the adductor longus and adductor brevis. The posterior division of the obturator nerve lies in the substance of the obturator externus, which supplies before it leaves the pelvis. The nerve then runs down the thigh on the adductor magnus and under the adductor brevis.

Vessels: The medial femoral circumflex artery passes around the medial side of the distal part of the psoas tendon.

Posterolateral Approach (Figs. 303 to 305)

Gibson first described the posterolateral approach and recommended by Kocher and Langenbeck.

Position of the patient: Patient is in lateral position.

Landmarks and Incision (Figs. 304A to D)

- Begin the proximal limb of the incision at a point 6–8 cm anterior to the posterosuperior iliac spine and just distal to the iliac crest, overlying the anterior border of the gluteus maximus.
- Extend it distally to the anterior edge of the GT and then further distally along the line of the femur for 15–18 cm.
- By blunt dissection, reflect the flap of the skin and subcutaneous fat from the underlying deep fascia a short distance anteriorly and posteriorly.
- Then incise iliotibial band in line with its fiber, beginning at the distal end of the wound and extending proximally to the GT.
- Next, abduct the thigh, insert the gloved finger through the proximal end of the incision in the band, locate by palpation the sulcus at the anterior border of the gluteus maximus muscle and extend the incision proximally along this sulcus.
- Then adduct the thigh, reflect the anterior and posterior masses and expose the GT and the muscles that insert into it.
- Next, separate the posterior border of the gluteus medius muscle from the adjacent pyriformis tendon by blunt dissection.
- Divide the gluteus medius and minimus muscles at their insertion, but leave enough of their tendon attached to the GT to permit easy closure of the wound.

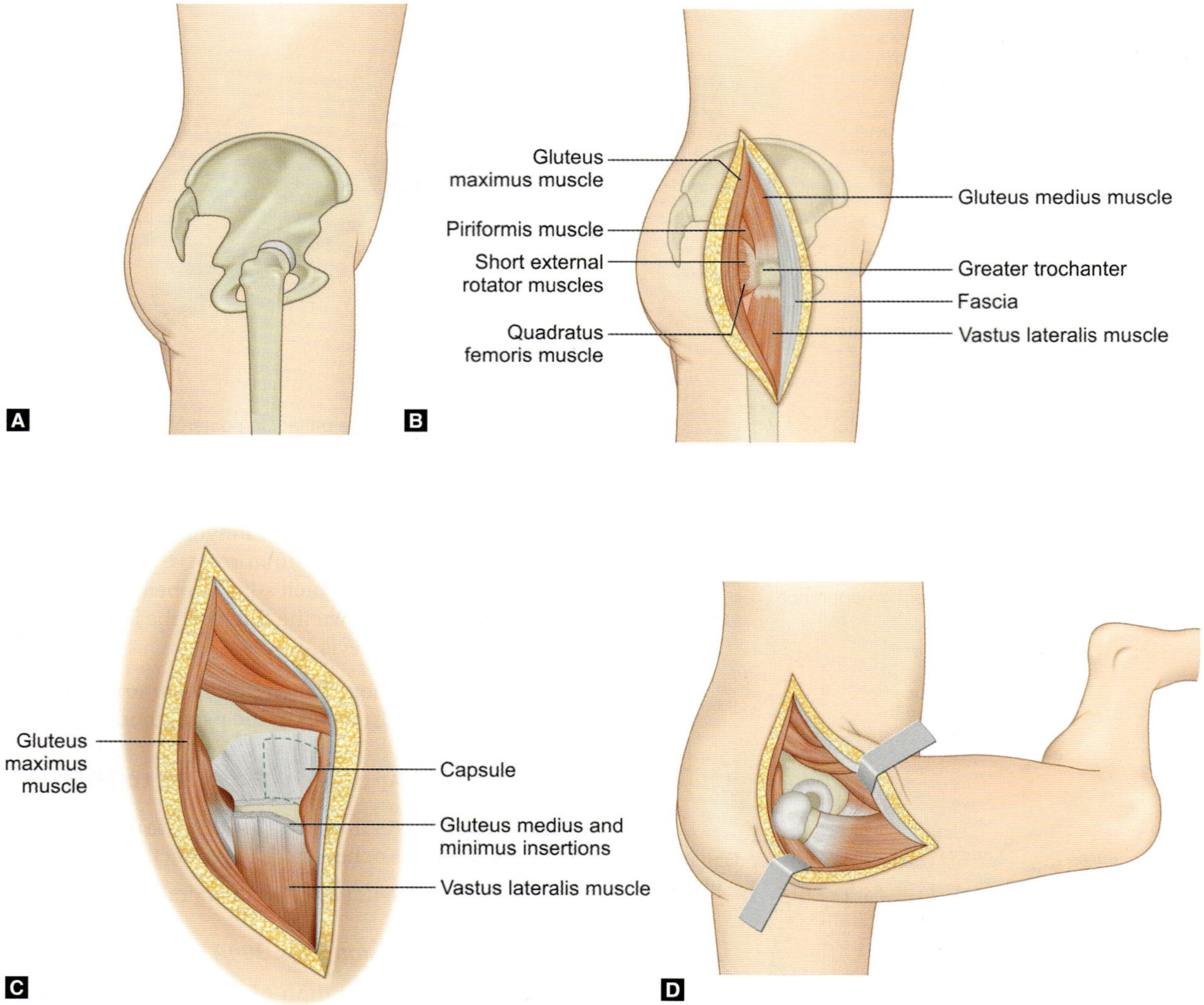

A

B

Gluteus maximus muscle

Piriformis muscle

Short external rotator muscles

Quadratus femoris muscle

Gluteus medius muscle

Greater trochanter

Fascia

Vastus lateralis muscle

C

Gluteus maximus muscle

Capsule

Gluteus medius and minimus insertions

Vastus lateralis muscle

D

Figs. 304A to D: Gibson posterolateral approach to hip joint—(A) Skin incision; (B) Anterior and posterior muscle masses have been retracted to expose greater trochanter and muscles that insert into it; (C) Gluteus medius and minimus have been near their insertion into greater trochanter and retracted incision in capsule is shown; (D) Hip joint has been dislocated by flexing, abducting and externally rotating thigh.

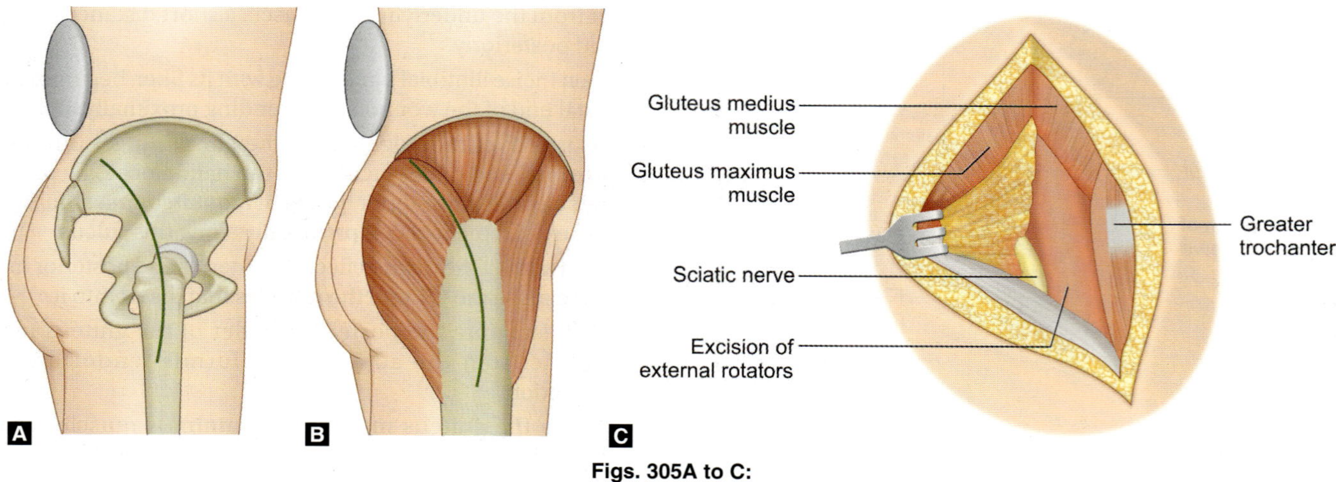

Figs. 305A to C: